Orthopaedic
Knowledge
Update 4

Home Study Syllabus

American Academy
of Orthopaedic Surgeons

Orthopaedic Knowledge Update 4 Home Study Syllabus

Published by the
American Academy of Orthopaedic Surgeons
6300 N. River Road
Rosemont, IL 60018
February 1993

The material presented in this *Orthopaedic Knowledge Update 4: Home Study Syllabus* has been made available by the American Academy of Orthopaedic Surgeons for educational purposes only. This material is not intended to represent the only, or necessarily the best, methods or procedures for the medical situations discussed, but rather is intended to present an approach, a view, statement, or opinion of the author(s) or producer(s), which may be helpful to others who face similar situations. Furthermore, any statements about commercial products are solely the opinion(s) of the author(s) and do not represent an Academy endorsement or evaluation of these products. These statements may not be used in advertising or for any commercial purpose.

Library of Congress Cataloging in Publication Data
88-645327
ISBN 0-89203-072-0

Acknowledgments

American Academy of Orthopaedic Surgeons
Thomas C. Nelson, Executive Director
Fred V. Featherstone, MD, Deputy Executive Director
Mark W. Wieting, Director, Division of Education
Marilyn L. Fox, PhD, Director, Department of Publications
Bruce Davis, Senior Editor

Ad Hoc Committee on Home Study
John W. Frymoyer, MD, Chairman
Peter C. Amadio, MD
Robert W. Bucholz, MD
Charles R. Clark, MD
Ralph W. Coonrad, MD
James H. Herndon, MD
Letha Y. Griffin, MD, PhD
Joseph P. Iannotti, MD, PhD
Bernard F. Morrey, MD
Raymond T. Morrissy, MD
Robert J. Neviaser, MD
James A. Nunley II, MD
David J. Schurman, MD
Marc F. Swiontkowski, MD
Hugh S. Tullos, MD

Contents

LOWER EXTREMITY

Contributors

	David J. Schurman, MD Stanford, California
Bone Metabolism and Metabolic Bone Disease	Thomas A. Einhorn, MD New York, New York
Arthritis	Thomas S. Thornhill, MD Boston, Massachusetts
	Jonathan L. Schaffer, MD Boston, Massachusetts
Muscle and Gait	Gunnar B. Andersson, MD, PhD Chicago, Illinois
Ligament Injury and Repair	Wayne H. Akeson, MD San Diego, California
	Malcolm H. Pope, DMSc, PhD Burlington, Vermont
	Bruce D. Beynnon, PhD Burlington, Vermont
Congenital Abnormalities	Lawrence I. Karlin, MD Boston, Massachusetts
Multiple Trauma: Pathophysiology and Management	Lawrence B. Bone, MD Buffalo, New York
	George Babikian, MD Portland, Maine
	John R. Border, MD Buffalo, New York
	Marc F. Swiontkowski, MD Seattle, Washington
Infection	John L. Esterhai, Jr., MD Philadelphia, Pennsylvania
Musculoskeletal Neoplasms	Stephen M. Horowitz, MD Philadelphia, Pennsylvania
Acute Pain Management	James N. Weinstein, DO Iowa City, Iowa
	Stephen D. Trigg, MD Jacksonville, Florida
Perioperative Management	Nancy E. Lane, MD San Francisco, California
	Douglas C. Bauer, MD San Francisco, California
Anesthesia for Orthopaedic Surgery	Denise J. Wedel, MD Rochester, Minnesota
	Nigel E. Sharrock, MD New York, New York
	E. Paul Didier, MD Rochester, Minnesota
	Beth A. Elliott, MD Rochester, Minnesota
	Teresa T. Horlocker, MD Rochester, Minnesota
	Diana G. McGregor, MBBS, FFARCS Rochester, Minnesota
	Steven H. Rose, MD Rochester, Minnesota
	Maria de Castro, MD Rochester, Minnesota
Blood Transfusion Medicine: 1993	Marie M. Keeling, MD Louisville, Kentucky
Microvascular Surgery	Gordon A. Brody, MD Stanford, California
Laser Surgery	Stephen J. O'Brien, MD New York, New York
	Stephen Fealy, BA New York, New York
Bone Grafts	Gary E. Friedlaender, MD New Haven, Connecticut

Prostheses: Materials, Fixation, and Design   Myron Spector, PhD
Boston, Massachusetts

Amputations and Prosthetics   Douglas G. Smith, MD
Seattle, Washington

Upper Extremity Task Force

Section Editors   Ralph W. Coonrad, MD
Durham, North Carolina
Bernard F. Morrey, MD
Rochester, Minnesota
Raymond T. Morrissy, MD
Atlanta, Georgia
Robert J. Neviaser, MD
Washington, DC
James A. Nunley II, MD
Durham, North Carolina
Hugh S. Tullos, MD
Houston, Texas

Shoulder: Pediatric   William J. Shaughnessy, MD
Rochester, Minnesota

Shoulder: Trauma   Joseph D. Zuckerman, MD
New York, New York
Kenneth J. Koval, MD
New York, New York

Shoulder: Instability   William J. Mallon, MD
Durham, North Carolina

Shoulder: Reconstruction   Gary M. Gartsman, MD
Houston, Texas
Douglas A. Becker, MD
Rochester, Minnesota

Elbow and Forearm: Trauma   Earl A. Stanley, MD
San Antonio, Texas
Thomas L. Melhoff, MD
Houston, Texas

Elbow: Reconstruction   Shawn W. O'Driscoll, MD, PhD
Rochester, Minnesota

Wrist and Hand: Congenital Anomalies and
Pediatric Reconstruction   Irwin E. Harris, MD
Tucson, Arizona

Wrist and Hand: Trauma   Richard D. Goldner, MD
Durham, North Carolina

Wrist and Hand: Reconstruction   Edward A. Nalebuff, MD
Boston, Massachusetts
Gary G. Poehling, MD
Winston-Salem, North Carolina
David B. Siegel, MD
Winston-Salem, North Carolina
L. Andrew Koman, MD
Winston-Salem, North Carolina

Spine Task Force

Section Editor   Charles R. Clark, MD
Iowa City, Iowa

Cervical Spine: Pediatric   Peter D. Pizzutillo, MD
Philadelphia, Pennsylvania

Cervical Spine: Trauma   Martin H. Krag, MD
Burlington, Vermont

Cervical Spine: Reconstruction   Edward N. Hanley, Jr., MD
Charlotte, North Carolina

Thoracolumbar Spine: Pediatric   Randal R. Betz, MD
Philadelphia, Pennsylvania

Thoracolumbar Spine: Trauma — Ernest M. Found, MD
Iowa City, Iowa

Thoracolumbar Spine: Reconstruction — James N. Weinstein, DO
Iowa City, Iowa

Lumbar Spine — Gordon R. Bell, MD
Cleveland, Ohio

Lower Extremity Task Force

Section Editors — Marc F. Swiontkowski, MD
Seattle, Washington
Robert W. Bucholz, MD
Dallas, Texas

Hip: Pediatric Aspects — John H. Wedge, MD, FRCSC
Ontario, Canada

Pelvis and Acetabulum: Trauma — Joel M. Matta, MD
Los Angeles, California

Hip: Trauma — Joseph D. Zuckerman, MD
New York, New York
Kenneth J. Koval, MD
New York, New York

Hip: Adult Joint Reconstruction — Dennis K. Collis, MD
Eugene, Oregon

Femur: Trauma — Kenneth D. Johnson, MD
Nashville, Tennessee

Knee and Leg: Pediatric Aspects — Jon R. Davids, MD
San Diego, California
Dennis R. Wenger, MD
San Diego, California

Knee and Leg: Bone Trauma — Fred Behrens, MD
Newark, New Jersey

Knee and Leg: Soft-Tissue Trauma — Freddie H. Fu, MD
Pittsburgh, Pennsylvania
Vincent J. Silvaggio, MD
Pittsburgh, Pennsylvania

Knee and Leg: Reconstruction — Aaron A. Hofmann, MD
Salt Lake City, Utah
Harry E. Rubash, MD
Pittsburgh, Pennsylvania
Theodore W. Crofford, MD
Fort Worth, Texas
Frederick J. Fletcher, MD
Albany, New York
Lawrence S. Crossett, MD
Pittsburgh, Pennsylvania

Ankle and Foot: Pediatric Aspects — Alvin H. Crawford, MD
Cincinnati, Ohio
Dennis P. Devito, MD
Atlanta, Georgia

Ankle and Foot: Trauma — Bruce J. Sangeorzan, MD
Seattle, Washington

Ankle and Foot: Reconstruction — Mark S. Myerson, MD
Baltimore, Maryland

Preface

In the 12 years encompassed by four Orthopaedic Knowledge Updates, major advances have been made in the capacity of orthopaedists to diagnose and treat more effectively a multitude of musculoskeletal disorders. At the same time, major scientific discoveries have been made, particularly in molecular biology. These advances are detailed throughout this latest edition, and form the major content of *Orthopaedic Knowledge Update 4*. As in all previous editions, we have made every effort to produce a balanced and unbiased accounting of core information and new knowledge necessary to diagnose and treat the spectrum of musculoskeletal disorders.

In parallel with these clinical and scientific advances, the environment in which the orthopaedist practices is changing rapidly. New applied research agendas are taking shape. "Quality," "clinical epidemiology," "outcome studies," "cost-effective treatment," and "small population variation analysis" are but some of the techniques now being used by orthopaedists to analyze the clinical and socioeconomic impact of our diagnostic and treatment methods. These techniques are the outgrowth and manifestations of broader societal forces deeply concerned about the costs and quality of health care. It is the belief of the editorial board that learning these new techniques will be of increasing and vital importance to practicing orthopaedists and residents in training. For that reason, this edition includes a new section that details this new information.

All previous editors, and I, fully recognize the enormous energy and devotion that lead to the successful production of a new Orthopaedic Knowledge Update. The individual contributors, section editors, and board of editors listed on the preceding pages have labored for over two years to produce this volume. The contents of this volume are the result of that energy and devotion. Academy staff, including Mark W. Wieting, Marilyn L. Fox,

PhD, Bruce Davis, Joan Abern, Jane Baque, Loraine Edwalds, Monica M. Trocker, Geraldine Dubberke, Em Lee Lambos, Sophie Tosta, and Sharon Duffy, have worked tirelessly to organize and manage the publication schedule and provide superb copyediting.

Last year all of us involved in this project faced an unexpected and tragic interruption with the untimely death of Wendy O. Schmidt, senior editor at the Academy. Since *Orthopaedic Knowledge Update 2*, Wendy had, in the words of Robert Poss, MD, editor of *OKU 3*, deserved "recognition for her overall management of the editorial process and superb editing." I found this same level of skill and commitment to *OKU 4*, and counted heavily on her for her professional skills and knowledge, organizational skills, and good humor.

Her death was a tragic loss for her family, professional associates, friends, and the Academy. It is a tribute to the Academy staff that they picked up the project and moved it forward without visible interruption. Their professionalism at a time of significant loss was truly magnificent.

Finally, all editors of Orthopaedic Knowledge Update have recognized the solid foundations laid by their predecessors, Marc A. Asher, MD, Robert H. Fitzgerald, Jr., MD, and Robert Poss, MD. Bob Poss, in particular, was invaluable in preparing me for the challenges and pitfalls which face all editors engaged in a project of this magnitude. Like my predecessor, I feel privileged to have been associated with all who made Orthopaedic Knowledge Update possible, and to present this fourth volume to the fellows of the American Academy of Orthopaedic Surgeons. I sincerely hope this home study syllabus will provide new information that will help all of us continue to improve on the care we render to patients with musculoskeletal disorders.

John W. Frymoyer, MD
Editor

I
Epidemiology

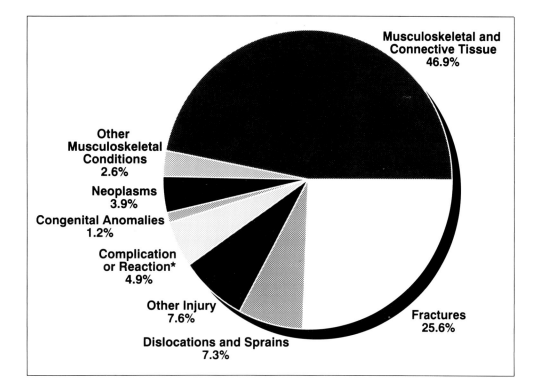

1

Clinical Epidemiology

A knowledge of epidemiologic concepts and the methodologies used by epidemiologists can enable the orthopaedist to interpret the published literature in an informed and critical way; to undertake further studies, if necessary; and, thus, to function more effectively in the challenging task of providing high quality care for increasingly complex medical problems using advanced technology.

Epidemiology is the study of the distribution and determinants of disease in populations. Originally developed to investigate epidemics of infectious diseases, its scope has widened in recent years to answer the following questions: What grouping of clinical and laboratory findings best defines a particular disease? What is the etiology of that disease? What patient characteristics are associated with an increased risk of acquiring the disease? Once acquired, what is the prognosis? What is the best treatment? What is the best way to prevent the disease or its complications?

These questions can rarely be answered on the basis of the clinical experience of individual physicians, most of whom see a limited range of patients with a particular disease. The most seriously affected patients are most likely to be attended, especially in referral practices, while mildly affected individuals may never be diagnosed. Further, patients may be selected for study on the basis of socioeconomic or geographic factors that could be related to the likelihood of acquiring the disease. Generally, a physician will see only small numbers of patients with any specific disease, and these cases may be seen over a period of many years, during which time the natural history of the disease could be changing. Finally, few physicians will have a normal or "control" group for comparison. As a result of these problems, individual physicians rarely acquire the needed knowledge through their own experience, but must rely on the work of others who have carried out specific studies of a problem. The literature on most subjects is extensive and often contradictory, with wide variation in quality and reliability, and it is essential that orthopaedists be able to evaluate the quality of this literature.

Epidemiologic View of Disease

Definition of Disease

The clinical definition of disease may not be straightforward. If the "disease" is defined on the basis of a specific pathophysiology, manifestations may vary. Thus, *Staphylococcus aureus* can have a range of manifestations from mildly symptomatic bone and joint infection to death. If defined on the basis of a specific manifestation, on the other hand, varied pathophysiology can be involved. Infective arthritis, for example, can be caused by *S aureus* (an aerobic bacterium), *Myxovirus parotitis* (a virus), or *Borrelia burgdorferi* (a spirochete). Additionally, diseases may be "discrete" (ie, either present or absent), such as hip fractures, or they may span a continuum from normal to abnormal, rendering classification somewhat arbitrary.

Regardless of how a particular disease is defined, gradation in severity of its manifestations is a general phenomenon. Because our definitions of disease are imprecise, and because humans are biologically variable, manifestations of any "disease" can vary widely. This concept is called the clinical spectrum of disease (Fig. 1). Frequently, only the most seriously diseased portion of the population is recognized clinically.

Patterns of Disease Occurrence

The basic premise of epidemiology is that disease occurs, not randomly, but in patterns that reflect the operation of the underlying causes. Clues to etiology, then, can be derived from the answers to three basic questions: Who is and who is not affected (person)? Where does disease occur and not occur (place)? When does it occur and not occur (time)? Thus, the prevalence of radiographically defined osteoarthritis of the hip is lower in blacks, while osteoarthritis of the knee may occur more frequently in black women. The latter finding, observed in Jamaica, implicates the rough footpaths over which people walk as a causative factor. Closer to home, age-adjusted incidence rates for hip fractures show a distinct north to south gradient, with higher rates in the southern United States. Soft and fluoridated water, poverty, reduced sunlight exposure, and rural location are associated with an increased risk of hip fracture. Interest in such geographic epidemiology is growing, especially in health services research that examines variations in resource utilization.

Measuring Disease Frequency

The fact that 22 patients died during a surgery for a particular condition at one center, compared with four patients at another center, has no meaning in the absence of information about the total number of patients who underwent surgery and how case severity and related factors differed between the two centers. Therefore, epide-

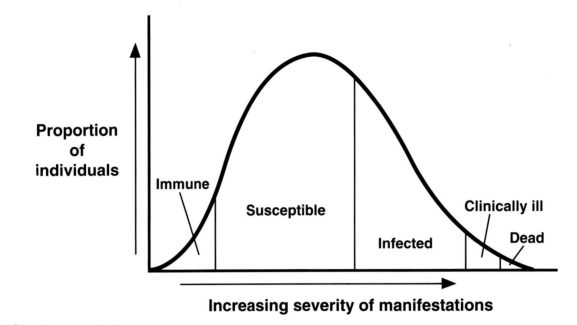

Fig. 1 Clinical spectrum of disease.

miologists use rates, rather than numbers, for a more accurate assessment of risk.

Incidence Rate

The single most important measure in epidemiology, the incidence rate (IR), is defined as follows:

$$IR = \frac{\text{Number of new cases of a disease in given period}}{\text{Population at risk in that time period}} \times \text{``factor''}$$

The numerator consists of only the new cases that arose from the denominator population at risk during the given period of time, usually one year. The denominator may be a fixed geographic population or, if a cohort of subjects is being followed, the denominator may be in "person-years." This accounts for subjects entering and leaving the study at different times and being under observation for unequal periods. Thus, one individual followed for ten years contributes ten person-years, as do ten individuals observed for one year each. Dividing the numerator by the denominator results in a fraction that is then multiplied by some "factor" (usually 100,000) to allow presentation of the result in a more convenient form. Thus, the incidence of initial traumatic shoulder dislocations in Olmsted County, Minnesota, during the period 1970-79 was 7.5 per 100,000 population per year.

Incidence rate (and other rates, too) usually are calculated and examined in terms of the three fundamental factors of interest to epidemiologists: who (person), where (place), and when (time). Examination according to specific characteristics, such as age, sex, or race, usu-

ally provides more information about disease occurrence than does a single summary statistic. For example, while the overall incidence of initial shoulder dislocations in Olmsted County, Minnesota, during the period 1970-79 was 7.5 per 100,000 per year, the rate for men (10.6 per 100,000 per year) was more than twice as high as the (sex-specific) rate for women (4.8 per 100,000 per year).

Incidence rates are used (1) to study the relationship between etiologic factors and disease, (2) to estimate an individual's risk of acquiring a particular disease, (3) to assess the effectiveness of preventive efforts, and (4) to describe trends in disease frequency over time.

Prevalence Rate

If the incidence rate, determined at intervals over a long period, can be likened to a motion picture, the prevalence rate is like a snapshot view. The prevalence rate (PR) is defined as follows:

$$PR = \frac{\text{Number of cases of a disease EXISTING at a given time}}{\text{Population at that time}} \times \text{``factor''}$$

The numerator consists of all cases, new and old alike, existing in the denominator total population at a particular time. The time can be a period, such as a year (period prevalence), or a specific date (point prevalence). The "factor" is for convenience, as before, and is usually 1,000 or 100 (percent), because prevalence generally is calculated only for common conditions. For example, to assess the prevalence of vertebral fractures, researchers surveyed a sample of women living in Rochester, Minnesota, in 1980; 53 of 200 women aged 50 years and older were found to have one or more vertebral fractures, a prevalence rate of 26.5%.

Prevalence rates primarily measure the disease burden in the community and are, hence, used for planning and prioritizing health services. Although they are used occasionally for etiologic studies when incidence rates cannot be determined, prevalence rates are less desirable for this purpose because they are affected not only by changes in the frequency of disease occurrence but also by changes in case ascertainment, by survivorship, and by migration of patients into and out of the study population. The introduction of such poorly understood variation renders interpretation of any results much more difficult.

Relationship of Incidence and Prevalence Rates

The prevalence rate of a disease is approximately equal to the product of the incidence rate and the average duration of the disease. Multiplying the latter two allows one to estimate the prevalence of the disease in the community (if incidence and duration are stable over time). Conversely, dividing the prevalence rate by the average duration of the disease theoretically provides one with an estimate of the incidence rate. Because of the problems mentioned above, however, such an estimate is unlikely to be accurate.

Mortality rate

The mortality rate (MR) is defined as follows:

$$MR = \frac{\text{Number of deaths in given period}}{\text{Population during that time period}} \times \text{"factor"}$$

The numerator is the number of deaths that occur in the denominator population during a given period time, usually one year. The convenience "factor" used is typically 1,000 for total deaths or 100,000 for deaths due to specific causes. For example, the mortality rate from motor vehicle accidents in the United States dropped from 23.3 to 19.5 per 100,000 population per year during the period 1950 to 1987.

Mortality rates are used in epidemiologic studies when morbidity (incidence and prevalence) rates are not available. Because deaths generally come from the serious end of the disease spectrum and may be influenced by factors that have little to do with disease etiology, mortality rates usually do not provide an accurate picture of the occurrence of disease in the population.

Mortality rates are often confused with case-fatality rates (surgical mortality rates). The case-fatality rate (CF) is defined as follows:

$$CF = \frac{\text{Number of patients with given disease who died}}{\text{Number of patients with that disease}} \times 100$$

In the motor vehicle accident example above, a case-fatality rate would calculate the proportion of patients who died after admission to a hospital following a motor vehicle accident. The case-fatality rate, therefore, provides no information about the frequency of deaths from the disease in the general population. It is, however, a clinically useful measure of the effectiveness of treatment for serious diseases that have a substantial early mortality.

Standardization of Rates

A problem arises when rates for different populations have to be compared. If the incidence (or prevalence or mortality) rates vary with age, race, or sex, the distribution of these factors in the population will affect the overall rate observed. Overall incidence rates, for example, might appear different in two populations, even if no real difference exists between comparable subpopulations. The solution is to make the comparison fair by "adjusting" (reweighting) the rates. Two approaches are available, the details of which are described in most textbooks on epidemiology.

With the direct standardization approach, the incidence (or prevalence or mortality) rates found for each study population subgroup (eg, white females 20 to 29 years old) are applied to a standard population (eg, U.S. residents in a particular year), and the rate is recalculated for the standard population. Thus, the incidence of initial traumatic shoulder dislocation among Olmsted County, Minnesota, residents was 8.2 per 100,000 per year when directly age- and sex-adjusted to the population structure of the United States in 1980.

With the indirect standardization approach, rates from an external population (usually the national population) are applied to the age, sex, and race distribution of the study group. This is done most often for mortality data, where the number of deaths actually observed is compared with the expected number (Standardized Mortality Ratio, SMR). The standard population is considered to have an SMR of 100; values above 100 indicate higher mortality rates, and vice versa. For example, applying England and Wales data on mortality caused by motor vehicle accidents, the Northern English region was noted to have an SMR of 94, while the SMR in East Anglia (a region in the south of the country) was 126. The reasons for the variation are not known but could reflect road conditions or driving habits.

Evaluating Disease Associations

The scientific method dictates that the results of study be used to develop an improved or more specific hypothesis and that this hypothesis, in turn, be tested in subsequent studies. A problem in clinical research often comes to light from reports of unusual cases or rapid changes in disease frequency. A case report is a detailed presentation of a single case or a few cases and focuses attention on a particular subject, most often an unusual one. Case reports should not be accepted as truth and the basis for action but, instead, as observations that may merit further investigation. Thus, isolated reports of malignant tumors associated with joint replacements led to an investigation by the Editor of *The Journal of Bone and Joint Surgery (Br)*, who asked for all such cases to be reported to *The Journal*. A similar response should be made to case series, which usually evaluate a procedure in a particular disease by comparing results with historical data, for example, from patients left untreated, or with series from elsewhere.

Unfortunately, the tendency has always been to try to use case reports and case series to determine etiology or the efficacy of treatment. The potential distortion caused by limiting a study to a portion of the clinical spectrum, such as hospitalized cases, should be obvious. Yet, this is commonly done and is of special significance because of the great volume of clinical research reported from teaching centers, where this problem is most acute (see selection bias later).

Sampling

Although epidemiologists are interested in populations, it is not always possible or necessary to study the population. Instead, a sample often is selected. To ensure that the findings can then be extrapolated to the population (external validity, which is the degree to which the results are correct for the sample), the sample studied must be representative of the population. This is accomplished by formal sampling procedures that permit the use of standard statistical methods for unbiased estimates, for measures of the precision of these estimates, and for significance testing. Some important rules for sampling from a human population include the following: (1) The population to be sampled must be well defined and all members of that population identifiable. This was not always the case. In an analysis of papers published in *The Journal of Bone and Joint Surgery (Br)* in 1984, about half of the papers lacked information on the source of the study sample, with a resultant loss of external validity. (2) The sampling mechanism must be such that, for every member of the population, the probability of that person's inclusion in the sample is known and not zero (probability sampling). This can be undertaken by various sampling strategies: random, systematic, stratified random, and staged (cluster) sampling. Studies that do not obtain samples in this way, a common practice in clinical research, suffer from selection bias (discussed later) that causes difficulty in interpreting results. (3) The sampling plan, which defines these probabilities, must be carried through exactly as planned, without changes that might be tempting for the sake of convenience. Therefore, it may be advisable to have an unbiased person draw the study sample. For example, in a randomized controlled trial to assess the effectiveness of geriatric rehabilitative care of elderly women who had proximal femoral fractures, patients were allocated in random sequence determined before the study began. The allocations were held

in sealed envelopes by the departmental secretary. (4) Conclusions may be restricted to the sample studies, unless proper sampling procedures are followed. For example, reports of hospitalized patients found that pelvic fractures were associated with severe trauma in young people and that the risk of associated pelvic organ injury was high. A population-based study, on the other hand, showed that most pelvic fractures in the community occurred in older women following minor injury; such fractures were unlikely to be associated with urologic or vascular complications. The findings of the hospital case series applied to the population of hospital patients but not to the general population; their use might have led to health care policy that was inappropriate for society at large.

Study Design: Observational Studies

Evaluation of the relationship (or association) between various patient characteristics (or exposures) and the development of disease (or outcome) is accomplished with three basic epidemiologic study designs: cross-sectional studies, cohort studies, and case-control studies. All of these are observational studies, insofar as the investigator has no control over the exposure status of different groups of subjects. By contrast, in experimental studies, the investigator randomly assigns the exposure factor being evaluated.

Cross-sectional Studies (Prevalence Studies)   A random sample of the general population to be studied is drawn, and each person in the sample is classified as having or not having the disease and as manifesting or not manifesting the risk factor of interest. The distinctive feature of a cross-sectional study is that this information is obtained at only one point in time. Thus, a study to ascertain the association between degenerative knee joint disease and previous meniscectomy seeks to identify subjects with either or both of these conditions. Subsequent analysis assesses the degree of association between exposure and disease by examining the null hypothesis that no difference exists in the proportion of exposed patients (those who had meniscectomy) and unexposed patients (those with intact menisci), all of whom have degenerative arthritis.

If the general population is sampled, this type of study allows estimation of the prevalence of disease and also the prevalence of exposure in the population. If the study is not population-based, these advantages do not accrue. The relative frequencies of exposure to the factor in the diseased and nondiseased groups can be estimated and used to determine the probabilities of exposure factor and disease occurring together. These data do not, however, provide an estimate of the risk of subsequent disease given exposure to the factor.

This method is very inefficient if either the risk factor or the disease are rare or if they are so common that unexposed or nondiseased subjects are rare. Then the total sample, even though large, provides little information on the association between the factor and the disease. Sampling from the general population is also difficult and is likely to be costly. As prevalence cases are examined, cases of long duration will be overrepresented (eg, early deaths will be missed). Also, it may not be possible to tell whether exposure preceded or followed the onset of disease.

Case-control Studies (Retrospective Studies) A sample of persons with a particular disease and a second sample of persons free of the disease are identified, and each member of the two groups is then classified with respect to exposure to the risk factor of interest. Much of what is known about chronic disease epidemiology has been derived from case-control studies, and such studies are usually the first approach to testing an etiologic hypothesis. For example, to examine the role of regular exercise and high calcium intake in reducing hip fractures, researchers undertook a case-control study in England. Three hundred of the 473 patients aged 50 years and older who were sequentially hospitalized with hip fractures were compared with 600 community controls. All subjects were interviewed to ascertain their recent calcium intake and level of physical activity. The risk of fracture increased significantly with lower levels of physical activity for both men and women. There was no change in fracture risk with increasing calcium intake among women, but there was a fall in risk among men.

The relative importance of a putative risk factor (the strength of its association with the disease) usually is estimated in a case-control study by the odds ratio (Fig. 2), defined as the odds that a case was exposed divided by the odds that a control was exposed. The odds ratio is an estimate of the relative risk of disease (see below) in exposed compared to unexposed persons as obtained from a cohort study. However, the odds ratio is an accurate estimate of relative risk only under the following conditions: (1) the disease group is representative, at least in terms of exposure, of all cases of the disease; (2) the control group is representative, at least in terms of exposure, of the general population of undiseased people; and (3) the incidence rate of the disease in the population is relatively small. Unfortunately, cases of the disease in question usually are obtained from hospitals or clinics, while controls often are chosen from other classes of hospital or clinic patients. However, population-based case-control studies can be conducted in which the cases represent a sample of all cases from the community and controls are sampled from the same community.

Efficiency in a case-control study can be enhanced by matching. This technique ensures that, for each subject in the study group, there is at least one subject in the comparison group with the same characteristics, except for the risk factor of interest. Matching usually is undertaken for important but extraneous variables, such as age and sex in studies of hip fractures. Thus, in the example cited earlier, community controls were matched individually to the hip fracture patients in the study group by sex

	DISEASE		
FACTOR	Present	Absent	
Exposed	a	b	a + b
Nonexposed	c	d	c + d
	a + c	b + d	

Cohort Study

Relative risk = $\dfrac{a/(a+b)}{c/(c+d)}$

Case-control study

Odds ratio = $\dfrac{\dfrac{a/(a+c)}{c/(a+c)}}{\dfrac{b/(b+d)}{d/(b+d)}} = \dfrac{a/c}{b/d} = \dfrac{ad}{bc}$

Fig. 2 Calculation of risk from cohort and case-control studies.

and by age within four years. Subjects can be matched for other significant factors, but matching for a variable precludes assessment of its effect on the outcome. Additionally, matching for many factors creates the practical problem of finding enough control subjects who meet all of the criteria. If not undertaken carefully, matching can introduce problems. For example, if cases and controls are matched on a variable related to the exposure, the exposure's effect on disease risk may be underestimated (overmatching).

A further requirement for a valid case-control study is that exposure be assessed accurately and equivalently for cases and controls. Most often, exposure is determined by interview; this may lead to a bias, if recall of the exposure is influenced by occurrence of the disease (memory bias). Consequently, validating exposure data (eg, by reviewing prior medical records) is generally a good idea.

Case-control studies are relatively inexpensive, and the results may be obtained within a short time. Often they are possible when other study designs are not feasible. Indeed, this may be the only way to study rare (ie, most) diseases. Case-control studies allow data to be collected and analyzed for a variety of exposures and are, thus, a powerful design for evaluating multiple risk factors. The case-control approach is especially useful in seeking out heretofore unsuspected risk factors.

Case-control studies are subject to Berkson bias when samples are drawn from hospital or clinic patients whose selection from the general population may be influenced by the factor of interest, to interviewer bias if study personnel are not blinded and systematically search harder for exposure data among the cases, and to memory bias if the occurrence of disease influences the likelihood of remembering the exposure. If exposure data are collected from previous records, the presence or absence of the factor in question may not have been collected at all, or inconsistent definitions may have been used. If information is obtained only from those living with the disease, the elimination of patients already dead may introduce serious bias. In addition, direct estimates of disease incidence in the exposed and unexposed groups cannot be obtained from a case-control study.

Cohort Studies (Prospective or Follow-up Studies) A sample of the disease-free population exposed to a factor and a second sample of persons not exposed to the factor are identified from the same population. Each member of the two samples (or cohorts) is followed for a specified period and observed for development of the disease. To establish a positive (or negative) association between exposure to the factor and occurrence of the disease, it is necessary to show that the incidence of disease is significantly higher (or lower) in those exposed than in those not exposed. With equal periods of observation in the two groups, this can be done by comparing the proportion of diseased patients among those exposed with the proportion in the unexposed group.

Cohort studies usually are undertaken to verify an association found in cross-sectional or case-control studies. For example, to study further the role of dietary calcium and physical activity in hip fractures, the same researchers (as in the example in the case-control study) followed 1,419 randomly selected people aged 65 years and older, 44 of whom sustained hip fractures during a 15-year follow-up period. Although the number of cases was small, elderly individuals with reduced physical activity had a higher risk of hip fracture, but calcium intake at baseline had no influence on fracture risk.

The ratio of the incidence of disease in exposed persons to the incidence in nonexposed persons is expressed as the relative risk (Fig. 2). Relative risk measures the potency of a particular risk factor and is important in assessing the etiologic role of that factor in disease causation. Thus, the larger the relative risk, the stronger the association between the factor and the disease. In the example cited earlier, the risk of hip fracture was 3.9 times higher in women who had a low outdoor activity index (less than 44 as derived from a series of questions) compared to those with a high activity index (57 or more). Usually, if the relative risk is greater than 2.0, which indicates a doubling of the likelihood of developing the disease on exposure to the factor, it is considered important.

A comparison also can be made in terms of the difference in incidence rates of exposed and nonexposed persons. The difference provides the attributable risk (incidence among exposed persons minus incidence among unexposed persons), which measures the practical importance of the factor in producing the disease in the population if the relationship is causal. Attributable risk indicates the amount by which the disease burden might be reduced if the causative factor could be eliminated

from the population. It is, thus, an important measure from a public health perspective.

Cohort studies provide direct estimates, with measurable precision, of relative risk, which answers the clinical question: How much is the risk of the disease increased by this exposure? This type of study is optimal only when one main risk factor is being evaluated and is especially valuable when multiple disease outcomes need to be assessed. Errors caused by misclassification of exposure status usually are minimized in a cohort study, because exposure can be assessed directly, thus eliminating memory bias. Further, information regarding the exposure is recorded without bias attributable to knowledge of the final outcome (ie, the disease that develops later cannot affect the determination of the presence or absence of the factor), as may occur in case-control studies. Cohort studies also allow for calculation of incidence rates of the disease.

This method provides a direct estimate of the frequency of exposure only if the study begins with a general population sample subsequently classified as exposed and not exposed to the factor of interest. If the disease is rare, efficiency may be very low, as large numbers of people have to be recruited for study in order to observe a sufficient number of outcome events. Even if the disease is not rare, the problem of identifying and sampling the exposed and unexposed groups is difficult and often expensive. In addition, it may be difficult and expensive to maintain follow-up on the cohorts if the time required to develop the disease is long. Finally, if the study period is prolonged, scientific advances may invalidate the original study question.

It is sometimes possible to overcome the disadvantage of prospective follow-up if one can locate records containing the needed information regarding exposure recorded at some time in the past. In this case, the previously existing population is identified, and the disease experience of the exposed and unexposed groups is ascertained up to the present time (retrospective cohort study). An obvious difficulty in using the retrospective approach is the frequent inability to relocate all of the subjects in the original samples for follow-up.

Comparison of Observational Study Designs The salient features of the three main designs for observational epidemiologic studies are summarized in Table 1.

Study Design: Experimental Studies

In studying the relative importance of exposure to some factor in influencing the occurrence of a disease, the ideal method of investigation is an experimental one. In its purest form, a sample from the general population free of the disease and not yet exposed to the factor is divided randomly into two groups of similar composition, one of which is exposed to the intervention being evaluated. The two groups may be matched (or balanced) by age, race, sex, and other characteristics thought to be of importance in the disease, but randomi-

Table 1. Salient features of cross-sectional, case-control, and cohort studies

Cross-sectional	Case-control	Cohort
Begins with defined population	Population at risk not defined	Begins with defined population
Useful for developing an etiologic hypothesis	Usually the first approach to testing an etiologic hypothesis	Best for a precisely formulated etiologic hypothesis
Exposure and disease measured simultaneously	Disease measured before exposure	Exposure measured before disease
Tests whether suspected factor and disease occur together	Tests whether suspected factor occurs more frequently in those with disease	Tests whether disease occurs more frequently in those exposed to suspected factor
Incidence and risk of disease cannot be measured	Incidence cannot be measured; risk estimated by odds ratio	Incidence and risk can be measured directly
Can be undertaken quickly	Can be undertaken quickly	Takes time, especially prospective
Can assess multiple diseases	Can assess one disease	Can assess multiple disease outcomes
Can assess multiple exposures	Can assess multiple exposures	Can assess one exposure
Not suitable for rare diseases	Ideal for rare diseases	Not suitable for rare diseases

zation also controls for the effects of other, unknown factors that may influence the outcome. Each group is followed for an appropriate period of time, during which every effort is made to ensure compliance in the exposed group while the comparison group is kept from all such exposure. The relative frequency of occurrence of the disease in the two groups is then observed. This is the principle of the randomized clinical trial, where the ability of some therapeutic maneuver to prevent disease (or to prevent complications or death) is evaluated.

Randomized controlled clinical trials usually are undertaken to evaluate two or more treatments that have different outcomes but are perceived by some physicians to be of equal value to the patient. For example, care of elderly patients with hip fractures was assessed by a randomized trial following reports that collaboration between orthopaedic surgeons and physicians in geriatric medicine shortened hospital stay, improved the patients' personal independence at discharge, and reduced the level of care they needed after discharge. One hundred and eight elderly patients with hip fractures were randomized to a treatment or control group; the treatment group was supervised extensively by a geriatrician in addition to receiving physiotherapy and other services. At discharge, patients in the treatment group had been hospitalized for a shorter time and were significantly more independent in terms of activities of daily living.

Blinding (or masking) often is used to enhance the internal validity of such studies. It is most necessary when the reporting of the outcome under consideration might be influenced by knowledge of the treatment. A study may be single-blind (subjects do not know if they are in the treatment or the control group), double-blind (neither the subject nor the investigator knows the group), or triple-blind (neither the subject, the investigator, nor the analyst knows which treatment the subject is receiving). In the example quoted above, neither the staff nor the patients were blinded to the trial. Therefore, the findings may have been biased, especially since a similar study from a different center reported contrary

results. Blinding is not always an option in surgical research, and, in such studies, it may be useful to have an independent clinician evaluate the results.

An experiment is the most powerful design for establishing a causal association or the superiority of one treatment regimen over another. It may be the only acceptable design for some research questions, and certainly for evaluating the usefulness of expensive or high risk technology. Experiments also provide for valid probability statements that require minimal assumptions.

Apart from ethical concerns, experiments often are difficult and expensive to carry out. Moreover, despite their apparent simplicity, experiments are subject to significant biases in the selection of study subjects and specification of the population to which study results are referable (referent population), in the allocation and compliance with the randomized treatment, and in the equal assessment of outcomes in treated and untreated groups. For example, whether the results of a randomized clinical trial apply to the general population with the particular condition depends on how study subjects were selected. Thus, results of surgery from a tertiary referral center may not be applicable to orthopaedic practice in the community, because patients seen at the referral center are not typical of such patients in general and are operated on by experts. Randomized clinical trials may be difficult to undertake in orthopaedic surgery because of problems related to the nature of surgery; ie, irreversibility of the procedure, comparability of surgeons, and the long follow-up required to determine outcome.

Interpreting Epidemiologic Data

Hypothesis Testing

The result of many epidemiologic studies is a series of associations between the disease in question and various potential risk factors. Such associations can be examined by stating and testing hypotheses. In the statistical analysis of epidemiologic data, a null hypothesis (Ho) usually is stated, and an attempt is made to disprove it in favor of an alternative hypothesis (Ha) as follows: suppose the null hypothesis were true that there is no real relationship between the exposure and the disease. What, then, is the probability of observing an effect as strong as that seen in the study if, in fact, there is no real effect? If the probability is small, reject the null hypothesis and conclude that the evidence supports the alternative (that an effect exists). The familiar p-value is a statement of the probability that observed differences in a particular study could have happened by chance alone. The p-value measures the likelihood of an alpha (α) error; ie, the error of saying that there is a difference when there is not. It is customary to accept values less than 0.05 as significant, the implication being that such an occurrence would arise by chance alone in fewer than one in 20 observations and is, therefore, unlikely to be due to chance.

However, if the probability is not small, the null hypothesis cannot be rejected. This raises the possibility of a beta (β) error; ie, the error of concluding that an effect does not exist when it does. This possibility must be considered whenever a study results in a finding of "no difference," but especially when the study is small. The probability that a study will find a statistically significant difference when a difference really exists is called statistical power and is expressed as 1 minus the probability of beta error.

Chance Association

As is obvious from the preceding discussion, the relationship between exposure to some factor and disease may be on the basis of chance alone. Even if the exposure and the disease are uncommon, some individuals will be found with both simply by chance; this is the problem in interpreting case reports. One main purpose of statistical analysis is to identify and eliminate this sort of association.

Whether chance can account for the observed differences depends on the following:

Size of the Sample   Sample size is guided by the magnitude of the difference to be detected. Assuming that everything else is equal, detection of small differences requires a large number of patients. For example, researchers in Sweden calculated that 2,960 patients were required to demonstrate a significant difference (p<0.05) in loosening probability between two types of total hip prostheses, assuming a probability of failure of 5% and 3%, respectively. Multicenter research was suggested to obtain such a large sample.

Alpha Error   Although it is customary to set alpha at 0.05, the acceptable size for alpha error is a value judgment. However, to ensure only a small risk of concluding that a particular treatment is useful when it is not, alpha should be small. If, in the above example, a one in 20 risk were too high, the investigators could set alpha at one in 100 or p<0.01. Assuming 80% power ($\beta = 0.20$), the

sample size required would now be 4,416 patients, 2,208 in each treatment group.

Beta Error   By convention, beta often is set at 0.20; ie, a 20% chance of missing a true difference in a particular study of a given size. The study in such a case is said to have 80% power for detecting a difference of the magnitude specified. Again, a decision has to be made by the researcher on where to set the limit. In an example quoted earlier, in which only 44 cases of hip fracture were identified in the cohort of 1,419 men and women, the researchers acknowledged the low power of their study to detect an effect of calcium intake on the risk of hip fracture.

Of late, there has been some concern about the use of p-values in reporting research findings. The use of confidence intervals has been urged instead, because investigators and users of the findings need to know the size of the difference between groups, not simply whether the difference is statistically significant. Confidence intervals give an indication of the precision of the study value as an estimate of the true difference in the population. Thus, in the cohort study example, the relative risk of hip fracture in women with limited outdoor activities (index of <44) was 3.9, but the 95% confidence interval varied from 1.4 to 10.9. Although the relative risk was thus higher than 1.0, the value under the null hypothesis, there was considerable uncertainty about the exact figure. On this basis, the reader can make a more informed judgment about the reliability of the result.

Spurious Association (Bias)

Even if not due to chance, the relationship between the exposure and the disease may be spurious because of some bias (or systematic error) in data collection or some defect in study design. Biases produce results that differ systematically from the true values. Bias and chance can coexist in the same study. There are seven stages of a case-control study: (1) reading up on the field, (2) specifying and selecting the study sample, (3) executing the experimental maneuver, (4) measuring exposures and outcomes, (5) analyzing data, (6) interpreting the analysis, and (7) publishing the results. Fifty-seven different types of bias or spurious association have been listed that may occur in one or another of these seven stages. One of the main roles of epidemiologic analysis is to identify and minimize spurious associations.

Orthopaedists need to be aware of the following four broad categories of bias:

Selection bias   Selection bias was alluded to earlier in describing pelvic fractures. Bias occurs because the patients studied may be different in important ways from the larger population to whom the study results may supposedly apply. Berkson bias is a type of selection bias that is especially relevant to clinicians conducting case-control studies of patients drawn from a hospital. False conclusions result from over- or underrepresentation of different combinations of disease and exposure caused by hospital or patient characteristics that determined why some patients chose the particular hospital.

Measurement bias Measurement bias results from systematic variation in study instruments (measurement variation), study subjects (biologic variation), or in the way measurements are made (intraobserver and interobserver variation). For example, poor agreement between observers on radiographic signs of union of scaphoid fractures has a bearing on treatment and prognosis and may have medicolegal implications. Standard definitions may reduce these variations. Thus, to allow meaningful comparisons between different investigators reporting results of total hip arthroplasty, the Hip Society has produced a standard system of terminology, and its use has been advocated by the American Academy of Orthopaedic Surgeons.

Response bias Response bias is systematic error occurring when subjects respond inaccurately to the question either by design or by accident. Memory or recall bias, referred to earlier (see case-control study), occurs because those with the disease are generally more likely to recall an antecedent exposure than those who do not have the disease. To avoid memory bias, researchers in the cohort study example calculated calcium intake from a seven-day dietary record kept by the patients rather than from the 24-hour recall used in a similar study in California.

Hawthorne effect Hawthorne effect refers to the fact that people, on learning that they are the subjects of a study, often change their behavior. This is difficult to avoid. Thus, in the study to assess the effectiveness of geriatric care on hip fractures, patients' awareness of the study may have led them to make an extra effort in order to please their physicians, creating a bias. The role of blinding in experiments is to ensure that any effect of this sort is similar in the treatment and comparison groups.

Indirect Association (Confounding)

A relationship between the exposure and the disease can also exist because both treatment and comparison groups are related to some other underlying condition or factor that has not been taken into consideration. This underlying factor is called a confounder. For example, in the case-control study described earlier, body mass index, cigarette smoking, alcohol consumption, history of stroke, and use of steroids were possible confounding variables, and the researchers adjusted accordingly for these variables in examining the relationship between physical activity and risk of hip fracture. An alternative to adjustment during analysis is matching. The reader will recall that controls were matched to patients by age and sex.

The possibility that a confounder exists is an important concern in all studies and dictates that other plausible

explanations for the findings be considered in addition to the obvious one of a direct causal association. In another example, long distance runners were more likely to have radiographic signs of hip joint disease than were bobsleigh riders or controls, but they were also older. Age, therefore, could have caused the association indirectly, and researchers age-adjusted their data accordingly in estimating the risk of degenerative hip joint disease associated with prolonged long-distance running.

Direct Association

Finally, the disease and the exposure may truly be related. However, the factor could be an effect as well as the cause of the disease, so further study of this point is required before causality can be assumed. In order to be considered causally associated, a particular exposure factor must, alone or with other "causes," produce the disease in question. To be considered causal, a putative risk factor should meet the following criteria:

Strength The stronger the association, in terms of risk, the more likely it is that the relationship is causal.

Consistency The association should hold up in repeated studies undertaken in different places and under different circumstances by different investigators.

Specificity The presence of the exposure should predict the disease as uniquely as possible, although other factors may be required for disease production and although a single factor may be associated with more than one disease.

Temporality The presumed causal exposure factor should precede the development of the disease in time.

Biological gradient The likelihood of causality is improved if an increase in the "dose" of the exposure factor leads to an increased risk of the disease.

Plausibility The relationship should make sense in terms of present biologic knowledge.

Coherence The proposed cause and effect should not seriously conflict with generally known facts about the natural history and biology of the disease.

Experiment There is experimental evidence (in animals, perhaps) that directly tests the nature of the relationship.

Analogy Instances may be known in which relationships similar to the one in question have been proven to exist.

Inference from Epidemiologic Studies

The results of a study may apply to the sample or to the entire population, depending on the study's validity. However, the interpretation of validity must be made on a number of levels.

Statistical judgment Statistical judgment is required to determine whether the observed associations are caused by chance or, alternatively, how much confidence we have that the results are not caused by chance. This is accomplished through statistically adequate study design and analysis, including p-values, confidence intervals, and other such measurements.

Epidemiologic judgment Epidemiologic judgment contributes by ensuring epidemiologically valid design in the first place and by assessing whether uncontrollable biases, rather than true relationships, may have produced any statistically "significant" associations that are observed.

Clinical judgment Clinical judgment is the most important contribution. Clinical judgment leads to the decision that the question is important and that the study is worth doing in the first place. Clinical judgment is essential to interpretation by distinguishing what is statistically and epidemiologically significant from what is clinically significant and useful.

Future Opportunities

Overall, orthopaedic surgery is a relatively young specialty. Its research base is, therefore, small. Although major advances in medical technology and in surgical and anesthetic techniques have been made in recent years, additional research is required (some of it urgently) in almost all areas from disease definition to outcome measurement. The burden of orthopaedic conditions, their frequency, their costs (both to the patient and to society), and the clinical and social sequelae of these diseases need study. Better disease definitions are required for epidemiologic studies, which can help examine natural history as well as trends in incidence and prevalence rates for specific disorders. Etiologic hypotheses need testing so that preventive strategies can be formulated. Criteria for surgical interventions need to be developed, and the interventions need to be subjected to randomized control trials for proper evaluation of their cost and risk. The ultimate aim of treatment must be improvement in the patient's quality of life. In this respect, outcomes assessment is an area that has been neglected. There is a need for better methodology to measure functional disability, cost of care, and quality of life for the orthopaedic patient.

Annotated Bibliography

Altman RD: Criteria for classification of clinical osteoarthritis. *J Rheumatol* 1991;27(suppl):10-12.

  To permit uniform reporting, the American College of Rheumatology has developed classification criteria for symptomatic osteoarthritis of the knee, hip, and hand. Specific criteria based on clinical, laboratory, and radiographic findings are recommended for population surveys and reporting results.

Apley AG: Malignancy and joint replacement: The tip of an iceberg? *J Bone Joint Surg* 1989;71B:1.

  Following case reports of malignancy associated with joint replacement, the Editor of *The Journal* exhorts orthopaedic surgeons to report any such cases to *The Journal* in order to help clarify the issue.

Chang RW, Falconer J, Stulberg SD, et al: Prerandomization: An alternative to classic randomization: The effects on recruitment in a controlled trial of arthroscopy for osteoarthrosis of the knee. *J Bone Joint Surg* 1990;72A:1451-1455.

  Because of physicians' concerns about a compromised physician-patient relationship, difficulty with attaining informed consent, and dislike of discussions of uncertainty, enrollment for randomized control trials can be problematic. A design that overcomes these difficulties is described.

Cooper C, Barker DJ, Wickham C: Physical activity, muscle strength, and calcium intake in fracture of the proximal femur in Britain. *Br Med J* 1988;297:1443-1446.

  This case-control study demonstrates an increased risk of hip fracture in less physically active elderly persons who also have reduced grip strength. The importance of being active in old age is emphasized.

Davis MA, Ettinger WH, Neuhaus JM, et al: Knee osteoarthritis and physical functioning: Evidence from the NHANES I Epidemiologic Followup Study. *J Rheumatol* 1991;18:591-598.

  To describe the patterns of physical difficulty ten years after the diagnosis of radiographic knee OA, National Health and Nutrition Examination Survey (NHANES) 1971-75 and NHANES Epidemiologic Study Follow-up data were analyzed. Persons with radiographic knee OA reported more difficulty with physical functioning, including activities of daily living, compared with persons without knee OA. Persons who had knee pain and OA at the first examination had more subsequent disability, and these factors can indicate the likelihood of deterioration in physical functioning.

Day SJ, Graham DF: Sample size and power for comparing two or more treatment groups in clinical trials. *Br Med J* 1989;299:663-665.

  A nomogram to calculate the sample size required when comparing up to five parallel groups is described. The nomogram also can be used determine the power of a study given the sample size.

Deyo RA, Cherkin D, Conrad D, et al: Cost, controversy, crisis: Low back pain and the health of the public. *Annu Rev Public Health* 1991;12:141-156.

This review discusses some pertinent issues relating to low back pain, the direct personal medical care costs of which were $12.9 billion in the United States in 1977 (1988 estimate = $17.9 billion); the condition affects 70% to 80% of adults at some time during their lives. There is considerable variation in the management of patients with low back pain, with a high failure rate of surgical treatment. Due regard to social and economic factors that influence the outcome of back pain, effective prevention programs at the work place, and education may help to reduce the burden on the health care system and society at large.

Dias JJ, Taylor M, Thompson, J, et al: Radiographic signs of union of scaphoid fractures: An analysis of inter-observer agreement and reproducibility. *J Bone Joint Surg* 1988;70B:299-301.

Poor observer agreement on what constitutes a radiologically united scaphoid fracture may have clinical implications and medicolegal significance.

Dobbs HS: Survivorship of total hip replacements. *J Bone Joint Surg* 1980;62B:168-173.

Using the method described by Armitage, metal-on-plastic prostheses were demonstrated to perform better than metal-on-metal. Loosening was the predominant failure mode, and the rate of loosening increased with increasing follow-up period.

Felson DT: The epidemiology of knee osteoarthritis: Results from the Framingham Osteoarthritis Study. *Semin Arthritis Rheum* 1990(suppl 1);20:42-50.

By examining the Framingham Heart Study cohort, the prevalence of osteoarthritis of the knee was found to increase gradually with age, and this rise was more marked in women. Obesity, previous knee injury, chondrocalcinosis, and occupational knee bending and physical labor were important risk factors associated with OA of the knee.

Fletcher RH, Fletcher SW: Clinical research in general medical journals: A 30-year perspective. *N Engl J Med* 1979;301:180-183.

The frequency of published studies of weak research design increased during the period from 1946 through 1976. Such studies can cause misleading conclusions, as witnessed in many instances in which subsequent studies with more powerful design were undertaken.

Fowkes FG, Fulton PM: Critical appraisal of published research: Introductory guidelines. *Br Med J* 1991;302:1136-1140.

This paper describes the various study designs and how to critique them. Essentially, the appraisal involves ruling out chance, bias, and confounding as causes of an observed association. The guidelines can help readers to determine the quality of the published literature.

Friedman GD: Medical usage and abusage: "Prevalence" and "incidence." *Ann Intern Med* 1976;84:502-504.

After starting with ". . .the easiest way to distinguish a clinician from an epidemiologist is by the clinician's incorrect use of the term 'incidence,' Dr. Friedman explains what the terms

mean. A better understanding of these terms would help improve communication with others.

Gardner MJ, Altman DG: Confidence intervals rather than P values: Estimation rather than hypothesis testing. *Br Med J* 1986;292:746-750.

The emphasis on hypothesis testing and the use of p values in the medical literature allows little useful interpretation of study results. The size of the difference of a measured outcome between groups is of more interest to practitioners than whether a difference is statistically significant. This can be determined by estimation and confidence intervals. Methods for calculating confidence intervals are given and their use is urged.

Gartland JJ: Orthopaedic clinical research: Deficiencies in experimental design and determinations of outcome. *J Bone Joint Surg* 1988;70A:1357-1364.

Authors, journals, program committees, and professional societies are blamed for poor study design in orthopaedic research. The common deficiencies in ten follow-up studies of patients with total hip arthroplasty are described, along with suggestions on how to improve the present state of affairs.

Haralson RH III: Computerized information retrieval and medical education for orthopaedists: Current concepts review. *J Bone Joint Surg* 1988;70A:624-629.

Information retrieval has become much easier with computer technology. Various ways of accessing information are described.

Haynes RB, McKibbon KA, Fitzgerald D, et al: How to keep up with the medical literature: I. Why try to keep up and how to get started. *Ann Intern Med* 1986;105:149-153.

Haynes RB, McKibbon KA, Fitzgerald D, et al: How to keep up with the medical literature: II. Deciding which journals to read regularly. *Ann Intern Med* 1986;105:309-312.

Haynes RB, McKibbon KA, Fitzgerald D, et al: How to keep up with the medical literature: III. Expanding the number of journals you read regularly. *Ann Intern Med* 1986;105:474-478.

Haynes RB, McKibbon KA, Fitzgerald D, et al: How to keep up with the medical literature: IV. Using the literature to solve clinical problems. *Ann Intern Med* 1986;105:636-640.

Haynes RB, McKibbon KA, Fitzgerald D, et al: How to keep up with the medical literature: V. Access by personal computer to the medical literature. *Ann Intern Med* 1986;105:810-824.

Haynes RB, McKibbon KA, Fitzgerald D, et al: How to keep up with the medical literature: VI. How to store and retrieve articles worth keeping. *Ann Intern Med* 1986;105:978-984.

This series is good, perhaps essential, reading for beginners. The self-explanatory titles should help in deciding.

Herberts P, Ahnfelt L, Malchau H, et al: Multicenter clinical trials and their value in assessing total joint arthroplasty. *Clin Orthop* 1989;249:48-55.

Proper evaluation of total joint replacement requires large numbers of patients, and multicenter trials can help achieve the required sample size.

Hill AB: The environment and disease: Association or causation? *Proc Roy Soc Med* 1965;58:295-300.

This classic paper describes the nine criteria used to evaluate causality against which a putative factor must be measured. It plays down the role of formal tests of significance in answering the questions: Is there any other way of explaining the set of facts before use? and Is there any other answer equally or more likely than cause and effect?

Kennie DC, Reid J, Richardson IR, et al: Effectiveness of geriatric rehabilitative care after fractures of the proximal femur in elderly women: A randomised clinical trial. *Br Med J* 1988;297:1083-1086

Elderly women with hip fractures had a better outcome if they were transferred to the care of physicians with an interest in care of the elderly following initial management, including surgery.

Kurland LT, Molgaard CA: The patient record in epidemiology. *Sci Am* 1981;245:54-63.

The central recordkeeping system at the Mayo Clinic allowed the development of an epidemiologic laboratory and made possible the study of many diseases. Much of the data on the incidence of various fractures in the United States comes from studies undertaken here. The article describes the uses and limitations of studies based on clinical records.

Melton LJ, Riggs BL: Epidemiology of age-related fractures, in Avioli LV (ed): *The Osteoporotic Syndrome; Detection, Prevention and Treatment.* New York, Grune & Stratton Inc, 1983, pp 45-72.

The importance of epidemiologic data on age-related fractures lies in their use for generating and testing hypotheses, for predicting prognosis in individual patients, and for designing efficient preventive strategies. The need for such data is obvious considering the extent of mortality, morbidity, and costs associated with these fractures. Using epidemiologic principles, people at risk of developing fractures can be identified and remedial action undertaken.

Morris RW: A statistical study of papers in the *Journal of Bone and Joint Surgery (Br)* 1984. *J Bone Joint Surg* 1988;70B:242-246.

The statistical quality of original articles published in *The Journal of Bone and Joint Surgery (British volume)* in 1984 was found wanting overall, thus casting doubts on researchers' understanding of study design and their ability to analyze data and interpret results. This paper contains a useful checklist for assessing statistical aspects of scientific papers.

Motulsky AG: Sounding board: Biased ascertainment and the natural history of diseases. *N Engl J Med* 1978;298:1196-1197.

How selection bias influences the published data on the natural history of disease and the prognosis and surgical treatment of conditions is explained clearly.

O'Brien PC, Shampo MA: Statistics for clinicians. *Mayo Clin Proc* 1981;56:47-49,126-128,196-197,274-276,324-326,393-394,452-454,513-515,573-575,639-640,709-711,753-754,755-756.

In a series of papers, the authors describe the elementary concepts and methods of statistics. Descriptive statistics for describing a data set (mean, median, standard deviation) are followed by inferential statistics used in estimating population characteristics from random sample studies. Topics of interest include evaluation of new diagnostic procedures, determination of normal values, description of survivorship, and use of sequential methods. Altogether, this is a useful guide for the beginner.

Raskob GE, Lofthouse RN, Hull RD: Methodological guidelines for clinical trials evaluating new therapeutic approaches in bone and joint surgery: Current concepts review. *J Bone Joint Surg* 1985;67A:1294-1297.

Potentially serious implications of the premature introduction of a new therapy can and should be avoided by properly conducted trials. These trials should meet certain study design criteria, which are described. The use of these criteria is required in resolving controversial management issues, such as conservative versus surgical treatment for knee ligament injuries.

Riihimaki H: Low-back pain, its origin and risk indicators. *Scand J Work Environ Health* 1991;17:81-90.

The exact pathologic condition in patients with low back pain is difficult to determine, because pain can arise from various sites, and because there is poor correlation between imaging findings and symptoms. This review discusses the various occupational and personal factors associated with the risk of developing low back pain. The article provides a very useful reference list.

Rudicel S, Esdaile J: The randomized clinical trial in orthopaedics: Obligation or option? *J Bone Joint Surg* 1985;67A:1284-1293.

Randomized clinical trials, the scientific gold standard for research designed to answer questions regarding medical therapy, are not always an option in orthopaedic surgery. Four common biases (susceptibility, performance, detection, and transfer) limit the usefulness of the randomized control design in orthopaedic surgery. Problems such as surgical ethos, surgeons favoring one operation over another, and different skill in performing different operations suggest that an alternative to the randomized clinical trial may be the randomized surgeon design, which is then described.

Sackett DL: Bias in analytic research. *J Chronic Dis* 1979;32:51-63.

With the proliferation of case-control studies over the last few decades, readers must be aware of the pitfalls in such study design. This excellent paper catalogs the various biases that can occur at each stage of a study.

Wickham CA, Walsh K, Cooper C, et al: Dietary calcium, physical activity, and risk of hip fracture: A prospective study. *Br Med J* 1989;299:889-892.

The role of physical activity in protecting the elderly against hip fractures was confirmed in this cohort study.

2
The Epidemiology of Orthopaedic Practice

Introduction

This chapter begins by presenting a very different application of epidemiologic data. The discussion moves from a literal presentation of musculoskeletal incidence, utilization, and cost data to an in-depth analysis of the utilization patterns of musculoskeletal care by orthopaedists and their patients. When these studies are undertaken, what appears to be straightforward data reveals instead major inconsistencies in orthopaedic practice.

The chapter goes on to present important and useful epidemiologic data on the volume, categories of conditions, and cost impact of musculoskeletal disease and injury in the United States for the year 1988. These data provide important information concerning many aspects of health care policy and planning, including orthopaedic and ancillary manpower, hospital and health-care resources, costs of illness and injury, and strategies for injury prevention and treatment.

Small Area Analysis

In 1973, Wennberg and Gittelsohn described an important new concept in medical epidemiology. Using hospital discharge data, they developed the concept of small area analysis and practice pattern variations. Their work demonstrated for the first time marked variations in the provision of health care in the United States and other countries.

Using basic epidemiologic principles, Wennberg and Gittelsohn applied the technique of population-based analyses to the utilization and consumption of health care in hospitals. In retrospect the idea is simple, but no one had ever done it before, and what they learned about present-day medical care has led to a major reassessment of the practice of medicine in the United States and beyond.

The essential element in epidemiologic analyses is the calculation of population-based rates of care. One needs the numerator (the number of people treated), and the denominator (the population that might have been treated). Dividing the numerator by the denominator yields a rate, usually expressed as the number of cases per 1,000, 10,000, and so on. Numerator data are familiar to all of us. We usually know how many patients we see in our offices, how many we hospitalize, and the number of operations we perform. However, we rarely know the population base from which those patients are drawn, and so "rates" of care are unknown.

If rates of various kinds of medical care were the same across states and regions of the country, the information would be of general interest to health planners and payers, but it would not be of concern or particular interest to clinicians. However, what Wennberg and Gittelsohn discovered is of tremendous importance to all physicians and has changed medical practice in a fundamental way. They demonstrated that, for essentially all types of medical care, both medical and surgical, population-based rates reveal significant variations in utilization of medical services from one area to another. As these differences in rates of care have become apparent, they have sparked major interest and debate among the parties interested in health care. The term applied to this epidemiologic technique is "small area analysis" and the results are known as "small area variations."

Essential to small area analysis is the availability of a medical data base. At present, approximately 30 of the 50 states collect a standardized discharge data set on every patient discharged from an acute care hospital. The information collected is similar to that contained on the medical record discharge face sheet and provides essential demographic, diagnostic, and procedural data about each patient. It is computerized, processed, and maintained in a data base, usually in the public sector under the control of a state agency. Other large data bases, including Medicare, Medicaid, and private insurance, use claims data. Certain epidemiologic studies can also be carried out using this information.

Utilization of health care is calculated on the basis of location of residence of patients rather than on the location of the institution or provider. Using computer technology and zip codes of residence, it is possible to construct hospital service areas, also known as small areas. These are geographic locations in which the majority of residents are treated in hospitals located within the area. For most areas, the majority of residents receive medical care at hospitals within that area.

Although service areas are always developed around hospitals, it is important to note that a patient's admission is always counted based on his or her area of residence rather than where treatment is provided. A patient who leaves service area A for treatment at a facility in another area is counted back to his home area (A), whereas if a person residing in area B comes to an area A hospital for treatment, the case would be counted in area B. This methodology adjusts for the problem known as border crossing. Because there may be differences in population demographics, each area rate is adjusted for age and sex.

Analysis of data is carried out by calculating the state-wide utilization rate for a condition or procedure and then calculating the rates for the same procedure in each hospital service area. The average utilization rate for the whole state can be used as a reference point, and a ranking of rates for the individual service areas can be established. If there were consistency in how physicians treat patients, one would expect small area utilization rates to cluster around the state rate. It is important to note that the state average rate is not held out to be the "right rate." It simply represents the average utilization in that state for the year being measured. With adequate data, similar analyses can also be carried out across states, regions, and even between different countries.

As Wennberg and Gittelsohn began these kinds of analyses—initially in Vermont and later in Maine—they noted striking differences in per capita rates of utilization of health care. As previously noted, after appropriate statistical adjustments, one might expect that the rates of hospitalization for medical care would be fairly similar across a state or region. The likelihood of patients undergoing such procedures as joint arthroplasty and lumbar spine surgery should be roughly equal regardless of patients' residence. In fact, for a few conditions such as hernia repair, appendectomy, hip fracture, and a few others that is what happens. Per capita hospitalization rates for these conditions are quite similar and stable across small areas.

However, researchers have discovered that for most of medical care, utilization rates vary widely, occasionally by as much as ten fold or more from one area to another. In orthopaedics these include hip and knee replacement surgery, arthroscopy, and spinal procedures, among others. While surgical procedures demonstrate significant variations, medical causes of hospitalization vary even more extensively than surgery. Because of their increased frequency, these variations have much greater financial implications.

Causes of the Variations

There are a number of potential explanations for variations. Medical coding systems are used to gather and input data, and errors in coding can occur. These problems are diminishing with modern medical record and computer systems, but they do occur and must be considered and assessed.

Next, unrecognized (and therefore uncorrected) real differences in disease rates, environmental conditions, and demographic characteristics of populations can produce variations. All of these possibilities must be carefully evaluated in analyzing this kind of epidemiologic data. For instance, although hospitalization for hip fracture across small areas shows little or no variation, recent publications have demonstrated as yet unexplained regional variations across large areas of the United States.

Other factors considered in explaining variations include patient demand for medical care, physician supply and practice style, and hospital capacity. Patient demand is difficult to measure, and little is known about it. Physicians can influence demand by the way in which they present treatment options to patients. Other sources of information, such as publications and television, may influence the kind and volume of care patients request. However, if a patient learns of a new therapy and asks the physician to use it, one would hope that the treatment would be used only if it were appropriate and indicated for that patient. If physicians are consistent in medical decision making, then patient demand should have little effect on utilization.

Hospital capacity (or the number of beds per capita) appears to have a strong effect on hospitalization, but only as relates to medical admissions and not to surgical admission. In Maine, admissions for medical conditions such as pulmonary disease are much higher in rural areas of the state where there are high bed-to-population ratios and occupancy rates are low. In urban areas, where there are fewer beds per capita and hospital occupancy is high, discretionary admissions occur much less frequently. Residents of the city of Boston use 50% more health-care resources than residents of New Haven, all for discretionary medical admissions such as pneumonia, gastroenteritis, and medical back conditions. There are 4.5 beds per 1,000 residents in Boston and 2.9 in New Haven. There are 50% more beds available in Boston, and discretionary medical admissions rate 50% higher for Bostonians—a striking correlation (Table 1).

Although the hospital capacity issue appears to be very important for medical admissions, it plays a very small role in surgery. Thus, for orthopaedic practice variations we must look further for explanations. Physician supply may have a strong impact on per capita utilization and variation, but it is not consistent. One would anticipate that a high ratio of providers to patients would result in higher utilization rates. For example, the ratio of orthopaedic surgeons to the population in one hospital service area of Maine is 1:19,000; in another the ratio is 1:8,500. One area has more than twice as many orthopaedists per capita as the other. If the supply theory held, one would expect higher rates of orthopaedic procedures in the area with more available physicians. In fact, that is not the case. Surgical rates are essentially the same in both areas. However, there are examples in Maine where the volume of surgery does seem to relate more directly to the numbers of available surgeons.

Decision Making

There remains one major source of practice pattern variations, and for surgery and orthopaedics it is the most important. It relates to the way in which physicians make decisions and recommendations in clinical practice. As we know, orthopaedists undergo fairly standardized

Table 1. Comparison of utilization of hospital beds between Boston and New Haven (major surgical rates between the two cities are the same)

	Boston/New Haven Ratios			Excess Boston beds
Type of Service	Discharges/ 1,000	Length of stay	Days/ 1,000	
All cases*	1.34	1.07	1.44	739
Adult medical cases	1.49	1.09	1.64	527
Low variation	1.06	1.11	1.17	
High variation	1.56	1.11	1.74	
Pediatric medical cases	1.47	1.16	1.70	35
Surgical cases				
Minor	1.38	1.17	1.61	89
Major	1.00	1.13	1.13	88

*Excluding discharges for deliveries (DRGs 370-384), neonatal care (DRGs 385-391), and mental disorders (DRGs 424-432).
(Reproduced with permission from Wennberg JE, Freeman JL, Culp WJ: Are hospital services rationed in New Haven or over-utilised in Boston? *Lancet* 1987;1:1185-1188.)

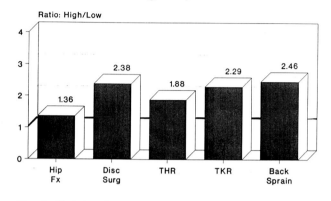

Fig. 1 Variations in orthopaedic procedures across four large United States geographic regions.

undergraduate medical education, residency training, in-service training exams, fellowships, board certification, and continuing medical education. The goal of these activities is to produce a standardized core of basic knowledge, diagnostic and therapeutic skills, and clinical information. Certainly, we would anticipate that a patient with a minor toe fracture would not expect orthopaedist A to recommend a comfortable shoe and crutches while Dr. B suggested amputation of the digit.

Most orthopaedists would likely assert that our approach to various clinical problems will be fairly consistent, but the variation phenomenon makes it clear that, like most doctors, we develop very different practice styles. As illustrated in Figure 1, there are significant differences in utilization rates across the four large national geographic regions. Not unexpectedly, hip fractures vary minimally, apparently as a function of a true regional variation in incidence. On the other hand, total hip replacements vary by a factor of 1.9, knee replacements by 2.3, and disk procedures by 2.4.

If we appear to agree about clinical issues, why do the rates of surgery vary? There is agreement on broad general concepts about hip replacement and many other orthopaedic procedures, but within these broad parameters there is much room for differences in decision making, and it is here that the variations surface. Thus, a patient with hip arthritis might consult two orthopaedists. The symptoms and findings are identical, but one doctor feels the patient should have surgery and the other does not.

Factors That Influence Decision Making

The factors that influence one physician to recommend surgery while another does not are poorly measured or articulated in the basic assessments and indications we all agree upon. It seems probable that there is a much more subtle force at work in medical decision making. The term "physician uncertainty" has been applied to this phenomenon. It appears to be the greatest source of surgical variations. One might be inclined to attribute differing practice styles to the desire of individual physicians to maintain or gain certain levels of income. While this factor may play a role on occasion, there is evidence to the contrary. Small area variation studies have been carried out in many settings, including countries such as England and Norway, as well as in the Veterans Administration and health maintenance organizations in the United States. The fact that significant practice pattern variations occur in all of these health care systems provides substantial evidence that the reimbursement system plays a small role, if any, in explaining this phenomenon.

Paralleling "uncertainty" is a finding known as the "surgical signature." Analysis of practice patterns over time shows that there can be significant differences in utilization rates within a community. For one procedure the rates may be above average; for another, they may be below. These rates tend to be stable over time. Surgeons who perform a procedure more frequently do so year after year. Likewise, surgeons operating at low rates maintain that pattern consistently.

This combination of "physician uncertainty" about the most appropriate way to treat many conditions and the "surgical signature" phenomenon seems to indicate that current knowledge and practice allow for markedly different practice patterns and that, once developed, doctors tend to maintain these practice styles over time.

Physician Response to Variations

The study of practice pattern variations has resulted in two major responses. First, work in Maine has demonstrated that when physicians have the opportunity to learn about and analyze variations, they have responded almost consistently by reducing apparent high rates of utilization. Second, the fact that variations appear to be the result of uncertainty about the most effective methods of treatment has produced a national initiative in outcomes research.

Physicians in Maine have developed a series of specialty study groups within an organization known as the Maine Medical Assessment Foundation (MMAF). Groups of specialists have analyzed and responded to hospital discharge data relevant to their practices. Several lessons have been learned. First, until this type of epidemiologic data is presented to physicians, they have no idea of their rates of practice. Doctors and hospitals may be aware of how many patients are admitted, treated, and operated on, but the denominator of the equation, the population base they serve, remains unknown. Second, physicians tend to be defensive about their practice patterns and initially, at least, may feel threatened when presented with this type of information. Third, once practitioners understand the validity and importance of small area variations, they tend to become eager participants in the process of data analysis and discussion of its significance. The effect of this educational feedback process has been to decrease rates of treatment where they appear to be excessive.

For example, the MMAF Orthopaedic/Neurosurgical study group has been interested in variations in surgical rates for lumbar disk herniation for a number of years. Figure 2 shows that disk excision rates in one city and three surrounding smaller communities rose rapidly from the state average rate in 1983. Careful study of the underlying data and review by the study group revealed that the only apparent explanation for the change was the fact that three new surgeons had moved to the community in 1982.

This information was provided to the study group, which included participants from the area where rates had risen. The issues surrounding disk surgery were thoroughly discussed. Although absolute information was not available, it was the impression of most of the surgeons in attendance that the surgical rates in the city under focus were higher than they should be. The graph illustrates that disk excision rates began to drop toward the state average, where they have remained. This effect has been repeated for other procedures by other study groups.

We have concluded that, particularly for elective surgery, informing physicians in an educational feedback mode has a powerful effect. Regardless of their belief in the appropriateness of their medical decision making, physicians appear uncomfortable as "outliers" and alter their practice patterns quite consistently when they are confronted with this type of data.

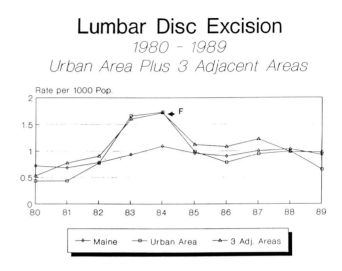

Fig. 2 A sudden increase in lumbar disk surgery occurred in one Maine city and three surrounding communities. Analysis revealed that three surgeons had established practice in the city. Feedback by the study group (arrow) produced a prompt change in practice behavior.

Appropriate Rates of Surgery

The question is frequently raised about low surgical rates and whether or not they should be increased. That situation could certainly occur. There are areas of under service and lack of access to care, and they can be identified by this technique.

It is important to stress that there is nothing inherent in the methodology of small area analysis that establishes what the "right rate" ought to be. The statewide average is used as a baseline from which to measure variations, but that average is not held out to be the proper or desirable rate. The fact that no one knows the correct rate for almost anything we do in medicine further reinforces the degree of uncertainty in medical care. The fact that surgeons in Maine have felt that some rates of surgery in their specialty are too high is entirely a function of the study group process and the judgment of those participants. We have never encountered the situation in which surgeons have decreased rates of activity and then reported to the study group that they are withholding care from their patients or offering medical care of lesser quality.

Additional evidence that higher rates of treatment may be inappropriate is buttressed by the fact that the United States has the highest rates of some kinds of health-care utilization in the world. For example, analysis of international rates of spine surgery for a number of nations indicates that the United States has the highest rate of spinal surgery measured—twice as many procedures as Australia and ten times as many as Scotland. Also, there are

Table 2. Number of restricted activity days and bed days for selected impairments: United States, 1988 (in thousands)

Type of Impairment	Restricted Activity Days	Restricted Activity Bed Days/Impairment	Bed Days Per Year	Bed Days Per Impairment
Hearing impairment	10,357	0.5	989	0.045
Visual impairment	46,213	5.5	15,614	1.9
Speech impairment	11,462	4.3	2,118	0.8
Musculoskeletal impairment	382,203	12.8	124,003	4.2
Back or spine	185,542	12.0	83,165	5.4
Lower extremity	147,228	13.2	31,284	2.8
Upper extremity	49,433	14.9	9,554	2.9
Paralysis	51,308	39.6	8,435	6.5
Absence of major extremity	22,909	15.1	3,932	2.6

Source: National Center for Health Statistics, National Health Interview Survey, 1988.

striking variations in the rates of spinal surgery across geographic regions of the United States. At the present time, we do not have enough information to indicate which of these remarkably different rates of spine surgery is most appropriate, but a ten-fold difference does not appear logical. The questions raised by these kinds of analyses should heighten interest and be a cause for concern among surgeons in all countries.

Societal Impact of Musculoskeletal Impairment and Treatment

Musculoskeletal conditions, which are among the most frequently occurring medical conditions, have a substantial impact on the health and quality of life of the population as well as on the utilization of health resources. The impact of musculoskeletal conditions includes three major categories: (1) the physical and social impact resulting from increased pain, limitations on mobility and activities of daily living, loss of independence, and a reduced quality of life; (2) direct expenditures for the diagnosis and treatment of musculoskeletal diseases and trauma; and (3) the indirect economic loss associated with reduced labor force participation, productivity, and wages, which result from activity limitations induced by musculoskeletal impairment and disability.

The impact of musculoskeletal conditions is, in large part, a function of their prevalence in the population. Among impairments, which are defined as a chronic or permanent defect representing a decrease or loss of ability to perform various functions that are identified in the National Health Interview Survey, musculoskeletal impairments are the most frequently reported. Approximately 29.9 million were reported in the United States in 1988. Musculoskeletal impairments are widely distributed in the population and are also the most frequently reported among both sexes and among major racial groups.

In the United States, musculoskeletal impairments occur at a rate of approximately 124.0/1,000 population. Back or spine impairments—the most frequently reported subcategories—represent 51.7% of musculoskel-

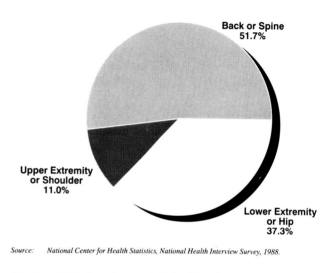

Source: National Center for Health Statistics, National Health Interview Survey, 1988.

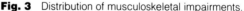

Fig. 3 Distribution of musculoskeletal impairments.

etal impairments (Fig. 3). Musculoskeletal impairments are a leading cause of activity limitation (Table 2) and in 1988 alone, resulted in over 382.2 million restricted activity days including 124.0 million bed days. Almost half (48.5%) of the restricted activity days resulted from back or spine impairments; 38.5% were from lower extremity or hip impairments. Of bed days, 67.1% were attributed to back or spine impairments, 25.2% to lower extremity or hip impairments, and 7.7% to upper extremity impairments.

Musculoskeletal conditions result in a significant use of health care resources. In 1988, there were approximately 3.5 million hospitalizations for musculoskeletal conditions—12.8% of all hospitalizations. Musculoskeletal conditions ranked second only to diseases of the circulatory system in overall frequency (Fig. 4). Table 3 shows that musculoskeletal diseases and connective tissue disorders account for the largest number of hospitalizations, including 459,000 for arthropathies and related disorders and 417,000 for intervertebral disk disorders. Fractures resulted in 899,000 hospitalizations; dislocations,

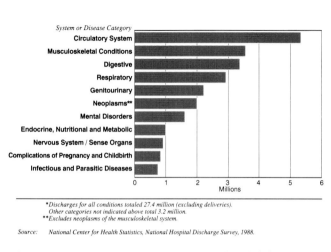

System or Disease Category

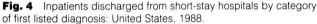

*Discharges for all conditions totaled 27.4 million (excluding deliveries).
Other categories not indicated above total 3.2 million.
**Excludes neoplasms of the musculoskeletal system.

Source: National Center for Health Statistics, National Hospital Discharge Survey, 1988.

Fig. 4 Inpatients discharged from short-stay hospitals by category of first listed diagnosis: United States, 1988.

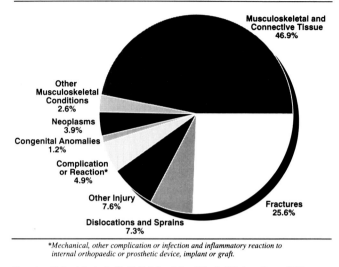

*Mechanical, other complication or infection and inflammatory reaction to internal orthopaedic or prosthetic device, implant or graft.

Source: National Center for Health Statistics, National Hospital Discharge Survey, 1988.

Fig. 5 Distribution of hospitalizations resulting from musculoskeletal conditions: United States, 1988 by aggregate category.

sprains, and other injuries resulted in an additional 526,000.

Musculoskeletal diseases and connective tissue disorders account for almost half of hospitalizations associated with musculoskeletal conditions (Fig. 5). Trauma accounts for an additional 40.5%. Complications or reactions, such as infection or inflammatory reactions to internal orthopaedic or prosthetic devices, implants, or grafts, account for about 5%. Smaller percentages result from neoplasms and congenital anomalies.

In 1988, over 3.0 million operations were performed on the musculoskeletal system. Operations on the musculoskeletal system account for 10.6% of all inpatient procedures and constituted the fourth largest procedure category (Fig. 6). Almost 40% of musculoskeletal procedures involve reduction of fractures (631,000) or arthroplasties (522,000). Arthroplasties include 251,000 joint replacements primarily involving the hip (129,000) and knee (105,000).

Musculoskeletal conditions also result in significant use of ambulatory/outpatient care. The most recent data available (1985) showed that musculoskeletal conditions accounted for 13.8% of all office visits and were the largest anatomic or disease category (Fig. 7). Approximately 87.5 million patient visits to office-based physicians resulted from musculoskeletal conditions.

A significant source of disability, resultant health care utilization, and productivity loss is injuries occurring in the workplace. In 1988, more than 6.2 million occupational injuries were reported to the Bureau of Labor Statistics for the private sector. Of these, almost half resulted in lost work time or restricted work activity. An additional 116,000 cases were reported for disorders associated with repeated trauma. Economy-wide, there were an estimated 1.93 million severe workplace inju-

Table 3. Hospitalization resulting from musculoskeletal conditions: United States 1988 by aggregate category

Musculoskeletal diseases and connective tissue disorders	1,647,000	
Arthropathies and related disorders		459,000
Intervertebral disk disorders		417,000
Other back disorders		178,000
Fractures	899,000	
Fracture of neck of femur		254,000
Dislocations and sprains	258,000	
Sprains and strains of the back		97,000
Other injuries	268,000	
Complications or reactions*	172,000	
Congenital anomalies	41,000	
Neoplasms	136,000	
Other musculoskeletal conditions	92,000	
Total, all musculoskeletal conditions	3,513,000	

*Mechanical, other complication or infection and inflammatory reaction to internal orthopaedic or prosthetic device, implant or graft.
Source: National Center for Health Statistics, National Health Interview Survey, 1988.

ries, injuries that resulted in three or more lost work days, in 1987. Of these, 31% required hospitalization, and 11% resulted in permanent disability. Among severe injuries by type, sprains and strains accounted for 47%, fractures and dislocations 12%, and severe contusions (excluding skull or head injuries) 12%. By anatomic site, lower back injuries account for 27% of severe injuries.

Musculoskeletal conditions have an enormous impact on the population of the United States. They rank highest among disease groups when indicators for the quality of life, such as impairment, disability, or limitation of activity are considered. Musculoskeletal conditions also rank first in frequency of visits to physicians, second in frequency of hospitalizations, and fourth in frequency of surgical procedures performed within hospitals. With the

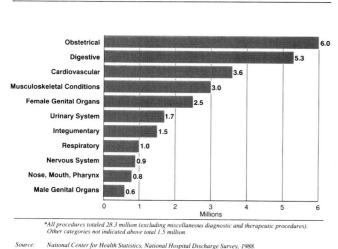

*All procedures totaled 28.3 million (excluding miscellaneous diagnostic and therapeutic procedures).
Other categories not indicated above total 1.5 million.*

Source: *National Center for Health Statistics, National Hospital Discharge Survey, 1988.*

Fig. 6 All listed procedures for inpatients discharged from short-stay hospitals: United States, 1988.

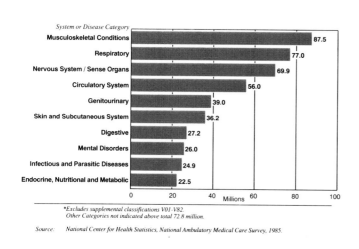

*Excludes supplemental classifications V01-V82.
Other Categories not indicated above total 72.8 million.*

Source: *National Center for Health Statistics, National Ambulatory Medical Care Survey, 1985.*

Fig. 7 Office visits by category of first listed diagnosis: United States, 1985.

aging of the population, the relative impact of musculoskeletal conditions will, in all probability, increase. The number of people aged 65 years and older is increasing two and one half times faster than the overall population. Individuals aged 85 years and older, who have the highest rates of musculoskeletal impairments and hospitalizations, are increasing six times faster than the population.

Cost of Musculoskeletal Conditions in 1988

The impact of musculoskeletal conditions in the United States involves the medical resources used for care, treatment, and rehabilitation; reduced or lost productivity; and the pain and suffering of patients, their families, and

friends. These conditions impose a substantial burden on the individual and on society as a whole. This burden must be translated into economic terms to better understand its magnitude compared with that of other major chronic illnesses so that informed decisions about health care policy can be made.

Total Economic Impact

Musculoskeletal conditions imposed a burden of almost $126 billion on the United States economy in 1988 (Table 4). Women accounted for 54% of these costs. The 45 to 64 year age group accounted for the largest share of costs, 37%, followed closely by the 65 years and older age group, which accounted for 35% of the total, reflecting the high prevalence of musculoskeletal conditions in these age groups.

Direct Costs

Direct costs for persons suffering from musculoskeletal conditions totaled almost $61 billion in 1988, or 12.7% of total personal health care spending for all illnesses in that year. About 36% ($22.1 billion) of the direct costs are expenditures for hospital inpatient care; an additional 9% ($5.6 billion) are for hospital outpatient care, including ambulatory surgery, physical therapy, rehabilitation, emergency rooms, and outpatient departments. Thus, hospital inpatient and outpatient care totaled $27.7 billion or 45% of direct costs.

Other treatment costs include $7.2 billion for physician inpatient and outpatient services and $2.5 billion for additional professional services, including private duty nurses, chiropractors, podiatrists, social workers, physical and occupational therapists, clinical psychologists, naturopaths, and others. Nursing home expenditures for persons with musculoskeletal conditions amounted to $12.4 billion. Prescription drugs were estimated at $680 million. The net cost of private insurance and administrative costs amounted to $2.9 billion. Non-health sector costs, including transportation to and from physicians' offices, extra household help, special diets, retraining and education, and alterations to living quarters, are estimated at $7.6 billion.

Indirect Costs

Morbidity Musculoskeletal morbidity costs, the value of reduced or lost productivity, amounted to $59.6 billion, 92% of the total indirect costs and 47% of total costs. These costs reflect the prevalence of musculoskeletal conditions in the population. For example, the National Health Interview Survey reports a total of 31.2 million persons with arthritic conditions, as well as 2 million with gout, 4.3 million with intervertebral disk disorders, 2.5 million with bone spur and tendinitis, and 1.5 million with disorders of bone or cartilage. Many persons with these musculoskeletal conditions are unable to work or carry on their major activity. Morbidity costs are slightly higher for women than for men, $30 billion and $29.7

Table 4. Estimated cost of all musculoskeletal conditions by age and type of cost, 1988 (in millions)

Type of Cost	Total	Younger than 18	18-44	45-64	65 & older
Total	$125,962	$3,579	$32,464	$46,481	$43,438
Direct costs, totals	60,987	3,357	13,294	12,287	32,049
Hospital inpatient	22,137	1,338	5,568	5,074	10,157
Hospital outpatient	5,600	338	1,409	1,283	2,570
Physician inpatient	3,159	241	952	727	1,239
Physician outpatient	4,008	521	1,579	1,079	829
Other practitioners	2,507	326	987	675	519
Drugs	680	15	145	261	259
Nursing home care	12,391	—	365	1,071	10,955
Prepayment	2,934	161	640	591	1,542
Nonhealth sector	7,571	417	1,650	1,525	3,979
Indirect costs, total	64,975	222	19,170	34,194	11,389
Morbidity	59,619	—	16,821	32,112	10,686
Mortality[1]	5,356	222	2,349	2,082	703

[1]Present value of lifetime earnings discounted at 4%.

Table 5. Mortality from all musculoskeletal conditions: Number of deaths, person-years lost, and discounted productivity losses by age and gender, 1988

Patients	Number of Deaths	Person-Years Lost Number (in thousands)	Per Death	Productivity Losses[1] Amount (in millions)	Per Death
Both sexes	44,787	701[2]	15.7[2]	$5,356[2]	$119,582[2]
Younger than 15	440	31	70.2	222	503,470
15-44	3,585	157	43.8	2,349	655,154
45-64	9,176	210	22.8	2,082	226,935
65 and older	31,586	304	9.6	703	22,259
Males	20,326	316[2]	15.5[2]	3,174[2]	156,174[2]
Younger than 15	223	15	67.0	126	566,048
15-44	1,992	82	41.1	1,508	757,009
45-64	4,911	102	20.9	1,254	225,241
65 and older	13,200	117	8.8	287	21,725
Females	24,461	385[2]	15.8[2]	2,181[2]	89,176[2]
Younger than 15	217	16	73.5	95	438,981
15-44	1,593	75	47.2	841	527,836
45-64	4,265	107	25.1	829	194,341
65 and older	18,386	187	10.2	416	22,642

Note: Numbers may not add to totals due to rounding.
[1]Discounted at 4%.
[2]Excludes deaths with age not stated.

billion, respectively. Morbidity costs for the 45 to 64 year age group are the highest and comprise more than half the total musculoskeletal morbidity costs. The high costs for this age group reflect both the prevalence of these conditions among this population group and their high earnings.

Mortality   In 1988, a total of 44,787 deaths were caused by musculoskeletal conditions. These deaths represent 0.7 million person-years lost, or 15.7 years per death and a loss of $5.4 billion to the economy at a 4% discount rate, or $119,582 per death (Table 5). Deaths resulting from musculoskeletal conditions comprised 2.1% of the 2.2 million deaths in the United States in 1988 and 2.0% of the total person-years lost and of the total productivity losses.

Musculoskeletal Injuries

Musculoskeletal injuries include injuries related to fractures, dislocations and sprains, open wounds and crushing injury, traumatic amputation, and other selected injuries affecting the musculoskeletal system. The cost of these injuries amounted to $26.1 billion in 1988 (Table 6). About 86% of the total are direct costs; the remaining 14% are indirect costs. Of the indirect costs, 83% are morbidity costs. The rest are mortality costs. Mortality costs for musculoskeletal injuries are low because only 8,346 deaths from injuries could be identified as musculoskeletal deaths. The National Center for Health Statistics only codes injury deaths according to the external causes of death, and the vast majority of injury deaths in 1988 could not be identified according to body system. Thus the mortality costs associated with musculoskeletal injuries reported here are clearly an understatement.

Table 6. Estimated cost of musculoskeletal injuries by age and type of cost, 1988 (in millions)

Type of Cost	Total	Younger than 18	18-44	45-64	65 & older
Total	$26,107	$2,010	$8,567	$4,318	$11,212
Direct costs, totals	22,498	1,990	6,155	3,412	10,941
Hospital inpatient	9,170	754	2,533	1,389	4,494
Hospital outpatient	2,320	191	641	351	1,137
Physician inpatient	1,309	134	434	198	543
Physician outpatient	1,701	344	816	348	193
Other practitioners	1,064	215	510	218	121
Drugs	229	10	75	84	60
Nursing home care	2,830	—	86	236	2,508
Prepayment	1,083	95	296	165	527
Nonhealth sector	2,792	247	764	423	1,358
Indirect costs, total	3,609	20	2,412	906	271
Morbidity[1]	3,003	—	2,101	716	186
Mortality[2]	606	20	311	190	85

[1]Includes morbidity due to fractures, dislocations, sprains, and strains.
[2]Present value of lifetime earnings discounted at 4%.

Table 7. Estimated cost of selected musculoskeletal conditions by type of cost, 1988 (in millions)

Type of Cost	Arthritis	Fractures	Hip Fractures	Osteoporosis	Neoplasms	Congenital Musculoskeletal Deformities
Total	$54,589	$20,101	$8,728	$4,283	$5,918	$717
Direct costs, total	12,749	16,491	7,053	4,283	2,382	614
Hospital inpatient	2,621	7,185	3,077	1,813	1,233	198
Hospital outpatient	663	1,818	778	459	312	52
Physician inpatient	349	997	385	234	168	35
Physician outpatient	581	463	18	16	37	29
Other practitioners	363	290	11	10	22	20
Drugs	145	66	5	5	7	4
Nursing home care	5,831	2,830	1,565	1,008	193	171
Prepayment/administration	613	794	339	206	116	28
Nonhealth sector	1,583	2,048	875	532	294	77
Indirect costs, total	41,840	3,610	1,675	na	3,536	103
Morbidity	41,597[1]	3,003[2]	1,415	na	na	na
Mortality[3]	243	607	260	na	3,536	103

[1]Includes morbidity for persons reporting arthritis and other musculoskeletal conditions.
[2]Includes morbidity due to fractures, dislocations, sprains, and strains.
[3]Present value of lifetime earnings discounted at 4%.
na—not available.

Selected Musculoskeletal Conditions

The costs of selected musculoskeletal conditions, including arthritis, fractures, hip fractures, osteoporosis, neoplasms, and congenital musculoskeletal deformities are shown on Table 7.

Arthritis Arthritis is the second most prevalent chronic condition (sinusitis is first) reported by respondents to the National Health Interview Survey. In 1988, 31.3 million conditions were reported, a rate of 130 per 1,000 persons. The prevalence of arthritis increases with age, rising from 34 per 1,000 persons younger than 45 years of age, to 257 per 1,000 persons 45 to 64 years of age, and 486 per 1,000 persons 65 years and older. Arthritis is the leading chronic condition reported for the elderly. The high prevalence of arthritis in the population is reflected in high costs. In 1988, the total cost of arthritis was estimated at $54.6 billion, constituting more than two fifths

of the total cost of all musculoskeletal conditions. The debilitating and disabling effects of arthritis are seen in its high morbidity costs, amounting to $41.6 billion or three quarters of total direct costs related to arthritis. Included in the morbidity costs are persons reporting arthritis and other chronic musculoskeletal conditions. Direct costs of arthritis totaled $12.7 billion in 1988. Expenditures for nursing home care amounted to $5.8 billion. Almost one out of five nursing home residents report rheumatoid arthritis, osteoarthritis and allied disorders, and other arthritis or rheumatism upon admission to the nursing home. Hospital inpatient care totaled $2.6 billion, more than one fifth of direct costs. The National Hospital Discharge Survey reports about 2.9 million days of care for patients hospitalized for arthritis and related disorders.

Fractures The total costs of fractures were estimated at $20 billion in 1988, of which direct costs constitute more than four fifths of total expenditures. Of the total direct costs of $16.5 billion, hospital costs rank highest, $7.2 billion. Almost 900,000 persons were hospitalized for fractures, with an average length of stay of 8.8 days, a total of 7.9 million days. The second highest category of direct costs, nursing home care, amounts to $2.8 billion. About 120,000 residents were admitted to nursing homes in 1985 with fractures, comprising 8% of total nursing home residents. Outpatient hospital care for fractures, the third highest direct cost, amounts to $1.8 billion.

Indirect costs are estimated at $3.6 billion, of which $3.0 billion are morbidity costs. Morbidity costs are based on bed disability days associated with acute conditions reported in the 1988 National Health Survey and include fractures, dislocations, sprains, and strains. Therefore, morbidity costs for fractures may be slightly overstated. A total of 34.1 million bed days, or 93,292 person-years, were reported.

Hip Fractures The total cost of hip fractures was estimated at $8.7 billion, 43% of the total costs of fractures. Direct costs of hip fractures constitute four fifths of the total. Hospital inpatient care amounted to $3.1 billion. A total of 253,796 persons were hospitalized for hip fractures in 1988, of whom 85% were aged 65 years and older. Average length of stay for all inpatient hospital discharges was 13.4 days. The cost of nursing home care is second highest, amounting to $1.6 billion. The National Nursing Home Survey reported 66,300 admissions in 1985 for hip fracture, 4.4% of total admissions.

Osteoporosis The total direct costs of osteoporosis were estimated at $4.3 billion in 1988. Indirect costs of this musculoskeletal disorder were not estimated because reliable data were not available on which to base the estimates. Hospital inpatient costs constituted more than two fifths of the total direct costs of osteoporosis. A total of 2.0 million days of inpatient care were reported for this condition, of which more than three fourths were for persons 65 years of age and older.

Neoplasms Included in this category are malignant and benign neoplasms of the musculoskeletal system such as bone and articular cartilage, connective and other soft tissue, multiple myeloma and immunoproliferative neoplasms, and other malignant lymphomas. Total costs of neoplasms of the musculoskeletal system are estimated to be $5.9 billion, excluding morbidity costs, which could not be estimated because reliable data on morbidity were not available. Two fifths of the total costs are direct costs, and three fifths are mortality costs. Hospital inpatient care totaled 1.4 million days, at an estimated cost of $1.2 billion. A total of 26,783 deaths caused by neoplasms of the musculoskeletal system occurred in 1988. These

deaths represent 440 million person-years lost, or a loss of $3.5 billion to the economy.

Congenital Musculoskeletal Deformities The total cost of musculoskeletal deformities is estimated at $717 million, excluding morbidity costs. Again, these costs could not be estimated because of the lack of reliable data on which to make estimates. Congenital musculoskeletal deformities clearly result in illness, disability, and reduced productivity. Thus, the total costs reported here are an underestimate. Direct costs are estimated at $614 million, of which hospital inpatient costs comprise 32%, and nursing home costs 28%.

Conclusion

The epidemiologic studies of small area analysis and practice pattern variations begun by Wennberg have been carried on and repeated by others. There is no doubt that there are marked variations in medical and surgical utilization patterns, and evidence is growing that much of this utilization is highly discretionary and may involve care that may have been unnecessary or could have been rendered in a less expensive setting.

There is also good evidence that, when approached in a reasonable way, physicians will participate eagerly in the processing of analyzing this kind of data, and that rates of care will often decrease if they appear to be excessive. Epidemiologic analyses of this kind also provide the opportunity to identify areas of under service.

The variations issue and identification of underlying physician uncertainty has become the stimulus for another new and exciting dimension in medical care—the need for Outcomes Research. Small area analysis has identified the problem. Outcomes research offers the opportunity to find answers, eliminate uncertainty, reduce variations, and improve the quality of medical and orthopaedic care.

The total cost of musculoskeletal conditions to society in terms of resources used and in lost productivity are high, estimated at $126 billion in 1988. As noted earlier, this figure does not include costs associated with pain and suffering.

Acknowledgments

The latter part of this chapter is excerpted from *Musculoskeletal Conditions in the United States*, Praemer, Furner, and Rice, American Academy of Orthopaedic Surgeons, 1992. Complete descriptions of data sources and methodologies used can be found in the original publication.

Annotated Bibliography

Jacobsen SJ, Goldberg J, Miles TP, et al: Regional variation in the incidence of hip fracture: US white women aged 65 and older. *JAMA* 1990;264:500-502.

Analysis of Health Care Finance Administration and Veterans' Administration data bases demonstrated a significant difference in the incidence of hip fracture in women aged 65 and older. Higher rates occur in the Southern United States, especially from the Texas panhandle east to Arkansas, Mississippi, Alabama, and Georgia.

Keller RB, Soule DN: Main Medical Assessment Foundation Annual Report: 1991. Manchester, ME, Maine Medical Assessment Foundation, 1991.

Report of study group activities of this Foundation, discussing causes of variations, physician response, and other factors, such as resource allocation and hospital capacity.

Keller RB, Soule DN, Wennberg JE, et al: Dealing with geographic variations in the use of hospitals: The experience of the Maine Medical Assessment Foundation Orthopaedic Study Group. *J Bone Joint Surg* 1990;72A:1286-1293.

A discussion of the epidemiologic principles and methodologies of small area analysis. Studies of practice pattern variations by Maine orthopaedic surgeons indicated significant differences in hospital use and treatment of musculoskeletal conditions. Feedback on these data reduced variations.

McPherson K, Wennberg JE, Hovind OB, et al: Small area variations in the use of common surgical procedures: An international comparison of New England, England, and Norway. *N Engl J Med* 1982;307:1310-1314.

Small area variation analysis of these three international regions demonstrates differences in utilization for discretionary conditions, while non-discretionary procedures show little per capita variation.

Wennberg JE, Barnes BA, Zubkoff M: Professional uncertainty and the problem of supplier-induced demand. *Soc Sci Med* 1982;16:811-824.

Large differences in per capita use of common surgical procedures in three New England states demonstrates physician uncertainty in decision making about discretionary procedures. The concept of the "surgical signature" is discussed.

Wennberg JE, Freeman JL, Culp WJ: Are hospital services rationed in New Haven or over-utilised in Boston? *Lancet* 1987;1:1185-1189.

Epidemiologic analysis of hospital utilization by residents of Boston and New Haven revealed marked differences between the two cities, with much higher hospital utilization for Bostonians. Despite marked differences in rates of orthopaedic procedures between the two cities, admissions for medical services rather than surgery account for the largest differences in utilization and cost.

Wennberg J, Gittelsohn A: Small area variations in health care delivery. *Science* 1973;182:1102-1108.

This original article describes the concept and methodology of small area analysis and gives the results in Vermont.

3

Quality Assurance/Quality Improvement

Introduction

Whether the topic is cars, computers, or cardiac surgery, quality appears to be a buzzword for the 1990s. This chapter reviews the evolution of the quality movement, its key concepts, its relevance to current orthopaedic practice, and likely directions for the future.

Definitions

Quality Quality is defined in this context as the value of a product or service to its recipient or customer. A doctor's recipients include not only patients but also coworkers, referring doctors, and third party payers.

Quality Assurance Quality assurance is the measurement of a given activity, such as complication rates or waiting time, against a minimum standard, with the goal of assuring a minimum level of quality.

Quality Improvement Quality improvement refers to the concept of continuous improvement of quality. In this context, a minimum standard becomes less important, and the target becomes zero defects or problems. This produces a motivation to continuously improve the output of a process in search of perfection.

History of the Quality Movement

The quality movement in medicine is not new; both in medicine and in industry the first efforts began in the early 1900s. One of the real pioneers in this movement should be familiar to most orthopaedists—Ernest A. Codman, whose classic book, *The Shoulder*, was envisioned by the author as a means of disseminating his idea of end-results, which was "the common sense notion that every hospital should follow each patient it treats long enough to determine whether or not the treatment has been successful, and then to inquire 'If not, why not?' with a view to preventing a similar failure in the future." Codman's first efforts at what would now be considered outcome research were also the first examples of hospital-based quality assurance—the measurement and monitoring of clinical results.

Codman began his efforts before World War I. In 1917, through Codman's prompting, the American College of Surgeons started its Hospital Standardization Program. In 1951 this program evolved into the Joint Commission for the Accreditation of Hospitals, when the American Medical Association, the American Hospital Association, and the American College of Physicians joined the American College of Surgeons to establish minimum standards for certification of hospitals. This organization, now called the Joint Commission for the Accreditation of Healthcare Organizations, continues to monitor hospitals and other health facilities in the field of quality assurance.

Roughly concurrent with Codman's efforts in medicine, American industry was attempting to deal with the variable quality of the output of its assembly lines. In the 1930s, Walter Shewhart devised a system of statistical process control, which for the first time used statistical sampling methods to analyze the large outputs of factories. Briefly stated, a process is considered to be in statistical control if the mean value of a random sample of the output of that process falls within the 99% confidence limits (three standard errors) of the mean, calculated from a large series of such random samples (Fig. 1). Processes in control cannot be improved further without changing the entire process; variations within the control limits are assumed to be random, and, thus, inherent in the process itself. Observations outside the control limits are assumed to have special causes, because, by defini-

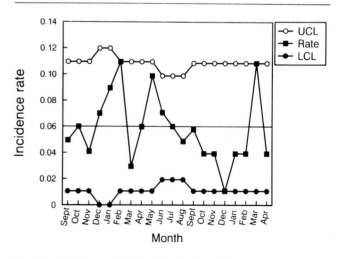

Fig. 1 A simple control chart. Each data point represents the mean of a series of observations. The upper (UCL) and lower (LCL) control limits are determined by first calculating the mean and range of each subgroup. Control limits represent plus or minus three standard errors of the mean. In this example, three data points intersect the control limits; investigation of those time periods may show some specific problems (key employee out sick; machine broken).

tion, the likelihood of such an observation lying outside the 99% confidence limits by chance alone is less than 1%. Efforts to bring processes under statistical control should focus, therefore, on any special causes that might be identified. These causes might, for example, be related to such problems as equipment failures or faulty training of individual workers. It is important to remember that a process in control does not necessarily mean a process that is good. It only means that the process is consistent. It may be consistently bad. Once a process is brought under statistical control, it can be improved only by changing the basic process itself. For example, consider a process that requires a report to be carried from one side of the hospital to another. There is wide variation in the time it takes for a report to get from point A to point B, because some of the messages get lost. This process can be brought under control by giving the messengers maps. Better results might be obtained by improving the process itself, for example, by sending the report electronically.

The distinction between random variation within control limits and special cause variation is critical to any discussion of quality assessment. Consider, for example, a hospital in which the quarterly fatal pulmonary embolism rate increased from 0.5% to 2%. Has something gone wrong, or is this a part of the normal fluctuation in this complication rate? The answer depends on the track record of pulmonary embolism rates. It may be that these rates are quite variable, ranging from 0% to 5%. If so, the increase in this example lies comfortably within the control limits. The quarter in question may seem unusual, but it is not. Efforts to track down a special cause are likely to be fruitless. Now, consider a case in which the rate varies little from quarter to quarter, and the control limits are very tight—perhaps the upper limit is 1.5%. In this case, it is highly likely that a 2% rate does represent a specific problem; investigation for a special cause is worthwhile. Thus, it is not only one observation and its change from a prior time period, but the history built up through a series of observations that is critical in determining whether a specific problem might explain the variation of one data point from another. Such special causes are unlikely—the most likely explanation for wide variability between pulmonary embolism rates is that the hospital in question does not have a very good system to address this problem. There may be an inconsistency in the definition or documentation of this complication, or there may be some inconsistency in applying prophylaxis to patients at risk. Such generic issues bring the entire system into question and call for an investigation not of the quarter in question but of the process itself. Most experts consider that special causes can be implicated only 10% to 20% of the time. Most improvement comes from addressing the process or system itself.

Shewhart's ideas were widely used in the United States during World War II. After that war ended, one of Shewhart's associates, W. E. Deming, brought these ideas to Japan, where the opportunities these ideas created for the continuous improvement of industrial processes were widely implemented. Deming emphasized that the opportunities for greatest improvement in quality usually existed in the planning phase of the new process, that is, it is cheaper to eliminate defects before they occur than it is to correct them later.

Other quality gurus have helped spread the message throughout the world. Although each "school" differs slightly from the rest, they share a number of features. These include a commitment of top management and leadership; empowerment of employees to effect change; use of statistical tools and techniques; quality throughout the organization—not just the function of a separate department; and the fact that the vast majority of quality problems relate to the basic structure of processes themselves, and not the failures among individual workers. All these experts agree that good quality is cost effective. The streamlining, simplifying strategies that improve quality also reduce cost. Also, all of them emphasize the cost of poor quality in terms of re-work (or work that shouldn't have been done in the first place), employee morale, and customer dissatisfaction. The Cleveland Clinic has estimated that each dissatisfied patient results in a loss of three future referrals as a result of negative word-of-mouth comments. Only 4% of dissatisfied patients actually expressed their dissatisfaction in the form of a complaint to their doctor; thus each complaint received may represent as many as 75 lost referrals.

Organizations that have implemented continuous quality improvement have learned several things. First, the theory works—profit, market share, and efficiency all improve. Second, in order for the system to work, the frontline employees must be treated with respect, and given the power to change the processes in which they work, for it is at their level that often the most critical insights regarding opportunities for improvement will arise. Third, several basic tools are critical for the analysis of data from which opportunities for improvement arise.

Basic Quality Improvement Tools

There are seven basic quality improvement tools. In general, these represent either simple organizational or statistical methods to deal with the data collected and, of course, problem analysis and problem solving.

Probably the most basic tool is the *Pareto diagram*, named for the Italian statistician who first described it. The diagram, which is simply a histogram sorted by order of frequency, is used to identify the "vital few" among all the potential sources of the problems at hand, and it thereby serves to focus attention and resources where the most effect can be had. A rule of thumb is that 20% of the problem sources will be responsible for 80% of the problem.

Once key problem areas have been identified, the processes in question can be mapped on *flow charts*. Often this mapping is instructive in itself—some systems have

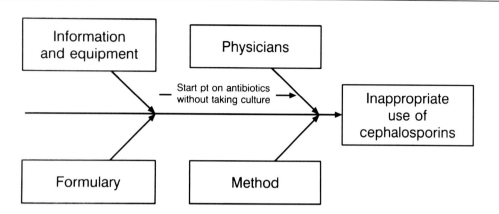

Fig. 2 Cause and effect, or "fishbone" diagram. Major causes of the end result, in this case "inappropriate use of cephalosporins," are mapped with arrows. The relative importance is signified by the location of the arrows; in this example physicians are considered a more important or significant cause than, for example, the formulary.

developed so haphazardly that the mere construction of a flow diagram of the current process will point to the need for a total system overhaul.

After the basic process at hand has been diagrammed and essential information has been collected, a *cause-and-effect diagram*, or "fishbone," can be developed (Fig. 2). The fishbone diagram seeks to map all possible causes for the major problems that were documented in the Pareto analysis and points the way for further data collection. A key organizational feature at this step is that the group charged with analyzing and correcting the problem should include representatives from each group affected by the process. For example, for an operating-room problem, the group should probably include surgeons, anesthesiologists, nurses, operating room technicians, and administrators. Workers on the "front lines," who deal with the process daily, are most likely to be aware of problems, and often have the best suggestions for improvement. Construction of a cause-and-effect diagram typically takes place during a *brainstorming* session of this group.

Once all the potential causes of the problem have been identified, they can be analyzed to determine which ones are, in fact, responsible. Analysis is done with such simple statistical tools as *run charts* (basically a control chart, such as the one shown in Fig. 1, but without the control limits), *scatter diagrams*, and *histograms*.

Once a problem's causes have been identified, solutions can be designed to correct it. This process often results in a redrawing of the initial process flow diagram, in an effort to reduce the number of steps and therefore the number of opportunities for problems to arise. If the solution corrects the problem, the new steady state can be monitored. As can be seen, these steps become a continuous loop—the plan, do, check, act, or PDCA cycle, which is also called the Shewhart cycle or Deming wheel (Fig. 3).

F ind a process to improve

O rganize a team that knows the process

C larify current knowledge of the process

U nderstand the causes of process variation

S elect the process improvement

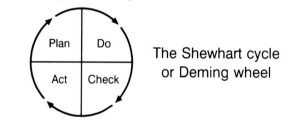

The Shewhart cycle or Deming wheel

Fig. 3 The plan, do, check, act cycle (Shewhart cycle or Deming wheel). The simple mnemonic F-O-C-U-S helps get the cycle started.

Quality and Medicine

On the medical front, Avedis Donabedian began to reorganize thinking on medical quality in the 1960s. Donabedian emphasized that there are three components of any activity that can be analyzed for opportunities for improvement: structure, process, and outcome. The structure of an activity relates to the equipment and personnel needed to produce it, and includes such things as machinery and training. Process, which refers to the actual steps taken by the structural elements, consists of inputs, actions, and outputs. Outcomes are the results produced by the activity. More recently, it has been pointed out that the structure of a system includes not only its physical infrastructure, knowledge base, and information systems, but also the cultures and values shared by the members of the organization in question.

Most recently, the role of customers has been emphasized in the definition of quality. Their role is particularly important in service industries, but in reality all types of organized activities have customers—those who receive the output, or the product that has been made. Customers may be internal if they are a part of the same organization as the producers of the service or product. For example, an orthopaedist may be an internal customer for a radiologist at a hospital. Customers are external if they are not a part of the same organization; in medicine, typical examples of external customers include patients, referring physicians, and third-party payers. Quality is defined as meeting or exceeding the expectations of the customer. This in turn implies that the expectations of the customer are known, and that they can be measured and specified.

B.C. James has further separated quality into two components: content and delivery. Content quality is the functional quality of the service itself. Was the radiograph in focus? Was the blood test result accurate? Did the wound heal without infection? Did the patient go back to work? Delivery quality focuses on such aspects of the customer/supplier interaction as courtesy and promptness. In medicine, it may also be appropriate to divide quality in another dimension, between operational and clinical activities, each of which, in turn, has content and delivery components.

Operational Activities

Operational activities are those typically associated with the medical institution, such as billing systems, scheduling systems, laboratory services, or imaging services. One may think of this side of quality as doing things right. In many ways, this is the more industrial side of medicine. Traditionally, it is more automated, and the industrial model of quality improvement and quality management discussed above has typically been first applied here, especially to measure operational content quality. It tends to be data driven and to rely on statistics (How long does it take for a bill to be mailed? How many radiographs have to be repeated?). Operational delivery quality has also been measured with satisfaction surveys.

Clinical Activities

Clinical activities and clinical decision making have been less subjected to quality improvement concepts, particularly in the realm of content quality. If operational quality improvement seeks to do things right, clinical quality improvement attempts to do the right things. Traditionally, this aspect of medical care has been monitored by a variety of regulations, in the form of quality assurance, recertification, and practice guidelines. Such mechanics are frequently based more on political judgment or opinions than on scientific research. Such regulations run several risks. If they are too rigid, they will stifle innovation. If they are too vague, they serve little practical purpose.

Also, because they often represent opinion, or other arbitrary judgment, they may not be accepted by their target group as relevant.

The classic measure of clinical science—the randomized, double-blind trial—is too slow and expensive a method to use in analyzing and improving clinical decision making. Instead, a new approach has been applied, which uses the same quality improvement tools used in industry. Outcomes research, which measures the product of clinical activity in terms of patient function and well-being, is a part of this new approach. Outcomes research can be used to measure the appropriateness and effectiveness, or content quality, of clinical activity. Delivery quality, or patient compliance, can also be measured. To achieve this, however, requires access to clinical data on large volumes of patients, which can then be analyzed to identify control limits, search for and identify causes of variation, and seek improvements. Several large data bases are already available, such as those used by the Health Care Finance Administration to compare Social Security mortality lists with Medicare Diagnostic-Related Group billing information. Other clinical data points, such as whether an operation was performed, are also readily retrievable from insurance files. This information has already been used to document wide variations in medical practice from community to community, and even between practitioners within the same community. Often these variations involve large differences in cost, but no apparent differences in outcome. As discussed elsewhere in this section, such variations suggest opportunities to improve practice—opportunities to which scientific methods can be applied. More details will clearly permit further analysis, and this has been the basis for the call for an automated or electronic medical record.

Quality Improvement in Medicine

Newer ideas regarding customer relationships have put a new face on quality as it relates to medical practice. The traditional model of minimal standards, or quality assurance, required by the triennial Joint Commission for the Accreditation of Healthcare Organizations reviews, is by now fairly well-known. These reviews have in turn become more important as reimbursement by third parties has been linked to certification by the Joint Commission and similar state accrediting bodies. D.M. Berwick has characterized this traditional model as the theory of bad apples: quality by inspection; quality by eliminating poor performance. As Berwick points out, this type of quality conception has several drawbacks. First, it addresses only a small part of the overall process or system—the part that fails to meet expectations or specifications (Fig. 4). In the Shewhart-Deming model, these are the special cause variations. Correcting them brings the system back into statistical control, but does nothing to improve the basic efficiency or appropriateness of the system. Second, those being inspected respond in a characteristic way, especially when they know that the purpose of in-

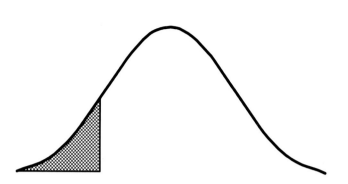

Fig. 4 The theory of bad apples. Only the shaded area is addressed; most production is unaffected by this sort of intervention.

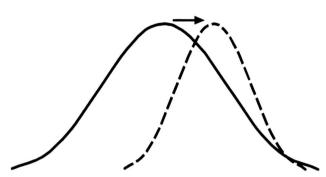

Fig. 5 The theory of continuous improvement. By reducing variation and improving overall quality, all aspects are improved.

spection (substitute recertification, the threat of malpractice, or third party authorization as needed) is to punish deviation from the standards. Characteristic responses include antagonism toward the regulator, floods of paperwork to give the appearance of compliance, and, when all else fails, the identification of a scapegoat. A third drawback, which arises in part out of the adversarial relationship between inspector and worker, is that the minimum standards rapidly become ceilings. Workers spend so much time trying to avoid being singled out that there is no time left to consider ways to improve.

Berwick and others have proposed an alternative to quality assurance and the theory of bad apples. This new approach has been called total quality management or continuous quality improvement. In this conception, the goal is not to eliminate the poor quality outliers but to improve the quality and reduce the variability for all of the outputs (Fig. 5). Experience in industry has shown that 80% to 90% of all quality problems do not result from individual bad apples, but, instead, from poor system design, limited understanding of basic systems, poor leadership, and lack of vision or focus. Therefore, the goal of the theory of continuous improvement is to truly understand the workings of basic systems. Deming calls this profound knowledge. P.M. Senge has called this understanding "the fifth discipline" of learning. P.B. Batalden stated that this profound knowledge consists of four dimensions: knowledge of the organization as a system; knowledge of the variations within a system; knowledge of intrinsic motivation of the workers, or industrial psychology; and an underlying theory or approach to continuous quality improvement. In addition, it is important to identify one's customers, to learn the customers' expectations and to focus on them. Finally, leadership must be harnessed to achieve these goals.

Again, a variety of educational programs have emphasized various portions of the continuous improvement concept, but there are certain basic features: (1) The analysis of health care, like any industry, is best carried out by examining the individual processes involved in a

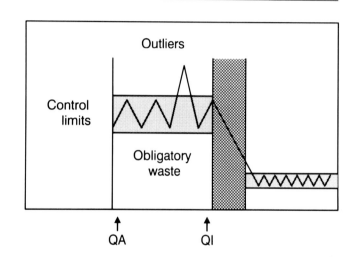

Fig. 6 Control charts can be used to document quality improvement. In this example, the process is "in control," but inefficient. There is considerable waste, and variation is high. After intervention, waste and variation are both reduced. This representation of process improvement is commonly referred to as the Juran trilogy, after Joseph Juran, the quality expert who popularized it.

service or product. Problems are usually caused by flawed processes, not flawed people. (2) The evaluation of processes requires the identification of suppliers and customers, who can be internal or external to the organization. Customer satisfaction defines quality. (3) Scientific methods are applied to the analysis of processes, both support or operational processes and clinical decision-making processes. People directly involved with the processes are in the best position to examine them. Because many processes cross departmental boundaries, cross-functional groups must be formed to fully understand, analyze, and improve these processes. (4) All processes can be improved. An organization must focus attention and resources on areas where the improvement will achieve the greatest benefit (Fig. 6). (5) Regarding clinical processes, comprehensive patient care data must be collected and used to identify practice activities associated with improved outcomes and optimal use of resources.

Future Directions in Quality Improvement

Combining operational and clinical quality improvement in a system for "doing the right things right" is the goal of clinical quality improvement in medicine. The informational needs are massive, and it is likely that the necessary systems will be phased in over in the next decade or so. We already have in place what one could term a clinical indicator system—the partially automated, often retrospectively collected, labor intensive "dip-sticks" that can give us infection rates, mortality rates, and the like, at most hospitals. In the next level of sophistication, clinical pathway systems, the entry of further electronic data will enable us to map the flow of patients through the medical system. To do this, data points will have to be timed as they are collected. This will permit more sophisticated retrospective data analysis and should provide sufficient information to develop treatment guidelines based on real clinical data. The third step toward an electronic medical record will likely be the development of on-line clinical advisory systems, with real-time feedback on such things as drug-drug interactions, interaction of antibiotic sensitivity information with antibiotic ordering, and drug-test relationships. These systems will highlight do's and don'ts for physicians, nurses, and other health care practitioners. Some of these advisory systems are already in place—Latter Day Saints Hospital in Salt Lake City and Children's Hospital in Boston both have pilot advisory systems already on-line.

The future is likely to see continued change in the area of quality definitions, tools, and techniques. The basic focus, however, should remain constant: to bring more resources to bear, more efficiently, in order to improve the quality of medical care for all patients.

Annotated Bibliography

Batalden PB: Organization wide quality improvement in health care. *Topics Health Record Management* 1991;11:1-12.

Quality improvement requires "system thinking;" Batalden reviews Deming's latest concepts here.

Berwick DM: Continuous improvement as an ideal in health care. *N Engl J Med* 1989;320:53-56.

An excellent overview of continuous improvement, in which Berwick expounds his "theory of bad apples."

Berwick DM, Godfrey AB, Roessner J: *Curing Health Care: New Strategies for Quality Improvement.* San Francisco, Jossey-Bass Publishers, Inc., 1990.

This publication includes a number of examples of quality improvement initiatives taken by hospitals around the country.

Brassard M: *The Memory Jogger: A Pocket Guide for Continuous Improvement.* Methuen, MA, GOAL/QPC, 1988.

An excellent pocket-guide, which summarizes the philosophy and techniques for quality improvement. It is meant to be used, and it makes the statistical methods of quality improvement easily understandable with simple examples.

Brown-Lawrence M: Experience of a concurrent screening quality assurance program on a vascular surgical unit. *Aust Clin Rev* 1989;9:17-26.

Donabedian A: The end results of healthcare: Ernest Codman's contribution to quality assurance and beyond. *Milbank Q* 1989;67:233-256.

This is an excellent summary of the history of quality improvement, and in particular, E.A. Codman's contribution to it.

Donabedian A: The quality of care: How can it be assessed? *JAMA* 1988;260:1743-1748.

In this paper Donabedian summarizes his concepts of structure, process, and outcome as they relate to medical care, the evaluation of quality, and the cost-benefit relationship.

Goldfield N, Nash DB (eds): *Providing Quality Care.* Philadelphia, American College of Physicians, 1989.

This slim volume published by the American College of Physicians provides an excellent reference and resource on quality improvement concepts, including a glimpse at the future of the automated medical record.

James BC: *Quality Management for Health Care Delivery.* Chicago, American Hospital Publishing, 1990.

This excellent volume outlines the success of the Intermountain Health Group in Salt Lake City in instituting quality improvement in their hospital system. Most of the examples relate to improvements in length of stay and resource utilization for prostate surgery, but the principles are easily adapted to orthopaedics as well.

Kritchevsky SB, Simmons BP: Continuous quality improvement: Concepts and applications for physician care. *JAMA* 1991;266:1817-1823.

This is a superb review of continuous improvement theory, with many excellent and easily understandable examples, from Semmelweiss, who used simple run charts to show that puerperal fever rates were higher for physicians than for midwives, through modern medical detectives who used control charts to pinpoint a cluster of "mercy killings" in a hospital ward.

Laffel G, Blumenthal D: The case for using industrial quality management science in health care organizations. *JAMA* 1989;262:2869-2873.

Industry both in the U.S. and abroad has significantly improved productivity by applying quality management principles. These principles can also be applied to medical practice, especially operational activities, to eliminate waste, rework, and unnecessary work.

Lohr KN, Schroeder SA: A strategy for quality assurance in Medicare. *N Engl J Med* 1990;322:707-712.

This proposal from the National Academy of Sciences proposes doubling the Medicare QA budget to investigate not only overuse but also underuse of procedures, and medical decision-making.

Luecke RW, Rosselli VR, Moss JM: The economic ramifications of client dissatisfaction. *Group Practice J* 1991;40:8-18.

This report from the Cleveland Clinic puts a dollar value on patient dissatisfaction. The authors estimate that each dissatisfied patient results in a loss of $10,000 in "hard" income and over $200,000 in "soft" income (due to loss of patient referrals).

Roberts JS, Coale JG, Redman RR: A history of the Joint Commission on Accreditation of Hospitals. *JAMA* 1987;258:936-940.

Surgeons often think that hospital certification is something which has been thrust upon them by some external organization, but this history clearly points out the seminal role of physicians in general and the American College of Surgeons in particular in creating the hospital certification process.

Roper WL, Winkenwerder W, Hackbarth GM, et al: Special article: Effectiveness in healthcare: An initiative to evaluate and improve medical practice. *N Engl J Med* 1988;319:1197-1202.

Using coronary artery surgery as an example, the authors review HCFA's efforts to improve the quality of medical care. Activities include increased monitoring and especially data analysis.

Sanazaro PJ, Mills DH: A critique of the use of generic screening in quality assessment. *JAMA* 1991;265:1977-1981.

Generic screens are not very sensitive (70% to 80%) or specific (20% to 70%) in identifying problems in medical care. Among the reasons are: errors in coding; lack of specificity; and difficulty in definition of problem cases. Focused or tailored reviews are generally more rewarding. Such focused studies require physician input as to goals, design, and implementation.

Senge PM: *The Fifth Discipline: Mastering the Five Practices of the Learning Organization*. New York, Doubleday, 1990.

This book outlines a management approach that includes many quality improvement concepts. It emphasizes "systems thinking," an approach that looks at problems not in isolation but as parts of systems which can be improved.

Walton M: *The Deming Management Method*. New York, Putman Publishing Group, 1986.

This highly readable book explains in simple terms Deming's philosophy and basic principles.

4
Practice Guidelines

Introduction

Practice guidelines (also known as clinical policies, practice policies, practice parameters, protocols, medical necessity guidelines, clinical indicators, algorithms, review criteria, and preferred practice patterns) have attracted considerable attention in recent years among physicians and other individuals concerned with delivery of health care. The interest of medical organizations, insurance companies, patient groups, and the government has been stimulated by many factors: significant variations in resource utilization with possibly high levels of unnecessary care, medical care price inflation, advances in medical technology and their rapid and at times relatively untested application in clinical settings, and an increasing focus on good quality care. Because these factors are largely influenced by the decisions of physicians, practice guidelines may improve patient care and contain costs by coordinating these decisions. But are practice guidelines the panacea for the problems facing health care systems?

Practice guidelines have been defined as "preformed recommendations issued for the purpose of influencing decisions about health interventions" and as "standardized specifications for care developed by a formal process that incorporates the best scientific evidence of effectiveness with expert opinion." Practice guidelines have been variously classified as standards, guidelines, and options, depending upon the intended degree of flexibility during their use. Standards define correct practices that must be followed and are thus inflexible. Guidelines, on the other hand, serve as reference points, and should be followed in the majority of instances. Options are very flexible and indeed may provide no guidance to a decision. The term "practice guidelines" in this chapter is intended to encompass all three. These practice guidelines may be pathway guidelines (or protocols or algorithms) that direct the physician along a preferred management path or boundary guidelines (or criteria) that define the limits of proper practices. By making unambiguous recommendations, such guidelines aim to help physicians and healthcare providers manage particular clinical problems.

The concept of practice guidelines is not new. Statements in the medical literature regarding indications, contraindications, drugs of choice, and recommended or standard practices have informed medical decision-making in the past. The current emphasis on practice guidelines reflects a shift away from viewing such statements simply as passive aids and toward consideration of practice guidelines as active management tools. Considerably more emphasis is now being placed on the development of formal methods for the generation of scientifically valid guidelines and their proper dissemination and implementation.

Purposes of Practice Guidelines

Perspectives of the Medical Community

Given the ultimate objective of achieving the most favorable outcome for a patient, the physician must consider a number of issues in determining the best form of management with the resources available. Physicians make decisions on the basis of personal experience and the experience of peers reported in formal publications and meetings. Using this information, physicians exercise clinical judgment. However, an individual physician may have limited clinical exposure to many medical conditions, may have little experience with most of the various management options, and may have inadequate follow-up and outcome data from his or her own practice. Therefore, depending on the situation, a physician may be ill-equipped to make the most appropriate decision. Practice guidelines can help solve this problem by providing a systematic approach to management of specific conditions.

Practice guidelines should discuss each stage of the management of a particular condition: the type of investigation(s) necessary for diagnosis, the indication(s) for surgery, the appropriate preoperative evaluation, and the postoperative follow-up care. The task of the physician, who no longer has to weigh each option, is made easier. In the absence of options or when some intervention may be inappropriate, practice guidelines become standards of care. When acceptable alternatives exist, guidelines define the range of interventions given the patient's characteristics and preferences. Ultimately, practice guidelines aim to improve the quality of patient care by ensuring appropriate and effective use of interventions. Finally, practice guidelines are viewed by the American Academy of Orthopaedic Surgeons (AAOS) as valuable in defending clinical decisions challenged in litigation.

Perspectives of Third-Party Payers and Health-Care Managers

Concern with health-care effectiveness and costs has prompted third-party payers to attempt to use practice guidelines in determining the coverage eligibility of medical services. Such third-party guidelines are either adopted from existing practice guidelines or are formulated de novo. In general, practice guidelines for established, high-volume technologies are adopted from external sources, while those for new and evolving technologies tend to be developed internally by the payers themselves.

Payer-sponsored technology assessment ideally involves an open and rational decision-making process. It should include a broad consideration of the relevant literature, as well as accommodating a variety of perspectives of professional opinion. When applicable for drugs, biologics, and medical devices, the assessment should include a consideration of the approved indications or restrictions on use. Criteria used for the assessment process, as well as any data and information considered in the decision itself, should be documented and available for outside review. Often, the assessment will employ specialized methods, such as meta-analysis and cost effectiveness analysis.

Once a technology is generally recognized as established, it is difficult for a payer to redefine appropriate use unilaterally, regardless of whether the evidence supports such a position. In this regard, payers usually must rely on their ability to document that a reasonable and discernible consensus exists within the medical profession to ensure that established practices can be linked to reimbursement eligibility. Conversely, the absence of coverage precedent and of broadly experienced use allows a payer to specify that new technologies must be proven safe and efficacious before being deemed reimbursable. Over time, as evidence allows, a set of approved and, therefore, covered indications may evolve for a new technology, while other investigative indications remain excluded from coverage. An administratively derived practice guideline comprises such a set of evolving indications. To the extent that a patient's coverage is tied to compliance, these guidelines may exert a significant influence over actual practice.

To the degree that most health-care costs result from the use of already established technologies, payers have shown increasing interest in the development of practice guidelines specifying appropriate indications for common, routine services. Practice guidelines developed by professional and academic medical interests thus have the potential for being adopted by payers and used to review actual practice. However, with the exception of moderately costly, elective procedures, practical administrative considerations make it unlikely that most guidelines could be used on a preprocedure or prepayment basis. Most practice guidelines are more easily adopted for the use on a postpayment basis, to review targeted samples of utilization. The results of such review might be used for network selection or for contract negotiation and settlement issues.

Relatively expensive, high-volume elective procedures are the most frequent targets of preprocedure review by payers. The challenge for the payer has been to facilitate a timely, efficient, and relatively unobtrusive review of proposed indications resulting in a defensible determination of appropriateness. One solution has been to incorporate practice guidelines into an interactive computerized decision-tree format, enabling nurse reviewers to assess the appropriateness of procedures by phone contact with physician clinics. Orthopaedic procedures that have been considered for this type of review include lumbar laminectomy, spinal fusion, knee arthroscopy, and carpal tunnel release.

Development of Practice Guidelines

Selection of Practice Guideline Topics

The choice of subject for the development of a practice guideline is determined by the purpose of the guideline. The usual approach is to target high-volume, high-cost, or high-risk procedures, especially if there is much variation in utilization or a lack of consensus about appropriateness.

The Consensus Development Program of the National Institutes of Health (NIH), one of the early organized attempts at formulating guidelines, was set up to address biomedical technologies that affected a large percentage of the population and that had influence on morbidity, mortality, or health-care costs. The initial emphasis on emerging technologies, however, rapidly shifted to existing ones when it became apparent that the safety and efficacy of many technologies already in use had not been adequately evaluated. The Agency for Health Care Policy and Research (AHCPR), recently established by the federal government, targets conditions that account for a significant portion of Medicare expenditure or have a significant variation in frequency or type of treatment provided.

When applied to common conditions and to high-volume procedures, guidelines have the potential for benefiting a large number of people. Thus, total hip arthroplasty was the subject of consensus development early in the NIH program. Presently, rates of complication following total joint arthroplasties vary among centers. In order to facilitate research in this area, the Hip Society recently produced guidelines for recording data for patients with total hip arthroplasty. The American Society of Anesthesiologists has developed guidelines (actually standards) that are intended, in part, to help manage malpractice risks and reduce premiums. Legal or economic considerations are, however, rarely the sole reason for developing guidelines.

Participants in Practice Guideline Development

Practice guidelines have been developed by individual physicians, professional organizations, hospital committees, pressure groups, insurance companies, and the government, usually independently. There are, however, concerns with guidelines developed by a particular group that has not consulted with other parties who may be affected by them. Practice guidelines developed by specialty organizations using their members only may introduce procedural-use bias and thus be criticized for being self-serving. Similarly, third-party payers who develop guidelines may be accused of ignoring the reality of practicing medicine, where many patient considerations influence choice of therapy. Accusations of cost containment may be leveled at a governmental agency developing guidelines. Guidelines developed by various agencies in isolation also may recommend different management options for the same patients and thus be in conflict with each other. Such conflict not only leaves physicians confused but also subjects some patients to the risk of inappropriate treatment and leads to loss of credibility of the organizations concerned.

The provision of health care is a highly interdependent, multiprofessional community activity. If practice guidelines are to be regarded as objective standards for quality of care, they should be developed in consultation with all parties who have a legitimate interest in the assessment of medical practice and improvements. In addition to physicians, patients, and health care organizations, many others (eg, social scientists, health economists, ethicists) have a valuable insight and contribution to make. The active participation of physicians in the production, dissemination, and assessment of guidelines is, however, paramount.

Guidelines that are not developed by physician organizations may lack professional and scientific credibility and have little influence on physician behavior. If developed by a specialty, on the other hand, the guidelines are likely to reflect the difficulties its members face in altering practice and may have a greater impact on changing medical care patterns to optimize patient outcomes. For example, although both multispecialty guidelines and specialty surgical society guidelines may label as "inappropriate" a selected indication for which no information is available regarding effectiveness, the implementation of such guidelines may be more efficient in terms of changing physician behavior through the specialty society that represents those physicians who actually perform the intervention in question.

Selected Methods of Practice Guideline Development

Historically, practice guidelines were not specifically designed but rather evolved through publications and meetings. By this slow evolutionary process, those practices that stood the "test of time" became the guidelines. Based on the experience of large numbers of practitioners, such guidelines described what was considered acceptable and thus became standard practice. Guidelines generated in this way, however, have been criticized for three reasons. First, so-called standard practice varies across geographic regions. Second, such guidelines ignore the fact that their promulgators often did not explicitly examine the evidence supporting their use or determine costs and benefits. Third, such guidelines have a way of persisting in textbooks as acceptable options, of-

ten long after scientific evidence suggests that they are no longer valid.

Obviously, in deciding on which intervention to recommend, the best method would be to conduct a randomized trial and compare the outcomes of the various treatment strategies. Such trials, however, are time-consuming and costly and are best reserved for resolving issues that have a major impact in terms of outcomes or costs. In the absence of definitive randomized trials that can be generalized to the management issues under consideration, practice guidelines can be formulated based on the use of published literature and expert opinion. The use of published data for developing guidelines, however, can be criticized for several reasons. The available evidence may be limited, and the studies may be methodologically unsound. In addition, there is often a time lag between completion of research and date of publication; thus, the information may be out of date, and developments that are at the cutting edge of technology may be missed. Finally, there is a publication bias that favors the reporting of positive rather than negative studies. However, newer techniques of information synthesis, such as meta-analysis, can provide some useful information from published literature. Similarly, the opinions of experts may be subjective and limited to their own experience. Given the above concerns, most approaches to guideline development involve some combination of quantitative literature synthesis and expert opinion.

The Consensus Development Program of the NIH that was initiated in the 1970s proceeds with development of a consensus statement through identification of advances and gaps in knowledge on a particular subject. This evidence is presented to a selected panel of experts at a consensus development conference. After the conference, the panel prepares a report with recommendations. The report is then presented for discussion to a multidisciplinary audience, including the public. These discussions are taken into account when a consensus statement is formulated.

In contrast, the Clinical Efficacy Assessment Project (CEAP) of the American College of Physicians (ACP) relies on scientific evaluation of a medical practice by analysis of published literature through quantitative methods, such as meta- and decision-analysis and cost-effectiveness analysis. Simultaneously, a position paper is developed. Both the evaluation and position paper are then subjected to extensive review by practicing physicians and the relevant specialties and subspecialties. Their views are incorporated into the guidelines. Subsequent publication of the guidelines in the *Annals of Internal Medicine* allows further debate. This project, which began in 1981, seeks to develop methods, assess medical practices and technologies, and secure physicians' acceptance of the findings.

The RAND Corporation uses a process of guideline development involving an exhaustive literature review to evaluate the benefits and risks of management options for specific clinical indications. After agreeing on definitions and the structure of the indications, a multidisciplinary panel of experts rates the appropriateness of each indication on a 9-point scale, with 1 = extremely inappropriate (risks greatly exceed benefits), 5 = equivocal (benefits and risks are about equal), and 9 = extremely appropriate (benefits greatly exceed risks). After two rounds of ratings, each indication is classified as being appropriate, inappropriate, or equivocal according to its median rating and the extent of agreement among panel members. Ultimately, a procedure is considered appropriate if the expected health benefits to an average patient (increased life expectancy, prevention of complications, relief of pain, reduced anxiety, increased functional capacity) exceed the expected health risks (mortality, morbidity, pain) by a sufficiently wide margin to ensure that the procedure is superior to alternative treatments (including no treatment).

The use of group techniques, particularly those that require group consensus, has drawbacks. The final conclusions may be influenced by the manner in which its members interact; how the chairperson conducts the business; dominance by more articulate or forceful speakers; deference to authority, power, or prestige; and other factors. Two techniques, Nominal Group Technique and Delphi Technique, however, can overcome these drawbacks. The interaction among participants is restricted, but each has an opportunity to be informed of the opinions of the others, which can be taken into account before the final judgment of each participant.

Originally developed as a method of involving disadvantaged citizens in community action agencies, the Nominal Group Technique has been recommended for seeking professionals' perceptions of health-care problems. Although this is a group technique, it should be noted that participants actually speak to each other only during certain periods. Five to nine participants, led by one individual, address a question in a session of approximately 60 to 90 minutes in duration. After introducing the questions, the leader invites all participants to write their ideas down on a worksheet. The leader then queries each participant, in turn, and notes their ideas on a blackboard or flipchart. Until this stage, no discussion is allowed. Each idea is then discussed to clarify issues and air points of view. Differences of opinion are left unresolved. From this long list, each participant chooses a specified number of ideas (six to eight) and ranks them on cards. The cards are collected and shuffled to maintain anonymity, and votes are recorded on the flipchart. Brief discussion of the voting pattern is permitted for additional clarification but not with a view to changing votes. Final voting is then conducted, and the most important items again may be ranked or may be given ratings on a scale from 0 (unimportant) to 10 or 100 (very important).

The Delphi Technique was first used to estimate which atom bomb targets might be selected by a potential enemy of the United States and how many bombs would be needed. Later, the technique came to be used extensively

Outline 1. Specific tasks for formulating practice guidelines

Identification of important health outcomes
Analysis of the effect of available practices on these outcomes
Estimation of benefits and harm
Comparison of benefits and harm
Estimation of costs
Comparison of health outcomes with costs
Comparison of alternative practices to determine priority

(Adapted with permission from Eddy DM: Practice policies: Where do they come from? *JAMA* 1990;263:877-878,880,1265-1269,1272,1275, and 264:389-391.)

in the health-care field. Face-to-face contact among participants is not required. Instead, a series of questionnaires is used, each one sent out after the results of the previous one have been analyzed. The process is continued until a consensus is reached. This procedure allows participants to contribute ideas, clarifies the reasons for any differences, and provides a chance for participants to revise their views. Modern communication methods can reduce considerably the time required for the Delphi Technique.

More recently, Eddy has proposed seven key tasks for formulating a guideline (Outline 1). Based on the explicitness with which these tasks are performed, he distinguishes four methods of developing a guideline:

Global Subjective Judgment   In this approach, the tasks are performed subjectively. The views of a group of experts are ascertained to identify a standard and acceptable practice, which is then adopted as the guideline. This approach has been used by many consensus programs and specialty societies. The advantages are the relative ease, speed, and low cost of developing a guideline.

Evidence-Based Approach   The evidence pertaining to a guideline is examined to ascertain that the practice is safe and effective. No precise quantification, however, is made of the anticipated outcomes of alternative practices.

Outcomes-Based Approach   Explicit estimation of the outcomes of alternative practices is undertaken. Resource requirements for developing a guideline in this way depend on the method used to estimate the magnitudes of outcomes. Subjective estimation of an outcome requires little additional effort, while formal quantitative estimation requires quantitative analytical skills and takes time.

Preference-Based Approach   This, the most complete approach, requires explicit performance of all tasks, including incorporation of patient-based utility estimates for various possible outcomes of a given condition. The approach, however, is in its infancy.

The choice of method for developing guidelines is governed ultimately by the complexities of the health problem; the quality and quantity of available evidence, especially relating to outcomes; and the difficulty of the value judgments. Minimal requirements of a process, however, are explicit descriptions of the assessment problem, the evidence, and the outcomes of different options. Ultimately, the aim should be to produce practice guidelines that are clinically relevant and comprehensive and include all key indications for the use of a given procedure; specific, in that they clearly describe the exact conditions for which the procedure is recommended; sufficiently detailed to identify clinical characteristics and tests required for decision-making and to discriminate between patients who will benefit from the procedure and those who will not; indicative of the appropriateness of a procedure; manageable; and readily usable.

Effectiveness of Practice Guidelines

There has been a plethora of practice guidelines in recent years. Some have been developed after exhaustive examination of practices and have optimized medical care quality and efficiency when they have been applied. Examples include guidelines for the use of preoperative chest radiology developed by the Royal College of Radiologists in the United Kingdom and, more recently, guidelines in the United States for skull radiography for patients with head injuries. However, the intuitive assumption that guidelines always modify physician behavior and result in improved quality of care is not borne out by examination of practice. The published evidence reflects inconsistent results with respect to the effect of the implementation of many guidelines on actual medical practice. For example, guidelines recommending a decrease in the use of cesarean section for breech presentation, previous cesarean section, and dystocia failed to alter physician practice in Canada, although physicians perceived that their practices had changed. Similarly, nationally developed guidelines for the management of breast, colorectal, and ovarian cancers had little impact on the care of patients with these malignancies in Italy.

In the United States, evaluation of the impact of the NIH consensus statements has been disappointing. Little change in practice has occurred, even in those regions that are highly familiar with the guidelines. For example, only 10% of women who had had a cesarean section underwent vaginal delivery during subsequent live births after the American College of Obstetricians and Gynecologists declared that previous cesarean section was not necessarily an appropriate indication for repeat cesarean section.

There are some examples, however, where guidelines have affected practice. Adoption of guidelines by the American Society of Anesthesiologists for monitoring during general anesthesia prevented the occurrence of hypoxic brain damage and led to a reduction of malpractice insurance fees for anesthesiologists in Massachusetts. Following examination of their practice, orthopaedic surgeons in California were able to reduce both average length of stay and cost, with no untoward loss of quality, for patients receiving total hip arthroplasty.

The overall dearth of evidence demonstrating the effectiveness of guidelines may stem from the relative absence of evaluation of guidelines in general. Considerations of design complexity, cost, legal liability, and credibility have been used to explain the reluctance of organizations to evaluate guidelines. Lack of proper conceptualization in the development of guidelines also may account for the reluctance of medical organizations to use them. Although it may be unrealistic to evaluate each guideline, the evaluation of a selected few may enhance understanding of the limiting factors. In this respect, the requirement for the United States Public Health Service to evaluate the impact of its first three guidelines by 1993 may provide useful information.

Apart from lack of evaluation, other reasons exist for the absence of demonstrated effectiveness of practice guidelines. First, physicians may have been reluctant to use them because of concerns that they are based on weak scientific evidence, preach "cookbook" medicine and stifle innovation, may be used as evidence in lawsuits, are "bland generalities," and represent compromises forced on physicians in an effort to reach consensus. There is also a concern that the use of guidelines may divide the profession by pitting physicians engaged in community practice against academically based physicians and physicians against managers and payers. In the future, better methods of development of more effective guidelines may overcome these concerns. The General Counsel's Office of the American Medical Association reassures physicians that practice guidelines may not be adopted by courts as inflexible standards of care, with failure to comply leading to loss of a lawsuit. Guidelines are placed alongside textbooks, journal articles, and other such evidence currently used by the courts; failure to follow them does not constitute negligence per se.

Second, equally important patient and manager concerns might have limited the use of guidelines in practice. Guidelines calling for restricted use interventions may not appeal to some patients, while "liberal" guidelines (those recommending more care than is being delivered) may disturb managers. In this respect, guidelines actually may be educational for patients and managers.

Third, guidelines may fail to modify physician behavior because relevant information has not reached individual physicians. The NIH distributes consensus statements and supporting material through its own channels, medical journals, the public media, professional organizations, and health systems agencies. Specialty guidelines often are published in specialty journals, sent to the members, and also made available on request. Guidelines developed by third-party payers, on the other hand, are usually kept secret by those payers, especially if they are used for screening insurance claims. There is, however, little evaluation of the dissemination process overall. In other fields, especially AIDS health education, evidence exists that information fails to reach a significant portion of the audience for which it is intended. Similarly, despite ensuring a distribution mechanism that was perceived to be adequate, 37% of the residents in English region hospitals did not receive guidelines for the management of head-injured patients.

Fourth, the resources for implementing guidelines often are inadequate. Guidelines by themselves have little impact on physician behavior unless they are supported by proper training in their use, along with systems support and monitoring. Strong continued commitment from the leaders also is necessary to ensure sustained changes in practice.

Fifth, there may be a lack of incentives for the use of guidelines. Linking guidelines to methods of reimbursement can be a strong incentive, and third-party payers have ensured physician compliance with their guidelines by refusing payment for certain procedures. Specialty-developed guidelines that give the profession ownership may provide an additional incentive. Another argument put forth is that social rather than scientific forces play a central role at each stage of the evolution of practice guidelines and lead to errors in reasoning and research. In addition to appropriate research methodology, due consideration of social forces is necessary to ensure the effectiveness of guidelines.

Status of Practice Guidelines in Orthopaedic Surgery: An International Perspective

To place this topic in perspective, four countries' approaches, differing in terms of their maturity, emphasis, and social context, will be discussed.

United States

To date, more than 1,100 practice guidelines have been developed by various medical specialty societies in the United States. In response to Dr. Roby Thompson's presidential address, which pointed out the need for flexible standards of practice to enable orthopaedists to exercise good clinical judgment and guide public and health care providers on proper standards of care, the Board of Directors of the American Academy of Orthopaedic Surgeons, in 1986, charged the Coordinating Committee for Health Policy with determining a process to allow the Academy to prepare guidelines of quality care. The Coordinating Committee subsequently developed an orthopaedic model for writing "clinical policies" and demonstrated its feasibility in a pilot study in 1987. A written clinical policy was described as "nothing more than a statement of the accepted collective actions physicians take when making patient care decisions," and clinical policies are viewed as connecting day-to-day practice with the latest research and judgments of experts. In developing the model, the committee placed great emphasis on flexibility of guidelines and supported practice decisions with literature citations and expert opinion. The

committee also decided to develop diagnosis-based rather than procedure-based policies.

Using the orthopaedic model, 16 clinical policies were developed by 1988 in consultation with the Board of Councilors and the Council on Medical Specialty Societies (COMSS). In presenting the results of this project, the Coordinating Committee for Health Policy recommended constitution of a Committee on Clinical Policy with representatives of various practice patterns and specialty interests of the Academy with the charge to review, update, and evaluate existing clinical policies and to develop new ones. In response, a task force was set up to select a sample from the 16 policies and refine their contents, using outside sources and a representative sample of the membership. Six policies, on carpal tunnel syndrome, Colles' fracture, femoral neck fracture, herniated lumbar disk, osteoarthritis of the hip, and tear of the medial meniscus, were published by the Academy in 1989.

The task force submitted that the clinical policies represented statements of broad principles of acceptable care for the given diagnoses and could provide the basis for more specifically derived practice guidelines. A commitment to the development of practice guidelines was seen to strengthen the Academy's position with other medical associations, such as the Joint Commission on Accreditation of Healthcare Organizations and the American Medical Association, as well as with the federal government, and collaboration with these agencies in developing practice guidelines was recommended. The importance of educating Academy fellows on an ongoing basis about the development of practice guidelines, both by and outside of the Academy, also was stressed.

Currently, the clinical policies project of the Academy is directed by the Sub-Committee on Clinical Policies. The sub-committee has updated the six policies published in 1989 and produced four new ones on De-Quervain's stenosing tenosynovitis (sprains/strains), low back musculoligamentous injury, spinal stenosis, and ulnar collateral ligament injury of the thumb.

Great Britain

In the United Kingdom, the British Orthopaedic Association (BOA) has produced guidelines for the prevention of cross-infection between patients and staff in operating rooms, with special reference to HIV and the blood-borne hepatitis viruses, as well as advisory booklets on the management of trauma. Work is presently ongoing to produce guidelines for the maintenance of allograft bone banks. No guidelines, however, have yet been developed for clinical management of specific conditions. Furthermore, there is no commitment to produce clinical guidelines in the foreseeable future. The BOA's view is shared by associations in New Zealand and South Africa. The orthopaedic associations in these countries do not perceive a need for guidelines in the practice of orthopaedic surgery. With the recent National Health Service reforms and emphasis on contracts for services and medical audit (peer review), this position may change in the future. Some orthopaedic surgeons already have suggested guidelines for reducing variations in clinical decisions and for reducing the number of inappropriate referrals to orthopaedic outpatient clinics. At a local level, guidelines recently were developed for the management of ankle injuries in an emergency room in an English hospital. Subsequent evaluation showed high compliance with the algorithm by the staff and a reduction in the number of patients undergoing radiography. A reduction in the number of patients subsequently attending a fracture clinic for review by an orthopaedic surgeon was, however, achieved at the expense of an increase in the number of patients being followed up in emergency rooms and in soft-tissue trauma clinics.

In contrast to the status of guidelines in orthopaedic surgery, the United Kingdom has been at the forefront of development of practice guidelines in other areas. Of specific relevance to the practice of orthopaedic surgery are guidelines for the management of patients with head injuries and the use of preoperative chest radiography.

Italy

The guidelines movement in Italy is still in its infancy. While the Italian health-care system is facing a somewhat radical structural and organizational change, attempts are being made to introduce new policy decisions based on scientific findings produced through quality assurance activities, particularly at the level of hospital care delivery. In this climate of increased attention to quality and appropriateness of care delivered, such tools as consensus conferences and practice guidelines are becoming popular and are generally welcomed with great enthusiasm, despite an increased awareness that they can be misused. In the country as a whole, only a few examples of the production of practice guidelines can be cited from inside the medical profession (eg, in oncology, cardiology, gastroenterology). Similar activities in the field of orthopaedics have been initiated only recently, and the first structured example concerns the management of low back pain.

Attention to the management of low back pain has been motivated by several concurrent considerations, such as its public health burden and the interest of specialists other than orthopaedic surgeons (eg, anesthesiologists, physical therapists, pharmacologists). The effort presently sponsored by the Italian Association of Orthopaedics (IAO) takes the form of a long-lasting and coordinated attempt to integrate the traditional consensus conference approach with the more explicit and time-consuming methods piloted in some experimental efforts aimed at producing treatment guidelines. After a multidisciplinary group of experts was identified that eventually will act as a consensus panel, a series of four working groups was appointed focusing respectively on epidemiology, diagnostic techniques, pharmacologic treatments and surgical techniques, rehabilitation, and physical therapies. These groups will be working to produce both

a thorough quantitative and qualitative review of available evidence and a series of tentative statements to be discussed on a preliminary basis with local panels and practitioners identified through ad hoc surveys carried out under the aegis of the IAO. The material produced through this process will be presented at the first meeting of the consensus panel, where an open discussion will take place allowing different groups to react to the content of the proposed statements. Resulting changes and proposed modifications will be sent back to the working groups, which will discuss whether and how the proposal can be accepted both among themselves and, if needed, through further consultation with local practitioner groups. Approximately one year after the inception of the whole process, the final consensus meeting will be held, and a document including the conclusions reached by each working group will be submitted. As part of their activity, the consensus panel also will appoint a working group charged with drafting the content of a series of practice guidelines.

As can be seen, the IOA is one of the first scientific associations in Italy to take the challenge of consensus building and practice guidelines diffusion seriously. At the same time, it is easy to see how this process might suffer many of the common pitfalls in the guidelines development process that are identified here. Although there is considerable enthusiasm in Italy for the potential impact of practice guidelines as effective educational instruments, there is also concern within the IOA that efforts such as those described in this chapter be integrated with proper incentives, and that their impact be assessed through evaluations aimed at identifying the positive (effective) and negative (ineffective) aspects of the guidelines production process.

Sweden

In 1975, the Swedish government established a program of developing condition-specific practice guidelines, including several conditions commonly managed by orthopaedic surgeons, with the stated goals of improving the quality of care and lowering costs. Many of these guidelines were well received by physicians and were judged to be effective in improving the overall level of care received for the conditions targeted by the guidelines. Subsequently, several factors contributed to a gradual abandonment of practice guideline use and, finally, to the recent discontinuation of the practice guideline program itself.

First, the relatively formal and cumbersome structure of the guideline development process made it difficult to update guidelines to reflect technical innovations and improvements in knowledge. Often, it took two years to update a guideline. Second, the guideline development process relied on consensus techniques that did not clearly emphasize distinctions between professional judgment and scientific fact. This sometimes led to an erosion of the guideline's credibility. Third, the structure of the Swedish health-care system, with physicians paid fixed salaries regardless of practice style, provided no economic incentive for compliance. Although the Swedish Council on Technology Assessment has issued several reports summarizing current scientific knowledge regarding the management of conditions, including a report in 1991 on back pain, the governmental program for development of specific guidelines has essentially been suspended until, as one of the initiators in the Swedish program described, the utility of practice guidelines can be demonstrated adequately by the United States.

The Swedish experience provides an example of some of the impediments likely to be encountered in practice guideline development and use. The current American approach to practice guidelines differs from the Swedish experience in several important aspects. First, the availability of information through electronically accessible media has been enhanced greatly and should lead to more efficient generation and updating of guidelines. Second, consensus building methods also are much improved, yielding a more timely and credible result. Finally, the American ability to monitor compliance is well developed and closely tied to economic and structural incentives traditionally used to encourage adherence to guidelines.

The Future of Practice Guidelines in Orthopaedic Surgery

A commitment to practice guidelines in orthopaedic surgery appears to be firmly entrenched in a number of health-care policy arenas in the United States. The U.S. government has already shown its commitment by mandating the development, dissemination, and evaluation of practice guidelines by the Agency for Health Care Policy and Research. Integrated efforts by physicians and other health-care professionals, payers, government, and the public ultimately are required if practice guidelines are to achieve their objective.

Some evidence for the effectiveness of guidelines does exist. If the primary goal of practice guideline development is to optimize patient outcomes, more research is needed to understand the attributes of practice guidelines that are associated with actual medical care practice change.

Annotated Bibliography

American Medical Association, Office of Quality Assurance: *Attributes to Guide the Development of Parameters*, Chicago, American Medical Association, 1990.

This brief but comprehensive document outlines the general attributes and characteristics that should be expected in a practice guideline development process. It is a useful tool with which to compare and contrast different practice guideline development activities, including those sponsored by governmental agencies, third-party payers, academic consortia, and individual specialty societies.

Audet AM, Greenfield S, Field M: Medical practice guidelines: Current activities and future directions. *Ann Intern Med* 1990;113:709-714.

This study found substantial support for guidelines among eight organizations prominent in the field of guideline development. However, lack of agreement on methods of development, assessment of contents, and evaluation of guidelines to ascertain their impact on physician behavior, outcomes, and health-care costs were identified as weaknesses of the current initiatives.

Brook RH: Practice guidelines and practicing medicine: Are they compatible? *JAMA* 1989;262:3027-3034.

Brook argues that several factors (increased financial pressures on the health system, accelerated introduction of technology, and data suggesting high levels of inappropriate care) will drive the development and implementation of practice guidelines. He contends that guidelines can enhance the health of the public as well as improve physician satisfaction with clinical practice.

Brook RH, Chassin MR, Fink A, et al: A method for the detailed assessment of the appropriateness of medical technologies. *Int J Technol: Assess Health Care* 1986;2:53-63.

In this early paper, investigators from the RAND Corporation describe their method of synthesizing expert medical opinion on appropriateness of medical interventions. Applying the methodology to six medical and surgical conditions, they demonstrate the feasibility of the method.

Chassin MR: Standards of care in medicine. *Inquiry* 1988;25:437-453.

In this comprehensive discussion, Chassin defines and explores operational requirements for effective guideline development. Configuration, context, scope, and continuity of the guideline development process are emphasized, using recent examples of successfully implemented practice standards. A discussion of caveats, limitations, and political considerations follows. The associated commentary by Dans and Bouxsean is of further interest.

Dixon AS: The evolution of clinical policies. *Med Care* 1990;28:201-220.

Dixon argues that social rather than scientific forces play a central role at each stage of the evolution of practice guidelines and lead to errors in reasoning and research. Four stages (development, diffusion, domination, and disillusionment) are identified in the evolution of clinical policy. In addition to appropriate research methodology, consideration of social forces is necessary to ensure the effectiveness of guidelines.

Eddy DM: Clinical decision making: From theory to practice: Practice policies: What are they? *JAMA* 1990;263:877-878,880.

Eddy defines practice policies as "preformed recommendations issued for the purpose of influencing decisions about health interventions" and uses the term to encompass options, guidelines, and standards. He discusses the various advantages of practice policies and traces their evolution from statements in textbooks to present practice guidelines that are being developed as active management aids by formal methods.

Eddy DM: Practice policies: Where do they come from? *JAMA* 1990;263:1265,1269,1272.

The traditional formulation of practice policies through continuous tracking of common practices and reinforcement via textbooks, journals, and other communications media is no longer acceptable because standard practice can vary tremendously. He describes four approaches to formulating policies with examples and list their advantages and disadvantages.

Eddy DM: Clinical decision making: From theory to practice: Practice policies: Guidelines for methods. *JAMA* 1990;263:1839-1841.

The choice of the method for developing a policy rests with the policy makers. Given that a policy must be accurate, accountable, predictable, defensible, and usable, an outcome-based approach with explicit assessment of patients' performance may be desirable. Irrespective of the method used, there is an onus on the policy makers to state the method for review by others. Full discussion of the method is also desirable, as practice policies come to be used in malpractice cases.

Eddy DM: Clinical decision making: From theory to practice: Resolving conflicts in practice policies. *JAMA* 1990;264:389-391.

Conflicting policies do not help anyone; resolution of conflict is a priority. The preferred approach is to identify conflicts quickly and resolve them through an orderly process before they become embedded and cause damage. Sources of conflict are described, along with ways of resolving differences.

Eddy DM: *A Manual for Assessing Health Practices and Designing Practice Policies*. Philadelphia, American College of Physicians, 1991.

The Council of Medical Specialty Societies, in its role as an agent for encouraging and promoting the development of practice guidelines, produced this manual under the direction of Eddy. The Manual clarifies the "jargon" and describes the steps and methods for developing guidelines.

Eiseman B, Wotkyns RS (eds): *Surgical Decision Making*. Philadelphia, WB Saunders, 1978.

The authors have made an attempt to facilitate surgical decision making by the use of algorithms. The breadth of subjects covered allows only a superficial examination of each, limiting its usefulness for the specialists.

Fowkes FR, Davies ER, Evans KT, et al: Multicentre trial of four strategies to reduce use of a radiological test. *Lancet* 1986;1:367-370.

Four strategies to examine compliance with the Royal College of Radiologists' guidelines on the use of preoperative chest radiography (POCR) showed that all had an impact in terms of reducing utilization when compared with that of a control hospital. The best results, however, were obtained by the appointment of a utilization review committee, which displayed the guidelines in surgical wards (8.5 POCRs per 100 operations against the recommended 12 per 100). Information feedback on the use of consultants also produced a consistent reduction from 29.4 to 13.3 POCRs per 100 operations. The remaining two strategies (the introduction of a new chest radiograph request form and concurrent review of request by a radiologist) had only a moderate and intermittent effect.

Hirshfeld EB: From the office of the General Counsel: Practice parameters and malpractice liability of physicians. *JAMA* 1990;263:1556,1559-1562.

This paper, from the office of the General Counsel of the American Medical Association, addresses physicians' concerns that practice guidelines may be adopted by courts as inflexible standards of care and that failure to follow them may lead to loss of a lawsuit. Describing the process of a malpractice suit, Hirshfeld places guidelines alongside textbooks, journal articles, and other such evidence currently used by the courts and points out that nonadherence to guidelines does not constitute negligence per se. He further argues that practice guidelines may indeed make results of malpractice litigation more fair.

Kelly JT, Swartwout JE: Development of practice parameters by physician organizations. *J Quality Assurance* 1990;16:54-57.

In this commentary, Kelly and Swartwout from the American Medical Association's Office of Quality Assurance acknowledge the benefits of practice parameters and recommend five principles to guide their development: (1) practice parameters should be developed by or in conjunction with physician organizations; (2) reliable methodologies that integrate relevant research findings and appropriate clinical expertise should be used to develop practice parameters; (3) practice parameters should be as comprehensive and specific as possible; (4) practice parameters should be based on current information; and (5) practice parameters should be widely disseminated.

Lomas J, Anderson GM, Domnick-Pierre K, et al: Do practice guidelines guide practice? The effect of a consensus statement on the practice of physicians. *N Engl J Med* 1989;321:1306-1311.

This study in Ontario showed that, despite awareness of and favorable attitudes toward guidelines recommending a decrease in the use of cesarean section for breech presentation, previous cesarean section, and dystocia, little actual change had occurred following distribution of a nationally endorsed consensus statement. Physicians' perceptions of altered behavior were in contrast to their actual clinical practice. Potential administrative, educational, patient-centered, or economic barriers to implementation of practice guidelines must be addressed to ensure behavior change.

Lowry RJ, Donaldson LJ, Gregg PJ: Variations in clinical decisions: A study of orthopaedic patients. *Public Health* 1991;105:351-355.

Clinical review of patients in an orthopaedic department suggested variations in the threshold for surgical interventions and, perhaps, inappropriate use of specialist hospital facilities. The medical profession was urged to develop a consensus approach to the management of common conditions.

Masters SJ, McClean PM, Arcarese JS, et al: Skull x-ray examinations after head trauma: Recommendations by a multidisciplinary panel and validation study. *N Engl J Med* 1987;316:84-91.

Guidelines for management after head injury were formulated by a multidisciplinary group of medical experts in the United States after two groups of patients were identified: those at high risk of intracranial injury and those at low risk of such injury. Subsequent study of 7,035 patients in 31 hospital emergency rooms showed that no intracranial injury was discovered among any of the low-risk patients, concluding that skull radiography may be omitted for low-risk patients to reduce unnecessary radiation exposure and costs.

Packer GJ, Goring CC, Gayner AD, et al: Audit of ankle injuries in an accident and emergency department. *Br Med J* 1991;302:885-887.

A locally developed algorithm for the management of ankle injuries was tested in this study of patients visiting an emergency room in an English hospital. There was high compliance with the algorithm, which reduced the number of patients undergoing radiography. The reduction in the number of patients attending a fracture clinic subsequently for review by an orthopaedic surgeon was achieved at the expense of an increase in the number of patients seen in emergency rooms and at soft-tissue trauma clinics.

Perry S: The NIH Consensus Development Program: A decade later. *N Engl J Med* 1987;317:485-488.

The Consensus Development Program is defended by Dr. Perry, who comments on progress made in the decade since its inception. He describes ways in which the program could become more effective, especially in the field of information dissemination.

Roland MO, Porter RW, Matthews JG, et al: Improving care: A study of orthopaedic outpatient referrals. *Br Med J* 1991;302:1124-1128.

Orthopaedic surgeons in an English hospital rated nearly 43% of the patient referrals to them by their general practitioners to be inappropriate referrals and recommended using referral guidelines to make more efficient use of hospital services.

Royal College of Radiologists: Preoperative chest radiology. *Lancet* 1979;2:83-86.

This landmark study by the Royal College of Radiologists examined the use of preoperative chest radiography (POCR) for elective nonpulmonary surgery in a number of centers in the United Kingdom. Almost 30% of the patients had received a POCR, but half of the patients with serious cardiopulmonary diseases had not. A radiologist's report was not available in 25.7% of those who had a POCR. The chances of a patient receiving inhalation anesthesia were independent of POCR and any radiologic abnormality. The high costs of a procedure of doubtful effectiveness culminated in guidelines for the use of POCR. Routine POCR was considered unjustified. POCR was recommended for patients with acute respiratory symptoms, possible metastasis, or suspected or established cardiorespiratory disease with no chest radiograph in the last 12 months, as well as for recent immigrants from places where tuberculosis was endemic.

Sommers LS, Schurman DJ, Jamison JQ, et al: Clinician-directed hospital cost management for total hip arthroplasty patients. *Clin Orthop* 1990;258:168-175.

Adoption of locally produced guidelines for the management of patients receiving total hip arthroplasty in California achieved a significant reduction in costs and in the average length of stay for patients. The reductions did not influence readmissions following surgery or increased nursing home placements.

Swedish Council on Technology Assessment in Health Care. *Back Pain: Causes, Diagnosis, Treatment*. Sweden, 1991.

This report from Sweden summarizes current scientific knowledge on the causes, diagnosis, and treatment of back pain. The discussion includes consideration of laminectomy, fusion, and chemonucleolysis, as well as many of the conservative methods for initial treatment and long-term palliation. A perspective on the psychosocial aspects of treatment and rehabilitation also is included.

Uhthoff HK, Sarkar K: An algorithm for shoulder pain caused by soft-tissue disorders. *Clin Orthop* 1990;254:121-127.

Soft-tissue disorders account for a significant proportion of painful shoulders. This paper argues that the diagnosis and management of shoulder pain can be assisted by following an algorithm.

5

Outcome Studies in Orthopaedic Surgery

Introduction

Outcomes research extends traditional clinical research on efficacy of medical interventions in research settings to their effectiveness in uncontrolled settings, considering a broader range of outcomes focusing on patient-centered and societal concerns. This chapter reviews the basic strategies, terminology, and issues in outcomes research and illustrates the points wherever possible by orthopaedic examples.

Outcomes research was dubbed the "third revolution in medical care" in an editorial of the *New England Journal of Medicine* in 1988, but a general surgeon started the revolution almost 60 years earlier. Then, Ernest Codman's term for outcome was end-result, and he urged the profession to follow up the results of its interventions in a systematic manner.

Outcomes research in the 1990s is distinguished by four features. The first is a view of end-results that measures not only technical success but patient satisfaction, as well as the patient's ability to function physically, emotionally, and socially. The second is the systematic study of cohorts to understand the clinical course of patients treated by conservative and surgical approaches. The third is the use of administrative data, such as Medicare billing information, for clinical research on effectiveness and efficacy. The fourth is the focus on information diffusion and the development of guidelines for clinical practice.

Outcomes research has had unprecedented growth. A new federal agency, the Agency for Health Care Policy and Research, has been established to fund research in delineating the effectiveness of medical interventions and developing guidelines for medical practice. Patient Outcome Research Teams (PORTs) that incorporate many aspects of outcome research have been initiated; four are in orthopaedic problems (low back pain, total knee arthroplasty, total hip arthroplasty in hip fractures, and carpal tunnel syndrome). The Joint Commission on the Accreditation of Healthcare Organizations is moving from its traditional emphasis on structural measures. The cornerstone of its future strategy for monitoring hospitals will be quality assessment based on outcomes, adjusted for severity of illness.

The increased emphasis on outcomes has its origins in three historical trends. The first is the fear that strategies to contain the escalating costs of health care would affect the quality of care. Second, outcomes research is seen as a means of assessing the relative effectiveness of different interventions to eliminate unnecessary and ineffective services or treatment. Third, outcomes research parallels the increased competitiveness of organized health care and the need of payers of health care to identify and buy "value."

Quasi-experimental Study Designs

Longitudinal Observation Studies

The "new" outcomes research model is distinguished by its emphasis on the use of longitudinal observational studies. Each study design has advantages and disadvantages and is more or less appropriate, depending on the state of knowledge (Outline 1). Clinical knowledge frequently begins with a case report or case series that reports observations on one or more patients. Such reports are appropriate in the formative evaluation of new procedures or techniques in which the investigator is interested in refining the technique and its indications and in estimating its usefulness. Such studies are frequently single-observer, single-institution studies that fail, unfortunately, to define the outcome precisely, quantitatively, or

Outline 1. Criteria for evaluating longitudinal cohort studies

Sampling
Information on potential biases should be given
  How was group assembled?
  How were members of cohort defined? Are specific diagnostic or operative criteria given?
  Are patients selected for any special characteristics?
  Critical descriptive information, such as age, gender, race, socioeconomic status, and comorbidity, should be described.

Description of intervention
  Are operative indications described?
  Is the technique described in sufficient detail?
  Is perioperative management (co-therapies) described?
  Is postoperative management described?

End points
  Measured in an objective, blinded manner (not by operating surgeon)?
  Measured by protocol (including frequency)?
  Measured with standardized, validated technique?
  Have outcome measures been checked for reliability if multiple observers involved?
  Do measures include complications, etc, ascertained in objective, active, and protocolized manner?

Completeness of follow-up
  Reports of dropouts, lost to follow-up, death
  Attempt to evaluate magnitude of bias on conclusion
Analysis
  Is there adjustment for baseline characteristics?
  Does analysis account for varying length of follow-up by life-table analysis?

objectively (blinded). Case series with variable lengths of follow-up are the dominant design in evaluating the effectiveness of orthopaedic procedures. Two reviews of evidence supporting the efficacy of total hip arthroplasty, by Gartland and by Gross, highlight these deficiencies.

Randomized Controlled Trials

The paragon of clinical research is the randomized controlled trial, in which eligible subjects are divided randomly into two groups, one of which receives the intervention and the other an alternative intervention or a placebo. Endpoints or outcomes are evaluated in an objective, blinded manner according to protocol, and patients are followed for a predefined time or to a predefined endpoint. Clinical trials are true experiments and are the most rigorous way to evaluate clinical effectiveness, but they have their limitations. These include high cost, the difficulties or ethics of randomizing patients, the specification of objective endpoints, blinding, and entry criteria that may preclude studying patient groups as heterogeneous as those seen in normal practice. Logistic, ethical, and medicolegal considerations sometimes limit the types of patients studied. For example, studies that exclude the elderly, patients with significant comorbid conditions, and women of childbearing age are of limited usefulness. Randomized trials define the efficacy of an orthopaedic procedure under the most controlled circumstances with selected patients, but a procedure's efficiency can be studied only under realistic conditions of practice.

Observational Cohort Design

The observational cohort design is an extension of the case series, studying patients treated in various ways at many health-care centers over an extended period of time and, ideally, using standardized outcome measures, including patient-oriented measures. Multivariate techniques can be used to identify patient characteristics or details of surgical technique associated with the better results. Its limitations are also its strengths. Studying patients from different sites increases the numbers and types of patients studied and the ability to evaluate an intervention in actual practice, but these same attributes can make the definition of the condition, the precise indication for a surgical procedure, the surgical technique itself, and the pre- and postsurgical care "nonstandard," which may pose a problem in interpreting the results.

For example, of the 11 published evaluations of decompressive laminectomy for degenerative lumbar stenosis reporting success rates of 64% to 95%, only two include explicit criteria and only three incorporate the opinion of the patient. A report on the results in 88 consecutive patients using standardized outcome assessment by an independent assessor and a self-administered questionnaire revealed that after an average of 4.4 years of follow-up, 17% had repeat operations because of instability or stenosis, and 30% had severe pain.

Expanded View of Endpoints

Function

Impaired physical, social, and emotional functioning is often the end result of acute and chronic musculoskeletal conditions and is a principal concern for the medical and surgical treatment, and rehabilitation, of arthritis and musculoskeletal disorders. Over the last 15 years, our ability to assess physical function through self-administered patient questionnaires has expanded tremendously. These tools are reliable and valid measures.

The new instruments build on three distinctions used to assess the impact of illness on the individual. (1) Impairment is a demonstrable anatomic loss or damage, a physiologic state. Examples include a limited range of motion or a radiograph that shows advanced structural joint damage. (2) Impairment need not cause functional limitations; for instance, a patient with joint space narrowing of the hip may not have problems walking. (3) Disability is the functional limitation caused by impairment(s), which limit(s) what a patient needs or wants to do. Physical function is a complex integrated ability that depends on the physical integrity of the joints and neuromotor system and on the patient's motivation to perform tasks of daily living, self-care, and work. When the activities of daily living are extended to essential activities in the home and community, the term "instrumental activities of daily living" is used. These include such vital tasks as using a telephone and shopping for groceries, the lack of which suggests a need for special services. Health status or quality of life, a more difficult concept, includes the dimensions of social and emotional function in addition to physical function.

Function is a complex phenomenon. Disability arises when there is a discrepancy between ability and need so that one's physical abilities are not sufficient for independence. Function changes over the course of a person's development in terms of that person's capabilities, wishes, and needs. In children, rapid change caused by maturation of cognitive, behavioral, emotional, and psychological functions is the rule, whereas in adult life those functions are stable, but life circumstances may change.

Self-administered questionnaires that quantitatively measure function and quality of life have gained wide usage. They have the properties of a quantitative scale: validity (ability to measure what the instrument purports to measure), reliability (reproducibility between raters and by one rater from one administration to another), and sensitivity to clinically important changes. The options for measuring both function and quality of life are vast. Studies indicate that the measures are interchangeable to a large degree, although certain instruments are able to measure subcomponents of function in a more sensitive manner.

For patients of working age, work status is important in characterizing function, as it may relate to disease severity or patient motivation. Improved work status is also a critical outcome, reflecting both improved function and increased economic productivity resulting from an intervention. Nevertheless, the effect of orthopaedic procedures on work status cannot be the only criterion for success, because many patients with musculoskeletal diseases are not part of the work force. Work status is multifactorial, depending in part on one's capacity to perform the task but also on factors such as motivation, the availability of work, and the inability to work because of lack of control over the pace of work. Inability to work because of orthopaedic condition must be differentiated from voluntary retirement and from inability to work because of other conditions, such as cardiovascular disease or stroke.

Health Status

In outcome studies, a person's general health can be viewed as the outcome or as a covariate that can affect operative results and overall quality of life. Self-administered questionnaires to measure general health status and health-related quality of life are as reliable, valid, and sensitive as traditional measures of operative success. During the 1970s, new measures were developed to evaluate other domains of health status: physical, social, and emotional status. These measures are particularly important in chronic diseases in which life expectancy is not markedly decreased, and morbidity and quality of life are the principal concerns. They have been used to evaluate health in populations and individuals, as well as the effectiveness of a wide variety of medical and surgical interventions, including total joint arthroplasty.

Health status and quality of life measures can be generic or disease-specific. Generic instruments permit comparisons across interventions and diagnostic conditions and capture the effects of treatment and comorbid conditions more accurately. Disease-specific measures, which can focus on particular functional areas, may be more responsive to disease-specific interventions.

Recently, investigators have attempted to increase the usefulness of these measures by developing short instruments. Preliminary evidence suggests that these shorter instruments are as able to discriminate changes in clinical status as are the longer instruments.

Pain

Relief of pain is one of the primary reasons for performing orthopaedic surgery. Various techniques are used to measure pain. Limitation of function and extent of involvement are reliable ways of assessing pain in musculoskeletal disease. A simple numerical or adjectival scale is easily administered in a standardized format. Visual analogue scales are less convenient to score, and respondents tend to use only a portion of the range. A notation of the use of analgesics, anti-inflammatory agents, and assistive devices that affect the level of pain and function can be useful in interpreting patient responses.

Patient Satisfaction/Expectations

Although objective measures of pain and function are critical parameters in the assessment of orthopaedic procedures, the extent to which the operation meets the patient's expectations or goals is also important. One study found that expectations were met fully in only 55% of patients who had undergone hip arthroplasty. This study also found that over 90% of patients expressed satisfaction with total hip arthroplasty; dissatisfaction was due primarily to persistent pain or poor walking capacity. Measurement of patients' expectations, their individual preferences for particular clinical states, and their satisfaction with the operation will improve patient selection and provide a greater understanding of the outcome of orthopaedic surgeries.

The best way to measure patient preferences and priorities has yet to be determined. There is little information comparing different ways of assessing preferences and understanding how the method may drive the response. Patient preferences have been measured by willingness-to-pay, time tradeoff, and standard gamble.

Inasmuch as quality of life and function are best understood relative to the individual, so are the values or preferences placed on aspects of health status and function. The priorities expressed by healthy individuals are not those of the sick and anxious, and preferences of the sick and anxious may alter as the illness waxes and wanes. Values change with time as people learn, adjust, or accommodate over the course of their lives. No system of patient preference measurement takes into account this dynamic state.

Complications

Outcome assessment should evaluate both positive and negative aspects of an intervention to determine the net benefit to the patient. Perioperative complications are defined as those that occur during the operation, the postoperative hospitalization, and up to two weeks after the operation. Complications must be assessed actively and by explicit ascertainment procedures to avoid the bias of studying only those patients who do well or who return for follow up. With the numerous options available, the practical problem is to pick measures for a particular application. The investigator should review the available options and choose the most appropriate measures.

Before choosing measures, one must understand the types and range of benefits and adverse effects that might be expected, as well as the best measure for each positive and negative attribute of an intervention. Traditional anthropometric devices that emphasize the measurement of impairment should be supplemented by the newer instruments that look at patient-centered concerns. The battery should include a general health status measure, particularly if the results are to be used for a social and health policy analysis. If available, disease- or joint-specific functional measures also should be used. The evaluation should include a measure of whether patients are satisfied with their status and global evaluations of whether they feel better and whether the treatment was worthwhile in view of the positive and negative effects. These assessments should be performed independently of the person who is providing the intervention.

There is limited comparative information to aid in the selection of outcome instruments. One study compared five instruments using joint replacement as a model. The Sickness Impact Profile, the Index of Well-Being, the Functional Status Index, the Arthritis Impact Measurement Scale, and the Modified Health Assessment Questionnaire correlate highly with one another and demonstrate important change. Of the five instruments, the Functional Status Index probably has the most missing data. The Arthritis Impact Measurement Scale, the Functional Status Index, and the Sickness Impact Profile are equally efficient in detecting improved mobility, but the Health Assessment Questionnaire and the Index of Well-Being are only about half as efficient as the other three instruments. For pain, the Arthritis Impact Measurement Scale is more sensitive than the Health Assessment Questionnaire. The Index of Well-Being and the Sickness Impact Profile do not have pain subscales. With regard to social function, the Sickness Impact Profile, the Index of Well-Being, and the Health Assessment Questionnaire are more sensitive than the Arthritis Impact Measurement Scale. For overall function, the Sickness Impact Profile, the Arthritis Impact Measurement Scale, and the Index of Well-Being are more efficient than the Functional Status Index and the Health Assessment Questionnaire.

Cost Effectiveness, Cost-Benefits

The cost of health care is an inescapable aspect of modern medical practice and, as such, should be considered in any evaluation of effectiveness. Costs of medical services are the economic resources (ie, equipment, supplies, professional labor) consumed in the provision of services. These costs are also termed direct medical costs. Indirect medical costs are income lost because of illness as measured by the difference between expected and actual earnings. The opportunity cost of a resource is the value of benefits foregone by failing to apply the resource to the most productive alternative use.

Cost-effectiveness and cost-benefit analyses are related but different approaches to the evaluation of an intervention. Cost-benefit analysis compares expenditures on different programs or interventions and values all outcomes, including morbidity and death, in the same economic or monetary terms. This has been done, for instance, by computing years of life saved, quality-adjusted life years, or quality of life expected in monetary terms. The major problem with the cost-benefit model is the requirement that lives saved or quality of life be valued in monetary units. This is not only difficult methodologically but ethically suspect.

Cost-effectiveness evaluation, by contrast, is the ratio of costs to benefits, but it requires that health outcomes be measured in some quantitative way and be expressed in commensurate units. Cost-benefit analysis, however, allows that costs be subtracted from benefits, which can express the net benefit for each intervention or program evaluated. It does not require knowledge of the cut-off level or the point on a list of programs at which available resources are exhausted or at which one is no longer willing to pay the price for the benefits documented. In both cost-effectiveness analysis and cost-benefit analysis, benefits and costs to individuals must be aggregated.

Factors Explaining Differences in Outcome

Measuring relevant outcomes in the evaluation of surgical procedures is only a part of the problem for improving patient care. It is also necessary to collect information that might explain the differences in surgical results (also called covariates).

An example of how difficult it is to explain why one group of patients does better than others is a recent report describing an investigation of excess perioperative infections after total knee replacement. It illustrates that even with a "hard" end point, such as joint infection, the reasons for the variation can be difficult to isolate, even with detailed study of the multiple factors involved. The following section details those variables that are thought to have general effects on the results of both medical and surgical interventions.

Variables

Age   Age is an important factor in a patient's general health, functional ability, and functional goals and requirements. One study of Medicare data showed an unusually high mortality rate after all types of elective operations, including total hip arthroplasty. These results are related to case-mix and disease severity, both of which are associated with advanced age.

Race   Membership in a minority group is associated with increased morbidity and mortality in most conditions studied and is also linked to decreased health-care utilization and access to health-care. These relationships are complex and may be confounded by socioeconomic status; lower socioeconomic status correlates with worse outcomes in virtually every medical and surgical condition studied.

Socioeconomic Status   Poor health outcome in virtually every medical and surgical condition studied is closely associated with low income or low educational attainment. Low socioeconomic status may affect access to health care, compliance, patient satisfaction, nutrition, housing conditions, employment opportunities, employment skills, and resourcefulness in the face of adversity.

Social Support   Social support refers to resources in the environment that meet an individual's interpersonal needs. The presence of social support has a good influence on health status and the ability to modify stress. Strong social support improves recovery from myocardial infarction, survival chances in cancer patients, and functional status in elderly patients with osteoarthritis.

Primary Diagnosis Another factor that influences outcome is the nature of the disorder for which treatment is being sought. For example, a patient with longstanding rheumatoid arthritis is less likely to have a good outcome from hip surgery than a patient whose only medical problems is in the hip. Also, medications used in the treatment of the disorder may alter outcome. Corticosteroids used to treat rheumatoid arthritis suppress the immune response and impair wound healing.

Comorbidity Concurrent active medical or surgical problems may be associated with pain or functional loss, potentially confounding outcomes of orthopaedic surgery. Several instruments are available for quantifying comorbid conditions and are probably interchangeable. Most require a trained individual or physician to make a judgment.

Risk of Infection Specific factors that may predispose the patient to postoperative infection should be documented carefully. These include previous operations; poor nutrition; steroid therapy; diabetes mellitus; sites of preexisting infection, such as the oropharynx or urinary tract; areas of skin breakdown; carious teeth; and urinary tract infection.

Factors Related to Surgeons and Their Support Teams
The skill of surgeons and their support teams appears to be a general factor for surgical outcomes. It is likely to be an important determinant of in-hospital mortality rates associated with coronary artery bypass grafting (CABG)—even more important than disease severity. Limited study in orthopaedic procedures suggests the same for perioperative mortality; whether other outcomes, such as functional outcome, are related to surgical skill is unstudied.

In one study of surgeons performing CABG in Maine, New Hampshire, and Vermont, investigators prospectively evaluated 3,055 patients who underwent CABG between 1987 and 1989. An analysis adjusted for age, sex, comorbid conditions, reoperation, ejection fraction, emergent versus scheduled surgery, and other factors showed a 2.5-fold difference in mortality rates among medical centers (2.3% to 5.8%) and a 4.2-fold difference among surgeons (2.2% to 9.3%).

In a study of CABG surgery performed at five major Philadelphia teaching hospitals between 1985 and 1987, investigators drew similar conclusions. Adjusted in-hospital mortality rates ranged from 4.4% to 9.9% among 12 surgeons studied. Mortality rates by surgeon did not correlate with surgical volume. When surgeons moved from one hospital to another, their mortality rates remained about the same, even if other surgeons in the new hospital had quite different rates.

Other investigators have shown that the volume of operations at a hospital is a strong determinant of mortality from total hip arthroplasties; it is likely that volume also correlates with differences in operative results and complications. The relationship between volume and outcome is not altogether clear, because many surgeons with large volumes are treating patients with complications who have been referred by other surgeons. The results of surgeons who do revisions would not be expected to be the same as those who do only primary total hip arthroplasties. The availability of a skilled rehabilitation staff might affect the functional results and length of stay, as might laminar flow and isolator systems, which may reduce postoperative infections. Another investigator suggests that perioperative total parenteral nutrition in patients with some degree of malnutrition possibly increases infectious complications.

Identifying and standardizing the critical determinants of outcome is a methodologic and political challenge, and the orthopaedic community has provided strong leadership. Parameters for outcome evaluation are completed for total hip arthroplasty and in advanced stages for carpal tunnel syndrome, knee arthroplasty, and low back pain. These parameters incorporate the dimensions discussed above. Some consolidation will eliminate redundancy, and measures should look at groups of joints rather than at a specific procedure. More similarities than differences exist in outcome measures for a weight-bearing joint—be it hip, knee, or ankle—and it would be well to merge the instruments. To do so would parallel the actual clinical evaluation, in which patients with one joint involved must have their other joints evaluated. It is important to remember that outcome measures can be used for the evaluation of any treatment, not simply surgical management. From the policy perspective, the utility of surgery over watchful waiting or conservative management is the key question.

Use of Administrative Data for Research
Recent efforts to understand utilization of health-care services have been heavily influenced by the work by Dr. John Wennberg and others. This research demonstrated striking variations in the rates of hospital admission and surgical procedures across geographic regions, using large databases collected for administrative purposes (Outline 2). As discussed in chapter 2, variations appear to be greatest when indications and expected results are least clearly defined.

Research using Medicare billing information, with particular emphasis on geographic variations and assessment of outcomes, is ongoing in a variety of orthopaedic conditions and procedures, including low back pain, total hip and knee arthroplasty, and carpal tunnel syndrome. Medicare data tapes contain information on 28 million aged and 3 million disabled beneficiaries and include 11 million inpatient bills (Medicare Part A) and 360 million ambulatory physician and supplier bills (Medicare Part B). The data also include information from hospital outpatient visits, home health agencies, skilled nursing facilities, and the endstage renal disease program. Outline 2 presents other national data sets that have been or could be used for research. In addition, at least 30 states have information on hospital discharge diagnosis. Thus, a rich source of data for epidemiologic studies on variation of health resource utilization exists.

Because these data sets were amassed primarily for billing purposes, a variety of practical, logistic, and scientific problems are involved in using them in epidemiologic studies. Foremost is the accuracy of the diagnostic procedural codes that are captured. Medicare tapes include claims that have not been fully adjudicated and reflect a wide range of coding practices and diagnostic criteria. The most appropriate utilization rate cannot be deduced from the data tapes alone. Vital information, such as outcome, comorbid conditions, functional status, and severity of illness, is not routinely available. Studies also indicate that the Medicare population represented on the data tapes differs from the general population in important sociodemographic characteristics. Finally, differences in diagnostic and procedural codes among regions can have a number of explanations, none of which are mutually exclusive.

Dissemination Research

On its face, research into the dissemination of research findings has great appeal. The half-life of medical information is getting shorter, and the sheer volume of new information makes it difficult to distinguish significant findings from all the rest. The traditional means of disseminating new research findings to practitioners have proven unwieldy and ineffective. Publication in medical journals has little or no immediate effect on practice. Continued medical education too frequently dwells on controversies and the latest biology, rather than on communicating developments that would affect patient outcomes.

One strategy in dissemination is to provide practice guidelines, particularly in commonly used and/or expensive technologies. Practice guideline development in many areas is confounded by a lack of data, but this is seen as even more reason to come to grips with medical uncertainty and to develop reasonable guidelines for practice. These topics are dicussed further in chapter 4.

In the past, summarizing the literature in a field was most commonly done by a qualitative synthesis. Meta-analysis, a technique used in formal practice guideline development, attempts a quantitative synthesis. Used originally in the social sciences and epidemiology, meta-analysis is increasingly used in the medical literature to resolve conflicting or inconclusive studies, particularly those that studied too few subjects to allow any firm conclusion. By pooling studies and summarizing their results statistically, useful insights as to the true effect of an intervention can be gained. Another use of meta-analysis is to evaluate more precisely the incidence of a side effect or complication.

The principles of meta-analysis are simple, but its execution is difficult. A "good" meta-analysis follows six major steps. The first step is to develop a protocol for including and excluding studies. A thorough literature search, frequently assisted by computerized bibliographic techniques, generates a list of studies to be analyzed. The second step is to present the criteria by which the studies are pooled, so that others can determine whether these criteria are reasonable. In the third step, the individual studies are extracted in a blinded manner. The fourth step involves pooling the result effects to assess the degree to which given effects or outcomes are present in the population (the effects size) and calculating the statistical error and confidence intervals. In the fifth step, the studies are screened on the basis of their adherence to study design principles, such as success of the randomization and blinding. This often is referred to as a "quality score" for an individual study. In the sixth step, a sensitivity analysis is performed to evaluate the impact of varying assumptions or findings on the end result of the meta-analysis. This frequently identifies critical assumptions that might affect the final conclusions for which future studies must be directed.

Decision analysis is a way of making decisions under uncertainty. First used in business and military applications, decision analysis was designed to show how varying probabilities can affect the outcome of a given problem. It does this by specifying critical points and their probability of occurrence and by identifying data that would be necessary to increase the reliability or accuracy of a given decision. Previously a laborious computation, software is now available that makes this accessible.

Another goal of outcome studies is to provide consumers of health services with information on benefits and risks. A striking example is the interactive computerized video for patients considering prostatectomy surgery. The video allows patients to query a data base on prostatectomy, including complications such as impotence, to prioritize their preferences for various outcomes, and to obtain estimates of the probability of these outcomes based on real and local experience. It is unlikely that such programs can be developed for every decision in medicine, but they show great promise for common medical interventions and surgical procedures. Also, by collecting the kind of information patients seek and having the ability to update probabilities of various outcomes, this educational device serves as a research tool for understanding the basis on which patients make decisions.

Patient Outcome Research Teams (PORT) are, in a sense, the culmination of these research strategies. A synthesis of the published literature on outcomes for a condition is produced by meta-analysis and decision analysis and provides a range of estimates of various outcomes and the critical probabilities that drive the end result. Small area variation of surgical procedures is studied through Medicare billing tapes or other administrative data sets to identify variations in resource utilization and, where possible, to link that variation with outcomes. The typical PORT also assembles cohorts of patients treated surgically or nonsurgically with a variety of techniques to track their health status function over time. Groups of physicians and consumers are involved with the review of such data and the development of practice guidelines based on data from the studies. Finally, after dissemination of findings, variation and outcomes are studied to see whether changes of variation have any demonstrable effect on outcomes.

Conclusion

Outcomes research in orthopaedic surgery is not new, but the standards by which efficacy is measured have been immutably transformed. They now encompass a richer array of outcome measures that are more patient-centered (physical and emotional function, social activity, return to productive work, patient satisfaction) and include parameters (costs, cost-benefit, cost-effectiveness, cost-utility) to inform the debate on how to reduce the costs of care without compromising the quality or humanity of care in an era of growing consumer expectations and unparalleled explosion of health-care technology. Orthopaedic surgery, with a tradition of evaluation since the days of Codman, is uniquely positioned to lead the way.

Whether the results of outcomes research will change the way medicine is practiced and contribute to the rationalization of health care and the resolution of the health-care financial crisis is moot. The cynic will say that research on effectiveness is slow to change practice, unable to keep up with new practices, and unable to study all of the questions. Abuses of the system occur not because of lack of data but because of lack of integrity. Rising health care costs are fueled by administrative waste, malpractice litigation, unrealistic expectations of patients, and lack of societal will to make choices.

No complicated social problem can be solved by research alone, and it is likely that outcomes research, too, will fall short of achieving the ambitious goals of its proponents. However, the conduct of objective studies has an inherent relevancy to scientific medicine on its own merit.

Annotated Bibliography

Charlson ME, Pompei P, Ales KL, et al: A new method of classifying prognostic comorbidity in longitudinal studies: Development and validation. *J Chronic Dis* 1987;40:373-383.

This study describes a method for classifying comorbid conditions.

Connell FA, Diehr P, Hart LG: The use of large data bases in health care studies. *Ann Rev Public Health* 1987;8:51-74.

The authors review the advantages and disadvantages of research done on large data sets.

Detsky AS: Parenteral nutrition: Is it helpful? *N Engl J Med* 1991;325:573-575.

Parenteral nutrition is not helpful in surgical patients and may increase infections and complications.

Ellwood PM: Shattuck Lecture: Outcomes management. A technology of patient experience. *N Engl J Med* 1988;318:1549-1556.

Ellwood urges the standardization of outcomes measures.

Epstein AM: The outcomes movement: Will it get us where we want to go? *N Engl J Med* 1990;323:266-270.

This is an editorial on the historical determinants of outcomes management and its key features.

Fisher ES, Whaley FS, Krushat WM, et al: The accuracy of Medicare's hospital claims data: Progress has been made, but problems remain. *Am J Public Health* 1992;82:243-248.

The percentage of agreement between the principal diagnosis on a reabstracted record and the original hospital record, when analyzed at the third digit ICD-9 CM code, improved from 73.2% in 1977 to 78.2% in 1985. Analysis of 1985 data demonstrated that the accuracy of diagnosis and procedure coding varies substantially across conditions.

Gartland JJ: Orthopaedic clinical research: Deficiencies in experimental design and determinations of outcome. *J Bone Joint Surg* 1988;70A:1357-1364.

Gartland provides a critique of the literature involving the efficacy of total hip arthroplasty.

Gordon SM, Culver DH, Simmons BP, et al: Risk factors for wound infections after total knee arthroplasty. *Am J Epidemiol* 1990;131:905-916.

An epidemic of infections after total knee arthroplasty was attributed to multiple patient, surgical, and perioperative factors.

Green J, Wintfeld N, Sharkey P, et al: The importance of severity of illness in assessing hospital mortality. *JAMA* 1990;263:241-246.

This study shows that case-mix is critical to understanding hospital mortality rates.

Gross M: A critique of methodologies used in clinical studies of hip-joint arthroplasty published in English-language orthopaedic literature. *J Bone Joint Surg* 1988;70A:1364-1371.

Gross develops a critique of literature showing the deficiencies of study design.

Katz JN, Lipson SJ, Larson MG, et al: The outcome of decompressive laminectomy for degenerative lumbar stenosis. *J Bone Joint Surg* 1991;73A:809-816.

Example of a cohort study using standardized patient-centered outcomes that suggests that previous reports may overestimate usefulness. Uses multivariate approaches to identify potential factors linked to better results.

Kay A, Davison B, Badley E, et al: Hip Arthroplasty: Patient satisfaction. *Br J Rheumatol* 1983;22:243-249.

The authors undertook a study asking patient expectations and satisfaction in evaluating hip arthropathy. Although 90% were satisfied, only 55% had all their expectations met.

Liang MH, Fossel AH, Larson MG: Comparisons of five health status instruments for orthopedic evaluation. *Med Care* 1990;28:632-642.

This is the only long-term study comparing five health status measures in total joint arthroplasty. The authors found that instruments correlated highly and pain and mobility subscales were more sensitive than social and global function. The tables provided for sample size estimates.

Lubitz J, Riley G, Newton M: Outcomes of surgery among Medicare aged: Mortality after surgery. *Health Care Financing Rev* 1985;6:103-114.

Increased postsurgical mortality was observed in aged population.

Luft HS, Bunker JP, Enthoven AC: Should operations be regionalized? The empirical relation between surgical volume and mortality. *N Engl J Med* 1979;301:1364-1369.

Lower surgical volume was associated with higher perioperative mortality for many surgical procedures.

O'Connor GT, Plume SK, Olmstead EM, et al: A regional prospective study of in-hospital mortality associated with coronary artery bypass grafting: The Northern New England Cardiovascular Disease Study Group. *JAMA* 1991;266:803-809.

Mortality after cardiac surgery in New England states influenced by technique and aftercare.

Stroup NE, Freni-Titulaer LW, Schwartz JJ: Unexpected geographic variation in rates of hospitalization for patients who have fracture of the hip: Medicare enrollees in the United States. *J Bone Joint Surg* 1990;72A:1294-1298.

Hospitalization for fractured hip was thought to be nondiscretionary, but this study suggests that the base rate driving hospitalization may actually vary.

The Glossary Committee (American College of Rheumatology): Health status measurement in *Dictionary of Rheumatic Diseases*. Bayport, NY, Contact Associates Int. Ltd., 1988, vol 3.

This is an excellent review of instruments available to measure pain, function, quality of life, and other factors. Addresses where instruments can be obtained are given.

Williams SV, Nash DB, Goldfarb N, et al: Differences in mortality from coronary artery bypass graft surgery at five teaching hospitals. *JAMA* 1991;266:810-815.

Mortality after cardiac surgery in Philadelphia teaching hospitals influenced by surgical technique.

6

Technology Assessment: A Case Study in Diagnostic Imaging

Advances in medical technology are expected to improve the quality of patient care. In order to ascertain whether a given technology improves patient care, however, one must be able to evaluate its efficacy. This is particularly true for new technologies that significantly change the way in which a disease is diagnosed. Three of these advances, computed tomography (CT), magnetic resonance imaging (MRI), and radionuclide imaging, have had a major impact on the diagnosis of musculoskeletal disorders. These imaging modalities have been employed sufficiently to merit a critical evaluation of their relative efficacies in the examination of a range of clinical disorders. Their assessment should ascertain safety, reliability, informational value, clinical utility, and cost-effectiveness. A given modality, for example, may provide accurate information but may have little impact on patient care. Efficient use of these diagnostic procedures will be possible only if controlled studies document their relative value.

In order to evaluate the quality of the literature published to date on a particular technology as well as to conduct studies of that technology, the orthopaedic surgeon must understand the terminology used by epidemiologists and statisticians in studying patient populations in relation to diseases as well as the diagnosis and management of these diseases.

This chapter focuses on the assessment of a specific subset of technologies—those associated with diagnostic imaging. Many of the concepts reviewed here may also be applied to the evaluation of new drugs, surgical procedures, implants, and other devices.

Factors to Consider in the Assessment of Diagnostic Technology

Efficacy

Efficacy refers to the potential benefit for a defined patient population of a procedure used for a specific clinical problem under ideal conditions. The efficacy of a procedure is measured in terms of safety, technical quality, accuracy, therapeutic impact, and patient outcome. Effectiveness refers to the potential patient benefits of a procedure in a noncontrolled environment.

Safety and Technical Quality The first step in assessing the efficacy of a new procedure is to determine the examination's safety. Safety must be demonstrated through experimentation before the technology is used on human beings. Technical evaluation of diagnostic imaging, for

Table 1. Fourfold Table of Examination Results Compared to a Definitive Reference

		Disease State	
		Patient With Disease	Patient Without Disease
Results	Positive Result	True Positive A	False Positive B
	Negative Result	False Negative C	True Negative D

(Adapted with permission from Haynes R.: How to read clinical journals: To learn about a diagnostic test. *Can Med Assoc J* 1981;124:703-710).

$$\text{Sensitivity} = \frac{A}{A+C}$$

$$\text{Specificity} = \frac{D}{B+D}$$

$$\text{Positive Predictive Value} = \frac{A}{A+B}$$

$$\text{Negative Predictive Value} = \frac{D}{C+D}$$

$$\text{Accuracy} = \frac{A+D}{A+B+C+D}$$

$$\text{Disease Prevalence} = \frac{A+C}{A+B+C+D}$$

example, initially includes experimentation on animals and cadavers to determine how well a new examination is able to display the anatomy of various regions of the body. If it appears to provide new diagnostic information, descriptive studies are initiated. These studies determine the appearance of various pathologic states using the new diagnostic examination but do not establish its clinical value.

Diagnostic Accuracy The diagnostic accuracy or value of an imaging examination or other procedure lies in its ability to detect the presence or absence of disease in a particular clinical setting. Diagnostic accuracy can be expressed statistically by a number of probability indices (Table 1).

Sensitivity is the probability of a positive examination result in diseased patients. Specificity is the probability of a negative examination result in normal patients. Sensitivity and specificity are considered intrinsic properties of a procedure. The indices do not depend upon the prevalence of a disease in the study population and can, therefore, be compared between different study groups.

Sensitivity and specificity are constant only if an examination is performed and interpreted the same way by different examiners. If different examiners use different criteria for what constitutes a positive or negative examination, each examiner will obtain a different set of values for its sensitivity and specificity. Receiver operating curve (ROC) analysis currently is employed to circumvent this problem by determining the strengths of a test independent of decision threshold effects. There has been recent concern that even ROC analysis may not circumvent these problems.

The sensitivity and specificity of a particular examination are established against a definitive reference (an independent gold standard) that determines the presence of disease. The sensitivity of an examination does not necessarily measure its ability to predict the patient's true state; it merely measures its ability to predict the results of the gold standard. It is, therefore, extremely important to assess whether the choice of a particular gold standard is appropriate for the disease being evaluated. A gold standard may be difficult to establish for many clinical studies. Tissue or organ histology frequently is used as a gold standard, but it provides only a qualitative diagnosis (cancer versus inflammation). The gold standard may not reflect the extent of disease or the rate of disease progression. In many instances, anatomic extent or growth rate may be more predictive of the patient's outcome than histologic appearance. If a gold standard is an invasive procedure (eg, biopsy), its use may not be equally applicable to the entire study population.

Most research attempting to determine diagnostic accuracy (the sensitivity and specificity of an examination) is performed in a controlled clinical setting. The anatomic extent of a disease is vital when determining accuracy. The examination may be less sensitive in detecting a disease at an earlier stage than at a later stage. Consideration of the dynamics and nature of the disease is necessary in assessing the value of diagnostic examinations.

Predictive value is another of the probabilistic indices. Positive predictive value is the probability that a disease is present given a positive result on examination. Negative predictive value is the probability that no disease is present given a negative result on the examination. Predictive value is directly affected by the prevalence of disease in the study population.

Overall accuracy is the number of correct examinations divided by the total number performed. Overall accuracy is not a useful probabilistic index to apply to examination results in clinical situations, because it includes the results of both diseased and nondiseased patients in the same equation.

Bias

Bias is any systematic error arising from the design or performance of a study that may compromise its validity. Bias does not suggest willful manipulation of the data, but it often results in limiting implementation of the results of the study. Many types of bias are reviewed in chapter 1. In addition to those types, there are certain forms of bias that are of particular importance in technology assessment. These are reviewed below.

Verification or Work-up Bias Verification bias occurs when the results of an examination influence the application of a diagnostic gold standard. Overestimation of the sensitivity of an examination may occur if patients with positive test results are more thoroughly evaluated than those with negative results. True positive cases are more likely to be categorized correctly than false negative cases. Verification bias can lead to overestimation or underestimation of an examination's specificity, depending on the way patients with negative test results and no definitive diagnosis are analyzed. Studies that require an examination to have a definitive diagnosis may grossly underestimate the examination's specificity. To avoid verification bias, all patients in a study need to undergo a definitive reference test by having the gold standard applied. If this is not feasible (because of invasive nature of the reference test), long-term follow-up evaluations of all patients with unverified disease must be performed to detect misclassifications.

Examination Review Bias A critical feature of many clinical evaluations, including radiologic imaging, is the inherent subjectivity of interpretation. Examination review bias (test review bias) may arise if an examination is interpreted after the definitive diagnosis has been established, which might influence interpretation of the examination, and lead to inflated estimates of its efficacy. In examination review bias, the nonblinded observer is inclined to miscategorize false negative cases as true positive and false positive cases as true negative. This miscategorization leads to overestimation of both the sensitivity and specificity of the examination. Even apparently quantitative determinations of discrete factors such as signal intensity can be subject to examination review bias if they depend on the examiner to locate the cursor for the intensity measured. Such bias can be eliminated by providing appropriate blinding conditions for the interpreters.

Diagnostic Review Bias Diagnostic review bias occurs when the diagnosis of the disease is made by someone who know the results of the examination being tested. The potential of generating this type of bias increases when surgical or pathologic findings are ambiguous and the results of prior diagnostic examinations are known. The result may be an overestimation of both the sensitivity and specificity of an examination.

Lead Time and Length Bias Because of the dynamic nature of disease, a modality that provides earlier disease detection does not necessarily have a positive effect on patient outcome. In assessing the value of a new diagnostic examination, it is necessary to determine whether lead time or length biases account for an apparent improvement in patient outcome. Lead time bias refers to the comparison of examinations that do not account for the temporal history of disease. Length bias refers to the comparison of examinations that do not account for the variable rate of disease progression.

Comparison Bias A study comparing the accuracy of two different technologies may be biased if the results are not interpreted independently by equally qualified individuals. Avoidance of comparison bias also requires a gold standard independent of the technologies being compared.

Susceptibility Bias If two prognostically dissimilar groups are chosen for evaluation at the time of patient selection, the study may be flawed by susceptibility bias. For the results of an efficacy study to be relevant in different clinical situations, the spectrum of patients evaluated must be similar. A common problem associated with application of a new diagnostic examination is that it may be accurate in a well defined clinical setting, but have a low positive predictive value when patients are tested in less controlled environments. Susceptibility bias may occur for two reasons. First, the examination may be applied to a new population of patients with a lower prevalence of the disease than that in the original test population. Second, the practicing clinician may be inclined to change the interpretation criteria regarding what constitutes a positive examination if the original study does not clearly define this information. This change may increase the sensitivity of the examination at the cost of generating an increased number of false positive results.

Performance Bias Unequal performance and unequal interpretation of an examination by clinicians with different levels of skill result in performance bias. A well-constructed study will have as many readers as possible and an adequate number of cases per reader to ensure that between-reader effects can be analyzed. The inherent subjective assessment of imaging procedures in particular naturally results in interobserver variation. It is important to distinguish between a situation in which two readers may be equally accurate in their assessment of a diagnostic examination but may classify their findings differently, and a situation in which one reader is more accurate than the other. To assess interobserver variation, several different evaluators must interpret the same examination independently. To assess intraobserver variation of an imaging modality, for example, readers must read the same images more than once without knowledge of their own prior interpretations. In addition, many efficacy studies are performed in academic medical centers, where the skill of the clinicians interpreting the studies may differ from that of clinicians in nonacademic locations. The excellent results of the initial efficacy studies may be difficult to duplicate outside of this controlled environment. The same may be said, of course, for a new operation reported initially by the surgeon who devised

it; his skill and interest may not be easily duplicated by others. Finally, the bias interest of a proprietary interest in a new technology should go without saying.

Clinical Trials
A clinical trial frequently is undertaken to determine the efficacy of a new diagnostic imaging study. Ideally, prospective, randomized, double-blinded studies should be performed to assess the usefulness of a new diagnostic examination. To date, such studies have been inherently difficult to implement. With a prospective study, a representative sample of both diseased and nondiseased patients can be tested, and inclusion and exclusion criteria for cohort selection can be stated specifically. The limitations of prospective, randomized, double-blinded trials include high costs, rapidly changing technology, the large size of the study population, and limited application of results. Most studies that have reported on the value of new techniques, be they surgical procedures or diagnostic imaging, have been retrospective in nature. One of the primary limitations of retrospective studies of diagnostic accuracy is that patients are selected on the basis of events that led to the diagnostic examination. These patients may not be representative of the diseased patients who are ordinarily tested in clinical situations. In addition, control subjects in retrospective studies may not be representative of patients outside of the study who are tested because of clinical findings suggesting disease.

Diagnostic and Therapeutic Impact
A new diagnostic imaging examination may offer significantly useful clinical information, but its impact on the improvement of patient outcome may be limited initially by a lag in the improvement of treatment methods. Therefore, determining the effects of diagnostic examinations on the quality of health care may be more difficult than evaluating new medical or surgical therapeutic regimens, where specific criteria can be established more easily.

New diagnostic technology frequently has the greatest impact on clinical situations in which a physician is uncertain of the presence of disease. Because existing diagnostic examinations may provide much of the information needed by the clinician, the incremental diagnostic information of new studies should be assessed independently. Comparing the frequency of false negative and false positive results in two or more examinations provides the necessary data for a decision-making model that will indicate which examination is preferred. Instead of replacing an existing procedure, the new examination may be used in combination with the existing one. The new combination also should be evaluated. Other variables to be considered in evaluating an imaging examination include the psychological dependence of patients and physicians on examinations, the expense of the work-up of false positive results, the natural history of the disease, and the benefits and risks of alternative treatment chosen on the basis of the examination's results.

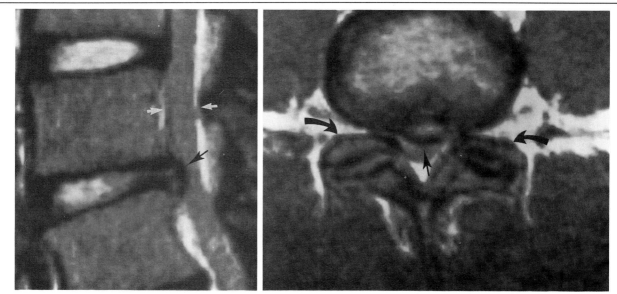

Fig. 1 On the sagittal **(left)** and axial **(right)** T_1-weighted images, a posterior-contained disk herniation (black arrow) is identified at the L4-L5 disk level causing moderate thecal sac effacement. The degree of thecal sac effacement is amplified because of a developmentally small central spinal canal. The developmental sagittal diameter (white arrows) measures 12 mm. On the axial image **(right)**, the facet joints (curved arrows) are prominent, but there are no facet degenerative changes. (Reproduced with permission from Herzog RJ: Magnetic resonance imaging of the spine, in Frymoyer JW, Ducker TV, Hadler NM, et al (eds): *The Adult Spine: Principles and Practice*. New York, Raven Press, 1991, vol 1, chap 23, pp 457-510.)

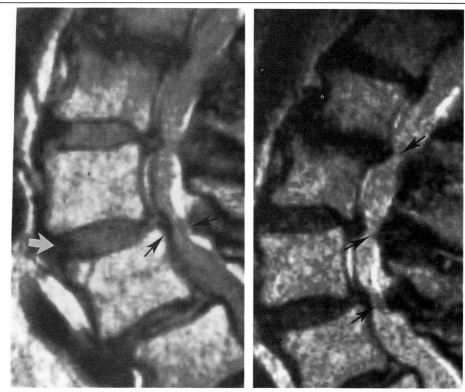

Fig. 2 Multilevel degenerative changes associated with an anterior degenerative spondylolisthesis at the L3-L4 and L4-L5 disk levels. On the sagittal proton-density weighted image **(left)**, multilevel degenerative changes are identified. A degenerative anterolisthesis is present at the L3-L4 disk level (white arrow), causing moderately severe central canal stenosis (black arrows). On the sagittal T_2-weighted image **(right)**, disk degeneration and loss of signal intensity are identified at all disk levels. Increased signal intensity in the thecal sac facilitates evaluation of the degree of multilevel central canal stenosis (arrows). (Reproduced with permission from Herzog RJ: Magnetic resonance imaging of the spine, in Frymoyer JW, Ducker TV, Hadler NM, et al (eds): *The Adult Spine: Principles and Practice*. New York, Raven Press, 1991, vol 1, chap 23, pp 457-510.)

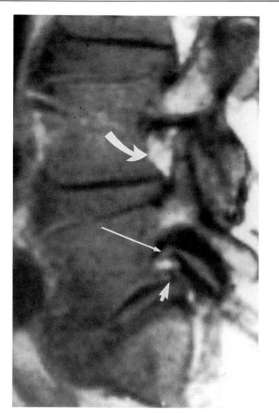

Fig. 3 Multilevel intervertebral canal stenosis. On the sagittal proton-density weighted image, stenosis of the intervertebral canals is identified secondary to end-plate spurs (curved white arrows), disk herniations (long black arrows), and hypertrophied facet joints (straight white arrows). (Reproduced with permission from Herzog RJ: Magnetic resonance imaging of the spine in Frymoyer JW, Ducker TV, Hadler NM, et al (eds): *The Adult Spine: Principles and Practice*. New York, Raven Press, 1991, vol 1, chap 23, 457-510.)

Similarly, new therapeutic technology will have its greatest impact when no previous effective treatment exists. When other effective treatments do exist, the incremental benefit of the new technology must be assessed in relation to existing therapies.

Cost-Effectiveness Analysis

The Office of Technology Assessment defines cost-effectiveness analysis as a comparison of the positive and negative economic consequences of using alternative technologies. It is difficult to determine the cost-effectiveness of a new technology if clinical efficacy has not been established. A technology that increases both cost and benefit may or may not be considered cost-effective, depending on its cost-effectiveness ratio (CER), defined as the marginal cost divided by the marginal benefit.

Case Studies of Technology Assessment: Analysis of Efficacy of CT, MRI, and Radionuclide Imaging Examinations

Before the efficacy of new diagnostic examinations can be compared, the intrinsic properties that enable them to evaluate a broad spectrum of diseased and nondiseased patients must be established (Figs. 1-3). Studies designed to evaluate new technologies can be divided into those reporting on their development and those assessing their clinical value.

Studies reporting on the development of technologies can be further categorized into those addressing their invention, their description, and their standardization. Studies about the invention of particular technologies include accounts of the development of new procedures or instruments. Descriptive studies address the subjective characterization of morphologic findings obtained with the new procedures. These studies frequently are correlated with surgical or pathologic findings, but their methodology precludes drawing conclusions regarding the clinical value of the morphologic descriptions. Before the implementation of CT, MRI, and radionuclide imaging, it was necessary to demonstrate that their respective images accurately portray normal anatomy and structural pathology. This was accomplished by scanning phantoms, cadavers, laboratory animals, and surgical specimens.

Studies assessing the clinical value of new technologies address issues of validation (determination of the diagnostic accuracy of an examination measured by its sensitivity, specificity, and predictive value). Recent criticisms have been leveled at the quality of studies reporting on the clinical efficacy of diagnostic imaging. In 1988, Cooper noted the poor use of statistical methods, incomplete use of gold standards, and overall inadequate research methodology in 54 studies utilizing MRI. In 1990, Holman reviewed 540 original reports published between January and June 1989 in the radiologic literature of which a radiologist was a first author. He assessed the nature and quality of current radiologic research and found that 79% of these reports dealt mainly with the development of technology. Significantly fewer reports assessed the clinical value (test accuracy, patient outcome) of diagnostic imaging modalities. Only 24% had a cohort group of more than 20 patients and a control population, and only 6% were prospective with more than 50 patients and a control group. Only 4% of the reports focused on patient outcome and less than 1% on cost analysis.

A review of some frequently quoted efficacy studies on CT, MRI, and radionuclide imaging is presented below. The purpose of this review is to demonstrate that these efficacy studies have limited value because of flaws in their methodologies or because many of them are merely descriptive. Similar flaws mar clinical research with many other medical technologies as well.

MRI in the Evaluation of Low Back Pain

One recent study reported on the value of MRI in the evaluation of disk degeneration in 75 male patients who had low back pain and a control group of 34 healthy male volunteers, both groups having an average age of 20 years. Magnetic resonance imaging examinations were performed on all patients using a 0.02-T ultralow field resistive magnet; T_1- and T_2-weighted sagittal sequences were performed, but no axial images were obtained. Magnetic resonance images (MRIs) were evaluated both visually and with intensity measurements. On the visual assessment performed by two radiologists, an abnormal disk was defined as a disk with decreased signal intensity on the T_2-weighted sequence. The intensity calculations of each disk were determined using a region-of-interest cursor.

In the 75 patients with low back pain, 57% demonstrated one or more abnormal lumbar disks on the MR study, compared with 35% of the controls who had abnormal disks. The difference was statistically significant. The authors concluded that patients with low back pain had an increased rate of degenerative disk disease and that MRI served as a noninvasive and highly sensitive method for evaluating the presence of incipient disk degeneration.

The study contained methodologic flaws that limited the relevance of its findings. There was no gold standard to determine whether the abnormal disk on MRI represented a degenerative disk or whether it was the actual cause of the patient's symptoms. The study focused on signal intensity changes only and did not include an evaluation of the morphologic abnormalities, such as compressive neuropathy, that are important determinants in explaining the etiology of spinal symptoms. The study did not indicate whether the MR evaluations of symptomatic or control subjects were performed in a blinded fashion. The fact that 35% of the asymptomatic controls had abnormal disks on MR study suggests that the positive predictive value of an abnormal disk signal intensity may be limited.

Evaluation of Spondylolysis Using CT or MRI

Spondylolysis frequently is included in the differential diagnosis of young patients presenting with low back pain. The largest series of CT evaluations of spondylolysis was reported in a study of 253 patients with lumbar pars interarticularis defects detected by high resolution multiplanar computed tomography (CT/MPR). In this retrospective study, the investigators described the appearance of spondylolytic defects along with concomitant pathology. The study demonstrated the ability of CT to delineate a spondylolytic defect, but it made no attempt to evaluate the diagnostic accuracy or value of the examination in detecting spondylolysis in patients presenting with back pain. The investigators did not determine whether the spondylolysis was the cause of the patient's symptoms, or whether the diagnosis of spondylolysis established on the CT examination had any impact on patient care or outcome.

In two recent reports MRI is evaluated for its ability to detect spondylolytic defects identified on CT or plain films. The investigators reported on the MR findings in 14 patients with spondylolisthesis. Seven of these pa-

tients had a proven spondylolysis as a cause of the olisthy. The MR examination was considered positive for pars defect if there was a break in continuity of the marrow signal. MRI suggested "an abnormality of the pars interarticularis in all seven cases with confirmed spondylolysis" and also suggested "the presence of an abnormality in six of the seven cases that had no spondylolysis." The authors concluded that "much information can be gleaned from the routine sagittal MR." Given the small number and limited spectrum of patients studied, the high false-positive rate, and the fact that no statistical evaluation was presented, the study has little relevance in determining the value of MRI in the detection of lumbar spondylolysis.

In a retrospective analysis of 160 MR examinations of the lumbar spine in patients presenting with back pain, eight patients were found to have spondylolysis. The defect in the pars interarticularis was best delineated on a T_1- or proton-density-weighted sagittal image. The presence of spondylolysis was corroborated by plain radiographs in six cases and by CT in three. The number of false negative MR studies was not determined. Even though MRI was capable of delineating a spondylolytic defect, the authors correctly concluded that determining the role of MRI in the detection of isthmic spondylolysis would require a detailed comparative evaluation with plain radiographs and CT. The value of this study lies in its demonstration that MRI is capable of detecting a morphologic abnormality. The study did not establish the intrinsic value of MRI in detecting a spondylolytic defect, nor did it determine the role of MRI in the evaluation of patients with back pain.

Lumbar Disk Disease and Spinal Stenosis: CT Versus Myelography

Investigators reported on their comparison of metrizamide myelography and CT in the diagnosis of a herniated lumbar disk and spinal stenosis. One hundred twenty-two patients with surgically confirmed pathology, consisting of either herniated lumbar disk, spinal stenosis, or both, were included in the study. For each level and side surgically explored, an assessment was made as to whether the spine nerve was compressed. If there was no evidence of neural compression, the level was considered to be normal. If compression of the spinal nerve was present, the etiology of the compression (disk herniation or stenosis) was reported. Both CT and myelography were interpreted without knowledge of the patient's clinical or operative findings or knowledge of the results of other examinations.

The accuracy of CT and myelography in the prediction of a surgically confirmed herniated disk was 83% for myelography versus 72% for CT. The authors concluded that the study showed a metrizamide myelogram to be more accurate than CT in the diagnosis of herniated lumbar disks. Limitations in the study's protocol preclude an accurate comparison of the two modalities. Their criterion for diagnosing a disk herniation (compression of spinal nerve) is not the only basis for diagnosing a herniation on CT examinations. A herniation may be present, particularly at the L5-S1 disk level, without neural compression. By excluding herniations that are not compressing nerve roots, the study increased the apparent accuracy of myelography, which detects only herniations that compress the opacified thecal sac or nerve root sleeves. The study did not clarify whether the decision for surgery was related to the results of the myelographic or CT evaluations, thereby possibly introducing work-up and diagnostic review bias. Furthermore, the number of lateral herniations present in patients who had surgery was not noted. The apparent sensitivity of myelography in the detection of lumbar disk herniations would have been improved had there been no lateral herniations. In addition, the study included only patients with surgically confirmed lumbar disk herniations or spinal stenosis. These inclusion criteria preclude determination of the specificity or positive and negative predictive value of the imaging exams.

In their assessment of spinal stenosis, the authors concluded that metrizamide myelography was more accurate than CT in the diagnosis of spinal stenosis and that it remained the diagnostic examination of choice. Although the authors stated that "a painstaking attempt was made to describe precisely both the exact nature of the surgical findings as well as the exact nature of the preoperative myelogram and CT scan interpretations," they relaxed these criteria significantly in order to demonstrate differences between myelography and CT in diagnosing stenosis. When the two modalities were compared at a specific disk level, there was no statistically significant difference between diagnostic results. Only when a global approach to diagnosing stenosis was used were the myelographic results significantly more accurate than the CT examination. The authors justified the use of a global analysis because of the global nature of spinal stenosis. They also made the unsupported statement that a more global interpretation of an examination simplifies the statistical analysis of the data.

A major limitation of the study's methodology for the evaluation of stenosis is that intervertebral canal stenosis—lateral stenosis—was not evaluated as part of the stenotic process. Given myelography's insensitivity to intervertebral canal stenosis, the examination's accuracy in detecting stenosis will be greater if the diagnosis of intervertebral canal stenosis is not included.

Because intervertebral canal stenosis is an important cause of radiculopathy and failed spine surgery, it is not clear why this diagnosis was omitted in the evaluation of patients with stenotic symptoms. Because the preoperative diagnosis of intervertebral canal stenosis can alter significantly the surgical approach and type of decompression performed, it is critical that detection of the presence of intervertebral canal stenosis be included when comparing the efficacy of imaging examinations.

In one frequently quoted study comparing MRI to CT in the detection of lumbar disk herniation or spinal stenosis, the investigators prospectively studied 60 patients from 1984 to 1985 who were presumed to have a herniated disk, lumbar spinal stenosis, or both. The patients were included in the study on the basis of their clinical history and physical examination and with the probability that they would require surgery. MRI using surface coils, CT, and/or myelography were performed on all subjects. Forty-eight patients underwent lumbar surgery at 62 levels, and the surgical findings represented the gold standard for the study. There were no negative explorations.

MRI and CT criteria for diagnosis of disk herniations were similar, involving identification of a focal extension of the disk margin beyond the peripheral rim of the vertebral body endplate, resulting in epidural fat, nerve root, or thecal sac displacement. On the MR study, there was no evaluation of alterations in the disk signal intensity. At operation, 32 disk herniations were reported. The herniation was correctly detected by MRI in 88% of the cases, by CT in 86%, and by myelography in 84%. The authors concluded that technically adequate MR examination was equivalent to CT and myelography for the detection of disk herniations.

Several areas in the study's design limit its clinical application significantly. The patient inclusion criterion (high probability of a patient undergoing surgery), is not representative of the population of patients typically evaluated by MRI and CT for low back pain. The MR and CT studies were interpreted independently, but with the knowledge that the patient population had a strong probability of disk disease or stenosis. This knowledge could easily affect interpretation of the studies and increase the number of positive readings. The study does not report whether the surgeon knew the results of the imaging studies when the surgical findings were reported, but the fact that 12 patients without disk herniation or stenosis did not undergo operations and that there were no negative explorations strongly suggests that the results of the imaging studies directly affected the decision for surgery.

Knowing the results of the imaging studies may introduce work-up and/or diagnostic review bias, which would increase the sensitivity of the examinations. The outcomes of the 12 patients not operated on were not included in the data analysis, a fact that also could skew the results.

In patients who underwent surgery, the diagnosis of stenosis determined at surgery agreed with the finding on MRI in 77%, on CT in 79%, and on myelography in 54% of the cases. The diagnosis of stenosis made from the imaging studies was based on a subjective assessment of the distortion of epidural fat or diminution in the size of the neural foramina, central canal, and/or thecal sac. A significant drawback in the study's design is that there was no objective grading system for the surgical findings or for interpreting the imaging studies. Also, there was no testing of inter- or intraobserver variability using the subjective criteria. In addition, both central and intervertebral canal stenoses were grouped under the general heading of stenosis. If the surgical description was intervertebral canal stenosis, the imaging examination was considered correct, even if it detected only central canal stenosis and not intervertebral canal stenosis. This type of data analysis could result in an increased number of true positive findings and an inflated examination sensitivity.

The results of this study established that MRI is equal to CT in detecting morphologic abnormalities of the disk and in distinguishing stenosis in a very select group of patients. With the potential biases in the study, it is difficult to determine the efficacy of the imaging examinations, even in this group of patients.

Postoperative Evaluation of Recurrent Disk Herniations of the Lumbar Spine

Before the development of CT, the use of myelography to diagnose a postoperative recurrent disk herniation was an arduous task. In two reports the authors described excellent results with intravenous contrast-enhanced CT to distinguish between a recurrent disk herniation and postoperative fibrosis. Few investigators have been able to replicate these results with CT. Several recent studies employing MRI have shown that both standard and gadolinium-enhanced MR examinations can distinguish a recurrent disk herniation from postoperative fibrosis. One investigator recently reported on 193 postoperative patients who had MRI of the lumbar spine with and without the administration of gadolinium. The study group included 27 patients who had repeat surgery at 31 levels. The surgical diagnosis differed from the MR diagnosis in two patients at two levels. When results of this study were combined with results of those of the authors' previous study, the accuracy of MRI in differentiating postoperative scar from herniated disk in 44 patients was 96%.

Several aspects of the study may have biased the results. Because only 27 of the initial 193 patients underwent operations, the accuracy of gadolinium-enhanced MRI in this patient population cannot be determined. In all cases, the surgeon was aware of the preoperative MRI findings, thereby potentially introducing diagnostic review bias. The fact that only 14% of the patients underwent operations suggests work-up bias. Given that a diagnosis of "only scar" from the MR study decreased the likelihood of surgery, the number of false negative MR examinations for disk herniation cannot be evaluated accurately. The results of this study do not disclose the efficacy of gadolinium-enhanced MR examinations. Knowledge of the efficacy of gadolinium-enhanced MR examinations is important information, considering its extra cost and potential risks.

Spinal Inflammation: MRI Versus Radionuclide Imaging

Before the development of MRI, bone scintigraphy was the optimal examination to detect the presence of spinal infection. Although CT can detect cortical destruction, it is relatively insensitive in detecting an inflammatory pro-

cess in the early stages, when only the cancellous bone is involved. With the excellent capacity of MRI to detect abnormalities of cancellous bone, it was quickly applied to the investigation of spinal infection. One team of investigators reported on the prospective assessment using MRI, plain film radiography, and radionuclide examinations of 37 patients clinically suspected of having vertebral osteomyelitis. Of the patients, 23 were found to have osteomyelitis on the basis of a final clinical evaluation or microbiologic or histologic diagnosis. The imaging examinations were reviewed independently by investigators blinded to the final diagnosis. MRI had a sensitivity of 96%, a specificity of 92%, and an accuracy of 94%. Combined gallium and bone scan evaluations had a sensitivity of 90%, a specificity of 100%, and an accuracy of 94%. Bone scans alone had a sensitivity of 90%, a specificity of 78%, and an accuracy of 86%. Plain radiographs had a sensitivity of 82%, a specificity of 57%, and an accuracy of 73%. The authors concluded that the appearance of vertebral osteomyelitis on MRI was characteristic, and that MRI was as accurate and sensitive as radionuclide scanning in the detection of osteomyelitis.

Several facets of the study must be considered before the significance of these results can be determined. Eighty-two percent sensitivity on plain radiographs indicated a relatively advanced inflammatory process that would likely increase the sensitivity of both MRI and radionuclide examinations. Of the 23 patients considered to have a positive diagnosis of osteomyelitis, all were evaluated with plain radiographs, 22 with technetium examinations, and only 13 with MRI. It is, therefore, difficult to compare the relative accuracy of the studies, given that MRI was used in only 57% of the patients. Because no control group was included in the study, the specificity of MRI as a screening modality for osteomyelitis cannot be determined. In addition, the patients in the study were a highly select group. There was strong clinical suspicion of vertebral osteomyelitis in all of the patients based on symptoms, laboratory abnormalities, suspicious plain radiographs of the spine, and such predisposing factors as surgery, diabetes mellitus, and drug use. The study is valuable primarily for its description of the MR findings for vertebral osteomyelitis. However, without a prospective study of a large patient population representing many stages of vertebral osteomyelitis, one cannot determine the relative efficacy of MRI compared with bone scintigraphy in the diagnosis of this disorder.

Spinal Metastatic Disease: MR Versus Radionuclide Imaging

Investigators recently reported on the detection of spinal vertebral metastases in patients with normal radiographs, CT, and radionuclide bone scans. Forty-seven patients with known primary tumors and progressive back pain, who were suspected of having spinal metastatic disease, underwent MR examinations of the thoracic and lumbar spine. Conventional radiographs and CT scans of the spine were all normal. Radionuclide bone scans were equivocal. In 21 patients, focal or diffuse vertebral abnormalities were detected on the MR examination and a needle biopsy confirmed the presence of malignancy in all 21 patients. In this study, the authors make the important point that T_1-, proton-density, and T_2-weighted images were needed to detect the abnormalities in this group of patients. For these results to be reproduced, similar imaging sequences are needed if an equivalent sensitivity is what one hopes will be achieved.

When discussing the sensitivity of MRI in the detection of spinal metastasis, authors have not addressed the question of the natural history of the metastatic process. Lead time bias and length bias must be assessed to determine whether a more sensitive examination, with the capability of early detection of the disease, actually improves patient outcome. The increased cost of MRI versus bone scintigraphy also should be addressed. In addition, even though MRI has a high sensitivity for detecting metastatic deposits, it has a low specificity in determining the etiology of abnormal vertebral body marrow. Additional tests frequently are required to categorize further the abnormality detected on an MR examination. These costs must be included in any cost-benefit analysis. It is also important that all patients evaluated in the study of spinal vertebral metastases had primary tumors, progressive back pain, and were thought to have metastatic disease. Therefore, it is not possible to determine the relative efficacy of MRI versus radionuclide imaging when screening patients with back pain to rule out the possibility of metastatic disease, a broader application than that of this study.

General Considerations

Few studies of the efficacy of new imaging examinations assess the impact of the number of examinations that cannot be interpreted or performed. Successful MR studies are more difficult to achieve than are CT studies, because of the patient's claustrophobic and inadvertent motion. In addition, MR examinations are degraded more frequently than are CT examinations, because of such artifacts as truncation errors, physiologic motion, ferromagnetic artifacts, chemical shift errors, and magnetic susceptibility. In contrast to MR studies, CT studies are not operator-dependent, and the quality of CT examinations tend to vary little from one institution to another. The main limitations of radionuclide imagings are its poor spatial resolution, low specificity, and frequently long examination times.

Conclusion

The ideal imaging modality should identify accurately the presence or absence of a disease. When a disease is present, the modality should define its location and extent. With a precise diagnosis, a clinician can be more selective in choosing the appropriate therapeutic regiment and assessing its efficacy.

CT, MRI, and radionuclide imaging are excellent diagnostic tools, but until well-controlled prospective studies comparing the efficacy of these modalities are completed, it will not be possible to determine which examination is ideal in different clinical situations. New therapeutic technologies must also be evaluated by these rigorous standards. In addition to investigating the relative accuracy of new technology, studies assessing their short- and long-term effects on patient outcome and their cost effectiveness must be undertaken. Without such information, it will be impossible to know if any new technology is being overused, underused, used properly, used improperly, or even whether it ought to be used at all.

Annotated Bibliography

Assessment of Diagnostic Technologies

Efficacy

Black WC: How to evaluate the radiology literature. *AJR* 1990;154:17-22.

The author discusses methods of assessing an examination's accuracy. Because diseases are dynamic processes rather than static entities, accuracy must be qualified by the anatomic extent of a disease. Retrospective studies may not include representative samples of diseased patients who are ordinarily tested. The process of patient selection determines to whom the study results might apply. The way the selected patients are evaluated in the study determines the accuracy of the test for that selected group. The author describes the various biases that may affect the validity of a test and discusses the cost-effectiveness and clinical usefulness of new tests. A test useful in a controlled clinical environment may have a low positive predictive value in routine diagnostic screening, resulting in a high number of false positive cases.

Brismar J, Jacobsson B: Definition of terms used to judge the efficacy of diagnostic tests: A graphic approach. *AJR* 1990;155:621-623.

The authors present a graphic approach to understanding the probabilistic indices of sensitivity, specificity, and predictive value. Their approach facilitates a conceptual understanding of the way in which the prevalence of disease can affect the results of the different indices.

Gelfand D, Ott DJ: Methodologic considerations in comparing imaging methods. *AJR* 1985;144:1117-1121.

Current methods for evaluating and comparing imaging technologies may be inadequate in several important respects. Prospective investigations often fail to provide uniform conditions for data collection, because the skills of the physicians performing the studies vary. Uncontrolled variables inherent in skill-dependent procedures may affect either prospective or retrospective investigations. When comparing different studies, it is frequently difficult to determine whether investigation, patient selection, and examination techniques are similar. The authors discuss various statistical methods used to evaluate test results. Any diagnostic method compared with the reference examination is always shown to produce inferior results, if the reference examination is considered infallible. Because of the difficulty in assessing the impact of imaging studies, there is a need to create improved investigational designs and statistical analyses to determine the efficacy of diagnostic imaging studies. Skepticism should be exercised before accepting claims of a sensitivity much greater than 85% for a skill-dependent examination.

Hanley JA, McNeil BJ: The meaning and use of the area under a receiver operating characteristic (ROC) curve. *Radiology* 1982;143:29-36.

An in-depth evaluation of ROC curve analysis is provided in this article. ROC curves are used to assess the information content of a variety of imaging systems. The most common quantitative index describing a ROC curve is the area under the curve. This provides a quantitative index for assessment of the diagnostic accuracy of a test. The area under the ROC represents the probability that a random pair of normal and abnormal images will be ranked correctly as to their disease state.

Harrington M: Some methodological questions concerning receiver operating characteristic (ROC) analysis as a method for assessing imaging quality in radiology. *J Digital Imaging* 1990;3:211-218.

This paper raises five methodologic issues concerning receiver operating characteristic analysis. (1) Using ROC analysis, all radiologic findings must be scored unambiguously, which may not reflect accurately the methodology of interpretation used in everyday imaging procedures. (2) ROC analysis does not deal effectively with false negatives, despite their importance. (3) ROC analysis depends on a confidence criterion but does not account for a shift in the meaning of this criterion, both within and among radiologists. (4) There is no way to assure that the criterion will be applied reliably, even if uniformly understood. (5) The factors producing a given confidence level also may change in different clinical settings. The author provides a cogent discussion about whether a confidence criterion can be applied to diagnostic interpretation.

Metz CE: ROC methodology in radiologic imaging. *Investigative Radiol* 1986;21:720-733.

The author presents an in-depth analysis of ROC methodology as the only known basis for distinguishing between the tendencies of radiologists to underread or overread examinations. If the performance of a diagnostic imaging system is to be evaluated objectively and meaningfully, one must compare image-based diagnoses by radiologists with actual disease states. The requirements of a valid ROC study and data analysis are presented. ROC analysis provides the capacity to compare the performance of two diagnostic systems, even though each system may involve different confidence thresholds in disease diagnosis. The relationships between ROC curves and cost-benefit analysis also are presented. Examples of ROC analysis used to evaluate the performance of a broad range of diagnostic systems is presented (eg, chest radiography, mammography, CT, ultrasound, radionuclide imaging). The author concludes that, although the practicality of ROC methodology is questioned because it requires diagnostic truth to be established in large numbers of patients, diagnostic truth and adequate sample sizes are requirements of any objective method.

Phillips WC, Scott JA, Blasczcynski G: Statistics for diagnostic procedures: I. How sensitive is "sensitivity": How specific is "specificity"? *AJR* 1983;140:1265-1270.

The authors discuss the various terms used in medical decision-making (eg, accuracy, sensitivity, specificity, predictive value). These indices, which are used to evaluate the reliability of diagnostic information, presuppose that the true presence of a disease must be established by a gold standard (eg, pathologic or bacteriologic data, surgical findings, long-term patient follow-up, comparison with other tests that have a well-established track record). The authors discuss how the ability of a procedure to detect or exclude disease depends on these indices. A discussion of the inappropriate use of the term "accuracy" in the evaluation of diagnostic tests is included.

Phillips WC Jr, Scott JA: Medical decision making: Practical points for practicing radiologists. *AJR* 1990;154:1149-1155.

The authors discuss the definition of terms used in medical decision-making. Sensitivity indicates how accurate a test is among diseased patients and specificity how accurate the test is among nondiseased patients. The prevalence of a disease is defined as the number of patients in the test population who actually have the disease. Knowledge of sensitivity, specificity, and prevalence permits the calculation of other factors, such as positive and negative predictive values, which delineate how well a test should work in the screening situation. The importance of the prevalence of disease in clinical practice and the impact of prevalence on test application is discussed. Accuracy, the proportion of correct results, frequently is not a useful term when applied to the results of tests in clinical patients. This is because the term describes the test's reliability in two groups of patients, diseased and nondiseased, at the same time. Accuracy does not indicate the relative balance between false positive and false negative errors.

Bias

Begg CB, McNeil BJ: Assessment of radiologic tests: Control of bias and other design considerations. *Radiology* 1988;167:565-569.

Methods in the design and analysis of efficacy studies of diagnostic tests are the subject of this article. The author discusses the risk of bias as an inherent problem in studies of diagnostic test efficacy, which results in limitations to study implementation. A number of sources of bias are discussed (eg, verification of disease, test interpretation, incomplete verification of sample of patients tested, handling of uninterpretable results, disease spectrum, interobserver variation, absence of a definitive reference test). There may be a learning curve for new technologies, so patients investigated early in the application of a new technology may have to be excluded in the evaluation of a test's efficacy. Biases are best offset by a careful follow up of all patients and judicious blinding of study interpreters.

Black WC, Ling A: Is earlier diagnosis really better? The misleading effects of lead time and length biases. *AJR* 1990;155:625-630.

After clearly defining lead time bias and length bias, the authors provide an excellent graphic description of the impact of these biases on evaluation of the presence of disease. They stress that new radiologic techniques should not be used in routine practice solely because they appear to improve cure rates, except when the examination's efficacy has been adjusted for anatomic extent and rate of disease progression. The ability of an exam to detect disease at an earlier state increases the chance that treatment will benefit patients with clinically significant disease, but at the cost of increasing the proportion of diagnosed patients who have clinically significant disease.

Ransohoff DF, Feinstein AR: Problems of spectrum and bias in evaluating the efficacy of diagnostic tests. *N Engl J Med* 1978;299:926-930.

Methods of obtaining statistical rates of efficacy are discussed in this article. The authors define the efficacy of a diagnostic test as its ability to indicate the presence or absence of a disease. Statistical rates of efficacy establish the likelihood of a test's usefulness in diagnosis. A high sensitivity and high accuracy for negative prediction suggest that the test is valuable for ruling out disease. A high specificity and a high accuracy for positive prediction suggest that the test is valuable for ruling in disease. The authors present a variety of biases that can affect test interpretation and the establishment of diagnoses (eg, work-up bias, diagnostic-review bias, test review bias, incorporation bias). They stress that the study population must consist of a broad spectrum of patients if the efficacy of a diagnostic test is to be evaluated.

Clinical Trials

Rudicel S, Esdaile J: The randomized clinical trial in orthopaedics: Obligation or Option? *J Bone Joint Surg* 1985;67A:1284-1293.

The authors initially present four types of biases (susceptibility, performance, detection, and transfer bias) that present difficulties in the implementation of clinical studies. The importance of randomized clinical trials is discussed, along with the ethical implications of undertaking them. The essential strength of a randomized clinical trial is its potential for limiting bias. The authors define bias as any systematic error arising from the design or implementation of a study. Bias does not suggest prejudice or willful manipulation of data. A design that randomizes the use of surgeons is presented as an alternative to the classic randomized clinical trial. In this type of trial, a surgeon is assigned to a treatment group according to expertise. Patients are still randomized, but rather than being randomized to a procedure, they are allocated to a surgeon or group of surgeons who perform only one of the procedures. This allows surgeons to remain committed to their favorite therapeutic regimens. It allows them to project confidence to their patients and to perform the surgical procedures at which they are most skilled. The surgeon-patient relationship is, therefore, impaired. As in the classic randomized clinical trial, the randomized allocation of patients protects against susceptibility bias.

Diagnostic and Therapeutic Impact

Abrams HL, Hessel S: Health technology assessment: Problems and challenges. *AJR* 1987;149:1127-1132.

This article provides a useful overview of health technology assessment. The role of the Office of Technology Assessment in the investigation of medical technology is discussed. Some of the problems of collecting primary data and analyzing it are considered, as is the way in which information from prospective studies should be assessed. The authors present the concept of "marginal information increment," which is the diagnostic data that a new technology adds to the process of establishing a clinical diagnosis. They provide guidelines for technology assessment: Does the new technology change physician habits? Is it incorporated into usage? How is bias overcome? Has the technology diffused appropriately? Is the cost of the examination justified by its incremental value?

Abrams HL, McNeil BJ: Medical Implications of computed tomography ("CAT scanning"): Part I and Part II. *N Engl J Med* 1978;298:255-261:310-318.

Even though this article was published in 1978, it provides useful insights on the difficulty of determining whether a new technology, CT, is clinically efficacious. A new technology's accuracy and its ability to yield additional significant clinical information must be assessed. In addition, an evaluation must be made as to whether it will supplant existing diagnostic methods. The value of a new diagnostic technology is determined by its effect on the diagnostic process, on therapy, on the course of disease, and on patient outcome. Outcome analysis must include both short- and long-term evaluation. The authors discuss determination of the cost of a new diagnostic procedure and the importance of comparing its cost to that of conventional examinations.

Ellwood P: Shattuck lecture: Outcomes management: A technology of patient experience. *N Engl J Med* 1988;318:1549-1556.

The concept of outcomes management as a means of assessing health care is introduced in this article. Outcomes management has important implications in the assessment of new diagnostic technologies. The author stresses the importance of accurate and complete data collection. He notes the need for participation and cooperation of the entire health care system in the evaluation of patient outcomes. Not only could outcomes management improve the quality of health care; it might allow for sound economic choices to be made at both the personal and societal levels. The author states that the centerpiece and unifying ingredient of outcomes management is the tracking and measurement of function and well-being or quality of life. Therefore, quality of life must be defined before outcome analysis can be implemented.

Cost-Effectiveness Analysis

Abrams H, McNeil BJ: Computed tomography: Cost and efficacy implications. *AJR* 1978;131:81-87.

The authors provide a comprehensive analysis of the assessment of a particular diagnostic test, computed tomography. On average, new and improved technologic services, procedures, and techniques are responsible for 50% of the rise in hospital care costs. The efficacy of any new diagnostic test must be determined through prospective studies and compared with that of competing examinations.

Cravalho EG: Pitfalls and biases in evaluating diagnostic technologies, in McNeil BJ (ed): *Critical Issues in Medical Technology*. Westport, CT, Greenwood Publishers, 1981, pp 67-69.

The author presents several clinical examples in which technological improvements are not necessarily translated into more accurate diagnoses. The author discusses a study comparing computed tomography and radionuclide brain scanning in the diagnosis of cerebral tumors. The costs of the study were high ($2.2 million), and the total number of patients entered was large (nearly 3,000), but the total number of available patients for final analysis was small (only 136). The cost of a patient's entering the original study was about $765, but the cost per patient used for final analysis was $16,500. The interpretation of cost-effectiveness calculations can be problematic. Although a new technology may increase the percentage of patients with disease who are identified, frequently the number of patients tested also will be increased, thereby increasing total diagnostic costs.

Leaf A: Cost effectiveness as a criterion for Medicare coverage. *N Engl J Med* 1989;321:898-900.

The author discusses difficulties encountered in applying cost-effectiveness analysis to patient care. It is frequently difficult to quantify costs and accurate measurements of benefits to patients, because economic effects are often elusive and imprecise. One limitation of such analysis is that the goals of our health care system have not been clearly defined. The author discusses the difference between optimization of life and prolongation of life as the appropriate goal for health care system evaluation.

Petitti D: Competing technologies: Implications for the costs and complexity of medical care. *N Engl J Med* 1986;315:1480-1483.

Two technologies compete when they are used for the same purpose (eg, when the use of one precludes use of the other in the same patient, or when no data exist to establish the superiority of one over the other). Technologies do not compete if each makes an independent contribution to a component of the patient's care, regardless of the size of the contribution. Competing technologies represent a problem because they (1) increase the cost and complexity of medical care, (2) may introduce additional risks to the patient, and (3) may lead to inappropriate utilization due to an incomplete assessment of their efficacies. The author presents examples of competing technologies in a variety of medical subspecialties and discusses the need to eliminate the redundancy of competing technologies, especially at the hospital level.

Analysis of Efficacy Studies of CT, MRI, and Radionuclide Exams General Considerations

Abrams HL: Research in diagnostic radiology: A holistic perspective. *Clin Radiol* 1981;32:121-128.

A broad perspective of the radiologic process is presented. The process begins with the request for an examination and proceeds through the generation, enhancement, perception, and interpretation of the image. Assessment of the cost-effectiveness and clinical impact of a study is discussed. Radiology offers some of the most sophisticated and advanced tools for detecting disease, and the author stresses the importance of interfacing future radiologic research with research in other disciplines.

Cascade PN: Quality improvement in diagnostic radiology. *AJR* 1990;154:1117-1120.

In this article, factors are discussed that determine the assessment and improvement of the quality of diagnostic imaging exams. The author defines factors that are the best indicators of quality and specifies exactly what standards and thresholds should be set. Most research in radiology is directed toward the advancement of diagnostic and therapeutic knowledge and the comparative assessment of imaging technologies. The author stresses the importance of a coordinated effort among researchers in radiology, economics, statistics, computer science, public health administration, and the behavioral sciences and provides a comprehensive evaluation of research programs assessing the quality of diagnostic imaging technologies. The importance of a national data base for analysis of the impact of diagnostic studies on clinical outcome also is discussed.

Cooper LS, Chalmers TC, McCally M, et al: The poor quality of early evaluations of magnetic resonance imaging. *JAMA* 1988;259:3277-3280.

The authors report on the quality of early clinical research on magnetic resonance imaging and present limitations in the research methodology. No studies included blinded readers, discussion of observer error, randomization of imaging procedures, or appropriate statistical analysis of the distribution of quantitative readings. A gold standard was used in only 22% of the evaluations and a prospective design in one evaluation; comparison studies were made in 63% of the evaluations. Even though the criticism is directed at 54 evaluations of MR studies performed early in the development and implementation of this technology, the article is helpful in identifying criteria needed in the assessment of new technology.

Fineberg HV, Hiatt HH: Evaluation of medical practices: The case for technology assessment. *N Engl J Med* 1979;301:1086-1091.

Even though this article was published in November 1979, it provides an excellent discussion of the need for technology assessment. The author addresses the contribution of new technology to rising medical costs and its effect on hospitalized patients. With the application of new technology, hospitalized patients may have shorter stays but more intense use of resources during hospitalization. The increased consumption of resources more than offsets any savings realized from shortened stays. Advances in equipment design may improve efficiency, but potential savings can be offset by overutilization or other induced costs. The author also discusses the difficulty of establishing the value and measuring the effects of new technologies. Relatively few medical interventions are designed to save life. Rather, most are intended to improve its quality. Even when an evaluation convincingly demonstrates that an existing technology is ineffective, or reveals potential savings at little or no sacrifice in quality, changes in practice may be long in coming. Many forces other than results of objective evaluations affect the rate and extent to which a medical technology is used more often or is abandoned. These include the severity and urgency of the problem addressed by the technology, the availability and suitability of alternative approaches, financial and other advantages to the physician or hospital, compatibility of a new technology with current style of practice, the status and reputation of its advocates, promotional efforts of manufacturers, and the channels through which the physician or medical administrator learns about it.

Haynes R: How to read clinical journals: To learn about a diagnostic test. *Calif Med Assoc J* 1981;124:703-710.

The author provides an algorithmic approach to assess whether or not a journal article describing a new diagnostic test is useful. This systematic approach facilitates a quick, efficient screening of articles that is extremely helpful, considering the number of journals currently published.

Hendee WR: Technology assessment: The contribution of professional organizations. *AJR* 1990;154:647-651.

The author discusses the evolution of the evaluation of health care delivery and reimbursement, including the period of expansion, the era of cost-containment, and the current emphasis on assessment and accountability. A brief description of technology assessment by randomized controlled clinical trials, decision modeling, case series, case studies, meta-analysis, consensus development, and opinion surveys is presented. The article concludes with a discussion of organizations currently performing technology assessment. The Office of Technology Assessment (OTA) was established by Congress to study the ways in which technology affects people's lives. The Federal Office of Health Technology Assessment (OHTA) addresses questions about coverage of new technologies under Medicare. Technology assessments are performed by OHTA for HCFA, the federal agency responsible for Medicare reimbursement policies. Such assessments often require two to three years from the time a request is made to HCFA to culmination in an OHTA report. The author presents several factors that influence the decision by HCFA and OHTA to consider evaluating a particular technology. A discussion of reimbursement policies by private sector third-party carriers also is included. A recommendation for reimbursement by the national Blue Cross and Blue Shield Association usually requires that a technology satisfy five criteria: (1) The technology must have final approval from appropriate governmental regulatory bodies, (2) scientific evidence must support conclusions concerning the effect of the technology on health outcome, (3) the technology must improve the net health outcome, (4) the technology must be at least as beneficial as all established alternatives, and (5) the benefit must be attainable outside of an investigational setting.

Holman BL: The research that radiologists do: Perspective based on a survey of the literature. *Radiology* 1990;176:329-332.

This is an excellent follow-up article to Cooper's criticism of MRI. The author evaluates the nature of radiologic research as conducted by both radiologists and nonradiologists and reported clinical studies in during the first six months of 1989. Most of the research by radiologists as primary investigators first involved technology development, ie, invention (12%), standardization (35%), and description (32%). Most radiologic studies involved development of morphologic criteria to assess pathophysiology. Studies by nonradiologists more frequently assessed pathophysiology by functional criteria. There were few patient outcome or cost-related articles. The author concludes that research performed by radiologists relates primarily to technology development; few studies discuss cost analysis or patient outcome. The author believes that the low frequency of outcome studies results from several factors: (1) adequate validation studies are difficult to orchestrate and are fraught with pitfalls, (2) technologies often undergo rapid and fundamental changes before validations can be completed, (3) the radiology faculty often lacks the expertise to carry out adequate clinical trials, and (4) participation in multicenter clinical trials may not be attractive to faculty members in terms of career advancement or scientific creativity.

Sox H, Stern S, Owens D, et al: *Assessment of Diagnostic Technology in Health Care: Rationale, Methods, Problems, and Directions*. Washington DC, National Academy Press, 1989.

This excellent monograph by the Council on Health Care Technology covers all facets of technology assessment. Chapter titles include (1) The Historical Development of Health Care Technology Assessment; (2) The Rationale for Assessment of Diagnostic Technology; (3) The Use of Diagnostic Tests: A Probabilistic Approach; (4) Assessment: Problems and Proposed Solutions; (5) Primary Assessment of Diagnostic Tests: Barriers to Implementation; (6) Costs and Sources of Funding; (7) A National Program for Assessing Diagnostic Technology; and (8) Problems with Multi-institutional Studies. The authors stress that a responsive and well-developed system of technology assessment can provide a strong impetus for rapid application of essential technologies and prevent the wide diffusion of marginal methods. The need to judge the effects of technology from the patient's, society's, and the physician's perspectives is stressed.

Case Studies

Avrahami E, Tadmor R, Dally O, et al: Early MR demonstration of spinal metastases in patients with normal radiographs and CT and radionuclide bone scans. *J Comput Tomogr* 1989;13:598-602.

The authors report on the successful MR detection of spinal vertebral metastases in patients with normal radiographs, CT, and radionuclide bone scans. In 21 patients, focal or diffuse vertebral abnormalities were detected on the MR examinations that were not diagnosed by other imaging modalities.

Bell GR, Rothman RH, Booth RE, et al: A study of computer assisted tomography: II. Comparison of metrizamide myelography and computed tomography in the diagnosis of herniated lumbar disc and spinal stenosis. *Spine* 1984;6:552-556.

This reports presents a comparison of metrizamide myelography and computed tomography in the diagnosis of a herniated lumbar disk and spinal stenosis. The authors conclude that a metrizamide myelogram is more accurate than CT in the diagnosis of herniated lumbar disks and spinal stenosis. Considering the study's methodologic limitations, however, these conclusions must be seriously questioned.

Grenier N, Kressel HY, Schiebler ML, et al: Isthmic spondylolysis of the lumbar spine: MR imaging in 1.5T. *Radiology* 1989;170:489-493.

The authors demonstrate that MRI is capable of imaging spondylolytic defects, but the study does not establish the intrinsic value of MRI in detecting spondylolysis as a screening examination for patients with back pain.

Johnson DW, Farnum GN, Latchaw RE, et al: MR imaging of the pars interarticularis. *AJR* 1989;152:327-332.

The authors discuss MR findings in 14 patients with spondylolisthesis. Seven of these patients had spondylolysis as a cause of the olisthy. Results of the MR examination suggested an abnormality of the pars interarticularis in these seven patients. Due to the small number of cases and the high false positive rate, however, it is difficult to determine the efficacy of MRI in the evaluation of spondylolysis.

Modic MT, Masaryk T, Boumphrey F, et al: Lumbar herniated disk disease and canal stenosis: Prospective evaluation by surface coil MR, CT, and myelography. *AJR* 1986;147:757-765.

The authors report on a comparison of MRI, CT, and myelography in the diagnosis of lumbar disk herniation of spinal stenosis. They conclude that an MR examination was equivalent to CT and myelography for the detection of disk herniations and spinal stenosis. Several methodologic drawbacks in the study make it difficult to determine whether MRI or CT is optimal in the evaluation of these clinical conditions.

Modic MT, Feiglin DH, Piraino DW, et al: Vertebral osteomyelitis: Assessment using MR. *Radiology* 1985;157:157-166.

The authors report on prospective assessment using MRI, plain film radiography, and radionuclide imaging for 37 patients clinically suspected of having vertebral osteomyelitis. They concluded that the appearance of vertebral osteomyelitis on MRI is characteristic, and that MRI is as accurate and sensitive as radionuclide scanning in the detection of osteomyelitis. The methodology of the study significantly limits the significance of these conclusions. There was a strong clinical suspicion of vertebral osteomyelitis in all of these patients; therefore, it is not possible to determine the true efficacy of MRI as a screening examination for osteomyelitis.

Paajanen H, Erkintalo M, Kuusela T, et al: Magnetic resonance study of disc degeneration in young low-back pain patients. *Spine* 1989;14:982-985.

The authors report on the value of MRI in the evaluation of disk degeneration in young patients with low back pain. They concluded that patients with low back pain have an increased rate of degenerative disk disease, and that MRI serves as a highly sensitive noninvasive method for evaluating the presence of incipient disk degeneration. This study contains many methodologic flaws limiting the relevance of its findings.

Ross JS, Masaryk TJ, Schrader M, et al: MR imaging of the postoperative lumbar spine: Assessment with gadopentetate dimeglumine. *AJR* 1990;155:867-872.

The authors report on the differentiation of disk herniations from postoperative fibrosis in patients with failed spine surgery. The accuracy of MRI in differentiating postoperative scar, using gadolinium, from a herniated disk was 96%. Even with these excellent results, it is not possible to determine the efficacy of gadolinium-enhanced MR examinations because of the study's protocol design. Only 27 of 193 patients evaluated underwent operations; therefore, a comprehensive assessment of the efficacy of gadolinium-enhanced MRI cannot be determined. In addition, the surgeons were aware of the preoperative MR findings, thereby potentially introducing diagnostic review bias and work-up bias.

Rothman SL, Glenn WV Jr: CT multiplanar reconstruction in 253 cases of lumbar spondylolysis. *Am J Neuroradiol* 1984;5:81-90.

This is the largest series on the CT evaluation of spondylolysis using high resolution multiplanar computed tomography. This retrospective study describes the appearance of spondylolytic defects along with concomitant pathology, but it makes no attempt to evaluate the diagnostic accuracy or value of the CT exam in detecting spondylolysis in patients presenting with back pain.

II
General Knowledge

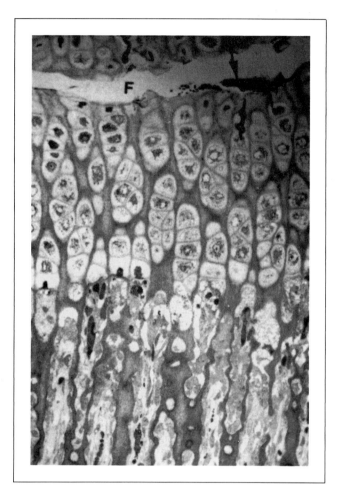

7

Bone Metabolism and Metabolic Bone Disease

Bone is vital, dynamic, connective tissue that: (1) supports mechanical loads, (2) protects vital organs, (3) contributes to ionized mineral homeostasis, and (4) plays a role in hematopoiesis and the synthesis of the paracrine and autocrine factors that regulate tissue development, remodeling, and repair. The study of bone metabolism defines the role of bone in the body's endocrine system. When the normal hormonal and molecular control of bone fails, some form of metabolic bone disease or impairment in bone remodeling and repair will result.

Cellular Control of Bone Metabolism

Bone metabolism is regulated by bone cells, which respond to various environmental signals, including chemical, mechanical, electrical, and magnetic stimuli. In general, specific responses are governed by cellular receptors found on the membrane of the cell or within its cytoplasm. Cell membrane receptors bind the exogenous signal and transfer the information across the cell's cytoplasm to the nucleus through a series of interactions that involve at least one additional messenger. Cytoplasmic (or cytosolic) receptors bind the stimulus (usually a steroid hormone, which has crossed the cell membrane and entered the cell) and then translocate that effector to the nucleus where it binds to a specific DNA promotor sequence of a gene. Three cell types are found in bone—osteoblasts, osteoclasts, and osteocytes.

Osteoblasts, generally regarded as bone-forming cells, govern bone metabolism. Their most obvious function is to synthesize osteoid, the protein component of bone tissue, but they also initiate bone resorption by elaborating various neutral proteases. The proteases remove surface osteoid, after which other cells participate in bone resorption. Because osteoblasts contain the receptors for most chemical mediators of bone metabolism including bone resorption, they play a critical role in the regulation of bone turnover.

Osteoclasts, the active agents in bone resorption, are ultimately responsible for the remodeling of bone. They are found at the apex of the classical "cutting cone" seen in histologic sections of bone reparative processes, and they create the resorptive cavities, known as Howship's lacunae, seen on bone surfaces undergoing active remodeling. Osteoclasts are multinucleated, but their progenitors are hematopoietic mononuclear cells. Differentiations toward an osteoclastic phenotype occurs early in the development of these cells.

Osteocytes are abundant in mineralized bone matrix, but their function is poorly understood. Recent evidence suggests that they may receive mechanical input signals and transmit these stimuli to other cells in bone. Osteoblasts and osteocytes are both derived from the same mesenchymal stem cell precursor (found in bone marrow stroma, periosteum, soft tissues, and possibly peripheral blood vessel endothelium). Osteoclasts arise from hematopoietic mononuclear cells.

Osteoblasts and Osteocytes

As the mesenchymal stem cell develops, it reaches a stage at which it becomes differentiated or committed as an osteoprogenitor cell. It is not known what signal induces these cells to express an osteoblastic phenotype, but factors such as bone morphogenetic protein and related substances may participate in the process.

Bone surfaces are lined by osteoblasts with small intercellular gaps between cells and their cytoplasmic processes. The endosteal surface is connected with the Volkmann canals of the Haversian systems via canaliculi. The cellular layer "protects" the bone from the extracellular fluid space, but the osteocytes within the mineralized bone maintain contact with the osteoblasts on the surface through these canaliculi and cytoplasmic processes. This organizational structure is consistent with the concept that bone cells are in intimate communication with each other.

Under electron microscopy, the cellular membranes of bone cells have a typical trilaminar appearance. During calcification of the extracellular matrix, osteoblasts may elaborate portions of this cell membrane to form vesicularized structures known as matrix vesicles. These submicroscopic (30 to 100 nm) bodies may serve as initial sites of calcification in newly formed bone, growth plate cartilage, and dental matrix. Their high electronegative charge allows matrix vesicles to bind cations, such as calcium, during transport. In addition, the matrix vesicle membrane contains phosphatases (alkaline phosphatase, adenosine triphosphatase, pyrophosphatase) and neutral proteases, which hydrolyze phosphodiester inorganic substrates and protein polysaccharide components in the matrix, respectively. These enzymes remove calcification inhibitors and also provide the phosphate ions that allow mineral precipitation to take place. Although matrix vesicle biogenesis and function is important to bone matrix mineralization, it may not be the only mechanism by which mineralization occurs. Several lines of evidence suggest that calcium phosphate deposits can be precipitated directly on collagen fibrils in osteoid.

Of the nonhormonal responses observed in bone, bioelectricity is among the most widely studied. The electrical potentials in bone are of two types: piezoelectric and bioelectric. Piezoelectric effects are produced by stress and do not depend on tissue viability. Essentially, they convert mechanical energy to electrical energy, using bone as the medium. Bioelectric effects are dependent on cellular function and are independent of stress. The ability of bone to act as a tissue that develops, produces, and transmits electrical signals depends on the function of its cells, matrix, and mineral phase. The mechanism by which electrical stimuli produce their effects is presently unclear.

Osteoblasts have several functions, and their microanatomic structure and shape change, depending on their mode of activity. The tall plump osteoblasts that line bone surfaces are metabolically active and are dedicated to bone matrix (osteoid) synthesis. On other bone surfaces, where bone is not being formed actively, osteoblasts are elongated, flat, and metabolically quiescent. These osteoblasts are called resting osteoblasts. Evidence suggests that resting osteoblasts may produce enzymes such as collagenase, collagenase inhibitor, and plasminogen activator that are involved in bone matrix degradation, which is the initial step in bone resorption.

The specific receptor-effector interaction in osteoblasts are exemplified by responses to parathyroid hormone, prostaglandin, 1,25-dihydroxyvitamin D, and glucocorticoids. Parathyroid hormone and prostaglandin bind to cell surface-associated receptors, where they trigger the intracellular signal transduction pathways that bring about the cellular response. One such mechanism involves the attenuation or amplification of the stimulus by guanine nucleotide-binding proteins in the membrane, followed by induction of the enzyme adenylate cyclase, which triggers cyclic AMP production. Other mechanisms activate phospholipase C, which catalyzes the phosphotidylinositol pathway, and an increased influx of Ca^{++} ions, which trigger the calcium messenger system. The 1,25-dihydroxyvitamin D and glucocorticoids diffuse across the membrane and bind to cytosolic receptors, which translocate to the nucleus of the cell and interact with nuclear DNA. Recent evidence suggests that osteoblasts also contain receptors for estrogen and that these also are cytosolic steroid receptors. The function of these estrogen receptors and the resultant osteoblastic responses in osteoclastic bone resorption remains unknown.

Physical and chemical signals activate osteoclasts and osteoblasts to states of high metabolic activity. Activation of osteoclasts at specific bone sites is thought to occur only after disruption of the osteoid layer that covers the bone surface (a process mediated by resting osteoblasts), and by the contraction of osteoblasts in response to stimulation by specific hormones. This contraction allows osteoclasts access to the mineralized bone. The hormonally stimulated osteoblasts may also elaborate signals to the osteoclast, telling it to resorb bone. Osteoclastic bone resorption may then activate specific molecules buried within bone matrix. These molecules, such as transforming growth factor beta (TGF-β), may stimulate bone formation by osteoblasts or signal the osteoclasts to decrease bone resorption. As such, they may regulate bone homeostasis by coupling bone formation and resorption.

Osteoclasts

Osteoclasts, the multinucleated giant cells responsible for bone resorption, derive from the same hematopoietic precursors that give rise to monocytes and macrophages. Monocytes are mononuclear cells, and macrophages and osteoclasts are formed from the fusion of monocytes. Osteoclasts differ from macrophages in that they are able to resorb bone and express certain cell surface markers and tartrate-resistant acid phosphatase activity.

The two intracellular areas of the osteoclast involved in bone resorption are the clear zone and the ruffled border. The clear zone is the part of the osteoclast that attaches to the bone surface. Evidence suggests that attachment of the osteoclast to bone is mediated by the interaction between receptors on the osteoclast known as integrins, and specific molecules found in bone matrix. Once osteoclasts have attached to bone, the clear zone surrounds and seals off the area where bone is to be resorbed, the area known as the subosteoclastic space. Bone resorption takes place in a concerted fashion whereby intracellular carbonic anhydrase degrades carbonic acid to produce free protons (hydrogen ions). Because this area of the bone is isolated beneath the osteoclast, these protons accumulate until the pH of this microenvironment reaches a level low enough (between 3 and 4) to dissolve the mineral phase and activate the osteoclastic hydrolytic enzymes. Lysosomal enzymes, including cathespin B, are then released across the ruffled border, a complex of plasma membrane infoldings. These enzymes are the actual agents that degrade the organic matrix and dissociate the mineral phase. Evidence suggests that some of the free mineral crystals and matrix components are phagocytized back into the cell and that vacuoles within the cell degrade them further.

Because bone remodeling is a specific spatial process, resorption occurs under close local control, possibly through the facility of other cells in bone and bone marrow. Because the predominant bone-resorbing hormones, such as parathyroid hormone, 1,25-dihydroxyvitamin D, and prostaglandin E, do not have receptors on osteoclasts, their action to increase bone resorption is mediated through other cells, such as osteoblasts, which do have receptors for these agonists. Other cells may also participate in the bone resorption process. For example, mast cells release heparin, an agent that enhances collagenase activity and may have a resorptive effect on bone matrix. Monocytes and lymphocytes may modulate bone remodeling through the release of local regulatory cytokines. At present, the regulation of bone resorption is an area of active investigation.

Bone Composition

Bone is composed of mineral, water, and matrix. By weight, approximately 70% of the tissue is mineral or inorganic matter, water comprises 5% to 8%; and the organic matrix makes up the remainder. Approximately 95% of the mineral phase is hydroxyapatite; impurities make up the remaining 5%. Ninety-eight percent of the organic matrix is composed of collagen and noncollagenous proteins; the cells make up only 2%.

Inorganic Phase The inorganic component of bone is principally calcium phosphate, in the form of the calcium hydroxyapatite crystal, together with small amounts of other calcium precipitates, such as octacalcium phosphate and brushite. Hydroxyapatite is present as platelike crystals, which are 20 to 80 nm long and 2 to 5 nm thick. Newly formed woven bone is not as well mineralized as mature lamellar bone and contains particles with a smaller average crystal size. Impurities, such as carbonate (which can replace the phosphate groups) or chloride and fluoride (which can replace the hydroxyl groups), may alter the crystal's solubility and certain other physical properties. These altered properties may impart biologic effects critical to normal function.

Organic Phase The organic matrix of bone, osteoid, consists of proteins synthesized and secreted by osteoblasts. Approximately 95% of osteoid is type I collagen; the remaining 5% is composed of various large and small proteins. The larger molecules are generally structural proteins, such as proteoglycans and glycosaminoglycans. The low molecular weight species may be growth factors, attachment proteins, or inductive proteins. In addition, other molecules, such as osteonectin, osteopontin, osteocalcin, bone sialoprotein, lipoproteins, and phosphoproteins, are a small part of the overall volume and weight of the tissue, but make a major contribution to its biologic function.

Collagen is the major structural component of the matrix. A ubiquitous protein of extremely low solubility, it consists of three tropocollagen polypeptide chains composed of approximately 1,000 amino acids each. Bone collagen is a linear molecule 300 nm long in the form of a triple helix of two α1(I) chains and one α2 chain crosslinked by hydrogen bonding. Each molecule is aligned with the next in a parallel fashion to produce a collagen fibril, and the collagen fibrils are grouped in bundles to form the collagen fiber. Within the collagen fibril, the gaps between the molecules are called hole zones. In addition, there are pores between the sides of parallel molecules (Fig. 1). These spaces are probably occupied by either noncollagenous proteins or mineral deposits, depending on the state of mineralization of the matrix.

Collagen molecules are synthesized both within the cell and in the matrix, by both posttranslational and postsecretory processing. In the cell, almost half of the proline and lysine residues are hydroxylated. These reactions are followed by glycosylation of the hydroxylysine residues to form the triple helical procollagen molecule—the secreted form. Once outside the cell, the amino terminals are cleaved enzymatically to form the tropocollagen molecule. These modifications are then locked in extracellularly by interchain aldehyde crosslinking, which decreases the solubility of the molecule and increases its tensile strength.

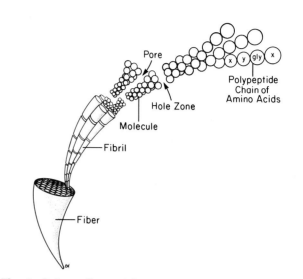

Fig. 1 Collagen fiber and fibril structure showing putative locations of pores and hole zones.

One of the more extensively studied noncollagenous proteins in bone is osteocalcin or bone gamma carboxyglutamic acid. In this small (5.8 kD) protein, three glutamic acid residues are carboxylated as a result of the vitamin K-dependent post-translational modification of the peptide. The carboxylation of these residues allows the molecule to bind to calcium. Osteocalcin accounts for 10% to 20% of the noncollagenous protein present in bone and is closely associated with the mineral phase. While its function is not known, osteocalcin is thought to play a role in attracting osteoclasts to sites of bone resorption. It may also regulate the rate of mineralization or the final shape assumed by crystals. Synthesis of osteocalcin is enhanced by 1,25-dihydroxyvitamin D and inhibited by parathyroid hormone and corticosteroids. Osteocalcin is the only protein made by osteoblasts exclusively.

Levels of osteocalcin and other gamma carboxylated glutamic acid-containing proteins (Gla proteins) have been shown to be elevated in the serum and urine of patients with Paget's disease, primary hyperparathyroidism, renal osteodystrophy, and high-turnover osteoporosis. Although this increase could be caused by either increased osteoblastic activity or increased resorption with release from bone, these levels are generally associated with bone formation.

Other noncollagenous proteins found in bone may also be involved in calcium-binding. Osteonectin, a 32-kd protein secreted by osteoblasts and platelets, binds both collagen and hydroxyapatite. Osteonectin may potentiate calcium phosphate nucleation, stabilization, or the organization of mineral within the matrix framework. Sialoproteins, proteoglycans, and other phosphoproteins thought to be synthesized by osteoblasts have also been identified. Phosphoproteins may be localized in the "hole zones" of collagen fibrils. Their phosphate groups attract calcium to the area and may have a role in nucleation during the initial stages of mineralization.

As indicated above, many other noncollagenous proteins have been isolated from bone, including bone morphogenetic protein (BMP), transforming growth factor-beta (TGF-β), and other growth factors. These proteins may be exposed during osteoclastic bone resorption, and their local and systemic release may have important autocrine and paracrine effects on the functions of osteoblasts, osteoclasts, osteocytes, and other mesenchymal cells found in bone.

Mineralization of the organic matrix of bone is a complicated process that is not fully understood. Osteoblasts regulate the concentration of calcium ions in the matrix through the release of calcium from intercellular compartments, primarily mitochondria. Osteoblasts also secrete macromolecules, as indicated above, that determine the site and rate of calcification. Proteoglycans and glycosaminoglycans probably control the sequence, rate, and degree of mineralization, and phosphoproteins, phospholipids, and other related peptides are thought to facilitate the nucleation process that initiates mineralization. The temporal sequence by which osteoblasts synthesize and release these protein products may be regulated by local and systemically produced factors that regulate growth, differentiation, and cellular function.

Mineral Metabolism

The extracellular calcium concentration is an important regulator of neural, muscular, and cardiovascular function, as well as being an intracellular second messenger in almost every cell in the body; therefore, regulation of intra- and extracellular calcium is vital. At the macroscopic level, calcium homeostasis is maintained by three organ systems—the intestines, bone, and kidneys.

All calcium intake is from the diet. Calcium absorption varies with the perceived systemic requirements and is under complex hormonal regulation. Approximately 20% of dietary calcium is absorbed; the remainder is either not absorbable or not absorbed and is excreted in the stool. Under normal conditions, urinary excretion of calcium balances the amount of calcium absorbed. Absorption of calcium from the gut and excretion from the urine averages 150 to 200 mg per day.

In the intestines, calcium is actively transported across the duodenum in association with a calcium-binding pro-

Table 1. Daily calcium requirements

Status and Age	Elemental Calcium (mg/day)
Youth (1 to 10 yrs.)	800 to 1,000
Young adult (11 to 15 yrs.)	1,200
Premenopausal (26 to 49 yrs.)	1,000
Postmenopausal (50 yrs. and older)	1,500
Pregnancy	1,500
Lactation	1,500 to 2,000
Fracture healing	1,500

tein. With low calcium diets, most dietary calcium is taken up by this active absorption mechanism. However, in the jejunum, there is passive diffusion of calcium.

It is estimated that, in Western countries, 900 mg of calcium per day must be ingested to maintain calcium balance. Significant variations exist between individuals, however, and dietary requirements of calcium are higher in both the very young and older patients (Table 1).

Children require significantly more calcium until they achieve their peak level of bone mass between the second and third decades of life. During growth, the minimal amount of calcium required is not known. Later in life, it is necessary to increase dietary calcium intake in order to counteract the effect of calcium lost to increased bone resorption. Pregnant women, lactating women, adolescents, and post-menopausal women have the greatest calcium requirements—1,500, 2,000, 1,300, and 1,500 mg per day, respectively. Unfortunately, the average American diet provides only 450 mg of calcium per day. Recent data show that adolescents consume only 430 mg of calcium per day. This calcium deficiency during growth can adversely affect the peak bone mass attained and, thus, increase that individual's risk of developing osteoporosis in the future.

The normal blood level of calcium is 9 to 10 mg/dl; approximately one half is bound to plasma protein (primarily albumin), a small fraction is associated with phosphate or citrate, and about 45% exists in the form of free calcium ions. Ionized, free calcium is critical for maintenance of membrane electrical potentials, blood coagulation, and most functions of living organisms. The ionized calcium concentration is maintained within very narrow limits, and, when necessary, bone mineral is sacrificed to maintain the ionized calcium level in the physiologic range.

Endocrine Function

Regulation of bone homeostasis depends on the delicate balance between the functions of several endocrine organs. These include the skin, parathyroid gland, liver, kidney, gonads, adrenals, and thyroid. In addition, in certain pathologic states, pituitary and hypothalamic function also affect bone physiology. The activities of the endocrine system as they apply to bone are to maintain normal serum calcium levels for the organism.

Vitamin D

Vitamin D modulates calcium homeostasis, either directly or by affecting various calcium-regulating cell systems. When skin is exposed to ultraviolet light, vitamin D_3 (cholecalciferol) is formed endogenously from 7-dehydrocholesterol. In Caucasians, 15 minutes per day of exposure to bright sunlight on the hands and face produces enough vitamin D_3 to provide the minimum requirement (10 mg) of cholecalciferol. Dark-skinned people may require longer exposure. The major source of vitamin D is the diet, which provides ergocalciferol, or vitamin D_2. These two isomeric forms have the same endogenous function and differ biochemically at only one carbon on the molecule. Both metabolites are stored in several tissues. The highest concentrations are found in adipose tissue and muscle. All vitamin D metabolites are fat-soluble vitamins. Because some individuals lack sufficient exposure to sunlight and dietary intake of vitamin D-contained nutrients, most milk in the United States is supplemented with vitamin D_2. The only significant natural source of vitamin D is cod-liver oil.

In vitamin D metabolism, precursor molecules are converted to the active form. After 7-dehydrocholesterol has been converted to cholecalciferol (vitamin D) in the skin, the cholecalciferol circulates to the liver, where it is hydroxylated to produce the major circulating pro-hormone, calcifediol, or 25-hydroxyvitamin D_3. This step is catalyzed by two vitamin D 25-hydroxylases, which are located in hepatic microsomes. Once formed, 25-hydroxyvitamin D_3 becomes the major circulating vitamin D metabolite and is transported bound to an α-globulin. Conditions that affect hepatic function, or drugs that induce P-450 microsomal enzymes, for example, phenytoin, interrupt this conversion pathway and lead inactive polar metabolites of cholecalciferol. These conditions can lead to various forms of osteomalacia.

The next step in the metabolism of vitamin D is the 1-α-hydroxylation of 25-hydroxyvitamin D_3 to form 1,25 dihydroxyvitamin D_3 (calcitriol)—the physiologically active form of the vitamin. Hydroxylation at this C-1 position is the rate-limiting step in the production of this biologically active form, and the hydroxylase enzyme for this reaction, located in the mitochondria of renal tubular cells, is activated by parathyroid hormone. In the presence of low parathyroid hormone levels and high calcitriol levels, alternate hydroxylation of calcifediol occurs at the 24-position, yielding 24,25-dihydroxyvitamin D_3. Recent evidence suggests that 24,25-dihydroxyvitamin D may play a role in cartilage differentiation. The only other tissue that participates significantly in this metabolic pathway is the placenta, where another 1-α hydroxylase has been found. Moreover, although parathyroid hormone is the major molecule that controls 1-α hydroxylase function, phosphate, ionized calcium, and specific levels of 1,25 dihydroxyvitamin D itself can regulate this activity.

The major target tissues of 1,25-dihydroxyvitamin D are kidney, bone, and intestine. In the kidney, it increases proximal tubular reabsorption of phosphate. It also increases 24-hydroxylase activity and reduces 1-α hydroxylase activity, thereby acting as a feedback regulator of its own formation. In the intestine, calcitriol induces production of the critical calcium-binding protein responsible for active calcium transport. When calcitriol levels increase, or when calcitriol is administered exogenously, the first effect observed is an increase in intestinal calcium absorption, leading to increased serum calcium levels.

Although bone is the major target tissue for calcitriol, the physiologic role of vitamin D in bone is less well understood. Studies of monocytes and macrophages indicate that calcitriol promotes the differentiation or fusion of osteoclast precursors to osteoclasts. At pharmacologic doses, it accelerates bone resorption by increasing the activity and number of osteoclasts. Calcitriol also alters phospholipid metabolism by osteoblast-like cells. Because vitamin D receptors are not known to exist in the cytoplasm of osteoclasts but have been demonstrated in osteoblast-like cells, calcitriol probably modulates bone physiology by acting on the osteoblast. Consequently, activities related to mineralization, bone resorption, and cellular differentiation may be osteoblast-regulated.

Circulating levels of the pro-hormone calcifediol decrease with age. In addition, aging may reduce the activity of 1-α hydroxylase because of impaired renal function, reducing calcitriol levels. These alterations in vitamin D metabolism may account for decreases in fractional calcium absorption observed in the elderly.

Parathyroid Hormone

Parathyroid hormone and vitamin D together form a parathyroid hormone/1,25-dihydroxyvitamin D axis, which is the major metabolic regulator of calcium and phosphate fluxes in the body. The three major target organs of parathyroid hormone are bone, kidney, and intestines.

In bone, parathyroid hormone is regarded as a bone-resorbing hormone. However, receptors for parathyroid hormone are found not on osteoclasts, but on osteoblasts, osteoblast precursors, and very early osteoclast precursors. Parathyroid hormone causes osteoblasts to: (1) stimulate the release of neutral proteases, which degrade surface osteoid and initiate the bone-remodeling cycle, (2) stimulate the release of unknown factors from osteoblasts, which stimulate osteoclasts to resorb bone, and (3) stimulate osteoblasts to synthesize osteoid and form bone.

The rate of synthesis and release of parathyroid hormone is related to the extracellular ionized calcium concentration. Intact parathyroid hormone is relatively short-lived once it enters the circulation. The liver and kidney rapidly cleave the circulating intact molecule into amino-terminal (N-terminal) and carboxy-terminal (C-terminal) fragments. Both the biologically active N-terminal fragment and the intact hormone have a circulating half-life shorter than that of the C-terminal fragment.

When kidney function is impaired, clearance of the inactive carboxy fragment slows and levels increase, which confounds the ability of C-terminal assays to determine parathyroid hormone function in renal failure patients. The N-terminal fragment, which has a short half-life, is a more accurate measure of parathyroid hormone activity in the absence of renal function.

Secretion of parathyroid hormone is a tightly regulated but sensitive process. A decrease in ionized calcium concentration as small as 0.3 mg/dl will stimulate release of the hormone from the parathyroid gland. The adenylate cyclase/cAMP system regulates that secretion. An increase in calcium flux inhibits cAMP formation and decreases the amount of hormone secreted. Hormone release is stimulated by hypocalcemia, prostaglandin E secretion, and β-adrenergic agonists. Propranolol has the ability to block parathyroid hormone release. Some studies indicate that the parathyroid gland has specific β_2 receptors.

In the kidney, parathyroid hormone activates adenylate cyclases distributed along the length of the renal tubule. In the proximal tubule, parathyroid hormone decreases reabsorption of phosphorus. Distally, parathyroid hormone increases the reabsorption of calcium. Consequent to the activation of tubular adenylate cyclase, cAMP content in the urine is increased. Therefore, nephrogenous cAMP is a good indicator of circulating parathyroid hormone levels.

Increased levels of parathyroid hormone have been noted in the elderly, possibly because of a decrease in fractional calcium absorption in the intestine. Nephrogenous cAMP levels are increased in these patients, as is tubular excretion of phosphorus. These findings support the conclusion that the parathyroid hormone/1,25-dihydroxyvitamin D axis may aggravate the progressive loss of bone mass in the aged.

Calcitonin

Calcitonin is an important calcium-regulating hormone whose exact physiologic role remains controversial. It does not regulate directly the functions of parathyroid hormone or vitamin D metabolites, but its ability to modulate serum calcium and phosphate levels is significant.

Calcitonin is produced and secreted mainly by the C cells (parafollicular cells) of the thyroid gland. These cells originate in embryonic neural crest tissue. Small amounts of calcitonin are found in the thymus, pituitary, gut, liver, and cerebrospinal fluid. Whether or not it is specifically produced by these tissues and what its function may be at these sites is unclear.

The major target tissues for calcitonin seem to be bone, kidney, and the gastrointestinal tract. In bone, the major defined action is the inhibition of osteoclastic bone resorption. In vitro, osteoclasts have been shown to lose their ruffled borders and clear zones and undergo considerable contraction within 15 minutes after exposure to calcitonin. Therefore, although osteoclasts do not pos-

sess specific receptors for parathyroid hormone and 1,25-dihydroxyvitamin D, they do for calcitonin. Specific receptors in the kidney decrease the tubular reabsorption of calcium and phosphate. In the gut, pharmalogic doses of calcitonin increase the secretion of sodium, potassium, chloride, and water and decrease the secretion of acid.

Calcitonin binds to specific membrane receptors and activates adenylate cyclase, which increases intracellular cAMP. Secretion of calcitonin is controlled by serum calcium levels. Hypercalcemia stimulates secretion; low calcium levels suppress its release. Other divalent cations influence secretion only at superphysiological levels. In addition, β_2-adrenergic receptors are believed to exist in certain tissues, and their stimulation elicits release of calcitonin, an effect that can be blocked by hydrochlorothiazide. Pharmacologic doses of the intestinal hormones gastrin, cholecystokinin, and cerulein also stimulate calcitonin release, which raises the possibility that calcitonin is in some way involved with gastrointestinal function. It is possible that the major role of calcitonin in these tissues is to control the rise in serum calcium levels after ingestion of a calcium-rich meal. In this way, calcitonin's ability to regulate serum calcium levels would limit the confounding immediate effect that food ingestion could have on the parathyroid hormone/1,25-dihydroxyvitamin D axis.

Salmon calcitonin, which is available as a drug, differs from human calcitonin at sixteen different amino acid positions. This alteration is large enough to cause it to be immunogenic. Interestingly, the salmon calcitonin form is several times more potent than human calcitonin in the treatment of patients.

Calcitonin deficiency has not been demonstrated to cause a specific metabolic disorder, despite its important physiologic role in calcium homeostasis. Calcitonin does have proven pharmacologic value and is used to treat Paget's disease, prevent disuse osteoporosis, and lower serum calcium in severe hypercalcemic states. It has recently been shown to have an important prophylactic role in postmenopausal osteoporosis. Some evidence suggests that calcitonin may have a specific analgesic effect in controlling the pain in patients with vertebral crush fractures.

Estrogens and Corticosteroids

The association between bone loss, fracture risk, and a postmenopausal state (naturally occurring or surgically induced) is well-known. Many studies have shown that bone loss is accelerated after menopause, and, when ovarian hormone production ceases and circulating levels fall to 20% of previous levels, this bone loss can be reversed only by administration of estrogen. In addition, it has been shown that obesity can protect against this bone loss, probably because of higher circulating levels of estrogen metabolites produced from precursor molecules stored in adipose sites. Although estrogens are known to inhibit bone resorption, the mechanisms responsible for this effect are not understood. Only recently has the presence of specific estrogen receptors in osteoblasts been confirmed. Although the level of such receptors is very low, the fact that they appear to be active in osteoblasts and osteoblast-like cells provides the first real evidence that bone is a target tissue for estrogen action. Preliminary evidence also suggests that osteoclasts possess estrogen receptors. If this is true, estrogen may exert direct control over both bone formation and resorption.

Both men and women experience age-related bone loss, particularly from cortical bone. In women, the rate of trabecular bone loss increases in the first few years after menopause, and this is the bone loss that is associated with a decrease in endogenous estrogens. Not only does estrogen replacement block this bone loss in the early postmenopausal years (years three to six), but a decrease in fracture rates in the appendicular skeleton has also been documented. When used alone, 0.625 mg of conjugated estrogen per day is the lowest effective dose for retarding bone loss. When combined with calcium supplementation, some studies have suggested that 0.3 mg may be equally effective.

Patients who undergo bilateral oophorectomy before natural menopause also respond to estrogen therapy. This group is especially at risk for developing osteoporosis because the number of years spent with low estrogen levels is greater. To obtain maximal benefit from estrogen replacement therapy, it should be started as soon as possible after surgical or natural menopause. Although it has been said that estrogen therapy is of limited benefit if not started within the first five to ten years after menopause, this statement is based not on a loss of tissue responsiveness but rather because by this time, significant bone loss has already taken place.

Numerous studies have demonstrated an association of estrogen therapy with an increased risk of cerebrovascular accident, thrombosis, fluid retention, gallbladder disease, and uterine bleeding. More importantly, studies have demonstrated a potentially higher risk of breast cancer and endometrial cancer in women taking estrogens. Although the information reported in these studies is valuable, some of the studies have suffered from specific methodological flaws. It is, however, well accepted that any factor that increases a patient's exposure to estrogen (early menarche, late menopause, estrogen replacement therapy) can increase the risk of breast or endometrial cancer. Combined cyclical estrogen-progestin therapy is believed to decrease the occurrence of endometrial but not breast cancer. In patients who have undergone hysterectomy, unopposed estrogen treatment is indicated.

The most important factors to consider in determining whether a patient should or should not take estrogen is the relative risk/benefit ratio. In general, patients with a strong family history of breast cancer or endometrial cancer, who have smoked or who have heart disease may be at increased risk for developing cancers or stroke as a result of estrogen treatment. In addition, the use of estrogen is known to exacerbate benign breast diseases and

cholecystitis. On the other hand, estrogen is strongly beneficial not only in the prevention of osteoporosis and hip fractures but in the prevention of heart disease in females.

Orally administered estrogens have been shown to increase high-density lipoproteins and lower low-density lipoproteins. However, progestogens decrease high-density lipoproteins and increase low-density lipoprotein levels. Thus, cyclical oral estrogen/progestogen therapy may have a net neutral effect on serum lipoproteins, deter bone loss, significantly reduce the risk of endometrial carcinoma as a result of estrogen use, and have an unclear effect on the incidence of breast cancer. Any form of estrogen is contraindicated in patients with hypertension or a history of congestive heart failure because its effect on the renin/angiotensin axis is to increase the degree of sodium retention.

Corticosteroids can cause bone loss by inhibiting directly calcium absorption, increasing renal calcium excretion, and stimulating indirectly secondary hyperparathyroidism. Their principal effects are to decrease production of the intestinal-binding proteins required for calcium absorption. Very high doses of steroids decrease both bone formation and resorption. Even with doses as low as 10 mg of prednisone per day, significant bone loss has been shown to occur. Alternate-day treatment programs may have less potential to affect bone mass.

Thyroid Hormones

Thyroid hormones resemble steroid hormones in that they interact with specific cell receptors, eventually binding to nuclear DNA. The thyroid gland produces two hormones, thyroxine (T4) and 3,5,3'-triiodothyronine (T3). Both hormones are bound to proteins in the plasma.

Patients with hyperthyroidism or exogenous thyroid treatment may develop osteoporotic bone disease. Both bone resorption and formation are stimulated, but resorption seems to occur at a slightly faster rate than formation. The radiographic findings may be indistinguishable from those of idiopathic osteoporosis. High levels of thyroid hormones, particularly when produced pharmacologically, can affect bone metabolism disproportionately. Consequently, chronic thyroid supplementation may contribute to osteoporosis. Thyroid-stimulating hormone stimulation tests, including measurement of thyroid-stimulating hormone levels, can identify patients who are receiving excessive thyroid supplementation.

Bone Biomechanics in Relation to Bone Metabolism

The biologic factors involved in forming, modeling, and remodeling the skeleton give bone important structural and mechanical properties. Because the skeleton supports mechanical loads; serves as a reservoir for calcium, phosphate, magnesium, other trace elements; and is a major site of hematopoiesis, the interaction between bone biomechanics and metabolism is complex.

Bone, a composite material, consists of two biomechanical phases—osteoid and hydroxyapatite mineral. Osteoid provides predominantly tensile strength; hydroxyapatite mineral provides tensile stiffness and compressive strength. Bone is also a composite structure. The structural parameters of bone consist of cancellous and cortical envelopes; the spongy (trabecular) and compact parts, respectively. At the microscopic level, mature cancellous and cortical bone are arranged in a lamellar fashion. For cortical bone, the primary structural unit is the osteon; for cancellous bone, it is the trabeculum. Biomechanical testing of these individual subunits yields similar structural properties for each. It is the macroscopic arrangement of the microscopic units that gives cortical and cancellous bone their markedly different mechanical properties.

Cortical bone displays the unique feature of mass conservation in relation to function by being highly resistant to torsional and bending moments using relatively small amounts of tissue. Cancellous bone differs by being arranged in a lattice-like framework, with vertical struts interconnected by horizontal plates. Its structure enables it to accept and transmit compressive and shear forces.

The relationships between bone biomechanics and bone metabolism are seen in the interactions of cellular events and the resultant structural forms. Cortical bone has a low surface-to-volume ratio and is composed of a system of osteons, each of which has a central blood vessel known as a Haversian canal. Osteoclasts and osteoblasts create cutting cones in bone as osteoclasts remove and osteoblasts replace cortical bone. New osteonal systems are formed during bone remodeling, a process termed "tunneling resorption." Trabecular bone, although largely lamellar, differs from cortical bone by virtue of its high surface-to-volume ratio. Remodeling in trabecular bone occurs on the surface, not by tunneling resorption. Osteoclasts carve out Howship's lacunae, and osteoblastic bone formation fills these lacunae.

Two processes, modeling and remodeling, govern the development of structural properties in bone. In modeling, appositional growth occurs on the surface of the loaded bone at the greatest distance from its epicenter. In this type of growth, bone resorption does not precede bone formation. Instead, bone formation in modeling bone occurs primarily. A good example of modeling bone is illustrated by periosteal bone formation after bones are injured or stressed. It is also observed during the process of "creeping substitution" which occurs when osteonecrotic bone serves as a dead trabecular scaffold for the deposition of new appositional bone.

In remodeling, existing bone is removed and replaced with new bone. During remodeling, porosities are formed by resorptive cells and their subsequent reossification creates tissue that may be mechanically deficient. This remodeled bone is similar to a concrete wall in which holes or microcracks are plugged or repaired by fresh concrete. Such a wall can never be as strong as the original structure, and bone, too, can be weakened by the remodeling and repair process. Under normal metabolic conditions, bone turnover serves to protect bone's mechanical structure by limiting the remodeling process to a homeostatic level. However, increased remodeling producing micro-weakness is exemplified by hyperparathyroidism, high turnover osteoporosis, hyperthyroidism, or even Paget's disease, in which hyper-remodeling states lead to a high incidence of stress fractures. Trabecular bone, with its high surface-to-volume ratio, is more significantly affected by hypermetabolic states than is cortical bone, which remodels more slowly. In osteoporosis, resorption of bone exceeds bone formation and, thus, the remodeling process becomes uncoupled in favor of bone loss. Moreover, weakening of the mechanical properties of bone during remodeling can contribute significantly to skeletal fragility. This may be one reason why measurements of bone density in patients do not always correlate with fracture risk.

Bone's material properties are governed by its microdensity. In a homogeneous material, the compressive strength is proportional to the square of the density. When a tissue is not homogeneous, its weakest point is in the area of least density. At the structural level, bone geometry determines bone strength. For example, the tensile strength of a solid rod is the same as that of a hollow tube of the same diameter. Although the tube uses less material, the properties of area moment of inertia and polar moment of inertia dictate that the material farthest from the central axis of rotation or bending does the most to resist the applied load. During aging, endosteal and outer periosteal diameters increase as a protective mechanism. As the bone mass shifts farther from the epicenter, skeletal strength is maximized despite a decrease in bone mass. In this way, remodeling compensates for losses in bone mass in the tubular portion of the skeleton (diaphyseal bone). Similar protective phenomena do not occur in areas of cancellous bone (the vertebrae, proximal femur, distal radius, etc), however, and because these areas of the skeleton are not protected during aging they are more likely to fracture. In addition, certain parts of the skeleton, such as the femoral neck, may be deficient in periosteum and unable to compensate for loss of endosteal bone by periosteal bone formation (appositional bone formation), which may partially explain the increased frequency of fractures of the femoral neck in elderly women.

Cortical bone provides protection against torque and bending loads. Cortical bone forms slowly, and its dimensions develop in response to a long history of specific recurring stresses. The vertebral body consists of an outer cortical shell and a large trabecular interior. Removing the cortex of the vertebral body lessens the compressive strength by only 7%. Consequently, 93% of the compressive strength of the vertebral body is maintained by trabecular bone. This same phenomenon has been observed in the subchondral area of the femur and the proximal tibia. The femoral neck, which has little trabecular bone and depends on cortical bone for its integrity, fails mainly in torque and bending modes.

Several laboratories have provided important information on the role of mechanical forces in dictating alterations in skeletal form. In an adult avian ulnar model, osteoblasts were shown to respond within 24 hours of dynamic loading by increasing their production of ribonucleic acid. Within seven days, an active periosteal surface developed on the stress side of the ulna. In a canine model, application of a known stress to a region of cancellous bone led to a biphasic response in which an initial peak of activity by eight weeks led to the production of an abundant but unorganized bone tissue. However, after 18 to 22 weeks, the trabeculae had become better organized and could more efficiently transmit applied loads to the tissue. This response was closely related to the strain energy density. Because bone responds to specific loads in terms of their frequency, duration, intensity, and dose, investigation into the transduction of mechanical forces into biological responses will be an important area of future research.

Metabolic Bone Diseases

Metabolic bone disease results from some failure in the normal processes of bone formation, mineralization, and remodeling. It can be broadly divided into osteopenic conditions; those such as osteoporosis and osteomalacia that result in low bone mass or insufficiently mineralized bone; and osteosclerotic conditions; those such as Paget's disease and osteopetrosis that result in increased amounts of bone due to abnormal bone remodeling. Several forms of osteopenic and osteosclerotic conditions have been identified. This section discusses the four metabolic conditions most commonly encountered in orthopaedic practice.

Osteoporosis

Osteoporosis is an age-related bone disorder characterized by decreased bone mass and an increased susceptibility to fracture. Currently 15 to 21 million people in the United States are afflicted, resulting in approximately 1.5 million fractures per year. More than one third of women over the age of 65 have suffered vertebral crush fractures, and it is estimated that of individuals living to the age of 90, 32% of women and 17% of men will have sustained one hip fracture. The mortality rates for patients sustaining hip fractures is 12% to 20% higher than for individuals who have not. Fewer than 30% of patients with hip fractures return to a lifestyle comparable to the one they had before they sustained the fracture. The economic impact of osteoporosis may be as great as ten billion dollars per year.

All men and women lose bone as they age, but not everyone has osteoporosis. Osteoporosis is associated with certain risk factors and systemic or environmental

conditions. One major risk factor is a sensitivity of the skeleton to estrogen withdrawal, whether as a result of a natural or surgically induced menopause. In addition, impaired metabolism, long-term calcium deficiency, secondary hyperparathyroidism, and decreased activity levels have also been implicated. Other risk factors include genetic predisposition (individuals who are fair skinned, small, have hypermobile joints, are of Northern European ancestry, or who have scoliosis), cigarette smoking, or excessive alcohol intake. Cigarette smokers show significantly increased incidences of bone loss and of hip and vertebral fractures, which may be caused, in part, by abnormal systemic handling of certain estrogen metabolites. Heavy alcohol users may develop osteoporosis as a result of either calcium diuresis or a direct depressive effect of alcohol on osteoblast function.

Osteoporosis can be divided into primary and secondary forms. Primary osteoporosis, also known as involutional or idiopathic osteoporosis, occurs in certain individuals as they age or after they go through menopause and is unrelated to any specific endocrinopathy or other disease state. Secondary osteoporosis occurs in association with an endocrinopathy, neoplastic disease, hematologic disorder, mechanical disorder, metabolic collagen disturbance, or nutritional aberration. These conditions must be addressed adequately before any attempt is made to therapeutically address a patient's impaired bone metabolism.

Most individuals attain their level of peak bone mass between the ages of 16 and 25. This is the greatest amount of bone that the individual will ever have, and the higher this value is, the better the chance is of avoiding osteoporosis. The reason for this is that the amount of bone present before bone loss begins determines how quickly any specific rate of bone loss (from whatever cause) will reduce bone mass to a critically low level. In men, normal bone loss occurs at a rate of 0.3% per year. In women, it can be as high as 0.5%. The accelerated bone loss, which occurs at the rate of 2% to 3% per year, begins after natural or surgical menopause and may last from six to ten years. Because of this link with menopause, osteoporosis is much more common in women.

For the purposes of description and understanding of the disease, osteoporosis has been categorized into two distinct syndromes. Type I, known as postmenopausal osteoporosis, occurs most commonly in women within 15 to 20 years after menopause. It most often affects trabecular bone and is clinically associated with vertebral crush and distal radius fractures. Type II osteoporosis, known as senile osteoporosis, occurs in men and women over the age of 70, with a female-to-male ratio of 2:1. It affects cortical and trabecular bone equally and is associated with multiple vertebral wedge, femoral neck, pelvic, proximal humeral, and proximal tibial fractures. Thus, in type I osteoporosis, estrogen deficiency plays a primary role; in type II osteoporosis, aging and long-term calcium deficiency are more important (Table 2).

Table 2. Types of involutional osteoporosis

Factors	Type I (Postmenopausal)	Type II (Senile)
Age (years)	51 to 75	>70
Sex ratio	6:1	2:1
Type of bone loss	Mainly trabecular	Trabecular & cortical
Fracture site	Vertebrae (crush)	Vertebrae (multiple wedge)
	Distal radius	Hip (mainly femoral neck)
	Hip (mainly intertrochanteric)	Proximal humerus
		Proximal tibia
Main causes	Factors related to menopause	Factors related to aging

(Modified with permission from Riggs BL, Melton LJ: Involutional osteoporosis. *N Engl J Med* 1986;314:1676-1686.)

Clinical Presentation and Diagnosis In general, osteoporosis is a silent and progressive disorder that is only brought to the attention of the patient or the physician after an acute painful fracture. Occasionally, the condition may be recognized by asymptomatic thoracic wedge or lumbar compression fractures on a routine lateral chest radiograph. Before bone loss can be detected on radiographs, anywhere from 30% to 50% of the bone mineral must be lost. The differential diagnosis of radiographic osteopenia is based on disorders of bone marrow, endocrinopathies, primary or secondary osteoporosis, or osteomalacia (Outline 1).

Patient Evaluation The evaluation of the patient with osteopenic disease is designed to arrive at a diagnosis as well as to stage the condition for treatment purposes. The components of the work-up include the history, serum and urine biochemical tests, radiographic procedures, bone densitometry, and when indicated, a transilial bone biopsy.

Medical History The medical history documents past and present illnesses, medications, surgery, occupational exposure, nutrition, family history, and social habits, all of which are used to formulate an understanding of the patient's disease risk (Outline 2). Particular attention to specific risk factors, causes of secondary osteoporosis (Outline 3), and known causes of osteomalacia (Outline 4) can be very useful in directing further diagnostic tests. In addition, identification of certain iatrogenic conditions, such as drug-induced hyperthyroidism and steroid treatment, can lead to a reappraisal of the patient, a reduction in the use of particular pharmacologic agents, and an improvement in bone mass.

Biochemical Test Serum and urine tests are done routinely to establish the biochemical status of a patient's condition. A complete blood count and a routine analysis of serum biochemical levels will reveal the presence of hematologic disorders, mineral and electrolyte imbalances, and underlying, unrecognized systemic disease. Renal function is screened by measuring the serum creat-

Outline 1. Differential diagnosis of osteopenia

Primary osteoporosis
   Type I, postmenopausal
   Type II, senile
Osteomalacia
   Impaired vitamin D metabolism
   Malabsorption
   Vitamin-D resistant rickets
   Aluminum intoxication (hemodialysis patients)
Endocrine disorders
   Cushing's disease
   Diabetes mellitus
   Estrogen deficiency
   Hyperparathyroidism
   Hypogonadism
   Iatrogenic glucocorticoid treatment
Disuse disorders
   Prolonged immobilization
   Paralysis
Neoplastic disorders
   Leukemia
   Multiple myeloma
Nutritional disorders
   Anorexia nervosa
   High protein diet
   High phosphate diet
   Low calcium diet
   Alcoholism
Hematologic disorders
   Sickle cell anemia
   Thalassemia
Collagen disorders
   Homocystinuria
   Osteogenesis imperfecta

Outline 2. Osteoporosis risk factors

Genetic and biological
   Caucasian race
   Fair skin and hair
   Northern European heredity
   Scoliosis
   Osteogenesis imperfecta
   Early menopause
   Slender body build
Behavior and environmental
   Cigarette smoking
   Alcohol excess
   Inactivity
   Malnutrition
   Caffeine use
   Exercise-induced amenorrhea
   High fiber diet
   High phosphate diet
   High protein diet

inine levels. Hepatic function is assessed using the aspartate amino transferase, alanine amino transferase, alkaline phosphatase, and gamma-glutamyl transpeptidase values. If the alkaline phosphatase level is elevated, fractionation of this enzyme is helpful, because isoenzymes are secreted by several tissues, including bone, liver, kidney, and intestine. If malabsorption is suspected, the serum carotene test is a quick screening method. If positive, a more complete malabsorption work-up is indicated.

Outline 3. Causes of secondary osteoporosis

Thyroid excess
Parathyroid excess
Hypothalamic hypogonadism
Diabetes mellitus
Steroid exposure (endogenous, iatrogenic)
Multiple myeloma
Leukemia

Outline 4. Causes of osteomalacia

Vitamin D deficiency
  Dietary
    Malabsorption
      Intestinal disease
      Intestinal surgery
    Insufficient sunlight
Impaired vitamin D synthesis
  Liver disease
  Hepatic microsomal enzyme induction
    Anticonvulsant
  Renal failure
Metabolic acidosis
  Fanconi's syndrome (renal tubular defect)
Hypophosphatemia
  Malabsorption
  X-linked hypophosphatemic rickets
  Oncogenic
  Oral phosphate-binding antacid excess
Mineralization inhibition
  Disphosphonate
  Aluminum
  Fluoride
  Iron
  Hypophosphatasia

For many years, 24-hour urine collection was used to monitor bone resorption. One metabolite measured by this test was the amino acid, hydroxyproline. However, because only 15% of the hydroxyproline excreted in the urine is derived from the turnover of bone type I collagen, this test lacked sensitivity. More recently, newer tests for bone collagen degradation have been developed. Pyridinoline and deoxypyridinoline, two crosslinks of collagen molecules, are referred to collectively as pyridinium crosslinks. Found in several connective tissues, they are most abundant in bone and cartilage. They are excreted in large quantities in the urine during bone resorption, and their measurement is a sensitive indicator of bone turnover.

Apart from markers of bone collagen turnover, calcium excretion remains an important means of determining the rate of bone loss in patients. Here the 24-hour urine collection is used to determine calcium and phosphorus balance. If calcium excretion in the urine increases, treatment aimed at increasing total body calcium retention may be indicated. Thiazide diuretics have been shown to be effective in maintaining total body calcium levels. If calcium excretion is low, there may be insufficient calcium ingestion, defective calcium absorption, or vitamin D deficiency. Phosphorus excretion is indicative of the effects of parathyroid hormone on the kidney and

is usually elevated when the parathyroid hormone activity is high.

Another important marker of bone turnover is the measurement of gamma-carboxyglutamic acid in the serum or urine. This molecule, sometimes referred to as osteocalcin or bone glycoprotein (BGP), is a low-molecular-weight protein synthesized only by osteoblasts and secreted directly into the circulation. Although the osteocalcin bound to bone matrix is released from bone during bone resorption, high levels of this protein in serum or urine are more indicative of bone formation. High levels suggest a metabolic disorder in which bone is being actively formed and degraded, such as high-turnover osteoporosis, renal osteodystrophy, or Paget's disease.

In the past, measurements of specific calciotropic hormones, such as parathyroid hormone and the different vitamin D metabolites, were a standard component of the routine work-up for metabolic bone disease patients. Recently, because limited funds are available for healthcare programs, these expensive tests are reserved for patients in whom a specific abnormality is suspected. Therefore, after the above routine tests have been performed, patients in whom hypercalcemia has been detected should undergo a workup for primary or secondary hyperparathyroidism. This requires obtaining the measurement of serum parathyroid hormone as well as vitamin D levels. Although several tests can be used to measure parathyroid hormone, assay of the intact molecule, as opposed to the carboxy or amino terminals, is most appropriate. Patients with hypocalcemia, hypophosphatemia, or evidence of renal failure should be worked up for vitamin D deficiency by assays for 25-hydroxyvitamin D and 1,25-dihydroxyvitamin D.

To complete the biochemical evaluation, measurements of plasma cortisol and a dexamethasone suppression test are done to rule out a cushingoid cause of bone loss, and a serum protein electrophoresis is performed to rule out an occult lymphoproliferative malignancy such as myeloma. If there is an elevated gamma-globulin region, a serum immunoelectrophoresis is ordered to look for a monoclonal immunoglobulin spike. A urine immunoelectrophoresis may demonstrate the presence of a Bence Jones protein to confirm a diagnosis of multiple myeloma (Outline 5).

Radiologic Assessment Two forms of radiography are used to evaluate metabolic bone disease: plain radiographs and densitometric scans. In the work-up of patients suspected of having osteoporosis, anteroposterior and lateral radiographs of the thoracic and lumbar spines are standard. Because the vertebral bodies are the skeletal elements most at risk of fracture in this disease, documentation of the status of the vertebrae at the onset of treatment establishes a method for assessing the clinical outcome of any treatment protocol.

Perhaps the greatest contribution to diagnostic efforts in metabolic bone disease has come through bone densitometry studies. Noninvasive methods have been devel-

Outline 5. Laboratory tests

Routine
  Complete blood count
  Electrolytes, creatinine, BUN, calcium, phosphorous, protein, albumin, alkaline phosphatase, liver enzymes
  24-hour urinary calcium
  Serum protein electrophoresis
  Thyroid function tests
Special
  25-hydroxyvitamin D_3
  1,25-dihydroxyvitamin D_3
  Intact parathyroid hormone
  Osteocalcin (bone Gla protein)
  Urine pyridinium crosslinks
Recommended panels for further work-up based on initial history:
GI (malabsorption)
Serum carotene
Endocrine
  Thyroid function tests
  Plasma cortisol
  Dexamethasone suppression test
  Serum testosterone (men)
Other
  Urine immunoelectrophoresis
  Bence Jones protein

oped, which can be repeated at 6- to 12-month intervals. At present, the most widely tested and clinically useful methods are single and dual photon absorptiometry (SPA and DPA), single and dual energy quantitative computed tomography (QCT), and dual x-ray absorptiometry (DXA). Important considerations in deciding which of these methods to use are the anatomic sites available for study, the radiation dose to the patient, and the precision and accuracy of the test. Precision is the coefficient of variation (standard deviation divided by the mean) for repeated measurements over a short period of time. Accuracy is the coefficient of variation for measurements in a specimen whose mineral content has been determined by other means, such as measurement of ashed weight.

In photon absorptiometry, either one or two gamma ray sources, a detector, and system of electronics are employed to measure beam attenuation through a section of bone. This method can be applied to the radius, hip, calcaneus, spine, or whole body with a relatively low radiation dose (10-20 mrem). For single photon absorptiometry, precision and accuracy are 1% to 3% and 5%, respectively. For dual photon techniques, these parameters are 2% to 4% and 4% to 10%. Quantitative computed tomography (QCT) uses a mineral calibration phantom in conjunction with a computed tomography scanner. A lateral computed tomographic scan localizes the midplane of two to four lumbar vertebral bodies. Quantitative readings are then obtained from a region of trabecular bone in the anterior portion of the vertebra. Computed tomographic determination of density in the vertebra is then compared to known density readings of solutions in the phantoms. The measurements of the vertebrae are then averaged and used to calculate the density of the trabecular bone expressed as mineral equivalents of K_2HPO_4 (mg/cm²). The radiation dose is 100-200 mrem, approximately one-tenth of that used in a routine computed tomographic study. Recently, it has been shown that QCT measurements can be used to estimate vertebral strength as well as fracture risk. Although experimental protocols have measured QCT at the hip, this method is only available clinically for measurements of spinal bone mass. Precision and accuracy for QCT are 2% to 5% and 5% to 20%, respectively.

The most recent advances in bone densitometry technology have been the use of lateral photon densitometry and a new measuring system called dual energy x-ray absorptiometry (DXA). In lateral densitometry, the same system used in dual photon absorptiometry is applied to the vertebral bodies; however, the beam is aimed in a lateral direction instead of an anteroposterior one. The advantage here is that attenuation of the beam is specifically related to mineral density in the vertebral bodies and is not perturbed by calcifications in the large vessels of the trunk or the posterior elements of the spine. In DXA, an x-ray tube emits an x-ray beam the attenuation of which is detected by an energy discriminating photon counter. It is similar to photon densitometry, except that it uses an x-ray beam rather than a photon beam, and it provides greater precision and accuracy and a lower radiation exposure (1-3 mrem). In addition, the average scan time for the spine is five minutes with DXA. Photon absorptiometry and quantitative computed tomography (QCT) require a minimum of 40 and 20 minutes, respectively. DXA can be used to measure bone mass at the radius, calcaneus, hip, spine, or total body, and precision and accuracy are 0.5% to 2% and 3% to 5%, respectively.

Bone Biopsy   An extremely useful test in certain metabolic bone disease work-ups is the transilial bone biopsy. Although invasive, it is associated with little pain and inconvenience to the patient, can be performed on an ambulatory basis, and has an extremely low complication rate. It is used to establish a diagnosis in the patient in whom osteomalacia or an occult malignancy is suspected, to distinguish between osteomalacia and osteitis fibrosa cystica in certain dialysis patients, or to elucidate the cause of severe osteopenia in patients with inconclusive blood and urine test results.

The biopsy is taken from a point 3 cm posterior and 3 cm inferior to the anterior superior iliac spine. The instrument used should produce a cylindrical specimen at least 6 mm in diameter, containing two cortices and an intervening marrow space. Once obtained, the specimen is embedded in methylmethacrylate and is cut, processed, and stained using an undecalcified technique. Unstained sections are examined by fluorescence microscopy to determine the dynamic properties of bone. This is made possible by the presence of the tetracycline labels. The cellular parameters of bone turnover are assessed by light microscopic examination of hematoxylin- and eosin-stained sections. The technique involves preoperative administration of oral tetracycline in two doses separated in time by a specified number of days.

Differentiation of mineralized from unmineralized osteoid is achieved through the use of a salt stain such as Von Kossa, in which calcium and phosphorus salts appear dark and unmineralized osteoid appears pale (Fig. 2). Through the use of a computer-assisted calculating system, an optical drawing tube, and an integrated eyepiece, a large number of quantitative parameters of bone statics and dynamics are measured. This technique, known as histomorphometry, enables the clinician to diagnose the disorder accurately and to determine to what extent resorptive or blastic activities are influencing the disease. In patients with renal disease, special stains are used to identify the presence of aluminum in bone as a cause of osteomalacia. This technique is particularly important, because dramatic clinical improvements have been reported after removal of this metal from the bone.

Osteoporosis Treatment Regimens Various treatments have been proposed for osteoporosis. At present, the goals of therapy are to prevent further deterioration of the skeleton, manage symptoms, and improve function. To this end, patient management involves a combination drug therapy, physical therapy, and rehabilitation and is based on the specific needs of the patient as determined by the work-up outlined above.

Drug therapy can be broadly divided into anticatabolic and formation-stimulation therapies. Anticatabolic therapies include the use of estrogen, calcitonin, and bisphosphonates. These methods are aimed at producing a direct or indirect reduction in osteoclastic resorbing activity. The formation-stimulating therapies include sodium fluoride, coherence therapy (phosphate/calcitonin or phosphate/bisphosphonate), and parathyroid hormone/1,25 dihydroxyvitamin D_3.

A recent report has shown that an adequate dietary calcium intake in premenopausal women, does not, in itself, protect women against the development of osteoporosis. However, in older postmenopausal women (six years or more after menopause), supplementing the diet with calcium can protect against bone loss. Moreover, the role of dietary calcium supplementation in the prevention of osteoporosis appears to be most critical during childhood and adolescence when peak bone mass is being built. An adequate dietary calcium intake is required at all times, however, to prevent the adverse skeletal effects of secondary hyperparathyroidism. For this reason, all patients under treatment for osteoporosis should take 1.5 g of elemental calcium daily, plus one or two multivitamins containing 400 units of vitamin D each. Studies are in progress to determine the best preparation of oral calcium to use in order to enhance intestinal calcium absorption (calcium carbonate, calcium citrate, calcium citrate malate, etc). Any calcium compound is best absorbed when taken with meals.

The goal of any osteoporosis treatment regimen is to prevent further bone loss. Presently, there are no well-

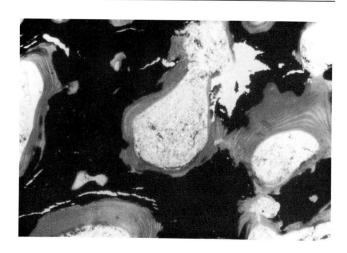

Fig. 2 Low power view of osteomalacic bone from a 25-year-old male with metabolic acidosis. Note that mineralized bone appears dark; unmineralized osteoid does not take up the stain and appears pale (Von Kossa, x25).

accepted treatment protocols that can be shown to safely increase bone mass. To improve the treatment of osteoporosis, the preferred approach is to custom design therapies for each patient. After tests are completed and the history is incorporated into the total evaluation, the patient is treated according to the following plan. If a patient has active osteoporosis, indicated by biochemical or histologic evidence of osteoclastic activity, estrogen replacement may be introduced. If the patient has no history of breast, heart, thromboembolic, or endometrial disease, and such therapy is approved by her gynecologist, this therapy is currently thought to be safe. The notion that estrogen therapy must begin within five years after menopause is no longer considered valid. As long as serum or urine biochemical tests or bone biopsy show that bone turnover is still active, hormonal therapy will be effective. A regimen recommended by several physicians is: conjugated estrogen (0.625 mg/day) for days 1-25, progesterone (10 mg/day) for days 16-25, and neither medication from day 25 to the end of the month. A gynecologic examination is required at the onset of treatment, and endometrial biopsies are obtained at six and 12 months. If these show no unusual activity within the first year of treatment, no further biopsies are required. However, a yearly mammogram is strongly recommended.

If the patient is unable to use estrogen, calcitonin therapy at a dose of 50-100 units per day, injected subcutaneously, can be prescribed. This drug is directly toxic to osteoclasts and is therefore an effective anticatabolic agent. Its drawbacks are that currently it can only be administered by injection, there is a possibility of an allergic hypersensitivity reaction, and the drug's high cost. In the near future, a nasal spray form will be available that will resolve some of these problems.

Recently, etidronate disodium, a bisphosphonate with a long history of therapeutic use in patients with Paget's disease, has been shown to prevent bone loss and provide a small (3% to 5%) increase in bone mass in postmenopausal osteoporotic women. In two studies, one from Denmark and the other from the United States, a significant increase in vertebral bone mass accompanied by a significant reduction in the incidence of new vertebral fractures was demonstrated. Because the major concern of etidronate therapy has been the development of osteomalacia after chronic use or with high doses, the recommended regimen for using this drug is 400 mg administered cyclically. This would mean 400 mg per day for two weeks followed by a ten-week period with no medication, and a continuous repetition of this cycle. Since etidronate is very poorly absorbed from the gut, it is critical that patients take this drug at least one hour before or two hours after a meal. Preferably, it should be taken in the morning, at least one hour before breakfast, with only a glass of water.

Although no major side effects have been reported regarding the short-term (less than two years) use of cyclical etidronate in postmenopausal women, the results of long-term studies have not been determined. For this reason, use of this drug beyond two years is not recommended at this time.

Finally, if a hypercalciuric component accompanies the active osteoporotic state, one to two daily doses of thiazide is given to increase total body calcium retention.

Inactive osteoporosis can be difficult to treat. Combination therapy with calcium, sodium fluoride, and vitamin D_2 is probably the only treatment that has been shown consistently to increase bone mass. The use of sodium fluoride, however, is associated with clinical problems such as gastritis and lower extremity pain syndrome. In addition, not all patients respond to this therapy. In a recent four-year, double-blind, randomized, placebo-controlled study in 202 osteoporotic women, this drug was shown to increase spinal bone mass and, to a lesser extent, bone mass in the femoral neck and intertrochanteric region. However, it leads simultaneously to a small decrease in appendicular bone mass. Of great concern, however, are the findings that these increases did not reduce the incidence of spinal compression fractures, and that the number of fractures in the appendicular skeleton increased. At present, sodium fluoride should not be used clinically except as part of an approved experimental protocol. Other forms of formation-stimulating therapies, such as phosphate/calcitonin and PTH/1,25-dihydroxyvitamin D_3, are considered to be too experimental for widespread use at this time. Presently, only conjugated estrogen and calcitonin have been approved by the Food and Drug Administration for use in the management of osteoporosis.

At the onset of therapy, a bone densitometry examination is done to provide a baseline to assess response to treatment. Subsequent bone density measurements can be made at six- to twelve-month intervals.

Perhaps the best form of symptomatic relief is achieved through physical therapy and rehabilitation. In those patients who, after careful evaluation, are deemed able to withstand some low-level spinal stresses, a program of back extension and deep breathing exercises is begun. Occasionally, external support in the form of a back support or bivalved custom polypropylene body jacket is useful. In addition, counseling and instruction are provided to all patients on the subjects of correct posture and body mechanics in order to prevent further pathologic fractures and the propensity to falls.

Menstrual Function, Exercise, and Bone Homeostasis   In young women, there is a correlation between abnormal menstrual function and low bone mineral density. This phenomenon is observed with irregular menses and, especially, with amenorrhea. Several factors can contribute to the development of amenorrhea. Runners who begin training on or before the onset of menarche have a higher rate of amenorrhea. Other factors include low body-fat composition, nutritional status, and weekly mileage. One third of highly competitive female athletes have some form of an eating disorder, and there is a correlation between low calorie intake and amenorrhea. A correlation between anorexia nervosa, amenorrhea, and low bone mineral density has been well established.

Osteomalacia, Renal Bone Disease, and Hyperparathyroidism

Osteomalacia is a metabolic disorder marked by inadequate mineralization of newly formed osteoid. It can result from vitamin D deficiency, vitamin D resistance, intestinal malabsorption disorders, acquired or hereditary renal disorders, intoxication with metals such as aluminum or iron, and other assorted etiologies as listed in Outline 4. To obtain a correct diagnosis, all these potential causes must be considered. The childhood form of osteomalacia, rickets, also has multiple causes. Rickets of the developing and growing skeleton caused by dietary deficiency of vitamin D has become rare now that most dairy products are supplemented with vitamin D.

The clinical diagnosis of osteomalacia is often difficult. Patients usually have nonspecific complaints, such as muscle weakness or diffuse aches and pains. Radiographic evidence of osteomalacia often mimics other disorders, including osteoporosis. However, the presence of pseudofractures or Looser's transformation zones is good evidence that some degree of osteomalacia is present. Looser's zones are radiolucent areas of bone that are the result of multiple microstress fractures that have healed by the formation of unmineralized osteomalacic bone.

Biochemically, different forms of osteomalacia may present in different ways. However, the orthopaedist is usually alerted to the present of this disease by elevated alkaline phosphatase, low serum calcium, or low inorganic phosphorus levels. Assays for specific vitamin D metabolites, such as 25-hydroxyvitamin D or 1,25-dihydroxyvitamin D, can further elucidate an abnormality.

In most patients, transilial bone biopsy is necessary to confirm the diagnosis. The histologic hallmark of osteomalacia is an increase in the width and extent of osteoid seams, with evidence of decreased rates of mineral apposition as determined by tetracycline labeling. In normal bone, tetracycline labels show discrete uptake of tetracycline only at times when mineral is being deposited. In osteomalacic bone, these labels are not separated in time, because of the slow rate of mineralization, and the test results have a smudged appearance.

Classic osteomalacia is caused by a decrease in the vitamin D content in the diet. These patients are easily identified because of such dietary habits as strict vegetarianism or a diet extremely low in fat. Typically, classic osteomalacia is seen in elderly patients. It has been proposed that the mild malabsorption of the elderly predisposes these patients to bone disease. This disorder is easily treated with vitamin D.

Outline 4 lists the causes of osteomalacia. Among the more common of these are gastrointestinal abnormalities, blind loops, malabsorption, or surgically induced malabsorption as a result of intestinal bypass surgery. In addition, the widespread use of anticonvulsant drugs such as phenytoin has been shown to cause osteomalacia by inducing the P-450 mixed function oxidases in hepatic cells, and thus converting vitamin D to inactive polar metabolites. The reduced production of 25-hydroxyvitamin D leads to insufficient quantities of the 25-hydroxyvitamin D substrate which is needed for renal conversion to the active 1,25-dihydroxyvitamin D metabolite.

In 1948, Albright described a disorder termed "distal renal tubular acidosis." It has a dominant mode of inheritance with variable penetrance. Patients usually show at least one of the three major features: renal stones, hypophosphatemia, and osteomalacia. High doses of vitamin D and sodium bicarbonate are used to treat this condition. It has been suggested that vitamin D deficiency and subsequent osteomalacia occur because of damage done to the renal tubular cells by calcium deposits within the kidney.

Osteomalacia is commonly seen in patients on hemodialysis therapy for chronic renal failure. Although it was originally presumed that the cause of this condition was an inability to form 1,25-dihydroxyvitamin D in the absence of renal function, treatment with 1,25-dihydroxyvitamin D does not usually correct this defect. Instead, the major cause of the osteomalacia in patients undergoing hemodialysis therapy is the intoxication of the skeleton with aluminum. Aluminum is presented to the body in the form of aluminum-containing phosphate binding antacids which are used to control phosphate accumulation in patients with renal failure. Phosphate accumulation lowers the serum calcium level, causing the parathyroid glands to respond (secondary hyperparathyroidism). This can lead to osteitis fibrosa cystica. Recent efforts to develop other drugs, such as calcium carbonate, to control serum phosphate levels may reduce the occurrence of this complication. However, if aluminum-containing phosphate binding antacids must be used, aluminum levels can be intermittently controlled with the aluminum chelating agent deferoxamine. It is important to note that, in some cases of severe renal secondary hyperparathyroidism, bone pain can be excruciating, serum parathyroid hormone levels can be difficult to control, and brown tumors can occur (although it is more common to see brown tumor in primary hyperparathyroidism). In this situation, a parathyroidectomy (partial or total) may be indicated. If aluminum is present in bone at this time, the resultant decrease in bone turnover caused by parathyroid down-regulation may facilitate aluminum accumulation and exacerbate or cause an osteomalacic state. For this reason, bone biopsy with aluminum staining should be done in hemodialysis patients before performing a parathyroidectomy. Moreover, patients who undergo parathyroidectomy after severe skeletal involvement may develop the so-called hungry bone disease, a condition in which skeletal sites of previously active resorption act like a calcium sink and rapidly draw calcium out of the vascular space. Serum calcium levels must be closely monitored for several days after surgery to avoid life-threatening hypocalcemia.

There are several known hereditary renal causes of rickets in growing children. If the disorder is detected early in life, the skeleton may develop normally. Treatment with phosphate and 1,25-dihydroxyvitamin D can usually maintain normal growth in such disorders as sex-linked dominant hypophosphatemic rickets. Recently, a new hereditary syndrome of hypophosphatemic rickets has been described that is unusual in that symptoms include hypercalciuria and a normal serum calcium level. High 1,25-dihydroxyvitamin D levels and hyperabsorption of dietary calcium distinguish this new disorder from the more common X-linked familial hypophosphatemic rickets, in which defective 1,25-dihydroxyvitamin D production is the usual feature. It is probably that both X-linked and hypophosphatemic forms have a similar renal tubular defect in phosphate reabsorption.

Table 3 outlines the treatment strategies for different forms of osteomalacia. Note the use of different vitamin D metabolites, either alone or in combination with each other, as well as the supplementation of the treatment regiment with other metabolic modifiers (bottom of the table).

Although a diagnosis of osteomalacia requires that, on bone biopsy, more than 10% of the bone volume be unmineralized, milder forms of this condition, known as hyperosteoidosis, are not uncommon in certain patients with osteoporosis. Hyperosteoidoses can occur in the elderly if the diet is deficient in vitamin D, if there is insufficient exposure to sunlight, or if the patient is experiencing mild chronic renal failure. It is recommended that these individuals take prophylactic doses of between 400 and 1,000 units of vitamin D daily.

Table 3. Treatment of osteomalacia*

Disorder	Vitamin D$_2$ (U)	25(OH)D$_3$ (μg)	1,25(OH)$_2$D$_3$ (μg)
Nutritional vitamin D deficiency	50,000 3-5 x/week		
Malabsorption	50,000/day	20-200/day	
Anticonvulsant-induced osteomalacia	50,000/day	20-100/day	
Renal osteomalacia**			1-2/day
Metabolic acidosis+	50,000/day		1-2/day
X-linked hypophosphatemia++			2-3/day until healing then 0.5-1.0/day

*All patients receive 1.5 g elemental Ca/day.
**Renal patients with bone A1 may require deferoxamine.
+To correct acidosis, titrate blood pH with sodium bicarbonate.
++Add 1-2 g/day of phosphorus.
(Reproduced with permission from Einhorn TA: Evaluation and treatment methods for metabolic bone diseases. *Contemp Orthop* 1987;14:21-34.)

Paget's Disease of Bone

Paget's disease of bone is a relatively common disorder characterized by excessive bone resorption and formation. The incidence of this disease varies by geographic location. It is most common in the United Kingdom and is less common in Scandinavia, Africa, the Middle East, and the Far East. It is currently estimated that as many as 4% of the Anglo-Saxon population of the world older than 55 years of age have Paget's disease. Interestingly, although it is uncommon on the African continent, its prevalence is as high as 1.3% in the black population of South Africa.

Studies have failed to detect a genetic predisposition or an HLA-antigen association type in Paget's disease. However, a viral etiology was proposed in 1974, when virus-like inclusion bodies were found in osteoclasts from affected bone. Since then, researchers have focused on a slow virus as the causative agent. Measles virus, the cause of subacute sclerosing panencephalitis (SSPE) may be the etiologic agent. The most recent finding of interest is a higher incidence of Paget's disease in dog owners. Scientists hypothesize that the canine distemper virus may be the cause of Paget's disease in these individuals. However, until definitive studies are done to show that a virus can be isolated from patients with Paget's disease and can be transfected into a normal organism, causing it to develop Paget's disease, the viral etiology will remain hypothetical.

Histologic analyses of specimens of pagetic bone have shown extensive osteolysis by large numbers of active osteoclasts. This is followed by activation of osteoblasts and the production of a woven-type bone. The new bone is produced in abundance and contains widened lamellae and disorganized cement lines—the characteristic "mosaic pattern" appearance of pagetic bone. Concomitant with these cellular activities, the normal fatty or hematopoietic marrow spaces are replaced by loose, highly vascularized fibrous connective tissue. Ultimately, both the osteoclastic and osteoblastic activities decrease, resulting in a "burned-out" stage, with enlarged and deformed bones that are densely sclerotic.

The radiographic appearance of Paget's disease is closely correlated with the histologic course. Initially, the osteolytic stage is seen as discrete areas of bone lysis. Subsequent activation of endosteal erosion leads to expansion of the bone with the compensatory formation of subperiosteal new bone. Treatment at this stage with an anti-osteoclastic agent, such as calcitonin or a bisphosphonate, may transform the lytic pagetic bone into dense bone, providing radiographic evidence of therapeutic success.

Biochemically, the rate of bone turnover in Paget's disease results in an immediate increase in the excretion of type 1 collagen breakdown products, such as hydroxyproline. The compensatory osteoblastic state is marked by an increase in alkaline phosphatase activity. These two markers, serum alkaline phosphatase and urinary hydroxyproline, are used to follow the course of the disease and its response to treatment. It is predicted that the recently available urine pyridinium crosslink assays will replace the less sensitive hydroxyproline test.

Paget's disease is often discovered as an incidental finding on radiographic examinations. Consequently, clinical experience has shown that most patients afflicted by this condition are asymptomatic. Patients who are symptomatic describe bone pain and joint pain and, later in the disease, may show deformities. One of the most common presentations occurs in patients with low back pain who on radiographic examination show pagetic involvement of the spine. The technetium 99m MDP bone scan is an excellent method for screening areas of pagetic involvement. For patients known to have Paget's disease, a technetium bone scan should be done before obtaining any further radiographs. Areas that show increased isotopic uptake may require radiographic examination to determine the extent and nature of involvement of that part of the skeleton.

Most patients with Paget's disease do not need pharmacologic treatment. Unless there is pain or significant abnormalities in urinary collagen breakdown products or serum alkaline phosphatase, patients may be followed without the use of drugs. For those patients who do have increased pain and poorly controlled biochemical indices of bone turnover, three classes of drugs are available for use—nonsteroidal anti-inflammatory drugs, calcitonin, and the bisphosphonates. The use of other agents, such as plicamycin, is indicated in severe states of the disease, when there is spinal cord compression or hearing loss. For the management of mild symptoms related to Paget's disease, indomethacin and other related nonsteroidal anti-inflammatory agents have been shown to be useful clinically. Although they do not specifically target metabolic activities, patients experience pain relief if the symptoms are reasonably moderate. Patients with abnormally high alkaline phosphatase activities that are within 100% to 300% of control values may be managed with a bisphosphonate. The only bisphosphonate currently available and approved by the United States Food and Drug Administration is etidronate disodium. The mechanism of action of etidronate is unknown, but it is believed to interfere with both the ability of osteoclasts to resorb bone and the mineralization of newly formed woven bone. The latter effect is considered potentially detrimental in that long-term use of this agent may lead to osteomalacia. For this reason, most patients treated with etidronate are placed on cyclical programs in which they are on the drug for several months at a time and then taken off the drug for long periods of rest. Any patient using etidronate who sustains a long bone fracture should be taken off this drug until the fracture has healed. This avoids development of a nonunion, which might otherwise occur because etidronate inhibits the mineralization of newly formed fracture callus matrix.

Newer bisphosphonates currently under study, such 3-amino-1-hydroxypropyl-idene, 1-bios-phosphonate (APD), and amino hydroxybutane bisphosphonate, appear highly promising for future use. These agents are more potent than etidronate and have a lower toxicity. Therefore, a lower dose can be used to achieve a greater antiresorptive effect, at the same time showing little or no inhibition of mineralization.

Calcitonin is probably the most effective agent used to treat patients with Paget's disease. This naturally occurring hormone acts via direct inactivation of osteoclasts. However, approximately 60% of patients given this drug develop antibodies. As a result, the agent may lose its effectiveness after a time. Currently, the most potent preparation is salmon calcitonin. Interestingly, human calcitonin is less effective. The present method of delivery is by subcutaneous injection, but, in the future, a nasal spray may be available. Early studies suggest that nasal spray calcitonin leads to fewer side effects and is better tolerated. The most common side effect of this drug is an allergic reaction manifested in the form of nausea, flushing, and the occasional development of a rash. Patients indicated for treatment with calcitonin should receive the first injection under the supervision of a physician, to prevent potentially disastrous side effects from a true anaphylactic reaction. These reactions, however, are rare.

Many patients suffering from Paget's disease in the vicinity of joints develop degenerative joint disease. This may be caused by the biomechanical alteration of subchondral bone as a result of the sclerotic phase of this condition. Treatment of degenerative joint disease may involve hip or knee replacement arthroplasty. A ten-year follow-up study of total hip arthroplasty in patients with degenerative coaxarthrosis secondary to Paget's disease showed the rate of revision was not statistically higher than in patients without Paget's disease. Aseptic loosening made revision necessary in approximately 15% of the cases.

Orthopaedically, patients undergoing fracture management should be taken off of etidronate and placed on calcitonin until fracture healing is completed. In pagetic patients undergoing joint replacement surgery, it has been suggested that high-dose etidronate (20 mg/kg/day) be used for one month before and three months after the procedure in order to prevent heterotopic ossification. However, there have been no well-conducted, well-designed clinical trials to support this contention. The use of perioperative calcitonin may also be beneficial, particularly with regard to reducing the blood loss possibly associated with highly vascular pagetic bone.

Polyostotic Paget's disease typically involves the pelvis and spine. Pelvic lesions are well tolerated unless the acetabulum is involved. Spinal involvement is not as well tolerated. Low back pain is a frequent complaint and is often associated with symptoms of spinal stenosis. The affected spinal segment may become progressively deformed, leading to a narrowing of static canal measurements and resulting in spinal stenosis. These patients often respond well to pharmacologic therapy, but patients who do not respond to medical management may require decompressive laminotomy.

Sarcomatous degeneration occurs in less than 1% of patients with active Paget's disease. Those with the polyostotic form are at greatest risk but it is not uncommon for patients with monostotic Paget's disease to develop malignant degeneration as well. Osteogenic sarcoma is the most common type of sarcoma. Fibrosarcomas and chondrosarcomas, as well as malignant giant cell tumors, have also been reported in this condition. Any increase in pain secondary to Paget's disease is strongly suggestive of the development of a sarcoma. Radiographs combined with technetium and gallium bone scans, as well as magnetic resonance imaging, may be useful in detecting malignant degeneration. A carefully planned biopsy confirms the diagnosis. The treatment of a sarcoma is surgery, and if possible, chemotherapy. The survival rate for Enneking stage IIB disease is 15%, with appendicular lesions having the best prognosis.

A benign tumor associated with Paget's disease was described by Mirra. Intranuclear inclusion bodies similar to those seen in non-neoplastic pagetic tissue were demonstrated in the nuclei of giant cells associated with this tumor. The epidemiologic aspects of this tumor demonstrate that most cases can be traced to a small town in

Italy, Avellino. This finding further supports an infectious etiology for this condition.

Osteopetrosis

Osteopetrosis (Albers-Schönberg disease or marble bone disease) is a rare metabolic bone disease characterized by a diffuse increase in skeletal density and obliteration of marrow spaces. Histologically, the skeleton shows cores of calcified cartilage that are surrounded by areas of new bone indicating normal bone formation but deficient bone and cartilage resorption. Osteoclasts may or may not be present, but those that are are deficient in some way, possibly lacking in a functional ruffled border.

In humans, osteopetrosis has traditionally been diagnosed as being either the congenital (juvenile, malignant, or infantile form) or the adult (tarda) form. In the juvenile form, the mode of transmission is autosomal recessive and this condition is characterized by severe anemia, hepatosplenomegaly, thrombocytopenia, cranial and optic nerve palsy, and a compromised immune system. Death usually occurs at a young age secondary to overwhelming anemia and sepsis.

Treatment for infantile or juvenile osteopetrosis is by bone marrow transplantation at a young age with an appropriately matched donor. Mismatched transplants are unsuccessful in 30% of cases. A successful transplant may resolve the hematologic abnormalities, including the defect in the immune system, and can result in a gradual restoration of patent marrow cavities. A few isolated reports have suggested that high dose 1,25-dihydroxyvitamin D therapy and a low calcium diet can also treat this condition. While the mechanism is unclear, it is possible that 1,25-dihydroxyvitamin D either stimulates the development of a normal ruffled border in osteoclasts, or, more likely, increases the fusion of mononuclear osteoclast progenitor cells to multinucleated bone-resorbing osteoclasts.

A syndrome consisting of osteopetrosis, renal tubular acidosis, cerebral calcifications, and minimal hematologic abnormalities has been described. This is also inherited as an autosomal recessive trait, and the defect has been traced to a deficiency of a carbonic anhydrase isoenzyme.

The adult or tarda form of osteopetrosis is inherited as an autosomal dominant trait, but some investigators report that autosomal recessive forms of this disease exist as well. Although this condition is much less severe than the infantile form, a lifelong history of fractures usually characterizes the clinical picture. Two distinct phenotypes of adult osteopetrosis exist: Type 1 is characterized by sclerosis of the entire skull, minimal involvement of the spine, and a high incidence of conductive hearing loss. Type II shows radiographic evidence of sclerosis, primarily at the base of the skull, increased radiographic densities of the vertebral endplates ("Rugger-Jersey" spine) and the appearance of a "bone within a bone" in the pelvic ring. Serum acid phosphatase levels are increased in type II patients.

Recent reports in patients with adult osteopetrosis have demonstrated the presence of viral inclusion bodies in osteoclastic nuclei as well as molecular biological evidence for the existence of retroviral DNA in the osteoclast genome. The notion that osteopetrosis occurred as a result of retroviral insertion of DNA which was subsequently passed on from generation to generation by standard Mendelian patterns seems plausible.

Annotated Bibliography

Cellular Control of Bone Metabolism

Boskey AL: Noncollagenous matrix proteins and their role in mineralization. *Bone Miner* 1989;6:111-123.

This is a review of the current knowledge of bone matrix proteins and their role in mineralization.

Horton MA, Davies J: Adhesion receptors in bone. *J Bone Min Res* 1989;4:803-808.

This is a review of the recent knowledge regarding integrins and extracellular matrix proteins and how they interact with each other to enhance cellular adhesion and attachment.

Lian JB, Gundberg CM: Osteocalcin: Biochemical considerations and clinical applications. *Clin Orthop* 1988;226:267-291.

This is a comprehensive review of the chemistry and clinical significance of this unique bone matrix protein.

Skerry TM, Bitensky L, Chayen J, et al: Early strain-related changes in enzyme activity in osteocytes following bone loading in vivo. *J Bone Min Res* 1989;4:783-788.

This report shows that intermittent loading of bone produces strain-related biochemical effects on osteocytes and suggests that osteocytes may be important sensors of mechanical input during done remodeling.

Vaes G: Cellular biology and biochemical mechanism of bone resorption: A review of recent developments on the formation, activation, and mode of action of osteoclasts. *Clin Orthop* 1988;231:239-271.

The author reviews recent literature on osteoclast-mediated resorption and the factors and cells that regulate osteoclasts.

Mineral Metabolism

Eastell R, Riggs BL: Calcium homeostasis and osteoporosis. *Endocrinol Metab Clin North Am* 1987;16:829-842.

This is a recent review of calcium homeostasis as it relates to osteoporosis.

Hurley DL, Tiegs RD, Wahner HW, et al: Axial and appendicular bone mineral density in patients with long-term deficiency or excess of calcitonin. *N Engl J Med* 1987;317:537-541.

The nonrole of calcitonin in calcium homeostasis is examined through patient studies.

Ott SM: Bone density in adolescents. *N Engl J Med* 1991;325:1646-1647.

This review indicates that the most critical time for ensuring adequate calcium intake is during adolescence, when peak bone mass is being developed.

Endocrine Function

Colditz GA, Stampfer MJ, Willett WC, et al: Prospective study of estrogen replacement therapy and risk of breast cancer in postmenopausal women. *JAMA* 1990;264:2648-2653.

A prospective study of up to 14 years conducted in 121,700 female nurses between the ages of 30 and 55 showed that, in current uses of estrogen, there is a 30% increased risk of breast cancer. However, long-term use is not related to an increased risk.

Eriksen EF, Colvard DS, Berg NJ, et al: Evidence of estrogen receptors in normal human osteoblast-like cells. *Science* 1988;241:84-86.

Ettinger B, Genant HK, Cann CE: Postmenopausal bone loss is prevented by treatment with low-dosage estrogen with calcium. *Ann Intern Med* 1987;106:40-45.

This two-year follow-up study demonstrates the protective effects of low-dosage estrogen (0.3mg/day conjugated estrogen) plus calcium in postmenopausal bone loss.

Komm BS, Terpening CM, Benz DJ, et al: Estrogen binding, receptor mRNA, and biologic response in osteoblast-like osteosarcoma cells. *Science* 1988;241:81-83.

These two articles were published simultaneously and provided the first evidence that bone cells indeed have receptors for estrogen. This suggests that estrogen's action to influence bone homeostasis may be via a direct effect on osteoblasts.

Silverberg SJ, Shane E, de la Cruz L, et al: Abnormalities in parathyroid hormone secretion and 1,25-dihydroxyvitamin D_3 formation in women with osteoporosis. *N Engl J Med* 1989;320:277-281.

Evidence for an abnormality in parathyroid hormone secretion in addition to a decline in 1,25-dihydroxyvitamin D_3 responsiveness in the elderly is presented.

Steinberg KK, Thacker SB, Smith SJ, et al: A meta-analysis of the effect of estrogen replacement therapy on the risk of breast cancer. *JAMA* 1991;265:1985-1990.

This meta-analysis of 16 studies shows a 30% increased risk of breast cancer with or without estrogen use. This risk was higher among women with a family history of breast cancer.

Osteoporosis

Dawson-Hughes B, Dallal GE, Krall EA, et al: A controlled trial of the effect of calcium supplementation on bone density in postmenopausal women. *N Engl J Med* 1990;323:878-883.

A study conducted in healthy older postmenopausal women showed that daily calcium intake of less than 400 mg leads to bone loss, that intake above 800 mg tend to maintain bone mass, and that calcium citrate malate was more effective than calcium carbonate.

Johnson CC, Slemenda CW, Melton LJ: Clinical use of bone densitometry. *N Engl J Med* 1991;324:1105-1109.

This is a current concept review of bone densitometry methods.

Kiel DP, Felson DT, Anderson JJ, et al: Hip fracture and the use of estrogens in postmenopausal women: The Framingham study. *N Engl J Med* 1987;317:1169-1174.

Estrogen supplementation affected the hip fracture rate in the Framingham study.

Prince RL, Smith M, Dick IM, et al: Prevention of postmenopausal osteoporosis: A comparative study of exercise, calcium supplementation, and hormone-replacement therapy. *N Engl J Med* 1991;325:1189-1195.

This study showed that exercise plus calcium supplementation was as effective as estrogen replacement therapy in retarding bone loss.

Prior JC, Vigna YM, Schechter MT, et al: Spinal bone loss and ovulatory disturbances. *N Engl J Med* 1990;323:1221-1227.

Decreases in spinal bone density in female athletes correlated with asymptomatic disturbances of ovulation and not with physical activity.

Raisz LG: Local and systemic factors in the pathogenesis of osteoporosis. *N Engl J Med* 1988;318:818-828.

This is an excellent review of the role of local bone factors in the etiology of the metabolic bone disorders of osteopenia.

Riggs BL, Hodgson SF, O'Fallon W, et al: Effect of fluoride treatment on the fracture rate in postmenopausal women with osteoporosis. *N Engl J Med* 1990;322:802-809.

This study showed that sodium fluoride increases spinal bone mass, decreases appendicular bone mass, has no effect on spinal fracture incidence, and may increase fractures in the peripheral skeleton.

Rigotti NA, Neer RM, Skates SJ, et al: The clinical course of osteoporosis in anorexia nervosa: A longitudinal study of cortical bone mass. *JAMA* 1991;265:1133-1138.

Anorexia nervosa leads to decreased bone mineral density. Bone mass may not be restored to normal when anorexia is reversed.

Riis B, Thomsen K, Christiansen C: Does calcium supplementation prevent postmenopausal bone loss? A double-blind controlled clinical study. *N Engl J Med* 1987;316:173-177.

Calcium may have had a minor effect on the loss of cortical bone, but it has no effect on trabecular bone when used alone in the prevention of postmenopausal osteoporosis.

Storm T, Thamsborg G, Steiniche T, et al: Effect of intermittent cyclical etidronate therapy on bone mass and fracture rate in women with postmenopausal osteoporosis. *N Engl J Med* 1990;322:1265-1271.

This report documented the potential use of this biphosphonate in the prevention of bone loss in postmenopausal women.

Uebelhart D, Gineyts E, Chapuy MC, et al: Urinary excretion of pyridinium crosslinks: A new marker of bone resorption in metabolic bone disease. *Bone Miner* 1990;8:87-96.

This is a preliminary report describing the use of these two new urinary excretion metabolites which appear to hold great potential for enhancing the sensitivity of clinical assays of bone resorption.

Watts NB, Harris ST, Genant HK, et al: Intermittent cyclical etidronate treatment of postmenopausal osteoporosis. *N Engl J Med* 1990;323:73-79.

This report documented the potential use of etidronate in the prevention of bone loss in postmenopausal women.

Paget's Disease

Gabel GT, Rand JA, Sim FH: Total knee arthroplasty for osteoarthrosis in patients who have Paget disease of bone at the knee. *J Bone Joint Surg* 1991;73A:739-744.

The presence of bone with Paget's disease did not affect blood loss or rate of loosening. However, multiple technical difficulties resulting in suboptimum varus or valgus alignment were encountered.

McDonald DJ, Sim FH: Total hip arthroplasty in Paget's disease: A follow-up note. *J Bone Joint Surg* 1987;69A:766-772.

A presentation of the long-term follow-up of total hip arthroplasty in patients with Paget's disease.

Osteopetrosis

Kaplan FS, August CS, Fallon MD, et al: Successful treatment of infantiles malignant osteopetrosis by bone-marrow transplantation: A case report. *J Bone Joint Surg* 1988;70A:617-623.

Five-year follow-up data for a patient who received a bone marrow transplant for osteopetrosis and review of the subject.

Mills BG, Yabe H, Singer FR: Osteoclasts in human osteopetrosis contain viral-nucleocapsid-like nuclear inclusions. *J Bone Min Res* 1988;3:101-106.

This report suggests that, as in Paget's disease, viral inclusions are found in the nuclei of osteoclasts from patients with benign osteopetrosis and that these may be related to the disease.

8

Arthritis

Advances in the diagnosis and treatment of arthritis include the identification of biochemical markers of normal and abnormal physiologic states, the continued development of anatomic imaging studies, and the evolution of function-associated treatment. The discussion of normal joint physiology has progressed from gross anatomy to cellular structure and function. Application of new findings in molecular biology to osseous and cartilaginous structures may lead to development of new treatments for arthritis. The widespread acceptance of magnetic resonance imaging has increased knowledge of intra-articular anatomy in the various stages of arthritis, and advances in total joint replacement for all forms of end-stage arthritis have continued.

Normal Joint Physiology

Synovial joints are composed of cartilage, bone, and synovial tissue. This discussion covers the contributions of each of these components as they act together, rather than in isolation. Normal synovial tissue provides the necessary lubrication to assist in decreasing the friction of the moving joint surfaces. Subchondral bone provides the foundation of support for the articular surface. The articular surface is an avascular, aneural, hypocellular, and alymphatic tissue composed of articular cartilage. The chondrocytes are encased by an extensive mass of extracellular matrix, which is a superhydrated material (approximately 75% water) composed predominantly of proteoglycans and type II collagen. The matrix provides articular cartilage with its material and structural properties and many of its characteristics. Although articular cartilage has little ability to repair itself, it functions well for an entire lifetime if the physical demands placed upon the joint are not excessive.

Cellular Metabolism

Chondrocytes Chondrocytes are metabolically very active cells that produce the collagenous and proteoglycan elements of the extracellular matrix as well as the enzymes necessary for the synthesis, maintenance, and degradation of cartilage. These cells range from 3 to 40 microns in cross section. Less than 5% of the volume of articular cartilage contains chondrocytes, which are nested as single cells within lacunae. Once embedded within the lacunae, mature chondrocytes under normal conditions are incapable of mitosis. Although the individual cells are physically isolated from each other, they

are very responsive to various physical, pharmacologic, and hormonal perturbations.

Articular cartilage is composed of four zones—superficial, transitional, deep (or radial), and calcified—characterized by morphologic changes in chondrocytes as well as by a transition in chondrocyte metabolism. The superficial zone, the outermost and thinnest layer, contains densely packed chondrocytes oriented parallel to the joint surface. These chondrocytes are elongated ovoid cells that have the largest amount of rough endoplasmic reticulum area per unit volume, the smallest amount of proteoglycans, and the fewest intracytoplasmic filaments among the cells of all zones. At the microscopic level, the normal articular surface is not smooth; it contains many surface elevations, representing the superficial chondrocytes covered by a layer of collagen fibrils, and relative depressions that provide an additional mechanism for joint lubrication. From the superficial zone through the top half of the calcified zone, the chondrocytes are more spheroidal and have increasing amounts of endoplasmic reticulum, Golgi apparatus, mitochondria, lysosomes, and intracytoplasmic filaments, indicative of increased metabolic activity. The calcified zone provides the attachment site of cartilage to bone and is separated from the other noncalcified layers by the tidemark. The fiber framework in this zone is oriented perpendicular to the joint surface and subchondral plate, possibly indicating a structural role. In the bottom half of the calcified zone, the number of intracellular organelles is decreased, indicating a decrease in metabolic activity.

Articular cartilage chondrocytes depend principally on diffusion of small (<100 kd) molecules for nourishment and intercell communication. The small molecules are derived from a plasma transudate from the synovial vessels and, to a lesser extent, the subchondral bone plate. Because chondrocytes are physically isolated and totally dependent on diffusion mechanisms, their juxtacellular microenvironment is markedly different from those of most other cells. Chondrocytes are maintained in a higher level of carbon dioxide and a lower level of oxygen, allowing them to survival after extended periods of diminished or absent blood flow to a limb. When the pH is artificially increased or decreased from the normal value of 7.4, a variety of degradative processes are initiated. The chondrocyte differentiation pattern changes as a function of the chondrocyte age.

Chondrocytes respond to a number of growth factors, interleukins, pharmaceutical agents, and mechanical perturbations. Growth hormone, insulin, calcitonin, and androgens stimulate chondrocyte proliferation as well as the synthesis of type II collagen and proteoglycans. Dexamethasone decreases the cellular volume and the organelle content. Nonsteroidal antiinflammatory agents reversibly decrease both proteoglycan synthesis and its secretion in cartilage explants and chondrocyte monolayer cultures. Cartilage-derived growth factor can increase hyaluronate synthesis while decreasing synthesis of sulfate glycosaminoglycans. Transforming growth factor beta, a local autocrine factor, stimulates proteoglycan synthesis. Insulin-like growth factor 1, a modulator of anabolic and catabolic cartilage metabolism, stimulates the proliferation of postnatal chondrocytes to a greater extent than it does fetal chondrocytes. Interleukin-1, a small molecular messenger synthesized by macrophages and leukocytes, stimulates chondrocytes to degrade their own matrix by releasing a variety of collagenolytic and proteoglycanase products. Chondrocyte adenylate cyclase is activated by histamine through a type II receptor and is more responsive to histamine than are synovial fibroblasts. Under dynamic, intermittent compression, the loss of macromolecules from cartilage is greater than that observed with a static compressive load. Further, chondrocyte synthesis of glycosaminoglycans under intermittent compression differs from that under static or no compression. Physiologic hydrostatic pressures have been shown to stimulate matrix synthesis as a function of the pressure, time of application, and the position of the joint. The dynamic compression of cartilage in vitro at physiologic forces can accelerate the synthesis and release of matrix proteoglycans through physical phenomena, including tissue strain and fluid flow. Exposure to air reversibly decreases the glycosaminoglycan content of cartilage and leads to histologic and ultrastructural changes.

Extracellular Matrix   The extracellular matrix is composed of the chondrocyte products, type II collagen, proteoglycans, noncollagenous proteins, glycoproteins, and water. Cartilage is a biphasic material composed of 80% water and 20% organic solid. The mechanical properties of articular cartilage are determined by individual mechanical and material properties of each of these macromolecules as well as by the highly ordered structure formed in the composite material. Water molecules are trapped within the collagen-proteoglycan complex by hydrostatic forces. The concentration of water is greatest at the superficial zone, decreasing from 80% there to 65% in the calcified zone. The articular surface, the initial contact point for the resistance of tensile stresses, is stiffer than the deeper zones, reflecting a higher degree of collagen fibril orientation.

Collagen molecules are composed of three polypeptide chains in a triple helix conformation. The amino acid sequence of collagen imparts a unique three-dimensional stability to the triple helix. Every fourth amino acid is proline or hydroxyproline, both of which have large ring structures as side chains. Every third amino acid is a glycine residue that has a small single hydrogen atom side

chain. Type II collagen, a triple-helix molecule with excellent tensile strength, is ubiquitous in all hyaline cartilage and makes up 95% of the fibrillar network of articular cartilage. Small amounts of minor types IX, X, and XI short-helix collagen are also present. Type X collagen, usually present in the hypertrophic zone of the growth plate, has been found in the calcified zone of articular cartilage, appearing just before mineralization. Type II collagen is secreted by chondrocytes as a precursor procollagen molecule that forms microfibrils and, subsequently, fibrils. Interfibrillar cross-linking is thought to be facilitated by the minor collagen types IX and XI. Other minor types of collagen, such as type V and VI, may be responsible for the control of fibril diameter, fibrillogenesis, and fibril cross-linking.

Collagen cross-linking determines the tensile strength of the extracellular matrix. These covalent cross-links, which are formed by the aldehydes produced by the reaction of lysine or hydroxylysine side chains with lysyl oxidase, increase the mechanical strength of the fibrils. In lathyrism this cross-linking mechanism is inhibited. The degradation of the cross-links produces an increase in urinary pyridinoline, a clinically useful indicator of bone turnover that is more sensitive than urinary hydroxyproline.

Proteoglycans, accounting for 5% to 10% of the wet weight of articular cartilage, are complex anionic glycoproteins that, in concert with the collagenous network, determine the load-bearing ability of the joint surface. Proteoglycans are made up of the glycosaminoglycans chondroitin 4 sulfate, chondroitin 6 sulfate, and keratosulfate, which combine with a core protein to form the monomer, and are attached to a long hyaluronic acid chain by link protein. The proteoglycan monomer is synthesized as a precursor that has a low affinity for hyaluronic acid. The end of the core protein farthest from its link to the hyaluronic acid is made up of a C-terminal globular domain. Adjacent to this, there is a large region of the core protein to which chondroitin sulfate attaches at right angles; next, there is a region to which keratan sulfate attaches; finally, there is a small, 50-kd hyaluronate-binding region. This region has few or no glycosaminoglycan chains and is a globular domain that mediates binding to the hyaluronic acid in conjunction with link protein. Proteoglycan aggregates typically stimulate the formation of type II collagen fibrils, and nonaggregating proteoglycans retard the formation of type II collagen fibrils except early in life when they strongly stimulate fibril formation in cartilage.

The distribution and structure of the proteoglycans in articular cartilage is heterogenous and nonuniform. Variations in the amounts, chain length, degree of aggregation, and distribution are observed in disease states and with aging. The superficial zone contains insoluble proteoglycan aggregates (multiple monomers on hyaluronic acid) that are attached to hyaluronic acid and are not readily diffusible. The deeper zones contain soluble hydrated proteoglycan monomers that, when not attached to the hyaluronic acid, can diffuse out into the synovial fluid and then into the bloodstream. The negative charge produced by the high concentration of monomers produces a very hydrated material with a high osmotic pressure, providing an expansive force on the collagenous framework. As compression decreases the volume of each aggregate, the electronegative forces resist further compression and decrease the flow of water within the structure.

The third major component of the extracellular matrix consists of noncollagenous proteins and glycoproteins. Some of these proteins, such as chondronectin, anchorin, and link protein assist in the aggregation and stabilization of the macromolecules and may participate in prevention of neovascularization and proteolysis.

Extracellular matrix homeostasis is controlled by the chondrocyte. Collagen turnover is relatively slow compared to that of the proteoglycans. In addition to synthesizing and secreting the synthetic elements of the matrix, chondrocytes synthesize and secrete the enzymes necessary for matrix degradation. The chondrocytes also produce protease inhibitors. These inhibitors are also produced by synovial tissue and normally are found in excess in synovial fluid and articular cartilage. The major neutral protease may be a metalloproteinase, secreted as a precursor, that is activated by an acidic environment. The metalloproteinases collagenase and stromolysin degrade both proteoglycans and collagen and are typically present in osteoarthrosis at concentrations that are 15% above normal. Investigators have postulated that specific events independently trigger the release of each of these seemingly conflicting agents.

Subchondral Bone Although osteoarthritis is thought to be primarily a cartilage disease, there is mounting evidence that the supporting subchondral bone plate plays a vital, if not central, role in the maintenance of healthy articular cartilage. The composite structure of the articular cartilage and supporting subchondral bone provides an ideal joint for locomotion and weightbearing. The subchondral bone, which is less resilient to pressure and friction than cartilage, is shielded from these forces by the articular surface. The thickness of articular cartilage is in direct proportion to the magnitude of the compressive forces in the subchondral plate. In most diarthrodial joints, there is a narrow range of normalized joint forces. The transmission of forces across the subchondral bone during normal daily activities is believed to be responsible for the maintenance of normal articular cartilage.

The architecture of the subchondral bone is influenced by those metabolic alterations that affect the supporting bone structures as well as by the calcified layer of articular cartilage. With damage originating in the underlying osseous structures, osteoclastic resorption proceeds, and there is an increase in vascularity and new bone formation. Normal aging and immobilization lead to increased vascularity and eventual remodeling. Resorption of subchondral bone is the hallmark of osteonecrosis with eventual collapse of the supporting structure. An investigation of the short-term immobilization of rabbit hind limbs demonstrated that subchondral vascularization and metaphyseal resorption precede the articular surface changes. In osteoarthrosis, the subchondral bone is stiffer, with an increased trabecular volume and subchondral plate thickness and decreased mineralization, leading some authors to conclude that the primary defect resides in the bone and not in the cartilage.

Damage to the articular surface alters the architecture of subchondral bone. At the site of cartilage damage, the underlying cancellous bone is replaced by vascularized dense bone. Transmission of excessive pressure to osseous structures causes cystic changes and growth of vascularized fibrous tissue in the bone. With normalization of the excessive joint forces, these cystic abnormalities are converted to bone. The anterior cruciate ligament resection model of osteoarthritis increases subchondral bone formation. Intra-articular injection of interleukin (IL-1), as a model of inflammatory arthritis, produces erosion of subchondral bone and of articular surface. The subchondral bone is invaded by vascular channels that proceed from the marrow through the subchondral plate. Tetracycline labeling experiments demonstrate new bone formation in the trabecular network in the marrow and along the joint periphery as the bone attempts to return the joint forces to normal. Radiographically, these sclerotic changes are observed in the subchondral plate and in periarticular osteophytes. New bone formation superficial to the subchondral plate, seen as replication of the calcified cartilage tidemark, occurs in osteoarthritis and can ultimately lead to articular cartilage detachment. The rate and magnitude of these changes can be altered by the mechanical environment.

Synovium and Synovial Fluid Synovium is a highly vascularized connective tissue that, although it lines the intra-articular cavity, does not have a basement membrane. Additionally, the synovial capillaries are fenestrated. The absence of any barrier between the synovial fluid and vasculature facilitates the diffusion of nutrients and waste materials. The synovial fluid is an ultrafiltrate of plasma with non-Newtonian characteristics, such that the shear rate and shear stress are not proportional. An increase in joint velocity is not accompanied by an increase in joint friction. A thin layer of fluid covers the articular surfaces under normal conditions; in diseased states, the volume of fluid increases. The diffusion rate to and from intravascular and intra-articular spaces is affected by many factors. Electrolyte and glucose concentration are typically identical to that of plasma, with glucose undergoing some form of facilitated diffusion. Large proteins are present in concentrations inversely proportional to their molecular size. Insulin-like growth factors are believed to be important regulators of synovial fluid proteoglycan synthesis.

The synovium is composed primarily of type A (phagocytic) and type B (secretory) cells with a smaller population of undifferentiated precursor cells. The cellular distribution increases from the capsular surface to the intra-articular surface and in those areas not subjected to mechanical stresses. The type A macrophage-like cells have prominent Golgi apparatuses and vacuoles, contain lysosomes, and have abundant intracellular cytoskeletal filaments. These cells phagocytize debris that is present at the interface of the synovial fluid and the cell. The lymphatic system can also participate in the removal of particulates and large macromolecules. The type B fibroblast-like cells contain large rough endoplasmic reticulum complexes and have been shown to synthesize degradative enzymes and cytokines. The synovial cells also secrete macromolecules, such as glycoproteins, that are important for joint lubrication and nutrition.

Physiologic Senescence   With advancing age, the ability of cartilage to withstand compression decreases. Age-associated changes occur at the cellular as well as the structural level. The senescent chondrocyte is typically larger than younger cells and has an intracellular concentration of degradative enzymes that exceeds that required for normal remodeling. These older cells do not synthesize DNA and do not proceed through the mitotic stages of the cell cycle. The matrix components also exhibit age-related phenomena. The cellularity and absolute amounts of collagen or glycosaminoglycans do not change with age. Protein content increases while water content, proteoglycan half life and subunit size, the ratio of chondroitin sulfate to keratan sulfate, and proteoglycan content all decrease with age. These age-related physiologic changes in normal articular cartilage metabolism lessen the once advantageous mechanical and material properties of cartilage. These changes differ from those seen with cartilage damage, in which both cell replication and matrix synthesis increase. Loadbearing and load history do not seem to be related to the onset of degenerative changes.

Structurally, with increasing age, the superficial layers of the cartilaginous surface become fibrillated. Fibrillation starts at the peripheral and superficial areas and proceeds centrally and to the deeper layers. The resultant surface irregularities can be observed arthroscopically as areas that lack the glossy finish of normal articular cartilage. Arthroscopic inspection with a probe reveals relatively softer areas of cartilage. The collagen concentration in these fibrillated areas does not vary; however, the concentration of glycosaminoglycans has been shown to be decreased, leading to a decrease in resilience and stiffness. Degenerated areas of cartilage may have a yellow discoloration that does not affect the material properties of the cartilage.

Biomechanics

Cellular   The cyclic mechanical stresses on the chondroosseous skeleton have been hypothesized to control skeletal morphogenesis, development, growth, regenera-

tion, maintenance, and degeneration. In turn, the structure and composition of the articular cartilage determine its capability to withstand these repetitive stresses. These repetitive intermittent loading signals provide a tissue stress history that is somewhat predictive of the biologic features of connective tissues. However, the exact mechanism by which these mechanical signals are transduced to cellular function within articular cartilage is not known. Experimental models of the mechanical forces relevant to joint function include those systems that provide shear, compression, and hydrostatic forces. For example, physiologic hydrostatic pressure on bovine articular cartilage slices, independent of other mechanical forces, stimulated the synthesis of extracellular matrix. Moreover, the magnitude of the stimulation was found to vary with the position of the articular cartilage within the joint.

Joint Function   Articular cartilage is a biphasic material that undergoes intermittent cyclic mechanical loading. When a load is applied, articular cartilage decreases the contact stresses by deforming its solid phase, thereby increasing the contact area and normalizing the stress per unit area. Additionally, joint fluid is dispersed during the load, diminishing the friction and wear.

During normal gait, the muscles and osseous structures surrounding a joint absorb most of the force. Coordinated motion of these structures is important for the protection of the articular cartilage under load. The external load imposed on the joint surface leads to a complex redistribution of the mechanical forces, which can be expressed in terms of the load's individual components with specific magnitude and direction. The major components are the hydrostatic stress and the tensile shear stress. If the compressive stress from all directions is equal, a state of pure hydrostatic stress is present. If the stresses are not equal from all directions, shear stresses are present also. Shear in articular cartilage is caused by tensile strain perpendicular to the primary direction in which the cartilage is being compressed. Although numerous mechanisms of joint lubrication have been discussed in the literature, fluid-film lubrication and boundary lubrication are the most important. With fluid-film lubrication, articular surfaces are separated by a thin film of minimally compressible synovial fluid. With boundary lubrication, the molecular composition of the articular surface produces a decreased coefficient of friction while the opposing surfaces are in contact.

The viscoelastic behavior of articular cartilage, permitting deformation under load and subsequent recovery, is similar to that observed with other polymeric systems. This sort of behavior is expected, because articular cartilage is a polymer of collagen fibers and proteoglycan molecules. Initially, there is distortion of the solid articular surface resulting from compression of the collagenous structure and the movement of water. The tensile strength of collagen is primarily responsible for resisting deformation, and the reorganization of the long-chain molecules generates intermolecular friction. The collagen fibrils deform and align with the axis of loading. This intrinsic property is independent of the fluid flow and depends on the stiffness of the collagenous network, the collagen content, and the ratio of collagen to proteoglycan. The resistance to compressive forces is under the control of the proteoglycan subunits. During the time-dependent deformation stage (creep phase) that follows, fluid flow and, thus, permeability are under the control of the proteoglycan subunits. The creep observed is a direct result of the fluid extravasation. Decreases in either water content or proteoglycan content, as seen with physiologic senescence, lead to a decrease in permeability. The interstitial fluid flow permits the indentation of the articular surface to increase under the constant load, normalizing the joint forces. The fluid is extravasated at the leading edge of the surface contact area and simultaneously reabsorbed at the trailing margin, producing another method of lubrication. Upon removal of the load there is an initial immediate recovery, followed by a long, sustained recovery to normal volume. In degenerative conditions, the collagenous framework is less organized, which decreases its ability to withstand deformation.

Degenerative Arthropathies

Osteoarthrosis

Osteoarthritis is commonly used to refer to a group of noninflammatory arthritides. However, because the suffix, -itis, means inflammation, it should not be used when speaking of noninflammatory conditions. While there is often an inflammatory component as part of the pathophysiology of this condition, it is generally agreed that the initiating events are mechanical, not inflammatory. The prevalence of osteoarthrosis generally increases with age. Osteoarthrosis is stratified into primary (idiopathic) disease and disease secondary to an associated factor. The most common of these associated factors is trauma, but there are many other associated factors, including congenital epiphyseal dysplasia, postinflammatory arthritis, acromegaly, hemochromatosis, ochronosis, and hyperparathyroidism.

Etiology   The etiology of osteoarthrosis is multifactorial. The theories can be stratified into two categories—excessive stresses on otherwise normal cartilage and the response of abnormal cartilage to normal forces. Aging has been shown to decrease the fatigue strength of articular cartilage and increase susceptibility to osteoarthrosis. Moreover, genetic and constitutional factors are involved in both damage to and attempted repair of the cartilage matrix.

Under normal conditions, articular cartilage is loaded at roughly 20 to 25 kg/cm². There is a narrow tolerance, because underloading reduces diffusion of cartilage nutrients and overloading enhances matrix breakdown. In a study of the effect of long-distance running on the devel-

opment of osteoarthrosis, it was felt that in the absence of other etiologic factors, recreational runners are not at risk for premature osteoarthrosis.

A canine model was used to examine osteoarthrotic changes after an acute transarticular load. In this study, an acute load (2,170 N) was applied to the patellofemoral joint of a dog. Within six months, characteristic changes of osteoarthrosis had occurred, including surface fissures, loss of safranin-O straining, fibrillation, and subchondral new bone formation. This study demonstrated the deleterious effects of a single transarticular load to the patellofemoral joint in a closed system, which may parallel the clinical syndrome of trauma-induced chondromalacia.

Experimental Osteoarthrosis   A widely used model for degenerative arthritis involves transection of the canine anterior cruciate ligament (ACL). Overt fibrillation can occur in the articular cartilage within six weeks, but in some cases only mild cartilage changes are noted after almost four years. Onset and severity of cartilage lesions depend on such factors as the breed of the dog, its age and weight, exercise, and surgical technique. A recent study demonstrated, however, that the in vivo reaction in this model differs markedly in different anatomic areas of the joint. The medial femoral condyle appears to have an exaggerated chondrocytic response leading to hypertrophic repair. In another study, there were interspecies variations in the intrinsic mechanical properties of the distal femoral condyle among five species. Additional differences depended on the site of the joint analyzed. For instance, the modulus was lowest in the anterior patellar groove, suggesting that this cartilage can undergo greater and more rapid compression. This lower modulus might be an adaptive change in the patellofemoral cartilage to adjust to the varying contact areas and variable loads as the knee is flexed and extended. The concerns involved in extrapolating experimental animal models to the human situation were pointed out.

Disruption of rabbit ACLs resulted in cartilage hypertrophy, reduced cell density, cystic lesions and enlarged perichondrocytic lacunae. In a canine model, there was a progressive and significant decrease in hyaluronic acid content seven to 14 weeks after disruption of cartilage in the weightbearing areas of the dogs' knees.

This loss of hyaluronic acid may lead to further alterations in proteoglycan aggregation. At least two types of proteoglycans aggregate with hyaluronate in adult articular cartilage. The larger proteoglycans are richer in chondroitin sulfate, and the smaller proteoglycans are richer in keratan sulfate, which may not be found in neonatal cartilage. Cartilage resulting from ACL disruption contains more of the large chondroitin sulfate-rich proteoglycans than cartilage in adjacent sites not involved with osteoarthrosis. Newly synthesized proteoglycans extracted from cartilage from dogs' osteoarthritic joints were larger than those from normal cartilage three weeks, three months, and six months after surgery. The chondroitin sulfate-rich proteoglycan region from joints with experimentally induced osteoarthritis was found to be slightly larger hydrodynamically than normal control tissue and to have higher uronate-protein and galactosamine-glucosamine ratios.

Much of the proteoglycan produced in early experimental osteoarthrosis is not incorporated into the cartilage matrix. Mature chondrocytes in culture have less capacity than immature chondrocytes to synthesize link protein and to assemble proteoglycan aggregates. Because it lacks sufficient link protein, mature cartilage with osteoarthrosis may not be able to stabilize proteoglycan subunits as aggregates and, thereby, incorporate them into a reparative matrix.

Interleukin-1 (IL-1), or catabolin, is released by various cells, including synoviocytes, monocytes, and, perhaps, chondrocytes. Because this multifunctional cytokine stimulates chondrocytes to release degradative enzymes that affect the cartilage matrix, it is likely that IL-1 plays a role in degenerative osteoarthrosis.

A cartilage matrix glycoprotein was found in the serum of dogs following ACL transsection. This protein, which was not present before ACL transection, may serve as a serum marker for osteoarthrosis.

In another study, glycosaminoglycan polysulfuric acid ester was injected into the knee joints of dogs following ACL transection. Cartilage from treated animals had less cartilage swelling, less metalloproteinase activity, and lower hystopathologic scores than were found in cartilage from saline controls. These data suggested that the protective effect of glycosaminoglycan polysulfuric acid ester was achieved by decreasing the synthesis of metalloproteinases or by inhibiting enzymatic activity rather than by increasing the synthesis of proteoglycans by the chondrocytes.

Pathophysiology   The earliest changes in osteoarthrosis (cartilage swelling, increased hydration) can be attributed to a breakdown of the collagenous frameworth that allows further hydration of the matrix. Synthesis of proteoglycans (especially those richer in chondroitin sulfate) increases early in osteoarthritis, presumably as an attempted repair mechanism. When mechanical overload persists, these repair mechanisms are overwhelmed, and overall proteoglycan degradation ensues. With further breakdown of the collagen framework and depletion of matrix proteins, structural changes, such as blistering, fibrillation, and fissuring, appear. There are concomitant changes in the subchondral bone, and, eventually, the articular surface is denuded.

The role of cytokines and growth factors in the pathogenesis of osteoarthrosis and in attempts to counteract the cartilage damage was recently investigated. These cytokines and growth factors appear to be involved both in normal matrix homeostasis and in osteoarthrosis. For instance, IL-1 and tumor necrosis factor alpha (TNF-α) stimulate chondrocytes and synovial fibroblasts to produce proteases, which can degrade matrix collagen and proteoglycans and suppress their synthesis. Moreover, growth factors such as transforming growth factor beta (TGF-β) can counteract the effect of the cytokines.

Diagnosis   Osteoarthrosis is a long-term process with patients seeking medical care at variable stages of the disease. It is questionable whether early diagnosis and institution of therapy will modify the disease. Elevated levels of keratan sulfate were found in the serum of 125 patients with osteoarthrosis. Although there was a great variability in serum keratan sulfate levels in this study, serial measurements in individual patients may be helpful in following disease progression and monitoring response to treatment.

In another study, conventional radiography was compared with computed tomography and magnetic resonance imaging to assess the extent and severity of osteoarthrosis. Magnetic resonance imaging was found to be more sensitive in detecting changes in the least involved compartment, presence of early osteophytes, and changes in the meniscal and ligamentous elements.

Treatment   The nonsurgical management of osteoarthrosis involves patient education, modification of function, weight reduction, and physical therapy. Careful use of isometric and isokinetic exercises can strengthen periarticular soft tissues and decrease stresses across the damaged articular surface.

The use of nonsteroidal anti-inflammatory drugs (NSAIDs) has not been shown to be chondroprotective in human osteoarthrosis. A recent study compared the NSAID ibuprofen with the analgesic agent acetaminophen. Patients with osteoarthrosis, who were treated for four weeks with ibuprofen in anti-inflammatory doses (2,400 mg/day) or analgesic doses (1,200 mg/day) were compared with a third group receiving acetaminophen (4,000 mg/day). There were no differences in pain, disability, walking distance, or physician assessment during this brief study.

Surgical treatment of osteoarthrosis depends upon the extent and pattern of the disease as well as the patient's symptoms. A recent review of the role of arthroscopy in osteoarthrosis pointed out the importance of deformity, loss of joint space, and symptoms of internal derangement in the outcome of this procedure. Patients with little varus or valgus deformity and only slight radiographic changes do quite well. In these circumstances, removal of unstable meniscal and chondral flaps, lavage, excision of intercondylar osteophytes, and drilling of areas of exposed bone less than 1 cm in diameter may provide symptomatic relief for up to 5 years for 60% to 80% of patients.

Tibial osteotomy remains the treatment of choice for single compartment osteoarthrosis of either the medial or lateral plateaus of the knee. In general, medial osteoarthrosis is treated by high tibial osteotomy, and lateral osteoarthrosis is treated by supracondylar femoral osteotomy. A long-term follow-up study of high tibial osteotomy for medial osteoarthrosis of the knee indicated that at 6 years, 50% of knees were good and over 75% were acceptable. At 11.9 years, 43% were good and 60% acceptable. The best results were obtained in patients with grade 1 (slight reduction in joint space) or grade 2 (obliteration of joint space) and if a mean angulation of 3 to 7 degrees of mechanical valgus was obtained postoperatively.

Unicompartmental knee arthroplasty (UKA) has been reevaluated in terms of its role in treatment of osteoarthrosis. Parallel survivorship curves comparing unicompartmental and total knee arthroplasty show that at 10 years, survivorship is better in total knee arthroplasty. Analysis of the failures of unicompartmental knee arthroplasty show that most result from poor patient selection, errors in surgical technique, and poor prosthetic design. Unicompartmental knee arthroplasty is contraindicated in patients with inflammatory arthritis, subluxation of the tibia on the femur, significant articular chondrocalcinosis, nonarticular deformity, and obesity. In one institution, the percentage of osteoarthrosis patients undergoing unicompartmental versus total knee arthroplasty has decreased from 40% to 9% in the past eight years. Total knee arthroplasty continues to provide excellent results in over 90% of patients at 10 years. Marked deformity, bone loss, flexion contracture, and previous surgery present specific technical problems in performing total knee arthroplasty in patients with end-stage osteoarthrosis.

Inflammatory Arthropathies

Immunogenetic Basis of Inflammatory Arthropathy

The pathology of most inflammatory arthritides results from the challenge of an immunogenetically susceptible host by a relevant antigen. The evidence for genetic susceptibility to most inherited diseases is seen in their widespread occurrence throughout affected families as well as by the presence of disease susceptibility markers on the major histocompatibility complexes (MHC) of affected individuals.

Studies of families and of identical and fraternal twins suggest there is a genetic influence on susceptibility to diseases such as rheumatoid arthritis, systemic lupus erythematosis, ankylosing spondylitis, and Sjögren's syndrome. These diseases are more likely to appear in first-degree relatives of affected patients than in the general population. Moreover, these diseases appear more frequently in monozygotic (identical) twins than in dizygotic (fraternal) twins, suggesting a stronger genetic than environmental association. Their lack of full penetrance in monozygotic twins demonstrates the environmental influence on the development of inflammatory arthropathies.

In humans, the MHC resides on the short arm of chromosome 6 and has three major loci. Class-I loci consist of three related types of molecules, called HLA-A, HLA-

Table 1. Common association of class-I and class-II alleles with rheumatic diseases

Disease	HLA Alleles	Relative Frequency
Ankylosing spondylitis	B27	69x
Reiter's syndrome	B27	37x
Psoriatic arthritis	B27	11x
	B38	10x
Systemic lupus (SLE)	DR2	2.3x
	DR2	2.5x
Rheumatoid arthritis	DR1	1.4x
	DR4	2.7x
Sjögren's syndrome	DR2	5.2x
	DR3	3.6x
Lyme arthritis (chronic)	DR4	4x

B, and HLA-C. Class-I antigens are found on all cells except red blood cells and early embryonic tissue and are the primary factors in self-recognition and the development of tolerance. Class-I antigens are responsible for graft rejection.

The class-II (IA) loci encode for molecules termed HLA-DR, -DQ, and -DP. These molecules are involved in antigen presentation to helper/inducer T-lymphocytes (also called T cells) and are present on B-lymphocytes (also called B cells), macrophages, and activated T cells. Class-III loci are between the class-I and class-II loci in chromosome 6 and encode for soluble proteins that are involved primarily in the complement cascade.

Several rheumatic diseases have been associated with MHC, class-I and class-II alleles. This association is defined by the relative risk, the increased chance that an individual with a disease-associated HLA antigen has of developing the disorder when compared with an individual lacking that antigen, and the absolute risk, the chance a patient with a disease-associated HLA antigen has of actually developing the disease. Table 1 summarizes the common associations of MHC (class-I and class-II alleles) with common rheumatic diseases. These associations vary when studied in different populations. The presence of an association between a known infectious arthritis such as Lyme disease and a class-II HLA-allele DR4 underscores the interaction of environmental and genetic factors in the development of rheumatic diseases.

The association of class-II antigens with rheumatic disease is logical in that the receptors for these antigens on the presenting cells are the class-II molecules. Processed antigen binds to these receptors and is then recognized by helper T cell receptors complementary to the MHC-antigen complex. Most patients with rheumatoid arthritis carry DR1, DR4, or both. There is evidence that the presence of DR4 not only is involved in programming susceptibility to rheumatoid arthritis, but also relates to disease severity.

The mechanism by which DR4 and DR1 can share responsibility for susceptibility to rheumatic arthritis is best understood by the concept of shared epitopes. Recombinant DNA technology has led to a better understanding of class-II MHC molecular structure encoded on chromosome 6. Genes that code for the HLA-DR subregion include one alpha chain and several polymorphic beta chains. This allelic variability produces five subtypes of DR4 (Dw4, Dw10, Dw13, Dw14, and Dw15). The two subtypes (Dw4 and Dw14) of DR4 responsible for promoting susceptibility to rheumatoid arthritis share an epitope from amino acids 70 to 74 in the third hypervariable region of the beta chain. Subtypes of DR4 that do not have this specific amino acid sequence have no associated relative risk for the development of rheumatoid arthritis. Similar shared epitopes present on the DR1 subtypes may be responsible for conferring disease susceptibility. These new technologies should further elucidate the genetic control of disease susceptibility in rheumatic conditions.

Rheumatoid Arthritis

The cause of rheumatoid arthritis is unknown. Many putative agents have been associated with this disease and implicated in its etiology. Epstein-Barr virus, human T cell lymphotrophic virus type-I, rubella virus, cytomegalovirus, and herpesvirus have all been proposed as etiologic agents in rheumatoid arthritis. The identification of mycoplasma in a rheumatoid-like arthritis in gorillas as well as in pig erysipelothrix arthritis has caused speculation as to the association of these agents in rheumatoid arthritis. Although parvoviruses and other viral-related proteins have been identified in the synovium of patients with rheumatoid arthritis, no investigators have fulfilled Rivers' postulates, a series of requisites that must be met before a virus can be associated with disease etiology.

The association of mycobacteria with rheumatoid arthritis has been postulated because these bacteria express heat shock proteins that are identical to the arthrogenic factors in a rat arthritis model. Moreover, elevated levels of antibodies to heat shock proteins from recombinant mycobacteria have been found in patients with rheumatoid arthritis.

Most investigators agree that altered immune reactivity or autoimmunity plays a major role in the progression of rheumatoid arthritis. There is less agreement as to whether autoimmunity has a role in causing it. Most theories of autoimmunity in rheumatoid arthritis implicate the development of autoantibodies towards collagen, proteoglycan, and/or IgG.

The role of collagen autoimmunity in rheumatoid arthritis is demonstrated in a rat model in which intraperitoneal injection of denatured type-II collagen produces a rheumatoid-like condition. Moreover, elevated titers of antibody to both native and denatured type-II collagen have been reported in the serum of patients with rheumatoid arthritis. There is no evidence, however, that these antibodies precede the clinical onset of the disease, suggesting that the cartilage destruction exposes previously sequestered epitopes on degraded portions of collagen as an epiphenomenon of the disease. These collagen-antibody complexes precipitate within the superficial layers of cartilage and may serve as a chemoattractant for the invading pannus tissue.

Rheumatoid factor was first described in 1947. This class of antibodies is directed against antigenic determinants in the Fc region of IgG. Rheumatoid factors have been identified among IgM, IgA, IgG, and IgE classes of immunoglobulin. The classic latex fixation test identifies the presence of IgM rheumatoid factor in the serum of patients. Approximately 80% of patients with rheumatoid arthritis have rheumatoid factor in their blood. The presence of this factor is associated with increased morbidity and nodule formation, and is considered and amplifier of the inflammatory response. The immune complexes produced by these factors can activate complement and serve as chemoattractants. In recent years, genes capable of encoding rheumatoid factors have been identified in humans. The presence of these genes has been associated with an increased risk (2.8 times) of the individual developing rheumatoid arthritis.

Diagnosis   Rheumatoid arthritis is diagnosed on the basis of clinical criteria and not laboratory findings. These clinical criteria include: (1) morning joint stiffness lasting at least one hour; (2) periarticular soft-tissue swelling around three or more joints; (3) swelling of the proximal interphalangeal, metacarpo-phalangeal, or wrist joints; and (4) symmetric arthritis. These symptoms must be present for at least six weeks. The presence of subcutaneous nodules, a positive test for rheumatoid factor, and radiographic evidence of joint erosions and/or periarticular osteopenia in the hands and wrists confirm the diagnosis. When these criteria are used, the diagnosis of rheumatoid arthritis can be confirmed with a 91% to 94% sensitivity and a 89% specificity. The diagnoses most likely to be confused with rheumatoid arthritis early in the course of the disease include systemic lupus erythematosus, psoriatic arthritis, ankylosing spondylitis, mixed connective tissue disease, Reiter's syndrome, polymyalgia, Sjögren's syndrome, crystal deposition disease, and septic arthritis.

Laboratory tests alone cannot confirm the diagnosis of rheumatoid arthritis. Rheumatoid factors can be present (usually in low titers) in normal individuals and in association with other disease states. Common laboratory findings in rheumatoid arthritis include decreased hemoglobin, elevated acute phase reactants (sedimentation rate, C reactive protein), elevated serum cryoglobulins, and precipitating antibodies to soluble antigens.

Disease Stage and Pathophysiology   Rheumatoid arthritis has been divided into five clinical stages based on pathology as well as symptoms, signs, and radiographic findings. Stage I refers to the asymptomatic patient in whom a relevant antigen has been presented to an immunogenetically susceptible host. Stage II is characterized by B cell and T cell proliferation and synovial angiogenesis. Patients in stage II have symptoms of malaise and stiffness as well as early periarticular swelling. There are no radiographic changes at this point.

Angiogenesis is essential for synovial proliferation, and it is controlled mainly by growth factors released from activated cells. Other factors, such as plasminogen activator, facilitate the invasion of newly formed vessels by activating the major metalloproteineases—collagenase and stromolysin.

During neovascularization of the synovial membrane, circulating lymphocytes adhere to and migrate through the walls of the newly formed vessels. The presence of certain cytokines, interferon gamma, interleukin-1 (IL-1) tumor necrosis factor alpha (TNF-α), enhances lymphocyte adhesiveness. There are more T-lymphocytes than B-lymphocytes in the synovial membrane, and the helper/inducer T-lymphocytes adhere better than the cytotoxic/suppressor subset. The predominance of helper/inducer T cells intensifies the immune response. The activated T cells cause B cell proliferation into antibody-secreting cells under the control of a variety of cytokines including interleukin-2. These combined B cell and T cell functions direct the humoral and cellular events leading to destruction of the rheumatoid joint.

Stage III is marked by a continuation of synovial cell proliferation and accumulation of neutrophils in the synovial fluid. Patients have increased constitutional symptoms as well as more soft-tissue swelling and evidence of synovitis. Radiographically, these patients demonstrate soft-tissue swelling.

In stage III disease, the complex interaction of cytokines becomes more evident. Different cytokines can stimulate proliferation of cells under some conditions and inhibit them in others. Cytokine interactions may be synergistic, additive, or inhibitory. They may act at the level of cell-cell interaction or directly on gene expression. The interleukins-2, -3, and -4 as well as gamma interferon are produced by T cells and act in the stimulation and amplification of cellular and humoral immune responses. Interleukin-1 and -6, colony-stimulating factor-1, and TNF-α are synthesized primarily by macrophages and fibroblasts. Their major effects are on cell proliferation, prostaglandin production, matrix degradation, and bone resorption.

Not all cytokines found in rheumatoid arthritis are destructive. Transforming growth factor beta (TGF-β) counteracts many of the effects of IL-1, IL-6, and TNF. It suppresses the production of collagenase by synovial cells and enhances the biosynthesis of matrix proteins. Moreover, identification of cytokine inhibitors in synovial tissue of patients with rheumatoid arthritis suggests that these effects could be downregulated.

Published reports on the role of cytokines in rheumatoid arthritis are confusing. This confusion is fostered by the cytokines' complex interactions as well as by the fact that they were usually named for their biologic effect or the target organ. A cytokine might be called by more than one name, and cytokines that are active in synovium were frequently named for their nonsynovial action(s).

Reports of recent studies of cytokine messenger RNA (m-RNA) from patients with rheumatoid arthritis indicate that IL-6 was found in highest concentration in synovial tissue followed by IL-1β, TNF-α, colony-stimulating factor, gamma interferon, and IL-2.

The fact that neutrophils are found in high concentrations in synovial fluid of patients with rheumatoid arthritis, but rarely in the synovial membrane, suggests that the principal chemoattractants for neutrophils are in the joint space. These include an activated component of complement (C5a), leukotriene B4, and platelet-activating factor. The neutrophils are activated by phagocytosis of cellular debris and immune complexes. This activation results in the release of metalloproteinases, activation of arachidonic acid metabolism to produce prostaglandins, and production of superoxide anions. These and other events in the joint fluid produce inflammation, amplify the response, and induce matrix degradation. Other processes include the activation of the complement system, production of vasoactive kinins by kallikrein, and activation of the clotting cascade.

Stage IV disease is marked by the initiation of the enzymatic degradation of cartilage. Patients become more symptomatic and magnetic resonance imaging shows evidence of pannus formation and of periarticular osteopenia. Stage V disease is marked by further erosion of subchondral bone as well as by radiographic evidence of joint destruction with narrowing of the joint space. Clinically, patients develop deformity because of cartilage loss and ligamentous laxity. There is limited range of motion, and flexion contractures develop.

Treatment The multiple mechanisms and the complex interaction of events leading to cartilage destruction in rheumatoid arthritis explain why a single agent is incapable of blocking these events. Appropriate treatment requires the physician to classify the clinical stage of the disease as well as to develop objective criteria to evaluate disease activity.

Self-management programs are useful in the early stages of the disease. Patients should be educated as to the flares and remissions characteristic of rheumatoid arthritis as well as to means of protecting joints while sustaining muscle strength. A balance must be sought between activity, mobility, and strengthening to maintain muscle tone and preserve range of motion versus overactivity with the resulting accelerated joint damage.

Drug therapy can be divided into first-line and second-line agents. The first-line agents, salicylates and nonsteroidal anti-inflammatory drugs (NSAIDs), block cyclooxygenase and are therefore anti-inflammatory. There are no clinically approved first line drugs that block the lipoxygenase wing of arachidonic acid metabolism. Aspirin is a particularly useful therapy, but it has lost favor in recent years with the proliferation of NSAIDs. Aspirin is inexpensive, easy to measure, and the associated gastric distress often can be controlled by dosing around meals and/or with the use of carafate and H2 antagonists. All of the NSAIDs are capable of producing gastric distress as well as renal toxicity. Care should be taken in prescribing NSAIDs in association with warfarin therapy or for people with renal dysfunction, ulcer disease, or advancing age.

Most rheumatologists use first-line therapy in treatment of patients with rheumatoid arthritis. There is a trend toward early institution of a second-line drug if symptoms are not controlled. The mechanism of action of the second-line agents is unknown. The major second-line agents (and their proposed actions) include: antimalarials (stabilize lysosomal membranes, inhibit IL-1), gold salts (inhibit monocyte function), methotrexate (anti-folate, immunosuppressive activity), d-penicillamine (modulate lymphocyte function), azathioprine (immunosuppressive), and sulfasalazine (anti-folate activity). Sulfasalazine is not yet approved by the FDA for treatment of rheumatoid arthritis. The relative roles and timing of second-line agent use in rheumatoid arthritis are still evolving. The antimalarial, hydroxychloroquine sulfate, is frequently the first of the second-line agents to be used. The major side effect is macular degeneration, and patients on this drug should have an ocular examination every six months. Gold salts continue to be used, but patients require careful monitoring of blood and urine to identify potential toxicities such as thrombocytopenia, neutropenia, or proteinuria. Oral gold salt therapy is less toxic, but does not appear to be sufficiently efficacious to replace the injectable preparations.

In recent years, low-dose methotrexate (5 to 15 mg, once weekly) has been used as a second-line agent. Patients on methotrexate must be followed by a rheumatologist to monitor such potentially serious side effects as hepatic and pulmonary toxicity. Drugs that cause potentially harmful interactions when taken at the same time as methotrexate include trimethoprim-sulfamethoxazole (bone marrow suppression) and probenicid (blocks tubular secretion of methotrexate). There are no guidelines about the perioperative administration of methotrexate during total joint arthroplasty. In general, it is prudent to withhold therapy during the perioperative period, because fluid shifts and alterations in renal blood flow can alter methotrexate levels.

Corticosteroid administration is reserved for patients whose disease is refractory and those with severe nonarticular manifestations of rheumatoid arthritis. While these agents block many of the pathologic events in rheumatoid arthritis, harmful side effects mitigate against their routine usage.

In patients with persistent synovitis without joint space narrowing, synovectomy may control symptoms in a specific joint. Surgical synovectomy can be performed either by open or by arthroscopic techniques. Radiation synovectomy has been used in multiple joints to control synovial proliferation. The efficacy of dysprosium (Dy 165) ferric hydroxide macroaggregate in controlling symptoms and retarding disease progression in rheumatoid joints recently has been examined. These techniques do not work if there is significant cartilage destruction with the joint space narrowing. Early results suggest that the symptoms are controlled, but the long-term benefits in terms of disease progression are uncertain.

The role of total arthroplasty in the treatment of stage V disease is well established. Patients with rheumatoid arthritis require special consideration when total joint arthroplasty is contemplated. The presence of nonarticular manifestations, such as vasculitis, neuropathy, and pulmonary involvement, increase perioperative risk and may affect ultimate function. The polyarticular nature of rheumatoid arthritis often makes it difficult to assess which of the involved joints most affects patient function. Moreover, involvement of other extremities can influence postoperative physical rehabilitation. In general, multiply involved ipsilateral joints should be corrected from a proximal to distal direction; that is, total hip before total knee and total shoulder before total elbow. Fixation of implants is often difficult in rheumatoid patients and implants frequently must be cemented. In most cases, however, the prostheses function well and are protected by the physical limitations dictated by other manifestations of the disease. The reduced activity of most patients with stage V rheumatoid arthritis allows successful arthroplasties of the shoulder, elbow, and ankle, which would have a higher failure rate in the more active individual with osteoarthritis.

Procedures such as hemiarthroplasty, osteotomy, and unicondylar knee replacement are not indicated in patients with rheumatoid arthritis, because those procedures do not influence the destructive interaction between the synovium and the remaining cartilage.

Patients with rheumatoid arthritis require specific anesthetic considerations. Micrognathia and cervical spine stiffness make these individuals difficult to intubate. Moreover, instability in cervical vertebral C-1 and C-2 increases the risk of spinal cord injury. Recent advances in epidural and other regional anesthetics have reduced the risk in patients who often face multiple surgical procedures.

Juvenile Rheumatoid Arthritis

Juvenile rheumatoid arthritis affects 60,000 to 200,000 children in the United States. There are three specific subtypes of juvenile rheumatoid arthritis—systemic onset (Still's disease), polyarticular onset, and pauciarticular onset.

Approximately 20% of children with juvenile rheumatoid arthritis have systemic onset. The ratio of boys to girls is equal. Clinical manifestations include fever, rash, lymphadenopathy, hepatosplenomegaly, and pericardial or pleural effusions. Leukocytosis and anemia are common, but antinuclear antibodies and rheumatoid factor are generally absent. Chronic polyarthritis develops within weeks to months in many individuals. About 25% of patients develop a severe chronic arthritis.

Polyarticular juvenile rheumatoid arthritis occurs in approximately 40% of patients. These children have constitutional symptoms, growth retardation, low grade fever, mild organomegaly, adenopathy, and anemia. Cervical spine involvement, particularly at C-2 and C-3, is common in this form. Polyarticular juvenile rheumatoid arthritis can occur at any age; girls are affected more often than boys by a ration of two to one. Latex fixation is positive in only 15% of children with polyarticular onset; in general, these children have a worse prognosis than those who are latex negative.

Pauciarticular onset disease occurs in 40% of children with juvenile rheumatoid arthritis. These patients often have serum antinuclear antibodies, but are rheumatoid factor negative. Inflammation of the anterior uveal tract (iridocyclitis) develops in 10% to 50% of children with pauciarticular disease; these patients require regular slit-lamp examinations by an ophthalmologist.

Although early diagnosis and appropriate therapy are important, the prognosis for most children with juvenile rheumatoid arthritis is quite good. At least 75% of patients enter a long period of remission and have little or no residual disability.

The goals of therapy in juvenile rheumatoid arthritis are relief of symptoms, maintenance of joint motion, and preservation of function. Salicylates remain the basic anti-inflammatory medication in these patients. NSAIDs that have been approved for use in children are used for patients who cannot tolerate aspirin. Gold salts are as effective in the treatment of juvenile rheumatoid arthritis as in the adult disease; antimalarials and penicillamine do not work as well in juvenile rheumatoid arthritis. Corticosteroids are contraindicated in the treatment of juvenile rheumatoid arthritis except in a crisis situation. Iridocyclitis can usually be managed with topical steroid preparations and dilating agents. Other second-line therapies remain experimental.

Synovectomy does not appear to benefit the course of the disease, but may be helpful in controlling symptoms. Total joint arthroplasty has proven to be beneficial in rheumatoid arthritis but requires special consideration in juvenile rheumatoid arthritis. Total hip arthroplasty is often complicated by excessive coxa valga, anteversion, and a narrow isthmus. Total knee arthroplasty may require posterior cruciate ligament substitution to decrease severe flexion contracture. This procedure requires careful preoperative consideration, and frequently requires the use of modular or custom components.

Seronegative Spondyloarthropathies

These conditions include ankylosing spondylitis, Reiter's syndrome, psoriatic arthropathy, arthritis associated with intestinal bowel disease, juvenile ankylosing spondylitis, and reactive arthropathy.

Ankylosing spondylitis involves the sacroiliac joints, the spine, and to a lesser extent, the peripheral joints. Current studies indicate more uniform gender distribution for this disease, which once was considered to be predominant in men. Although women have less progressive spinal disease, they are more likely to have peripheral joint manifestation. The disease's association with HLA-B27 antigen is presented in Table 1.

A recent report reviewed 29 hip replacements performed in 19 patients with ankylosing spondylitis. While pain relief and functional improvement were significant at a mean four-year follow-up, 23% of the hips developed Brooker class III or class IV heterotopic ossification. Another report of 53 total hip replacements in 31 patients with ankylosing spondylitis (mean follow-up, 6.3 years) reported excellent durability with conventional cemented arthroplasty. Of these patients, 11% developed class III and class IV heterotopic ossification. Significant heterotopic ossification occurred only in those patients with previous hip surgery, postoperative infection, or complete preoperative ankylosis. Prophylactic radiation was recommended for those patients who developed heterotopic ossification on the contralateral hip or were undergoing a reoperation.

Corrective spinal osteotomy was reported in 21 patients with ankylosing spondylitis treated over an eight-year period. The average correction for rigid thoracic kyphosis treated with at two-stage anterior and posterior procedure was 36 degrees. Single-stage lumbar osteotomy with Harrington compression resulted in an average 30-degree correction. All but one patient in this series had improvement in pain and spinal alignment. There were no perioperative deaths and no permanent neurologic abnormalities. Patients with ankylosing spondylitis are reported to have a higher incidence of spinal fracture with minimal trauma. These fractures are associated with a higher risk of severe spinal cord injury and permanent neurologic deficit.

Systemic Lupus Erythematosus

Systemic lupus erythematosus (SLE) is a chronic inflammatory disease resulting from abnormal immunoregulation. Its etiology, like that of rheumatoid arthritis, is unknown, but both genetic and environmental factors are probably involved. SLE has a marked female predominance (greater than 9 to 1). It is more common among African-Americans and certain Asian populations, with a prevalence reported to be from 2.9 to 400 per 100,000. The disease affects many organ systems, including bones, joints, tendons, skin, heart, kidney, and the central nervous system. The diagnosis is made on the basis of clinical findings and a variety of laboratory tests. Patients are generally anemic and have elevated acute-phase reactants. The fluorescent anti-nuclear antibody test is positive in most patients, with a homogeneous pattern indicating antibodies to nucleoprotein or a rim pattern indicating anti DNA antibodies. Antibodies to double-stranded DNA or identification of extractable nuclear antigen may aid in the diagnosis. Treatment of the disease is related to its activity and the target organ. NSAIDs, corticosteroids, antimalarials, and immunosuppressive agents all have a role in the treatment of SLE. Patients with SLE require careful monitoring by a rheumatologist.

The orthopaedic treatment of patients with SLE generally revolves around joint involvement and/or osteonecrosis. Patients undergoing total joint arthroplasty for SLE have increased perioperative risks, including infection. Ligamentous balance is more difficult because of soft-tissue involvement with SLE. Disease activity and corticosteroid therapy frequently produce osteopenia and predispose a patient to loosening and possible fracture.

A review of the use of bipolar hemiarthroplasty in patients with osteonecrosis secondary to SLE revealed a higher incidence of failure, leading to the recommendation for primary total hip arthroplasty in these patients. This higher incidence of failure presumably is caused by lupus synovitis.

Crystal Arthritis

Gout The diagnosis of gouty arthritis is both overused and, at times, overlooked. Gout cannot be diagnosed purely on the basis of clinical findings. Podagra, pain in the first metatarsophalangeal joint, is common in gout but not specific for that diagnosis. Moreover, gout may present in many joints, either as an acute event or as chronic arthritis. The diagnosis is confirmed by the identification of sodium urate crystals located within neutrophils in synovial fluid. These needle-like crystals are negatively birefringent when viewed with a polarized microscope and a first-order red compensator. Those crystals parallel with the compensator will appear bright yellow. This is in direct contrast to the short, rhomboidal calcium pyrophosphate crystals of chondrocalcinosis, which are weakly birefringent and appear blue when parallel to the compensator. Sodium urate crystals may also be identified in tophi. Early tophi may be detected on examination of the extensor surface of the elbow and particularly the pinna of the ear, aiding in the diagnosis of gout. Patients with an established diagnosis of gout should be monitored by a rheumatologist. The treatment of asymptomatic hyperuricemia is controversial. This condition is more common in patients on thiazides or in association with alcohol consumption; moreover, it is seen with higher frequency in conditions such as psoriasis, a variety of hematologic conditions, renal disease, and hyperlipidemia.

Patients with hyperuricemia should undergo a 24-hour uric acid determination, because the risk of uric acid stones is closely related to urinary uric acid excretion. Of patients with urinary uric acid excretion over 1,100 mg per day, 50% will ultimately develop renal stones and should receive chronic long-term treatment. A recent study suggests that patients with gout produce a urate crystal promoter, or perhaps lack an inhibitor of crystal formation. This may explain why some hyperuricemic individuals develop gout and others remain asymptomatic.

Acute gout may be confused with other acute arthritides, including infection. Although major joints are frequently involved, the acute presentation can even be that of infectious tenosynovitis. If gout is suspected, a tissue specimen should be fixed in ethanol, because standard formalin fixation dissolves the sodium urate crystals.

Acute gouty attacks can be treated with NSAIDs, adrenocorticotropic hormone (ACTH) (40 IU, IM), or colchicine (0.6 mg) given one tablet every two hours until diarrhea, nausea, or vomiting occurs. Alternatively, colchicine can be given as two to three tablets followed by one tablet twice daily until side effects occur. Colchicine should not be given intravenously because it is known to cause marrow depression, local venous irritation, and potential cardiotoxicity. Because of colchicine's side effects, most clinicians prefer ACTH or NSAIDs. In a prospective comparison of 100 patients treated for one year with either a single intramuscular injection of ACTH (40 IU) or oral indomethacin (40 mg, four times daily with meals) until the acute attack subsided, improvement in symptoms occurred much more rapidly with the ACTH (average 3 hours) than with indomethacin (24 hours). None of the patients receiving ACTH developed side effects, whereas more than 50% of those receiving indomethacin developed gastrointestinal disturbance, headaches, or other central nervous system symptoms.

Long-term treatment of patients with recurrent gouty episodes may prevent recurrent attacks. It is important to identify whether the patient is an underexcreter of uric acid (85% to 90% of primary gout) or an overproducer (10% to 15% of primary gout). These patients are generally managed with uricosuric agents (probenecid, sulfinpyrazone) or allopurinol, respectively. The frequency of side effects of these agents is similar, but those to allopurinol are more severe. The allopurinol hypersensitivity syndrome is characterized by fever, eosinophilia, leukocytosis, impaired renal function, hepatocellular injury, and rash. These reactions are severe and may be fatal. For this reason, allopurinol use should be carefully monitored but still may be indicated in patients with tophi, renal insufficiency, a history of uric acid stones, and in those individuals with a 24-hour urinary uric acid over 1,100 mg.

Chondrocalcinosis Chondrocalcinosis, or calcium pyrophosphate dihydrate deposition disease, has many clinical patterns, including asymptomatic calcium pyrophosphate dihydrate deposition disease, pseudogout, pseudorheumatoid arthritis, and pseudoosteoarthritis. The orthopaedic surgeon sees this disease most commonly either as an asymptomatic finding in association with arthritis or as an acute postoperative inflammatory arthritis. Calcium pyrophosphate dihydrate deposition disease is more common in patients with gout, rheumatoid arthritis, hemochromatosis, Wilson's disease, and hyperparathyroidism. The diagnosis is confirmed by identification of weakly positive, short, rhomboidal crystals of calcium pyrophosphate dihydrate seen in neutrophilic leukocytes.

The identification of calcium pyrophosphate crystals embedded in articular cartilage at the time of surgery is a relative contraindication of both osteotomy and unicondylar knee replacement. These crystals are believed to dessicate the articular cartilage and render it more susceptible to wear at normal loads. Moreover, significant chondrocalcinosis is often associated with a reactive synovitis that might persist after osteotomy or unicondylar replacement.

Pseudogout is often confused with infection and, in fact, a report indicated that 14 of 93 acute inflammatory pseudogout attacks were misdiagnosed as septic arthritis. Pseudogout tends to occur with greater frequency in the postoperative period. The diagnosis is confirmed by joint aspiration and crystal analysis. Aspiration of the involved joint and steroid injection, once the diagnosis of infection has been excluded, will usually control symptoms. Alternatively, NSAIDs may be used to control acute attacks.

Infectious Arthropathies

The advent of antibiotic therapy has decreased the destructive effects of acute septic arthritis. In a *Staphylococcus aureus* infectious knee arthritis model in rabbits, prompt antibiotic therapy reduced but did not eliminate cartilage wear. In this model, untreated animals lost more than half of the glycosaminoglycan in articular cartilage by three weeks. Antibiotic administration one day after experimental infection reduced the overall loss of cartilage by 37%. This study underscored the importance of prompt diagnosis and early treatment.

Arthroscopic lavage was used to treat 46 cases of septic arthritis of the knee. Fifteen of the cases were secondary to puncture and 20 resulted from postoperative infection. Positive cultures were obtained in only 63% of the cases. Treatment included arthroscopic lavage and prolonged antibiotic therapy (average two months). In this series, there were 36 cures (78.3%), five failures (10.9%), and five recurrences (10.9%) after apparent initial success. The role of arthroscopic lavage in the treatment of acute septic arthritis may be joint specific and related to the extent of synovitis. The knee seems most suitable for this form of treatment, because the surgery is easily performed and the results can be followed by physical examination; however, its role in the treatment of other major joint infections in adults is unclear.

A review of septic arthritis and osteomyelitis of the hand outlines both the surgical and medical management of these infections and the importance of prompt and adequate treatment to prevent osteomyelitis and other late complications. The need for proper diagnosis and therapy is emphasized in a review of acute septic arthritis in infancy and childhood that also covers the changing patterns of bacterial pathogens in this condition. A dosage schedule for commonly used antibiotics is included.

Hemophiliac Arthropathy

Patients with severe hemophilia have a higher incidence of early arthritis of major joints. The most frequently involved joints, in order, are knees, ankles, elbows, shoulders, and hips. The mechanism of arthritis in hemophiliacs is controversial, but most investigators agree that recurrent hemoarthrosis with subsequent free-radical formation predisposes the articular surface to injury. Patients with severe hemophilia can generally be maintained at home on factor VIII therapy. Factor VIII concentrates prepared from pooled donors are no longer used because of the high risk of HIV and non-A, non-B hepatitis. Preparations prepared by heat, detergent, and solvent therapy carry a lower risk of viral transmission. Newer agents, such as monoclonal affinity column purified factor VIII and pasteurized, heat-treated factor VIII concentrate, are costly, but carry a low risk of viral transmission. Recombinant factor VIII is currently undergoing clinical trials.

Factor VIII levels of patients undergoing joint replacement surgery for hemophilic arthritis must be carefully monitored in the perioperative period. This monitoring should be done in consultation with the hematologist, but, generally, administration of one unit of factor VIII per kg of body weight will raise the level by 2%. It is generally recommended that factor VIII levels be maintained at 100% to 130% of normal for the first two to three days after surgery and at 50% to 60% of normal for the first 14 days. For six weeks the patients are maintained between 30% and 50% of normal, depending on their physical therapy and response to treatment. Patients known to have inhibitors to factor VIII should not undergo elective orthopaedic surgery.

Seventy percent of hemophiliacs who have received pooled untreated factor VIII preparations are HIV positive, and as many as 90% of severe hemophiliacs are HIV positive. The T4 (helper/inducer T cell subset) counts of these patients are carefully monitored, and AZT therapy is often begun when the T4 count falls below 500. The increased risk of infection in patients with low T4 counts makes elective total joint arthroplasty in this situation questionable.

Good to excellent results were reported for 13 of 19 total knee arthroplasties performed for hemophilic arthropathy, with an average follow-up of 9.5 years. Complications, including deep infection, superficial skin necrosis, nerve palsy, and postoperative bleeding, occurred in ten of the 19 knees. One hundred percent factor VIII coverage was needed in the perioperative period.

Annotated Bibliography

Normal Joint Physiology: Cellular Metabolism

Archer CW, McDowell J, Bayliss MT, et al: Phenotypic modulation in sub-populations of human articular chondrocytes in vitro. *J Cell Sci* 1990; 97:361-71.

The morphology and temporal expression of the chondrogenic phenotype in the depth dependant subpopulations of chondrocytes varies as a function of the culture type, monolayers, or suspension over agarose. The cartilage was separated into surface (15% of tissue depth) and deep (remaining tissue) zones and the chondrocytes released by enzymatic digestion.

Collier S, Ghosh P: Comparison of the effects of non-steroidal anti-inflammatory drugs (NSAIDs) on proteoglycan synthesis by articular cartilage explant and chondrocyte monolayer cultures. *Biochem Pharmacol* 1991;41:1375-1384.

Nonsteroidal antiinflammatory agents were administered to articular cartilage explant and confluent chondrocyte monolayer cultures. Cell culture proteoglycan production was maximal early in the culture period, although the explants increased proteoglycan production as a function of time. Explant proteoglycan production was retained in the matrix, whereas the proteoglycan produced by cell cultures was secreted into the medium. Most NSAIDs inhibited proteoglycan secretion by both cell and explant cultures. In the cell cultures, inhibition was reversed after the NSAIDs were discontinued.

Franchimont P, Bassleer C: Effects of hormones and local growth factors on articular chondrocyte metabolism. *J Rheumatol Suppl* 1991;27:68-70.

Hormones such as growth hormone, calcitonin, and androgens and parahormones such as insulin-like growth factor I and epidermal growth factor stimulated chondrocyte proliferation and collagen type II and proteoglycan synthesis.

Lefebvre V, Peeters-Joris C, Vaes G: Production of collagens, collagenase and collagenase inhibitor during the dedifferentiation of articular chondrocytes by serial subcultures. *Biochim Biophys Acta* 1990;1051:266-275.

Progressive changes in the differentiated phenotype of rabbit articular chondrocytes monolayer cultures in monolayer were followed from passage to passage. Cell densities in confluent cultures decreased between the primary culture and the second or third subculture. Collagen synthesis, but not that of other proteins, decreased sharply with a smaller proportion of collagen being incorporated into the matrix. There was a shift from the cartilage-specific collagens, types II and XI, which were mostly deposited in the matrix, to synthesis of collagen types I and III, with subsequent release into the culture medium. The production of the collagenase inhibitor TIMP (tissue inhibitor of metalloproteinases) increased from passage to passage.

Livne E, Weiss A and Silbermann M: Articular chondrocytes lose their proliferative activity with aging yet can be restimulated by PTH-(1-84), PGE1, and dexamethasone. *J Bone Miner Res* 1989;4:539-548.

Age-related changes in the proliferative functions of chondrocytes and their potential for hormonal response were examined in a mouse mandibular condyles model that spontaneously develops degenerative changes by six months of age. Although older cells demonstrated an age related decrease in labeling index of the articular cartilage, DNA synthesis resumed following in vitro treatment with PTH-(1-84), PGE1, and dexamethasone, indicating a direct stimulatory effect on senescent chondrocytes.

Osborn KD, Trippel SB, Mankin HJ: Growth factor stimulation of adult articular cartilage. *J Orthop Res* 1989;7:35-42.

An adult bovine articular chondrocyte organ culture system demonstrated the capacity to augment both mitotic and differentiated cell functions in response to growth factors.

Redini F, Daireaux M, Mauviel A, et al: Characterization of proteoglycans synthesized by rabbit articular chondrocytes in response to transforming growth factor-beta (TGF-beta). *Biochim Biophys Acta* 1991;1093:196-206.

A rabbit articular chondrocyte culture was used to demonstrate that the extracellular matrix is altered in response to TGF-β. Confluent cells increased proteoglycan production, but not release, in response to TGF-β with the cell layer distribution decreasing in response to increasing serum concentration. The relative distribution of disaccharide 6- and 4-sulfate in GAG chains was altered by TGF-β with a decrease in chondroitin 6-sulfate and an increase in chondroitin 4-sulfate.

Smith RL, Palathumpat MV, Ku CW, et al: Growth hormone stimulates insulin-like growth factor I actions on adult articular chondrocytes. *J Orthop Res* 1989;7:198-207.

In an in vitro model of adult bovine articular chondrocytes plated at high density, growth hormone alone did not have any metabolic effect while insulin-like growth factor 1 stimulated chondrocyte DNA and proteoglycan synthesis. There was a synergistic effect of insulin-like growth factor 1 and human growth hormone in stimulating chondrocyte extracellular matrix synthesis.

Speer KP, Callaghan JJ, Seaber AV, et al: The effects of exposure of articular cartilage to air. A histochemical and ultrastructural investigation. *J Bone Joint Surg* 1990;72A:1442-1450.

The effects of exposure of articular cartilage to air and the potential for reversibility of the histologic and ultrastructural changes that were produced in the knee joint of the rabbit by this exposure were investigated. The articular cartilage in 45 rabbits was exposed to air for one, two, and three hours, and the reversibility of the histological and ultrastructural changes that were produced by this exposure were assessed. After one hour of exposure to the ambient atmosphere, the matrix glycosaminoglycans were depleted and ultrastructural changes were observed throughout the full thickness of articular cartilage. These changes became more pronounced with the time of exposure, but were reversible.

Normal Joint Physiology: Subchondral Bone

Chai BF: Subchondral bone tissues in osteoarthritis of knee joint: A tetracycline labelling study. *Chung Hua Wai Ko Tsa Chih* 1991;29:305-307.

Tetracycline labeling in patients with late osteoarthritis of the knee joint was administered prior to high tibial osteotomies or knee replacements. The findings suggested that the formation and deposition of new bone was initiated in the marrow interstices and along the periphery of the trabeculae. These two areas of bone formation fused, increasing the bone mass as indicated by the sclerotic changes in proximal tibia and distal femur.

de Vries BJ, van den Berg WB: Impact of NSAIDS on murine antigen induced arthritis: II. A light microscopic investigation of antiinflammatory and bone protective effects. *J Rheumatol* 1990;17:295-303.

The effects of nonsteroidal antiinflammatory drugs and prednisolone on the mouse knee joint in a model of antigen-induced arthritis were examined by light microscopy. Synovium and joint cavity inflammatory cell infiltrates were decreased in mice treated with prednisolone but not with the NSAIDs. Osteocyte death was confined to the tibial subchondral bone. Prednisolone was the most effective antiinflammatory and arthroprotective agent.

Gevers G, Dequeker J, Martens M, et al: Biomechanical characteristics of iliac crest bone in elderly women according to osteoarthritis grade at the hand joints. *J Rheumatol* 1989;16:660-663.

Examination of postmortem iliac crest trabecular bone specimens and compression testing were compared to trabecular bone volume and width histomorphometric measurements and radiographic grading of osteoarthritis of carpal joints. Those specimens with frank osteoarthritis had stiffer bone, an increased compressive strength value, and a higher trabecular bone volume and trabecular width as compared to those specimens with minimal or no osteoarthritis. The authors concluded that the primary defect in osteoarthritis is in the subchondral bone and not in the articular cartilage.

Layton MW, Goldstein SA, Goulet RW, et al: Examination of subchondral bone architecture in experimental osteoarthritis by microscopic computed axial tomography. *Arthritis Rheum* 1988;31:1400-1405.

The subchondral bone changes in osteoarthritis were evaluated with microscopic computed axial tomography of the femoral heads from a guinea pig model of osteoarthritis. The subchondral trabeculae were thicker and had less porosity indicating a possible role of trabecular remodeling as an early event in this model of osteoarthritis.

Smith RL, Thomas KD, Schurman DJ, et al: Rabbit knee immobilization: bone remodeling precedes cartilage degradation. *J Orthop Res* 1992;10:88-95.

Subchondral vascular eruptions were observed after short-term immobilization of the right hind limbs of postadolescent and mature rabbits. The femoral metaphyseal bone density decreased while calcein green fluorescence increased 1.9-fold in the metaphyseal trabeculae of immobilized femurs. No changes in glycosaminoglycan and hydroxyproline levels were found; however, sulfate and thymidine incorporation into femoral cartilage glycosaminoglycan increased. These results indicated that bone loss and remodeling preceded erosive cartilage degradation.

Normal Joint Physiology: Synovium and Synovial Fluid

Schalkwijk J, Joosten LA, van den Berg WB, et al: Insulin-like growth factor stimulation of chondrocyte proteoglycan synthesis by human synovial fluid. *Arthritis Rheum* 1989;32:66-71.

Synovial fluid from patients with rheumatoid arthritis and from control patients stimulated chondrocyte proteoglycan

synthesis in a bovine articular cartilage explant culture system. Monoclonal antibodies directed against insulin-like growth factor-1 (IGF-1) completely blocked the stimulatory action of synovial fluid. The synovial fluid levels of IGF-1 were lower than the serum level for both patient groups, but no differences in the serum levels of IGF-1 between either patient population were found.

Normal Joint Physiology: Physiologic Senescence

Brandt KD, Myers SL, Burr D, et al: Osteoarthritic changes in canine articular cartilage, subchondral bone, and synovium fifty-four months after transection of the anterior cruciate ligament. *Arthritis Rheum* 1991;34:1560-1570.

The anterior cruciate ligament transection model of osteoarthritis results not only in osteophyte formation but also in morphologic, metabolic, biochemical, and biomechanical changes in the articular cartilage. At sacrifice, full-thickness articular cartilage ulceration was observed on the medial femoral condyle and tibial plateau of the unstable knee. There was also an increased subchondral bone volume. In contrast, hypertrophic cartilage repair was observed in other areas of the ipsilateral as well as the contralateral knee. Although only three dogs were used in this study, the long-term effects of ACL transection are progressive and mimic those observed in osteoarthritis.

Brand HS, de Koning MH, van Kampen GP, et al: Age related changes in the turnover of proteoglycans from explants of bovine articular cartilage. *J Rheumatol* 1991;18:599-605.

In explant cultures of mature and immature bovine articular cartilage, the mature cartilage had longer chondroitin sulfate chains, a shorter half-life, a lower ratio of 6-sulfated over 4-sulfated disaccharides of both proteoglycans, and a higher proportion of ^{35}S-sulfate incorporation in the small proteoglycan.

Chandrasekhar S, Harvey AK, Hrubey PS, et al: Arthritis induced by interleukin-1 is dependent on the site and frequency of intraarticular injection. *Clin Immunol Immunopathol* 1990;55:382-400.

Injection of rat knee joints either with a single dose of interleukin-1 or with an equivalent dose divided into three injections resulted in varying degrees of inflammatory changes. There was an age-associated inflammatory response, with the older animals generating a greater response. Multiple dose administration resulted in a greater inflammatory response than did a single intra-articular injection. Although a single injection led to a mild volume increase initially, no discernible change was observed at the end of seven days. When an identical dose was administered in three divided doses, a dramatic increase in joint volume persisted for at least three weeks. Histologically, the divided-dose knee joints developed marked acute synovitis, fibroplasia, loss of proteoglycans and chondrocytes, resorption of subchondral bone, and transition of hematopoietic marrow cells into cells of mesenchymal morphology. Single-dose knees had a mild and transient inflammatory response that resolved by two weeks and progressive focal loss of chondrocytes and proteoglycans of the knee joint cartilage, indicative of degenerative changes.

Hardingham T, Bayliss M: Proteoglycans of articular cartilage: changes in aging and in joint disease. *Semin Arthritis Rheum* 1990;20:12-33.

This review paper discusses proteoglycan structure and the alterations observed in aging and degenerative joint disease. Although structural damage of cartilage proteoglycans is a primary event in osteoarthritis and changes the tissue's material properties, the exact nature of the pathologic process and the biochemical mechanisms are poorly understood.

Melching LI, Roughley PJ: A matrix protein of Mr 55,000 that accumulates in human articular cartilage with age. *Biochim Biophys Acta* 1990;1036:213-220.

Articular cartilage contains a Mr 55,000 protein which is present in the adult and absent in newborn cartilage. In 4 M guanidinium chloride extracts, this protein is one of the most abundant noncollagenous, nonproteoglycan molecules, and although it is synthesized by chondrocytes, it may accumulate with increasing age and not be a significant synthetic product.

Rosenthal AK, Cheung HS, Ryan LM, et al: Transforming growth factor beta 1 stimulates inorganic pyrophosphate elaboration by porcine cartilage. *Arthritis Rheum* 1991;34:904-911.

Transforming growth factor beta 1 (TGF-β1) alone and in concert with epidermal growth factor or TGF-α stimulates inorganic pyrophosphate production by articular cartilage organ and monolayer cultures. The increase levels of inorganic pyrophosphate produced by chondrocytes may be be relevant in the intrarticular formation of calcium pyrophosphate dihydrate crystals and the development of pseudogout or chondrocalcinosis.

Biomechanics

Hall AC, Urban JP, Gehl KA: The effects of hydrostatic pressure on matrix synthesis in articular cartilage. *J Orthop Res* 1991;9:1-10.

The hydrostatic pressure effects on articular cartilage matrix synthesis vary as a function of the pressure level and the time at that pressure. Physiologic pressures (5 to 15 MPa), applied continuously for two hours or intermittently, stimulated the incorporation of $^{35}SO_4$ and [^3H] proline into adult bovine articular cartilage slices in vitro. With intermittent pressure, the response was stimulatory from 5 to 15 MPa; with continuous pressure the incorporation was reversibly decreased above 20 MPa. The stimulation also varied with position along the joint and among different animals.

Kiviranta I, Jurvelin J, Tammi M, et al: Weight bearing controls glycosaminoglycan concentration and articular cartilage thickness in the knee joints of young beagle dogs. *Arthritis Rheum* 1987;30:801-809.

Immobilization of articular cartilage leads to decreased local proteoglycan content. Right knee joints of young beagle dogs were casted for 11 weeks. The glycosaminoglycan concentration of the uncalcified articular cartilage decreased 48% while the increased weightbearing in the contralateral limb led to a 25% to 35% increase in glycosaminoglycan concentration in all zones of cartilage and an increase in uncalcified cartilage thickness. The glycosaminoglycans were decreased primarily in the superficial cartilage zone, and no change in the thickness of the uncalcified cartilage was observed. However, the calcified cartilage under the tidemark was thinned at the femoral condyles.

Sah RL, Kim YJ, Doong JY, et al: Biosynthetic response of cartilage explants to dynamic compression. *J Orthop Res* 1989;7:619-636.

Physiologic dynamic compression of calf articular cartilage explants was evaluated over a extensive range of amplitudes, waveforms, and frequencies. A specially designed culture chamber provided uniaxial, radially unconfined compression. The compression accelerated the synthesis and release of matrix proteoglycans through physical phenomena including tissue strain and fluid flow. There was no compression-induced depletion of total glycosaminoglycan content with any of the compression routines.

Osteoarthrosis

Campion GV, McCrae F, Schnitzer TJ, et aL: Levels of keratan sulfate in the serum and synovial fluid of patients with osteoarthritis of the knee. *Arthritis Rheum* 1991;34:1254-1259.

The authors report their use of an assay system for keratan sulfate in patients with osteoarthritis. In their study, 125 patients with osteoarthritis were found to have a mean level of serum keratan sulfate of 393 ng/ml (significantly higher than controls). The large variations in these values suggest that the test may not be of diagnostic significance but individual serial monitoring may be useful in determining disease progression and response to therapy.

Dandy DJ: Editorial: Arthroscopic debridement of the knee for osteoarthritis. *J Bone Joint Surg* 1991;73B:877-878.

This editorial reviews the history, published results, and the author's opinion of the current indications for arthroscopic debridement of the knee in osteoarthritis. It points out the importance of radiographic severity, angular deformity, and the presence of internal derangement of the knee in determining indications for this procedure.

Chan WP, Lang P, Stevens MP, et al: Osteoarthritis of the knee: Comparison of radiography, CT and MR imaging to assess extent and severity. *Am J Roent* 1991;157:799-806.

The authors compared MR, CT, and plain radiographs in the evaluation of osteoarthritis. They report MR to be more sensitive, especially for evaluating the least involved compartment, the presence of osteophytes, and damage to meniscal and ligamentous structures.

Pelletier JP, Roughley PJ, DiBattista JA, et al: Are cytokines involved in osteoarthritic pathophysiology? *Sem Arthritis Rheum* 1991;20:12-25.

The role of IL-1 and TNF-α in osteoarthritis is discussed. The cytokines recognize receptors on chondrocytes in synovial fibroblasts and act to produce matrix proteases and to inhibit synthesis of collagen and proteoglycan. Cytokines and cytokine interactions do occur in osteoarthritis, both to cause destruction of cartilage and to block repair. Moreover, growth factors such as TGF-β can counteract the effect of cytokines by stimulating synthesis or by producing inhibitors to the degradative enzymes.

Moskowitz RW, Boja B, Denko CW: The role of growth factors in degenerative joint disorders. *J Rheumatol Suppl* 1991;27:147-148.

The authors discuss the relative role of cytokines and growth factors in the maintenance of cartilage and in the pathophysiology of osteoarthritis (OA) and diffuse idiopathic skeletal hyperostosis (DISH). In patients with osteoarthritis, insulin like growth factor (IGF-1) was decreased as compared to non-arthritic controls. While levels of insulin and growth hormone were elevated in DISH, IGF-1 levels were normal. These data suggest a role of growth factors in the pathophysiology of osteoarthritis and differences in patients with OA and DISH.

Fife RS, Brandt KD: Cartilage matrix glycoprotein is present in serum in experimental canine osteoarthritis. *J Clin Invest* 1989;84:1432-1439.

A cartilage matrix glycoprotein (CMGP) appears as cleavage products in the serum of dogs following ACL transsection. Detection of CMGP by monoclonal antibody may serve as a marker for OA in this model.

Ivarsson I, Myrnerts R, Gillquist J: High tibial osteotomy for medial osteoarthritis of the knee: A 5 to 7 and 11 year follow-up. *J Bone Joint Surg* 1990;72B:238-244.

This study reviews the long-term results of tibial osteotomy for medial OA of the knee. It points out that alignment and the loss of the joint space are important factors that predict outcome from this procedure.

Konradsen L, Hansen EM, Søndergaard L: Long distance running and osteoarthrosis. *Am J Sports Med* 1990;18:379-381.

Thirty long-distance runners were compared to age matched controls to study the effect of running on the development of osteoarthrosis. No differences in joint alignment, range of motion, or complaints of pain were found between runners and nonrunners suggesting that recreational runners are not at increased risk for developing premature osteoarthrosis.

Thompson RC Jr, Oegema TR Jr, Lewis JL, et al: Osteoarthrotic changes after acute transarticular load: An animal model. *J Bone Joint Surg* 1991;73A:990-1001.

The authors report on a closed model of osteoarthritis. In this study, a load was applied to the patellofemoral joint with resultant characteristic changes of OA. The closed nature of this model obviates the confounding bias of an open surgical procedure.

Adams ME: Cartilage hypertrophy following canine anterior cruciate ligament transection differs among different areas of the joint. *J Rheumatol* 1989;16:818-824.

The widely used canine anterior cruciate ligament resection model for OA produces changes that differ in various areas of the joint. This study underscores the importance of comparing results in this model from site specific areas.

Athanasiou KA, Rosenwasser MP, Buckwalter JA, et al: Interspecies comparisons of in situ intrinsic mechanical properties of distal femoral cartilage. *J Orthop Res* 1991;9:330-340.

This study compared the biomechanical properties of the knee joint in five species (bovine, canine, human, monkey, and rabbit). Differences were reported not only amongst species but also at differing sites. The lowest aggregate modulus and highest permeability occurred in the anterior patellar groove suggesting that this cartilage can undergo greater and faster compression. This would allow the patellofemoral articulation to compress more rapidly to maintain congruency.

Rheumatoid Arthritis

Westacott CI, Whicher JT, Barnes IC, et al: Synovial fluid concentrations of five different cytokines in rheumatic diseases. *Ann Rheum Dis* 1990;49:676-681.

Synovial fluid samples of 68 patients with rheumatic diseases were assayed for IL-1β, IL-2, TNF-α, α-interferon, and gamma interferon. IL-1β was higher in patients with rheumatoid arthritis compared to osteoarthritics. While IL-2 and TNF-α were lower in the rheumatoids, distinct cytokine patterns were observed in the different rheumatic disease suggesting a role of these peptides in the pathophysiology of the disease process.

Harris ED Jr: Rheumatoid arthritis. Pathophysiology and implications for therapy. *New Engl J Med* 1990;322:1277-1289.

This excellent review summarizes the recent data on the etiology, pathogenesis, and treatment of rheumatoid arthritis.

Crystal Arthritis

McGill NW, Dieppe PA: Evidence for a promoter of urate crystal formation in gouty synovial fluid. *Ann Rheum Dis* 1991;50:558-561.

Serum and synovial fluid obtained from 12 patients with gout were compared with normal controls. Gouty synovial fluids promoted urate crystal formation significantly more than did controls and patients with either RA or CPPD. This may explain why some individuals with hyperuricemia develop gout while others remain symptomatic.

Seronegative Spondyloarthropathies

Walker LG, Sledge CB: Total hip arthroplasty in ankylosing spondylitis. *Clin Orthop* 1991;262:198-204.

THRs were performed in 19 patients (29 hips) with ankylosing spondylitis over a 13-year period. Complete pain relief was achieved in 97% of patients. Brooker class-III and class-IV heterotopic ossification developed in 23% of patients.

Kilgus DJ, Namba RS, Goreck JE, et al: Total hip replacement for patients who have ankylosing spondylitis: The importance of the formation of heterotopic bone and of the durability of fixation of cemented components. *J Bone Joint Surg* 1990;72A:834-839.

THRs were performed in 31 patients (53 hips) with ankylosing spondylitis with an average follow-up of 6.3 years. Brooker class-III and class-IV heterotopic ossification developed in 11% of patients. The authors recommend heterotopic prophylaxis in those patients who have had previous surgery on the hip, have a history of infection, or have a complete ankylosis preoperatively.

Bradford DS, Schumacher WL, Lonstein JE, et al: Ankylosing spondylitis: Experience in surgical management of 21 patients. *Spine* 1987;12:238-243.

Twenty-one patients with ankylosing spondylitis underwent spinal osteotomy between 1976 and 1984. At latest follow-up, all but one patient improved in pain and spinal alignment. There were no deaths and no persistent neurologic problems from these procedures.

Graham B, Van Peteghem PK: Fractures of the spine in ankylosing spondylitis. Diagnosis, treatment, and complications. *Spine* 1989;14:803-807.

This study underscores the increased incidence of fractures in patients with ankylosing spondylitis and the associated severe neurologic deficits (75% of cases). Although the fractures were unstable, nonoperative treatment was uniformly successful in achieving union.

Septic Arthritis

Shaw BA, Kasser JR: Acute septic arthritis in infancy and childhood. *Clin Orthop* 1990;257:212-225.

This review article points out the importance of early diagnosis and aggressive treatment. Moreover, it discusses pathologic organisms and appropriate treatment in a pediatric population.

Freeland AE, Senter BS: Septic arthritis and osteomyelitis. *Hand Clin* 1989;5:533-552.

This review article covers the pathophysiology, bacteriology, diagnosis, and treatment of septic arthritis and osteomyelitis of the hand.

Thiery JA: Arthroscopic drainage in septic arthritis of the knee: A multicenter study. *Arthroscopy* 1989;5:65-69.

In this study of 46 cases of septic arthritis, patients were treated by arthroscopic drainage and prolonged antibiotic therapy (average 2 months). Average follow-up was 7.1 months. There were 36 bacteriologic cures, 5 failures, and 5 recurrences of infection. Following a second therapeutic attempt in the failed group, there was an overall 89.2% bacteriologic cure.

9

Muscle and Gait

Introduction

Skeletal muscle constitutes almost 50% of the body weight and uses almost 50% of the body's metabolism. The human body contains about 400 muscles, each with a special function, but most generate moments about the joints. All are under the direct control of the voluntary (somatic) nervous system.

Structure

Each skeletal muscle consists of muscle bundles, and each of these bundles is composed of a variable number of muscle fibers (Fig. 1). The muscle fiber is the individual cell of the muscle and, like all cells, includes numerous components such as protoplasm, nuclei, mitochondria, glycogen, and adenosine triphosphate (ATP). The basic subcellular component that distinguishes skeletal muscle, the myofibril, consists of filaments of actin and myosin, the protein components responsible for muscle contraction.

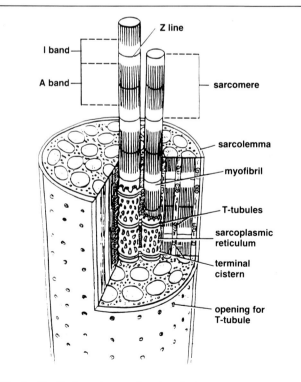

Fig. 1 Myofibrils and sarcoplasmic reticulum.

The contractile unit of the myofibril, the sarcomere, extends from one Z-line to the next Z-line (shown schematically, Fig. 2). Immediately inside the Z-line is a lighter I-band, composed only of the contractile protein actin. The darker A-band consists of interdigitating layers of actin and myosin, while the adjacent H-zone in the

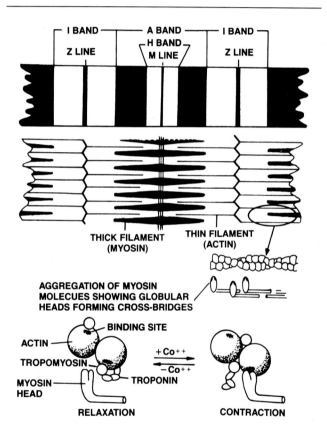

Fig. 2 **Top,** Relationship of cross banding to the thin and thick filaments. Shown enlarged is the interdigitation of thick and thin filaments and the relationship of muscle proteins to each other. (Reproduced with permission from Chaffin DB, Andersson GJ: The structure and function of the musculoskeletal system, in *Occupational Biomechanics*, ed 2. New York, John Wiley & Sons, 1991, p 32.) **Bottom,** Schematic representation of how Ca++ controls actin and myosin interaction in some muscles. On the left, in absence of Ca++, tropomyosin hides the binding site from myosin and the muscle is relaxed. On the right, in the presence of Ca++, calcium binds to troponin an the tropomyosin moves into the groove exposing the binding site, allowing interaction, and the muscle contracts. (Reproduced with permission from Rosse C, Clawson DK, in *Musculoskeletal System in Health and Disease*, New York, Harper & Rowe, 1980, p 46.)

center of the sarcomere represents an area where only myosin is present.

The muscle is covered by fascia, the epimysium. Connective tissue septa (perimysia) extend from the epimysium inward, subdividing the muscle into muscle fiber bundles, called fasciculi. Fasciculi are further divided into individual fibers, which are surrounded by connective tissue membranes, the endomysia. Just beneath the endomysium is a thin elastic membrane, the sarcolemma, which constitutes the muscle cell membrane. This membrane plays an important role in the activation of muscle. These connective tissue components serve as the pathway for nerves and blood vessels and contribute to the mechanical properties of the muscle. Because the connective tissue is more resistant to stretch than the muscle fibers, it determines the muscle's maximal deformation.

Muscle Contraction

The unique property of muscle, contractility, requires a mechanism for contraction, a method to stimulate and control that mechanism, and an energy source.

The Mechanism for Contraction and Types of Contraction

During contraction, the myofibril generates tension and shortens. The actin filaments slide over the myosin filaments, and the H-zone essentially disappears. It is likely that the disappearance of the H-zone is the result of coupling of the myosin cross-links. When the muscle relaxes, these cross-links uncouple. When the muscle is stimulated, the cross-links couple the actin with the myosin, and during contraction the cross-bridges swivel, sliding the myosin over the actin to effect shortening (decrease in the distance between Z-lines) and develop tension.

Muscles may contract isometrically, isotonically (concentrically), eccentrically, isokinetically, or isoinertially (Table 1). During an isometric (static) contraction, the external muscle length does not change. Because the muscle does not grossly move, no work is done, and power cannot be calculated. However, no contraction is completely isometric because within the fibril the distance between the Z-lines always shortens.

An isotonic contraction (also termed concentric or shortening) is one in which constant internal force is produced, and the muscle shortens. It can also be defined as a dynamic exercise with a constant load or resistance. Pure isotonic contractions are rare, because the moment arm and, therefore, the resistance changes as a function of the position of the limb segment. Because there is movement, measurable power and work are produced. As a rule, the maximum isotonic contraction is about 80% of the maximum isometric tension.

An eccentric (lengthening) contraction is one in which the external force is greater than the internal force of the muscle, which causes the muscle to lengthen while con-

Table 1. Characteristics of muscle contraction

Type	Action	Tension/ unit area	Metabolic Demand
Isometric	Tension but no motion	Medium	Related to intensity
Concentric	Moving a resistance while shortening (raising)	Low	High
Eccentric	Moving a resistance while lengthening (lowering)	High	Low

tinuing to maintain tension. In eccentric contractions, movement is controlled but not initiated. During an eccentric contraction, the muscle can sustain greater tension than it can develop in an isometric contraction at any given muscle length. Because greater tension is generated, these muscles are more vulnerable to rupture. The work performed during an eccentric contraction is often defined as negative.

Isokinetic contraction has been popularized as a method of measuring strength, as well as an exercise regimen. The term means "constant force" and typically is used to describe a dynamic exercise performed through the range of motion of a joint at a constant velocity. The equipment used in isokinetic exercises accommodates the exerted force to maintain the specified velocity throughout the arc of motion. Because velocity does not change, the kinetic energy remains constant. Isokinetic contractions are not part of normal physiologic muscle function.

Finally, isoinertial contractions define a situation where the muscle contracts against a constant load, but with variable internal force. If the torque generated by the muscle is larger than the resistance (load), the muscle's length will change and the additional torque will accelerate the body segment. This allows for measurements of acceleration and velocity.

The Stimulation and Control Mechanisms

Muscle contraction is initiated and controlled by the somatic nervous system. At the neuromuscular junction, each fiber is innervated by a terminal branch of an efferent nerve fiber. The motor unit is the functional unit of the muscle and represents a group of fibers innervated by branches of the same neural axon (Fig. 3). It varies in size (number of fibers) depending on the function of the muscle. Where precise control is important, the number of fibers is small. In large, coarse muscle, the number is greater. Because the muscle fibers of a motor unit are not in discrete bundles, but are distributed throughout the muscle, a large part of a muscle contracts when a single motor unit is stimulated.

Motor units act according to the law of "all or nothing." When a nerve impulse reaches a motor unit, all the muscle fibers in the unit contract almost simultaneously. An afferent feedback loop is initiated by muscle spindles, oriented parallel to the muscle fibers and anchored to the endo- and perimysium. Passive stretch results in tension

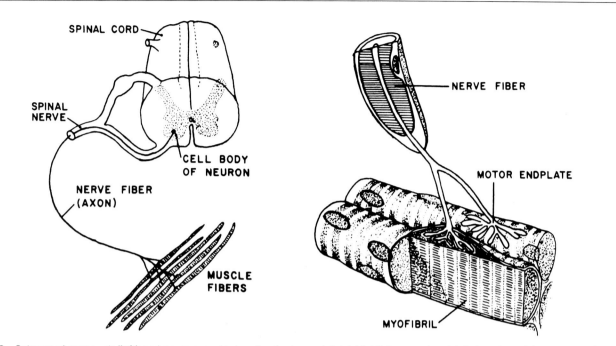

Fig. 3 Scheme of motor unit (**left**) and neuromuscular junction (motor endplate) (**right**) in a greater detail. A motor unit is one nerve fiber and all muscle fibers innervated by that particular fiber. (Adapted with permission from Basmajian JV, in *Muscles Alive*. Baltimore, Williams & Wilkins, 1978, p 8.)

of the spindle, while muscle contraction relieves that tension.

Contraction is initiated by a nerve impulse generated in the nerve axons. A change in the selective permeability of the neural membrane to different ions results in depolarization and generates an action potential transmitted along the axon to the motor endplates. At the motor endplate, neuromuscular transmission is chemically mediated. In the presence of calcium ions, acetylcholine (ACh) is released from the terminal branches of the nerve-axon causing the muscle fiber membranes to depolarize, resulting in a muscle action potential moving along the muscle membrane (sarcolemma).

Energy Sources

The contractile process requires energy (Fig. 4). The immediate source of energy is adenosine triphosphate (ATP), which is split to a lower energy form of adenosine diphosphate (ADP). Within less than a millisecond after a single contractile cycle ends, ADP is converted back to ATP by a reaction with phosphocreatine, another high-energy phosphate available in the muscle. The process described is useful only for brief contractions because ATP is not produced at a rate needed for sustained contraction. After 15 to 30 seconds of strenuous exertions, the phosphocreatine is depleted. In sustained contraction, resynthesis of ATP is necessary to provide continued energy. Two chemical mechanisms can become operational. One is anaerobic metabolism of glycogen, which

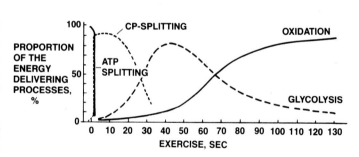

Fig. 4 Schematic representation of substrates supplying energy for muscle contraction at maximum voluntary contraction level. Stored ATP sources supply only immediate needs for initial few muscle contractions. The next source is creatinine phosphate, allowing 30-40 sec of muscular activity. As the creatinine stores become depleted, anaerobic glycolysis becomes the next major source of high-energy nucleotides. With progression of activity, oxidative metabolism of carbohydrates takes over as the major energy source. (Reproduced with permission from Keul J, Doll E, Keppler D: *Energy Metabolism of Human Muscle*. New York, S. Karger, 1972.)

is the primary source of energy in vigorous activity from 30 to 90 seconds, and produces lactate as its end product. The second is resynthesis through an oxidative aerobic metabolic process. This is the main energy source for contractions lasting 90 seconds and longer, and depends on the metabolism of carbohydrate, fat, and protein.

During moderate activity, the oxygen supply is often sufficient to allow the aerobic supply of high-energy phosphates (ATP) to occur. When an individual is working at such a level, a steady state results and muscle fatigue does not develop. At higher levels of activity, the oxygen supply is inadequate and the energy requirement to produce ATP must be met by the anaerobic process. This leads to an accumulation of lactic acid and an oxygen debt. If this oxygen debt is not repaid, muscle fatigue develops.

During exercise at the same intensity, physically trained individuals derive a much greater percentage of their energy from fatty acid oxidation than do untrained individuals. Increasing lipid oxidation during exercise slows the rate of glycolysis and inhibits lactate formation, thereby also influencing the muscle's respiratory capacity. Hence, the beneficial effects of training on endurance performance are not solely the result of increased Vo_2 max. Physical training also produces changes in muscle ultrastructure, capillarization, oxidative capacity, and substrate utilization, all of which may be major determinants of successful, prolonged performance.

Measurements of Muscle Strength

Strength is the ability of a muscle or group of muscles to exert force. By definition, strength is not limited to one particular type of muscle contraction. However, the type of contraction does influence the force output and, therefore, the measurement method must be described—isometric (static strength), isotonic (concentric strength), eccentric, isokinetic, or isoinertial (Table 2).

Maximum strength—the greatest force that a muscle can exert on the skeletal system under a given set of loading conditions—is used most frequently in clinical practice. Because strength varies as a function of joint angle, it is best defined graphically as the force output as a function of the joint angle, referred to as a strength curve. Strength curves can be generated by repeated isometric measures at different joint angles or by dynamic measures in which strength is recorded continuously as a function of the joint angle. Regardless of the method chosen, strength curves are affected by variables such as age, sex, subject motivation, pain, muscle and joint physiology and geometry, and also by the conditions of the exercise. A meaningful test report must define and record all of these parameters.

Men typically have greater muscular strength than women when unnormalized data are compared. Upper body strength in women is reported to be 56% of that in men, trunk strength about 64%, and lower body strength about 72%. When strength is normalized relative to lean body mass, these differences are less apparent. Upper extremity strength, as measured by the ability to do biceps curls, in women increases to 76% of that in men, bench press strength increases to 83%, and leg-press strength increases to 106%. When strength is examined relative to the cross-sectional area of muscle, it is equal in

Table 2. Definitions of muscle contractions

Isometric	The external length of the muscle does not change. Same as static.
Isotonic	The internal force of the muscle does not change but the muscle shortens. Same as concentric.
Eccentric	The external force is greater than the internal force of the muscle, causing a lengthening of the muscle.
Isokinetic	A dynamic exercise where the speed of motion is constant.
Isoinertial	Contraction against a constant load. The torque generated by the muscle causes acceleration.

men and women. Women respond the same as men to exercise and training.

Fiber Types and Response to Training

The function of muscles and their response to training are influenced, in part, by the fiber type, which is genetically determined and differentiated by the characteristics of myosin heavy chains and oxidative metabolism. Type I are slow-twitch fibers with low glycogen and glycolytic enzyme content. High concentrations of mitochondria and associated oxidative phosphorylation enzymes are present. These fibers are most important when there is the demand for high-repetition and low-load endurance activities.

Type II muscle fibers are better adapted for activities that require power and speed. Type IIA and type IIB fibers are differentiated by genetically distinctive heavy myosin chains. Type IIA fibers have a higher concentration of oxidative enzymes. Type IIC fibers contain both type IIA and IIC myosin heavy chains, whereas, type IIM fibers have a third genetically distinctive myosin heavy-chain protein, and are the fastest contracting muscle fibers.

Although all skeletal muscles require load to maintain and increase their functional capability, the fiber types have differing responses to exercise. Endurance training is described as high-repetition, low-load tension activity for a minimum of 30 to 60 minutes. This training regimen is most effective for type I fibers.

There also is a strong association between lactate threshold and ability to perform endurance exercise. The muscle's respiratory capacity has primary importance in determining when blood lactate accumulation begins during exercise. Muscle adapts to training by increasing the concentrations of mitochondria and the enzymes of oxidative metabolism, thus increasing the total oxidative potential of the muscle fibers. Muscle also responds to conditioning by an increased capillarization. Thus, increased fitness improves the body's ability to deliver metabolites to the muscle and the muscle's ability to utilize these metabolites.

The proportion of slow-twitch fibers also may play an important role in determining the relative lactate threshold. One study found the percentage and relative fiber area of slow-twitch fibers were significantly related to the lactate threshold. The ratio of slow-twitch to fast-twitch fibers may exert a genetic influence over the lactate threshold and may control the range within which the lactate threshold can shift. This finding supports a current concept that endurance athletes are born rather than trained.

The functional capacity of type II muscle fibers is increased best by a resistance training program. Progressive load increases are required during strength training to maximize its effects. When type II fibers are trained with high-tension and low-frequency loads, muscle hypertrophy results. The increased bulk represents an increase in the cross-sectional area of individual muscle cells, which is secondary to an increase in the number of myofibrils per fiber in each muscle cell. Although type I fibers undergo some hypertrophy with this type of training, the effects are far greater in type II muscle. However, strength training has minimal effect on capillary density, blood flow to muscles, or oxidative capacity.

Muscle Pain and Injury

Exercise-induced muscle soreness usually occurs 12 to 48 hours after heavy exercise, particularly when the activity involves eccentric exercise. In animal models, multiple cycles of eccentric contractions result in histologic evidence of muscle injury accompanied by a temporary reduction of the isometric strength. In comparison, repetitive isometric and concentric contractions appear to cause relatively minor fiber changes.

These observations have, in part, been confirmed in biopsies taken from marathon runners. Ultra-structural changes, consistent with cell damage and an inflammatory response, are diffuse throughout the muscles tested. However, these changes are temporary and appear to have no lasting negative effects on muscle function.

In comparison, clinically evident muscle strains are partial disruptions of the muscle-tendon unit in response to powerful eccentric contractions. Laboratory investigations confirm the usual site of disruption is at the musculotendinous junction followed by an intense inflammatory reaction and subsequent fibrosis. Magnetic resonance imaging of patients with significant muscle strains indicates a similar pattern of injury and repair in humans.

In laboratory studies, the force required to produce failure varies as a function of muscular strength and fatigue. A contracted muscle can absorb up to twice the energy of an uncontracted muscle before failure. Weak and fatigued muscles are characterized by diminished active force in muscle and can absorb less energy before failing.

Direct Muscle Injuries and Repair

Direct injury is the result of a laceration or a direct blow to the muscle; indirect injury is the result of a strain or muscle damage caused by excessive stretch, muscle contraction, or both.

Laceration

Few clinical and research studies have dealt with the recovery of muscle after laceration and surgical repair. Muscle tissue can be sutured if the connective tissues or tendons around the muscle provide enough holding strength for sutures. In very thin muscles, the defect may be bridged by normal muscle tissue. In larger muscles, healing usually occurs with a dense scar at the laceration site.

Following injury, the physiologic function, in part, is determined by the neural supply to the injured muscle segments. In one study, the portion of the muscle containing the motor point remained physiologically active, whereas the portion of the muscle separated from the motor point and from intramuscular innervation became fibrotic, with many histologic features of denervated muscle. However, the portion isolated from the motor point was able to transmit tension and shortening generated in the innervated portion. The extent of physiologic recovery also depends on the architectural arrangement of the muscle fibers. In general, the ability of muscle to produce tension is proportional to the cross-sectional area of muscle fibers, and the ability to shorten is relative to the length of the muscle fibers. Following disruption of a penniform muscle, only the muscle segment containing the nerve supply continues to function. Because only half of the muscle fibers are in this section, only half of the tension of the whole muscle can be generated. The intact fibers are their full original length and therefore shortening near the normal amount is possible when imposed loads are light. The distal segment becomes fibrotic and is able to transmit the tension in the proximal innervated segment. The distal segment remains viable if its blood supply is not destroyed, but it cannot function as active muscle if isolated from its nerve supply.

Blunt Trauma

Unlike laceration, blunt trauma produces muscle injury without disrupting the muscle belly. Blunt trauma can affect the deeper muscles in proximity to bone and can result in myositis ossificans. In the laboratory, standardized and controlled blunt trauma causes disruption of the muscle fibers similar to a laceration. There is an initial intense inflammatory reaction with eventual clearing of the necrotic muscle and formation of a dense connective tissue scar, which disrupts the continuity of the muscle fibers. Younger animals demonstrate more rapid and intense healing than older animals. The associated formation of heterotrophic bone following blunt trauma is variable, and appears to result from metaplastic ossification.

Repair

The events following muscle injury have been studied at the cellular and ultrastructural levels, most commonly in ischemic models of injury. Following an ischemic episode, there is early damage to muscle membrane, loss of sarcomeres and Z-bands, mitochondrial swelling, and nuclear pyknosis. If circulation is intact, macrophages then penetrate the basal lamina of the muscle cells and phagocytize the necrotic muscle fibers. As repair progresses, primitive muscle cells (myoblasts) appear within the remaining cell membrane to form a new myotube, which contains muscle fibers. Eventually, the central myoblastic cells migrate to the periphery of the newly formed muscle fiber to complete regeneration. Failure of muscle to regenerate after injury is associated primarily with overgrowth of fibrous connective tissue, which inhibits further regeneration and reformation of muscle tubules.

The innervation remaining to the injured muscle determines the type of muscle fiber formed during regeneration. Type II regeneration occurs when the motor nerves are type II. Similarly, type I muscle regeneration depends on type I motor nerve fibers.

Effects of Immobilization

The results of immobilization are muscular atrophy, often accompanied by joint stiffness and contracture. Depending on the position of the injured limb, sarcomeres are added or deleted primarily at the musculotendinous junction. These changes in sarcomere length accommodate the muscle length to the position of immobilization. Immobilization also accelerates the production of granulation tissue in injured muscle. In animal models, immobilization for as little as five days results in a contracting scar. Poor structural reorganization of muscle and scarring occurred after this brief period of immobilization. Muscle that heals in a shortened position is at greater risk for rerupture. In comparison, healing in a long position reduces the risk of reinjury.

Muscle Inhibition

Immobilization or injury can cause muscular inhibition, which is characterized by an inability of the nervous system to control the muscle and to recruit all the muscle fibers effectively. Even after arthroscopic knee surgery, the maximal muscle force is significantly and persistently reduced for days. A less dramatic but similar event occurs after the injection of saline into normal knee joints to simulate an effusion. The reduced ability of the quadriceps to produce force is thought to be secondary to nociceptors and other sensory receptors about the joint. Thus, there may be two very different effects on the muscle following immobilization and injury—the direct effect of immobilization and disuse and the effect of altered nervous system recruitment.

Electrical Stimulation

To overcome muscular inhibition and maintain muscle force, electrical stimulation has been used in immobilized limbs. Following electrical stimulation there are increases in muscle weight, fiber diameter, and ratio changes in fiber type. However, these effects are less than those produced by conventional isotonic contractions. An increase in capillary number, capillary density, and the ratio of capillaries to muscle fibers is observed, as well as a decrease in intercapillary distance.

Compartment Syndromes

Acute

Ischemia accompanied by increased pressure produces muscle injury more severe than that produced by ischemia alone. What constitutes the threshold of muscle and limb injury in the presence of increased compartment pressures is debated. Although absolute measurement of compartment pressures has been used in the past, many investigators believe relative values of intracompartmental pressures and perfusion pressures are more reliable. When the pressure difference between the compartment and arterial pressure is less than 30 mm Hg, the muscle is unable to maintain its normal metabolic state (Fig. 5). A larger pressure differential (at least 40 mm Hg) is required if there has been moderate trauma.

Because there are no absolutely established threshold values, debate continues as to when surgical decompression is required. Factors that must be considered include the magnitude of trauma to the muscle and the diastolic or mean arterial pressure as well as the compartment pressure.

Chronic

Persisting or recurrent pretibial pain after exercise may be caused by periostitis, superficial peroneal nerve compression, medial tibial syndrome, muscle hernias, and compartment syndromes. The criterion for the diagnosis of chronic, exertional compartment syndrome has been debated, and includes increased pressures before, during, and after exercise. In one report, only 25% of patients examined because of a possible diagnosis of lower leg chronic compartment syndrome eventually fulfilled the criterion.

In the lower extremity, the anterior compartment is most frequently involved and the superficial posterior compartment is least often involved. A fascial defect may be present in as many as 40% of patients, usually over the distal portion of the compartment where a branch of the superficial peroneal nerve penetrates the fascia. An accompanying superficial peroneal nerve entrapment is sometimes present.

The initial treatment of chronic lower extremity compartment symptoms requires modification of activity. If these measures fail, surgical fasciotomy of the involved

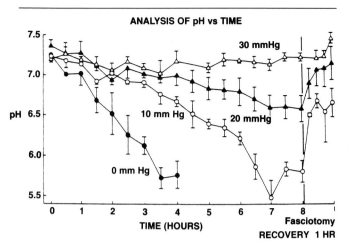

ANALYSIS OF pH vs TIME

30 mmHg

10 mm Hg   20 mmHg

0 mm Hg

Fasciotomy
RECOVERY 1 HR

Fig. 5 The mean intracellular pH is plotted as a function of time in groups with differences between mean arterial blood pressure and the compartment pressure. It is clear that with a pressure differential of 30 mm Hg, there is little effect on intracellular pH. The effect increases as the pressure differential is smaller. (Reproduced with permission from Heppenstall RB, Sapega AA, Scott R, et al: The compartment syndrome: An experimental and clinical study of muscular energy metabolism using phosphorus nuclear magnetic resonance spectroscopy. *Clin Orthop* 1988;226:138-155.)

compartment will generally allow athletes to return to their desired activity level. The success rate is best when the anterior compartment is involved. However, success rates are acceptable for exertional deep compartment syndrome. A complete surgical release of the posterior compartment fascia and the fascial covering of the tibialis posterior is required. Once a fascial defect is made it should never be repaired, because, after repair, an acute compartment syndrome can ensue, with catastrophic consequences.

A less common acute or chronic compartment syndrome has also been reported in the lumbar paraspinal muscles. The acute syndrome is characterized by severe back pain, muscle rigidity, elevation of muscle enzymes, and myoglobinurea. Enlargement of the paraspinal muscles is observed in MRI images. This rare condition is differentiated from idiopathic rhabdomyolysis. A chronic compartment syndrome has also been proposed as a cause of recurrent back pain after exercise. Although pressure measurements have established the normal behavior of a paraspinal compartment, currently there are no strict criteria to identify patients for whom this diagnosis might be entertained.

Normal Gait

Descriptions of how people walk are best done by describing the gait cycle, which begins when one foot strikes the ground and ends when it strikes the ground again. The gait cycle is divided into swing and stance phases. Swing phase, when the limb is unsupported, has been further divided into initial, mid-, and terminal thirds. Throughout swing, the pelvis rotates forward; the hip flexes to about 30 degrees; the knee flexes 60 degrees initially and extends terminally; and the ankle plantarflexes 10 degrees initially and becomes neutral terminally. The hip flexors are the main motors advancing the limb in the first two-thirds of swing. The ankle dorsiflexors assure clearance in the final two-thirds of swing. The hamstring muscles decelerate the thigh in the terminal one-third of swing.

Stance phase has five parts: contact, loading, midstance, terminal stance, and preswing. Throughout stance the pelvis gradually rotates backward and the hip extends. At initial contact, the knee is extended and the ankle is neutral (or slightly plantarflexed). During loading, the knee flexes 15 degrees while the ankle plantarflexes 15 degrees, which is an energy-conserving mechanism. By midstance the knee is extended and the ankle is neutral again. At preswing, the knee flexes 35 degrees and the ankle plantarflexes 20 degrees. In these last phases of stance, the toes, which have been neutral, dorsiflex at the metatarsophalangeal joints. Throughout the first phase of stance, the hamstrings and ankle dorsiflexors remain active. The quadriceps and gluteal muscles act during loading and throughout early midstance to maintain hip and knee stability. In midstance, the triceps surae acts to control tibial advancement.

Stance phase represents about 60% of the gait cycle, swing 40%. Double support, when both feet are in contact with the ground, lasts about 10% of the whole gait cycle. Normal gait is symmetric and, thus, the relationship between the swing and stance phases of each leg are consistent. Step length is the distance between two feet at stance, while one stride is the sum of the right and left step lengths—a full gait cycle. Cadence is the number of steps per unit time, and walking velocity is the step length times the cadence.

Normal gait requires stability in stance phase, a means of progression, and energy conservation. Stability requires constant balancing of the trunk over the base of support. During progression, potential energy is converted into kinetic energy. Much of the kinetic energy for the swinging limb is provided by inertia, which is augmented by the plantarflexors (85%) and hip flexors (15%). Energy is conserved by minimizing the movements of the center of gravity of the body, by controlling momentum, and by transfer of energy between body segments.

When analyzing gait, it is important to remember the dependence of time-distance, kinematic, and kinetic parameters on each other. Stride length, for example, varies with walking speed, although the relationship tends to be reproducible in a healthy individual. Joint angles and moments also vary with walking speed. To compare individuals, or the same individual on different occasions, walking speed must be taken into account.

Analysis of Gait

The sophisticated analysis of gait measures the kinematics of body segments in three dimensions, the ground reaction forces, muscle activity, and sometimes oxygen consumption. A variety of commercially available systems have certain commonalities including three-dimensional video cameras, foot force plates, and computer systems for processing generated data.

The three-dimensional cameras measure the kinematics of limb segments expressed as joint angles and velocity during each segment of the gait cycle. The foot force plates measure the direction, magnitude, and area of contact during the stance phase. In addition to displaying normal and abnormal force patterns, the force plate can also be used to assess the effects of walking aids and braces.

Calculations of the external moments about the hip, knee, and ankle joints requires synchronization of the force platform and motion data, and the integration of these data into biomechanical models. Joint moments are meaningful, because their magnitude and direction relate to muscular activities and joint loading. For example, the normal flexion-extension moment at the knee joint is biplane, oscillating about the 0 position. This corresponds to the location of the ground-reaction-force vector. For amputees, moment information for normal and prosthetic limbs allows immediate adjustments to the hydraulic mechanism so that optimal function can be determined objectively.

Dynamic electromyography provides information on when a particular muscle is activated, which normally is no more than 30% to 40% of the entire gait cycle. The timing of muscle activity within the gait cycle can be used to compare a given subject's performance with normal values. However, the magnitude of the myoelectric signal does not represent the absolute force of the muscle. Therefore, reliable comparisons cannot be made between individuals, or between an individual's performance at separate testing sessions.

Two electromyographic methods are employed commonly. The least invasive uses surface electrodes, which record electrical activity from more than one muscle. The more precise, but invasive, method uses bipolar wires inserted into the muscle. When the insertion site is selected properly, an accurate representation of the electrical activity of the entire muscle can be obtained.

Gait Abnormalities

Sophisticated gait analysis is used to assess abnormalities produced by neurologic, muscular, and arthritic disorders and to analyze the effects of surgery or nonsurgical treatment.

Arthritis

Gait analysis is used in patients with arthritis to determine the mechanical changes brought on by the disease, or injury. Characteristic adaptations of gait differ, depending on the joint(s) involved. The primary purpose of these adaptations is to reduce pain by reducing loading of the joint. In general, arthritic patients have significantly decreased walking velocity, cadence, and stride length. Of greater interest has been the effects of surgical interventions, particularly joint replacement. These data also allow a better understanding of the characteristics of joint loading, stress distribution, and the biologic response of bones to stress.

Comparisons have been made of cemented and noncemented total hip replacements. The gait variable that provides the best objective evidence of a change in a patient's ambulatory status is weightbearing capacity, not joint motion. Maximal vertical force and average velocity were the only variables that distinguished between the two prosthetic types.

Persistent abnormalities noted following total knee replacement include shorter than normal stride length, reduced midstance knee flexion, and abnormalities in the flexion-extension moment. These differences are observed even in patients who are asymptomatic and whose clinical result is rated excellent.

Neuromuscular Disorders

The characteristic gait abnormality of children with cerebral palsy is abnormal timing of muscle activity. Abnormalities are also identified in velocity, cadence, and stride length. These parameters change with age as they do in normal children. Stride length increases and stride frequency (cadence) decreases, although they never achieve normal values. Some of these characteristics are found in children with idiopathic toe walking. Idiopathic toe walkers also show abnormalities in muscle timing, similar to those seen in children with cerebral palsy and equinus deformities. However, the characteristic family history, predominance of males, and learning disabilities associated with idiopathic toe walking suggest that it is a distinct entity.

In the adult, hemiplegias secondary to stroke or head injury demonstrate characteristic abnormalities in gait. In the stance phase, there is an equinus deformity of the ankle and, sometimes, increased hip flexion. A further subclassification characterizes the gait as follows: In type I there is a compensated back-knee deformity and symmetric steps. In type II there is a hyperextension of the knee and increased stance flexion of the hip. The steps of the unaffected limb decrease to 50% of normal, and there are prolonged periods of double limb support. Type III produces such instability that the uninvolved limb cannot advance past the affected stationary limb. Circumduction of the affected limb is often required to achieve toe clearance.

The walking performance of selected hemiplegic patients often can be improved with orthoses or tendon surgery. Ankle-foot orthoses can increase walking speed. Key to the outcome is proper adjustment of plantarflexion. Improper adjustments can result in an exaggerated knee-flexion moment and produce greater knee instability.

It is estimated that 50% of hemiplegics can be improved by surgical interventions and can achieve brace-free function. The usual approach is lengthening of the Achilles tendon, often with split transfer of the anterior tibial tendon. Selective muscle releases may also benefit some patients. A successful outcome may allow the patient to achieve normal values for stance and for the double support phase of gait.

Sports Medicine
Gait Analysis in Athletes

Sophisticated gait analysis techniques are increasingly applied to athletes to more accurately define motion patterns, muscle actions, and forces occurring during sports activities. In these patients, deficits may only be apparent when the functional demands are high. For example, running requires greater muscular effort and larger arcs of joint motions, and it generates higher forces than walking. Also, there is no double support phase in running. The flexion moments about the knee joint become seven to eight times greater than those imposed by walking.

Studies of running, cutting, stopping, and jumping have helped determine the consequences of cruciate ligament tears, and the effectiveness of knee braces. Cutting, defined as a quick turn while running over an abruptly stabilized foot, imposes high loading and torsional forces on the knee. Although the running gait of an individual with an anterior cruciate tear may appear normal, these people often are unable to cut, or they perform a protective maneuver to reduce the vertical force and external torque. Following cruciate reconstruction, those classified as stable perform more normally than those classified as having residual instability. The results do not appear to be influenced by whether the repairs performed are acute or delayed. Braces provide little functional gain, other than reducing knee motion. Their effects on cutting performance are debated.

Patients with posterior cruciate ligament tears have been analyzed with or without surgical reconstruction using the medial head of the gastrocnemius. The untreated group walk more slowly, with less movement of the knee than the operated group. Although the pattern of muscle activity is generally similar to the normal pattern, floor-reaction forces are lower for the involved limb than the healthy one, particularly in the untreated group. These differences are thought to be an accommodation to a weak quadriceps and a way of guarding the posterior joint structures from stretch.

Annotated Bibliography

Muscle General

Caplan A, Carlson B, Faulkner J, et al: Skeletal muscle, in Woo SL-Y, Buckwalter JA (eds): *Injury and Repair of the Musculoskeletal Soft Tissues*. Park Ridge, IL, American Academy of Orthopaedic Surgeons, 1988, pp 213-291.

This is the definitive review of the nature of muscle injury and repair, summarizing current knowledge of muscle types and regeneration.

Sapega AA: Muscle performance evaluation in orthopaedic practice. *J Bone Joint Surg* 1990;72A:1562-1574.

This current concepts review focuses on the principles, advantages, disadvantages, and limitations of current methods to evaluate muscular performance. Basic concepts, current test methods, and interpretation of data from quantitative testing of muscular performance are critically reviewed.

Muscle Injury

Garrett WE Jr, Nikolaou PK, Ribbeck BM, et al: The effect of muscle architecture on the biomechanical failure properties of skeletal muscle under passive extension. *Am J Sport Med* 1988;16:7-12.

This study demonstrated the mechanism of failure of muscle in response to passive stretch. Failure occurred routinely near the myotendinous junction.

Garrett WE Jr, Safran MD, Seaber AV, et al: Biomechanical comparison of stimulated and nonstimulated skeletal muscle pulled to failure. *Am J Sports Med* 1987;15:448-454.

Rabbit hind limb muscles were strained to failure while the motor nerve was maximally stimulated to provide a model of eccentric contraction. The muscle did not tear at a significantly different length; its maximal force was slightly increased, but the energy absorbed before failure was much higher in contracting muscles than in passively stretched muscle.

Lieber RL, Fridén JL, McKee-Woodburn TG: Selective damage of fast glycolytic muscle fibers with eccentric exercise of the rabbit tibialis anterior. *Trans Orthop Res Soc* 1988;13:337.

This abstract clearly delineates selective damage to type II muscle fibers from eccentric exercise.

Lieber RL, Woodburn TM, Fridén J: Muscle damage induced by eccentric contractions of 25% strain. *J Appl Physiol* 1991;70:2498-2507.

Eccentric contraction of the rabbit tibialis anterior muscle resulted in significant muscle injury after even a brief period.

Risser WL: Musculoskeletal injuries caused by weight training: Guidelines for prevention. *Clin Pediatr* 1990;29:305-310.

Weight training for sports is used in the United States by a large number of children, adolescents, and young adults. Injury risks are surprisingly high but can be reduced by attention to technique, training routine, and equipment.

Effects of Immobilization

Booth FW: Physiologic and biochemical effects of immobilization on muscle. *Clin Orthop* 1987;219:15-20.

There are profound changes in muscle strength and in muscle fatigability after immobilization. Strategies to avoid these changes are presented.

Effects of Electrical Stimulation

Cabric M, Appell HJ, Resic A: Stereological analysis of capillaries in electrostimulated human muscles. *Int J Sports Med* 1987;8:327-330.

The effects of two different electrical stimulation protocols (50 Hz or 2 kHz, each for 21 days) were investigated by means of biopsy specimens taken before and after the study.

Snyder-Mackler L, Ladin Z, Schepsis AA, et al: Electrical stimulation of the thigh muscles after reconstruction of the anterior cruciate ligament. *J Bone Joint Surg* 1991;73A:1025-1036.

Neuromuscular electrical stimulation and exercise and exercise alone were compared in a group of patients after reconstruction of the anterior cruciate ligament. The patients who received stimulation had stronger quadriceps muscles and a more normal gait pattern.

Compartment Syndromes

Fronek J, Mubarak SJ, Hargens AR, et al: Management of chronic exertional anterior compartment syndrome of the lower extremity. *Clin Orthop* 1987;220:217-227.

Intramuscular pressures of 10 mm Hg or more at rest and/or 25 mm Hg or more five minutes after exercise was defined as abnormally increased in 18 patients with chronic compartment syndrome. Fasciotomy or reduction of exertional activities was found to be an effective treatment.

Heppenstall RB, Sapega AA, Scott R, et al: The compartment syndrome: An experimental and clinical study of muscular energy metabolism using phosphorus nuclear magnetic resonance spectroscopy. *Clin Orthop* 1988;226:138-155.

Experimental ischemic compartment syndrome was studied in dogs using nuclear magnetic resonance spectroscopy. The injury threshold was defined in terms of a pressure difference between the mean arterial blood pressure and the compartment pressure.

Pedowitz RA, Gershuni DH, Schmidt AH, et al: Muscle injury induced beneath and distal to a pneumatic tourniquet: A quantitative animal study of effects of tourniquet pressure and duration. *J Hand Surg* 1991;16A:610-621.

Two hours of continuous tourniquet application at clinically relevant cuff inflation pressures induced significant skeletal muscle necrosis beneath the tourniquet. The lowest possible inflation pressure and shortest possible time should be used to minimize the degree of injury.

Rorabeck CH, Fowler PJ, Nott L: The results of fasciotomy in the management of chronic exertional compartment syndrome. *Am J Sports Med* 1988;16:224-227.

Fasciotomy of the anterior compartment gave excellent relief of pain in 22 of 25 patients who had resting pressures in excess of 15 mm Hg and increased pressures after exercise with delayed normalization.

Styf J: Diagnosis of exercise-induced pain in the anterior aspect of the lower leg. *Am J Sports Med* 1988;16:165-169.

In a series of 98 patients chronic compartment syndrome was found to be an uncommon cause of chronic exercise-induced pain in the anterior compartment of the lower leg.

Gait

Andriacchi TP: Evaluation of surgical procedures and/or joint implants with gait analysis, in Greene WB (ed): *Instructional Course Lectures XXXIX*. Park Ridge, IL, American Academy of Orthopaedic Surgeons, 1990, pp 343-350.

This chapter describes how gait analysis has been used to evaluate surgical procedures and joint implants. It emphasizes the use of the joint moment as a method of analysis.

Gage JR: An overview of normal walking, in Greene WB (ed): *Instructional Course Lectures XXXIX*. Park Ridge, IL, American Academy of Orthopaedic Surgeons, 1990, pp 291-303.

This text describes normal walking and gait analysis comprehensively but in easily understandable terms.

Perry J: Pathologic gait, in Greene WB (ed): *Instructional Course Lectures XXXIX*. Park Ridge, IL, American Academy of Orthopaedic Surgeons, 1990, pp 325-331.

Principle gait deviations associated with pathologic gait are described.

Sutherland DH: Gait analysis in neuromuscular diseases, in Greene WB (ed): *Instructional Course Lectures XXXIX*. Park Ridge, IL, American Academy of Orthopaedic Surgeons, 1990, pp 333-341.

A summary of studies of gait in patients with neuromuscular diseases.

Instrumentation Systems

Claeys R: The analysis of ground reaction forces in pathological gait secondary to disorders of the foot. *Int Orthop* 1983;7:113-119.

The normal gait pattern is characterized by a marked population variability, a considerable step-to-step consistency, and symmetry of the forces from both feet. The force pattern in pathologic gait secondary to disorders of the foot also shows a marked repeatability but is characterized by a pronounced asymmetry. A specific disorder of the foot does not necessarily result in a typical corresponding force pattern.

Opila KA, Nicol AC, Paul JP: Forces and impulses during aided gait. *Arch Phys Med Rehabil* 1987;68:715-722.

The relative contributions of limbs and aids were quantified in three patient groups: those with total hip replacements, those with tibial fractures, and those with paraplegia. Results showed (1) variability in aid loadings among the subjects with total hip replacements and between ipsilateral and contralateral sticks; (2) symmetric restraining and propelling aid loadings in those with fractures; and (3) greater aid impulses medially than anteroposteriorly in four of seven subjects performing three-point gait.

Arthritis

Mansour JM, Pereira JM: Quantitative functional anatomy of the lower limb with application to human gait. *J Biomech* 1987;20:51-58.

The functions of muscles crossing the hip and knee joints were computed on the basis of the changing relative positions of joint centers and muscle origins and insertions during one gait cycle. The function of several of the major muscles crossing the hip and knee joints was recorded for the different limb positions corresponding to normal gait. The amount of force necessary to produce a given moment about a joint depended on the limb position. In addition, muscle function changed significantly with limb position.

Willmott M: The effect of a vinyl floor surface and a carpeted floor surface upon walking in elderly hospital in-patients. *Age Ageing* 1986;15:119-120.

Fifty-eight elderly hospital patients walked along a 20-m length of carpet corridor and 10-m length of vinyl-tiled corridor. Gait speed and step length were significantly greater on the carpeted than on the vinyl surface.

Cerebral Palsy

Gage JR: Computer based decision making, in Sussman MD (ed): *The Diplegic Child: Evaluation and Management*. Rosemont, IL, American Academy of Orthopaedic Surgeons, 1992, pp 187-201.

This chapter discusses the routine use of gait analysis in the management of gait problems.

Norlin R, Odenrick P: Development of gait in spastic children with cerebral palsy. *J Pediatr Orthop* 1986;6:674-680.

The gait of 50 spastic children, 3 to 16 years old, showed abnormal values for the basal parameters of phases of the stride. Although values for gait velocity and stride length were lower than normal, they increased with age. Stance phase was longer than in normal children, the same tendency shown by double support. Most changes with age were the same as those in normal children. The prolonged stance and double support suggest deteriorated postural control, resulting in an increased need for support.

Olney SJ, Costigan PA, Hedden DM: Mechanical energy patterns in gait of cerebral palsied children with hemiplegia. *Phys Ther* 1987;67:1348-1354.

The mechanical energy costs of walking were studied in ten children with cerebral palsy and hemiplegia to determine whether their values were substantially different from normal and, if so, to discover the movements responsible. A two-dimensional, sagittal-plane cinematographic analysis of the subjects' normal walking was undertaken. In most cases, the energy costs were above normal and were attributable to poor patterns of exchange between the potential and kinetic energy types of the head, arms, and trunk segment, to very low levels of kinetic energy that precluded exchange, or to both.

Rab GT: Diplegic gait: Is there more than spasticity? in Sussman MD (ed): *The Diplegic Child: Evaluation and Management*. Rosemont, IL, American Academy of Orthopaedic Surgeons, 1992, pp 99-110.

The unique nature of diplegic gait is confirmed through comparison with gait of spinal-cord injured patients.

Hemiplegia

Holden MK, Gill KM, Magliozzi MR: Gait assessment for neurologically impaired patients: Standards for outcome assessment. *Phys Ther* 1986;66:1530-1539.

The authors compared the time-distance gait values of two groups of neurologically impaired subjects with those of healthy subjects and analyzed the influence of nine clinical characteristics. Velocity, cadence, step length, stride length, and ratio of stride length to lower-extremity length were recorded for 37 subjects with hemiplegia and 24 subjects with multiple sclerosis. Time-distance values were well below normal values, even in functionally independent subjects. Overall, the subjects with hemiparesis had lower values than the subjects with multiple sclerosis.

Maležič M, Bogataj U, Gros N, et al: Evaluation of gait with multichannel electrical stimulation. *Orthopaedics* 1987;10:769-772.

Short, intensive multichannel electrical stimulation therapy was evaluated in 14 hemiplegic patients after stroke or head injury. The stimulation of the peroneal nerve and the soleus, quadriceps, hamstring, gluteus maximus, and triceps brachii muscles with individually preprogrammed sequences was applied by surface electrodes at the beginning of gait rehabilitation. The patients started walking with the support of a therapist, gradually increasing the walking distance. All achieved independent ambulation with a crutch after an average of 14 stimulation sessions.

Sports Medicine

Perry J: Gait analysis in sports medicine, in Greene WB (ed): *Instructional Course Lectures XXXIX*. Park Ridge, IL, American Academy of Orthopaedic Surgeons, 1990, pp 319-324.

This review article succinctly summarizes important information on sports medicine obtained in the gait laboratory.

10

Ligament Injury and Repair

Ligament Biomechanics

The basic processes involved in ligament injury and repair have received major attention in recent years. Most studies have involved the ligaments of the knee because of their clinical significance.

The anterior cruciate ligament (ACL) is a key structure in providing stability to the knee. To understand the biomechanical behavior of a normal anterior cruciate ligament or a soft-tissue graft, both structural and mechanical (material) properties must be appreciated. Structural failure properties describe the behavior of the femur-anterior cruciate ligament-tibia complex and are measured by the load-displacement response of a ligament specimen using a tensile load-to-failure test. These properties describe both insertion-site and midsubstance behavior

of the ligament, and they include linear stiffness, ultimate load, and energy absorbed at failure (Fig. 1).

Mechanical, or material, failure properties describe the behavior of the ligament substance isolated from the insertion-site effects and may also be measured by failure testing of isolated anterior cruciate ligament specimens. These properties include the tangent modulus, ultimate stress, and strain at failure (Fig. 1).

The structural failure properties of the anterior cruciate ligament have been shown to be affected by specimen orientation during failure testing. Tensile failure testing with the loading applied along a bony axis will produce different results from those of failure tests performed with load applied along the length of the ligament fibers. Animal studies of anterior cruciate ligament reconstruc-

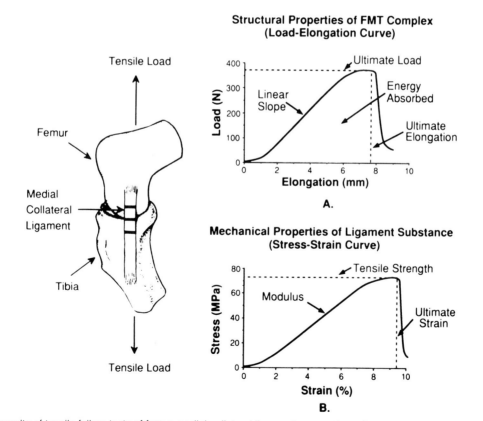

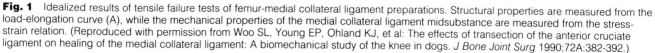

Fig. 1 Idealized results of tensile failure tests of femur-medial collateral ligament preparations. Structural properties are measured from the load-elongation curve (A), while the mechanical properties of the medial collateral ligament midsubstance are measured from the stress-strain relation. (Reproduced with permission from Woo SL, Young EP, Ohland KJ, et al: The effects of transection of the anterior cruciate ligament on healing of the medial collateral ligament: A biomechanical study of the knee in dogs. *J Bone Joint Surg* 1990;72A:382-392.)

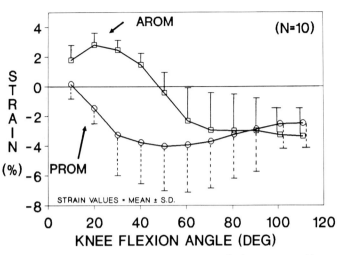

Fig. 2 Normal anterior cruciate ligament strain data measured in ten volunteers in vivo. Included are anterior cruciate ligament strain values for the seated subject extending the lower leg against gravity (active range of motion - AROM), and values derived from the investigator's coursing a subject's knee through the same range of motion without contraction of the lower limb musculature (passive range of motion - PROM). These PROM data are important criteria to reproduce at the time of anterior cruciate ligament reconstruction. (Reproduced with permission from Beynnon BD, Howe JG, Pope MH, et al: The measurement of anterior cruciate ligament strain in vivo. *Int Orthop (SICOT)* 1992;16:1-12.)

tion that report an inappropriately low failure strength value for the normal control will produce an inappropriately high operated-to-control failure strength ratio. The structural failure properties of the anterior cruciate ligament change as the specimen ages. There is also a higher incidence of ligament substance failures in older specimens, which suggests that the ligament substance deteriorates faster than the insertion sites as the specimen ages.

Measurement of the mechanical properties of cruciate ligament subbundles dissected from human cadaver specimens has shown that spatial variations in strain values exist along the length of the ligaments, with greater magnitudes of strain occurring at the insertion sites. Anterior ACL subbundles have significantly larger strain energy density and stress values at failure compared with posterior ACL subbundles. All ACL subbundles have similar maximum strain values at failure, indicating that each subbundle fails by a strain-dependent mechanism.

In vitro investigations have revealed that passive knee extension produces forces along the anterior cruciate ligament only during the last ten degrees of knee extension. At five degrees of hyperextension, the anterior cruciate ligament forces range between 50 and 240 newtons. Hyperextension of the knee develops much higher forces in the anterior cruciate than in the posterior cruciate ligament. These human cadaveric studies have suggested that the compressive joint load produced by body weight protects the anterior cruciate ligament from the high forces that are developed by applied anterior tibial shear force.

In vivo investigations of the strain behavior of the anteromedial portion of the normal anterior cruciate ligament have been performed in patient volunteers undergoing diagnostic arthroscopic surgery. These studies demonstrate that anteroposterior shear loading of the tibia relative to the femur at 30 degrees (the Lachman test) is a better examination technique than similar tests performed at 90 degrees of flexion (the drawer test). During isometric quadriceps contraction, values of anterior cruciate ligament strain measured at 30 degrees of knee flexion were significantly higher than those observed at 90 degrees, where the ligament remained unstrained with isometric quadriceps activity. These studies indicate that quadriceps activity with the knee in a flexed position may be considered a safe rehabilitation activity immediately after anterior cruciate ligament reconstruction. Active extension of the knee between the limits of 50 and 110 degrees does not strain the anterior cruciate; therefore, this activity presents minimal risk of overstraining an anterior cruciate graft (Fig. 2).

The anterior cruciate ligament does not remain an isometric, or constant length, structure as the knee is flexed and extended. Rather, the ligament increases in strain magnitude as the lower leg is passively extended, with the femur in a horizontal plane (Fig. 2). Consequently, reconstruction of the anterior cruciate ligament should not strive to achieve an isometric placement of the graft, but rather reproduce the strain behavior of the normal anterior cruciate ligament (Fig. 2).

Failure analysis of the inferior glenohumeral ligament has demonstrated that the ultimate stress at failure is significantly less than other soft-tissue structures such as the cruciate ligaments. This suggests that the inferior glenohumeral ligament may not be capable of independently stabilizing the glenohumeral joint.

Stress Deprivation Effects

The effects of immobilization without injury have been studied. Immobilization significantly decreases the strength and energy-absorbing capacity of rabbit bone-ligament-bone preparations. The effect is most obvious at the ligament-bone junction. A period of immobilization leads to an increased likelihood that failure in response to strain would occur at the junction. Under conditions of stress deprivation, there is increased osteoclastic activity at the junctional region of bone. Stress deprivation decreases strength in the ligament and in the junction. The effects are more pronounced at the junction, however, with functional failure becoming more likely with increased immobilization. This effect is reversible. After immobilization the junction regains its strength, although relatively slowly. Four to 12 months of recovery may be needed before the junction recovers its normal biomechanical characteristics.

The age of the animal is also important. For immature animals, failure occurs preferentially at the bone-ligament junction. After epiphyseal closure in rabbits, the site of injury shifts from the junction to the ligament substance. Maturation leads to increased strength of the ligament substance and the junction. Near the time of epiphyseal closure, junction strength exceeds that of the ligament substance. The strengths of both level off soon after skeletal maturity is reached.

Activity level and exercise have been shown to be important in ligament and junction biomechanics. Exercise has significant effects on the strength of bone-ligament-bone preparations. Ultrastructurally, these changes correlate with differences in the collagen fibrils. Rats subjected to intensive training demonstrate a decrease in the size of collagen fibrils and an increase in the number of fibrils. These changes are not associated with change in the tensile strength of the ligaments; however, the exercised ligaments are less stiff than controls.

The Biology of Repair

After injury, a ligament undergoes a reparative process similar to that of other healing tissues. The initial hematoma causes the associated blood-borne cells and injured tissue cells to secrete a number of active cytokines leading to inflammation. Capillary permeability and increased cellularity are the result of chemotaxis and differentiation of the incoming cells.

Cells from different ligaments behave differently after injury. The anterior cruciate ligament cells, for example, which are similar morphologically to fibrocartilage cells, migrate more slowly than medial collateral ligament cells. This cellular property may be an important factor in the poor healing characteristics of anterior cruciate ligament injuries.

Collagen synthesis and degradation proceed simultaneously, as in other types of wound healing, but collagen content increases. The initial collagen is type III, although later the composition changes to predominantly type I. Glycosaminoglycans also increase in the early phase of wound healing. With remodeling and maturation, the contents gradually return toward normal.

Injured ligaments sometimes demonstrate the ability to contract or to "tighten up." Rat medial collateral ligaments Z-lengthened are able to contract to normal tightness in three weeks. There is an associated increase in the amount of actin as measured by immunofluorescent staining. Actin is the same contractile protein found in the thin filaments of muscle sarcomeres and in the cytoplasm of mobile cells. It is interesting to consider that the repairing tissue has the ability to contract by a mechanism involving proteins and mechanisms similar to those in the contractile process of muscle.

Quantitative analysis of the collagen fibril diameter of anterior cruciate ligament autografts removed from human subjects nine months to six years after implantation have demonstrated that the remodeled grafts do not re-form the large diameter and tightly packed fibrils seen in the normal anterior cruciate ligament. Analysis of anterior cruciate ligament allografts has produced similar results. These findings may explain the decreased tensile strength of the grafts compared with the normal anterior cruciate ligament.

The Effect of Repair of the MCL

Isolated injuries to medial collateral ligaments in canine and rat models recover well without surgery. After simple sectioning with a scalpel cut, the results in surgically treated groups are not as good as the results obtained without surgery and without immobilization. Investigations that have combined a "mop-end" midsubstance tear with an insertion-site medial collateral ligament injury have not demonstrated a significant difference between surgical and nonsurgical treatment groups in structural or mechanical properties of the healing ligament.

The secondary restraints to valgus knee motion, especially the anterior cruciate ligament, are sufficient to maintain knee stability and to allow healing in the presence of unrestricted knee motion. When the secondary restraints are also injured, however, the medial collateral ligament recovery is not as successful and the ligament may heal in the lengthened position.

The Effect of Stress and Strain on Healing

Ligament repair progresses more rapidly and to a better mechanical and physiologic status if the repair is subjected to controlled stresses and strain during the healing process. A number of studies have demonstrated the beneficial effect of stress and strain on the actual recovery of the injured ligaments. It was once thought that early motion might benefit the articular cartilage, bone strength, muscular function, and other factors, but that it would compromise the healing of the injured ligament. Earlier ultrastructural investigation of skeletally immature rabbits showed that the mean matrix alignment of the healing medial collateral ligaments was better for immobilized animals compared with those with immediate mobilization. However, the bulk of recent evidence indicates that the ligament repair itself benefits from early exposures to stress and strain. These data must be interpreted cautiously in the clinical situation. Obviously, a healing ligament needs some protection from large deformations. At present there is much interest in determining how aggressive rehabilitation should be to obtain quicker and better healing without a high risk of reinjury to the repaired or reconstructed ligament. However, the magnitude of stress that is beneficial or deleterious to ligament or graft healing remains unknown.

Sensory Functions

Attention has been focused on the possibility that ligaments provide sensory data to the nervous system and may have a significant functional role in the detection of motion and pressure. Human anterior cruciate ligaments contain three morphologic types of mechanoreceptor and free nerve endings. Ligament and joint capsule receptors have been shown to have significant reflex importance in animal models. Joint motion leads to afferent signals from the receptors with a corresponding reflex muscular effect. The absence of sensory input can impair motor function in a manner separate from the effect on joint stability.

Annotated Bibliography

Ligament Biomechanics

Beynnon BD, Howe JG, Pope MH, et al: The measurement of anterior cruciate ligament strain in-vivo. *Int Orthop (SICOT)* 1992;16:1-12.

The Hall Effect Strain Transducer was used in a new arthroscopic technique to study the normal anterior cruciate ligament in vivo. Participants were patients who volunteered for the study. They had normal anterior cruciate ligaments and were undergoing diagnostic arthroscopic surgery. This research has demonstrated why the Lachman test is a better ACL examination technique than the drawer test. During isometric quadriceps contraction, values of anterior cruciate ligament strain measured at 30 degrees of knee flexion were significantly higher than those observed at 90 degrees. The anterior cruciate remained unstrained with isometric quadriceps activity performed at 90 degrees of knee flexion. These findings indicate that isometric quadriceps activity at 90 degrees of knee flexion can be prescribed for rehabilitation immediately after anterior cruciate ligament reconstruction. These data indicate that active extension of the knee between the limits of 5 degrees and 110 degrees and passive range of knee motion between 0 degrees and 110 degrees may be performed with minimal risk of strain to a reconstructive replacement. Investigation of the passive range of knee motion activity has demonstrated that the anterior cruciate ligament does not remain isometric, or the same length, as the knee is coursed through passive motion. Rather, the strain magnitude of the anterior cruciate increases as the knee is passively brought into full extension. These data are important standards by which to accept or reject tunnel position measurements made with commercially available isometer systems.

Bigliani LU, Pollock RG, Soslowsky LJ, et al: Tensile properties of the inferior glenohumeral ligament. *J Orthop Res* 1992;10:187-197.

The investigators studied the failure behavior of three different regions of the inferior glenohumeral ligament, including a superior band, an anterior axillary pouch, and a posterior axillary pouch. As with most soft-tissue structures, larger strain values occurred near the insertion sites. However, the mean stress at failure (5.5 MPa) was significantly less than other soft-tissue structures such as the anterior cruciate ligament and patella tendon. This finding led the authors to suggest that the inferior glenohumeral ligament may not be capable of independently stabilizing the glenohumeral joint. Three different failure sites were observed: the glenoid insertion (40%), the ligament midsubstance (35%), and the humeral insertion (25%). As with the anterior cruciate ligament, specimen age may influence the mechanical properties and failure site of the ligament.

Markolf KL, Gorek JK, Kabo JM, et al: Direct measurement of resultant forces in the anterior cruciate ligament: An in vitro study performed with a new experimental technique. *J Bone Joint Surg* 1990;72A:557-567.

This investigation introduced a new technique for measuring the resultant anterior cruciate ligament force in cadaver specimens. The tibial insertion of the anterior cruciate ligament was mechanically isolated with a coring cutter, and a biaxial load sensor was fixed to the tibial insertion so that the resultant anterior cruciate ligament forces were directly measured. Passive knee extension produced anterior cruciate ligament forces only during the last ten degrees of extension. At five degrees of knee hyperextension, the anterior cruciate ligament forces ranged between 50 and 240 N. Internal torque applied to the tibia produced greater anterior cruciate ligament forces than did external torque. With applied anterior translation of the tibia relative to femur, the load applied to the knee was approximately equal to the resultant anterior cruciate ligament load. A compressive joint load was applied to the knee to simulate body weight, and this was found to protect the anterior cruciate ligament from the high forces that are developed by applied anterior tibial force. No such protective mechanism was found for applied internal and external tibial torque.

Woo SL, Hollis JM, Adams DJ, et al: Tensile properties of the human femur-anterior cruciate ligament-tibia complex: The effects of specimen age and orientation. *Am J Sports Med* 1991;19:217-225.

The tensile structural failure properties of the anterior cruciate ligament, including both midsubstance and insertion site behavior, were found to be affected by specimen age and orientation during failure testing. The ultimate failure load, linear stiffness, and energy absorbed at failure were found to decrease significantly with specimen age. In the younger specimens, the mean ultimate failure load was 2,160 N and the linear stiffness was 242 N/mm when the femur-anterior cruciate ligament-tibia complex was tested with the failure load applied along the axis of the ligament in both the frontal and sagittal planes. These values were higher than those previously reported in the literature, demonstrating that the technique used to perform the failure test can influence the results. There was a higher incidence of ligament substance failures in older specimens, which the authors suggested was produced because with increasing age the ligament substance deteriorates more rapidly than the insertion sites.

Stress Deprivation Effects

Woo SL, Gomez MA, Sites TJ, et al: The biomechanical and morphological changes in the medial collateral ligament of the rabbit after immobilization and remobilization. *J Bone Joint Surg* 1987;69A:1200-1211.

Stress deprivation results in rapid deterioration of properties of the bone-ligament-bone complex of the knee. The deterioration occurs both in properties of the ligament substance and the insertion site. The recovery of ligament substance properties is seen in weeks, but those of the insertion site require many months for full recovery. These observations have implications for treatment and rehabilitation protocols.

Woo SL, Peterson RH, Ohland KJ, et al: The effects of strain rate on the properties of the medial collateral ligament in skeletally immature and mature rabbits: A biomechanical and histological study. *J Orthop Res* 1990;8:712-721.

In an effort to understand the importance of ligaments in providing joint stability during injury, the effect that the rate of applied failure load has on the structural properties (including ligament midsubstance and insertion sites) and mechanical properties (including only midsubstance behavior) of the rabbit medial collateral ligament were studied. For immature rabbits the structural properties significantly increased with the rate of applied loading, while the failure mode was ligament evulsion. For the mature animals there were increases in the structural properties found with the increased rate of loading, but these were smaller in magnitude than were those of the immature animals, while the failure mode was found to be within the ligament substance. The mechanical properties were only minimally affected by the rate of loading for both the skeletally mature and immature animals. Skeletal maturity was found to have more influence than the rate of applied load to failure on the biomechanical properties of the medial collateral ligament.

The Biology of Repair

Kwan MK, Sung KL, Akeson WH: Adhesion characteristics of human ligament fibroblasts. *Trans Orthop Res Soc* 1992;17:76.

The authors demonstrate that the adhesion strengths of ACL and MCL cells to fibronectin substrate differ. The adhesion strength in both types of cells varies according to concentration of the fibronectin substrate and to time of exposure to substrate. Overall, the MCL cells had higher adhesion strength than ACL cells. The functional differences in adhesion strength, along with previous observations of differences in phenotype and the slower mobility of ACL cells, suggest that these differences may play a role in the poor healing of the ACL universally observed after injury.

Lyon RM, Akeson WH, Amiel D, et al: Ultrastructural differences between the cells of the medial collateral and the anterior cruciate ligaments. *Clin Orthop* 1991;272:279-286.

Cells of the ACL and MCL have different morphologic characteristics. The appearance of the MCL cells is typical of fibroblasts in general. They possess long cytoplasmic processes extending distances many times greater than the length of the cell body. The cells of the ACL, in contrast, are rounded and possess only vestigial microprocesses. These cells resemble fibrocartilage cells. These characteristics may have a bearing on differences in healing between the ligaments.

Frank C, Woo SL, Andriacchi T, et al: Normal ligament: Structure, function, and composition, in Buckwalter JA,

Woo SL-Y (eds): *Injury and Repair of the Musculoskeletal Soft Tissues.* Park Ridge, IL, American Academy of Orthopaedic Surgeons, 1988, pp 66-82.

Collagen fibril diameters were quantitatively analyzed in autogenous anterior cruciate ligament grafts (including the patella tendon, hamstrings, and iliotibial tract) taken from human subjects nine months to six years after implantation. Large-diameter collagen fibrils (>100 nm) were found to form approximately 45% of the cross-sectional area in the normal human patella tendon at the time of harvest. In comparison, the normal ACL collagen fibers (<100 nm) were found to form 85% of the cross-sectional area. There was a predominance of small-diameter collagen fibrils (<100 nm) with poor packing and alignment in all of the autogenous anterior cruciate ligament grafts. The remodeled grafts did not re-form the large diameter and tightly packed fibrils seen in the normal anterior cruciate ligament. The authors indicated that this finding may help explain the experimental evidence of decreased tensile strength of the grafts compared with normal anterior cruciate ligament.

Shinko K, Oakes BW, Inoue M: Human ACL allograft: Collagen fibril populations studied as a function of age of the graft. *Trans Orthop Res Soc* 1990;15:520.

This study measured the collagen fiber diameters of ACL allografts (including Achilles tendon and tibialis tendons) taken from human subjects at various intervals after surgical reconstruction. Analysis six months after implantation revealed that the allografts contained predominantly small-diameter collagen fibrils (<60 nm), which were not as tightly packed as in the normal ACL. The loss of the large-diameter collagen fibrils and the predominance of the smaller diameter fibrils was thought to correspond to the dramatic reduction in the allograft strength seen over time.

The Effect of Repair of the Medial Collateral Ligament

Inoue M, McGurk-Burleson E, Hollis JM, et al: Treatment of the medial collateral ligament injury: I. The importance of anterior cruciate ligament on the varus-valgus knee laxity. *Am J Sports Med* 1987;15:15-21.

Although isolated MCL injuries have been observed to heal well without surgical repair, this paper emphasizes that the intact ACL partially compensates for the MCL in valgus rotation. Therefore, in the case of combined injuries of MCL and ACL, valgus rotation is less restrained, and treatment must be modified appropriately.

King G, Edwards S, Brunt N, et al: Intra-operative tensioning of rabbit medial collateral ligament autografts influences post-operative ligament laxity and strength. *Trans Orthop Res Soc* 1992;17:658.

The authors demonstrate that intraoperative tensioning of rabbit MCL grafts produces significant differences in laxity initially, but that these differences normalize during healing. The paper illustrates that ligament cells have ability within certain limits to adjust ligament tension after surgery or after injury.

Weiss JA, Woo SL, Ohland KJ, et al: Evaluation of a new injury model to study medial collateral ligament healing: Primary repair versus nonoperative treatment. *J Orthop Res* 1991;9:516-528.

Mop-end tears of the medial collateral ligament were combined with injury to the insertion sites in the rabbit model, and primary repair was compared with nonoperative treatment. Biomechanical evaluation of varus/valgus laxity and the structural and mechanical properties of the MCL showed no significant difference between the primary repair and nonoperative treatment modes. The ligament insertion to bone was reported to recover more slowly than did the ligament substance. Failure evaluation of the medial collateral ligament revealed that, by the 12th week after injury, the mechanical properties, or midsubstance behavior, of the healed ligament was significantly less normal than in the control.

Woo SL, Inoue M, McGurk-Burleson E, et al: Treatment of medial collateral ligament injury: II. Structure and function of canine knees in response to differing treatment regimens. *Am J Sports Med* 1987;15:22-29.

Isolated MCL injuries created by surgical transection were performed in canines to study the effect of surgical repair and rehabilitation. The varus-valgus joint laxity and structure behavior of the MCL in animals that had no repair and immediate mobilization were similar to the normal contralateral limb. In animals that underwent repair followed either by three or six weeks of immobilization, results were inferior compared with the contralateral normal limbs. The recovery of the midsubstance of material properties of the MCL was not complete by 48 weeks. This investigation confirms previous findings by demonstrating that immobilization has a deleterious effect on MCL healing and indicates that early mobilization is the treatment of choice in cases of isolated MCL.

Woo SL, Young EP, Ohland KJ, et al: The effects of transection of the anterior cruciate ligament on healing of the medial collateral ligament: A biomechanical study of the knee in dogs. *J Bone Joint Surg* 1990;72A:382-392.

The healing of injuries to the MCL with concurrent injury to the ACL were investigated using the canine model. An intact, partial transection of the MCL and complete transection of the ACL were compared. Healing of the transected MCL was found to be adversely affected by concomitant and complete transection of the ACL. These findings were consistent with previous clinical studies that showed an increase in valgus knee rotation after conservative management of a combined MCL and ACL injury. These findings led the authors to suggest that in patients with concomitant MCL and ACL injuries, conservative management with early mobilization should not be attempted.

The Effect of Stress and Strain on Healing

Frank C, MacFarlane B, Edwards P, et al: A quantitative analysis of matrix alignment in ligament scars: A comparison of movement versus immobilization in an immature rabbit model. *J Orthop Res* 1991;9:219-227.

Skeletally immature rabbits were used to investigate the fibrillar matrix alignment of healing MCLs treated with and without immobilization. A wire rupture injury was produced at the midsubstance portion of the MCL. The nonimmobilized scars were found to return to normal matrix alignment after 14 weeks of healing. The matrix alignment was superior in the immobilized group. This finding led the authors to suggest that active flexion/extension motion of the knee may not be required to achieve normal fibrillar alignment of the scar matrix during the healing process. This is an important finding, because the axis of fibrillar orientation in both normal and healing ligaments is thought to correspond to the direction of forces transmitted through the scar. This model did not determine if the force transmission properties (ie, mechanical and structural properties) are also similar for immobilized and nonimmobilized treatment. This work must be performed before these results are applied clinically.

Gomez MA, Woo SL, Amiel D, et al: The effect of increased tension on healing medial collateral ligaments. *Am J Sports Med* 1991;19:347-354.

The effect of joint motion and increased level of stress on the MCL were investigated using the rabbit model. Increased stress to the healing ligament, created by inserting a steel pin perpendicularly underneath the healing ligament, was found to result in improved biomechanical, biochemical, and morphologic properties over time. At six weeks after injury, isolated transection of the ligament produced a varus/valgus joint laxity twice that of normal, while joints with increased MCL stress during healing had a varus/valgus laxity 1.5 times that of the control limb. By 12 weeks, the joints with an increased MCL stress during healing had varus/valgus laxity similar to control values. In this group histologic improvements were also seen, including a longitudinal alignment of the collagen fibers and decreased cellularity.

Sensory Functions

Hoffman AH, Grigg P: Measurement of joint capsule tissue loading in the cat knee using calibrated mechanoreceptors. *J Biomech* 1989;22:787-791.

The mechanoreceptive sensory neurons in the posterior capsule of the cat were found to function as in vivo load transducers, from which it was possible to estimate loading of the posterior capsule. This investigation revealed that the capsule is very lightly loaded with knee extension and that only a fraction of the applied extension moment was sustained by the posterior portion of the joint capsule. This study represents a new and innovative in vivo approach to measuring the force behavior of the structures surrounding the knee joint. It should be mentioned, however, that the knee and surrounding soft-tissue structures of the cat are significantly different from those of the human.

Schutte MJ, Dabezies EJ, Zimny ML, et al: Neural anatomy of the human anterior cruciate ligament. *J Bone Joint Surg* 1987;69A:243-247.

The human ACL was investigated to define the neural anatomy. Two slow-adapting Ruffini-type mechanoreceptors were identified that were thought to sense the motion, position, and angle of knee rotation. A third group of rapidly adapting Pacinian corpuscle mechanoreceptors was defined and thought to signal joint acceleration at the initiation and termination of joint movement. A fourth group of free nerve endings responsible for pain were also identified. The combined four groups of neural elements comprised 1% of the total area of the ACL. This study indicates that a torn ACL not only leaves the knee without a strong stabilizing structure, but also results in the loss of a portion of the afferent neural system and in denervation of the joint.

Goertzen MJ, Dellmann A, Gruber J, et al: Neurovascular anatomy of anterior cruciate ligament allografts revealed by metallic impregnation and vascular injection techniques. *Trans Orthop Res Soc* 1992;17:666.

Revascularization of ACL allografts demonstrate a normal pattern one year after reconstruction in canine knees. At one year, viable mechanoreceptors and free nerve endings are present in the reconstructive ligaments. This information is important with respect to potential return of proprioceptive function of the ligament and to knee rehabilitation.

11
Congenital Abnormalities

Congenital abnormalities encompass many pathologic conditions present at birth. Obvious structural problems (such as clubfoot) already exist in some cases. In others, the disorder (such as muscular dystrophy) has not yet appeared. This section will review congenital defects and discuss representative problems that affect the musculoskeletal system. Isolated congenital malformations are discussed elsewhere in this book.

Etiology

While the exact cause of many congenital abnormalities is not known, most will fall under a general category (Table 1). Many abnormalities involve mendelian inheritance (autosomal dominant, recessive, or X-linked), which occurs on a familial basis or following spontaneous mutations. Chromosomal abnormalities result when either too little or too much chromosome is inherited, as in trisomy, deletion, or translocations.

One third of the most common birth defects have a multifactorial origin, a combination of multiple genetic and environmental factors. In general, the recurrence rate will be 3%, 0.7%, and 0.3% among first-, second-, and third-degree relatives, respectively. More severe malformations, such as congenital equinovarus, developmental dysplasia of the hip, and pyloric stenosis, have a high recurrence rate.

A teratogen is an environmental factor that produces an abnormality in form or function during embryogenesis. Teratogens are grouped into four general categories: (1) infectious agents; (2) physical agents (including mechanical factors such as heat, radiation, and crowding in utero); (3) drug and chemical agents; and (4) maternal metabolic and genetic factors. The effects on the fetus vary and depend on the time of exposure, dosage, host susceptibility, and other environmental factors. Factors causing fetal malformations in utero include crowding, breech presentation, and umbilical cord entanglement, as is seen in amniotic band syndrome.

Structural Defects Present at Birth

A knowledge of the cause of structural defects is essential in providing a prognosis, management plan, and, if necessary, genetic counseling. In many cases, the obvious deformity at birth is of relatively minor importance compared with less obvious but potentially more serious related problems, as when clubfoot is associated with camptomelic syndrome.

Table 1. Cause of congenital malformations

Cause	Approximate Percentage
Genetic abnormalities	
Chromosome abnormalities	6 to 10
Single gene abnormalities	3 to 8
Familial—uncertain pattern of inheritance	18
Multifactorial inheritance	20 to 30
Environmental factors	
Maternal conditions	4 to 5
Teratogens	3 to 4
Environmental exposures	1 to 2
Unknown cause	30 to 60

In general, there are three pathologic events that can lead to structural defects—malformation, deformation, and disruption. A malformation is a morphologic defect caused by an intrinsically abnormal developmental process in which the part never forms normally. Deformation involves a disturbance in form or position that is caused by an intrinsic or extrinsic mechanical force acting on a part that initially formed normally. Deformations are usually less severe, nongenetic, and more likely to respond favorably to treatment. A disruption is the breakdown of a previously normal tissue.

Any of these pathologic events can lead to a predictable pattern or sequence of multiple anomalies. Multiple anomalies that are not part of a sequence may be the result of multiple defects in one or more tissue—malformation syndromes are usually caused by a single factor. The presence of one malformation should lead to a search for others.

Prenatal Diagnosis

The number of congenital abnormalities identified before birth is increasing because of the success of prenatal diagnosis. Indications for such tests include: (1) advanced maternal age (generally accepted at 35 years or older); (2) history of chromosomal abnormality in a previous pregnancy; (3) parental genetic history of chromosomal abnormalities (such as balanced translocation); (4) family history of neural tube, metabolic, or biochemical defects; (5) abnormal X-linked genes (suspected carriers should determine the sex of an unborn child); (6) high-risk population with family history of inherited disorders. In approximately 90% of cases prenatal studies indicate no abnormality and serve to reassure the parents. Good screening programs lead to an increase in term births.

Several screening methods are currently available. Amniocentesis can be performed at 14 to 16 weeks of gestation. Cells obtained are cultured for chromosomal studies, and biochemical defects are diagnosed by assay of enzyme-specific activities.

Measurement of alpha-fetoprotein is important because low levels in maternal serum are associated with chromosome abnormalities in the fetus. Of the women screened, 5% will be affected; about half of these will require amniocentesis following ultrasonography. Only one in 40 of these will have a chromosomal abnormality. The relationship between increased levels of maternal alpha-fetoprotein and fetal mortality, recently studied, shows that fetal death may occur late in the pregnancy and can possibly be prevented by close monitoring of alpha-fetoprotein.

Chorionic villus sampling is done during the first trimester, and its use is presently limited. It has an increased complication rate, with an overall loss of 4%. Ultrasonography, which allows prenatal monitoring during amniocentesis and shows the size, age, and placental positions of the fetus as well as details of malformations, is safe and used extensively.

Connective Tissue Disorders

Connective tissue disorders all involve abnormalities of the same type of tissue, and it is not surprising that they often share common clinical features, such as ligamentous laxity; thin, distensible skin; easy bruisability; and poor scar formation. Within each disease, however, is a tremendous heterogeneity. The information available regarding the molecular basis of these disorders more clearly explains the broad phenotypic variation. In osteogenesis imperfecta, for example, the gene for type I collagen involves several expressed and nonexpressed DNA sequences. Mutations at numerous sites have been identified. This can lead to a wide range of abnormalities in the tropocollagen molecule and, hence, in the clinical expression.

Marfan's Syndrome

Marfan's syndrome is a serious, hereditary connective tissue disorder. Its incidence is unknown, because mild cases escape diagnosis, but a minimum estimate is four to six cases per 100,000 births. The mode of inheritance is autosomal dominant; however, 15% to 25% of patients represent new mutations. The gene for this disorder has been located on the long arm of chromosome 15 in a gene for fibrillin, a fibrillar protein found in the eye, aorta, and several connective tissues.

The disease is identified by its mode of inheritance and clinical features. To make a diagnosis, two or more of the following diagnostic criteria must be met: (1) positive family history; (2) cardiovascular involvement, which usually consists of dilatation of the ascending aorta and, in some cases, mitral valve prolapse; (3) superior disloca-

tion of the ocular lens; and (4) musculoskeletal disorders, including scoliosis, arachnodactyly, pectus excavatum, and joint laxity.

The usual ocular manifestation of Marfan's syndrome is bilateral superior subluxation of the lens, which is present in 50% to 80% of affected patients and is diagnosed at or shortly after birth. Iridodonesis, or tremor of the eye following sudden cessation of rapid eye movement, is caused by subluxation of the lens, because the iris lacks the posterior support usually provided by the lens. Myopia is often present and may be severe. Retinal detachment can occur in association with severe myopia, leading to partial or complete blindness. This is a treatable problem, and routine opthalmologic examinations are mandatory.

The cardiovascular manifestations are the most serious, causing 90% of the deaths. The major abnormality is dilatation of the ascending aorta, which usually begins in the intrapericardial portion and extends into or beyond the aortic arch. Dilatation at the level of the valve often results in aortic regurgitation. Radiographs of the chest are not reliable for early diagnosis of aortic dilatation, but early recognition is possibly with echocardiology. The dilatation is progressive and usually precedes aortic dissection and rupture. Dilatation and dissection of the descending abnormal aorta and other major arteries can also occur, but are rare. Mitral regurgitation secondary to mitral valve prolapse may also occur, and cardiac arrhythmias have been implicated as a cause of death. Newer medical and surgical techniques allow early diagnosis, improved care, and increased life expectancy (which previously was the early 40s).

The musculoskeletal manifestations, when prominent, are quite characteristic. Patients with Marfan's syndrome are tall, over the 90th percentile, with slender limbs that exaggerate their height. Relative disproportions have been identified but no one calculation is more accurate than another, and all can overlap with the general population. In 75% of involved patients, the normal upper to lower limb segment ratio is two standard deviations below the mean, reflecting the increase in length of the legs over the trunk. In these patients, arm span is significantly greater than height. Arachnodactyly is common. Pectus excavatum is the most common deformity of the chest wall.

Joint laxity is variable. Chronic and recurrent subluxation of the patella, shoulder, sternoclavicular joint, and metacarpophalangeal joints of the thumb are common. Genu valgum and recurvatum also occur. In general, soft-tissue surgery to correct joint laxity is unsuccessful, and the best treatment is therapy aimed at strengthening the muscle. Pes planovalgus, characterized by a long, thin foot with a disproportionately long great toe, and unstable ankle often make shoe-fitting difficult. These problems can be treated with orthosis and, rarely, arthrodesis.

Protrusio acetabulum is a peculiar finding in many patients and may be progressive, symptomatic, and accom-

Table 2. Classification of osteogenesis imperfecta

Type	Inheritance	Sclera	Clinical Features
I	Autosomal dominant	Blue	Fractures during childhood; hearing loss; subgroups with and without opalescent teeth; most common type
II	Autosomal recessive	Blue	Lethal in perinatal period; crumpled long bones; flattened vertebrae; very rare
III	Autosomal recessive	White	Birth fractures and progressive deformity; markedly short stature; subgroups with and without opalescent teeth; spinal deformity and costovertebral anomalies
IV	Autosomal dominant	White	Skeletal fragility; no hearing loss; moderate growth failure; may have opalescent teeth

panied by chondrolysis. Closure of the triradiate cartilage reportedly corrects the abnormality in symptomatic patients.

Scoliosis is quite common in Marfan's syndrome, but curvatures significant enough to require treatment occur in only 20% of patients. The scoliosis, which often occurs before the age of 10, may progress rapidly. Bracing is complicated by thoracic lordosis. Surgery may be indicated following cardiac evaluation. Spinal fusion is often complicated by pseudarthrosis. Dural ectasia and anterior myelomeningocele may be present and are thought to be caused by cerebrospinal fluid pulsations against a weakened dura. Progesterone and estrogen therapy to induce puberty and control progressive scoliosis has not been successful. High-grade spondylolisthesis is an additional spinal deformity that reportedly occurs with this syndrome.

Several conditions closely resemble Marfan's syndrome, including congenital contractural arachnodactyly, homocystinuria, Stickler syndrome, hypermobility syndrome, and mitral valve prolapse.

Osteogenesis Imperfecta

This group of disorders is characterized by variable bone fragility ranging from multiple fractures at birth that lead to perinatal death to osteoporosis in adults. The usual classification is based on clinical and genetic factors (Table 2), but biochemical analysis shows far greater heterogeneity. Most patients with osteogenesis imperfecta have mutations at either the gene for pro alpha I (I chain) or the gene for pro alpha II (I chain) of type I procollagen. Several different mutations have been identified, and two basic defects have been established. Quantitative defects occur when not enough structurally normal type I collagen is produced, which causes the mild form of the disease (type I). Qualitative defects produce structurally abnormal chains, leading to all forms of osteogenesis imperfecta, but usually types II, III, and IV.

Osteogenesis imperfecta in children is characterized by underlying connective tissue defects, such as ligamentous laxity, thin, distensible skin, easy bruisability, and poor scar formation. Blue sclera, when present, may not develop until several years after birth. Hearing defects secondary to inner and middle ear abnormalities may develop, and affected children require regular audiologic examinations. Abnormal tooth development occurs; the teeth appear opalescent and have a propensity for decay. Other classic findings include multiple fractures, scoliosis, long bone deformities, wormian bones in the skull, and small triangular face.

The orthopaedic consequences of osteogenesis imperfecta are the most striking. Multiple fractures are the primary source of morbidity. In the most severe form of the disease, multiple fractures of the long bones and ribs, with associated deformities, are present at birth. Over 90% of these patients die. Of those with less deformity, 90% survive, but many become wheelchair-dependent. In those without neonatal fractures, one third become wheelchair-dependent if the fractures occur before the child begins to walk. When fractures first appear after walking begins, most patients remain ambulatory with appropriate treatment. In general, most patients born with fractures have no family history for osteogenesis imperfecta. Weightbearing with lightweight, supportive bracing should begin as soon as possible in all patients.

Acute fractures usually heal promptly with apparently normal callus, but proper remodeling to lamellar bone does not occur and the likelihood of reinjury is increased. Nonunions occur in 20% of the patients and careful treatment of the fracture with reduction and immobilization is necessary. Hyperplastic callus and malignant degeneration have been reported.

Bone deformities caused by microfractures on the tension side of the bones are common. When severe enough to interfere with bracing or allow recurrent fractures, multiple realignment osteotomies fixed with expandable intramedullary rods should be performed. All substantial deformities should be corrected simultaneously to limit immobilization time. Postoperative bracing to avoid recurrent deformity must be considered. Fractures usually cease at puberty.

It may be difficult to distinguish osteogenesis imperfecta from child abuse. Children with multiple fractures and osteogenesis imperfecta may have a family history of skeletal fragility. In these cases, other identifying characteristics of osteogenesis imperfecta should be sought.

Scoliosis develops in over 50% of involved patients. Bracing is ineffective because of the plasticity of the chest wall. Surgical correction with posterior instrumentation is usually successful. Hooks may be reinforced with methylmethacrylate. Segmental instrumentation techniques have recently been used successfully. Vertebral compression of fractures caused by osteoporosis can occur at any age and may lead to symptomatic back deformities. Recent reports document the problems associ-

Table 2. Ehlers-Danlos syndrome

Type	Inheritance	Biochemistry	Major Clinical Features		
			Skin	**Joints**	**Other**
I Gravis	Autosomal dominant	Unknown	Fragile; hyperextensible; easily bruised	Laxity with dislocation	Scoliosis; varicose veins; hernia; premature birth
II Mitis	Autosomal dominant	Unknown	Moderately hyperextensible; mild bruising	Moderate laxity in hands and feet; no dislocations	——
III Benign hypermobile	Autosomal dominant	Unknown	Normal	Severe laxity; frequent dislocations	——
IV Ecchymotic	Autosomal dominant or autosomal recessive	Decreased type III collagen synthesis and/or secretion	Thin; severe bruising; deep tissues very friable	Laxity only in hands and fingers; occasional dislocations	Aneurysms; spontaneous artery rupture; rupture of uterus and colon; early vascular death
V X-linked	X-linked recessive	Deficiency of peptidyl lysine oxidase (?)	Strikingly hyperextensible; mild fragility and bruising	Minimal laxity; no dislocations	——
VI Ocular-scoliotic	Autosomal recessive	Deficiency of peptidyl lysine hydroxylase	Moderately hyperextensible; moderate fragility and bruising	Moderate laxity with dislocations	Severe scoliosis; ocular fragility; congenital clubfeet; "floppy baby"
VII Arthrochalasis multiplex congenita	Autosomal dominant and autosomal recessive	Deficiency of procollagen n-protease; resistant terminal cleavage site in procollagen 2	Moderate fragility and hyperextensibility	Severe laxity; frequent dislocations; bilateral congenital dislocated hips	Scoliosis; short stature; abnormal facies
VIII Periodontosis	Autosomal dominant	Protease-sensitive collagen (?)	Mild hyperextensibility; severe fragility	Moderate laxity, especially fingers; no dislocations	Periodontal disease with tooth loss
IX Occipital horns	X-linked recessive	Deficiency of peptidyl lysine oxidase and abnormal copper metabolism	More lax than hyperextensible	Hands and feet lax but elbows stiff	Widespread skeletal dysplasia; occipital bony exostoses; congenitally dislocated radial heads; urinary tract dysplasia
X Platelet dysfunction	Autosomal recessive	Abnormal fibronectin	Moderately hyperextensible; easily bruised	Laxity in hands and feet; no dislocations	Defect in platelet aggregation
XI Familial joint laxity	Autosomal dominant	Unknown	Normal	Severe laxity; frequent dislocations; patellar subluxation; congenital dislocated hip	——

ated with intramedullary rodding in long bone fractures. It appears as if the elongating rods, such as Bailey-Duboy and Sheffield, are superior to nonelongating ones. Many complications involving the instrumentation are technical and relatively easy to overcome. Crimping of the T-pieces will prevent dislodgement.

Ehlers-Danlos Syndrome

These genetically unrelated inherited disorders share certain clinical features. Again, there is remarkable phenotypic heterogeneity. To date, the classification involves 11 varieties based on clinical presentation, inheritance pattern, and specific biochemical abnormalities (Table 3). Many patients do not fall under one given category. The biochemical defects have been elucidated in only a few of the subgroups. Two forms of the disease are known to occur from mutations of collagen genes: type IV (from type III collagen defects) and type VII (from type I collagen defects).

Cutaneous manifestations are present in all forms. The skin is soft, velvety, and may be abundant over the hands and feet. It is hyperextensible, but returns immediately to normal configuration when released. It may be extremely fragile, splitting after insignificant trauma. The wounds are characterized by minor bleeding and dehiscence. Sutures may pull out of surgical wounds. Prolonged fixation of the skin edge with tape may alter the usual pattern of scarring, which is likened to cigarette paper or papyrus, and produce thin, shiny, broad atrophic and often hyperpigmented scars. Umbilical and inguinal hernias are additional findings.

The facies may be abnormal, with epicanthic folds, a high, arched palate, hyperextensible mucous membranes, and friable gums. Diverticulitis of the small and large intestines, bladder, and uterus may occur. Rectal prolapse in children has been noted; prolapse of the bladder and uterus in postpartum women is not uncommon. Spontaneous rupture of a hollow viscus and pneumothorax can occur. Life-threatening consequences result when the cardiovascular system is involved. The connective tissue that supports blood vessels is weak, leading to varicose veins and aneurysms. In type IV disease, the activities of daily living may provide enough stress to rupture large and medium-sized arteries. Mitral valve prolapse and, rarely, dilatation and dissection of the aorta can also occur.

Orthopaedic problems are related to joint hypermobility. Joint dislocation, which occurs in 25% of patients, may be present at birth or evolve as an acute or chronic problem. Joint effusions and arthralgias are common, and children are often misdiagnosed with forms of arthritis. Symptomatic shoulder dislocations are typically multidirectional. Subluxations and dislocations of the patella are very common and reducible, while radial head and medial sternoclavicular distractions are irreducible. Dislocations involving the interphalangeal, metacarpophalangeal, and carpometacarpal joints of the thumb can cause bothersome symptoms. In general, soft-tissue stabilizing procedures are doomed to failure as they stretch out over time because of the underlying collagen abnormality. Physical therapy and appropriate orthoses should be the first line of treatment, with arthrodesis reserved for selected cases. Stabilization of the hip requires correction of all deformities. In general, capsular repair must be combined with osteotomy of the femur, acetabu-

lum, or both. Clubfoot deformities are common. Treatment can be difficult, often requiring surgery. Scoliosis occurs and should be treated by bracing according to the criteria of an idiopathic curvature. The increased flexibility probably leads to a higher risk of progression in these patients, and early fusion may be indicated.

Skeletal Dysplasias

A dysplasia is a generalized developmental abnormality that occurs because of a pathologic organization of cells within a specific tissue type. Skeletal dysplasias include those disorders that result from abnormalities within the cartilage or bony tissues. They usually involve simple mendelian inheritance. The standard classification used is the International Nomenclature of Constitutional Disorders of Bone. However, because many disorders do not fit within this classification, at present most chondro-osseous dysplasias are named for the region of the bone affected roentgenographically.

Those dysplasias that involve the epiphysis of the long bones, such as pseudoachondroplasia and multiple epiphyseal dysplasia, result in joint deformities and precocious arthritis. Several mechanisms are involved. Delayed ossification leads to the loss of the osseous support in deformities secondary to mechanical forces. Additionally, alterations in the cartilage ultrastructure predispose the joints to degenerative changes. The surgical restoration of a normal mechanical axis may not alter the ultimate fate of the joint.

Achondroplasia

This disorder is single gene-autosomal dominant. The most common type of short-limbed dwarfism, it has a prevalence of 0.5 to 1.5 cases per 10,000 births. At maturity, the average heights of men and women with achondroplasia are 130 cm and 125 cm, respectively. At least 80% of cases result from random, new mutations. The underlying cause has not been confirmed, but the deficit is in endochondral ossification. The hypertrophic layer of the growth plate is incompletely developed and an alteration takes place in the normal processes of chondrocyte maturation, hypertrophy, and degeneration. An abnormality in the gene for type II procollagen has been identified in some patients. Recent studies have revealed defective oxidative energy metabolism in mitochondria.

Children with achondroplasia are recognizable at birth by several features, including rhizomelic short limbs and normal trunk height, prominent frontal bossing, depressed nasal bridge, midface hypoplasia, and relative mandibular prominence. The hands are short and broad. Fingers are three-pronged with a space between the third and fourth digits, producing the characteristic trident hand, a feature that is lost late in childhood. Characteristic radiographic findings are vertebral wedging at T-12 or L-1, short iliac wings and small sciatic notch, and progressive narrowing of the lumbar interpedicular distances.

Motor milestones are delayed and many children do not begin to walk independently until 2 to 3 years of age. Hypotonic ligamentous laxity, relatively large head, and disproportionate trunk and limbs may contribute to the problem. Intelligence is normal, but speech problems may exist because of tongue thrust, which usually resolves by school age. Maxillary hypoplasia may lead to dental crowding and malocclusion. Recurrent otitis media will lead to a higher incidence of conductive hearing loss in adults. Obesity is common.

At least 3% of affected individuals have hydrocephalus; detection is difficult because the head size normally runs above the 97th percentile. Specific growth curves of head circumference are available and allow detection of abnormal expansion, which must then be evaluated with computed tomography or magnetic resonance imaging. Significant respiratory problems develop in 10% of affected individuals because of an abnormal thoracic cage configuration, midfacial hypoplasia, upper airway obstruction, or spinal cord compression at the foramen magnum. Careful preoperative assessment and postoperative monitoring of pulmonary function are necessary.

The most common and potentially most disabling orthopaedic problems in achondroplasia are related to the deformities found throughout the axial skeleton. Thoracolumbar kyphosis, usually present in infancy, resolves in 90% of affected children as they begin to walk; however, if this disorder persists, it should be treated, if tolerated, with extension orthoses. Persistent angular thoracolumbar kyphosis with vertebral wedging of 40 degrees or more by age 5 should be aggressively treated with surgery, as significant correction cannot be anticipated. Combined anterior strut grafts and posterior fusions should be performed, with anterior decompression reserved for those patients with neurologic compromise. Instrumentation that affects the stenotic spinal cord must be avoided.

Spinal stenosis occurs in both the cervical and lumbar spine. The foramen magnum is small and misshapen and can compromise the neural structures, producing a wide range of symptoms; sleep apnea, respiratory dysfunction, cyanotic episodes, feeding problems, quadriparesis, and sudden death. Delayed ambulation, frequently occurring on a constitutional basis, may also be secondary to neurologic compression. Evaluation with computed tomography is indicated when compression is suspected. In some children, the stenosis will improve with growth of the foramen magnum, and a decision must be made whether or not to rely on apnea monitoring with these children or to perform suboccipital decompression. Decompression is often helpful, but significant complications are frequent enough that it should not be performed as prophylaxis. The decision to treat foramen magnum stenosis by observation or decompression may be aided by foramen magnum growth charts developed with CT scans.

Stenosis of the lumbar spine is circumferential because of short, thickened pedicles, narrowed interpedicular distances, thickened lamina, and inferior facets. Degenerative changes further compromise the spinal canal, leading to cauda equina or lumbar nerve root compressive symptoms in 40% to 50% of individuals. Conservative treatment consists of weight reduction and antilordotic exercises or bracing. Surgical treatment, which is often necessary, involves wide lumbar decompression and foraminotomies. The facets should be undercut to preserve them when possible. If the thoracolumbar kyphosis exceeds 40 degrees, progressive kyphosis will follow laminectomy. In these cases, fusion must accompany the decompression. Either a postoperative cast or pedicular fixation can be used. A sharply angled thoracolumbar kyphosis should be stabilized anteriorly and posteriorly. It is best to avoid fusions beyond L-4 to allow lumbosacral motion, which will benefit individuals with short arms and legs.

Angular deformities, which are common in both upper and lower extremities, presumably originate from the relative undergrowth of the thicker bones, the tibia and radius. Ligamentous laxity and obesity are contributing factors. In the lower extremity, genu varum and varus ankle deformities are found. Unlike dysplasias that involve the epiphysis, degenerative arthritis is rare, and prophylactic surgical correction of deformities is probably not indicated. Bracing is not beneficial because the orthosis often opens the joint medially, secondary to ligamentous laxity. Indications for surgical treatment are pain, progressive deformities, and lateral tibial shift. Corrective osteotomies will produce improvement and are usually performed proximally when ankle varus is not severe. Proximal and distal fibular epiphysiodesis is a less involved procedure and may allow gradual correction if the deformities of significant growth remains. In the upper extremity, elbow extension is often diminished and posterolateral radial head dislocation may occur. Shortening of the upper extremities such that the fingers reach the level of the hips may cause difficulty in hygienic care.

Limb lengthening techniques for treatment of skeletal dysplasias have been performed extensively in the former USSR and Italy. These procedures are especially useful for achondroplasia and hypochondroplasia, conditions in which the soft tissues initially appear too large for the short bones. Limb contour becomes more normal with lengthening. These procedures are contraindicated in dysplasias with epiphyseal involvement, which are at risk for articular damage secondary to mechanical forces. The callotasis method is preferred for lengthening, but significant and major complications continue to be an issue. Joint contractures require intensive physical therapy and occasional soft-tissue releases. Significant joint limitation occurs infrequently. To maintain proper proportions, both humeri are lengthened 8 to 10 cm.

Preliminary studies show a high percentage of patient satisfaction with these techniques. However, the ultimate height achieved is still well below that of the average adult, and whether or not functional benefits outweigh the considerable expense, morbidity, and risk is highly questionable at this time.

Pseudoachondroplasia

The pseudoachondroplastic dysplasias represent a heterogenous group characterized by disproportionate short-limbed dwarfism. There are moderate to severe epiphyseal, metaphyseal, and physeal abnormalities in long bones, as well as spinal involvement. Four subtypes have been proposed: two with autosomal inheritance (I, III) and two with recessive inheritance (II, IV). The subtypes are further differentiated by the severity of skeletal involvement, with type I the mildest and type IV the most severe. Dwarfism can easily be differentiated from achondroplasia by the normal face and skull, and the absence of interpedicular narrowing of the lumbar spine.

The condition is not recognized at birth, but growth retardation is apparent by the age of 2 or 3 years. At that time, rhizomelic shortening of the extremities is evident. The adult height ranges from 106 to 130 cm. The face and head have a normal appearance and the trunk is normal except for an exaggerated lumbar lordosis.

The long bones are characterized by epiphyseal, metaphyseal, and physeal changes. Precocious arthritis is a major complication, as in other epiphyseal dysplasias. The central portion of the physis seems to grow at a slower rate. This uneven growth leads to joint incongruity and malalignment. There is rhizomelic shortening, with flaring of the metaphysis and delayed ossification of the epiphysis. Angular deformities occur at the hip and knee.

Coxa vara is relatively mild but may lead to deformity, lateral subluxation, and incongruity. In planning corrective osteotomies, preoperative arthrography is necessary, because the correction of subluxation by varus osteotomy can lead to increasing incongruity. At the knee, genu valgum, varum, and windswept deformities occur because of bony abnormalities as well as ligamentous laxity. Bracing is not helpful. When the deformity occurs on either side of the joint, multiple osteotomies are required to realign the mechanical axis while maintaining the horizontal plane of the distal femoral condyles.

Progressive thoracolumbar kyphosis may occur but is much less severe than that seen in achondroplasia. Angular or vertebral wedging or a kyphosis may result from several less involved vertebral bodies. Odontoid dysplasia with atlantoaxial instability has been reported, and the generalized laxity of these children is considered to be a predisposing factor. When identified, such instability must be followed clinically until maturity.

Spondyloepiphyseal Dysplasia

This is a descriptive term for a group of disorders predominantly affecting the vertebra and the epiphyseal centers, resulting in short trunk disproportionate dwarfism. Included are: chondrodysplasia punctata, spondyloepiphyseal dysplasia tarda, and spondyloepiphyseal dysplasia congenita. These are generally transmitted as autosomal dominant traits, although most cases arise as random mutations.

Spondyloepiphyseal dysplasia congenita is the most severe variety. At birth, this disorder may be confused with achondroplasia because the symptoms in children are dwarfism, lumbar lordosis with protruberant abdomen, thoracic kyphosis, pectus carinatum, and a flattened midface. Many children also display hypotonicity. The eyes are wide set. Retinal detachment and severe myopia may occur in more than 50% of cases.

Atlantoaxial instability secondary to odontoid hypoplasia or osodontoideum is found in many patients and is responsible for myelopathy in up to one third. Instability may be anterior, posterior, or both. Symptoms include delayed developmental milestones, diminished endurance, and respiratory dysfunction. Reduction and fusion are indicated. Kyphoscoliosis may be encountered and should be treated as indicated with bracing or posterior instrumentation and fusion. Lumbar lordosis is usually secondary to hip flexion contractures.

The main problem in the lower extremity is coxa vara, which develops early and at times includes discontinuity of the femoral neck. Ossification of the capital femoral epiphysis is delayed and often does not appear until age 5 years. The combination of delayed ossification, highriding femur, and limited abduction often gives the false impression of a dislocated hip. Progressive subluxation can occur and may result in precocious arthritis. Valgus intertrochanteric osteotomy is indicated for a varus deformity of 100 degrees or less, progressive varus, high-grade epiphyseal angle, and the presence of an unossified triangular metaphyseal fragment in the femoral neck. Preoperative arthrography is necessary to determine the most congruent alignment.

Spondyloepiphyseal dysplasia tarda is usually transmitted as an X-linked recessive characteristic, remaining unrecognized until late in childhood. Many individuals exceed the third percentile for height. Significant joint deformities are uncommon but precocious arthritis may occur. Atlantoaxial instability has been described.

Multiple Epiphyseal Dysplasia

One of the more common skeletal dysplasias, multiple epiphyseal dysplasia, is usually inherited as an autosomal dominant trait. The pathologic abnormality is a disturbance in enchondral ossification of the epiphyses and physes. The ossific centers appear late and are fragmented and irregular. In general, individuals display mild to moderate short-limbed dwarfing with the adult height ranging from 145 to 170 cm, well above the third percentile.

The primary orthopaedic problem relates to precocious osteoarthritis predominantly involving the hips, knees, and ankles. Angular deformities are present, such as coxa vara at the hip, and coxa valga or, less often, genu vara at the knee. Most joints are usually involved symmetrically. The femoral head is flattened. Acetabular changes ranging from mild irregularity in ossification to severe dysplasia or protrusio acetabuli occur and help differentiate the disease from Legg-Calvé-Perthes disease. Avascular necrosis of the femoral head may also occur. Corrective osteotomies are indicated in symptomatic patients. Preoperative arthrography helps determine the orientation required to create optimal congruity. When possible, osteotomies are best performed close to skeletal maturity, as deformities tend to recur with growth. Spinal deformity, when present, is mild, usually consisting of insignificant end-plate irregularities of the thoracic spine.

The natural history of the hips is quite variable. It appears that the severity of the arthritis is reasonably constant within families. In isolated cases, a prognosis may be made radiographically. Precocious arthritis is more likely when the epiphyseal ossification is fragmented, the femoral head is deformed and poorly covered, and the acetabulum is dysplastic. While mechanical factors do play an important role, arthritis can also occur in congruent situations because of articular cartilage imperfections.

Shoulder disability is also related to the deformity. Minor epiphyseal abnormalities can lead to painful osteoarthritis, but severe deformity or "hatchet head" shoulder results in severe joint limitations at an early age.

Diastrophic Dysplasia

This is a rare skeletal dysplasia transmitted as an autosomal recessive trait and characterized by severe short-limbed dwarfism and striking orthopaedic abnormalities. The cause seems related to a defect in the structure or synthesis of type II collagen in the physis.

The presence of this disease may be recognized at birth by a narrow nasal bridge, broadened midnose, flared nostrils, and circumoral fullness. Fifty-nine percent of affected infants have a cleft palate. A peculiar ear deformity, cauliflower ear, occurs later in childhood because of a cartilage abnormality. Some infants with diastrophic dysplasia die of respiratory failure, but most have a normal life expectancy, assuming that a cardiopulmonary compromise secondary to severe scoliosis or quadriplegia secondary to cervical kyphosis do not occur.

These individuals have extremely short stature, with a mean adult height of 118 cm. Specific hand and foot abnormalities are nearly constant and quite characteristic. A severe, rigid equinovarus deformity usually requires surgery. Symphalangism of the proximal interphalangeal joints of the fingers, and an abducted "hitchhiker's" thumb are also present.

The long bones are shortened in a rhizomelic pattern. The epiphyseal ossification is delayed, resulting in flattening and irregularity. At the hip, dislocation or osteoarthritis are common sequelae of coxa vara and incongruity. Genu valgus deformities are common at the knees. Treatment is complicated by the severe flexion contractures that involve most joints. Thoracolumbar spine deformity occurs in 83% of patients, with scoliosis, kyphosis, or kyphoscoliosis usually developing before the age of 4 years. Early orthotic management is considered when the curves are flexible. Surgical treatment is required for curves that continue to progress. When present, cervical kyphosis may resolve or progress enough to result in quadriplegia. Surgery is indicated for continued progression or instability.

Multiple Cartilaginous Exostosis

This is one of the most common skeletal dysplasias, with an estimated incidence of nine cases per million. Its mode of inheritance is autosomal dominant and it displays a wide spectrum of involvement. Cartilaginous exostoses (osteochondromas) are found throughout the endochondral skeleton, predominantly involving the long bones, iliac crests, scapulae, and ribs. They arise from the metaphyses, point away from the epiphysis, and appear to extend down the diaphysis during growth. They increase in size and number with growth, and stabilize at skeletal maturity. Surgical excision of the entire cartilaginous cap is indicated when symptoms are caused either by pressure on contiguous structures such as peripheral nerves and vessels, or by interference with the gliding function of the tendons.

Stature may be somewhat affected. Seventy-five percent of involved individuals are below the mean height for their age, but are not considered dwarfs. Side-to-side differences in leg length are severe enough to require equalization procedures in half of the individuals.

Bones with the smallest cross sectional area at the epiphyses are more affected. In two bone extremities, differential growth results in angular deformities. In the upper extremities, shortening of the ulna leads to radial bowing, ulnar tilt at the distal radius, ulnar translation at the carpus, and radial head dislocations. Forearm rotation may be limited. In the lower extremity the fibula is more involved, resulting in a valgus ankle, diastasis of the ankle, and genu valgum. Corrective osteotomies, stapling, or lengthening procedures may be indicated.

The most serious orthopaedic problem is the development of chondrosarcoma, which occurs in approximately 1.3% of patients older than 21 years of age. A change in size of the exostosis or the onset of pain in an affected adult is cause for concern and investigation. Monitoring patients via annual bone scans has been recommended, but its efficacy remains unproven.

Treatment programs for ankle deformity have been established. Surgical indications include pain from trauma to the prominent masses, ankle pain associated with deformity, limited motion, and undesirable cosmesis. Excision of the osteochondroma alone is indicated for local symptoms or the development of angular deformity or length discrepancies in young patients. When tibiotalar valgus reaches 15 degrees, hemiepiphyseal stapling is performed. Fibular lengthening is done when the distal fibular physis is proximal to the distal tibial epiphysis. This single-stage lengthening is performed in conjunction with hemiepiphyseal stapling when valgus coexists with length discrepancy.

Metaphyseal Chondrodysplasia

The Schmid and McKusick types are the most common of a number of eponymic forms used to describe this heterogenous group of disorders. They are characterized by radiographic changes and the typical appearance of the metaphyses of the tubular bones. The mode of inheritance is usually autosomal dominant. The histologic defect appears to lie in the proliferative and hypertrophic zone of the physis.

The condition is first recognized in early childhood when children present with a waddling gait, exaggerated lumbar lordosis, genu varum, and short stature. The radiographic appearance of an enlarged metaphysis and widened cupped physis is similar to rickets. Coxa vara occurs without an associated bowed femur. It may be treated with valgus intertrochanteric osteotomy when progressive. Genu varum may be severe in the Schmid type. Surgical correction should be delayed until it is determined that spontaneous correction will not occur. Metaphyseal chondrodysplasia may be associated with neutropenia, lymphopenia, immune deficiency, pancreatic exocrine insufficiency, Hirschsprung's disease, and intestinal malabsorption.

Enchondromatosis

Enchondromatosis, or Ollier's disease, is a nonhereditary disorder characterized by linear masses of cartilage in the metaphysis and diaphysis of the long bones. The extent of the lesions varies greatly, and distribution is asymmetric and often unilateral.

The involved limbs are short and deformed. Pathologic fractures may occur. Lesions enlarge during growth, ceasing at puberty. Orthopaedic treatment is required to correct limb-length discrepancies and to realign the deformities. Epiphysiodesis can be used when the discrepancies are small. Callus distraction methods can be used both to lengthen and to realign the significantly shortened and deformed extremity.

Sarcomatous changes, often heralded by localized growth or pain in adults, occur in approximately 25% of cases. The chondrosarcomas that occur are usually low-grade.

Mucopolysaccharide Storage Disease

This group of disorders is characterized by a deficiency of specific lysosomal enzymes required for the degradation of glycosaminoglycans. The substances accumulate in tissues such as brain, viscera, heart, lung, and joints. Affected individuals are normal at birth but worsen as the disease progresses, producing the characteristic clinical course of normal beginning, plateau, and then downhill progression. With the exception of X-linked type II

Table 4. The mucopolysaccharidoses

Type	Syndrome	Biochemical Defect
I	Hurler; Scheie	α-L-Iduronidase
II	Hunter	Sulfoid uronate sulfatase
IIIA	Sanfillipo A	Heparan N-sulfatase
IIIB	Sanfillipo B	N-Acetyl-α-D-glucosaminidase
IIIC	Sanfillipo C	Acetyl CoA:α-glucosaminide-N-acetyltransferase
IIID	Sanfillipo D	N-Acetyl-α-D-glucoaminide-β-sulfatase
IVA	Morquio A	N-Acetylgalactosamine-6-sulfatase
IVB	Morquio B	β-Galactosidase
VI	Moroteaux-Lamy	Arylsulfatase B
VII	Sly	β-Glucuronidase

Hunter syndrome, all are inherited as autosomal recessive disorders. They are classified by the specific enzyme involved and the clinical course (Table 4). Different eponymic diseases may be caused by the same enzyme defect, and several enzyme defects can cause the same eponymic disease.

Affected children have a characteristic clinical appearance with coarse facial features and short stature. Radiographic findings include platyspondyly with an anterior tongue, broad medial end of the clavicle, and the characteristic pelvis with flared iliac wings, large capacious acetabula, and unossified femoral head cartilage with coxa valga.

The two most common varieties are mucopolysaccharidosis I (Hurler's syndrome, Scheie's syndrome) and mucopolysaccharidosis IV (Morquio's syndrome). Type I is the most severe mucopolysaccharide storage disease and causes cardiopulmonary complications that result in death within the first decade of life. The enzyme defect may be detected in the blood and on skin biopsy, which allows accurate diagnosis, carrier detection, and prenatal diagnosis. The course facial features and hepatosplenomegaly become apparent by the age of 18 months. Other characteristics include short stature, with a disproportionately short trunk, thoracolumbar kyphosis, and corneal opacities.

Children with Morquio's syndrome have normal intelligence and survive well into adulthood. The short trunk disproportionate dwarfism is established by the age of 2 or 3 years and progresses. Pectus carinatum is also apparent. The most severe orthopaedic problem is atlantoaxial instability, which is secondary to odontoid hypoplasia and ligamentous laxity. Myelopathy may occur at age 5 or 6 years, causing a gradual loss of walking ability. Spinal fusion may be necessary at an early age. The iliac crest has been shown to be a poor source of bone in these individuals. The occurrence of platyspondyly and thoracolumbar kyphosis may also lead to myelopathy. Severe genu valgus deformities result from significant ligamentous laxity.

Atlantoaxial instability has now been demonstrated in mucopolysaccharide storage disease type VII, and screening for instability is now suggested in this group as well as in types I and IV.

Chromosomal Abnormalities

Chromosomal abnormalities, including trisomy, deletion, and unbalanced translocation cause approximately 10% of all congenital malformations. Fifteen percent of moderate to severe retardation and 5% to 10% of fetal deaths beyond 20 weeks' gestation are associated with some form of chromosomal abnormality. As these entities tend to cause patterns of multiple abnormalities, karyotyping is indicated in the child who has two or more primary malformations that together do not fit into any recognizable syndrome.

Trisomy 21: Down Syndrome

Down syndrome occurs in approximately one of every 700 to 800 live newborns. It is the most common autosomal chromosome abnormality and the most common malformation-mental retardation syndrome known. The physical features are distinct enough to permit identification of the disorder in the newborn. Craniofacial abnormalities include brachycephaly, small ears, upslanted palpebral fissures, low nasal root, flat midface, full cheeks, and facial grimace while crying. Epicanthal folds and simian crease have only a 50% frequency of occurrence. Brachydactyly is commonly found in the hand. Hypotonia occurs in 90%.

Cytogenetic studies should be performed in all patients with the clinical phenotype of Down syndrome to determine the presence of chromosomal syndromes that mimic the syndrome, such as XXXXY, partial 10Q trisomy, and to determine in those with Down syndrome the type of chromosomal abnormality and the corresponding risk to the offspring. Of individuals with Down syndrome, 95% have an extra chromosome. Translocations account for 4% of the cases, and mosaicism approximately 1%. In those with the translocation variety, one third of the cases will have one parent as a carrier. The risk of recurrence with one carrier is 5% to 15% with maternal involvement, and 2% to 5% for paternal involvement. The prevalence of Down syndrome increases with advanced maternal age, and the risk of age 35 years is approximately one of 200 live births. The likelihood that a mother younger than age 35 years will have a second child with this deformity is 1%.

Growth and developmental retardation exist. Affected children are of short stature, with mean adult heights of 154 cm and 145 cm for men and women, respectively. There is disproportionate shortness of the legs. Nearly all have diminished intelligence, although the IQ range is quite wide. Social skills tend to be closer to the norm than performance skills. Factors influencing intellectual achievement include family background, early institutionalization, early intervention programs, presence of congenital heart disease, and physical abnormalities. Because 50% of children have some hearing loss that can affect intellectual development, audiology examinations are necessary. The onset of ambulation is delayed to between ages 2 and 3 years, and the characteristic gait consists of a broad base and side-to-side waddling.

Congenital heart defects are present in 30% to 50% of affected individuals. One third are endocardial cushion defects, and one third ventricular septal defects. Gastrointestinal malformations are present in 5% to 7%. The mortality rate is increased during the first ten years, even when deaths resulting from congenital heart defects are excluded. This problem is believed to be caused by infections. The increased susceptibility may be caused by abnormal function of the T-lymphocytes or to an anatomic abnormality of the respiratory system, such as gastroesophageal reflux, primary pulmonary hypertension, and obstructive sleep apnea. Ninety percent of children without significant congenital defects, however, will live to adulthood.

Individuals with Down syndrome are at increased risk for several other medical problems, including cataracts, juvenile onset diabetes mellitus, acquired thyroid conditions, and seizures. Leukemia is present in 1% of patients. Individuals seem to age prematurely, appearing older than their chronological age. Some develop a progressive dementia similar to Alzheimer's disease by the fourth decade.

Orthopaedic problems are predominantly related to the increase in ligamentous laxity. The most significant problem is atlantoaxial instability with an anterior C1-2 interval greater than 5 mm, which occurs in approximately 20%.

An idiopathic scoliotic pattern develops in 50% of involved individuals. It should be managed according to the usual criteria with bracing and posterior spinal fusion. Progression is most likely in institutionalized women.

In the lower extremity, the knee and hip are the most frequently affected. Recurrent subluxations of the patella occur in one third of the individuals, while 10% have frank dislocations. Physical therapy is difficult in these children, but surgical results will be compromised by recurrence caused by ligamentous laxity. One out of 20 children are affected with hip instability during the first decade. Acute dislocations, habitual dislocation, subluxation, and progressive instability and dysplasia may continue into adulthood. Treatment must be tailored to each anatomic problem, but soft-tissue procedures must be supplemented by correction of bony deformities to obtain stability.

Slipped capital femoral epiphysis may be seen in these individuals, and hypothyroidism should be looked for. Planovalgus deformities of the feet are common but rarely symptomatic. Metatarsus primus varus is often found and may result in a symptomatic hallux valgus deformity. Juvenile rheumatoid arthritis also seems to be linked to Down syndrome.

Recent reviews have demonstrated a very significant complication rate in cervical fusions for instability. Prophylactic fusion is not indicated. Fusions should be reserved for those with neurologic findings or severe instability approaching 1 cm of atlantoaxial displacement.

Turner's Syndrome

This syndrome of gonadal dysgenesis is found in women with a single X chromosome (45 XO), a mosaic pattern (XO/XX), or with deletions of a portion of the X chromosome. The clinical features involve short stature, sexual infantilism, web neck without bony abnormalities, and cubitus valgus. The ovaries are replaced by streaks of stromal tissue. Afflicted persons will be only 137 to 142 cm tall at adulthood.

Idiopathic scoliosis is the most critical orthopaedic problem and is quite common. It may begin early and has an extended period of progression, as skeletal maturation is delayed considerably in these individuals. Treatment of the growth retardation and sexual infantilism with estrogens, growth hormone, and androgen may accelerate curve progression. An additional unique finding in these individuals is a relative shortening of the fourth and occasionally the fifth metacarpal and, in some cases, the metatarsal.

Noonan's Syndrome

Individuals with this syndrome, which is phenotypically identical to Turner's syndrome, are males with a normal XY genotype and females with a normal XX genotype. Scoliosis occurs in 40% of those affected, along with a distinctive chest wall deformity with a pectus carinatum superiorly and pectus excavatum inferiorly. There is also a degree of mental retardation and right-sided congenital heart defects.

Children with Noonan's syndrome reportedly are at risk for malignant hyperthermia during surgery. In these reports, the individuals may have been confused with children with the King-Denborough syndrome, a rare myopathic form of arthrogryposis. Nevertheless, precautions against malignant hyperthermia should be used in individuals with Noonan's syndrome.

Malformation Caused by Teratogens

Malformations during pregnancy may be caused by maternal conditions, diseases, or infections, drugs taken during pregnancy, or exposure to heavy metals. Malformations are most likely to occur during the first trimester, although exposure to teratogens in the second and third trimester may be related to the development of microcephaly, growth retardation, and cognitive dysfunction.

Fetal AIDS

The human immunodeficiency virus (HIV) may be transmitted across the placenta. The median time after birth to the onset of symptoms in infants of high-risk mothers is four months. Sixty percent of affected individuals are diagnosed before the first birthday. The serologic response to HIV in children is weak and often falsely negative. Dysmorphic cranial and facial features that may indicate the presence of HIV include prominent, box-shaped forehead, wide-spaced eyes, growth failure, and microcephaly. Further indications of the disease are poor growth, lymphadenopathy, hepatosplenomegaly, frequent episodes of diarrhea, otitis media, rash, persistent oral thrush, and recurrent bacterial infections.

Fetal Alcohol Syndrome

There is a clear association between maternal alcohol use and fetal damage. Two drinks per day or periodic binges in the early stages of pregnancy may be associated with recognizable abnormalities. There is a 50% or greater risk of abnormalities in growth and performance in offspring of chronic alcoholics.

The children are small at birth, and height and weight remain below normal. These symptoms are often presented as a failure to thrive. Mental retardation, delayed developmental milestones, and hypotonicity or hypertonicity are common. Newborns characteristically are jittery and tremulous and a relative lack of coordination continues. The dysmorphic facies include a flat midface with narrow palpebral fissures, low nasal bridge, and short, upturned nose.

Orthopaedic problems are present in 50% of individuals. Joint motion is restricted, especially in the elbows and the metacarpophalangeal and interphalangeal joints of the hands. Hip dislocation is present in 10%. There may be cervical vertebral fusions, congenital scoliosis, and myelodysplasia. Upper extremity bone fusions involving a proximal radial ulnar synostosis and carpal bone fusions are encountered. Cleft palate and cardiac malformations also occur.

Neurocutaneous and Vascular Syndromes

Neurofibromatosis

Neurofibromatosis is the most common single gene disorder in humans. It is autosomal dominant, with a 100% rate of penetrance. Half of reported cases comprise a fresh mutation. The cause is unknown, although cells derived from the neural crest and their response to circulating substances have been implicated.

In neurofibromatosis, malignancies can occur in 5% to 15% of affected individuals. Neurofibromas in adolescence and adulthood may undergo malignant degeneration, or malignant neurofibrosarcomas may appear de novo. Other malignancies, including Wilms' tumor, leukemia, and rhabdomyosarcoma, are more likely to appear. Affected individuals tend to be short with large heads. They frequently experience precocious puberty. Seizures are another finding and varying degrees of intellectual deficiency are presented in 50%.

There are two forms of neurofibromatosis. Type I has a gene location on chromosome 17 and an incidence of one in 3,000 live births. It demonstrates the more typical skin changes. Type II, with a gene location on chromosome 22, is far less common, with an incidence of one in 50,000 births. It has fewer peripheral lesions but more significant intracranial ones, including bilateral acoustic neuromas and other tumors of the meninges and Schwann cells (Outline 1).

The clinical presentation of the disease varies widely, and many affected individuals appear normal at birth. Numerous organ systems are affected. In the more common type I neurofibromatosis, characteristic features are the cutaneous pigment changes of café-au-lait spots, axillary freckles, hyperpigmented nevi, and neurofibromas of the peripheral and central nervous systems. The café-au-lait spots are usually present at birth but may take up to a year or more to appear. Their number and size increase after their initial presentation, rendering inaccurate a diagnosis based on numbers and size during the first decade of life. The hyperpigmented nevus is often associated with a deep plexiform neurofibroma.

The typical neurofibromas begin to appear by age 10 years; they also increase in size and number during puberty. Lesions are composed of benign Schwann cells and fibrous connective tissue. They are either sessile or peduncular and may develop along the path of a peripheral nerve or motor root. They rarely cause neurologic deficit.

Plexiform neurofibroma presents a much more serious problem. They usually are present at birth and are characterized by a deep brown skin pigmentation with overhanging pendulous skin folds. Though histologically benign, they cause the significant problems of limb overgrowth and gigantism, infiltration of the neuraxis, and grotesque facial disfigurement. As the lesions are highly vascular, surgical removal is impractical.

Partial gigantism and macrodactyly are usually related to the plexiform neurofibromas. The overgrowth does not symmetrically involve all parts and the skeleton is often variably involved. Erosion and cystic changes may occur within bones and may mimic other diseases.

A major orthopaedic problem is present in at least 40% of these individuals. Neurofibromatosis must be considered when evaluating a patient with a significant scoliosis or spinal deformity, pseudarthrosis of a long bone, hypertrophy of a part, or an unusual radiographic lesion.

Scoliosis occurs frequently, and it may be the presenting symptom. Curvatures are either idiopathic and dystrophic. The dystrophic type is short (four to six spinal segments) and sharp. The classic radiographic findings are scalloping of the posterior vertebral body, enlargement of the neuroforamen, defective eroded pedicles, and thinning or pencilling of the ribs. The enlarged neuroforamen may occur with normal intraspinal contents, but may also be indicative of intraspinal tumor, dumbbell neurofibroma, dural ectasia, and lateral meningocele. The idiopathic variety is treated as such. Dysplastic curvatures are often progressive and refractory to brace treatment. Prompt surgical fusion is required. The

Outline 1. Criteria of NF-1 and NF-2

Criteria for NF-1 (2 or more of the following):
1. Six or more café-au-lait macules whose greatest diameter is 5 mm in prepubertal patients and 15 mm in postpubertal patients
2. Two or more neurofibromas of any type or one plexiform neurofibroma
3. Freckling in the axillary or inguinal regions
4. Optic glioma
5. Two or more Lisch nodules (iris hamartomas)
6. A distinctive osseous lesion, such as sphenoid dysplasia or thinning of long bone cortex, with or without pseudarthrosis
7. A first-degree relative (parent, sibling, or child) with NF-1 by the above criteria

Criteria for NF-2 (1 of the following):
1. Bilateral eighth nerve masses seen with appropriate imaging techniques (eg, computed tomography or magnetic resonance imaging)
2. NF-2 in a first-degree relative, and either a unilateral eighth nerve mass or two of the following: neurofibroma, meningioma, glioma, schwannoma, or juvenile posterior subcapsular lenticular opacity

(Reproduced with permission from Aoki S, Barkovich AJ, Nishimura K, et al: Neurofibromatosis types 1 and 2: Cranial MR findings. *Radiology* 1989;172:527-534.)

incidence of pseudarthrosis is very high. An associated kyphosis increases the risk of paraplegia and of pseudarthrosis following surgery. Anterior fusion combined with posterior instrumentation and fusion are indicated when the kyphosis exceeds 50 degrees or the scoliosis is greater than 80 degrees. The combined procedures do not guarantee stability.

Spinal stability is often lost because of the pedicular changes that lead to subluxations or dislocations throughout the spine. Cervical kyphosis is commonly associated with a dystrophic thoracic curve and must be evaluated before using endotracheal anesthesia.

Pseudarthrosis usually involves the tibia and appears in infancy with the classic anterolateral bow. The ulna, femur, clavicle, radius, and humerus may also be involved. The relationship of pseudarthrosis to neurofibromatosis is well established, but the mechanism remains unknown. The prognosis for establishing a solid union remains guarded.

Magnetic resonance imaging studies have demonstrated a high sensitivity and allow the detection of intracranial lesions and the differentiation of type I from type II neurofibromatosis. Such studies of the spine are mandatory before surgery to detect the intraspinal lesions of neurofibroma, dural ectasia, and meningocele can be undertaken.

Spinal dislocation with minimal or no neurologic defects can occur, because the dural ectasia causes significant erosion, leaving more space for the neural elements. Stabilization alone without reduction, which avoids dissection near the precarious neural elements, may reverse early neurologic findings in selected patients.

Congenital Vascular Malformations

Congenital vascular abnormalities are classified as telangiectasias and hemangiomas. Telangiectasias consist of blood vessels that are normal in number but are dilated. Hemangiomas are produced by the proliferation of endothelial cells. Some syndromes have no genetic basis while both autosomal dominant (blue rubber bleb nevus syndrome) and recessive (ataxia telangiectasia) modes of inheritance exist. Several types of hemangiomas exist and their clinical significance varies widely. Some have major orthopaedic considerations.

Klippel-Trenaunay Syndrome

This syndrome consists of the classic triad of cutaneous hemangiomas, varicose veins, and limb hypertrophy, though only the cutaneous hemangiomas may be noted at birth. These hemangiomas are of the port-wine variety and often follow a dermatomal distribution. Cavernous and capillary hemangiomas may also be present as well as malformed lymphatics. Stasis, ulceration, and focal thrombophlebitis are local problems.

Clinical outcome is usually related to the presence or absence of arteriovenous malformations. These may be so extensive as to cause high output cardiac failure and require amputation as a life-saving measure. Patients with functionally significant arteriovenous malformations are those most likely to develop gross limb hypertrophy.

The overgrowth, which involves both soft tissue and bone, follows a variable pattern, with involvement of a single digit, an entire limb, or multiple limbs in a contralateral or ipsilateral fashion. Surprisingly, the hypertrophy may involve an anatomic part remote from the vascular malformation. The variable amount of overgrowth adds to the confusion, and the soft tissue and bony hypertrophy may not involve corresponding parts. Loss of joint motion often accompanies overgrowth and is resistant to treatment. Torsional malalignments also occur. Orthopaedic treatment is difficult because there is no well established, successful treatment of a vascular malformation, although selective embolization may temporarily diminish blood loss during orthopaedic procedures. Inability to wear shoes may be treated with debulking procedures and epiphysiodesis, when the local vascular anatomy permits. Leg-length discrepancy may require an epiphysiodesis, but timing is difficult to determine, because the rate for overgrowth is often nonlinear. Often the most conservative treatment is amputation.

Maffucci's Syndrome

This skeletal dysplasia is characterized by the presence of both multiple enchondromas and cavernous hemangiomas. In 25% of patients, both are evident at birth or within the first year of life, and in most the diagnosis can be established by the age of 5 years. The hemangiomas are anatomically unrelated to the enchondromas and produce little disability. The enchondromas cause the disability. They can involve the entire appendicular and axial skeleton, but do show a predilection for the small bones of the hands and feet. More than half of the patients will have significant sequelae, including severe an-

gular deformities of limbs, leg-length discrepancy, scoliosis and stunting of stature, severe limb distortion, pathologic fractures, and neurologic symptoms.

Despite what can be a severely deforming orthopaedic condition, the major concern is the association with malignancy. Sarcomatous transformation within the enchondroma occurs in 30% of the patients. Malignant degeneration also occurs in other mesodermal tissue, as angiosarcoma and fibrosarcoma. Benign and malignant tumors are more likely to develop in the abdominal viscera and the central nervous system. Serial evaluation of the skeletal system, with technetium bone scan, and of the abdomen and central nervous system is indicated.

Miscellaneous

Hemihypertrophy

Most instances of asymmetric extremity enlargement are the result of localized, acquired causes such as inflammation, infection, trauma, neurologic abnormalities, and tumors. Some syndromes such as Beckwith-Wiedemann and Russell-Silver are associated with congenital hemihypertrophy, but the most common form is idiopathic hemihypertrophy. In these congenital forms, exactly half of the body is enlarged, including the upper and lower extremities as well as the trunk, face, and paired viscera. The skeleton is increased both in length and width and the enlarged limb always grows faster than the opposite side, resulting in an increasing leg-length discrepancy. Longitudinal growth studies are required and the usual treatment is an appropriately timed epiphysiodesis. The discrepancy in girth is untreatable at present. There are associated structural renal malformations and a 5% risk of development of an intra-abdominal malignant tumor, most commonly Wilms' nephroblastoma.

Arthrogryposis Syndromes

Arthrogryposis is characterized by congenitally deformed, fusiform, and creaseless limbs, and by rigid joints. This condition may be caused by intrinsic factors that work along the neuromuscular pathway and include lesions of the brain, anterior horn cells, peripheral nerves, motor endplates, and muscles or by extrinsic factors that include abnormalities of the fetal environment such as oligohydramnios. The most frequent pathologic finding is reduction of the number of anterior horn cells in the spinal cord. Local pathologic findings are a thickened joint capsule and the fibrocartilaginous replacement of atrophic muscle fibers.

There are well over 100 different clinical disorders that occur along with congenital contractures. These include random events as well as specific syndromes and chromosomal abnormalities. It is obvious that a specific diagnosis is necessary for proper treatment, planning, and counseling. Children with congenital contractures require a careful neurologic evaluation that includes neurometric and serum enzyme studies. Muscle biopsy should be delayed until after four months of age, as interpretation of specimens before this time is difficult. The risk of recurrence is 5% when no specific cause can be determined. Real-time ultrasound can diagnose multiple contractures in utero.

Arthrogryposis Multiplex Congenita

Arthrogryposis multiplex congenita, also known as amyoplasia, is the most common condition causing congenital articular rigidity. The disease is not genetic, and there are no diagnostic laboratory tests. The diagnosis is based on the presence of consistent clinical features: (1) characteristic symmetric limb posture; (2) typical facies; (3) absence of visceral abnormalities; (4) normal intelligence; and (5) absent family history.

Delivery may be difficult because of fetal joint stiffness and malpositioned limbs, resulting in a 25% incidence of fractures at birth. The face in infancy and childhood is typically oval and small, with a slightly upturned nose. A characteristic but inconsistent feature is a capillary hemangioma over the bridge of the nose, forehead, and eyelids. There is a 15% incidence of inguinal hernia secondary to muscular weakness. Survival during the first year of life is threatened by respiratory problems caused by positioning difficulties, but thereafter the life expectancy is unaffected.

About one third of these patients will have scoliosis of the typical neuromuscular pattern, which responds poorly to bracing and, if progressive, requires surgical stabilization. Congenital scoliosis is most unusual and its presence suggests the diagnosis of multiple pterygium syndrome.

The goal of treatment of the upper extremity is to maintain flexibility to allow self-care skills and increased mobility. Surgery should be delayed until at least the second year of life to allow a study of the functional capabilities of the hands. Procedures should be designed to improve function, and not merely to correct deformities.

The shoulders are typically held in internal rotation and adduction, and function may at times be improved with a derotation osteotomy. The elbow is extended and if adequate motion cannot be obtained conservatively, soft-tissue releases, tendon transfers, and distal humeral osteotomies may be helpful. The wrist is flexed and ulnarly deviated.

Knee deformities occur in 60% of involved individuals. Flexion and extension contractures occur, with flexion being more resistant to treatment. Extension contractures treated conservatively seem to have a high incidence of late arthritic radiographic changes, perhaps implicating overzealous manipulations. Femoral shortening

with hamstring release and quadriceps transfer has resulted in significant improvement in flexion deformities.

Multiple Pterygium Syndrome

This syndrome is autosomal dominant and is characterized by cutaneous webs across the flexor aspects of joints. In the more severe cases, webs may cross the flexor creases of the anterior and lateral neck, the popliteal space, and antecubital, axillary, and interdigital areas. When the webs are smaller, the condition may be mistaken for amyoplasia, but multiple pterygium syndrome can be differentiated by its associated orthopaedic problems: congenital vertical talus in 80% of involved individuals and congenital scoliosis with failures of segmentation in more than 50% of affected individuals. Surgical releases should be performed before adaptive bony changes, although the superficial location of the sciatic nerve at the knee must be kept in mind.

Congenital Constriction Band Syndrome

This syndrome represents a random, nongenetic disruption sequence that apparently occurs when strands of amniotic tissue wrap about previously formed portions of the fetus. The incidence is approximately one in 5,000 live births. Its association with neonatal death is well established.

The deformities have been classified as: (1) simple ring constrictions; (2) ring constrictions accompanied by fusion of the distal bony parts; (3) ring constrictions accompanied by fusion of the soft-tissue parts; and (4) intrauterine amputation. Distribution is random although the distal portions of the limbs are more usually affected. Bands may cross the face and trunk; however, this does not occur often. The amputations behave as acquired instead of congenital amputations and can be associated with the problems of appositional growth.

Associated anomalies include syndactyly in up to 50% of cases, clubfoot, cleft lip, cleft palate, and cranial defects. Proximal bands are more likely to be associated with neurologic defects. Leg-length discrepancy in excess of 2.5 cm occurs in 20% of the patients.

The treatment is essentially cosmetic, although it may be emergent if significant venous or lymphatic disturbances exist. Releases customarily have been formed via Z-plasties as a staged procedure.

When limbs are more proximally involved, there seems to be an incidence in the 20% range of neurologic deficits. Early detection with electrodiagnostic studies and early surgical treatment via neurolysis or grafting may improve the ultimate neurologic function. Additionally, single stage constriction band releases are reportedly safe.

Annotated Bibliography

General Considerations

Goldberg MJ: *The Dysmorphic Child: An Orthopedic Perspective*. New York, Raven Press, 1987.

The clinical features of the most common syndromes are presented in a thoroughly organized fashion with an emphasis on differential diagnosis.

Connective Tissue Disorders

Cohn DH, Byers RH: Clinical screening for collagen defects in connective tissue diseases. *Clin Perinatol* 1990;17:793-809.

The current molecular basis of the collagen diseases is reviewed followed by a description of the methods for prenatal screening.

Gamble JG, Strudwick WJ, Rinsky LA, et al: Complications of intramedullary rods in osteogenesis imperfecta: Bailey-Dubow rods versus nonelongating rods. *J Pediatr Orthop* 1988;8:645-649.

Significant complication rates were encountered with intramedullary roddings of long bone in children with this disease. The Bailey-Dubow rods had a lower rate of reoperation and replacement than nonelongating rods.

Prockop DJ: Mutations in collagen genes as a cause of connective-tissue diseases. *N Engl J Med* 1992;326:540-546.

This review article presents the latest knowledge of the molecular and genetic base of the connective tissue disorders.

Mucopolysaccharide Storage Disease

Pizzutillo P, Osterkamp JA, Scott CI Jr, et al: Atlantoaxial instability in mucopolysaccharidosis type VII. *J Pediatr Orthop* 1989;9:76-78.

A case of atlantoaxial instability with quadriparesis is reported in a 15-year-old boy with mucopolysaccharidosis type VII.

Skeletal Dysplasia

Ingram RR: The shoulder in multiple epiphyseal dysplasia. *J Bone Joint Surg* 1991;73B:277-279.

Analysis of patients with shoulder symptoms revealed two groups. Those with minor epiphyseal involvement developed painful osteoarthritis in middle age but retained shoulder motion until late in the clinical course. Those with "hatchet head" shoulders had symptoms in middle age but limited motion developed at an earlier stage.

Liu J, Hudkins PG, Swee RG, et al: Bone sarcomas associated with Ollier's disease. *Cancer* 1987;59:1376-1385.

Approximately 30% of patients presenting with Ollier's disease had malignant bone neoplasms. There were 12 chondrosarcomas, 2 differentiated chondrosarcomas, 1 chordoma, and 1 osteosarcoma. The prognosis is good for most patients.

MacKenzie WG, Bassett GS, Mandell GA, et al: Avascular necrosis of the hip in multiple epiphyseal dysplasia. *J Pediatr Orthop* 1989;9:666-671.

The changes of avascular necrosis, documented by plain radiographs, bone scintigraphy, and magnetic resonance imaging were observed in nine of 11 patients with multiple epiphyseal dysplasia.

Snearly WN, Peterson HA: Management of ankle deformities in multiple hereditary osteochondromata. *J Pediatr Orthop* 1989;9:427-432.

A surgical treatment of symptomatic ankle lesions and deformities is developed. Hemiepiphyseal tibial stapling is performed when the tibiotalar valgus exceeds 15 degrees. When the relative fibular shortening is significant, fibular lengthening is indicated.

Treble NJ, Jensen FO, Bankier A, et al: Development of the hip in multiple epiphyseal dysplasia: Natural history and susceptibility to premature osteoarthritis. *J Bone Joint Surg* 1990;72B:1061-1064.

Two types of immature hips were identified. Premature osteoarthritis was inevitable in those with incongruent hips. Similar clinical courses were found within families.

Vilarrubias JM, Ginebreda I, Jimeno E: Lengthening of the lower limbs and correction of lumbar hyperlordosis in achondroplasia. *Clin Orthop* 1990;250:143-149.

Lower limb lengthenings of over 30 cm are described and analyzed.

Chromosomal Abnormalities

Segal LS, Drummond DS, Zanotti RM, et al: Complications of posterior arthrodesis of the cervical spine in patients who have Down syndrome. *J Bone Joint Surg* 1991;73A:1547-1554.

Ten Down syndrome patients who had posterior arthrodesis of the upper cervical spine were reviewed. All had complications which included infection and wound dehiscence, incomplete reduction, instability of adjacent motor section, neurological problems, resorption of autogenous bone graft, and death in the postoperative period.

Tredwell SJ, Newman DE, Lockitch G: Instability of the upper cervical spine in Down syndrome. *J Pediatr Orthop* 1990;10:602-606.

Ligamentous laxity of the upper cervical spine was noted at more than one level. Instability at the atlanto-occipital area was common.

Neurocutaneous and Vascular Syndromes

Aoki S, Barkovich AJ, Nishimura K, et al: Neurofibromatosis types 1 and 2: Cranial MR findings. *Radiology* 1989;172:527-534.

Cranial magnetic resonance imaging in 53 patients with NF-1 revealed 19 with optic gliomas, eight with parenchymal gliomas, and 32 with areas of prolonged T2 images. In the NF-2 group of 11, all had acoustic neuromas; in addition, eight had cranial nerve schwannomas and six had meningiomas.

Crawford AH: Pitfalls of spinal deformities associated with neurofibromatosis in children. *Clin Orthop* 1989;245:29-42.

Of 116 children with neurofibromatosis, 64% had spinal deformities. Combined anterior and posterior procedures are recommended on dystrophic curvatures when kyphosis exceeds 50 degrees or scoliosis 80 degrees. Magnetic resonance imaging or computed tomographic myelography should be performed preoperatively to determine the presence of intraspinal pathology. Cervical spine deformities are frequently overlooked.

McGrory BJ, Amadio PC, Dobyns JH, et al: Anomalies of the fingers and toes associated with Klippel-Trenaunay syndrome. *J Bone Joint Surg* 1991;73A:1537-1546.

In a series of 108 patients with this syndrome, 29 had anomalies of the digits; macrodactyly, syndactyly, metatarsus primus varus, clinodactyly, polydactyly, camptodactyly, and congenital trigger finger. Thirty-three of the 126 anomalies were in extremities uninvolved with vascular changes or hypertrophy.

Winter RB: Spontaneous dislocation of a vertebra in a patient who had neurofibromatosis: Report of a case with dural ectasia. *J Bone Joint Surg* 1991;73A:1402-1404.

Osseous erosions from dural ectasia can produce significant instability. In this case the neurological deficits resolved after stabilization without reduction of the complete dislocation of the ninth or the tenth thoracic vertebrae.

Miscellaneous Syndromes

Muguti GI: The amniotic band syndrome: Single-stage correction. *Br J Plast Surg* 1990;43:706-708.

Two cases of amniotic band syndrome were treated by single-stage excision of the ring and multiple Z-plasty repair.

Sarwark JF, MacEwen GD, Scott CI Jr: Amyoplasia: A common form of arthrogryposis. *J Bone Joint Surg* 1990;72A:465-469.

The current knowledge of amyoplasia is reviewed.

Segal LS, Mann DC, Feiwell E, et al: Equinovarus deformity in arthrogryposis and myelomeningocele: Evaluation of primary talectomy. *Foot Ankle* 1989;10:12-16.

Primary talectomy for equinovarus deformity in a group of arthrogryposis patients produced better results, decreased recurrence rates, and resulted in less procedures per foot than posterior medial releases. Cavus and forefeet deformities did occur after primary talectomies, and the long term status of these feet is not yet known.

Södergård J, Ryöppy S: The knee in arthrogryposis multiplex congenita. *J Pediatr Orthop* 1990;10:177-182.

Both operative and nonoperative treatment of flexion and extension knee deformities were evaluated. The treatment of flexion contractures was more difficult and more often required surgery. The risk of degenerative arthritis was evaluated in the group with extension contractures.

12

Multiple Trauma: Pathophysiology and Management

Pathophysiology

A wound causes activation of the leukocyte system, which is composed of all the circulating leukocytes (including platelets), the endothelium, and certain tissue cells (eg, the basophil and the mast cell). Wounds may be either closed (without direct bacterial contamination) or open (with direct bacterial contamination). The volume of devitalized and marginally viable tissue may be small (incised wounds, either accidental or surgical), moderate (indirect violence fractures, either open or closed), or large (direct violence fractures, burns, blunt crushing or tearing wounds, pancreatitis, blunt multiple trauma). The devitalized tissue has no circulation and therefore has little immediate effect on the systemic injury response, whereas the marginally viable tissue, with its intact but limited circulation, has a significant effect on the systemic response from the very beginning. It is the total volume of marginally viable tissue in all wounds that is important, and this tissue produces the edema observed. Wounds cause hypovolemia by bleeding, by fluid sequestration as edema, and, with major trauma, by a generalized capillary leak syndrome. This loss of circulating volume causes a failure of oxygen transport, which, if severe enough, can have negative consequences for the heart as a propulsive organ and for the gut mucosa as a containment mechanism for bacteria and bacterial toxin. It is most important for the fate of the wound and the patient that oxygen transport be promptly restored to normal or, preferably, supranormal levels by volume restoration and cardiopulmonary support.

In all wounds, the devitalized tissue provides nutrients to support microbial growth if there is bacterial access. Hematoma is particularly important in all wound complications. Hematoma provides a particularly good nutrient source for bacteria because of its numerous binding sites and its iron content. Devitalized muscle is probably an equally good source of nutrients. Essentially all clinically important bacteria require iron for growth, and the iron-binding proteins are an important antibacterial mechanism in the normal human body. Because the iron in hematoma is complexed to hemoglobin and that in muscle to myoglobin, it thus is available only to those bacteria that have the proper iron-releasing enzyme systems. This feature restricts the types of bacteria that can grow.

The presence of bacteria in the devitalized tissue of a wound does not constitute an infection. An infection must be defined as the progressive invasion of viable tissue by bacteria; a process that occurs much more readily in marginally viable than in normally viable tissue. Because the diffusion barrier created by devitalized tissue generally excludes systemic antibiotics, the bacterial dosage within devitalized tissue can rapidly (three to ten days) reach concentrations that enable the microorganisms to invade the nearby viable tissue and produce an infection. For the infection to be ongoing, the bacteria must either contain iron-releasing enzyme systems or elicit from the responding leukocyte system materials that continue to kill tissue in order to provide nutrients which support bacterial growth. Only a few surgically important bacteria, such as streptococci and some clostridia, contain such enzyme systems. Most others kill tissue by eliciting the release of tissue-destructive agents from activated leukocytes. Antibiotics are clearly effective in treating infections to the extent that they have access to the bacteria where they are causing disease and are correctly chosen and administered in the right dosage. The devitalized tissue produced by bacteria and their toxins and by activated leukocytes always interferes to some degree with antibiotic access. It is the systemic escape of activated leukocyte agents that produces the septic response and the organ failures.

Blunt Multiple Trauma

So far, single major wounds containing large amounts of devitalized and marginally viable tissue have been considered. The patient with blunt multiple trauma may have a large amount of marginally viable tissue in several wounds. After a period of edema, most of this tissue will revascularize spontaneously with no lasting functional damage. The muscle injuries secondary to femur and upper extremity fractures are good examples, as are the nonbleeding liver or spleen wound, the pulmonary contusion, and even the myocardial contusion. In addition to this sort of marginally viable tissue, there will be a host of hematomas that contain devitalized tissue but do not have bacterial exposure. Pelvic and retroperitoneal hematomas may contain large amounts of devitalized tissue. Closed management of a fracture is also associated with the need to manage devitalized hematoma.

The essential point is that all of these different wounds produce leukocyte systems activation, which in sum total may be very large. Because of circulatory access problems, this activation occurs in two phases. In the first phase, the marginally viable tissue, because of its limited circulation, produces massive leukocyte system activation. Although that activation will cause some of the marginally viable tissue to become devitalized, in general, it will lead to revascularization and a return to normal of most such tissue. In contrast, with devitalized tissue, the leukocyte system initially has only surface access. The activation of the leukocytes by the devitalized tissue surface leads over time to reabsorption of that tissue in association with continued vascular invasion and with leukocyte activation to a much smaller degree but for a much longer time until all devitalized tissue has been removed. The point is that in the course of its revascularization, the marginally viable tissue will have immediate large-scale systemic effects leading to organ (especially pulmonary) failure, while the devitalized tissue, if it is not invaded by bacteria, will have more enduring but much smaller systemic consequences.

The normal business of the leukocyte system in most of the body is the clearance of devitalized and marginally viable tissue (with or without bacterial growth), followed by direction of wound healing, largely by the macrophages. The normal business of the leukocyte system in the gut is the clearance of bacteria and bacterial toxins that transgress the gut wall to enter the rest of the body. Endotoxin is a particularly good and common activator of the leukocyte system. The leukocyte system in the normal gut has a host of backup mechanisms that reduce the penetration of the gut wall by bacteria and their toxins and which provide follow-up clearance (hepatic leukocyte system) for any bacteria or toxins missed by the leukocytes of the gut submucosa. As a result of all of these systems, although the normal gut contains sufficient bacteria and bacterial toxins to kill the host millions of times over, these agents have little systemic consequence. This is not true of the critically ill patient, as discussed below in the section on the hidden gut wound.

Local Metabolic Response

The leukocyte system is normally activated in two stages. In the first, the endothelium and circulating leukocytes are primed by the splitting of complement to produce several products. The complement cascade comprises more than 20 serum proteins. (The term "complement" is derived from the observation that this system is complementary to leukocytes in the immune system's battle against foreign invasion and effete tissue.) The complement factors of crucial importance for leukocyte priming are activated complement 3 (C3a) and 5 (C5a). These may be produced in the presence of devitalized tissue with or without bacteria and in the gut submucosa in the presence of bacteria and their toxins. Split complement products also may be produced by tissue hypoxia with subsequent reperfusion. This reaction occurs via the endothelial xanthine oxidase system. In the presence of sufficient hypoxia, the adenosine in ATP is converted to xanthine and hypoxanthine, while xanthine dehydrogenase is converted to xanthine oxidase. With reperfusion, this change releases oxidants that prime and damage the endothelium while producing hemolysis (small amount) or fragile rigid red blood cells (large amount) and splitting complement to its active agents either directly or through oxidant effects on the damaged red cells. This

endothelial system is present in all tissues, but the magnitude and duration of the hypoxia required for its activation is variable. The system appears to be most sensitive to hypoxia in the gut mucosa. The split complement factors produced (C3a, C5a) then prime the circulating leukocytes and endothelium by binding to cell receptors. These primed cells are inactive briefly until a second exposure to split complement factors. Such cells are routinely observed in the venous blood with all major trauma and in essentially all critically ill patients.

This basic system allows a temporary ischemic insult to recruit the long-term, much more active, oxidant-generating system of circulating leukocytes. Recruitment of this system not only adds oxidant-generating capacity but also releases destructive lysosomal enzymes, which normally work with the oxidants. This oxidant-generating capability is based on a cell membrane enzyme system and NADPH, which can be generated in quantity by the phagocyte. The oxidant released is normally the superoxide anion. The toxicity of the oxidants can be greatly increased by the Haber-Weiss reaction with free iron to produce the hydroxyl radical. The toxicity of the hydroxyl radical can likewise be greatly increased by chain reactions that create alkoxyl and peroxyl radicals from cell materials. One example of this series of reactions is peroxidation of the polyunsaturated lipids in the cell membrane. This can injure the lipid membrane severely enough to destroy the cell or can generate arachidonic acid products that have great biologic potency, such as the leukotrienes, prostaglandins, and thromboxanes. Peroxidation can also damage the extracellular matrix of protein and glycoproteins. Because normal wound healing is the result of a variety of growth factors acting on a normal interstitial matrix, this disruption of the matrix by oxidants can impair wound healing.

The type of phagocyte active in the wound varies with time. At first, the primary phagocyte is the neutrophil. This cell is very good at releasing and using the tissue-destructive system of oxidants and lysosomal enzymes but has little or no capacity to release cytokines and wound-healing factors. In the neutrophil phagolysosome, the superoxide radical, in conjunction with the enzyme myeloperoxidase, generates the very powerful oxidizing agent hypochlorous acid. By 48 to 72 hours, the plasma monocyte has matured into the tissue macrophage. This cell has a great capacity to generate and use the tissue-destructive systems but also releases a large number of cytokines and growth factors that modulate the function of wound cells to produce immune suppression and wound healing.

This joint oxidant-generating system from the endothelium followed by the phagocyte is clearly active in a number of the experimental tissue injuries that accompany ischemia–reperfusion. Examples include certain gastric stress ulcers; injuries of the pancreas, gut mucosa, liver, kidney, or heart; compartment syndromes; and burns.

There are normal systems in vivo to limit oxidant damage. These range from enzymes (superoxide dismutase, catalase) to ingested reducing materials (alpha-tocopherol, vitamin C) to acute-phase proteins (ceruloplasmin), to normal intracellular materials (glutathione peroxidase). There are also a large number of materials that, used pharmacologically, interfere with oxidant damage. Mannitol is the agent most commonly used clinically. Other such agents are dimethylsulfoxide (DMSO), dimethylthiourea (DMTU), and iron-binding agents such as deferoxamine, which is used to prevent formation of the hydroxyl radical.

Excess circulating split complement products are deactivated by carboxypeptidase N by conversion to their much less active des Arg derivatives. These products are routinely observed with major trauma and critical illness. The priming of leukocytes by split complement creates a cell predisposed both to enhanced production of oxidants and release of lysosomal enzymes in response to a second stimulus and to exposure of hidden receptors that facilitate the second stimulus. Oxidant products, blocked lysosomal destructive enzymes, and rigid red cells are also routinely observed in venous blood after major trauma and during critical illness. The rigid red cells reflect lipid peroxidation and can reduce microcirculatory flow. The additional receptor components of this response are at least CR1 and CR3 (phagocytic split complement), CD11/CD18 integrin adhesive molecules, and receptors for priming exocytic triggering with adherence by cytokines (tumor necrosis factor-α, granulocyte—macrophage colony-stimulating factor [GMSF], and granulocyte colony-stimulating factor [GSF]). The CD11/CD18 leukocyte adherence factors are composed of a CD18 molecule (also known as lectin adhesion molecule 1, or LECAM-1) and the CD11 molecule, which confers β_2-integrin specificity for the interstitial tissue receptors. These receptors are bared by the endothelial cell retraction that occurs as a part of priming. This same endothelial retraction also contributes to the edema observed.

At the same time these events are taking place in the leukocyte, the endothelium is being primed by split complement products, lipopolysaccharide (endotoxin), interleukin-1β (IL-1β), tumor necrosis factor-α, or other cytokines to expose its receptors. The primed circulating leukocytes then bind to the receptors of the primed endothelium. Diapedesis through the vessel wall requires that the leukocyte receptor be internalized and discarded and that the endothelium receptors be exposed and bound to the interstitial receptors. This apparently is achieved via endothelial cell synthesis and release of the cytokine IL-8. An endothelial-interstitial tissue gradient of IL-8 plus the split complement products C3a and C5a and the cytokines IL-1β and tumor necrosis factor-α then modulate leukocyte movement into the wound. Many of these same cellular responses are also produced by local wound or endothelial release of arachidonic acid derivatives such as leukotriene B4 plus platelet-activating factor and the cytokines IL-6, GMSF, and GSF. The release of oxi-

dants plus other mechanisms supports the generation of arachidonic acid derivatives by the wound. Leukotriene B4 is particularly important in leukocyte invasion of the wound, while prostaglandin E2 is particularly important in the wound and in venous blood as a suppressive agent. Prostaglandin E2 suppresses lymphocyte production of both IL-2 and IL-2 receptors, thus impeding both macrophage antigen presentation and lymphocyte clone expansion.

In the wound, adherence to the interstitium magnifies the exocytic response of the neutrophil at least to tumor necrosis factor-α and GMSF. Adherence, therefore increases the local extracellular release by the leukocyte system of tissue-destructive oxidants and lysosomal enzymes and perhaps of other agents. This causes the neutrophil to behave much more like a macrophage relative to oxidant release during the first 24 to 48 hours after injury while monocytes are maturing into macrophages. Thereafter, the macrophage becomes the dominant phagocytic cell, even the master cell, in the wound, releasing at least 100 different materials.

The materials released by the activated leukocyte system (especially the macrophage) are present in high concentrations in the wound and have strong effects on the different cells there. These effects are generally considered to be either autocrine or paracrine. The autocrine effects are those within the same cell type and may involve the cell of origin (cell-associated cytokine) or cells of the same lineage being influenced through materials in solution (cell-free cytokine). The paracrine effects are those produced by cells of one lineage on the behavior of cells of different lineage via soluble mediators. Autocrine cell-associated materials may exert their effects by direct cell-cell interaction (eg, antigen presentation by the macrophage to the lymphocyte). Many of the cytokines are produced primarily by macrophages, lymphocytes, or endothelium in the wound or by intact circulating cells, so that plasma concentrations seldom reflect the true activity of these molecules. The production of cytokines normally is severely suppressed in all cells. However, once the factories begin operation in response to a first stimulus, a second rather mild stimulus can elicit abundant production of cytokines in almost any tissue. The tissue-destructive systems that are released can be very damaging, causing further damage to and devitalization of normal tissue. Endotoxin is an excellent stimulus for this system. If the damage to the gut mucosa allows entry of endotoxin, self-regenerating tissue-damaging systems can be established.

Systemic Response

Some of the primed leukocytes (neutrophils, platelets, and monocytes) do not bind locally but continue circulating singly and in aggregates to the next organ in the venous system. There have been many studies of these circulating venous blood cells, which in general have been interpreted to show suppression of function that correlated with the prostaglandin E2 level. However, this general interpretation is clearly in error for the neutrophil and monocyte, because both of these cells, despite reduced activity in the plasma, have enhanced interstitial functions. Suppressed immune actions of the plasma lymphocyte clearly exist and probably are caused by prostaglandin E2. It is not possible to extrapolate the function of circulating leukocytes directly to interstitial function because of the effect of autocrine and paracrine agents in the wound and because the circulating leukocytes include the immature cells being delivered to the wound from other sources.

If the endothelium in the next organ is not primed, the newly arrived leukocytes simply rest there until their priming dissipates (internalization of the C3a and C5a receptor complex) and then continue their normal function. If the endothelium in the next organ is primed (and it could well be because of escape of wound products that are not supposed to escape), then the sequence of events will be the same as in the wound.

The primed tissue-bound leukocytes are further activated by phagocytosis of any material (devitalized tissue, bacteria, even sterile latex beads) and by exposure to bacterial toxins. The activated leukocyte system then releases a whole variety of materials. These include the leukocyte tissue-destructive system (oxidants, lysosomal enzymes, complement and split products, agents that produce microvascular thrombosis), a variety of cytokines (some of which have been discussed above), and eicosanoic acid derivatives (eg, prostaglandins, leukotrienes), histamine, and bradykinin, among others.

The tissue-destructive system of the phagocytes is released both extracellularly and intracellularly (into the phagolysosome). In its extracellular function, the oxidants and lysosomal enzymes carry out surface digestion that bares C3b receptors to aid phagocytosis, splits complement to produce the products required to support phagocytosis, and produces microvascular thrombosis to aid in isolating the wound from the rest of the body. This process activates and consumes platelets and causes both release of such platelet products as thromboxane A2 and the activation of all the systems related to blood clotting. In their intracellular function, the oxidants and lysosomal enzymes kill bacteria and digest them and phagocytized devitalized tissue in the phagolysosome. The tissue-destructive agents released into the wound by the activated leukocyte system clearly can damage and devitalize normally viable tissue.

Many of the agents whose function in the wound is vital have highly damaging effects on the body if they escape into the circulation in too great a quantity (eg, invasion by leukocytes of the next organ in the venous circulation or alteration of metabolism). It is therefore very important that these agents be confined to the wound.

Neuroendocrine Effects

In contrast to these products that are relatively isolated in the wound, there are a variety of agents that must escape to modulate the systemic response to the wound. In fact, the wound acts as an endocrine organ that superimposes its control on the normal neuroendocrine system of the body. This control is exerted in part by mobilization of the catabolic neuroendocrine system, which is normally active with exercise, probably through release of IL-1 and tumor necrosis factor (or a product of these agents), which then act on the hypothalamus to increase the activation of the sympathetic nervous system, the adrenal medulla, and the adrenal cortex. Hypothalamus activation increases the plasma concentrations of glucagon, epinephrine, adrenal corticosteroids, and beta-endorphins. It also increases the effect of direct sympathetic innervation on the stomach and colon, liver and pancreas, arterioles, veins, heart, and a number of other organs. The collective result of these activities is reduced gastric and colonic motility plus mobilization of the energetic substrate such as glucose and its precursors and fatty acids from adipose tissue. These same events mobilize oxygen transport by increasing cardiac output (venous vasoconstriction, cardiac contractility, cardiac rate) and, concurrently, pulmonary oxygen transport. All of these changes occur normally with exercise.

A variety of other reactions produce protein breakdown in resting skeletal muscle to supply the amino acids that support a variety of synthetic needs. This occurs normally in the absence of exercise. A breakdown product of IL-1, called by Clowes the "muscle proteolysis factor" appears to be important in modulating resting muscle protein catabolism. The synthetic events supported by this increased oxygen transport and provision of larger quantities of synthetic and energetic substrate are also in part modulated by wound endocrine function. These events include cytogenesis (bone marrow via colony-stimulating factors, lymphocyte cytogenesis via IL-2 and IL-6 and other agents, enterocyte replication, all the elements of granulation tissue via products of the macrophage), cell hypertrophy (cardiac and respiratory muscle and liver, all because of the greater work demands), and increased synthesis and release of acute-phase plasma proteins (probably an effect of the hepatic Kupffer cell and IL-6). Interleukin-6 not only stimulates hepatic synthesis of acute-phase proteins but also stimulates B-lymphocyte proliferation and immunoglobulin synthesis. Another example of a systemic wound effect is a decrease in plasma iron and zinc. As noted above, the decreased plasma iron is an antibacterial mechanism.

All of these synthetic events together increase the rate of energy expenditure and therefore the rate of heat generation. The intensity of this fever is dependent on the reset of the thermoregulatory hypothalamic control unit by IL-1 and possibly tumor necrosis factor or a product of these agents. This unit modulates heat dissipation via its regulation of the arteriovenous shunts that control blood flow in the subcapillary venous plexus of the skin where heat dissipation occurs. The set of the hypothalamic thermoregulatory center controls the zone of thermoneutrality, which is the ambient temperature at which the rate of energy expenditure is minimal for a nude person lying quietly in the room. Energy expenditure increases for room temperature below this (cold exposure) and above this (heat dissipation). For normal individuals, the zone of thermoneutrality is set at about 27 C (80.6 F). Because this is above the usual room temperature, an individual lying quietly in the nude in a normal room is cold exposed. In an alert and oriented person this problem is corrected with clothes or bedclothes. In sickness, the thermoneutral zone is increased to between 30 C (86 F) and 34 C (93 F). It is this event that produces a fever by reducing heat dissipation relative to the heat generated by the enhanced synthetic activity. This occurs at the same time cerebration is obtunded and multiple physical examinations remove the bedclothes without proper replacement. These events can easily lead to prolonged cold exposure, which increases energy expenditure in an attempt to increase body temperature while in addition producing vasoconstriction in the heat-dissipating areas of the skin. Temperature maintenance is a problem, not only during long-term ICU care, but also during acute resuscitation, where hypothermia is very common.

For both emergency and elective surgery, the operating room is by far the most common cause of hypothermia. It is very important to recognize this, because as these patients rewarm, they will have vasodilation that causes a blood volume which was barely adequate during hypothermia to become grossly inadequate. The patient then is hypovolemic. In the ICU, after full resuscitation, the patient must be kept covered with adequate bedclothes to reduce cold exposure, energy expenditure, and protein catabolism. Temperature maintenance is most difficult to accomplish with any sort of traction device, because the extremities are sources of significant heat dissipation. Elevated body temperatures that do not exceed 104 F have no ill effect; indeed, they probably have a beneficial effect and should not be corrected because the fever is far too valuable an index of the patient's clinical condition.

The Wound and the Final Clearance of Wound Agents

The systemic elements of the metabolic response to trauma are very important in survival. The acute-phase response not only provides a variety of antienzymes that entirely or partially block the function of the destructive lysosomal enzymes which escape the wound, but concurrently provides other agents, such as ceruloplasmin, that act as antioxidants to the oxidants which also escape the wound. This is one of the backup mechanisms that helps to control the systemic effects of any damaging wound materials that escape.

There is another backup mechanism in the lung. The normal lung clears all embolic material (aggregates of primed leukocytes and platelets, fat emboli, bacteria) and in addition clears prostaglandin E2 and bradykinin almost completely. There are probably a variety of other materials cleared that are as yet unknown. Prostaglandin E2—normally released from most organs into the venous blood—is released in large amounts, depending on wound size, by the wound. A total absence of prostaglandin E2 in arterial blood is required if prostaglandin E2 is to perform its normal biochemical regulatory function in the tissues via a local generation washaway system. This zero concentration in the arterial blood is normally accomplished by the lung's almost total clearance of prostaglandin E2. In addition to these functions, the lung is the principal source of angiotensin II via its angiotensin-converting enzyme. This system is very responsive to hypovolemia. How well these functions are performed with the pulmonary failure of adult respiratory distress syndrome (ARDS) is unknown, but the capacity is probably diminished; and systemic function changes may result. In addition, ARDS, pulmonary contusions, atelectasis, and pneumonia will activate the pulmonary leukocyte system, with probable direct release into the arterial blood of damaging products.

Support of the Systemic Response: Catabolism

The problem with this whole system is that the essential protein synthetic activities are supported only by the relatively small mass of protein contained in resting muscle. Even this substrate is in part wasted, because the proteins being synthesized and the proteins being broken down contain different quantities of amino acids. All the amino acids not used promptly in the new protein are catabolized with the production largely of glucose and urea. It is this event that contributes to the rise in hepatic gluconeogenesis and ureagenesis, which increases the urinary nitrogen output, producing the characteristic negative nitrogen balance of the patient who lacks exogenous nutritional support. Gluconeogenesis is further increased by the wound's consumption of glucose with release of lactate and by glucose consumption in adipose tissue to support the increased recycling of fatty acids into and out of triglycerides with release of glycerol.

In these patients, support with exogenous glucose plus protein (or its equivalent as amino acids in a bottle) can increase the rate of protein synthesis, and that increase can be almost matched to the rate of protein breakdown if sufficient exogenous protein is given. The amount of protein nutrition required far exceeds normal demands. The resting muscle in injured patients is primarily in the muscles of ambulation, and use of this protein leads to the extreme weakness observed in convalescence. Finally, not only is the protein in resting muscle a limited source to support synthesis in the rest of the body (five to ten days with severe septic response), but the biochemical changes required to obtain it lead to a glutamine deficiency. The only other source of glutamine is the lung, which is largely shut off with ARDS. Glutamine is essential for cytogenesis, as a fuel for the gut mucosa, and as a support element for the major intracellular antioxidant system based on glutathione. The other important vascular fuel source for the gut mucosa is ketone bodies, and hepatic production of ketone bodies is also largely shut off with the septic response. Within five to ten days, these changes grossly reduce both the energetic and the synthetic substrate available to support the essential synthetic processes of cytogenesis in the bone marrow, lymph nodes, and gut mucosa.

Granted the essential nature of the synthetic responses for survival and the limited protein stores of the normal body, it is imperative that after adequate oxygen-transport resuscitation, sufficient exogenous protein be provided to patients who are going to be critically ill for more that a few days, preferably with added glutamine. Bottled amino acid products do not contain glutamine, which must be added separately. The amount required appears to be in the range of 6 to 18 g or more per day but has not been well defined. The amount of exogenous protein that is sufficient depends in part on the magnitude of the septic response, but certainly is at least 1.5 g/kg per day and may be as much as 2.5 g/kg or more per day. It must be understood that the body has no way to deal with inadequate supplies of protein but can easily manage excess protein and its amino acids. It is therefore important to err on the side of too much protein. The daily amounts per kilogram actually administered were 1.5 g minimum, 2.38 g mean, and 4 g maximum. The supplies of energetic substrate provided beyond the obligatory glucose catabolism target of 150 g per day plus a bit (up to 500 g) are much less critical, because the body can and does burn fatty acids, which are present in ample amounts in most patients. In fact, glucose in excess of 400 to 600 g per day is mostly converted to fats in the liver before it is burned, and excess glucose clearly contributes to fatty liver failure.

The Hidden Gut Wound

The Hidden Wound and ICU Care

There is a hidden wound associated with hypovolemia and resuscitation that admits the bacteria and bacterial toxins of the gut lumen to the rest of the body. How big a problem this gut wound is depends on the degree and duration of the hypovolemia and the adequacy of resuscitation. The latter, in turn, depends not only on volume but also on the presence or absence of preexisting or acute limitations of cardiopulmonary or hepatic function and their management. The hypovolemia associated with a hidden gut wound may persist for a long period in the ICU under standard care and is closely associated with late septic deaths. Present standard ICU care does not always disclose the presence of a hidden gut wound.

Systemic Consequences of the Hidden Wound

The essential point of the hidden gut wound, both acute and chronic, is not only the penetration of the gut mucosa to produce bacteremias and toxemias but, even more importantly, that the clearance of these agents by the leukocyte system of the gut submucosa will increase the release of all the leukocyte tissue-destructive products plus the associated cytokines and arachidonic acid derivatives

previously discussed. Moreover, this release takes place, not into a wound, where significant diffusion limitations restrict access to the blood, but directly or almost directly into the circulating blood. Therefore, agents normally confined to the wound have only the anti-agents of the plasma to reduce their activity. These destructive agents are then carried to the liver, where they clearly damage parenchyma and activate the already primed hepatic leukocyte system, especially the Kupffer cells. The activation of the Kupffer cells plus wound release of IL-6 changes the function of hepatic parenchymal cells while the Kupffer cells attempt to clear both the destructive materials released from the hidden gut wound and the damaged hepatic tissue created by that material. It is this combination of events that produces the changes in hepatic function observed in association with the inflammatory lesions of multifocal microvascular thrombosis observed in biopsy specimens or at autopsy. It will also cause the release of tissue-destructive products from the hepatic leukocyte system. The essential point for the lungs is that both the hidden gut wound and the known trauma wounds are associated with the release of tissue-destructive leukocyte products to damage the lung. This damage does not need to involve detectable bacterial toxins or bacteria in either portal or systemic venous blood.

Enteral Feeding and Multiple Systems Organ Failure

We may state the problem differently. In contrast to the evidence that broad-spectrum antibiotics do not help, and some evidence that they make the pulmonary failure of multiple systems organ failure worse, all the observations of which we are aware in patients and animals without preexisting cardiopulmonary or hepatic disease show that rapid enteral feeding reduces gut bacterial translocation, the septic response, and organ failure if sufficient total protein is delivered (1.5 to 2.5 g/kg or more per day). The evidence that inadequate total protein intake is associated with sepsis and organ failure began with the publication of Border and associates in 1976 and now derives from a large number of studies, all based on inadequate protein intake in patients in the enforced supine position for long periods. Those studies were able to predict accurately which patients would die of the septic response and organ failure (98% accuracy based on one plasma analysis taken an average of nine days before death). It continues on the basis of a randomized study in severely burned children reported in 1980. Burn patients, especially children, are normally much more mobile than patients with blunt multiple trauma who are receiving conservative fracture management. In that 1980 study, early enteral protein intake in excess of the then-conventional recommendations (which were not low) was associated with a definite decrease in septic behavior, organ failures, and mortality rate. These results were confirmed and greatly expanded in animal studies. The results of the clinical report were largely replicated by other investigators studying severely burned adults. In that study, increased enteral protein intake did not improve nitrogen balance but did improve certain aspects of immune function. In animals with experimental peritonitis receiving the same nutritional support, those that received it enterally had a much better survival rate than those that received it intravenously.

Trauma Management

In 1985, 2.1 million individuals sustained a traumatic injury that resulted in hospitalization. Hospital expenditures totalled $11.4 billion, inclusive of professional fees. Adolescents and adults between the ages of 15 and 44 years accounted for nearly half of all discharges and total hospital costs. The elderly, who represent only 12% of the population, accounted for an additional 25% of the total discharges and hospital costs. Nearly three quarters of the hospitalizations and half of the total expenditures were for minor injuries: only 12% of patients and 25% of trauma care dollars involved injuries sufficiently severe to require treatment at trauma centers.

These data reveal the magnitude of the trauma problem in the United States. The cost of medical care for the victims is extensive but can be reduced through proper preventive legislation such as requiring the use of automobile seat belts and of helmets for motorcycle riders. The medical costs of motorcycle accidents decreased almost 49% in California when mandatory helmet legislation was enacted. The length of hospital stay by accident victims decreased 37% and the need for a hospital stay of longer than 20 days declined by 80%. The cost of long-term disability (longer than 30 days) decreased by 81%. The use of helmets by motorcycle riders reduced the risk of head injury by a factor of two and the risk of fatal accidents by half.

Triage

The initial triage for trauma patients in the prehospital arena has improved with the revision of the trauma score to include the Glasgow Coma Scale and assessment of systolic blood pressure and respiratory rate and to exclude capillary refill and respiratory expansion, which are difficult to assess in the field (Table 1). Patients with a Glasgow Coma Scale Score of less than 13, a systolic blood pressure of less than 90 mm Hg, or a respiratory rate of greater than 29 or less than 10 per minute should be sent to a trauma center. The revised trauma score does not require computation and is therefore easier to implement. Using these guidelines, the specificity for selecting appropriate patients for the trauma center is 80%, and 97% of the patients who die from their injuries are selected for triage to the trauma center. Trauma scoring methods are discussed in greater detail below.

Airway Control

The establishment of endotracheal intubation in the emergency room to control a trauma patient's airway as well as to maintain proper oxygenation can be a lifesav-

Table 1. Evaluation with revised trauma score

Glasgow Coma Score	Systolic Blood Pressure	Respiratory Rate/Min	Coded Value*
13-15	>89	>29	4
9-12	76-89	10-29	3
6-8	50-75	6-9	2
4-5	1-49	1-5	1
3	0	0	0

*Patients with total score of 11 or less should be sent to a trauma center (Reproduced with permission from Champion HR, Sacco JS, Copes WS, et al: A revision of the trauma score. *J Trauma* 1989;29:623-629.)

ing procedure. However, the use of paralytic agents and intubation of the head-injured patient has the potential for further increasing the intracranial pressure. Nevertheless, when 100 consecutive trauma patients were evaluated after planned emergency intubation with muscle paralysis, no ill effects were found. These patients were intubated by either a surgeon or an anesthesiologist and paralyzed with either vecuronium or succinylcholine. Nasal intubation was used in 43 patients and oral intubation in 57 patients. Ninety-four patients with suspected head injuries had a CT scan performed. Fifty-five had a positive scan, and 15 required emergency neurosurgical intervention. No patient suffered any known ill effect from the emergency room intubation.

Fluid Resuscitation

Fluid resuscitation by the emergency medical technician has always been controversial. Prehospital administration of intravenous fluids is widely accepted as appropriate for trauma patients; however, its value has not been substantiated. Moreover, time lost placing intravenous catheters at the scene may delay definitive management of life-threatening hemorrhage and increase the mortality rate.

When prehospital fluid administration was compared with no fluid for its effect on the mortality rate, no difference was found. This study subdivided patients into those with an Injury Severity Score (ISS) of less than 25, 25 to 50, and more than 50. While the mortality rate rose with increasing injury severity, there was no difference between patients who received prehospital fluid and those who did not.

Ringer's lactate has remained the standard initial fluid for resuscitation in hemorrhagic shock. Its principal drawback is that large volumes need to be infused if there has been severe blood loss. The ideal resuscitation would be simultaneous replacement of the intravascular volume while minimizing cerebral edema in the head-injured patient. Recent animal studies have shown promise for the use of hypertonic (6.5%) saline to resuscitate the head-injured patient in that smaller volumes were required compared with Ringer's lactate for the resuscitation of the animals with or without brain injury. Moreover, the water content in the injured brain was less after the use of hypertonic saline resuscitation than after use of Ringer's lactate. These studies suggest that in the patient with a brain injury and hemorrhagic shock, resuscitation with hypertonic saline will cause a smaller increase in the intracerebral pressure than would Ringer's lactate.

Diagnosis

Head Injury Computed tomography is the gold standard for head injury evaluation, even with the more recent development of magnetic resonance imaging (MRI). A comparison of these two modalities has been published. When 170 patients with head trauma were studied by MRI within three days of injury, 177 lesions were demonstrated in 123 patients. In contrast, CT demonstrated 103 lesions in 90 patients. The MRI study was found to be superior to CT scanning in the diagnosis of nonhemorrhagic contusion, demonstrated as a high-intensity area on the T_2-weighted images. Magnetic resonance provided some information about the severity of diffuse accidental brain injury and also was helpful in predicting delayed traumatic intracranial hematoma. Logistic issues and cost are the factors responsible for the continued preeminence of CT scanning as the tool for head injury assessment.

Cervical Spine Significant difficulty remains in the diagnosis of fractures and dislocations of the cervical spine in patients who cannot provide clinical clues about their injury. How many radiographs are enough to clear the cervical spine of a motor vehicle crash victim? In a review of 110 patients who were thought to have cervical fractures or dislocations, 92 patients proved to have suffered a bony or ligamentous injury. Twelve of these injuries were wrongly diagnosed or not identified initially (false-negative radiograph). Eighteen patients suspected initially of having a cervical spine injury proved on review not to have an injury (false-positive study). When all data had been collected and the diagnosis made, a review of the lateral cervical spine radiographs with a swimmer's view, when necessary, showed a sensitivity for the injury of 83%, a specificity of 97%, a positive predictive value of 81%, and a negative predictive value of 98%, with an accuracy of 96%. With the addition of an anteroposterior and open mouth view of the cervical spine, the sensitivity rose to 100%. Outpatients responsive enough to report neck pain, tenderness, or other neurologic symptoms referable to the spinal cord or roots when the plain radiographs are normal should have further studies such as repeated plain films after the passage of several days or a CT scan directed to the level suggested by the clinical findings. Flexion extension views may be obtained if the above studies are normal.

Cardiac The diagnosis of blunt cardiac injury in traumatized patients is problematic, and the implications of such a diagnosis are not clear. Elevation of the MB fraction of creatinine phosphokinase (CPK-MB) to greater than 200 U/l, together with an abnormal EKG, accurately discriminated between patients who will develop cardiac complications requiring treatment and those who will not.

Traumatic rupture of the aorta is a lethal injury. The diagnosis must be made rapidly, followed by appropriate surgical intervention. Signs suggesting a ruptured thoracic aorta include a widened mediastinum, high rib fractures, and a deviated esophagus. The condition should be strongly suspected in those patients sustaining head-on, high-speed deceleration injuries. The use of CT for the diagnosis of injuries involving the abdominal cavity has increased; however, when this diagnostic modality was used to rule out thoracic aortic ruptures, an accuracy of only 52% was demonstrated. When clinical suspicion or radiographic suggestion of thoracic aortic rupture is present, arteriography remains the appropriate diagnostic method. Because of the implications of this injury, a negative study rate of 95% to 97% is desirable.

Abdomen The diagnostic peritoneal lavage (DPL) remains the gold standard for diagnosing operable intra-abdominal injury. When reviewed retrospectively, DPL on the patient sustaining blunt trauma has a sensitivity of 87%, a specificity of 97%, and an accuracy of 97%, a positive predictive value of 85%, and a negative predictive value of 97% for abdominal injuries requiring surgical repair. The diagnostic criteria for a positive peritoneal lavage in blunt trauma have included a red blood cell count of greater than $100,000/mm^3$, a white blood cell count greater than $500/mm^3$, an amylase content greater than 175 U/dl, and the presence of bile, bacteria, or intestinal contents in the lavage fluid or a hematocrit on spun fluid of greater than 1%. However, recent studies have shown a white blood cell count of $500/mm^3$ or more has a very low predictive value when used as the only criterion for laparotomy in the blunt trauma patient.

Computer tomography has become more widely used in abdominal evaluation but still is not as good as DPL, with a sensitivity of 74.3%, a specificity of 99.5%, and an accuracy of 92.6%. Moreover, the complication rate for DPL is 0.9% versus 3.4% for CT. In addition, DPL is associated with lower rates of preventable mortality than the CT scan in the evaluation of abdominal trauma.

The use of ultrasonography in the emergency room for diagnosing hemoperitoneum has become standard in Europe and Japan. It is less widely used in the United States. Studies from Japan have shown that such use of ultrasonography has a sensitivity of 86.7%, a specificity of 100%, and an accuracy of 97.2%. Ultrasonography is easily and quickly performed and is noninvasive. However, the accuracy of the study depends on the experience of the examiner, and the method is still undergoing clinical investigation in North America.

Greater acceptance of conservative management of blunt renal injuries has led to the use of CT for their accurate and detailed assessment. While there is general agreement that rapid surgical intervention is required in an unstable patient with renal injuries, a stable patient may often be observed. Computed tomography, particularly a dynamic study, has proved adequate for the assessment of the renal injuries in these patients. In addition, the CT scan has been found to be invaluable for the assessment of other retroperitoneal organs such as the pancreas and vascular structures.

Vascular Injuries Major blood vessels of the extremities have a high exposure to injury. Diagnosis of arterial injuries, however, has been controversial for those injuries without clear physical signs such as active hemorrhage, distal pulse deficit, large expanding or pulsatile hematomas, distal ischemia, bruits, or thrills. When such signs are not present, the arteriogram that is usually performed is an exclusion study based on the old premise of a penetrating injury in the proximity of a major vessel. A recent group of investigators has admitted these patients for observation for 24 hours, then followed them as outpatients, rather than exposing them to the invasive and expensive procedure of arteriography. When the patient with a potential vascular injury without clear physical signs was observed for 24 hours, there proved to be only two missed injuries (a false-negative rate of 0.7%). In follow-up, there were no deaths or morbidity related to this observation period.

The Doppler arterial pressure index is the systemic arterial pressure in the injured extremity divided by the arterial pressure in an uninjured arm. An index of less than 0.90 was found to have a sensitivity and specificity of 95% and 78%, respectively, for major arterial injuries. With the use of the Doppler arterial pressure index and a good physical examination to rule out clear physical signs of vascular injury, the need for exclusion arteriography for extremity vascular injuries can be greatly reduced.

Patients suffering blunt leg trauma resulting in below knee fracture, tibial artery injury, and soft-tissue damage are at significant risk for amputation. Among patients with severe lower-extremity trauma involving arterial injuries, those who require amputation have a significantly greater incidence of involvement of three or more fascial compartments in muscular injury, two or more injured tibial vessels, failed tibial reconstruction, a cadaveric foot at initial examination, and severe crush injury or muscle tissue loss. In one series, no extremity was salvaged when more than two of these factors were present, and a failed vascular reconstruction led to a limb amputation in all cases. Therefore, these factors mark an irretrievable extremity after blunt tibial arterial trauma, allowing amputation before life-threatening wound sepsis develops.

Missed Injuries

Priorities in the management of acutely injured trauma patients require rapid identification of all injuries in a timely fashion, often in a patient who is unable to cooperate because of neurologic injury or substance abuse. To achieve these goals, it is necessary to approach the patient in an organized fashion. Application of primary and secondary surveys, as outlined by the Advanced Trauma Life Support Course of the American College of Sur-

geons, is one approach to the trauma patient. Even with this organized approach, however, injuries can be missed because of the presence of multiple casualties, the need for emergency operations, or an unconscious patient. When a tertiary review is made, usually in a follow-up in-hospital assessment, as many as 10% of injuries in the blunt trauma patient may be found to have been missed. Missed injuries most commonly include fractures of extremities that were not studied radiographically or for which the films were poorly done or misinterpreted. While these injuries tend to be less severe, it is important that they be identified and managed appropriately. The multiply injured patient or the patient with altered levels of consciousness must be reevaluated at an appropriate time, both by physical examination and by review of radiographs.

Trauma Scoring Systems

Since 1984, the Injury Severity Score (ISS) has been the principal means of predicting trauma outcome. This score is computed from the Abbreviated Injury Scale (AIS) scores associated with individual injuries, which range from 1 (minor) to 6 (nearly always fatal). The ISS ranges from 1 to 75. Any patient with an AIS 6 injury is assigned the maximum ISS of 75.

Limitations of the ISS have recently been identified that call into serious question its continued use in traditional application. These limitations result from three factors. First, the ISS is based on at most the highest AIS score among the injuries in a body region. Thus, the ISS may underestimate the severity of the condition of patients with multiple injuries in one or more body regions. Second, diverse injury combinations with distinct survival probabilities can have the same or nearly the same ISS values. For instance, an AIS value of 5 for a head injury would give an ISS of 25, and an abdominal injury AIS of 4 plus an extremity injury of AIS of 3 (such as a liver laceration and an open fracture of a radius) would likewise equal an ISS of 25, yet the expected mortality rate for such patients differs substantially. Finally, the ISS gives equal weighting to injuries with the same AIS severity in different body regions.

Since 1982, the American College of Surgeons Major Trauma Outcome Study (MTOS) has been under way. Recent analysis of the data collected from 1982 to 1988 has been undertaken by Copes and Champion, who have developed an improved outcome concept characterized by using anatomic injury. The concept of a four-value ABCD description of injuries was introduced. The Anatomic Profile (AP) is a score in which A is a summary of the scores of all serious injuries to the head and neck region, B and C are analogous scores for the thoracic, abdominal, and pelvic contents and the other body regions, respectfully, and D is a summary score of all non-serious injuries (Table 2).

The data for developing the AP (the design set) and relating it and the ISS to the survival probability were derived from 20,946 patients 15 to 54 years of age consec-

Table 2. Logistic function coefficients for outcome prediction using Anatomic Profile Scale

	Injury Severity Score*	Anatomic Profile
Constant	4.3705	4.0801
ISS	-0.1064	—
A	—	-0.4914
B	—	-0.2066
B^2	—	-0.0161
C^2	—	-0.0351

*G (summary score) = $4.0801 + (-0.4914A) + (-0.2066B) + (-0.0161B^2) + (-0.0351C^2)$
(Reproduced with permission from Copes WS, Champion HR, Sacco WJ, et al: Progress in characterizing anatomic injury. *J Trauma* 1990;30:1200-1207.)

utively admitted before 1987 to the MTOS institution for treatment of blunt injuries. The MTOS uses the ICD-9 CM coding for injury, and extensive logistic regression and statistical analysis was made for AP and ISS for predicting outcome. The AP logistic function better discriminates between survivors and nonsurvivors by placing a greater weight on the head injury followed in order by injuries to the chest, abdomen, and pelvic contents. A one-value summary score is provided by the logistic regression relating AP component values to survivor probability. The summary is the value G obtained by summing the values of AP components multiplied by the appropriate coefficient. Smaller values of G indicate a more serious injury. The result is a more rational way to compare patient samples and to predict the outcome.

Evaluation and Outcome of Head Injuries

Further evidence of the importance of the skull and brain injury is shown when only two numbers are characterized for anatomic disruption: the maximum AIS for skull or brain injury and the maximum AIS for extracranial injury. When this analysis was performed in 16,524 patients with injuries to the brain and skull, there was an overall mortality rate of 18.2%, which was three times that in patients in whom no head injury occurred. The cause of death in the fatal cases was the head injury itself in 67.8%, extracranial injuries in 6.6%, and both in 25.6%. Head injury is thus associated with more deaths than all other injuries and causes almost as many deaths as do all extracranial injuries combined. Because of its high mortality rate, head injury is the single largest contributor to trauma center deaths and thus should have the most important role in computing injury severity and assessing the prognosis of the trauma patient.

A severity score to help in better predicting the mortality rate is the Glasgow Coma Scale, or GCS (Table 3). This method was compared with three other severity scores: the Acute Physiologic Score, the Simplified Acute Physiologic Score, and the Therapeutic Intervention Scoring System (TISS). The GCS was superior to all three in predicting outcome and was more specific and sensitive regarding the level of care needed by patients; that is, the need for trauma center referral.

Table 3. Glasgow Coma Scale*

Eye opening	
Spontaneous	4
To voice	3
To pain	2
None	1
Verbal response	
Oriented	5
Confused	4
Inappropriate words	3
Incomprehensible sounds	2
None	1
Motor response	
Obeys commands	6
Purposeful movement	5
Withdraw to pain	4
Flexion to pain	3
Extension to pain	2
None	1

*The most severe injuries have scores below 9.

In a review of head-injured patients, a good recovery was seen in 99% of 87 patients with a GCS score of 15 to 13. The recovery rate fell to 71% in 24 patients with a GCS score of 12 to 9. Among the 59 patients having a GCS score below 9, 41% died and an additional 17% had poor recovery, leaving only 35% with an uneventful outcome. By using the GCS in association with the ISS or AP score six hours after injury, physicians can more accurately predict outcomes for multiple-trauma patients with head injury.

Acute subdural hematoma continues to be one of the most lethal of all intracranial injuries. A review of 1,150 consecutive severely head-injured patients found 137 patients, or 12%, with subdural hematoma. Analysis was made of the outcome, morbidity, and mortality rate from the hematoma in which the mechanism of injury, age, neurologic presentation, postoperative intracranial pressure, and timing from injury to operative evaluation were considered. The only variables found to be statistically correlated with outcome were the neurologic condition (p=0.001) and a postoperative intracranial pressure greater than 45 mm Hg (p=0.001). The timing from injury to operative evaluation of the hematoma has previously been reported to affect outcome, but no statistical significance was found in this study (p=0.418).

Evaluation and Outcome of Chest Injuries

When major chest trauma was reviewed, multiple rib fractures (flail chest) were found to be an indicator of the severity of injury. The principal factors determining the need for ventilatory systems were an ISS of 23 or more, blood transfusion in the first 24 hours, moderately severe associated injuries (fractures, head injuries, or truncal organ requiring operation), and shock on admission. An adverse outcome ensued when ventilatory assistance was required for 14 days or more. Of interest was the higher incidence of a need for ventilatory assistance and the development of pneumonia in the group of patients with extrathoracic fractures. Three factors that were identified as increasing the incidence of need for long-term ventilatory support or of septic death were an ISS greater than 31, associated fractures or head or truncal injuries, and need for blood transfusions. This study further supports the present view that early total care of the multiply injured patient, including stabilization of major fractures within 24 hours, will reduce the incidence of pulmonary complications and the need for ventilatory support.

Evaluation and Outcome of Long Bone and Pelvic Fractures

A delay in femur fracture stabilization increases the incidence of ARDS and pulmonary shunt, especially in patients over the age of 50 years. This increased incidence of pulmonary failure has led to longer intensive care unit stays and hospitalization and higher cost of care. Similar findings have been reported with early fixation of major unstable pelvic fractures: a reduction in the number of complications, the blood transfusion requirement, and length of hospital stay was found when pelvic fractures were stabilized within eight hours of admission to the emergency room.

Reports of early total care of the trauma patient have shown significant decreases in morbidity and mortality rates, length of hospital stay, and cost. In the multiple injured patient with a significant head injury, however, there has often been a delay in the management of the non-life-threatening injury. In a comparison of head-injured patients with extremity trauma who underwent early total care under general anesthesia and head-injured patients who did not require general anesthesia for early surgery, no difference was found in the outcome of the head injury. Furthermore, there was no increase in morbidity or mortality rates associated with the general anesthesia required for the stabilization of major fractures, which has been found to be of such benefit in the multiply injured patient.

It is now clear that early total care of the multiply injured patient, including stabilization of fractures, improves the outcome. Fracture stabilization allows the patient to move out of the forced supine position into an upright chest position. Early enteral feeding augments this mobilization. A combination of fracture stabilization, mobilization, and enteral feeding significantly reduces not only respiratory failure, but also gut-origin septic response and multiple system organ failure.

Severe pelvic disruptions result from extreme force. These injuries can be life-threatening and are often associated with additional injuries to the extremities, torso, and head. In a review of more than 300 multiple trauma patients with major pelvic disruption, the associated injuries and mortality rate could be predicted by the mechanism of injury (i.e., the type of pelvic injury): anterior-posterior compression (APC), lateral compression (LC), or vertical shear, as well as the combined mechanism of injury (CMI). The high-grade lateral compression injury (grade 3) was associated with a large incidence of brain, lung, and upper-abdominal visceral

Table 4. Mangled Extremity Severity Score (MESS) for prediction of amputation

Variables	Points
Skeletal/soft-tissue injury	
Low energy (stab; simple fracture; "civilian" gunshot wound)	1
Medium energy (open or multiple fractures; dislocation)	2
High energy (close-range shotgun or "military" gunshot wound; crush injury)	3
Very high energy (above + gross contamination, soft-tissue avulsion)	4
Limb ischemia	
Pulse reduced or absent but perfusion normal	1*
Pulseless, paresthesias, diminished capillary refill	2*
Cool, paralyzed, insensate, numb	3*
Shock	
Systolic blood pressure always >90 mm Hg	0
Hypotensive transiently	1
Persistent hypotension	2
Age (years)	
<30	0
30-50	1
>50	2

*Score doubled for ischemia >6 hours
(Reproduced with permission from Johansen K, Daines M, Howey T, et al: Objective criteria accurately predict amputation following lower extremity trauma. *J Trauma* 1990;30:569.)

injuries. The APC injury showed a rising percentage of liver, spleen, bowel, and pelvic vascular injuries with increasing severity. In addition, there was a higher incidence of retroperitoneal hematoma, shock, sepsis, and ARDS, as well as a large increase in the need for volume replacement with an important incidence of brain and lung injuries. Organ injury pattern and percent mortality associated with a vertical shear were similar to those seen with severe grades of APC, but the combined injury had an associated organ injury pattern similar to that of a low-grade APC and LC fracture. Causes of death were different in the LC and the APC injury, with brain injury compounded by shock being a significant factor in the LC. By contrast, in APC injuries, there was a significant influence of shock, sepsis, and ARDS related to the massive torso force delivered, with large volume losses from visceral organs and the pelvis. These extensive data indicate that the type of mechanical force and the severity of the pelvic fractures are keys to the expected organ injury pattern, resuscitation needs, and mortality rate.

Objective criteria for predicting amputation after lower extremity trauma have been difficult to identify. Clinical decision-making in trauma victims with massive lower-extremity injury can be very difficult. Through retrospective analysis and a prospective trial, a Mangled Extremity Severity Score (MESS) has been developed as a simple rating scale for lower extremity trauma based on skeletal and soft-tissue damage, as well as on limb ischemia, shock, and age (Table 4). In retrospective and then in prospective studies, a MESS of 7 or greater predicted a need for amputation in 100% of patients. The use of this scale will be of significant benefit to the physician evaluating severely injured limbs.

Trauma Outcome

Mortality rate in trauma patients is a function of four factors: (1) injury severity; (2) host factors; (3) time to definitive care; and (4) quality of care. The most significant factor is obviously the injury severity. However, age has been shown to influence the mortality rate, and patients 65 years or older have higher fatality and complication rates and longer hospital stays than do younger patients. Preexisting conditions such as congenital coagulopathy, cirrhosis, ischemic heart disease, chronic obstructive pulmonary disease, and diabetes increase the mortality rate both in patients aged 65 years and older and in those between 45 and 65 years old.

The long-term recovery, rehabilitation, and return to function have recently been studied for the most severely injured patients, those with an ISS of 39 or greater and those with hospital charges of more than $100,000. In both studies, the majority (89.5%) of high-cost, severely injured patients survived and returned to productivity (54.5% in one study and 72% in the other). The main reasons for inability to work were brain and spinal cord injuries, blindness, and failure in reeducation. The severity of the injury predicted survival but not return to productivity.

These studies have shown that the treatment of even the most severely traumatized patients with multiple injuries is worth the cost and effort. The majority of these patients are returned to functional, profitable existence, benefiting society.

Annotated Bibliography

General Information

Border JR, Allgower M, Hansen ST Jr, et al (eds): *Blunt Multiple Trauma*. New York, Marcel Dekker, 1990.

An excellent comprehensive text on the pathophysiology and care of the trauma patient.

Fry DE: *Multiple System Organ Failure*. St. Louis, Mosby Year Book, 1992.

An in-depth look at the causes and management of multiple systems organ failure.

Bone LB: Emergency treatment of the injured patient, in Brower TD, Jupiter JB, Levine AM, et al (eds): *Skeletal Trauma*. Philadelphia, WB Saunders, 1992, vol 1, pp 127-136.

An organized, rational approach to the initial care of the multiply injured patient.

Emergency Treatment of the Injured Patient

Mackenzie EJ, Morris JA, Smith GS, et al: Acute hospital costs of trauma in the United States: Implications for regionalized systems of care. *J Trauma* 1990;30:1096-1103.

In 1985, 2.1 million individuals sustained a traumatic injury that resulted in hospitalization. Hospital costs totalled $11.4 billion. The elderly, who represent only 12% of the population, accounted for a quarter of the total discharges and hospital costs. Only 12% of patients and 25% of trauma dollars involved injuries requiring treatment at a trauma center.

McSwain NE, Belles A: Motorcycle helmets: Medical costs and the law. *J Trauma* 1990;30:1189-1199.

Without helmet laws, user rates drop from 99% to 50%. Non-helmeted riders have double the hospital stay, and fatalities increase to 6.2 per 1000 versus 1.6 with helmets. Accident rates are less with helmet legislation, 19% versus 48%. Medical costs decrease by 48.8%. Medical care and rehabilitation expenses per year were $120.8 million more as a direct result of nonuse of helmets.

Resuscitation

Champion HR, Sacco WJ, Copes WS, et al: A revision of the trauma score. *J Trauma* 1989;29:623-629.

A revision of the trauma score includes the Glasgow Coma Scale, systolic blood pressure, and respiratory rate.

Redan JA, Livingston DH, Tortella BJ, et al: The value of intubating and paralyzing patients with suspected head injury in the emergency department. *J Trauma* 1991;31:371-375.

One hundred consecutive trauma patients, of whom 94 had suspected head injuries, were intubated after being paralyzed in the emergency department, with no ill effects.

Diagnosis

Fabian TC, Cicala RS, Croce MA, et al: A prospective evaluation of myocardial contusion: Correlation of significant arrhythmias and cardiac output with CPK-MB measurements. *J Trauma* 1991;31:653-660.

Prospective evaluation of patients with blunt anterior chest injuries showed that serum CPK-MB levels correlated with significant dysrhythmias but were neither sensitive nor specific.

Gennarelli TA, Champion HR, Sacco WJ, et al: Mortality of patients with head injury and extracranial injury treated in trauma centers. *J Trauma* 1989;29:1193-1202.

Comparing mortality in head-injured patients with that of other injured patients showed a disproportionately high percentage (60%) of all deaths in the former group.

Henneman PL, Marx JA, Moore EE, et al: Diagnostic peritoneal lavage: Accuracy in predicting necessary laparotomy following blunt and penetrating trauma. *J Trauma* 1990;30:1345-1355.

In a retrospective review of 975 DPLs, initial DPL in 608 blunt trauma patients had a sensitivity of 78%, a specificity of 97%, an accuracy of 95%, and a positive predictive value of 97% for a need for operation.

McNutt R, Seabrook GR, Schmitt DD, et al: Blunt tibial artery trauma: Predicting the irretrievable extremity. *J Trauma* 1989;29:1624-1627.

Patients with major soft-tissue injury and fracture of the leg associated with an arterial injury had a significantly higher amputation rate if three or more fascial compartments were involved in muscular injury or there were two or more injured tibial vessels, failed vascular reconstruction, a cadaveric foot at initial examination, or severe crush injury or muscle tissue loss. No extremity was salvaged when two or more of these factors were present.

Pal J, Brown R, Fleiszer D: The value of the Glasgow Coma Scale and Injury Severity Score: Predicting outcome in multiple trauma patients with head injury. *J Trauma* 1989;29:746-748.

Using the GCS at five hours post injury, recovery was determined for head-injured patients with multiple injuries. Of the 59 patients having a GCS below 9, 41% died, and an additional 17% had a poor recovery.

Outcome

Champion HR, Copes WS, Sacco WJ, et al: The Major Trauma Outcome Study: Establishing national norms for trauma care. *J Trauma* 1990;30:1356-1365.

Using data collected by the MTOS, mortality rates for injury types are predicted using the Revised Trauma Score, ISS, patient age, and injury mechanism. The mortality rate was strongly related to the presence of serious head injury.

Copes WS, Champion HR, Sacco WJ, et al: Progress in characterizing anatomic injury. *J Trauma* 1990;30:1200-1207.

A three-valued description of anatomic injury is presented. Anatomic profile (AP) components A, B, and C summarize serious injuries to the head/brain or spinal cord, to the thorax or front of the neck, and all remaining areas, respectively. Relations between AP components and survival rate reaffirm the seriousness of head injury. The AP, which is based on the severity and location of all serious injuries, provides a more rational basis for comparing patient samples than the ISS.

Dalal SA, Burgess AR, Siegel JH, et al: Pelvic fracture in multiple trauma: Classification by mechanism is key to pattern of organ injury, resuscitative requirements and outcome. *J Trauma* 1989;29:981-1000.

In a study of 343 multiple trauma patients with major pelvic ring disruption, associated injuries, resuscitative requirements, and outcomes proved to be related to the type of pelvic fracture pattern (ie, the type of mechanical force).

Johansen K, Daines M, Howey T, et al: Objective criteria accurately predict amputation following lower extremity trauma. *J Trauma* 1990;30:508-572.

The MESS (Mangled Extremity Severity Score) is a rating scale for lower extremity trauma based on skeletal and soft-tissue damage, limb ischemia, shock, and age. In retrospective and prospective trials, a MESS value of ≥7 predicted amputation with 100% accuracy.

Kivioja AH, Myllynen PJ, Rokkanen PU: Is the treatment of the most severe multiply injured patient worth the effort? A follow-up examination 5 to 20 years after severe multiple injury. *J Trauma* 1990;30:480-483.

Ninety-two severely injured patients with injuries to at least four body regions and a mean ISS of 39 were examined five to 20 years after trauma. Almost three fourths (72%) had been able to return to work. The main reasons for inability to work were brain and spinal cord injuries and blindness. Most complaints arose from sequelae of brain, pelvic, and upper and lower extremity injuries.

Latenser BA, Gentilello LM, Tarver AA, et al: Improved outcome with early fixation of skeletally unstable pubic fractures. *J Trauma* 1991;31:28-31.

Early pelvic fracture fixation reduces hospital stay and long-term disability and may result in fewer complications, decreased blood loss, and better survival.

Morris JA, Sanchez AA, MacKenzie EJ, et al: Trauma patients' return to productivity. *J Trauma* 1991;31:827-834.

To help determine the cost effectiveness of treating the severely injured patient, a retrospective review was conducted of patients who had more than $100,000 in hospital charges. The majority of high-cost patients survived (89.5%) and returned to productivity (54.5%).

13

Infection

Introduction

During the past decade, orthopaedic surgeons and infectious disease specialists have confronted new clinical entities (toxic shock, lyme disease, and acquired immunodeficiency syndrome) and have faced problems with resistant organisms, including methicillin-resistant *Staphylococcus aureus* and coagulase-negative staphylococci. Prevention of infection was enhanced by improved staging systems for open fractures, identification of links between infection and operating room environmental factors, and perioperative antibiotics. More accurate differential diagnosis of infection was facilitated by studies using technetium, gallium, indium-labeled leukocytes, and magnetic resonance imaging. Basic science research has defined the way in which antibiotics penetrate bone. New families of antibiotics, second- and third-generation cephalosporins, and more cost-effective antibiotic delivery systems were evaluated clinically. Arthroscopy was used for drainage and debridement of pyarthroses. New emphasis was placed on the nutritional status of the patient. The emphasis on accurate and thorough debridement has remained constant, reaffirmed by work characterizing polysaccharide biofilms on implanted materials.

Microbiology

Staphylococci continue to be the most frequent cause of postoperative and posttraumatic musculoskeletal infections. Coagulase-negative staphylococci account for more than 50% of infections involving prosthetic valves, intravenous catheter tips, and sternal wound infections in some hospitals. Increasingly, these organisms are resistant to methicillin.

Anaerobic organisms are more prevalent in wounds of compromised hosts: elderly patients, those undergoing multiple revision surgery, patients with diabetes, and those whose conditions involve retained foreign bodies, necrotic tissue, or dead space. Optimal antibiotic treatment depends on prompt, accurate isolation of the organism and determination of its antibiotic sensitivity patterns.

Antibiotic resistance is increasing. Plasmids, packages of genetic material transferred from one bacterial cell to another by conjugation, transmit antibiotic resistance information. Resistance can be conferred by the production of an enzyme such as penicillinase, by an alteration in the cell wall protein binding site that prevents the antibiotic from attaching, or by a change in the cell wall that precludes antibiotic penetration.

The interactions of bacteria living in the same host can be complex. Parasitism means that one organism lives at the expense of another. Mutualism means that two organisms survive well together as commensals. Synergism means that the two organisms growing together do something that neither organism could do alone. There is good evidence that *S aureus* and Group A beta hemolytic streptoccoci act synergistically, such that the abscess or cellulitis is more severe than it would be if either organism was acting independently. The combination of a gram-positive bacterium, such as *S aureus*, and a gram-negative bacterium, such as *Pseudomonas aeruginosa*, frequently occurs in wounds, complicating open fractures. This combination is associated with a much more severe infection than would occur with either organism alone. Similarly, aerobic and anaerobic organisms in combination can cause resistant infections.

Toxic Shock Syndrome

This syndrome is characterized by fever, profound multisystem dysfunction, desquamative erythroderma, and minimal infection or colonization with *S aureus* occurring in previously healthy persons. Sixty-five percent of the isolates are nonsuppurative *S aureus*, Group I, phage type 29. The migmatoxin produced is similar to a combination of pyrogenic exotoxin Type C and enterotoxin Type F. Although no specific treatment has proved effective in resolving the altered microcirculation in the syndrome, drainage and irrigation of the surgical wound accompanied by systemic antistaphylococcal antibiotic seems appropriate.

Lyme Disease

Lyme disease is caused by the spirochete *Borrelia burgdorferi* carried by the deer tick, *Ixodes dammini*. Stage I Lyme disease becomes evident three to 30 days after the bite, with erythema chronicum migrans—an expanding red ring with central clearing and intermediate attacks of swelling in one or more joints. Stage II Lyme disease involves neurologic sequelae (frequently Bell's palsy) and cardiac abnormalities. Stage III Lyme disease involves arthritis, most frequently of the knee. In 90% of patients, the erythrocyte sedimentation rate is elevated. The sensitivity and specificity of the ELISA test for Lyme disease remain less than ideal. Treatment is phenoxymethylpenicillin (50 mg per kg of bodyweight per day) or tetracycline (30 mg per kg per day) for four weeks. If a patient fails to respond to this treatment regimen, penicillin G or ceftriaxone is administered intravenously.

Bacterial Resistance in the Presence of Foreign Material

Direct examination of tissue and biomaterials from infections related to prostheses, internal fixation devices, and percutaneous sutures has shown bacteria enveloped by extracellular material. This exopolysaccharide glycocalix protects the bacteria from host defense factors and accounts, in part, for their persistence and resistance to treatment. Factors that affect the way in which bacteria adhere include surface charge and surface free energy of the bacteria and biomaterial, extracellular components of the bacteria, bacterial interaction in mixed infections, alteration in host immune competence, and extracellular matrix. This extracellular glycocalix is composed of 24% protein and 40% carbohydrate. Slime-producing strains of *Staphylococcus epidermidis* produce more clinically significant infections than do non-slime producers. Because of the adherent growth of the organisms, accurate microbiologic sampling is difficult. Interactions between adherent organisms and nonadherent organisms are important, because such interactions promote the development of infection. Analysis of joint fluids, swabs of excised tissue, and prosthetic surfaces frequently yields only one species of organism from what is actually a polymicrobial population. The most accurate technique for obtaining information about a possible polymicrobial infection is to take several tissue samples for microbiologic analysis. Samples should be taken from different aspects of the wound, including involved bone, foreign body encapsulating scar tissue and glycocalyx, and involved synovium. If all of the organisms are not identified, the clinical infection may be suppressed, but a long-term cure will not be achieved.

Antimicrobial Agents

Open fractures following vehicular and industrial accidents are common and most, if not all, are contaminated. Surgical debridement and administration of antibiotics are considered standard treatment. Although some physicians refer to this use of antibiotics as prophylactic, it is, in fact, treatment of an incipient infection.

Antibiotics readily traverse the capillary membrane of normal and osteomyelitic bone. All agents studied to date attained bactericidal concentrations in the interstitial fluid space. These data refute the hypothesis of a capillary barrier to the passage of antimicrobials in bone tissue. Serum concentrations under steady state conditions accurately reflect the bone interstitial fluid concentration.

For prophylactic use to prevent infection in clean operative cases, antimicrobial agents are administered just before surgery and for 24 to 48 hours postoperatively. There are no controlled studies to demonstrate the effec-

tiveness of antibiotics administered for less than 24 hours, but it may be that a shorter period of administration would be equally effective. If so, continuation of administration for a long period of time not only is unnecessary, but, in fact, may be harmful because of increased incidence of toxicity from the agent, increased incidence of infection caused by changes in bacterial flora, and general increase in bacteria resistant to the antimicrobial agent.

In general, first generation cephalosporins are appropriate for prophylactic use. Second and third generation cephalosporins should be used only for organisms resistant to first generation cephalosporins. They are preferable to more toxic antibiotics such as aminoglycosides. First generation drugs are more effective against gram-positive cocci; more recent derivatives have increased gram-negative activity.

Antibiotic Toxicity

Patients with osteomyelitis or other types of musculoskeletal sepsis who require prolonged antibiotic therapy are more likely to develop toxic complications. Hypersensitivity reaction is the most common complication of penicillin and cephalosporin agents. If an agent to which a patient reports a sensitivity must be used, skin testing should be performed to verify the history. Patients can be desensitized as with other allergenic materials. Ototoxicity and renal toxicity remain the major complications associated with the aminoglycosides. These complications can be greatly decreased by establishing dosage regimens based on peak and trough serum levels measured once or twice a week and serum creatinine measured every other day. One of the first indications of renal toxicity is an increasing serum trough level. Should this occur, the dosage of antibiotics should be decreased, the time interval between doses increased, or both. Careful clinical history and examination should be repeated frequently to determine if the patient is developing signs of vestibular or auditory dysfunction. In those patients in whom toxicity is suspected, audiograms may be helpful. Significant bleeding problems have been associated with both carbenicillin and moxalactam.

Pseudomembranous enterocolitis is a feared complication of antimicrobial therapy. Although this complication was initially believed to be related to specific agents, such as clindamycin, careful screening has implicated a wide spectrum of antibiotics. The parenteral administration of antimicrobials disrupts the symbiotic microbial relationships of the gastrointestinal tract that promote the growth of *Clostridium difficile*. This organism produces a cytotoxin and an enterotoxin. The stool specimen can be analyzed for the toxin. Metronidazole is the drug of choice to eliminate *C difficile*. Should there be a relapse, vancomycin is the appropriate treatment drug.

Approval of new oral antibiotics by the Food and Drug Administration and continuing work on local medication delivery systems, such as osmotic pumps, antibiotic-impregnated methylmethacrylate, and home administration of intravenous antibiotics are shortening hospitalizations and decreasing the cost of care for many patients.

Ciprofloxacin

The fluoroquinolones have more complete gastrointestinal absorption, a broader antimicrobial spectrum, a lower incidence of resistance, and fewer adverse effects than the original quinolone, nalidixic acid. These drugs inhibit bacterial cell protein synthesis and DNA replication by preventing bacterial DNA-gyrase. Ciprofloxacin was the first fluoroquinolone antibiotic with systemic activity to be marketed in the United States. Ciprofloxacin, administered orally, is bactericidal against most gram-negative aerobic bacilli, including *P aeruginosa*. Activity against gram-positive organisms is more variable, but many strains of methicillin-susceptible and methicillin-resistant *S aureus* and coagulase-negative staphylococci as well as enterococci are inhibited by drug concentrations normally achieved in vivo. Activity against anaerobic bacteria is poor. Ciprofloxacin requires only twice daily oral dosing because of its serum half-life. Investigators have reported osteomyelitis arrest rates of 63% to 100% with ciprofloxacin.

Oral therapy offers major advantages over intravenous treatment, particularly in elderly patients and in intravenous drug abusers with venous access problems. Patients with infections complicating internal fixation of fractures can be treated orally, at home, over prolonged periods. The clinical signs of infection can be suppressed in some patients, thus allowing bone union before hardware removal.

Ciprofloxacin has two significant drug interactions. Antacids that contain magnesium or aluminum decrease its absorption by six- to tenfold, and ciprofloxacin increases theophylline serum concentrations more than twofold when the drugs are administered together. Therefore, the theophylline serum concentrations of patients receiving ciprofloxacin and theophylline should be carefully monitored. Compliance is essential to the success of oral antibiotic therapy. Candidates for outpatient management of osteomyelitis should be carefully selected because prolonged self-administration is difficult to maintain once the symptoms have cleared. Ciprofloxacin is not recommended for children because joint cartilage erosion has been documented in young experimental animals receiving the drug.

Antibiotic-Impregnated Methylmethacrylate

Local delivery of antibiotics to the site of infection has been facilitated by placing appropriate antibiotics in polymethylmethacrylate (PMMA). Antibiotics are released from the beads by diffusion. Local gentamicin concentrations of 200 to 300 g per ml have been recorded, with a concomitant serum concentration of 0.5 g per ml. The amount of antibiotic released is proportional to the surface area of the cement, the concentration of the antibiotic in the cement, and the amount of fluid around the cement. Local treatment with gentamicin-impregnated beads is not appropriate for osteomyelitis caused by anaerobic organisms or enterococci.

Insertion of antibiotic-impregnated PMMA beads is not a substitute for adequate surgical debridement. The goal is to remove all infected necrotic bone, scar, and foreign material. Careful wound closure with either local tissue or liquid impermeable synthetics is required to maintain the high local concentration of the antibiotic (Figs. 1 and 2).

There have been no published reports of ototoxicity or allergic reactions after implantation of as many as 540 beads in a single patient with chronic osteomyelitis.

Osmotic Pumps

Totally implantable pumps are used to deliver antibiotics locally in patients with chronic osteomyelitis. The pump has two chambers, which are separated by a flexible metal bellow. One chamber is the drug reservoir; the other holds the charging fluid in a completely sealed environment. The vapor pressure of the charging fluid exerts a constant pressure on the bellows, forcing the drug from the reservoir through an outlet filter and flow restrictor into a catheter for delivery to the selected body site. When the pump is filled, the increasing volume within the drug chamber exerts pressure on the charging fluid. The fluid vapor condenses to its liquid state, thereby storing energy for the next pumping cycle. Identical pumps have been used for several years to deliver drugs for treatment of cancer and for pain relief. Systemic antibiotics are used at the time of initial debridement to decrease the risk of pump-pocket infection.

Amikacin, a semi-synthetic derivative of kanamycin, is the antibiotic most frequently used with the implantable pump. Amikacin has been shown to maintain its stability in the pump. It inhibits protein synthesis in the bacterial cell and is bactericidal. Amikacin is active in vitro and in vivo against a wide variety of gram-positive and gram-negative organisms.

Contraindications to pump use include psychological intolerance to such a device, small body size and weight, allergic reactions to amikacin, and marked changes in altitude, such as might be experienced by frequent travelers.

Home Administration of Intravenous Antibiotics

Intravenous antibiotics can be delivered through either peripheral or central access. Catheters that provide central access require surgical placement in the operating room. The advantage for most patients is the ability to continue appropriate antibiotic therapy while at home with their families. Most insurance carriers recognize the cost-effectiveness of this home treatment program. Patients must be monitored for signs of toxicity, such as leukopenia, and, depending upon the antibiotic chosen, appropriate peak and trough levels must be maintained.

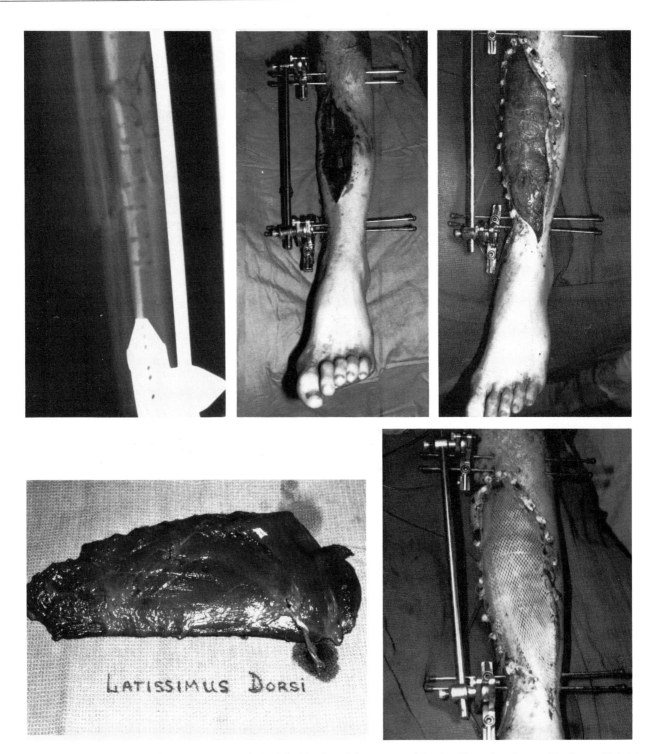

Fig. 1 **Top left**, Lateral radiograph of the midshaft of the left tibia of an eighteen-year-old male with acute osteomyelitis. The multiply injured patient had sustained a grade I open fracture of the tibia in a motor vehicle accident. Initial care had included DCP open reduction and internal fixation. A wound slough exposing plate and bone lead to an acute osteomyelitis. The hardware had been removed and an external fixator had been applied prior to transfer to a tertiary treatment center. **Top center**, Photograph of the left lower extremity after removal of necrotic, infected soft tissue and bone, prior to microvascular soft tissue-transfer. **Top right and bottom left**, Intraoperative photograph of latissimus dorsi with vascular pedicle prior to insertion into soft-tissue defect. **Bottom right**, Wound after insertion of latissimus dorsi and split-thickness skin graft.

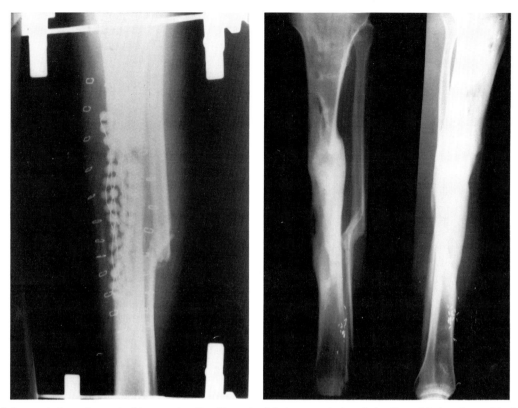

Fig. 2   Left, Anteroposterior radiograph of lower extremity with gentamicin-impregnated methylmethacrylate beads used for local antibiotic delivery. **Right,** Anteroposterior and lateral radiographs of left leg status post iliac crest bone grafting, healing, and initial remodeling of the fracture.

Oral Antibiotic Therapy for Children

Oral administration of antimicrobial agents to children with musculoskeletal infections has proven to be effective. Rigid criteria must be applied: adequate clinical response to parenteral therapy; bacterial sensitivity to the oral agent; patient tolerance of the oral antibiotic; adequate serum bactericidal activity (peak titer greater than one to eight with trough titer greater than one to two); and assurance of patient compliance.

Osteomyelitis

Prevention of osteomyelitis in patients with type III open fractures remains a challenge. There may be a significant benefit from aggressive early soft-tissue management. When free flap transfer was accomplished within 72 hours of injury, the flap failure rate was 0.75% and the infection rate was 1.5%.

Indium-labeled leukocyte scintigraphy and magnetic resonance imaging have made it possible to diagnose subclinical osteomyelitis and its extent within the medullary canal. Indium-labeled leukocyte scintigraphy is more accurate than plain technetium or sequential technetium-gallium imaging in suspected low grade infection of a

long bone or chronic musculoskeletal infection. Sequential technetium-gallium imaging is still preferred if the focus involves the vertebral column, because the hematopoietic nature of the vertebral marrow makes indium-labeled white blood cell scintigraphy images more difficult to interpret.

Magnetic resonance imaging is superior to indium-labeled leukocyte scintigraphy in defining the extent of infection. A magnetic resonance image is considered to be consistent with active osteomyelitis when an area of abnormal marrow with low signal intensity on T_1-weighted sequences corresponds to an increased signal intensity on the T_2-weighted image. Abnormal marrow caused by posttraumatic and postsurgical fibrosis and scarring is defined by a low marrow signal on T_1-weighted images with no evident increase in signal on T_2-weighted images. Cellulitis is defined by diffuse areas of intermediate signal in the soft tissues on T_1-weighted images, with similar soft-tissue areas displaying increased signal on T_2-weighted images. MRI cannot differentiate between edema and bacterially induced cellulitis.

The extent of intramedullary and extramedullary disease seen on magnetic resonance images correlated directly with that seen on serial sectioning of amputated specimens. Magnetic resonance imaging is not able to

Table 1. Osteomyelitis classification systems

System	Basis of System	Classification
Waldvogel	Etiology and region involved	Type 1: Hematogenous
		Type 2: Contiguous focus
		Type 3: Associated with major vessel disease
Kelly	Etiology and region involved	Type 1: Chronic hematogenous
		Type 2: Associated with fracture union
		Type 3: Associated with fracture nonunion
		Type 4: Posttraumatic or postoperative
		Type 5: Vertebral
		Type 6: Small bones of skull, face, hand, foot
Ger	Wound characteristics	Type 1: Single sinus
		Type 2: Chronic superficial ulcers
		Type 3: Multiple sinuses
		Type 4: Multiple skin-lined sinuses
Weiland	Extent of infection	Type I: Exposed bone with soft-tissue infection
		Type II: Circumferential, cortical, and endosteal infection
		Type III: Cortical and endosteal infection with segmental bone loss
Gordon	Severity of underlying bone damage	Type A: Tibial defect and nonunion without significant segmental loss
		Type B: Tibial defect >3 cm, fibula intact
		Type C: Tibial defect >3 cm, fibula fractured
University of Texas	Location of infection modified by immune system of host	Type I: Intramedullary
		Type II: Superficial
		Type III: Local
		Type IV: Diffuse, use with segmental bone loss
		Modifications: A, Normal immune system and adequate soft-tissue envelope. B, Local or systemic compromise or both. C, Requires immunosuppressive therapy or would be made worse by aggressive treatment.

differentiate clearly between areas of abnormal marrow resulting from chronic inactive osteomyelitis and marrow previously disrupted by trauma or surgery that has healed with fibrosis. MRI is unable to define the presence of a cortical osteomyelitis if there is no medullary involvement. Nonferromagnetic internal fixation devices located within the study area do not interfere significantly with image interpretation.

Comparison of published treatment results in osteomyelitis has been made more difficult by the lack of a uniform, widely accepted clinical staging system. Clearly all patients with osteomyelitis are not identical. Table 1 summarizes some of the classification systems.

Chronic Osteomyelitis

The cornerstone of surgical treatment of chronic osteomyelitis, thorough debridement, can be most difficult in chronically infected bone. Sepsis frequently recurs following curettage and bone scraping procedures. More radical localized surgical resection of infected and marginally vascularized tissues may be necessary to prevent recurrent sepsis.

Procedures are available that allow surgical reconstruction of defects following radical debridement. These include localized muscle flap, cancellous bone grafting, free tissue transfer (Figs. 1 and 2), and distraction osteogenesis (Fig. 3). When bony continuity is retained and the primary problem is residual dead space and soft-tissue loss, a local muscle flap or vascularized pedicle flap is used to repair the soft tissue.

Quantitative microbiologic techniques may provide an objective method upon which to base decisions regarding

wound closure and antibiotic therapy. Following debridement of the open wound, a 1-cc tissue specimen is submitted to the microbiology laboratory. For the immediate quantitative Gram stain smear, 0.01 ml of an undiluted homogenate is transferred onto a clean glass microscopic slide and spread in an area not exceeding 15 mm in diameter. After drying, the slide is gram stained. The entire smear is examined microscopically at a magnification of 1,000. The presence of a single organism in any field indicates a positive smear, suggestive of ongoing infection. The remainder of the tissue homogenate can be serially diluted in nutrient broth for quantitative culture. Cultures containing ten organisms per gram of tissue have a high probability of remaining infected if closed. The accuracy of quantitative microbiologic techniques has been reported to be 84% for Gram stain and 89% for culture.

The widespread recreational use of intravenous drugs by some members of society have led to gram-negative osteomyelitis and septic arthritis.

Hyperbaric Oxygen Therapy

Animal studies have suggested improved outcome in the treatment of gas gangrene and possibly chronic osteomyelitis when hyperbaric oxygen treatment is combined with other accepted methods of therapy. Although increased oxygen tension above 80 torr inhibits production of toxins by *Clostridium perfringens*, surgical excision of devitalized tissue remains of paramount importance.

In treating chronic osteomyelitis, hyperbaric oxygen may well be found to be most helpful in the Cierny-Mader class B host whose infection cannot be entirely re-

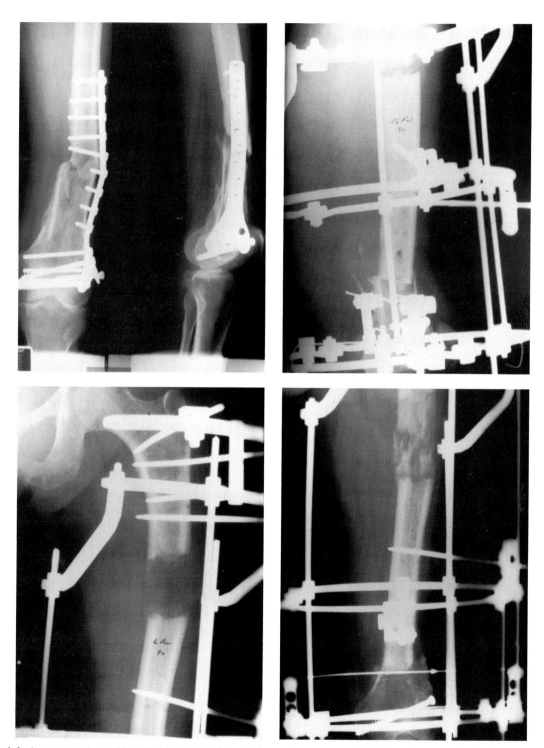

Fig. 3 **Top left,** Anteroposterior and lateral radiographs of the left femur of a young, multiply injured woman who had been struck as a pedestrian by a hit-and-run driver. The distal femur and condyles had been severely comminuted. In spite of meticulous care the patient developed an infection, which several attempts at local debridement had failed to eradicate. The patient had a nonunion complicated by extensive osteomyelitis and failure of the plate at the time of her transfer. **Top right,** Lateral radiograph of the distal femur after excision of 8.5 cm of necrotic infected bone, application of Ilizarov fixator, immediate intraoperative approximation of the remaining distal shaft to the condyles, and corticotomy. **Bottom left,** Anteroposterior radiograph seven weeks later. **Bottom right,** Anteroposterior radiograph of the femur four months after fixator application demonstrating recovery of 8 cm of length.

moved. The Cierny-Mader osteomyelitis classification system characterizes patients with regard to their ability to respond to treatment. Type A hosts have neither local soft-tissue compromise nor systemic illness that would be expected to jeopardize healing. Type B hosts have either local, systemic, or combined disease factors that would adversely affect healing. Local factors include chronic lymphedema, major vessel disease, venous stasis, extensive scarring, or radiation fibrosis. Systemic problems include malnutrition, malignancy, extremes of age, hepatic or renal failure, diabetes mellitus, and alcohol abuse. Type C hosts are sufficiently fragile that undertaking aggressive treatment could endanger the patient. Hyperbaric oxygenation has been found to be effective in radiation osteonecrosis and post-radiation chronic osteomyelitis of the mandible.

Septic Arthritis

Although there is general agreement that septic arthritis of the hip should be treated by immediate open drainage and appropriate antibiotics, there is ongoing controversy concerning the need for surgical treatment of pyarthrosis in most other joints. Any patient with the acute onset of monarticular arthritis should be approached as if he had bacterial septic arthritis. Septic arthritis may result from: hematogenous seeding secondary to bacteremia from distant infection or intravenous drug abuse; direct inoculation secondary to penetrating trauma, diagnostic or therapeutic joint aspiration; contiguous spread from soft-tissue infection; or joint contamination from periarticular osteomyelitis. Predisposing factors include: preexisting joint disease, especially rheumatoid arthritis; closed trauma to the joint; direct penetration of the joint; intravenous drug abuse; and impaired host defense mechanisms.

Infectious arthritis in rheumatoid patients has a worse prognosis than a similar infection would in other patient subgroups. One contributing factor to the poor outcome in rheumatoid arthritis patients is the delay in diagnosis that often accompanies these infections. The difficulty arises in distinguishing a rheumatoid flare from an acute infection. Pseudoseptic arthritis is well described in rheumatoid patients.

S aureus is the most common cause of nongonococcal septic arthritis. The knee is the most common joint involved with pyarthrosis, followed by the hip, shoulder, wrist, ankle, elbow, and hand. Work in animal models has documented lysosomal enzyme release within 24 hours of infection. Glycosaminoglycan depletion occurs by day 5. In vitro experiments have demonstrated that leukocyte proteinase can degrade cartilage. Sterile inflammatory synovial fluids have been shown to contain proteinase capable of destroying articular cartilage.

The coexistence of an acute bout of crystal-induced arthritis and septic arthritis can be overlooked, usually because of a failure to examine synovial fluid for bacteria or crystals if one or the other is found. Crystal-induced arthritis and septic arthritis may occur simultaneously secondary to the decreased joint pH associated with infection decreasing the solubility of urate. All patients with an acute arthritis should be screened for both infectious and crystal-induced causes. The presence of crystals does not rule out a bacterial arthritis.

The goals of treatment include: sterilization of the joint; decompression; removal of all inflammatory cells, enzymes, and debris of foreign bodies; elimination of destructive pannus; and return to full functional recovery.

The method by which drainage, decompression, and cleansing of the joint is best accomplished is highly debated. Dogmatic statements supporting either repeated arthrocentesis or surgical (arthroscopic or arthrotomy) drainage are found. Animal and retrospective clinical studies are cited to support either point of view. Advocates of repeated aspirations over arthroscopy or arthrotomy drainage cite extended hospitalization, wound management problems, and the need for anesthesia as reasons to avoid surgical intervention. Advocates of open drainage procedures describe the inability of arthrocentesis to deal adequately with purulent loculations and adhesions, pain of repeated arthrocentesis, possible iatrogenic inoculation of bone with the arthrocentesis needle, and difficulty in draining certain joints, such as the shoulder, wrist, and hip. Arthroscopy is not as reliable as open drainage in eradicating many infections.

Orthopaedic Infections in Pediatric Patients

Poor outcomes continue to occur in acute septic arthritis when the disease occurs during infancy, or as a result of delayed diagnosis, inadequate therapy, and associated osteomyelitis. In recent years significant advances have been made: recognition of changing patterns of causative organisms; development of new antibiotics and standards of therapy; and understanding of the inflammatory mediators of articular cartilage destruction.

Septic arthritis is more common and more commonly complicated by metaphyseal osteomyelitis in the neonate. Perhaps this is caused by the presence of transphyseal vessels, which disappear by six months of age, and by the synovial reflections, which extend over the metaphysis. In the older child, only the metaphyses of the hip, shoulder, and ankle remain intracapsular.

The knee (41%) and the hip (23%) are the joints most commonly involved. Pyarthrosis of the hip is the most devastating because of the risk of necrosis, growth arrest, and dislocation. The child usually has a swollen, painful joint and a temperature of 38 to 40 C. The classic physical signs—restriction of joint motion, tenderness, joint warmth, and effusion—may not be present in the neonate or infant. In this age group limited spontaneous movement or asymmetric posturing of the extremity may be the only clues.

The most important factors in determining outcome are timely diagnosis and appropriate treatment. Glycocosaminoglycan and collagen degradation begin within eight hours of infection. The erythrocyte sedimentation test is the most sensitive (elevated in 90% of patients). The serum leukocyte count is elevated in 30% to 60% and a shift to the left may occur in 60% to 70%. Blood cultures are positive in 40%. Radiographs may show joint-space widening, obliteration of fat planes, soft-tissue swelling, and after seven to 14 days, osteomyelitis. The definitive test is needle aspiration of the suspect joint. In the case of the hip, if no exudate is recovered, an arthrogram is performed to confirm needle placement.

The differential diagnosis can be difficult, including: juvenile rheumatoid arthritis, rheumatic fever, gonococcal arthritis, Lyme disease, trauma, cellulitis, osteomyelitis, sickle-cell crisis, hemophilia, and Schönlein-Henoch purpura. At the hip the differential diagnosis includes reactive transient synovitis; Legg-Perthes; slipped capital femoral epiphysis; femoral osteomyelitis; and pelvic, sacroiliac joint, and vertebral osteomyelitis. In the young patient with knee symptoms, the pain may be referred from the hip or related to other intrinsic knee pathology or osteomyelitis. With the exception of gonococcal arthritis, joint drainage is required to remove the organisms, host and bacterial enzymes, and particulate debris. Antibiotic therapy is begun as soon as blood, synovial fluid, and other appropriate cultures are obtained. The synovial fluid Gram stain is the best guide to initial antibiotic selection. If the Gram stain is negative, the antibiotic is chosen based on patient age, joint involved, local epidemiology, and the host's immune competency. Therapy in infants, which should cover staphylococci, streptococci, and gram-negative organisms, involves administration of a combination of oxacillin and gentamicin, or cefotaxime alone. Between the ages of six months and two years, *haemophilus influenzae* type B, staphylococci, and streptococci can be covered with cefuroxime (75 to 100 mg/kg/day). After four years of age, staphylococci and streptococci are the most prevalent. During adolescence *Neisseria gonorrhoeae* must be considered. Adjustments are made, as necessary, based on the results of culture and sensitivity testing and on the response to therapy.

Osteomyelitis continues to be a problem in children (Fig. 4). *S aureus* is the single most frequent identifiable cause. The etiology of a *Pseudomonas* osteomyelitis in childhood is puncture wound of the foot. The basic workup of a child with a clinical picture suggestive of osteomyelitis should include a complete blood count with differential, an erythrocyte sedimentation rate test, and a blood culture. If present, joint fluid should be aspirated and cultured. In children younger than three years of age, the urine should be screened for *H influenzae* type B capsular antigen. A bone aspirate should be obtained before beginning treatment. If frank pus is encountered in the diagnostic aspirate, surgical decompression

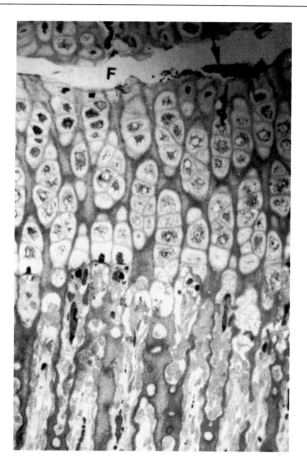

Fig. 4 Photomicrograph of injured physis, osteomyelitis rabbit model. The animal had had the intravenous injection of *S aureus* after traumatic disruption of the growth plate. The black arrow points to *S aureus* organisms in the growth plate fracture (F). None of the animals receiving intravenous injection of organisms without trauma developed infection.

through a cortical window is frequently required. Fluid and electrolyte therapy and analgesics should be given. Initial antibiotic therapy can be guided by the Gram stain result in 50% of patients, or it can be begun empirically, based on likely pathogens at various ages.

The minimum duration of treatment for successful eradication of infection is unknown. Each patient should be evaluated taking into account the speed of clinical response, radiographic findings, and whether surgical debridement was performed. The erythrocyte sedimentation rate is not a reliable means of monitoring treatment.

Nutritional Status

Complications can be decreased by maintaining appropriate patient nutritional status. The basal energy expenditure of a normal 70-kg man at rest is approximately 1,800 kilocalories per day. A patient with a major fracture or infection will have a significant increase in metabolic requirements. Liver and skeletal muscle glycogen stores, which are approximately 300 grams (1,200 kilocalories), can be depleted rapidly. Preoperative evaluation of the patient's nutritional status and appropriate supplementation is warranted.

Threats to Health Care Workers From Human Immunodeficiency Virus and Hepatitis B

Use of universal precautions and hepatitis B vaccine will help decrease the risk of life-threatening infections in health care workers. Universal precautions as recommended by the Centers for Disease Control include the following. (1) All health care workers should routinely use appropriate barrier precautions to prevent skin and mucous membrane exposure when contact with blood or other body fluids of any patient is anticipated. (2) Hands and other skin surfaces should be washed immediately after gloves are removed. (3) All health care workers should take precautions to prevent injuries caused by needles, scalpels, and other sharp instruments or devices. (4) Although saliva that is not contaminated with blood has not been implicated in HIV transmission, to minimize the need for emergency mouth-to-mouth resuscitation, bags or other ventilation devices should be available in areas in which the need for resuscitation is predictable. (5) Health care workers who have exudative lesions or weeping dermatitis should refrain from all direct patient care. (6) Pregnant health care workers should be especially familiar with and strictly adhere to precautions to minimize the risk of HIV transmission.

The Academy recommends the following precautions: double latex gloves, changed hourly, or a combination of cloth and latex; enclosed hoods and face mask and an operative isolator; knee length impervious gowns of high-count polyester weave or plastic-lined nonwoven spun lace polyester; waterproof shoe covers to the knee. All sharp instruments should be passed on trays. Suturing should be accomplished without hand contact with the needle, by one team member at a time. All punctures of the skin should be recorded to keep the operative team aware of contamination. Surgeons who are at risk for possible HIV contamination must convince their hospital administrators that it is the hospital's responsibility to provide the protective equipment required.

The following paragraphs are excerpted from the statement regarding the surgeon and HIV infection, which was approved by the American College of Surgeons Board of Regents in October 1991.

"In 1980, a new blood-borne viral infection was identified. Since that time, this newly discovered infection and its clinical entity (AIDS) has become a subject of major public and professional concern. Unfortunately, this serious infectious disease has attained a sociopolitical status that is resulting in some unusual reactions with significant consequences, particularly for the surgical community. Important virological information has

evolved from laboratory studies. However, important epidemiological information has not been readily accessible because of barriers to testing and because of the stigma and profound social and economic consequences that result when an individual tests positive. Consequently, important data for decision making are not fully available.

"We would emphasize that, to date, there have been no documented incidents of transmission of the HIV virus from a surgeon to a patient, and no transmission of the virus to a patient in a sterile operating room environment. This area has been investigated carefully, and despite testing of thousands of patients of HIV-infected surgeons, no evidence of transmission has been found.

"Guidelines published on July 12, 1991, by the Centers for Disease Control (CDC) and now widely distributed, are based on data that are not applicable to the surgical community; yet insurers, licensing bodies, government agencies, legislative bodies, and others are proposing rules based on these guidelines that will dramatically increase the cost of medical care and have a significant impact on the surgical community. We deplore these actions because they are not based on direct scientific data; they are not cost-effective; they are intrusive to the extreme; and they are unable to achieve their desired intent. Moreover, "risk-prone procedures" cannot be defined in any scientific or rational way. Because no procedure other than dental extraction has ever been shown to result in HIV transmission, this is the only procedure that can logically be called risk-prone. We feel that such a categorization would be irrelevant and counterproductive. In formulating these guidelines, the CDC ignored the overwhelming testimony of the scientific community, and the fact that all currently available data include that transmission from provider to patient in a hospital setting is, so far, a purely hypothetical event.

"Our paramount concern is to continue to minimize the risk. We believe that enforcing a high standard of infection control and universal precautions remains the best strategy for protecting patients from accidental exposure.

"Based on data currently available, we make the following recommendations: (1) Surgeons have the same ethical obligations to render care to HIV-infected patients as they have to care for other patients. (2) Surgeons should use the highest standards of infection control, involving the most effective known sterile barriers, universal precautions, and scientifically accepted infection control practices. This practice should extend to all sites where surgical care is rendered. (3) To date, there have been no documented incidents of transmission of HIV from a surgeon to a patient, and no transmission of the virus to a patient in a sterile operating room environment. Therefore, HIV-infected surgeons may continue to practice and perform invasive procedures unless there is clear evidence that a significant risk of transmission of infection exists through an inability to meet basic infection control procedures or unless the surgeon is functionally unable to care for patients. These determinations are to be made by the surgeon's personal physician and/or an institutional panel so designated for confidential counseling."

The AAOS extends those thoughts. The task force on AIDS and orthopaedic surgery recommends the following. (1) Orthopaedic surgeons have an ethical responsibility to know their own HIV status. (2) The HIV-positive physician has an obligation to inform the patient of his or her HIV status before performing an invasive procedure. (3) An HIV–positive surgeon generally should not perform invasive surgical procedures including injection, aspiration, creating an open wound, or changing the dressings on an open wound. (4) An HIV-positive orthopaedic surgeon should carefully consider the attributes of an exclusively office-based practice where less risk of HIV transmission would exist.

Hepatitis

The term "viral hepatitis" is commonly used for clinically similar diseases that are etiologically and epidemiologically distinct. Two of these, hepatitis A (formerly called infectious hepatitis) and hepatitis B (formerly called serum hepatitis) have been recognized as separate entities since the early 1940s. The third, currently known as non-A, non-B hepatitis, is probably caused by at least two different agents and is an important form of acute viral hepatitis in adults, currently accounting for most posttransfusion hepatitis in the United States.

The specific recommendations for hepatitis B prophylaxis after percutaneous exposure varies depending on whether the source is HBsAg-positive. If the health care worker is unvaccinated and the patient tests positive, one dose of hepatitis B immunoglobulin (HBIG) is given immediately and hepatitis vaccination is indicated. The first dose is given within one week of exposure and the second and third doses are given at one and six months, respectively. A health care worker who has already been vaccinated should be tested for anti-HBs. If the antibody titer is inadequate, the worker should receive one dose of HBIG immediately along with a hepatitis B vaccine booster dose.

Unlike hepatitis B, which is caused by a double-stranded DNA virus, hepatitis C is caused by a single-stranded RNA virus. Approximately 170,000 non-A, non-B hepatitis infections occur each year in the United States. Hepatitis C accounts for one half to two thirds of all non-A, non-B hepatitis (NANB). Intravenous drug abuse, blood transfusion, dialysis, and close personal contact with infected patients are the strongest risk factors accounting for 33%, 10%, 8%, and 7%, respectively. The most effective intervention to date for decreasing posttransfusion hepatitis has been the use of volunteer only donors. Non-A, non-B hepatitis results in a 50% incidence of chronic liver disease. Twenty percent of these patients develop cirrhosis. Although several studies have attempted to assess the value of immunoglobulin prophylaxis against non-A, non-B hepatitis, the results have been equivocal. NIH information suggests that the needlestick risk to medical personnel is low, with a 3.7% transmission rate recorded among 100 exposures. Treatment with interferon-α is effective in reducing serum transaminases and controlling liver inflammation in 50% of patients. Because this improvement is sustained after cessation of treatment in only 50% of these responders, treatment may need to be lifelong.

No evidence of HIV seroconversion has been observed among an estimated one million individuals who have been vaccinated against hepatitis B with plasma-derived vaccine. The recombinant vaccine is readily available, safe, and provides excellent active immunization. Those at high risk, including orthopaedic surgeons and operating room staff, should be vaccinated with recombinant vaccine.

Annotated Bibliography

Microbiology

Buck BE, Resnick L, Shah SM, et al: Human immunodeficiency virus cultured from bone: Implications for transplantation. *Clin Orthop* 1990;251:249-253.

The risk of cadaver-obtained donor tissue being contaminated with the HIV is approximately 1:1.6 million if the appropriate screening safeguards are employed.

Chang CC, Merritt K: Effect of *Staphylococcus epidermidis* on adherence of *Pseudomonas aeruginosa* and *Proteus mirabilis* to polymethylmethacrylate (PMMA) and gentamicin-containing PMMA. *J Orthop Res* 1991;9:284-288.

Biomaterial-centered infections produced by *S epidermidis* are difficult to eradicate, in part because of the extracellular glycocalyx formed by the organism, which changes the surface charge and surface free energy of the bacteria and biomaterial and forms a barrier against host defenses. *S epidermidis* biofilms, whether alive or dead, significantly increase the adherence of *Pseudomonas*. Adherence of *Proteus* was greater to dead biofilm than to live biofilm. Adherence of *Pseudomonas* and *Proteus* was found on gentamicin containing PMMA after preincubation with *S epidermidis*. Thus, once adherence of bacteria has begun, adherence of other organisms may be promoted, and the biofilm formed on PMMA-gentamicin may inhibit the ability of the antibiotic to kill other organisms.

Epps CH Jr, Bryant DD III, Coles MJ, et al: Osteomyelitis in patients who have sickle-cell disease: Diagnosis and management. *J Bone Joint Surg* 1991;73A:1281-1294.

Osteomyelitis is uncommon in patients who have sickle-cell trait. People with sickle-cell disease are at increased risk for bacterial infections secondary to infarcted tissue, splenic hypofunction, and defective opsonins. Although the world literature would suggest that patients who have sickle-cell disease are prone to infections with *Salmonella*, in the United States the association of sickle-cell with osteomyelitis is either unusual or under-reported. In this series, *S aureus* was isolated on culture of bone specimens in eight of 15 patients, *Salmonella* from six, and *Proteus mirabilis* from one. *Salmonella* may not be the most common organism involved in sickle cell-associated osteomyelitis in all populations.

Hoekman P, van de Perre P, Nelissen J, et al: Increased frequency of infection after open reduction of fractures in patients who are seropositive for human immunodeficiency virus. *J Bone Joint Surg* 1991;73A:675-679.

The relative frequency of postoperative infection was higher in patients who were seropositive and had associated clinical symptoms than in patients who were seronegative. Patients who developed infection responded to parenteral antibiotics. In this study 22% of the men and 11% of the women were seropositive.

Antimicrobial Agents

Bennett PB, Bove AA, Camporesi EM, et al: NHLBI workshop summary: Hyperbaric oxygenation therapy. *Am Rev Respir Dis* 1991;144:1414-1421.

The rationale for hyperbaric oxygen therapy is that a number of diseases have cellular oxygen deficiency as a major component. A workshop was held in September 1989 to review the physiologic basis of hyperbaric oxygen therapy and to make recommendations for future research. Defective wound healing is commonly associated with diabetes, peripheral venous stasis, arterial insufficiency, pressure, irradiation, collagen vascular disease, pulmonary disease, malnutrition, and sickle cell disease. While hyperoxia induces vasoconstriction and reduces blood flow in normal tissue, neoangiogenesis is enhanced at the margin of a wound if a steep oxygen gradient is provided by the breathing of oxygen at higher partial pressures. Direct exposure of healing tissues to topically administered oxygen suppresses wound angiogenesis, but epithelialization is usually increased. At the chemical level, oxygen is necessary for adequate leukocyte bactericidal activity. Leukocyte function is degraded at tissue oxygen partial pressures below 40 torr and improves through pressures up to 150 torr. The single most striking outcome of the workshop was the realization of the lack of basic knowledge about the pathophysiology of defective wound healing and recalcitrant infections.

Clarke HJ, Jinnah RH, Byank RP, et al: *Clostridium difficile* infection in orthopaedic patients. *J Bone Joint Surg* 1990;72A:1056-1059.

The appropriate test is a stool assay for *C difficile* toxin. Metronidazole should be the treatment of choice, rather than vancomycin, because of the large cost differential between the two therapies.

Lyons VO, Henry SL, Faghri M, et al: Bacterial adherence to plain and tobramycin-laden polymethylmethacrylate beads. *Clin Orthop* 1992;278:260-264.

Using a New Zealand white rabbit in vivo model, the authors demonstrated that tobramycin-sensitive bacteria did not adhere to tobramycin-laden beads. Therefore, implanted PMMA beads should contain antibiotic specific for the microorganisms under treatment. The beads should probably be removed once a significant amount of antibiotic elution has occurred to prevent future colonization of the PMMA.

Perry CR, Pearson RL: Local antibiotic delivery in the treatment of bone and joint infections. *Clin Orthop* 1991;263:215-226.

The authors report suppression of infection in 30 of 42 patients with resistant osteomyelitis, 30 of 37 patients with acutely infected total joint arthroplasties, and seven of ten chronically infected arthroplasties. There was a 7% pump site infection rate.

Osteomyelitis

Cattaneo R, Catagni M, Johnson EE: The treatment of infected nonunions and segmental defects of the tibia by the methods of Ilizarov. *Clin Orthop* 1992;280:143-152.

Twenty-eight patients with infected nonunion or segmental bone loss of the tibia were treated with debridement and internal bone transport or compression-distraction osteogenesis. Regenerate new bone formation averaged 6 cm (range 1.5 to 22 cm). All patients healed their bone defects without addition of soft-tissue transfers or cancellous grafting.

Fischer MD, Gustilo RB, Varecka TF: The timing of flap coverage, bone grafting, and intramedullary nailing in patients who have a fracture of the tibial shaft with extensive soft tissue injury. *J Bone Joint Surg* 1991;73A:1316-1322.

Of 43 patients with Type III-B open fractures of the tibial shaft, infection developed in two of 11 treated with early muscle flap coverage (five to ten days after injury), nine of 13 who were treated with a delayed flap, and ten of 19 who were managed with open care of the wound. Those who had bone grafting after complete wound closure and cessation of drainage had fewer infections than those who underwent grafting while traumatic wound drainage persisted—none of 16 versus four of 15. Delayed intramedullary reaming for rod placement was also associated with a high infection rate (nine of 19).

Gristina AG, Naylor PT, Webb LX: Molecular mechanisms in musculoskeletal sepsis: The race for the surface, in Greene WB (ed): American Academy of Orthopaedic Surgeons *Instructional Course Lectures, XXXIX*. Park Ridge, IL, American Academy of Orthopaedic Surgeons, 1990, pp 471-482.

Microbial adhesion affects pathogenesis and antibiotic resistance.

Gustilo RB, Merkow RL, Templeman D: The management of open fractures. *J Bone Joint Surg* 1990;72A:299-304.

The incidence of infection correlates with the soft-tissue damage associated with an open fracture: Type I, 0-2%; Type II, 2%-7%; Type IIIA, 7%; Type IIIB, 10%-50%; Type IIIC, 25%-50%.

McNeill TW: Spinal infections, in Greene WB (ed): American Academy of Orthopaedic Surgeons *Instructional Course Lectures, XXXIX.* Park Ridge, IL, American Academy of Orthopaedic Surgeons, 1990, pp 515-526.

The author discusses in detail the clinical features, appropriate diagnostic investigations, and treatment options. An initial biopsy is important for precise bacterial diagnosis. Although most infections respond to antibiotics and bed rest, emergency surgery is called for in the treatment of a symptomatic epidural abscess, and elective surgery is appropriate for drainage of paravertebral abscesses and late correction of spinal deformity.

Newman LG, Waller J, Palestro CJ, et al: Unsuspected osteomyelitis in diabetic foot ulcers: Diagnosis and monitoring by leukocyte scanning with indium-IN 111 oxyquinolone. *JAMA* 1991;266:1246-1251.

The prevalence of osteomyelitis in 35 diabetic patients who had a total of 41 foot ulcers was determined in a prospective study. Indium-labelled leukocyte scintigraphy was used to assist with diagnosis and treatment follow up. The sensitivity of the scan was 89%, specificity was 69%. The intensity of the leukocyte scan image began to decrease after 16 to 34 days of treatment and was interpreted as normal by 36 to 54 days of successful therapy.

Perry CR, Pearson RL, Miller GA: Accuracy of cultures of material from swabbing of the superficial aspect of the wound and needle biopsy in the preoperative assessment of osteomyelitis. *J Bone Joint Surg* 1991;73A:745-749.

Cultures of material obtained by superficial wound swab and needle biopsy did not identify all of the pathogens present in 60 patients who had posttraumatic or postoperative osteomyelitis. Aerobic, anaerobic, and fungal organisms were all missed when compared to specimens obtained in the operating room at the time of bone debridement. Similarly, six of nine patients in whom a negative needle biopsy had been obtained at the site of a tibial nonunion with possible persistent subclinical infection developed a postoperative exacerbation after reamed rodding.

Septic Arthritis

Lane JG, Falahee MH, Wojtys EM, et al: Pyarthrosis of the knee: Treatment considerations. *Clin Orthop* 1990;252:198-204.

The authors recommended open arthrotomy for immunocompromised patients, those infected with *S aureus* or gram-negative organisms, and those in whom there is a delay in treatment of more than three days.

Leslie BM, Harris JM III, Driscoll D: Septic arthritis of the shoulder in adults. *J Bone Joint Surg* 1989;71A:1515-1522.

Septic arthritis of the shoulder accounts for only 3% to 12% of all pyarthroses. The diagnosis was made within one week of onset in only five of 18 patients. Arthrotomy for drainage was superior to repeated attempts of arthrocentesis.

McCutchan HJ, Fisher RC: Synovial leukocytosis in infectious arthritis. *Clin Orthop* 1990;257:226-230.

Immunocompromised patients, such as those with neoplasms and those requiring systemic steroids or abusing intravenous drugs, may have a lower than anticipated synovial white blood cell count in the presence of a pyarthrosis.

Williams RJ III, Smith RL, Schurman DJ: Purified staphylococcal culture medium stimulates neutral metalloprotease secretion from human articular cartilage. *J Orthop Res* 1991;9:258-265.

Human articular cartilage released metal-dependent enzymes capable of degrading collagen after exposure to sterile, purified *S aureus* culture medium. The profile of enzymatic activity was comparable to that observed with interleukin-1. Activation could be due to an inactivation or decreased synthesis of an inhibitor such as tissue inhibitor of metalloproteinase (TIMP), direct stimulation of chondrocytes in vivo, or induction of IL-1 production by chondrocytes. Stimulation of neutral metaloproteinases by soluble staphylococcal factors may underlie cartilage destruction in *S aureus* septic arthritis.

Pediatric Infections

Choi IH, Pizzutillo PD, Bowen JR, et al: Sequelae and reconstruction after septic arthritis of the hip in infants. *J Bone Joint Surg* 1990;72A:1150-1165.

The authors define four classification groups on the basis of radiographic findings. Type I deformity hips had sustained transient ischemia of the epiphysis and did not need reconstruction. Type II hips had deformity of the epiphysis, physis, and metaphysis and required surgery to prevent subluxation. Type III deformity involved malalignment of the femoral neck or pseudarthrosis of the neck. These patients required realignment osteotomy or bone grafting. Type IV hips had destruction of the head and neck with severe leg length discrepancy and incompetence of the joint and required extensive surgery such as trochanteric arthroplasty, arthrodesis, and limb lengthening.

Faden H, Grossi M: Acute osteomyelitis in children: Reassessment of etiologic agents and their clinical characteristics. *Am J Dis Child* 1991;145:65-69.

One hundred thirty-five children with acute osteomyelitis were treated between 1980 and 1986. Ten different genera of bacteria were identified. *S aureus* was the most common pathogen (25%) in youngsters older than three years of age. Below three years of age, *H influenzae* type B was the most common etiology. The femur (29%), tibia (15%), foot (16%), and pelvis (7%) were the areas most frequently involved. Signs and symptoms at presentation included: pain (94%), fever (85%), local changes (69%), and irritability (12%). Positive soft-tissue cultures were obtained in 67%, positive bone cultures in 51%, positive joint fluid cultures in 37%, and positive blood cultures in 30%.

Katz K, Mechlis-Frish S, Cohen IJ, et al: Bone scans in the diagnosis of bone crisis in patients who have Gaucher disease. *J Bone Joint Surg* 1991;73A:513-517.

In patients who have Gaucher's disease, the symptoms and laboratory findings of crisis can be identical to those of acute hematogenous osteomyelitis. The rate of positive blood cultures in patients with osteomyelitis can be less than 50%. Technetium scintigraphy is not helpful in this context. A photon-deficient area may be seen on the delayed image of patients with Gaucher's or osteomyelitis. Therefore, if the clinical presentation, laboratory tests, and bone scan are inconclusive, additional evaluation with gallium-67, indium-labelled WBC scintigraphy, and aspiration of the involved bone should be obtained. Subsequent repeat CT and MRI may be needed to ensure that an abscess is not forming.

Shaw BA, Kasser JR: Acute septic arthritis in infancy and childhood. *Clin Orthop* 1990;257:212-225.

Optimal results require prompt diagnosis, adequate drainage, and appropriate antibiotic therapy. If aspiration/irrigation is to be used, the physician must document a satisfactory synovial fluid response. Pyarthrosis of the hip is a surgical emergency. Antibiotic therapy is usually continued for three to six weeks, depending on the clinical response. Oral therapy is appropriate if there has been an adequate response to initial parenteral therapy, the organism is sensitive, the patient is able to tolerate the oral medication, bactericidal titers can be obtained, and the patient and family are compliant.

Whalen JL, Fitzgerald RH Jr, Morrissy RT: A histologic study of acute hematogenous osteomyelitis following physeal injuries in rabbits. *J Bone Joint Surg* 1988;70A:1383-1392.

The effect of an intravenous injection of *S aureus* alone, or in combination with an injury to the physis, was studied in young rabbits. Metaphyseal osteomyelitis was seen by 48 hours in all rabbits that had bacteremia and traumatic growth plate disruption. An intravenous injection alone produced no osteomyelitis. A generalized lower resistance to infection seemed to be related to the trauma.

Threats to Health Care Workers

Hester RA, Nelson CL: Methods to reduce intraoperative transmission of blood-borne disease. *J Bone Joint Surg* 1991;73A:1108-1111.

The risk of contamination of skin and mucous membranes affects all surgeons. There are no perfect preventive measures. Improved methods of operative team protection increase the cost of providing surgical care. It is important that the principles be implemented during residency training, both to prevent current injury and to develop safer habits for the future.

Klein RS: Universal precautions for preventing occupational exposures to human immunodeficiency virus type I. *Am J Med* 1991;90:141-144.

To date, only 24 health care workers have proven seroconversions following exposure to HIV patients. None of the health care workers were surgeons, none were exposed to the operating room environment, and none were injured with solid bore needles.

Lau JY, Alexander GJ, Alberti A: Viral hepatitis. *Gut* 1991;Suppl:S41-S62.

There has been a significant increase in our understanding of viral hepatitis over the past 20 years. Five distinct viruses, designated as hepatitis A through E have been defined. The hepatitis B (HBV) genome, 3,200 base pairs in length, is the smallest known animal DNA virus. Immunization is the first line of defense for health-care workers. Universal precautions should help to diminish transmission. Treatment of chronic HBV infection with interferon-α (more that 5 million units/m^2 three times each week for three months) is effective in some patients.

Smith RC, Mooar PA, Cooke T, et al: Contamination of operating room personnel during total arthroplasty. *Clin Orthop* 1991;271:9-11.

Evaluation of the intraoperative contamination of the operating room team with blood and body fluids during total hip and total knee arthroplasty revealed that 100% of the surgeons and first assistants, despite protection by masks, hoods, eyewear, and moisture-repellent gowns, had skin contamination during the course of the surgery. Most of the exposure occurred on the forehead and neck related to pulsatile irrigation or bone fragments during osteotomy or reaming. Eighty-seven percent of the surgeons had contamination on their eyewear. Three percent had gross ocular contamination. During 60 consecutive total joint arthroplasties, the surgeon sustained a penetrating skin injury once and the first assistant, twice. The authors recommend wrap-around face shields, or helmets, fluid-impervious gowns, knee-high waterproof foot covers, and double or triple gloving.

14

Musculoskeletal Neoplasms

Initial Management of a Lesion

The basic approach to a patient with a bone or soft-tissue lesion begins with the history and physical examination. The goal of this initial approach to the bone or soft-tissue lesion is to determine the probable diagnosis and whether or not the lesion must be biopsied or treated further.

The age of the patient should be noted because certain lesions are characteristic in certain age groups. For example, Ewing's sarcoma is more common in children; malignant fibrous histiocytoma is more common in adults. It should be noted whether or not the lesion was discovered incidentally or discovered because it was painful, swollen, or accompanied by a pathologic fracture. Typically, painful lesions are usually discovered early and before fractures occur. A cartilaginous lesion with a benign appearance on radiographs that was discovered incidentally is much less worrisome than a similarly appearing lesion producing pain. During the physical examination, special attention must be given to the presence or absence of any mass. It is a good practice to record the location, size, and involvement of underlying structures, whether the mass feels superficial or deep, and if the mass is tender. Small (less than 5 cm), superficial lesion that are not increasing in size are much less likely to be malignant than larger, deep or growing lesions.

It is important to obtain high-quality plain radiographs at the patient's initial visit. A systematic approach should be taken in reviewing these studies. The examiner should note the location of the lesion, which bone is involved, whether or not the lesion is proximal or distal, and whether or not the lesion is eccentric or central, or on the surface of the bone. It should also be noted whether or not it is epiphyseal, metaphyseal, or diaphyseal. Attention should be given to the lesion's border, whether it is well-circumscribed, sclerotic, or not well delineated. The tumor matrix should be examined carefully for the presence of any calcification. It is also especially important that any periosteal reaction be noted.

From the history, physical examination, and review of the plain radiographs, the examiner should be able to formulate a reasonably good differential diagnosis. Small asymptomatic lesions with radiographic appearances characteristic of benign processes, such as a nonossifying fibroma or fibrous cortical defect, can frequently be safely observed with serial studies.

If there is any question as to the identity of the lesion, further radiographic studies should be performed. The bone scan is important in that it can rule out the presence

of other lesions, delineate whether or not the lesion is active, and give an idea of its extent. Computed tomography (CT) is excellent for delineating bone involvement, especially the presence of endosteal erosion. It is also useful in detecting calcification and can help differentiate a fibrous from a cartilaginous lesion. Magnetic resonance imaging (MRI) is particularly good for identifying soft-tissue extent and can also be used to identify the extent of the lesion in bone (Figs. 1-3). MRI also gives the examiner a good idea of the relationship between the lesion and the surrounding neurovascular structures and can help guide the biopsy as well as the resection. In addition, MRI has recently been demonstrated to detect the presence of skip metastases, which were not able to be identified on radiographs, isotope scan, or CT.

Whether the lesion is probably benign or metastatic, a biopsy and definitive treatment can frequently be done at the same time. If the lesion is most likely a sarcoma, most centers will perform the definitive treatment only after examination of the histologic material by an experienced pathologist.

Principles of the Biopsy

The biopsy is one of the most important procedures in managing patients with bone and soft-tissue tumors. Although some centers routinely perform needle biopsies on all sarcomas, most centers perform open biopsies. The advantages of the open biopsy are that it provides more tissue for diagnosis and is associated with a lower sample error. In a recent review, aspiration biopsy was found to have a diagnostic accuracy of only 72% in 31 patients who had a primary bone tumor that was suspected of being malignant. This indicates that aspiration biopsy may be inadequate in almost 30% of patients who are suspected of having a bone malignancy. In addition, this study also demonstrated an accuracy rate of just 23% in detecting those lesions suspected of being benign. If aspiration biopsy is performed, it should be done either by the surgeon who will do the resection or by a radiologist supervised by the surgeon because the needle will contaminate compartments that will then have to be excised at the time of tumor excision if a wide margin is to be obtained. If the biopsy tract is poorly placed or requires multiple aspirations that violate different compartments, the ability to perform a limb salvage procedure in the future may be compromised.

The placement of the incision for an open biopsy is of paramount importance. The type of limb salvage proce-

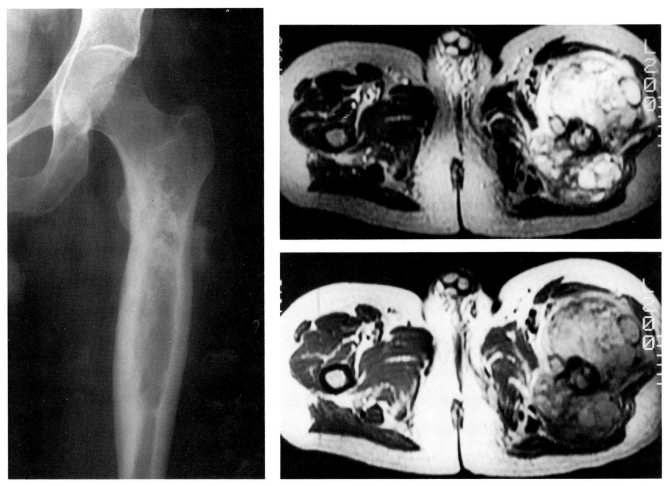

Fig. 1   **Left**, Lesion of proximal femur with permeative borders and periosteal reaction. Biopsy confirmed a diagnosis of osteogenic sarcoma. **Top right**, MRI demonstrating extensive soft-tissue mass surrounding femur and displacing the neurovascular structures. **Bottom right**, Marrow involvement in proximal femur is demonstrated by comparison of signal in the intramedullary canal of the involved side with that of the uninvolved side.

dure necessary if the lesion is a sarcoma must be considered before performing the biopsy. Transverse incisions on the extremities are contraindicated; the surgeon should try to violate as few compartments as possible. In the past, the poor placement of an incision for biopsy before the patient was referred to a center where sarcomas of the extremities are commonly treated was a frequent cause for amputation. Although still a problem, the more aggressive use of free and rotational flaps is allowing the salvage of extremities that would have previously required amputation because of the poor placement of an incision for biopsy.

Neurovascular structures should not be exposed at the time of biopsy so that they do not come in contact with tumor cells. If tumor cells are exposed to neurovascular structures, these structures will be contaminated, and it will not be possible to get a wide margin without removing them. At the time of resection, any tissue not in contact with the tumor cells must be removed, and this must be considered before performing the biopsy.

Postoperative hematoma formation can render a previously resectable lesion unresectable. An awareness of this potential problem at the time of biopsy is important. The surgeon must make every effort to keep bleeding to a minimum during the procedure and to keep the wound as dry as possible before closure. This often involves packing perforations in the bone with thrombin-soaked gelfoam or with polymethylmethacrylate to prevent postoperative bleeding. Most centers are now using drains postoperatively to help decrease the incidence of hematoma. Drains should be taken through the skin in line with the incision and close to the wound edge. Drain sites will be contaminated by tumor cells and must be removed at tumor excision. Frozen sections should be performed whenever possible at the time of biopsy to be certain that representative tissue is obtained. Cultures

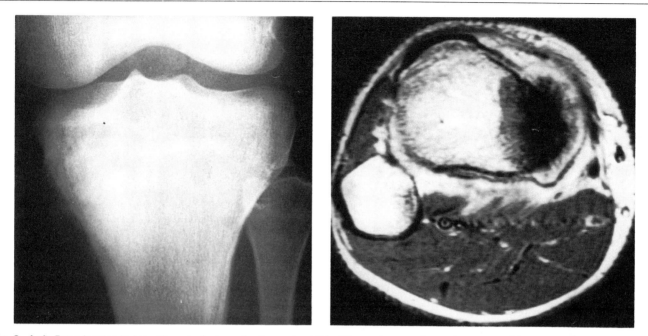

Fig. 2 **Left**, Bone-forming lesion with periosteal reaction in proximal tibia. Diagnosis was osteogenic sarcoma. **Right**, MRI demonstrates intramedullary involvement and soft-tissue mass.

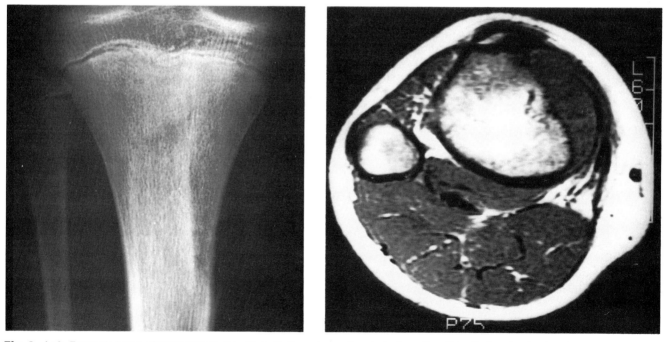

Fig. 3 **Left**, Eccentric lesion of tibial metaphysis with cortical erosion and periosteal reaction. Note Codman's triangle inferiorly. **Right**, MRI demonstrates that mass is contiguous with cortex but sparing medullary canal, characteristic of a periosteal or juxtacortical osteogenic sarcoma.

should always be taken at the time of biopsy to rule out the possibility of infection, and no patient should have preoperative antibiotics before being biopsied.

Current areas of research related to biopsy involve the use of flow cytometry to help determine which tumors may be better responders to certain chemotherapeutic agents before treatment. This would enable the physician to choose more specifically therapeutic agents and permit the exclusion of otherwise toxic agents that would not be beneficial.

Staging

The purpose of staging any tumor is to predict behavior and direct treatment. The most common staging system used for bone tumors was developed by William Enneking and involves the assignment of a Roman numeral to the histologic grade of the tumor, followed by an A or a B depending on whether the tumor is intracompartmental or extracompartmental. Stage I lesions are low grade, stage II lesions are high grade, and stage III are metastatic. This system has been found to be predictive of behavior in the majority of bone sarcomas and has also been used to stage soft-tissue sarcomas. In addition, the American Joint Commission (AJC) on cancer has its own staging system. The AJC system is based on tumor size, histologic grade, the presence or absence of lymph node involvement or the presence of distant metastases. A third system for soft-tissue sarcomas is the Hajdu system, which is based on the histologic grade, whether or not the tumor is deep or superficial, and whether or not the tumor is larger or smaller than 5 cm.

A recent review of patients with stage IIB osteogenic sarcoma and skip metastases revealed a poor prognosis similar to that of stage III osteogenic sarcomas. The survival of these patients was not improved by the use of adjuvant chemotherapy. For these reasons, it was recommended that the presence of a skip lesion be another criterion for considering an osteosarcoma to be a stage III lesion.

Primary Tumors

Osteosarcoma

Osteosarcoma is the most common primary bone sarcoma. Prior to 1971, the five-year survival of patients with osteogenic sarcoma was estimated to be 19.7%. At the present time, five- and ten-year disease-free survival is greater than 70% as reported in most studies. This survival is site-dependent. In a recent review of the three most common sites of involvement, humeral lesions had the best probability of survival (84% at ten years), followed by tibial lesions (81%) and femoral lesions (67%). In this study, histologic response to preoperative chemotherapy was the strongest predictor of outcome.

The increase in survival of patients with osteogenic sarcoma is related to improvements in surgical technique, early resection of lung metastases, and improvements in adjuvant chemotherapy. A recent multi-institutional study by the Musculoskeletal Tumor Society has determined that limb salvage surgery for osteogenic sarcoma at the distal end of the femur will result in a local recur-

rence rate and long-term survival is essentially the same as that of patients who have had above-knee amputations.

Patients who continue to have a very poor prognosis for survival despite chemotherapy include those with local recurrence and those with radiation-induced or pagetic sarcomas. In a recent review, only two of 18 patients with local recurrence were rendered long-term disease-free survivors. The five-year survival for radiation-induced and pagetic sarcomas is approximately 10% to 15% as reported in the most recent studies.

Ewing's Sarcoma

Traditionally, the treatment of Ewing's sarcoma has been chemotherapy and radiation therapy. Over the last few years, increased survival has been noted in patients treated by wide excision and chemotherapy when compared with those treated by chemotherapy and radiation therapy alone. In a recent review, 60% of the patients with Ewing's sarcoma treated with amputation or resection and radiotherapy were disease-free compared with 28% of those treated with radiation therapy alone at a minimum follow-up of five years. The local recurrence rate was 8% in the group treated with surgery or surgery and radiation compared with 36% in the group treated with radiation therapy alone. This and other studies have led to a trend at most institutions to treat Ewing's sarcoma more frequently with surgery when excision is possible.

Complications associated with the use of radiation therapy in the treatment of Ewing's sarcoma are not infrequent. These patients often suffer pathologic fractures through the area of radiation, especially if this is in a weightbearing bone. This complication may require prolonged immobilization or some type of surgical reconstruction for treatment. In addition, radiation therapy is associated with a significant risk for the development of secondary sarcomas.

Chondrosarcoma

If multiple myeloma is excluded, chondrosarcoma is second only to osteogenic sarcoma in frequency as a malignant tumor of bone. It compromises 17% to 22% of all primary tumors of bone. A primary chondrosarcoma can be defined as one that arises *de novo* in a previously normal bone. A secondary chondrosarcoma is a malignant cartilage tumor that arises from a benign cartilage tumor, usually an enchondroma or the cartilage cap of an osteocartilaginous exostosis. A dedifferentiated chondrosarcoma is a malignant cartilaginous tumor in which a component is of a different histologic type. This is most often an osteogenic sarcoma.

With the exception of some occasional dedifferentiated tumors, chondrosarcomas are highly resistant to chemotherapy. Because of this resistance, most surgeons recommend aggressive excision with a wide margin, especially for the intermediate and the high-grade tumors. In a recent review of chondrosarcomas of the spine, all patients who had an intralesional excision had progression of the disease and died.

Giant Cell Tumor

Giant cell tumor is one of the more common primary benign tumors of bone. The most common locations of this tumor are in the distal femur, proximal tibia, and distal radius. The radiologic hallmark of this tumor is extension into the subchondral bone.

Because of its proximity to the articular cartilage, it is difficult to do an intralesional excision of a giant cell tumor without leaving tumor cells behind, and the excision of giant cell tumors in the past has been associated with a high rate of local recurrence. Advances over the last ten years in the use of adjuncts to excision have been successful in decreasing this local recurrence rate. These have included the use of phenol, polymethylmethacrylate, and liquid nitrogen. The mechanism by which all these agents decrease local recurrence probably involves increasing the zone of necrosis at the periphery of the excision. Current areas of clinical investigation into the treatment of giant cell tumors involves answering the question of whether or not the polymethylmethacrylate cement used to fill the defect must eventually be removed and replaced with bone graft.

Unicameral Bone Cyst

Most centers treat this common bone lesion with aspiration and then injection of an agent to speed healing. This has traditionally involved the use of corticosteroids, but more recently, the use of bone marrow has also been found to improve healing. Whether the injection of the agent is the important component or whether just the needle aspiration itself leads to healing is a topic of discussion. Large lesions that remain unhealed after several attempts at aspiration and injection should be curetted out and bone grafted. If there is any question at all as to the diagnosis of this lesion, a biopsy should be performed and the specimen reviewed by an experienced pathologist.

In a recent retrospective study, the use of autographs and allografts for the treatment of benign bone lesions were compared with respect to time required and success of graft incorporation. Allografts were comparable to autografts when small volumes (less than 60 ml) were treated. Autographs were superior to allografts in the rate and completeness of healing for solitary large lesions.

Soft-Tissue Sarcomas

Whenever possible, obtaining a wide margin of excision is the recommended treatment of these lesions. These tumors frequently are in contact with neurovascular structures. Recent studies have demonstrated that local recurrence rates following marginal excision with preservation of these structures and the use of adjunctive radiation therapy yield local recurrence rates similar to more radical procedures. If the lesion is less than 3 cm and is superficial, most surgeons would recommend the performance of an excisional biopsy with removal of a cuff of uninvolved tissue surrounding the lesion. If the lesion is large or deep, or if the removal of this cuff of tissue may significantly impair function for the patient, an incisional biopsy is recommended. There have been several randomized trials in an attempt to determine if chemotherapy is of use in these sarcomas. Most of these trials have not been able to demonstrate an increase in patient survival with chemotherapy dosages that were in a tolerable range.

Several investigators over the last five years have reviewed the prognostic factors in survival and local recurrence for soft-tissue sarcomas. Tumor size greater than 5 cm, deep tumors, extracompartmental status, inadequate excision, and histologic high grade have all been determined to be unfavorable.

The treatment of aggressive fibromatosis has been a subject of much interest over the last five years. These lesions frequently present a challenge in management because of their extreme tendency to recur locally. The use of radiation therapy as an adjunct to surgical excision has become more popular. These tumors frequently involve neurovascular structures and have a tendency to infiltrate surrounding muscle. This characteristic makes it difficult to attain a wide margin in many cases without an ablative procedure. Because they do not in general represent a threat to the survival of the patient, most surgeons are hesitant to perform an amputation in order to gain local control. It is for these reasons that many centers are now using radiation therapy as an adjunct to surgical excision in the treatment of aggressive fibromatosis. In a recent review, 11 of 14 sites with presumed microscopic residual disease following excision and 14 of 16 sites with known grossly residual disease were locally controlled with the use of radiation therapy after more than five years of follow-up.

The treatment of aggressive fibromatosis in children is particularly difficult because of the problems associated with radiating an immature skeleton. Thus, there has been a significant interest in the development of chemotherapeutic protocols to treat this lesion. The early results have been encouraging, but further clinical trials are necessary to determine its efficacy.

Soft-tissue masses are frequently seen about the foot and ankle in the general orthopaedic practice. In a recent review, almost 90% of the masses around the foot and ankle were benign. The most common malignant tumor was the synovial sarcoma, which had a predilection for occurring in the ankle, heel, or dorsum of the foot.

Squamous cell carcinoma often presents in a pre-existing scar or draining sinus of an extremity. In a recent review, half of the patients studied developed metastasis to regional lymph nodes. Prognosis was uniformly poor for intermediate and high-grade lesions. The investigators recommended considering early amputation in those patients with high-grade lesions because wide excision is frequently difficult as the result of anatomy and tissue planes distorted by previous trauma or burns.

Metastatic Disease to Bone

Advances in chemotherapy have led to improved survival for patients with primary tumors outside the musculoskeletal system. Metastatic disease to bone is a frequent occurrence in these patients. The majority of patients who die from cancer have evidence of disease at autopsy. This has increased the need for the orthopaedic surgeon to become more familiar with managing metastatic disease to bone. The indications for internal fixation of tumors metastatic to bone have been outlined by Harrington and include a lesion that involves more than 2.5 cm of cortex, greater than 50% of the width of the bone, pain despite irradiation, and avulsion fracture of the lesser trochanter.

Deciding on a course of management of these patients frequently involves an appreciation of how long they can be expected to live. The survival for the patient following pathologic fractures depends on the type of tumor. A patient with carcinoma of the lung usually will not survive more than six months to one year following pathologic fracture; a patient with carcinoma of the thyroid will commonly survive five years or more. The recent advances in internal fixation that have included long-stem bipolar hip replacements and the use of proximal and distal interlocking nails have improved the orthopaedic management of these patients. Most centers now use additional polymethylmethacrylate to aid in fixation in areas where weak bone will not support the metallic device.

Limb Salvage Surgery

This has been an area of intense investigation over the last five years. The increasing interest in this type of surgery has resulted from several studies that have demonstrated little difference between patient survival and local recurrence rate for amputation versus limb salvage in certain anatomic locations. The basic criteria for performing a limb salvage procedure continue to be a recurrence rate and survival compatible with ablative surgery and function that is better than that with an amputation.

There continues to be great interest in the complications associated with limb salvage. The most common complication in limb salvage is wound necrosis leading to infection. There are three main reasons: (1) because the excision of the sarcoma usually requires the elevation of large flaps for exposure, which tends to devascularize the skin; (2) because it is necessary to excise the tumor with a cuff of uninvolved muscle in order to obtain a wide margin in a sarcoma with a soft-tissue mass, which further compromises the blood supply to the skin and will frequently place the allograft or prosthesis in a subcutaneous position, especially around the knee; and (3) because

of the use of chemotherapy, which is known to have a detrimental effect on wound healing.

In most centers, the high incidence of wound complications of ten years ago has significantly decreased as a result of improvement in surgical technique (the more aggressive use of free and rotational muscle flaps at the time of resection) and in the management of postoperative wound necrosis.

There have been several studies over the last five years of the use of allografts in limb salvage surgery. In a large retrospective review, the overall incidence of fracture of the allografts was determined to be 16%. The mean time to fracture was 29 months, with 55% of the fractures occurring within two years and 70% within three years. Most of the fractures did not occur within the first six months and no fracture occurred after four years. Another large retrospective study determined the incidence of infection in large allografts to be 11.7%, with 82% of these patients requiring amputation or removal of the graft to control infection. One advantage of using allografts over prostheses in limb salvage is that the former frequently provide an area for soft-tissue attachment that could improve function. In a recent series, osteoarticular allografts were used for reconstruction of the proximal humerus following excision for benign aggressive tumors or low grade sarcomas that did not require removal of a large soft-tissue cuff. Function was rated as good or excellent in more than half of these cases.

Ten years ago the problems of prosthetic breakage and wound necrosis were common when using prostheses for reconstruction in limb salvage. These problems have now become much less frequent because of improvement in the structure of the prostheses and the more aggressive use of soft-tissue procedures to improve coverage of these devices. The challenge of reconstructing these large defects around joints has led to innovations in prosthetic design. In a recent review, a prosthesis with a "ball-in-socket" articulation between the femoral and tibial components was used to reconstruct large defects created by extra-articular excision of sarcomas of the proximal tibia. This type of excision requires removal of the patella tendon insertion along with the proximal tibia. In an attempt to reconstruct the extensor mechanism, the patella remnant remaining after excision was attached directly to a porous pad on the surface of the tibial component. This procedure was successful in restoring active extension in the majority of patients. Overall, functional results using the rating system of the Musculoskeletal Tumor Society were good or excellent in the majority of cases.

One alternative to the use of prostheses or allografts to reconstruct large segmental defects around the knee is the van Ness rotationplasty. In this procedure, the tibia is turned 180 degrees on the femur so that the ankle functions as a knee joint. This allows a patient who would otherwise have had an above-knee amputation to have a functional below-knee amputation. In a recent review, functional testing demonstrated these patients to perform as well as those who had endoprosthetic replacement and better than those who had an above-knee amputation. It was also demonstrated to be an effective salvage procedure for failed endoprostheses.

Reconstruction following excision of malignant pelvic tumors continues to be a major challenge. In a recent review, the best functional and therapeutic results were in those patients in whom a wide margin could be obtained and femoral sacral continuity maintained or reconstructed.

The majority of patients will choose a limb salvage procedure over an amputation when given a choice in management of their sarcoma. Whether or not a limb salvage procedure provides any true psychologic advantage over that of an amputation has been a topic of interest. In a recent review, the emotional well-being of patients who had undergone either amputation, arthrodesis, or arthroplasty for tumors about the knees were compared. The patients who had the amputation were the least worried about damaging the affected limb but felt more isolated socially, found it more difficult to make friends, visited others less often, found that tasks involved extra effort, tired more easily, and did not enjoy things as much as those who had had an arthroplasty. However, they were not clinically depressed. The patients who had had an arthrodesis performed the most demanding physical work but had difficulty sitting and their feeling of emotional well being was not as strong as those who had had the arthroplasty, but stronger than those who had had an amputation.

Chemotherapy

The primary malignant tumors of bone that have been found to be most sensitive to chemotherapy include osteogenic sarcoma, Ewing's sarcoma, and malignant fibrous histiocytoma. Chondrosarcomas have been found to be relatively insensitive and are, in general, not treated with chemotherapy.

The majority of protocols for treating osteogenic sarcoma employ high-dose methotrexate, doxorubicin, and cisplatin. More recent protocols for osteogenic sarcoma also use ifosfamide with or without etoposide. Over the last several years, the use of intra-arterial chemotherapy has become more frequent because many investigators believe that it provides a more direct route of administration. The agent that has been found most effective in intra-arterial use is cisplatin. The protocol for treatment of metastatic osteogenic sarcoma involved chemotherapy with resection of the pulmonary lesions as well as the primary tumor. In patients with metastatic disease treated by the above protocol, 20% to 40% can be expected to survive more than five years.

The current five-year survival for patients with nonpelvic Ewing's sarcoma treated with chemotherapy, as reported in the literature, ranges from 57% to 70%. The agents include vincristine, actinomycin D, doxorubicin, and cyclophosphamide. Ifosfamide with or without etoposide is used for patients who have had a relapse after earlier treatment.

Chemotherapy in association with surgical excision has been demonstrated to improve survival for patients with malignant fibrous histiocytoma of bone. The regimens are similar to those used for osteogenic sarcoma. Unfortunately, at the present time there is no chemotherapeutic regimen currently available that has been demonstrated to be efficacious in treating chondrosarcoma. Research involves exploring the use of hormonal agents that have been shown to have an effect on cartilage growth. One such agent is somatostatin, which has been demonstrated to inhibit the growth of chondrosarcoma in rats.

The role of chemotherapy in the treatment of soft-tissue sarcomas remains unclear. The most commonly used agent in clinical trials is doxorubicin. Recently, ifosfamide has been tried in patients with advanced disease but has not been used in patients with localized disease. Chemotherapy has been found to improve survival in patents with childhood rhabdomyosarcoma. The protocols used currently employ vincristine, actinomycin D, and cyclophosphamide.

Bone Tumor Research

Unregulated growth is the hallmark of cancer. Understanding the mechanism by which cells become unregulated is the primary emphasis of much of cancer research. The loss of regulation may be a result of cellular defects at several levels. For example, the inappropriate production of a growth factor or the abnormal response of a cell receptor for the growth factor produced have both been demonstrated to lead to unregulated growth.

Platelet-derived growth factor (PDGF) is involved in regulating the growth of connective tissue cells. One mechanism of inappropriate growth in osteogenic sarcoma has been found to be related to inappropriate expression of the gene for PDGF. This leads to the production of a molecule that can bind to the cells' own receptor for PDGF and thus lead to uncontrolled growth.

Abnormal cytogenetics are characteristic of tumor cells. The majority of karyotypes or osteogenic sarcoma cells have been found to be abnormal, with an abnormal number of chromosomes per cell, as well as multiple translocations and deletions. In Ewing's sarcoma, the abnormal cytogenetics have been found to be remarkably consistent between different cell populations. The majority of cells have a translocation between chromosomes 11 and 22. This is found only in tumor cells and not in normal cells taken from the same patient. Current research in Ewing's sarcoma is directed toward understanding the significance of these consistent abnormalities, as well as the molecular cloning of the chromosomal breakpoints in the hope that the genes involved might be identified.

Individuals who suffer from hereditary retinoblastoma are 1,000 times more likely to develop osteogenic sarcoma than are unaffected individuals. This association has led to research that has identified a specific retinoblastoma gene. This gene is an anti-oncogene whose absence leads to the production of a retinoblastoma. Messenger RNA transcribed from the retinoblastoma gene has been found to be absent in some osteogenic sarcomas but present in others. This information has been used in the laboratory to determine if replacement of this missing gene may one day be effective in treating patients with osteogenic sarcoma. In one experiment, osteogenic sarcoma cells that did not express the retinoblastoma gene were transfected with a genetically engineered retinoblastoma gene. These transfected cells were demonstrated to revert to a nontransformed phenotype in culture. Transfection with a retinoblastoma gene in an osteogenic sarcoma cell line that expressed this gene normally had no effect. This indicates that loss of the retinoblastoma gene may be a primary event in the genesis of osteogenic sarcoma and that genetic replacement of this gene may some day be an element of treatment.

Annotated Bibliography

Biopsy

Dollahite HA, Tatum L, Moinuddin SM, et al: Aspiration biopsy of primary neoplasms of bone. *J Bone Joint Surg* 1989;71A:1166-1169.

Aspiration biopsy had a diagnostic accuracy of 72% in 31 patients who had a primary bone tumor that was suspected of being malignant and an accuracy rate of just 23% in those lesions suspected of being benign.

Osteogenic Sarcoma

Glasser DB, Lane JM: Stage IIB osteogenic sarcoma. *Clin Orthop* 1991;270:29-39.

The authors reviewed 271 consecutive patients treated for stage IIB osteogenic sarcoma from 1976 to 1986 at Memorial Sloan-Kettering Cancer Center. Disease-free survival for the entire group was 77% at five years and 74% at ten years. Humeral lesions had the best probability of survival (84% at ten years) followed by tibial lesions (81%) and femoral lesions (67%). Histologic response to preoperative chemotherapy was the strongest predictor of outcome. Local recurrence was a poor prognostic sign; only two of the 18 patients with local recurrence were long-term disease-free survivors.

Healey JH, Buss D: Radiation and pagetic osteogenic sarcomas. *Clin Orthop* 1991;270:128-134.

This retrospective review reveals a 15% five-year survival for radiation-induced and pagetic osteogenic sarcomas. Chemotherapy has not proven effective to date.

Wuisman P, Enneking WF: Prognosis for patients who have osteosarcoma with skip metastasis. *J Bone Joint Surg* 1990;72A:60-68.

The authors reviewed 23 patients with stage IIB osteosarcoma and skip metastases. All but one of these patients were dead at follow-up. The use of adjuvant chemotherapy did not improve the poor prognosis. In certain cases, MRI revealed a skip metatasis that had not been previously identified on radiograph, isotope scan, or computed tomography. The authors recommend that the presence of a skip lesion be another criterion for classifying an osteosarcoma as stage III.

Ewing's Sarcoma

Bacci G, Toni A, Avella M, et al: Long-term results in 144 localized Ewing's sarcoma patients treated with combined therapy. *Cancer* 1989;63:1477-1486.

The authors reviewed 144 cases of primary Ewing's sarcoma of bone. The minimum follow-up was five years. All patients received adjuvant chemotherapy. At a median follow-up of nine years, 41% of the patients were disease free. Three factors seem to correlate to prognosis: (1) the site of the lesion (pelvic lesions do worse than other locations); (2) the chemotherapeutic protocol; (3) the type of local treatment. Sixty percent of the patients treated with amputation or resection and radiotherapy were disease free compared with 28% of those treated with radiation therapy alone. The local recurrence rate was 8% in the group treated with surgery or surgery and radiation compared with 36% in the group treated with radiation therapy alone.

Chondrosarcoma

Shives TC, McLeod RA, Unni KK, et al: Chondrosarcoma of the spine. *J Bone Joint Surg* 1989;71A;1158-1165.

The authors reviewed the cases of 20 patients with chondrosarcoma of the spine treated at the Mayo Clinic between 1916 and 1981. All patients who had an intralesional excision had progression of the disease and died. The authors recommend an attempt at wide en bloc excision whenever possible.

Benign Lesions

Glancy GL, Brugioni DJ, Eilert RE, et al: Autograft versus allograft for benign lesions in children. *Clin Orthop* 1991;262:28-33.

This retrospective review of 54 patients with 61 benign lesions compares the efficacy of using autografts versus allografts with respect to time required and success of graft incorporation. Allografts were comparable to autografts when small-volume lesions (less than 60 ml) were treated. In that treatment of patients with solitary large lesions, autografts were superior to allografts in the rate and completeness of healing.

Soft-Tissue Sarcomas

Kirby EJ, Shereff MJ, Lewis MM: Soft-tissue tumors and tumor-like lesions of the foot: An analysis of eighty-three cases. *J Bone Joint Surg* 1989;71A:621-626.

The cases of 83 patients with soft-tissue masses in the foot were reviewed. Seventy-two (87%) were benign, with ganglion cysts and plantar fibromatosis being most common. Eleven were malignant, five (45%) of which were synovial sarcomas. Most of the malignant tumors, especially the synovial sarcomas, had a predilection for the ankle, heel, or dorsum of the foot. In patients between 30 and 70 years of age, 90% of all lesions in the sole were plantar fibromatosis.

Lifeso RM, Rooney RJ, El-Shaker M: Post-traumatic squamous-cell carcinoma. *J Bone Joint Surg* 1990;72A:12-18.

This is a retrospective review of 63 patients treated with squamous cell carcinoma that originated in a preexisting scar or sinus of an extremity. Forty-nine percent of the patients developed metastases to regional lymph nodes. Prognosis was uniformly poor for intermediate and high-grade lesions. The authors recommend local excision only for the patient with a low-grade lesion that can be closely followed. They recommend considering early amputation in those patients with a high-grade lesion because wide excision is frequently difficult due to distortion of the anatomy and tissue planes by previous trauma or burns.

Mandard AM, Petiot JF, Marnay J, et al: Prognostic factors in soft tissue sarcomas: A multivariate analysis of 109 cases. *Cancer* 1989;63:1437-1451.

Prognostic factors were reviewed in 109 soft-tissue sarcomas of the extremities, walls of the trunk, head, and neck. The following variables were determined as unfavorable: tumor size greater than 5 cm, deep tumors, extracompartmental status, inadequate excision, and histologically high grade.

McCollough WM, Parsons JT, Van Der Griend R, et al: Radiation therapy for aggressive fibromatosis: The experience at the University of Florida. *J Bone Joint Surg* 1991;73A:717-725.

The authors reviewed the cases of 29 patients (30 sites) with aggressive fibromatosis who were treated with radiation therapy; 76% of the patients were followed for more than five years. Eleven of 14 sites with presumed microscopic residual disease and 14 of 16 sites with known grossly residual disease were locally controlled. The authors state that radiation therapy alone is also an effective alternative to radical operation or when resection is not possible. There was no difference in local control between patients who were treated for primary aggressive fibromatosis and those who were treated after one or more local recurrences.

Limb Salvage

McDonald DJ, Capanna R, Gherlinzoni F, et al: Influence of chemotherapy on perioperative complications in limb salvage surgery for bone tumors. *Cancer* 1990;65:1509-1516.

The authors reviewed the influence of chemotherapy on the incidence of nonmechanical complications in 304 patients who underwent limb-salvage surgery. The most common complication was infection (12%), which led to amputation in three patients. Resections about the knee led to more complications than in other sites. Patients who did not receive chemotherapy had a 25% incidence of complications, those who received adjuvant treatment had a 33% incidence, and those who received neoadjuvant had a 55% incidence of complications.

Allografts

Berrey BH Jr, Lord CF, Gebhardt MC, et al: Fractures of allografts: Frequency, treatment, and end-results. *J Bone Joint Surg* 1990;72A:825-833.

This retrospective review of 274 patients who received massive frozen allografts revealed an overall incidence of fracture of 16%. The mean time to fracture was 29 months, with 55% of the fractures occurring within two years and 70% within three years. Most patients did not sustain fractures during the first six postoperative months, after which the likelihood of fracture sharply increased until it peaked between two and three years after the operation. No fracture occurred after four years. Most fractures could be effectively treated by reoperation, with good results, unlike the other complications of allografts, such as infection, which frequently leads to loss of limb.

Gebhardt MC, Roth YF, Mankin HJ: Osteoarticular allografts for reconstruction in the proximal part of the humerus after excision of a musculoskeletal tumor. *J Bone Joint Surg* 1990;72A:334-345.

This is a review of 20 patients who had resections of the proximal humerus for bone tumors. The majority of patients had either aggressive benign or low-grade malignancies. Patients with high-grade sarcomas were not given this treatment. Those selected for treatment had excision of the proximal humerus with preservation of the deltoid and rotator cuff. Function was graded as excellent in one, good in 11, fair in one, and poor in five. Twelve complications, including nonunion, instability, fracture, and infection, were related to the use of the allografts.

Lord CF, Gebhardt MC, Tomford WW, et al: Infection in bone allografts: Incidence, nature, and treatment. *J Bone Joint Surg* 1988;70A:369-376.

The authors reviewed the cases of 283 patients who had a massive allograft of bone and were followed for two years or more. Infection developed in 11.7%. Eighty-two percent of these infections required amputation of the limb or removal of the graft to control infection. The authors recommend that oral antibiotics be given for two to three months postoperatively, until the host's reaction to the graft has diminished and vascularization of the allograft has begun.

Tomford WW, Thongphasuk J, Mankin HJ, et al: Frozen musculoskeletal allografts: A study of the clinical incidence and causes of infection associated with their use. *J Bone Joint Surg* 1990;72A:1137-1143.

This is a retrospective review of 324 frozen bone and soft-tissue allograft operations; the allografts were supplied by the Massachusetts General Hospital bone bank over a two-year period. None of the small grafts, which consisted mainly of femoral heads, became infected. Large allografts had a 5% incidence of infection. This review does not discuss late infections (those that occur after the first few years postoperatively). In most patients, removal of the allograft was necessary to control infection.

Prostheses

Horowitz SM, Lane JM, Otis JC, et al: Prosthetic arthroplasty of the knee after resection of a sarcoma in the proximal end of the tibia: A report of sixteen cases. *J Bone Joint Surg* 1991;73A:286-293.

This is a retrospective review of 16 cases in which patients were treated with prosthetic arthroplasty of the knee after extra-articular resection of a sarcoma of the proximal tibia. A new prosthetic design that features "ball-in-socket" articulation between the femoral and tibial components is presented. Extensor mechanism reconstruction was performed by attaching the patella remnant to a porous surface on the tibial component. Functional results were good or excellent in the majority of cases, with an average follow-up of 63 months. Aseptic loosening occurred in three patients, all of whom had successful revision surgery.

Pelvis

O'Connor MI, Sim FH: Salvage of the limb in the treatment of malignant pelvic tumors. *J Bone Joint Surg* 1989;71A:481-494.

This article reviews the outcome of 60 patients treated from 1970 to 1985 by internal hemipelvectomy that salvaged the limb. The best oncologic and functional results were in those patients in whom a wide margin could be obtained and femoral sacral continuity maintained or reconstructed. Extension of the tumor into the sacrum was associated with a high rate of local recurrence.

Knee

Cammisa FP Jr, Glasser DB, Otis JC, et al: The van Ness tibial rotationplasty: A functionally viable reconstructive procedure in children who have a tumor of the distal end of the femur. *J Bone Joint Surg* 1990;72A:1541-1547.

This is a review of 12 patients with a malignant tumor of the distal end of the femur treated by resection and rotationplasty. Functional testing showed that these patients performed as well as those who had had endoprosthetic replacement and better than those who had had above-knee amputation. Rotationplasty may be used as a salvage procedure following failure of endoprosthetic replacement.

Harris IE, Leff AR, Gitelis S, et al: Function after amputation, arthrodesis, or arthroplasty for tumors about the knee. *J Bone Joint Surg* 1990;72A:1477-1485.

The functional results and emotional well being of seven patients who had an above-knee amputation were compared with nine who had a resection arthrodesis and six who had a replacement arthroplasty following excision of a malignant skeletal tumor adjacent to the knee.

Chemotherapy

Yasko AW, Lane JM: Current concepts review: Chemotherapy for bone and soft-tissue sarcomas of the extremities. *J Bone Joint Surg* 1991;73A:1263-1271.

This is an excellent review of current chemotherapy protocols used for the treatment of bone and soft-tissue sarcomas of the extremities.

Bone Tumor Research

Huang H-J, Yee J-K, Shew J-Y, et al: Suppression of the neoplastic phenotype by replacement of the RB gene in human cancer cells. *Science* 1988;242:1563-1566.

Cloned retinoblastoma genes were introduced into osteosarcoma cells via retroviral-mediated gene transfer. Expression of this exogenous antioncogene suppressed the neoplastic phenotype as reflected by morphology, growth rate, soft agar colony formation, and tumorigenicity in nude mice. This indicates that loss of the retinoblastoma gene may be a primary event in the genesis of osteogenic sarcoma and that the genetic replacement of this gene may some day be an element of treatment.

Turc-Carel C, Aurias A, Mugneret F, et al: Chromosomes in Ewing's sarcoma: An evaluation of 85 cases of remarkable consistency of t(11;22) (q24;q12). *Cancer Genet Cytogenet* 1988;32:229-238.

This study demonstrates that the majority of Ewing's sarcoma cells have a translocation between chromosomes 11 and 22. The breakpoint on chromosome 22q12 was the most consistently observed event (92% of cases).

Womer RB: The cellular biology of bone tumors. *Clin Orthop* 1991;262:12-21.

This is an excellent review of the recent developments in understanding osteogenic sarcoma and Ewing's sarcoma through the application of molecular biology techniques.

15

Acute Pain Management

One of the physician's primary obligations is to manage effectively the onset of acute pain resulting from trauma or surgery. Acute pain may be defined as an unpleasant, localized sensation in response to a noxious stimulus (trigger) that appears to be capable of producing tissue damage. Response to the acute pain includes retraction from the noxious stimulus, followed by a transitory period of guarding and protecting the affected part. In addition, the unpleasant sensation of pain produces an individually variable emotional response that depends on the physiologic, psychologic, cultural, and socioeconomic state of the patient. Postoperative pain and the temporary pain of recent injury both represent functional variants of the acute pain response.

Current understanding of the neuroanatomy and neurobiology of the pain sensory system has been reviewed extensively in *Orthopaedic Knowledge Update 3*. A working knowledge of this applied neurobiology is intrinsic to understanding, choosing, and implementing the alternatives available for pharmacologic management of acute pain. Moreover, as clinicians, we are concerned directly with any adverse physiologic or psychologic effects of pain, which by altering early responses to treatment or rehabilitation, can impede or prevent recovery.

Any significant degree of tissue damage, whether from injury or surgery, causes measurable systemic endocrine, metabolic, and immunologic changes referred to as the surgical stress response. The release mechanisms that initiate, amplify, and perpetuate the physiologic events that cause the surgical stress response have been localized experimentally to specific anatomic regions along the acute pain sensory system. Tissue damage at the site of injury stimulates peripheral nociceptors and causes the release of algogenic substances, such as bradykinin, potassium, prostaglandins, hydrogen ions, serotonin, and substance P, which further stimulate and sensitize the nociceptors.

The peripheral nociceptors transduce the stimuli into electrochemical impulses that are carried, via small myelinated A delta and unmyelinated C afferent fibers, to the dorsal horn of the spinal cord. The noxious impulses may stimulate dorsal horn neurons whose axons ascend within the spinal cord to areas in the midbrain, thalamus, and frontal cortex from which suprasegmental reflex and cortical responses arise. The impulses may also be influenced by modulating factors that alter further transmission, or they may pass to the anterior or anterolateral horns of the spinal cord where, by stimulating sympathetic preganglionic somatomotor neurons, they cause autonomic segmental (spinal) reflex responses. The segmental spinal and suprasegmental reflex responses result

in significant physiologic changes that affect the cardiopulmonary, gastrointestinal, urinary, endocrine, and immunologic systems.

Stimulation of neurons within the anterolateral horn produces segmental reflexive increases in heart rate, stroke volume, and myocardial oxygen consumption and decreases in gut motility (which can produce or contribute to postoperative ileus) and urinary output. Moreover, the nociceptor stimulation both sensitizes and reduces the threshold excitability of dorsal horn wide dynamic range neurons, which have been theorized to contribute to skeletal muscle spasms in areas of significant muscle tissue damage and to perpetuate focal pain, allodynia, hyperalgesia, and hyperemia at the site of injury or surgical procedure. Suprasegmental reflex responses produced by stimulation of the hypothalamus and medulla are characterized by hyperventilation, increased peripheral vascular resistance, an increase in the neuroendocrine secretion of catabolic hormones (cortisol, ACTH, cAMP, ADH glucagon, growth hormone), and a concomitant decrease in the secretion of anabolic hormones and insulin. These metabolic effects contribute to and amplify the effects of the spinal segmental reflexes on the myocardium, and they initiate an overall catabolic metabolism, the degree and persistence of which is directly related to the amount and type of initial tissue damage.

Less well understood are the cortex's contributions to surgical stress response. These are believed to begin with the individual's perception of pain, which evokes variable emotional responses characterized by anxiety and dread. The individual's perception and interpretation of the degree of pain have been linked to measurable increases in circulating catecholamines, cortisol, blood clotting time, fibrinolysis, and platelet aggregation. Surgical stress response also includes such alterations in the immune system as a nonspecific granulocytosis, decreases in T- and B-lymphocyte function, and leukocyte chemotaxis.

Although the presence of pain and the development of surgical stress response are clearly linked, only recently has investigation in the fields of anesthesia and pain research been directed toward determining the effect of perioperative analgesia on surgical stress response and, thus, on postoperative complications and rehabilitation. Experimental studies show that some methods of anesthesia (for example, epidural anesthesia) alter components of the surgical stress response by blocking nociceptive stimulation at specific sites along the pain pathway. Although at present no single prospective study has shown a clear causal relationship between effective blockade of the mechanisms that produce the surgical stress response and a measurable reduction in postoperative morbidity, numerous clinical studies have shown convincingly that patients who do not experience a prolonged degree of significant pain do better postoperatively (Outline 1).

This growing awareness of the short-term and potential long-term benefits to patients of effective analgesia in the early postoperative period has led researchers to investigate pain prevention rather than the traditional treatment-oriented approach to pain. Prevention calls for the use of anesthetic techniques that provide sustained or continuous analgesia in the early postoperative period, rather than an as-needed postoperative regimen, usually in the form of intramuscular injections. In addition to favorable clinical responses, the rationale for prevention of pain is validated by results of experimental research. Even brief periods of sustained noxious stimuli can produce prolonged changes within cells of the spinal cord pain pathway, allowing the pain response to be prolonged or persistent, and suppression of established pain is more difficult, requiring increased dosages of narcotics over longer periods. These data also affect the establishment of chronic pain syndromes.

Despite the growing body of clinical and experimental evidence that pain prevention has substantial benefits to the surgical patient, for the 23.3 million surgical procedures performed in 1989, the vast majority of postoperative analgesia orders were written on an as-needed basis. It has been conclusively indicated that traditional intramuscular opioid injection regimens fail to alleviate pain effectively in approximately half of all postoperative patients. This high rate of failure can be attributed to individual thresholds of perceived pain, variation in surgical procedures (and therefore narcotic requirements), variable rate of metabolic drug clearance, and the physical demands that such a regimen places upon available nursing staff. Recognition of these inadequacies in pain management has caused the United States Department of Health and Human Services' Agency for Health Care Policy and Research to publish "Clinical Practice Guideline for Acute Pain Management." This publication mandates that orthopaedic surgeons reexamine their current practices in postoperative pain management and consider implementing some of the newer, clinically proven pain-prevention oriented approaches. Newer techniques that are directly applicable to patients undergoing orthopaedic surgical procedures include: (1) increased use of oral and recently available injectable forms of nonsteroidal anti-inflammatory drugs (NSAIDs) alone or in combination with opioid medications; (2) increased use and reliance upon epidural, spinal, and regional anesthesia; (3) increased use of patient-controlled anesthesia devices; and (4) combination of analgesic techniques to provide multimodal treatment or balanced analgesia.

Outline 1. Adverse physiologic responses to pain affected by analgesic techniques

Pulmonary
  Improved results of pulmonary function tests and decreased incidence of pulmonary complications in patients receiving epidural analgesia versus intramuscular or intravenous analgesia.
Peripheral vasculature
  Decrease in incidence of pulmonary embolism after total hip arthroplasty.
  Increase in graft blood flow after vascular procedures in lower extremity.
Gastrointestinal
  Faster resolution of postoperative ileus with use of epidural analgesia.
Central nervous system
  Less postoperative sedation with use of epidural analgesia.
  Significantly better analgesia and substantial reduction in the need for systemic narcotics with use of epidural narcotics, local anesthetics, and intercostal nerve blocks.
Convalescence
  Earlier ambulation and earlier dismissal from the hospital with epidural analgesia than with systemic narcotics.

(Modified with permission from Lutz LJ, Lamer LT: Management of postoperative pain: Review of current techniques and methods. *Mayo Clin Proc* 1990;65:586.)

Postoperative Analgesia

NSAIDs have been used extensively to control the pain of arthritic and musculotendinous inflammatory processes. These drugs decrease the levels and effects of inflammatory mediators produced at the site of the injury. Oral NSAIDs alone may provide effective analgesia after minor surgical procedures. However, clinical studies indicate that oral NSAIDs used in combination with oral opioids provide greater analgesia than either class of drug used alone. Concurrent use of NSAIDs and opioids to control postoperative pain may have an opioid dose-sparing effect. A recently FDA-approved parenteral NSAID (ketorolac) has proven effective in controlling moderate-to-severe postoperative pain. Clinical trials are being developed to establish efficacy of this drug when used in combination with other medications to produce enhanced analgesia.

In the last decade, there has been a significant increase in the use of epidural anesthesia for surgery about the lower extremities. The clinical benefits of this form of anesthesia and analgesia have been seen most clearly in the elderly, in whom there has been a notable reduction in postoperative sedation caused by parenteral opioids as well as earlier mobilization after most procedures. In addition, short-term continuous epidural anesthesia has proven particularly effective with the increased use of continuous passive motion devices after total knee arthroplasty and has a high degree of patient acceptance. Epidural analgesia can be accomplished with infusion of either local anesthetics or spinal opioids. When administered for 12 to 72 hours after a wide variety of orthopaedic procedures, both classes of drugs provide more effective analgesia than parenteral narcotics. Administration of a dilute solution of local anesthetic or a precise dosage of either hydrophilic or lipophilic opioids by modern computerized infusion pumps minimizes excessive motor and sympathetic blockage caused by local anesthetics and the respiratory depression and urinary retention caused by spinal opioids. Moreover, spinal opioids and local anesthetics have pharmacologically dissimilar modes of action on different sites within the pain pathway, and a combination of these drugs (1 μg/ml of fentanyl with 0.1% bupivacaine) requires lower infusion rates than either drug used as a single agent. Preliminary clinical trials are currently underway on patient-controlled epidural anesthesia.

Regional anesthesia for surgical procedures about the upper extremities is gaining wider acceptance. This form of anesthesia allows early ambulation, improved vascular flow, and the possibility of prolonged sympathetic blockade. It results in greater patient acceptance of continuous passive motion, early postoperative mobilization, and physical therapy of the involved extremity. Special axillary catheters have been designed to permit prolonged anesthesia via intermittent bolus administration or continuous computerized infusion. With a dilute solution of bupivacaine (0.125% at 8 to 10 ml/hr), motor function is generally preserved while providing satisfactory analgesia.

Interscalene blockade of the brachial plexus is safe and effective for procedures about the shoulder and reduces postoperative narcotic requirements. Interscalene blockage also may be administered postoperatively in the recovery room after general anesthesia has worn off and neurologic function has returned to normal. Depending on the type and concentration of local anesthetic chosen, a single interscalene blockade may provide significant analgesia for up to 24 hours. Interscalene blockade has a higher degree of overall patient acceptance than intermittent intramuscular injections of opioids.

Numerous clinical studies indicate that up to half of all patients receiving intramuscular opioid narcotics, given every three to four hours on an as-needed basis, may not achieve adequate analgesia. Narcotic administered by this regiment may meet or exceed the minimal analgesia concentration for only 35% of the dosage interval (Fig. 1). Small doses of intravenous opioid narcotics provide more effective and rapid onset of analgesia than the intramuscular opioid injections. On-demand, patient-controlled anesthesia was made feasible with the development of programmable computerized dosage-delivery pumps. Typically, morphine sulfate and meperidine are used. After a bolus loading dose, the infusion pump is programmed to deliver a predetermined intravenous dose of the narcotic on an on-demand basis when the patient depresses a hand-held triggering device. Additional doses cannot be infused until a predetermined lock-out interval has elapsed. Although patient-controlled anesthesia has been in general use for a relatively

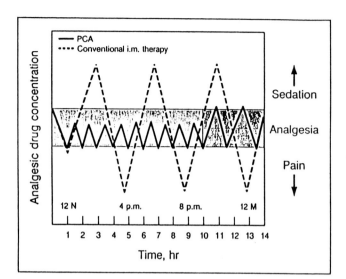

Fig. 1 Relationship among dose interval, analgesic drug concentration, and clinical effects in a comparison of patient-controlled analgesis (PCA) system and conventional intramuscular (i.m.) therapy. (Reproduced with permission from White PF: Use of patient-controlled analgesia for management of acute pain. *Semin Anesth* 1985;4:255-266.)

brief period of time, sufficient clinical data exist to show that this method of analgesia represents a major advance in the control of postoperative pain. Advantages of patient-controlled anesthesia include consistent efficacy over a wide range of surgical procedures, a high degree of patient acceptability, reduced demands on the nursing staff, generally low overall narcotic requirements, and few reported instances of narcotic-induced complications (for example, sedation and respiratory depression) when compared with traditional intramuscular narcotic regimens. This form of analgesia also has been shown to be effective and safe in children as young as 7 years of age. Whether or not its primary disadvantage, increased cost, will be offset by the potential advantages of reduced demands on nursing staff and earlier rehabilitation and hospital discharge remains under investigation.

Lastly, improvement in transdermal drug administration techniques has resulted in the development of transdermal narcotic (fentanyl) delivery that has been shown in preliminary clinical trials to provide sustained release of plasma concentrations that effectively relieve postoperative pain. This form of analgesia generally requires a systemic loading dose, followed by application of the transdermal patch two hours before the expected need. Transdermal narcotic administration may be particularly beneficial for use in very elderly or debilitated patients as well as in pediatric patients for whom patient-controlled anesthesia and other previously discussed methods of providing analgesia may not be applicable.

Management of Chronic Pain Syndromes

Both postoperative pain and the temporary residual pain of recent injury are physiologic (functional) variants of acute pain. Musculoskeletal surgeons generally have considerable clinical experience in dealing with a normal acute pain response and its variants by (1) providing proper care of the injured part, (2) administering appropriate analgesics, and (3) offering emotional support and counseling.

However, during the course of initial treatment or during subsequent rehabilitation, a patient's reported pain may be judged to be extreme with respect to the known degree of tissue damage, the location and quality of the pain may be poorly defined or nonspecific, or the pain may be abnormally prolonged. In these cases, the possibility of dysfunctional pain disorder must be considered after elimination of all plausible functional causes. An abnormal pain response is an unwelcome complication that often poses considerable challenges to the subsequent successful treatment and resolution of the original problem. Moreover, consternation and indecision regarding implementation of appropriate management often follow the recognition of dysfunctional pain. Such indecision is well founded because the historical details, nature, and occurrence of any one patient's dysfunctional pain pattern are unique, making clinical expertise difficult to achieve in normal practice. Furthermore, clinically useful information on chronic or abnormal pain disorders has been sparse in the musculoskeletal literature, and consists largely of anecdotal case studies. The more detailed descriptive reports dealing with this subject have been categorized collectively under a confusing array of terms (Outline 2).

Causalgia was defined by S. Weir Mitchell, a Union surgeon during the Civil War. He described a syndrome characterized by unrelenting intense burning pain of an affected extremity, hypersensitivity, vasomotor disturbances, overzealous guarding of the injured part, and consistent profound psychological changes. This syndrome was noted in a significant number of soldiers who sustained direct rifle ball wounds to major peripheral nerves. After the war, Mitchell and other noted physicians of the time continued research that was directed primarily toward elucidating neuropathophysiologic causes for the observed autonomic nervous system disturbances. Others proposed theories for a psychogenic basis of causalgia.

Most early investigative information on causalgia and related disorders was derived from the evaluation of patients who had sustained major violent injuries to the involved extremity. However, in 1953, Bonica proposed the term reflex sympathetic dystrophy (RSD) to define an abnormal pain syndrome of which sympathetic autonomic dysfunction was a major feature. Although clinically similar to causalgia, this syndrome was associated with an extremely varied range of etiologic factors. Such factors include major and minor trauma, multiple types

Outline 2. Chronic pain disorders

Causalgia
Mimocausalgia
Sympathetic dystrophy
Algoneurodystrophy
Chronic traumatic edema
Posttraumatic edema
Posttraumatic pain syndrome
Shoulder-hand syndrome
Sudeck's atrophy
Sympathalgia
Posttraumatic spreading neuralgia
Posttraumatic osteoporosis
Neurodystrophy
Reflex sympathetic dystrophy

of surgical procedures, and repetitive occupational activities, as well as a list of physiologically unrelated systemic diseases, including idiopathic case examples.

The confusing diversity of precipitating etiologic factors and the lack of reproducible laboratory models that explain either a pathophysiologic relationship or the relative causal importance of these factors to its clinical development have led to misuse of the term reflex sympathetic dystrophy. This term unfortunately has evolved both in general clinical correspondence and in the medical literature to become a generic term for any abnormal pain or prolonged extremity dysfunction, whether or not autonomic dysfunction exists. This confusion, as well as the generic use of the term with respect to the treatment of an individual patient, has resulted in lack of agreement regarding diagnostic criteria, natural history, and psychologic factors involved in the syndromes listed in Outline 2. These unresolved issues often have resulted in arbitrary evaluation and anecdotal treatment protocols.

The diagnostic criteria of all the various chronic pain syndromes, irrespective of the proposed etiologies or pathophysiologic factors, clearly have two common denominators: an abnormal pain response and dysfunction of the affected extremity. Recognition of the commonality of abnormal pain and extremity dysfunction among all the various pain syndromes has led to their being termed pain dysfunction syndromes. The term pain dysfunction syndrome is clinically descriptive and sufficiently broad to encompass the diversity of possible precipitating factors including individually variable signs and symptoms. Moreover, this term removes the requirement for sympathetic nervous system dysfunction that was implicit in the use of reflex sympathetic dystrophy. The latter term may be preferable when autonomic dysfunction is associated with chronic pain syndrome. However, the use of pain dysfunction syndrome as a clinically descriptive label allows the treating physician to objectively differentiate the possible causative factors and, thus, to design and implement an effective nonarbitrary treatment protocol.

When a noxious stimulus (mechanical, thermal, or chemical) is severe enough to produce tissue damage, local chemical mediators are released that cause focal edema, vasodilation, hyperpathia, and allodynia, which collectively make up the acute pain response. If there is no ongoing or irreversible tissue damage, both the cognitive perception of pain and the physiologic signs and symptoms of the acute pain response subside when the healing process is complete. The failure of any feature of the acute pain response to resolve normally becomes a matter of clinical concern. The abnormal persistence of pain may be caused by an unrecognized infection, tumor, or nerve entrapment. Furthermore, systemic factors such as rheumatologic disorders, endocrine or metabolic disorders (for example, diabetic neuropathy), and the collagen vascular diseases can alter normal pain sensation and delay healing. After functional causes for persistent pain have been excluded, particular attention should be given to reported changes in the intensity, quality, and location of the pain as well as to observations of persistent or disseminating focal edema, color changes, and vasomotor and thermoregulatory adaptations, because all of these are expected only initially and transiently as part of the acute pain response.

Sympathetic nervous system involvement in the pathogenesis of reflex sympathetic dystrophy has been demonstrated as follows. (1) Regional anesthetic blockage or interruption of the sympathetic nervous system relieves the pain. (2) Electrical stimulation of the sympathetic chain exacerbates the pain in many patients suspected of having sympathetically maintained pain. (3) In normal individuals, electrical stimulation of sympathetic outflow does not produce painful sensation, and regional sympathetic blockade does not alter normal pain sensation. Beyond these largely empiric clinical and experimental observations, there do not yet exist any definitive laboratory models to explain how the sympathetic nervous system alters, produces, or maintain the pain of reflex sympathetic dystrophy and related disorders, although numerous plausible hypotheses have been proposed. These hypotheses can be placed in two groups: adaptive central nervous system dysfunction primarily within the spinal cord or peripheral end organ (nociceptor) abnormalities.

The more accepted classification schemes for reflex sympathetic dystrophy have been based either on the natural history of signs and symptoms of the disorder or on the type and magnitude of the precipitating injury. Two distinct types of sympathetic dysfunction, based on the type of injury, have been proposed. The first, causalgia, caused by direct nerve injury, is further subcategorized into either major or minor causalgia depending on whether the injury is to a mixed or sensory nerve, respectively. The second type, traumatic dystrophy, is similarly subcategorized into major and minor subtypes. A minor traumatic dystrophy generally results from a less severe injury, such as a sprain or contusion, whereas a major traumatic dystrophy is secondary to a more extensive injury, such as a fracture. Many clinicians have pointed out that use of this type of classification scheme can be both confusing and imprecise because some cases of reflex sympathetic dystrophy have no clear traumatic etiology

and because some minor causalgia may prove to be more disabling than major causalgia.

Classification schemes based on the natural history of the clinically observed physiologic, morphologic, and functional changes observed in untreated reflex sympathetic dystrophy generally recognize three distinct stages: the acute stage (zero to three months), the dystrophic stage (three to six months), and the atrophic stage (six months and beyond). In the earlier phases, the pain described is often burning in character and more focal than diffuse, and the associated edema and vasomotor and thermoregulatory dysfunction usually are prevalent. In the later stages, the pain is more constant and poorly localized, and muscle atrophy, joint stiffness, or contractures may develop along with subcutaneous fibromatous organization and cyanosis of the skin. End-stage reflex sympathetic dystrophy is characterized by more permanent changes of the skin, blood vessels, and joints (ankylosis). Reflex sympathetic dystrophy is a dynamic process, and the above stages accurately describe in a general way the symptomatic and pathophysiologic changes that can occur in untreated cases. However, in any individual patient, there may be considerable temporal variability in the development of the characteristic signs and symptoms, and subtle and partial manifestations are generally the rule rather than the exception. Therefore, no classification scheme is wholly satisfactory.

Psychology of Pain and Dysfunction

The sensory neural mechanisms involved in the sensation of acute pain do not exist as an isolated physiologic event. The perception of a painful stimulus always yields an affective or emotional component that is individually variable and complex. The psychologic component of pain dysfunction syndrome may be quite pronounced, even becoming the dominant clinical feature. In the past, considerable clinical emphasis has been placed on the probability that there are definite psychogenic causes for some chronic pain disorders, in particular reflex sympathetic dystrophy. These clinical convictions probably arose from the early descriptive reports noting the profound psychologic changes, including bizarre ritualistic avoidance behavior described in classic examples of causalgia. The psychogenic basis for these disorders (even in less overt pain dysfunction syndromes) is based on the disparity between the physician's findings and the patient's degree of fear, anxiety, and reported discomfort. In the past, patients were described as "hysterical," "unstable," and "depressed." These terms implied the existence of a premorbid personality or, even, psychoses. Review of these early accounts clearly indicates that these psychologic assessments resulted largely from opinion rather than psychologic testing. Results of studies on chronic pain syndromes convincingly indicate that the observed personality and behavior changes are a consequence of prolonged suffering rather than the manifestation of a preexisting personality or psychologic disorder. Changes most frequently reported in persons living with chronic pain are persistent anxiety, reactive depression, dependency, and somatic preoccupation, all of which can impede the resolution of a pain dysfunction syndrome.

Psychologic components of a pain dysfunction syndrome must be differentiated from certain bona fide psychopathologic syndromes that often include decreased pain tolerance and/or increased pain susceptibility. These are somatization disorder, conversion disorder, malingering, and factitious injury disorders. Patients with a somatization disorder often describe chronic pain and have a history of recurrent multiple somatic complaints of long duration for which no physically diagnosable disorder can be found. These patients are convinced they are seriously ill and are not deterred by evidence of normal test results.

Patients with conversion disorder, formerly hysterical neurosis, often have a history of chronic intermittent pain, the source of which is not medically identifiable. Other common symptoms are: pseudoparalysis, nonanatomic sensory loss, and blindness. Posturing of the hand and upper extremity frequently is observed; persistence of this activity may result in fixed contractures. Onset of a conversion disorder usually is more sudden than that of a somatization disorder, and the physical manifestations of the disorder may unconsciously occur in reaction to a disturbing psychologic conflict.

Complaints of pain also commonly are associated with major depression (endogenous depression), hypochondriasis, factitious injury, and malingering. Major depression is characterized by malaise, a sense of hopelessness, vegetative symptoms (sleep alterations, poor appetite, fatigue) and, often, a preoccupation with pain, disease, and death. Hypochondriasis may be a symptom of major depression or exist as a separate disorder. Malingering is the conscious, willful misrepresentation of symptoms of illness to avoid obligation or to obtain secondary monetary gain. Factitious injury, when secondary gain is identifiable, represents a form of malingering.

Finally, orthopaedic surgeons are aware of socioeconomic and legal factors that can produce and perpetuate the psychologic components involved in a chronic pain syndrome. Workman's compensation laws, disability programs, and pending accident litigation all provide powerful disincentives to recovery from injury. Dealing with these impediments to the successful treatment of a musculoskeletal problem can be exasperating. Nonetheless, most patients initially have a legitimate claim of injury and a functional reason for pain. Often, during a prolonged rehabilitation from serious injury, the patient unconsciously loses the incentive to return to useful activity because of significant emotional, familial, and financial rewards for remaining disabled. Early settlement of compensation claims in such instances has had a positive effect on the overall recovery from a pain dysfunction syndrome.

Patient Examination and Diagnostic Studies

In most instances, diagnosis and treatment of a suspected pain dysfunction syndrome eventually becomes the responsibility of an orthopaedic surgeon. The first step is to obtain a detailed history including the events of the initial injury, if one is identifiable. The mechanism and site of injury are noted, as are the patient's recollection of the intensity and subjective quality of the initial pain or extent of extremity dysfunction. Details of the initial treatment and all subsequent treatment regimens are noted to establish the patient's assessment of the effectiveness of previous treatment as compared to clinical information in the medical records. Moreover, the patient's recollection of any signs or symptoms suggestive of autonomic dysfunction or of sympathetically maintained pain are noted and compared with the recorded data.

Work history, family setting, and job satisfaction should be investigated as part of the patient's assessment of how the injury and present dysfunction have affected family life, employment, and future goals. These data provide insight into the emotional and psychologic manifestations of the pain dysfunction syndrome. Any past or ongoing psychiatric treatment and/or present substance abuse, including prescribed medications, are relevant considerations. Finally, a detailed medical history is taken to discover any systemic diseases that may contribute to the existence or prolongation of chronic pain.

Often the degree of discomfort and level of anxiety impede the physical examination of a patient with pain dysfunction syndrome. The examination begins with observation of any pertinent visible signs. If an injury was sustained, the orthopaedist should note the posture and degree of protection of the injured part, the nature and extent of any wounds or surgical scars, the degree of edema or atrophy, and the presence of any characteristic signs of autonomic dysfunction including circulation differences, abnormal sweat patterns, and alterations of hair growth. During examination of the extremity, the location of the pain, presence of any spasm or cocontraction, range of motion measurements, reflexes, motor strength, and sensibility are recorded. Where pertinent, fracture reduction and healing are noted along with any associated joint swelling or synovitis that could trigger ongoing pain. Provocative maneuvers are performed to document any signs of a peripheral nerve injury or presence of a compressive neuropathy. After both extremities have been allowed to equilibrate to room temperature, the affected extremity can be compared with the contralateral side to assess thermoregulatory function. When thermal differences are noted, a more precise measurement can be accomplished by using special skin thermometers.

Musculoskeletal trigger points and irritability about peripheral nerves (particularly sensory cutaneous branches) commonly are found during the physical examination of patients with a pain dysfunction syndrome. Musculoskeletal trigger points, infrequently discussed in the orthopaedic literature, are described in literature of medical fields dealing with the treatment of chronic pain. Their etiology, however, remains controversial. Trigger points are localized areas of tenderness usually found about the origin and insertion of muscles, tendons, and ligaments; along fascial planes; and about capsular structures. They may or may not be related anatomically to the site of the original injury, and they often persist after the injury has healed and, thus, may perpetuate dysfunction. Irritability along cutaneous nerves is another common clinical problem found in pain dysfunction syndrome. This problem is often secondary to trauma, surgical procedures, and improper application of casts, and it can exist in the presence of prolonged focal edema. Like musculoskeletal trigger points, nerve irritability can persist for long periods, acting as a continued source of pain.

A step-wise, careful, selective injection of small amounts of a local anesthetic solution may aid in the localization of the sources of pain. This simple diagnostic procedure can also be used to help localize multiple adjacent trigger points.

Diagnostic tests should be ordered to provide further objective information. Current plain radiographs of the involved extremity can be compared with equivalent views of the contralateral extremity to detect any differences in radiographic bone density. Other studies including arthrograms, tomograms, computed tomography scans, magnetic resonance imaging studies, and electromyography and nerve conduction studies may yield useful formation or possible sources of pain and dysfunction. Radionuclide imaging may confirm a clinical diagnosis or can reveal previously unrecognized problems by localized increased radioisotope uptake. The three-phase bone scan technique has proven to be a particularly useful diagnostic tool in the evaluation of reflex sympathetic dystrophy, with a reported high degree of specificity in untreated cases.

Other diagnostic tests for reflex sympathetic dystrophy and autonomic dysfunction, including quantitative sweat production (Q-SART, Low), dynamic vasomotor reflex assessment, and cold stress thermoregulatory capacity, may add diagnostic information. The usefulness of thermography (infrared telethermometry) is controversial. Although all of these tests may be necessary in certain cases, the relief of pain in response to sympathetic blockade remains the single most useful and preferred test for the diagnosis of reflex sympathetic dystrophy.

As previously stated, the psychologic aspects of a pain dysfunction syndrome are variable in both degree and symptoms. Several standard personality, psychometric, and pain quantitation tests traditionally have been used to evaluate patients suffering from chronic pain and reflex sympathetic dystrophy. These include the Minnesota Multi-Phasic Personality Inventory, the McGill Pain Questionnaire, and the Dartmouth Pain Questionnaire. The Minnesota Multi-Phasic Personality Inventory, when properly interpreted, can provide useful information on the personality profiles for some chronic pain

states, although its importance as a predictor of treatment success has been debated. The McGill Pain Questionnaire is widely used to quantitate subjective pain intensity. This study and other visual quantification tools often are useful for assessing individual treatment progress.

Treatment Plan Design

Information gathered from a thorough history and physical examination and from appropriate diagnostic studies should allow the treating physician to identify accurately specific components involved in any pain dysfunction syndrome. These components are physical, systemic, psychologic, and autonomic nervous system dysfunctions that singly or in combination can initiate or perpetuate pain and extremity dysfunction. All the involved components must be treated if a complete and expeditious recovery from the pain disorder syndrome is to be expected. A prioritized outline should be constructed from which specific problem-oriented treatment regimens may be begun. Because the treatment of certain components of pain dysfunction syndrome is outside the domain of musculoskeletal surgery, consultation of other medical associates is required. Pain control specialists (anesthesiologists), physiatrists and physical therapists, and psychiatrists are consulted most often. Specialists in internal medicine, rheumatologists, neurologists, and endocrinologists may be required in specific instances. The primary physician generally yields to medical specialists' recommendations for specific treatment; however, the patient rightly expects that one physician will remain in charge. Failure in this area can result in disastrous treatment failures stemming from misunderstanding, disillusionment, and distrust.

The orthopaedic surgeon must identify any physical and anatomic problems that act as sources of continued pain and dysfunction. Fracture nonunions and malunions, offending internal fixation hardware, contractures, neuromas, painful constrictive scars, and traumatic arthritis are common examples of continued painful foci that are potentially correctable with surgical intervention. The surgeon should not be reluctant to perform corrective surgery, even in cases where there are recognizable extenuating problems, such as previous surgical failures, active psychologic dysfunction, and pending litigation.

The orthopaedic surgeon probably will be initially responsible for the form and direction of a physical therapy program. A close association with the therapist should be established early and maintained throughout rehabilitation. All involved components of a pain dysfunction syndrome should be discussed with the therapist to delineate the specific physical problems necessitating the referral and to identify any potential impediments to the success of subsequent treatment. There should be direct patient involvement in the design of any physical therapy program for pain dysfunction syndrome and in establishment of clearly defined treatment goals. Restoration of normal function involves both active and passive modalities. In the earlier phase of therapy, the degree of pain usually determines which modalities are to be used. However, active and active assist programs are generally most effective, because they allow the patient to have some control of his/her level of pain.

The orthopaedist may initiate pharmacologic pain management. Current rationale and guidelines are addressed in the section on Acute Pain Management. Other than for immediate postoperative medication, the use of narcotics should be avoided in the treatment of a pain dysfunction syndrome. Drug dependency and abuse may be associated with this disorder, and once identified, such problems require early referral for treatment. NSAIDs and other nonnarcotic drugs are allowable, and their use may facilitate participation in physical therapy and resumption of normal activities of daily living. When indicated, anesthetic injections of trigger points and injections of corticosteroids into joints and about inflamed musculotendinous structures are also effective and easily administered means of pain control.

The consultation of a pain control specialist is recommended for the treatment of refractory functional causes of pain and in all cases where autonomic dysfunction and sympathetically maintained pain exist. Pain control specialists may use oral, intravenous, and regional nerve blocks as well as adaptive therapeutic measures such as transcutaneous electric stimulation to control and treat chronic functional pain.

The sympathetic autonomic nervous system dysfunction of reflex sympathetic dystrophy is treated pharmacologically by blockade of abnormal sympathetic efferent activity. Multiple or continuous stellate ganglion blocks, continuous axillary blockade, end organ blockade by intravenous guanethidine, and systemic calcium channel blockers are used to provide this blockade. An interdisciplinary approach in which pharmacologic treatment is used with physical therapy and psychiatry may be initiated by the pain control specialist to treat all the manifestations of the disorder.

Measures to resolve the patient's pain are the first step in treatment of recognizable psychic disturbances. However, for any psychologic disturbance identified as a major feature of a pain dysfunction syndrome, psychotherapeutic consultation should be considered, even when the pain causes the disturbance. The patient may exhibit considerable reluctance, denial, and anger on mention of the possibility of associated psychologic factors, particularly when psychiatric referral is recommended. A confrontational manner should be avoided, and prior discussion with the psychotherapist may circumvent any potential negative consequences.

Relaxation therapy, hypnosis, biofeedback, distraction techniques, supportive psychotherapy, and psychotropic medications are effective measures in the management of the psychologic disturbances associated with chronic pain syndromes. The psychotherapist may help resolve familial, economic, and workmen's compensation issues. The early detection and prompt referral to psychotherapists for treatment of somatization disorder, conversion disorder, major depression, malingering, and factitious injury disorders is important to protect the individual from unnecessary surgery, possibly harmful diagnostic tests, and the potential for self-inflicted injury and unnecessary hospitalization and incurred medical costs.

Annotated Bibliography

Acute Pain Management

Agency for Health Care Policy and Research: *Clinical Practice Guideline for Acute Pain Management.* Washington, DC, United States Department of Health and Human Services (AHCPR Pub. No. 92-0032), Feb 1992.

This clinical practice guideline was compiled by a government-appointed interdisciplinary panel. It provides management guidelines based on studies suggesting inadequacies of standard practices of pain management. Sections on elderly and pediatric patients are included.

Woolf CJ: Recent advances in the pathophysiology of acute pain. *Br J Anaesth* 1989;63:139-146.

The present knowledge and theories of acute pain sensation are clearly discussed.

Postoperative Analgesia

Bonica JJ: Postoperative Pain, in Bonica JJ (ed): *The Management of Pain*, ed 2. Philadelphia, Lea & Febiger, 1990, pp 461-480.

The physiology and pathophysiology of postoperative pain as a variant of acute pain are discussed. Particular emphasis is placed on surgical biology and the surgical stress response. This is an excellent overview of the subject.

Kehlet H: Modification of responses to surgery by neural blockade: Clinical Implications, in Cousins MJ, Bridenbaugh PO (eds): *Neural Blockage in Clinical Anesthesia and Management of Pain*, ed 2. Philadelphia, JB Lippincott, 1988, pp 145-188.

The biology of the surgical stress response is discussed along with the implications for postoperative patient morbidity and rehabilitation.

Lutz LJ, Lamer TJ: Management of postoperative pain: Review of current techniques and methods. *Mayo Clin Proc* 1990;65:584-596.

A concise, current review of available anesthesia techniques applicable to postoperative pain management is presented. The rationale for each method is discussed and expected benefits are substantiated by extensive references.

Scott DB: Acute pain management, in Cousins MJ, Bridenbaugh PO (eds): *Neural Blockade in Clinical Anesthesia and Management of Pain*, ed 2. Philadelphia, JB Lippincott, pp 861-883.

This is a detailed chapter on the principles and techniques of acute and postoperative pain management. Most of the information is directly applicable to orthopaedic patients.

White PF: Use of patient-controlled analgesia for management of acute pain. *JAMA* 1988;259:243-247.

The rationale, development, and clinical experience with this form of analgesia are reviewed.

Chronic Pain Syndromes

Abram SE: Incidence - hypotheses - epidemiology, in Stanton-Hicks M (ed): *Pain and the Sympathetic Nervous System*. Norwell, MA, Kluwer Academic Publishers, 1989, pp 1-15.

Both the historic and current theories on the etiology of reflex sympathetic dystrophy and sympathetically maintained pain are presented. The entire book is an excellent current bibliographic resource on these subjects.

Amadio PC: Pain dysfunction syndromes. *J Bone Joint Surg* 1988;70A:944-949.

This is an excellent discussion on the clinical approach to patients with chronic pain who are encountered in orthopaedic practice. Diagnostic techniques and psychologic aspects of chronic pain are covered.

Dobyns JH: Pain dysfunction syndromes versus reflex sympathetic dystrophy: What's the difference and does it matter? *Am Soc Surg Hand Correspond Newslet* 1984;92.

This article introduces the term pain dysfunction syndrome and provides justification for its use as a clinical term. It also provides a simple, concise guideline for the clinical recognition, diagnosis, and management of patients with musculoskeletal chronic pain syndromes.

Haddox JD: Psychological aspects of reflex sympathetic dystrophy, in Stanton-Hicks M (ed): *Pain and the Sympathetic Nervous System*. Norwell, MA, Kluwer Academic Publishers, 1989, pp 107-224.

The psychologic aspects of chronic pain syndromes and reflex sympathetic dystrophy are presented. Particular emphasis is given to historic misconceptions of personality disorders. This chapter provides insight into the psychologic effects of pain.

Wilson PR: Sympathetically maintained pain: Diagnosis, measurement, and efficacy of treatment, in Stanton-Hicks M (ed): *Pain and the Sympathetic Nervous System*. Norwell, MA, Kluwer Academic Publishers, 1989, pp 91-123.

This is a comprehensive review of the diagnosis and treatment of reflex sympathetic dystrophy and related syndromes.

16

Perioperative Management

Assessment of Surgical Risk

General Considerations

Advances in surgical and anesthetic techniques have greatly reduced perioperative mortality. A number of factors do predict adverse outcomes, however, including advancing age, functional status, urgency of the procedure, and type of operation. Traditionally overall surgical risk has been assigned according to the classification system of the American Society of Anesthesiologists (ASA): class I, normal; class II, mild systemic disease (often includes neonates and those over 80); class III, severe systemic disease that limits activity; class IV, incapacitating systemic disease that is a constant threat to life; and class V, moribund and not expected to survive 24 hours.

In addition to ASA class, several other risk factors are worth noting. Age greater than 70 increases operative mortality four to eight times, presumably because of coexisting disease and reduced cardiopulmonary reserve. Emergency procedures double the surgical risk. Compared to such high-risk procedures as craniotomy and heart surgery, most orthopaedic procedures are considered intermediate risk. Although there are situations favorable to each, the type of anesthetic administered, either general or spinal, does not affect overall surgical risk.

Cardiac Risks

Because perioperative morbidity and mortality are largely a result of cardiorespiratory complications, a number of strategies have been developed to estimate the risk of adverse cardiac outcomes. The most widely used was developed through prospective documentation of the risk factors that predicted adverse cardiac outcomes in 1,001 patients undergoing noncardiac surgery. Eight factors were identified (Table 1) that increased the likelihood of a significant perioperative cardiac event, such as pulmonary edema, myocardial infarction, ventricular tachycardia, or death. On the basis of a "points" system, patients were stratified into four risk groups. For each of these categories, respectively, the risk of cardiac death or morbidity was: group 1, 0.9%; group 2, 7%; group 3, 13%; and group 4, 78%. Surprisingly, the risk of cardiac events is not increased by a number of factors, including stable angina, controlled hypertension, hyperlipidemia, smoking, diabetes, bundle branch blocks, nonspecific ST segment or T wave changes, and cardiomegaly. Prior cor-

Table 1. Calculation of multifactorial cardiac risk index

Variable	Points*
S3 gallop or jugular venous distention	11
Myocardial infarction in the past six months	10
Rhythm other than sinus or premature atrial contractions on last preoperative electrocardiogram	7
Age more than 70 years	5
Emergency operation	4
Intraperitoneal, intrathoracic, or aortic operation	3
Suspected critical aortic stenosis	3
Poor general medical condition+	3

*Operative risks, from lowest to highest, may be classified as: I (0-5 points); II (6-12 points); III (13-25 points); IV (>25 points).
+Electrolyte abnormalities (potassium <3.0 mmol/l or HCO_3 <20 mmol/l), abnormal arterial blood gases (PO_2 <60 mm Hg, or PCO_2 >50 mm Hg), renal insufficiency (blood urea >17.85 mmol/l (BUN >50 mg/dl), or creatinine >265 μmol/l) (>3.0 mg/dl), abnormal liver status (elevated transaminase, or physical signs of chronic liver disease), or patient bedridden.
(Adapted with permission from Goldman L: Cardiac risks and complications of noncardiac surgery. *Ann Intern Med* 1983;98:504-513.)

onary artery bypass graft reduces the cardiac risk in subsequent operations to nearly normal.

Patients with a recent infarction are at greatest risk for a postoperative infarction. After six months, the risk has dropped considerably, and it remains constant thereafter. The time of peak risk for a perioperative myocardial infarction is not during surgery, but on the third day after surgery, and many infarctions are clinically silent. At one time, the mortality rate for perioperative reinfarction was quite high, but recent advances in invasive monitoring and postoperative care have substantially reduced the risk of death.

Careful preoperative questioning and examination, specifically looking for an S_3 gallop or jugular venous distention, confirms the presence of congestive heart failure. Significant ventricular dysfunction places the patient at risk of postoperative pulmonary edema. Postoperative pulmonary edema occurs in as many as 30% of those with either an S_3 gallop or jugular venous distention, and occurs in up to 6% of those with compensated congestive heart failure. Postoperative pulmonary edema occurs both immediately after surgery, and one to two days later with increased fluid mobilization.

Preoperative auscultation should indicate the presence of significant valvular disease or cardiac arrhythmias. Aortic stenosis, typically indicated by a late peaking, harsh, systolic ejection-type murmur and delayed carotid upstrokes, is the most important valvular lesion to detect. Significant aortic stenosis is associated with a 20% incidence of new or worsening congestive heart failure postoperatively. Most arrhythmias detected preoperatively do not place the patient at high risk for an adverse outcome, and can be easily characterized by obtaining a 12-lead electrocardiogram (EKG) and rhythm strip.

Renal Risks

Most orthopaedic surgical procedures can be safely performed on patients with preexisting renal insufficiency. Significant azotemia and, to a lesser extent, proteinuria, are strong risk factors for perioperative renal complications. As the glomerular filtration rate approaches 25 ml/min, the complication rate increases. Other risk factors for postoperative renal failure include renal hypoperfusion, major trauma, diuretic use, sepsis, and nephrotoxins such as contrast dye studies, nonsteroidal anti-inflammatory drugs, myoglobin, and aminoglycoside antibiotics. In addition to careful monitoring of fluid and electrolytes in these situations, it is imperative to follow renal function serially, adjust the dose and frequency of drugs primarily excreted by the kidney, monitor volume status, and treat infections early.

Cost-Effective Preoperative Laboratory Evaluation

It is estimated that over 30 billion dollars are spent each year on preoperative laboratory testing. Concerns over cost and the lack of evidence that outcomes are improved have been published in several settings. There is an increasing consensus that preoperative laboratory testing is not essential for every patient undergoing surgery. The preoperative evaluation of the candidate for orthopaedic surgery often involves medical consultants and surgical house staff in addition to the orthopaedist and anesthesiologist, and each may view preoperative testing differently. Because the surgeon is primarily responsible for the preoperative evaluation, the orthopaedist should determine which preoperative tests are necessary for patients undergoing orthopaedic procedures.

The potential benefits of preoperative laboratory screening are limited to the identification of unsuspected disease that may adversely affect the operative or postoperative course. The results of screening tests are often ignored, even if abnormal, and rarely result in alteration of surgical or anesthetic management. Moreover, in addition to direct laboratory costs, the costs of preoperative screening include indirect costs for repetition of abnormal tests, last minute surgical cancellations, and reassuring the patient.

Chemistry and Hematologic Screening

A number of studies have examined the utility of routine chemistry screening before surgery. For several years, preoperative screening has been discouraged in other countries, such as Great Britain. A retrospective evaluation of 6,200 preoperative laboratory tests on 2,000 patients indicated that 60% were screening tests and 40% were ordered for specific indications. Tests surveyed included preoperative complete blood counts, differential

Table 2. Indication for preoperative tests

Test	Indications
Prothrombin time/ partial thromboplastin time	Known coagulation disorder, anticoagulant therapy, hemorrhage, anemia, liver disease, malabsorption, malnutrition, or other potentially relevant diseases (eg, systemic lupus erythematosus)
Platelet count	Known platelet abnormality, hemorrhage, purpura, hypersplenism, hematologic malignancy (eg, leukemia), radiation/chemotherapy, thrombosis, some anemias (eg, aplastic), other potentially relevant diseases (eg, systemic lupus erythematosus, paroxysmal nocturnal hemoglobinuria, or renal transplant rejection)
Hemoglobin	Potentially bloody operation (determined by need for preoperative crossmatch), chronic renal failure, known anemia, bleeding disorder, hemorrhage, hematologic malignancy, radiation/chemotherapy, or other potentially relevant diseases (eg, some infections, liver disease, or malnutrition)
White blood cell count and differential cell count	Infection, diseases of white blood cells, including leukemia, radiation/chemotherapy, immunosuppressive therapy, hypersplenism, aplastic anemia, or other potentially relevant abnormalities (eg, rheumatoid arthritis)
Six-factor automated multiple analysis	Age 60 years or over, diuretic usage, renal disease, other fluid/electrolyte abnormalities (eg, diarrhea, syndrome of inappropriate secretion of antidiuretic hormone, diabetes insipidus, or severe liver disease), or other potentially relevant abnormalities (eg, convulsions)
Glucose level	Diabetes mellitus, hypoglycemia, steroid treatment, pancreatic disease (eg, pancreatitis, carcinoma, or glucagonoma), pituitary disease (eg, acromegaly), hypothalamic disease, or adrenal disease

(Adapted with permission from Kaplan E, Sheiner L, Boeckmann A, et al: The usefulness of preoperative laboratory screening. *JAMA* 1985;253:3576-3581.)

blood counts, prothrombin times (PT), activated partial thromboplastin times (APTT), platelet counts, and determination of electrolytes, renal function, and glucose. A very small proportion of screening tests, 0.36%, indicated significant abnormalities. In addition only four tests (0.14% of the total) were of potential surgical significance, and chart reviews did not show any change in treatment or outcome. Similar results from a recent study of preoperative chemistry and hematologic tests from 3,782 surgical patients led to the conclusion that asymptomatic patients, typically ASA class 1, do not require preoperative chemistry and hematologic evaluations. Those patients with specific indications (Table 2) should have selected testing.

Preoperative screening of candidates for orthopaedic surgery for occult coagulopathies, typically with an APTT or a PT, cannot be justified. Postoperative hemorrhage is usually a result of anatomic abnormalities, concurrent treatment, or surgical technique, and not unsuspected coagulopathies. An adequate clinical assessment is sufficient to rule out congenital and acquired coagulopathies. This assessment should include inquiries about known personal or familial bleeding disorders, prolonged hemorrhage after minor injury or procedures, frequent or severe epistaxis or spontaneous bleeding, the recent use of anticoagulants (including aspirin), and a history of liver disease, malabsorption, or malnutrition. Physical findings of note include petechiae, ecchymoses, and hematomas. Patients without any of the above historical features or examination findings do not require screening coagulation tests.

Chest Radiographs

Routine preoperative chest radiographs on candidates for orthopaedic surgery are also unnecessary. Although asymptomatic abnormalities on preoperative chest films are common, particularly in the elderly, most of the abnormalities detected are not treatable and do not adversely affect surgical outcome. Because preoperative screening radiographs seldom enhance patient care, they should be obtained only for those patients with clinical evidence of active chest disease, regardless of age.

Urinalysis

Routine preoperative urinalysis is nearly universal in candidates for orthopaedic surgery. Unfortunately, many of the studies leading to the conclusion that preexisting urinary tract infection is associated with increased risk of surgical wound infection suffer from important methodologic flaws. A recent cost-effectiveness analysis of screening urinalyses in patients that were not candidates for prosthetics led to the conclusion that seeding from the genitourinary tract was exceedingly rare, that the aggregate costs of routine screening were $1.5 million per infection prevented, and that treating postoperative wound infections cost 500 times less than routine screening urinalyses. The data concerning the risk of postoperative seeding of prostheses from urinary tract infection are limited, but the potential for catastrophic infection is significant and until further studies clarify the situation, routine preoperative screening for urinary tract infections in patients receiving prostheses may be indicated. Patients with a history of certain genitourinary or systemic symptoms or diseases (Outline 1) should undergo preoperative urinalysis.

Electrocardiography

Another controversial preoperative test is the electrocardiogram (EKG). Abnormalities are common on routine preoperative EKGs, particularly with advancing age. The clinical significance of these abnormalities is less clear. Potential benefits of preoperative screening include recognition of previous myocardial infarction and of arrhythmias not apparent from the history or physical examination. However, even in a group at high risk for

Outline 1. Criteria for preoperative urinalysis

Urinary tract symptoms
Elevated levels of serum urea nitrogen or creatinine
History of renal disease
Systemic disease that may affect kidneys (eg, diabetes, hypertension, connective tissue disease, systemic infection)
Edema of unclear cause
Fever from sepsis of unclear source
Nephrotoxic drugs
Anticoagulants, coagulopathy
Pregnancy
Unexplained abdominal or back pain
Metabolic acidosis
Volume depletion: hyponatremia or hypernatremia

(Adapted with permission from Lawrence V, Gafni A, Gross M: The unproven utility of the preoperative urinalysis: Economic evaluation. *J Clin Epidemiol* 1989;42:1185-1192.

cardiac disease, such as men over age 75, the incidence of unrecognized myocardial infarction within the preceding six months has been estimated to be less than 0.5%. Similarly, most arrhythmias that adversely affect operative risk will be detected on physical examination. Available evidence does not support obtaining a preoperative EKG as a baseline for future comparisons. Potential negative effects of screening EKGs include the high incidence of clinically unhelpful or false-positive abnormalities that may delay surgery or require extensive evaluation. Preoperative EKGs may be useful in candidates for orthopaedic surgery who have historical or physical findings that suggest cardiac disease, and possibly in those with significant risk of unrecognized coronary disease, such as patients with hypertension, diabetes, or peripheral vascular disease. At this time there is no consensus on other indications for preoperative screening EKGs, and the surgeon should use clinical judgment rather than arbitrary guidelines.

Diabetes Mellitus

Surgical procedures cause a pronounced catabolic response, which is mediated by an excess production of glucagon, catecholamines, cortisol, and growth hormone and a relative deficiency of insulin. The magnitude of the catabolic response depends on the type and duration of the operation and the severity of the underlying clinical disorder. The cumulative metabolic alterations result in hyperglycemia resulting from gluconeogenesis and glycogenolysis and in mild (in noninsulin-dependent diabetes mellitus, NIDDM) to moderate (insulin-dependent diabetes mellitus, IDDM) ketosis resulting from lipolysis and ketogenesis. Patients undergoing surgery rarely will have hypoglycemia unless they have been treated with excessive insulin or they are affected by an erratic and unpredictable absorption of insulin administered subcutaneously before the procedure. Therefore, the major risk in both types of diabetes is dehydration and electrolyte imbalance caused by the hyperglycemia-induced osmotic diuresis. This can be associated with considerable hemodynamic changes, poor tissue perfusion, and organ ischemia. Should this state become complicated by notable ketoacidosis, especially in patients who are insulin-dependent, severe obtundation will occur. It is important to note that serious ketosis also may develop in severely stressed patients with NIDDM.

Preoperative evaluation should include a clinical assessment during an office visit preceding an elective procedure, and the type of diabetes should be identified. Twenty percent to 30% of patients that have NIDDM take insulin for adequate control of blood glucose levels. These patients tend to have increased peripheral resistance and reduced insulin secretion perioperatively; thus, their insulin needs are frequently greater than anticipated. Patients with IDDM should be given adequate insulin doses on a frequent schedule, every four to six hours, and the blood glucose cutoff for withholding an insulin dose should not be set too high. In general, an insulin infusion should be given unless the blood glucose levels fall to less than 100 mg/dl. All too frequently, patients with IDDM slip into ketoacidosis perioperatively because of the practice of withholding insulin until blood glucose values exceed 180 to 240 mg/dl. An insulin bolus should not be given intravenously because its biologic half-life is about 20 minutes; the effect dissipates rapidly and ketoacidosis can develop in the subsequent four to six hours.

The patient's level of glycemic control and the way the patient monitors blood glucose levels should be determined as part of the preoperative evaluation. The goal of the preoperative visit is to maintain the blood glucose between 100 and 180 mg/dl, because this level will reduce the morbidity from fluid and electrolyte imbalance, decrease the risk of infection, and, perhaps, increase the wound-healing rate. Close attention should be paid to diabetic complications such as nephropathy, autonomic neuropathy, hypertension, and coronary artery disease. Nephropathy aggravates fluid management, alters insulin pharmacokinetics (sustained effect), and necessitates a careful selection of antibiotics to avoid nephrotoxicity. Autonomic neuropathy modifies the cardiovascular response to surgery and anesthesia, producing a high risk of arrhythmia, urinary retention, and gastrointestinal disturbances that delay postoperative refeeding. Cardiovascular complications are the major causes of surgical mortality in diabetic patients.

Patients with IDDM and NIDDM who have fasting glucose levels greater than 180 mg/dl or glycosylated hemoglobin values of more than 10% should receive insulin during an operation. Patients with NIDDM who are within acceptable control (fasting blood glucose levels of less than 180 mg/dl and glycosylated hemoglobin between 8% and 10%) may not require insulin, but will need close perioperative monitoring with frequent blood glucose analyses.

Experience has shown that during surgery most patients with diabetes can be maintained in the blood glucose range of 120 to 220 mg/dl with regular insulin infu-

sion rates set between one and two units per hour. All patients with IDDM require more than 50 units of insulin per day. Insulin should be administered either by subcutaneous injection of 36 U/d with blood sugar monitored every six to eight hours or by intravenous drip of 1.5 U/hr with blood sugar monitored every four to six hours and glucose administered on a sliding scale to maintain a blood glucose level of 140 to 240 mg/dl. Patients with NIDDM treated by diet, oral agents, or insulin generally need less than 50 U/d. Insulin should be given by subcutaneous injection of 24 U/d or by intravenous drip of 1.0 U/hr with blood sugar monitoring and glucose administration as above to maintain a blood glucose level of 140 to 240 mg/dl. Conditions that are frequently associated with increased insulin requirements include: obesity, liver disease, severe infection, steroid use, general anesthesia, renal transplant, and coronary artery bypass graft. The insulin infusion should be started the night before the early morning procedures for patients needing improved glycemic control. Otherwise, patients take the usual evening dose of insulin or oral hypoglycemic agent. For those patients requiring insulin, the insulin infusion must be started at least two or three hours before the operation.

There are two basic regimens for administering insulin and glucose. The preferred method involves separate infusion of insulin and glucose, using dedicated pumps to allow independent adjustments of each infusion rate. The alternate method is to combine insulin and the maintenance fluids, preferably 5% dextrose in a solution of 0.5% saline, at a preestimated individualized concentration. This method lacks the flexibility frequently needed for a complicated operation; however, it is an acceptable method for an elective procedure. The success of either method of insulin-glucose infusion depends on hourly, accurate measurements of blood glucose levels. A bedside blood glucose monitoring system must be in place to guarantee optimal care during the perioperative period. Insulin given intravenously has a plasma half-life of five minutes and a biologic effect for about 20 minutes. Thus, even a brief period of insulin deficiency, especially in a patient with IDDM, may allow a rapid deterioration in metabolic control.

Because careful monitoring of potassium levels is needed during insulin and glucose infusion, maintenance fluids should contain at least 20 mEq of potassium per liter for patients with normal potassium values and should be modified in accordance with perioperative variation. The insulin infusion is continued until the patient tolerates oral feeding, and it is stopped after the first subcutaneous insulin injection. Blood glucose level should be measured before meals and at 10 PM and 3 AM, and when it is indicated, the patient should begin three meals and a before-bedtime snack (25 cal/kg).

Diabetic patients undergoing emergency surgery require close attention. The stress of the acute event frequently precipitates a deterioration in glycemic control, which can progress to diabetic ketoacidosis. Thus, the first priority is to assess the glucose control, level of hydration, and the acid-base status. Preoperative management will require an aggressive approach to correcting fluid and electrolyte imbalances, reversing acid-base disorders, and optimizing blood glucose levels. If ketoacidosis is present, the operation should be delayed four to six hours, when possible, while the patient is treated for that condition. A medical consultation for management of the ketoacidosis would be appropriate; such management requires higher fluid and insulin infusion rates. The infusion is generally preceded by an injection of 10 units of regular insulin. Adjustments are made according to hourly blood glucose levels. Adequate potassium replacement is critical, as are close monitoring of fluid and acid-base balance. Once a patient's condition is stable, the operation can be done safely.

For minor surgical procedures that do not require general anesthesia, patients with IDDM should be treated as follows: The morning insulin should be withheld for patients who are receiving nothing by mouth, and insulin cover should be provided on a subcutaneous insulin injection sliding scale that is adjusted for blood glucose values. If breakfast is allowed, the previously described insulin regimen is prescribed. Frequent determination of the patient's blood glucose levels will facilitate responses to avoid hyperglycemia or hypoglycemia. Patients whose diabetes is controlled by diet or oral hypoglycemic agents rarely need supplemental insulin injections for minor surgical procedures.

Patients Taking Steroids

Daily supraphysiologic doses of steroids, equivalent to more than 7.5 mg of prednisone, suppress the hypothalamic-pituitary axis (HPA). Such doses suppress the hypothalamic corticotropin-releasing hormone (CRH) and pituitary adrenocorticotropic hormone (ACTH). This suppression leads to decreased stimulation of the adrenal glands, reduced cortisol production, and glandular atrophy. Withdrawal of exogenous steroids leaves the patient with relative adrenal insufficiency which usually is not symptomatic, and such patients often remain unprepared for the stress of illness or surgery for a variable period of time.

Biologically short-acting steroids such as prednisone produce less HPA suppression than longer-acting steroids such as dexamethasone. A single dose of steroid administered early in the morning is less suppressive than steroid given later in the day or in divided doses. Alternate-day therapy, ACTH, and inhalants or topical steroids generally are not suppressive. Once suppressed, the HPA can take up to a year or more to recover, with recovery of the adrenal glands as the final step.

Various biochemical tests can be performed to evaluate the integrity of the HPA and to identify patients at risk for adrenal insufficiency. The metapyrone and insulin hypoglycemia tests evaluate the integrity of the entire HPA. However, these tests require careful monitoring to guard against hypotension in the case of the metapyrone test and against severe hypoglycemia in the case of the insulin test.

The cosyntropin test specifically measures adrenal function. Because the adrenal glands are the final part of the axis to regain responsiveness after suppression, it is reasonable to assume that a normal adrenal response to cosyntropin would imply that the entire HPA is intact. Cosyntropin is a synthetic polypeptide that stimulates the active portion of the ACTH molecule. A baseline plasma cortisol level is determined, 25 units of cosyntropin are injected parenterally, and 60 minutes later the plasma cortisol level is determined again. An absolute rise of 7 μg/dl, doubling of the baseline control value, or a stimulated value of greater than 18 μg/dl indicates normal adrenal responsiveness.

A careful history is the most important element in the preoperative evaluation of the patient who has taken exogenous steroids. It is imperative to ask about steroid use within the last year, the nature of the preparation, the dose and frequency of administration, the routine of administration, and the duration of therapy. Patients may give a history of vague malaise, low grade fever, nausea, arthralgia, and other nonspecific complaints that may suggest adrenal insufficiency. Signs of hypercortisolism on physical examination are helpful but need not be present for diagnosis. Posterior subcapsular cataracts and avascular necrosis of hips, cushingoid facies, and abdominal striae are peculiar to exogenous cortisol excess. A history of steroid use in supraphysiologic doses for more than two or three weeks within the preceding year should prompt the physician to check for suppression of the HPA. The patient can be tested with cosyntropin, or suspected decreased adrenal reserve can be treated empirically by administration of stress doses of steroids in the perioperative period. If emergency surgery is required, dexamethasone can be administered while the cosyntropin test is being performed. Dexamethosone will not suppress the HPA immediately and will not affect the measurement of plasma cortisol. Electrolyte levels should be measured in all patients.

Once it is determined that a patient has decreased adrenal reserve, a 100-mg dose of hydrocortisone hemisuccinate should be administered intravenously every six hours for 24 hours. Then the dose should be reduced by 50% per day until the patient's maintenance dose is reached. For minor surgery, a 100-mg dose of hydrocortisone is given parenterally before the procedure and every six hours thereafter for 24 hours. The maintenance dose of steroids is then resumed. The total dose of hydrocortisone approximates the output of the normal adrenal glands subjected to the stress of surgery. Other steroids can be substituted in equivalent doses, but intramuscular cortisone acetate should be avoided because of its uneven absorption. Protocols for instituting and tapering steroids in the perioperative period should be based on the nature of the procedure. Several such protocols have been recommended and published; however, common sense in the individual case should dictate how they are handled.

Although postoperative problems such as infection require longer therapy, steroids should be tapered as early as possible to minimize deleterious effects on wound healing and host defenses against infections. Blood pressure, blood glucose, and electrolyte levels should be followed. Antacids are frequently used to prevent presumed steroid-induced gastric ulceration, but data on the causative role of steroids are lacking.

Patients With Lung Disease

Pulmonary complications of surgery continue to be a significant source of perioperative morbidity and mortality. Preoperative evaluation should have as its goal the identification of risk factors related to the patient and the surgery, as well as a means to decrease the risk. On the day after upper abdominal surgery, forced vital capacity may decline to 40% of its preoperative value, returning to baseline during the next ten to 14 days. Functional residual capacity may decline to 60% of preoperative value, with gradual restoration to baseline by the seventh postoperative day. Atelectasis resulting from the decline in functional residual capacity produces physiologic shunting and associated declines in oxygenation. Other clinical features that increase the patient's risk include obesity, advanced age, the type of anesthesia (general versus spinal), the duration of surgery, baseline pulmonary dysfunction, and, in high-risk patients, the lack of preoperative pulmonary treatment.

The degree of abnormality in the pulmonary function tests of patients with chronic obstructive pulmonary disease has not been demonstrated to be a reliable way to quantitate their risk. In fact, no degree of abnormality on spirometric testing, down to a 1-sec forced expiratory volume of 450 ml, can be called "prohibitive" for nonlung resectional surgery. A PCO_2 of more than 45 to 50 mm Hg seems to be predictive of a high risk of morbidity and mortality, although measurement of PO_2 is not a reliable predictor. The incidence of pulmonary complication in patients with chronic obstructive pulmonary disease can be reduced by adjuncts such as deep-breathing maneuvers, chest physiotherapy, bronchodilators, and antibiotics. Preoperative initiation of the regimen is more effective than postoperative. Continuation of aminophylline into the postoperative period may be beneficial because it improves diaphragmatic function in the immediate postoperative period. Wheezing should be eliminated before surgery, and this may require the addition of steroids for several days preoperatively. Preoperative education on the importance of deep breathing, coughing, and the use of incentive spirometry is more effective than attempting to teach these principles in the presence of postoperative pain and analgesia.

Preoperative pulmonary function tests should be obtained in patients with any of the following characteristics: productive cough, 20 pack-year (1 pack/day for 20 years) or greater smoking history, obesity, or history or physical findings of cardiopulmonary disease. If moderate to severe abnormality is found on spirometry, arterial blood gases should also be obtained. Patients identified as being at increased risk because of abnormal pulmonary function tests or historic/physical examination findings of pulmonary disease should be considered for preoperative treatment beginning with discontinuation of smoking for at least eight weeks, treatment of intercurrent pulmonary infections, and treatment of any nutritional deficits. In the period 48 to 72 hours before surgery, the regimen should be more intensive, including bronchodilators, chest physiotherapy if indicated, and education on the importance of deep-breathing and coughing postoperatively. Postoperative adjuncts include judicious use of narcotics for pain relief, early ambulation, and removal of nasogastric tube as soon as is prudent. In addition, use of one of the prophylactic lung expansion maneuvers every one to two hours while awake during the first three to five days postoperatively should be prescribed for high-risk patients who are to undergo a procedure expected to last over three hours.

Hematologic Considerations

No empirical data clearly correlate the effect of hemoglobin level with the risks of anesthesia and surgery; however, in a number of studies, no surgical patient died who had a preoperative hemoglobin level above 8 g/dl and lost less than 500 cc of blood during surgery. Most patients with mild to moderate anemia (hematocrit 25% to 30%) tolerate major surgery well and do not require preoperative transfusion unless significant blood loss is anticipated. A hemoglobin level of 10 g/dl is the value usually quoted to ensure good tissue oxygenation. Patients who have chronic anemia and stable compensated intravascular volume can often safely be operated on when their hemoglobin levels are 7 g/dl. Higher preoperative hemoglobin levels are preferred in the following situations: old age and acute anticipated blood loss. Hemoglobin values are further reduced with intraoperative blood loss.

It is important to determine the etiology of an anemia because the underlying disorder may affect the patient's perioperative course. The history and physical examination and a few laboratory tests should define the etiology in most circumstances.

In patients with thrombocytopenias, the risk of bleeding is directly related to the platelet count. Bleeding time does not become prolonged until the platelet count is less than 100,000. Clinically significant bleeding is rare at counts of 50,000 to 100,000, although this may depend on the surgical procedure. Counts of 20,000 to 50,000 can be associated with surgical bleeding, although significant bleeding rarely occurs until the platelet count is less than

10,000, in which case platelet support is indicated. Quantitative platelet abnormalities should be considered in patients taking aspirin, nonsteroidal anti-inflammatory agents, dipyridimole, penicillins, beta-blockers, antidepressants, and alcohol. Aspirin has an irreversible effect on platelet aggregation that lasts seven to ten days. Prolonged bleeding time without thrombocytopenia suggests a qualitative platelet disorder. If a qualitative platelet defect is suspected, hematologic consultation and aggregration studies are indicated.

Coagulation disorders, including the prolongation of the prothrombin time (PT) or partial thromboplastin time (PTT), need to be interpreted in light of the patient's history, physical examination, and clinical situation. An 80% loss of coagulation factors is required to prolong PT or PTT. Isolated prolongation of the PT is rare and usually represents a specific deficiency of clotting factors. Acquired coagulation disorders are associated with multiple clotting factor deficiencies, and both PT and PTT are usually prolonged. These disorders include vitamin K deficiency, liver disease, and the use of anticoagulant drugs, "acquired anticoagulants," and disseminated intravascular coagulation. Preoperative therapy depends on surgical urgency. Vitamin K in doses of 10 to 20 mg, given subcutaneously or intravenously, usually corrects the coagulopathy over 24 to 48 hours. If surgery is urgent or bleeding is present, fresh frozen plasma should be slowly administered intravenously together with 20 mg of vitamin K. Intravenous vitamin K administration should be watched carefully because it has been associated with severe anaphylactic reactions. Additional fresh frozen plasma is usually required postoperatively. Whole blood transfusion may be necessary if the patient is bleeding actively.

Patients With Liver Disease

Operative morbidity and mortality in patients with liver disease usually results from postoperative gastrointestinal bleeding, hepatic encephalopathy, acute renal failure, and/or infection. Other perioperative considerations are altered metabolism of anesthetic drugs, coagulation defects, and potential contamination of surgical personnel with hepatitis virus. Preoperative assessment is aimed at estimating the degree of hepatic compromise and concomitant problems.

Surgery in patients with acute viral hepatitis has been associated with mortality as high as 10%, and major postoperative complications occur in 11%. If possible, surgery should be delayed until one month after the liver enzymes return to normal. This approach will also reduce the risk of infection in medical personnel. Hepatitis B surface antigen carriers pose a special problem of infecting surgical personnel and of contaminating hospital equipment; the risk is low for hepatitis A and is currently unknown for hepatitis C. For the asymptomatic carrier without evidence of active liver disease, there is no in-

creased risk for surgery nor is there any evidence of activation of the virus by anesthesia. Appropriate "secretions of body fluid precautions" should be maintained.

The risk of surgery in patients with other forms of liver disease is related directly to the degree of hepatic dysfunction. Bilirubin levels over 2 mg/dl, albumin less than 3 mg/dl, PT longer than 16 seconds, encephalopathy, and presence of varices or ascites all predict poor surgical risk and require vigorous preoperative preparation.

Nutritional Status

Inadequate nutrition can affect surgical outcome and increase the risk of complications. Caloric needs are generally increased after surgery. The rate of wound healing is also directly related to proper nutrition in the recovery period. A brief history of the patient's eating habits, an assessment of body habitus, and determination of serum levels of total protein, prealbumin, albumin, and transferrin can provide clues to inadequate nutritional status. Other significant factors include absolute weight loss of more than 10% in the previous six months, delayed hypersensitivity response to skin test antigens, and a total lymphocyte count of less than $1.5 \times 10^9/l$. If serious malnutrition is detected and it is safe to do so, surgery should be postponed until the individual's nutritional state can be improved. Current recommendations include a minimum of seven to ten days of preoperative nutritional repletion in the moderately malnourished patient. If surgery cannot be delayed and a prolonged interval without nutrition is entertained, parenteral or enteral hyperalimentation should be instituted.

Although there are no strict guidelines for initiation of hyperalimentation, in previously well-nourished patients who have suffered injury, burns, or sepsis, the goal is to minimize loss of lean body mass. Because nitrogen losses can reach levels of 15 to 40 g/day in severely stressed patients, full enteral or parenteral nutrition should be provided for patients who are not expected to return to adequate oral intake within a few days. Approximately 200 mg/kg/day of nitrogen should be provided. Equal amounts of fat and carbohydrates should constitute the nonprotein energy sources. When the patient becomes less hypermetabolic and hypercatabolic, both energy and nitrogen intakes can be increased to make up for previous losses.

Elderly Patients

The preoperative functional status of an elderly patient must be taken into account when planning postoperative rehabilitation. Given the high potential for mental status impairment in the elderly patient in the form of postoperative delirium or acute confusion, knowledge of baseline cognitive functioning is important in evaluating any acute deterioration in the postoperative period. Some clinical strategies for assessing mental status include: orientation to person, place, and time; the ability to list five items like cities, fruits, and vegetables; and the ability to remember and recall three objects after a short period.

Postoperative confusion resulting from the residual effect of anesthetics, analgesics, fever, and electrolyte disorders is more common in elderly patients. The stress of surgery and unfamiliar surroundings are also frequent precipitating causes. Because of the frequent occurrence of orthostatic hypotension, orthostatic blood pressure and pulse readings should be checked before ambulating elderly patients who have been at bed rest for more than two to three days. Pressure sores, incontinence, and aspiration pneumonia may also occur, as a result of immobility. The elderly patient's functional status and mental status may be enhanced by simple encouragement, early mobilization, and social interaction.

Monoarticular Arthritis

Acute attacks of gout or pseudogout can occur in the postoperative period. The onset is sudden, and the patient complains of severe pain in the affected joint. The metatarsophalangeal joint of the big toe is most commonly involved in gout, while the knee is most commonly involved in pseudogout. Erythema over the affected joints can mimic the appearance of cellulitis. The specific procedure to establish the diagnosis of acute gouty arthritis is the examination of the synovial fluid by compensated polarized microscopy.

The treatment of these crystal-induced arthritides that occur in the postoperative period includes the choice of oral or intravenous colchicine and/or nonsteroidal anti-inflammatory drugs. If the patient is unable to take an oral medication, intravenous colchicine is a good alternative. Recently, a new nonnarcotic analgesic medication, ketorolac tromethamine, has become available. It is a nonsteroidal anti-inflammatory agent that is approved for intramuscular administration. Ketorolac can be given for acute pain and has the advantage of having no narcotic-related side effects. It has proven useful in the treatment of acute gout and pseudogout in the postoperative setting.

Urinary Tract Infections

The presence of bacteria in the urine of patients undergoing orthopaedic surgery is quite common. Greater than 10^3 colony-forming units, either in males or females, is considered significant bacturia. Bacturia is nearly universal after several days of an indwelling Foley catheter. Asymptomatic bacturia is characterized both by the lack of inflammation, with little or no pyuria, and by the absence of typical voiding symptoms, such as urgency and dysuria. There is no evidence that treatment of asymptomatic bacturia is necessary, unless prosthetic devices are involved or the patient is immune-compromised. Although fever is common in true infections, bacteremia is rare unless an anatomic abnormality or obstruction exists. Symptomatic bacturia, with or without evidence of inflammation, should be treated with antibiotics. If infection develops in a patient with an indwelling catheter, the catheter should be removed as soon as possible.

Venous Thromboembolic Disease

Venous thromboembolic disease (VTED) is a common and serious complication of major orthopaedic surgery. Intraoperative disturbances in venous flow, systemic release of thrombogenic material, and femoral vein damage, as well as prolonged postoperative bed rest, may predispose patients to VTED. Although the exact timing of perioperative deep venous thrombosis (DVT) is uncertain, it is clear that a number of thromboses occur intraoperatively and in the immediate postoperative period. VTED also has been documented to occur days to weeks after surgery. The incidence of DVT is 40% to 50% after total hip replacement and may be even higher after total knee replacement and after hip fracture. Although DVT is associated with local complications such as the postphlebitic syndrome and stasis ulceration, its most important sequela is pulmonary embolism. Without prophylaxis, pulmonary embolism occurs in 1% to 2% of patients after total hip replacement and in up to 5% of patients after hip fracture.

Factors that increase the risk of thromboembolism include advanced age, hereditary deficiencies of coagulation inhibitors, oral contraceptives, paralysis, previous DVT, and, possibly, obesity, varicose veins, and coexisting cancer or congestive heart failure. Risk factors specific to patients undergoing orthopaedic surgery need further research, but some studies have suggested that general anesthesia, compared to regional, and the use of uncemented prostheses increase the risk of VTED.

Prophylaxis of VTED

Major Joint Replacement   Warfarin, typically begun the evening before surgery and adjusted to maintain a slightly prolonged prothrombin time (PT), is clearly effective in preventing perioperative DVT. The optimal duration of warfarin prophylaxis remains controversial, but it typically is used for one to three weeks postoperatively. Less intense anticoagulation, striving for a PT that is 1.3 to 1.5 times normal, has become accepted practice; nevertheless, the major disadvantage of warfarin therapy continues to be hemorrhage, both at the operative site and from other sites. Fixed-dose heparin, despite its proven utility in treatment of medical conditions and of patients undergoing general surgery, is ineffective in patients undergoing orthopaedic surgery and should not be used to prevent perioperative DVT. Adjusted dose heparin, however, is effective in patients undergoing total hip replacement when begun two days before surgery and given in split doses to maintain an activated partial thromboplastin time (APTT) in the high normal range.

The risk factors for bleeding complications in patients undergoing orthopaedic surgery who are on warfarin therapy have not been well studied. However, age over 65, history of stroke or gastrointestinal bleeding, serious comorbid disease, and atrial fibrillation are all associated with an increased likelihood of serious bleeding when warfarin is given in other settings. Daily monitoring of the PT and appropriate dose adjustment are mandatory for the safe use of warfarin. Contraindications to the use of anticoagulants include a recent cerebrovascular accident or gastrointestinal bleeding (within three months).

Although a number of antiplatelet agents have been proposed as prophylactic agents in patients undergoing orthopaedic surgery, their use is limited. A recent NIH Consensus Conference concluded that aspirin alone is inadequate for preventing VTED in patients undergoing total hip or knee replacement. Because of these problems, low molecular weight dextran is preferred. Dextran sulfate, a carbohydrate with antiplatelet properties, appears to be effective, but it can cause allergic reactions and volume overload, particularly in the elderly.

Vasoactive agents have also been used for VTED prophylaxis. Several investigational agents appear useful in preventing VTED, particularly low molecular weight heparin (LMWH). Although not approved for clinical use in this country, LMWH has been available overseas for some time and has been reported to be effective in reducing perioperative VTED with a low incidence of bleeding.

Mechanical measures to prevent VTED after joint replacement have included graduated elastic stockings, pneumatic compression stockings, and, in patients undergoing total knee replacement, continuous passive motion devices. Several studies have demonstrated that elastic stockings, although widely used, are ineffective in preventing DVT. There is some evidence that thigh-high intermittent pneumatic compression (IPC) stockings can reduce the incidence of DVT after hip or knee replacement, but the data are inconclusive. Presumably, IPC prevents lower extremity stasis and may potentiate thrombolytic mechanisms. There are no known complications of IPC stockings, and most patients tolerate them quite well. IPC can be started intraoperatively.

Several studies have examined the efficacy of IPC. In a randomized study of patients undergoing total hip replacement, proximal DVT was found in 14% of the IPC group, compared with 27% in the untreated controls. Venograms or bilateral duplex ultrasound examinations performed before discharge on 177 patients who had total hip replacements and were randomly allocated to either IPC, IPC and low dose warfarin, or IPC and aspirin indicated a 10% overall incidence of proximal DVT. The incidence among the three groups was not statistically different. In another group of patients undergoing total knee replacement, the incidence of DVT was 6% in the IPC group and 66% in the untreated group, a risk reduction of 90%. IPC has been found to be more effective than aspirin in preventing DVT in patients having total knee replacement.

Continuous passive motion devices have been advocated in the prevention of VTED after total hip replacement. The rationale for their use is that continuous postoperative movement would stimulate venous and lymphatic flow and would maintain range of motion of the joint. Although several studies have suggested these devices may be efficacious, results of a well-designed, randomized study in which continuous passive motion after total knee replacement was compared with untreated controls, indicated similar rates of DVT (nearly 40%) in both groups.

Hip Fracture   The risk of VTED with hip fracture may begin at the time of the fracture, not at surgery, and prophylactic measures that are useful in joint replacement may be ineffective. Low-dose warfarin reduces the risk of perioperative VTED by 40% after hip fracture, but is often associated with a significantly increased risk of bleeding.

Diagnosis of VTED

A number of techniques are available to diagnose postoperative DVT. The venogram remains the standard, but it is invasive, painful, and involves contrast dye. Noninvasive techniques to diagnosis DVT, which have become increasingly popular, suffer from a number of problems. Fibrinogen scans, which required exogenous plasma, could potentially transmit blood-borne pathogens and are no longer available. Impedance plethysmography is very useful in the diagnosis of proximal DVT in patients with medical problems but is surprisingly inaccurate in patients after orthopaedic surgery. The most promising noninvasive tests for DVT are ultrasound techniques that involve Doppler or real time (B mode) techniques.

Ultrasound has several advantages over venography. It is safe, rapid, noninvasive, and less expensive than venography. Portable units are available for bedside examinations. The interpretation of ultrasound studies is subjective and requires an experienced technician for satisfactory accuracy. Ultrasound has been found to be highly sensitive (85% to 90%) and specific (85% to 99%) in the diagnosis of proximal DVT, but is generally inaccurate for isolated calf DVT.

Despite DVT prophylaxis, a significant number of DVTs occur after joint procedures on the lower extremity, and some authors have recommended routine surveillance with ultrasound after all major orthopaedic surgical procedures. Although isolated calf DVT is not well identified by ultrasound screening, it rarely results in pulmonary emboli.

Pulmonary emboli are very difficult to diagnose on clinical grounds alone. Embolization should be suspected after surgery in patients with unexplained dyspnea, tachypnea, tachycardia, and pleuritic chest pain, particularly if there are no corresponding abnormalities on chest radiographs. The electrocardiogram may be useful in differentiating between pulmonary emboli and myocardial infarction, but it is often normal. Unexplained hypoxia is suggestive of pulmonary emboli, but normal arterial blood gases do not rule out the diagnosis.

The diagnostic test of choice in those patients suspected of having pulmonary emboli is the lung perfusion scan. Significant embolism can be ruled out if the perfusion scan is normal. If abnormal, a lung ventilation scan is indicated, and large mismatched defects strongly suggest embolization. Small or matched ventilation and perfusion defects are nondiagnostic, and additional testing, such as pulmonary angiography, is required. Pulmonary angiography is highly accurate and generally safe if performed by an experienced radiologist.

Treatment of VTED

In the absence of contraindications, proximal DVT, including asymptomatic disease, should be treated with prolonged anticoagulation to prevent further extension of the thrombus and reduce the risk of embolization and local complication. Because warfarin requires several days to achieve an adequate state of anticoagulation, intravenous heparin should be started immediately. Typically, heparin is begun with a bolus of 5,000 to 10,000 units followed by a continuous drip at 1,000 units per hour, with serial monitoring of the partial thromboplastin time to achieve a value 1.5 to two times normal. Significant bleeding at the operative site is unlikely if the patient is more than two days postoperative and not on antiplatelet therapy. Warfarin can be safely started concurrently with heparin, typically with an oral loading dose of 10 mg followed by 5 mg daily, and adjusted to maintain the prothrombin time (PT) at 1.3 to 1.5 times normal. After at least three days of adequate combined therapy with heparin and warfarin, and if the PT is in the therapeutic range, heparin may be discontinued. The initial therapy for documented pulmonary emboli is similar to that for DVT.

The management of isolated calf DVT remains controversial. If the thrombus remains in the calf, the risk of embolization is very low, but asymptomatic proximal propagation may occur. Some advocate anticoagulation for isolated calf DVT, regardless of symptoms, but a reasonable alternative approach is conservative therapy with heat and elevation plus careful serial noninvasive monitoring for proximal extension. Alternative therapies for VTED are limited. If there are absolute contraindications to anticoagulation, significant pulmonary emboli can be prevented with vena caval interruption, often by percutaneous placement of a filter device. Thrombolytic therapy, which actively dissolves thrombi, may be indicated for massive pulmonary emboli with hypotension or profound hypoxia. Unfortunately, thrombolytic therapy is frequently associated with serious hemorrhaging, particularly postoperatively, and is rarely indicated for patients who have DVT after orthopaedic surgery.

Annotated Bibliography

Preoperative Laboratory Evaluation

Goldberger AL, O'Konski M: Utility of the routine electrocardiogram before surgery and on general hospital admission: Critical review and new guidelines. *Ann Intern Med* 1986;105:552-557.

This critical review of the usefulness of preoperative electrocardiograms concludes that an EKG is not routinely indicated before noncardiac surgery.

Kaplan EB, Sheiner LB, Boeckmann AJ, et al: The usefulness of preoperative laboratory screening. *JAMA* 1985;253:3576-3581.

This retrospective study of 6,200 lab tests on 2,000 preoperative patients at a single teaching hospital in 1980 concluded that 60% were ordered without clear indications. When action limits for each test were defined, 3.4% exceeded the action limit, but only a small proportion were unsuspected. Four tests (0.14% of total) were of potential surgical significance but chart review did not reveal any change in treatment or outcome. The authors conclude that preoperative testing should be done only for specific indications.

Lawrence VA, Gafni A, Gross M: The unproven utility of the preoperative urinalysis: Economic evaluation. *J Clin Epidemiol* 1989;42:1185-1192.

This study is a cost-effectiveness analysis of routine urinalysis before nonprosthetic knee procedures. The authors conclude that 4.6 wound infections/year would be prevented by routine urine screening, at a cost of $1.5 million per infection.

Narr BJ, Hansen TR, Warner MA: Preoperative laboratory screening in healthy Mayo patients: Cost-effective elimination of tests and unchanged outcomes. *Mayo Clin Proc* 1991;66:155-159.

This is a retrospective review of 3,782 ASA class 1 surgical patients during 1988 at the Mayo Clinic. Only 4% (160 patients) had abnormal tests. None delayed surgery, and in ten the treatment changed. No preoperative laboratory abnormality predicted an adverse outcome.

Suchman A, Griner PF: Diagnostic uses of the activated partial thromboplastin time and prothrombin time. *Ann Intern Med* 1986;104:810-816.

This paper summarizes the studies suggesting routine screening for coagulation abnormalities is unjustified, and gives elements of the preoperative history and physical examination that might suggest an increased risk of bleeding.

Tape TG, Mushlin AT: The utility of routine chest radiographs. *Ann Intern Med* 1986;104:663-670.

This critical review of literature regarding preoperative radiographs concludes that routine preoperative chest radiographs are not indicated, even in the elderly.

Cardiovascular

Goldman L: Cardiac risks and complications of noncardiac surgery. *Ann Intern Med* 1983;98:504-513.

This is a classic review of cardiac risks in noncardiac surgery.

Renal

Beck LH: Perioperative renal, fluid, and electrolyte management. *Clin Geriatr Med* 1990;6:557-569.

This article covers the normal physiologic changes of aging that increase the likelihood of renal-electrolyte disorders in the elderly surgical patient.

Diabetes Mellitus Management

Gavin LA: Management of diabetes mellitus during surgery. *West J Med* 1989;151:525-529.

This article extensively reviews surgery in patients with diabetes. Management of the diabetic undergoing surgery is methodically examined with special emphasis on how to avoid problems.

Surgical Patients on Corticosteroids

Reding R, Michel LA, Donckier J, et al: Surgery in patients on long-term steroid therapy: A tentative model for risk assessment. *Br J Surg* 1990;77:1175-1178.

The effect of long-term steroid therapy on morbidity was determined by retrospectively reviewing the perioperative course of 55 steroid-treated patients. The authors conclude that bronchopulmonary disorders requiring a long duration of steroid therapy are associated with a higher risk of steroid-related complications after surgery. A convenient mathematical model is proposed, which may allow preoperative assessment of surgical risk, using steroid dose and duration of treatment.

Pulmonary Disease

Biery DR, Marks JD, Schapera A, et al: Factors affecting perioperative pulmonary function in the acute respiratory failure. *Chest* 1990;98:1455-1462.

This study retrospectively examined the magnitude, duration, and associated factors of perioperative changes in pulmonary function in 145 patients who required preoperative mechanical ventilation for acute respiratory failure. The authors conclude that the majority of patients did very well and recommended that necessary surgery not be postponed because of concern that pulmonary function will be worsened by surgery and anesthesia.

Hematologic System

Consensus development conference. NIH consensus statement on perioperative red cell transfusions. *Bull Pan Am Health Organ* 1989;23:356-357.

This review gives current recommendations on perioperative red cell transfusions.

Hepatologic Status

Gholson CF, Provenza JM, Bacon BR: Hepatologic considerations in patients with parenchymal liver disease undergoing surgery. *Am J Gastroenterol* 1990;85:487-496.

This review article covers the deleterious effect of anesthesia on hepatocellular function. Altered drug pharmacokinetics, aberrant hemostasis, postoperative encephalopathy and infection, with multiorgan failure, all contribute to perioperative morbidity and mortality. Recommendations are that a preoperative evaluation and risk assessment is imperative. Identification and correction of reversible risk factors via meticulous preoperative definition of the etiology, chronicity, and severity of the patient's liver disease within the confines of surgical urgency is the goal of the preoperative hepatology consultation.

Nutritional Status

Meguid MM, Campos AC, Hammond WG: Nutritional support in surgical practice: Part I. *Am J Surg* 1990;159:345-358.

This review article examines the issues regarding nutritional support in patients undergoing surgery for cancer, trauma, or burns. The authors conclude that enteral nutrition appears to be as effective as parenteral nutrition in improving operative outcome, as compared with ad libitum nutrition. Postoperative enteral nutrition and parenteral nutrition are equally effective in reducing postoperative complications.

Special Considerations in the Elderly Surgical Patient

Gordon M: Restoring functional independence in the older hip fracture patient. *Geriatrics* 1989;44:48-59.

The older patient requiring major orthopaedic surgery for a hip fracture is at risk of poor outcome if special precautions are not taken during the perioperative period. Close attention must be paid to associated medical problems and use of medications, especially during the postoperative period.

Tavani CA: Perioperative psychiatric considerations in the elderly. *Clin Geriatr Med* 1990;6:543-556.

This article deals with common issues encountered in elderly persons who are medically ill. Agitation and delirium, including alcohol withdrawal syndrome, are frequently encountered problems, and useful intervention and strategies are presented. Principles of pharmacotherapy in the elderly are reviewed.

Thromboembolism

Becker DM, Philbrick JT, Abbitt PL: Real-time ultrasonography for the diagnosis of lower extremity deep venous thrombosis: The wave of the future? *Arch Intern Med* 1989;149:1731-1734.

A review of published studies of ultrasonography and DVT. The reported sensitivity for proximal DVT ranged from 92% to 100% (mean 96%), and the specificity ranged from 96% to 100% (mean 99%). Discusses the strengths and weaknesses of ultrasonography.

Haas SB, Insall JN, Scuderi GR, et al: Pneumatic sequential-compression boots compared with aspirin prophylaxis of deep-vein thrombosis after total knee arthroplasty. *J Bone Joint Surg* 1990;72A:27-31.

This study was a randomized trial of intermittent pneumatic compression (IPC) compared to aspirin in 119 patients undergoing total knee replacement. Venograms were done on postoperative day four to five. In those patients undergoing unilateral total knee replacement, DVT occurred in 22% of the IPC group and 47% of the aspirin group.

Woolson ST, McCrory DW, Walter JF, et al: B-mode ultrasound scanning in the detection of proximal venous thrombosis after total hip replacement. *J Bone Joint Surg* 1990;72A:983-987.

This study of 143 patients who had both ultrasonographic and venographic studies following total hip replacement concluded that ultrasonography is accurate and compares favorably with venography for detection of DVT after total hip replacement.

17
Anesthesia for Orthopaedic Surgery

The growing trend toward subspecialization in the practice of anesthesia has resulted in benefits to the specialty, the surgeon, and the patient. The specialty of orthopaedic anesthesia is a logical outgrowth of this trend. Although candidates for orthopaedic surgery vary in age from infants to the extreme elderly, surgical procedures involving bone, muscle, and related soft tissues require similar anesthetic approaches to monitoring, intraoperative management, and postoperative pain management. Specific areas of concern to orthopaedic anesthesiologists include patient positioning, the advantages of regional versus general anesthesia, management of the difficult airway, the risk of susceptibility of malignant hyperthermia, special considerations in the patient undergoing spinal surgery, management of pediatric and outpatient populations, and concepts of postoperative pain management.

Preoperative Evaluation

Before a surgical procedure, an anesthesia plan is formulated based on the physical condition of the patient, the requirements of the surgeon and the surgical procedure, and the wishes of the patient. The plan is devised after review of the medical history, physical examination, and laboratory tests; the anesthesiologist's interview; and the surgeon's description of the objectives, risks, and outcome of the surgical procedure. Physical limitations that might affect airway management, positioning, and postoperative care must be integral to the anesthesia plan.

Routine preoperative laboratory testing in fit patients has been greatly diminished recently as a result of several studies that indicate such testing is of little value. Current recommendations for screening tests before surgery in healthy individuals are shown in Table 1. Patients with significant disease or those undergoing more hazardous surgery often require more extensive testing.

Positioning

Proper positioning of patients for orthopaedic surgery can be challenging; no surgical posture is immune from the potential for morbidity. Positioning patients with arthritic involvement of multiple joints, traumatic injuries, or external fixation devices may require some modification of the standard positions to accommodate their special needs. Adequate padding must be placed to avoid

Table 1. Recommended preoperative screening in healthy patients

Age (years)	Tests Required
Under 40	None
40-50	Electrocardiogram
	Creatinine/glucose
Over 60	Complete blood count
	Electrocardiogram
	Chest radiograph
	Creatinine/glucose

skin breakdown or peripheral nerve compression during prolonged surgery in one position.

When moving or turning patients, care should be taken to avoid hyperextension of the joints, particularly the neck, and to see that extremities are not compressed, allowed to hang unsupported, or placed in any nonanatomic or compromised position. Changes in head elevation, such as from supine or sitting, should be done slowly to allow hemodynamic reequilibration. Alterations of myocardial contractility, stroke volume, cardiac output, and autonomic tone occur in response to postural changes affecting the gravitational distribution of the intravascular blood volume. These alterations may be exaggerated by the hemodynamic effects of general or major regional anesthesia.

Most perioperative morbidity resulting from positioning involves the upper extremity. The brachial plexus is subject to injury from stretch, compression, and ischemia. Consequently, the arm should never be abducted beyond 90 degrees, should be level with the operating table, and should never be allowed to hang off the edge of the table. The head should remain in a neutral position to avoid excessive stretch on the upper brachial plexus. The elbow should be padded to protect the ulnar nerve, and the humerus protected to avoid radial nerve compression.

The lateral decubitus and prone positions are notorious for resulting in such ophthalmic injury as corneal abrasion or, less commonly, retinal ischemia due to compression. Despite careful preoperative positioning, any movement during surgery may cause the patient to shift and result in an injury. Frequent reevaluation of the eye during the surgical procedure is warranted when the patient is in either of these positions. Anterior spinal fusion in the lateral decubitus position often includes the use of a kidney rest to increase the degree of lateral flexion. In the proper position for this procedure, the patient's bony pelvis is placed over the kidney rest, allowing the pelvic brim to rotate away from the rib cage. If the kidney rest is placed under the flank or lower ribs, the resulting compression can jeopardize pulmonary function and risks vena caval obstruction.

The orthopaedic fracture table provides a unique positioning challenge to the surgical care team. The keys to success are familiarity with the given table and its operation and coordination of efforts. Because of the somewhat precarious position of the patient, sufficient personnel must be present to assist with lifting and stabilization. The perineal post should be placed in such a way as to avoid compression of the genitalia or the pudendal nerves.

Shoulder surgery is typically performed with the patient in a semisitting or "beach chair" position, and shifted toward the side of the table to allow relatively free access to the shoulder. It is important to assure that the patient is firmly secured in this position, because tugging on the arm could cause a further shift toward the edge of the table or even the floor. Whenever the operative site is higher than the heart, the potential for venous air embolism exists. This is widely held to be of theoretic concern only for patients undergoing shoulder surgery; however, it is actually a greater concern for patients having back surgery in the prone position.

Regional Versus General Anesthesia

Many factors must be considered before choosing a given anesthetic technique, including the patient's medical history, the procedure, the anticipated length of the procedure, the intraoperative position of the patient, the likelihood of significant blood loss, medications the patient is receiving, the experience of the anesthesiologist, and the patient's consent. Selection of the best anesthetic for any given patient and any given procedure is fraught with complexity and the absence of clear outcome data to legitimize the choice.

An issue of considerable interest and importance to orthopaedic anesthesiologists and their patients involves the selection of regional and/or general anesthesia. Regional anesthesia is well suited to the needs of many patients undergoing orthopaedic surgery. Carefully conducted regional anesthesia avoids the need for airway instrumentation, provides excellent postoperative analgesia, has a lesser incidence of nausea and vomiting, provides sympathetic blockade, allows communication with the patient, and facilitates recovery. Regional techniques also have problems and limitations, and they may be absolutely or relatively contraindicated (Outline 1).

Spinal and epidural anesthesia clearly are associated with significantly less blood loss than general anesthesia for a number of procedures including total hip arthroplasty. Perioperative thromboembolic complications (deep venous thrombosis/pulmonary thromboembolism) are fewer in patients receiving regional anesthesia, particularly in patients undergoing total hip or knee arthroplasty. However, because the studies establishing these

Outline 1. Preoperative assessment for regional anesthesia

Relative Contraindications

Progressive neurologic disease (for example, multiple sclerosis)
Aortic or mitral valve stenosis (central neural blockade)
Severe or unstable psychiatric disease
Severe emotional instability
Clotting disorders (uncompensated)

Medical Conditions That May Affect Anesthetic Choice

Stable preexisting neurologic disease (for example, documented peripheral neuropathy, cerebral vascular accident)
Diabetes mellitus
Medications (for example, antihypertensives and antiplatelet drugs)
Cardiovascular disease
Stable psychiatric and/or emotional disorders

(Reproduced with permission from Prithvi R P (ed): *Clinical Practice of Regional Anesthesia.* New York, Churchill Livingstone, 1991, p 512.)

claims were conducted mostly with patients who received no pharmacologic antithrombotic prophylaxis, they are difficult to interpret in contemporary practice. Regional anesthesia has been associated with decreased hospital stays and lower costs in some studies, but only in high-risk patients. Postoperative cognitive performance (except shortly after the procedure) does not differ between patients who have received regional or general anesthesia.

Regional anesthesia does profoundly alter the "stress" response to surgery, but the clinical significance of this alteration remains to be fully elucidated. The metabolic and endocrinologic response to surgery is markedly reduced by regional anesthesia in comparison to most forms of general anesthesia. Despite these differences, cardiovascular outcome has been shown to be similar after regional or general anesthesia except in high-risk patients in whom a combination of the two techniques may be beneficial. Mortality has not been shown to differ significantly between matched patients receiving regional or general anesthesia for hip fracture surgery. Regional anesthesia is often selected for patients with pulmonary disease to avoid intubation (a potent stimulus of bronchospasm) and the respiratory depression associated with general anesthesia. Some studies suggest improved perioperative pulmonary function with regional techniques but no major differences are proven.

Local Anesthetics

Local anesthetics are drugs that block the generation and propagation of impulses in excitable tissues. Their site of action is probably specific receptors inside cells associated with sodium channels. Local anesthetics are broadly classified into two main groups, esters and amides, based on the composition of the intermediate chain between the lipophilic benzene ring and the hydrophilic quaternary amine. Considerable differences exist between local anesthetics regarding potency, solubility, protein binding, expected duration, and toxicity. Table 2 lists several important clinical features of commonly used local anesthetics.

Table 2. Clinical features of commonly used local anesthetics

Local Anesthetics	Usual Clinical Uses*‡	Usual Concentrations (%)	Duration	Maximum (Minutes) Dose (mg)+
Esters				
2-chloroprocaine	I	1	30-60	1000**
	P	2	30-60	1000**
	E	2-3	30-90	1000**
Procaine	I	1	30-60	1000
	P	1-2	30-60	1000
	S	10	30-60	200
Tetracaine	T	2	30-60	80
	S	0.5	120-240	20
Amides				
Bupivacaine	P	0.25-0.5	4-12 hrs	200**
	E	0.25-0.75	120-240	200**
	S	0.75	120-240	20
Etidocaine	P	0.5-1	3-12 hrs	300**
	E	1-1.5	120-240	300**
Lidocaine	T	4	30-60	500**
	I	0.5-1	60-120	500**
	IV	0.25-0.5		500
	P	1-1.5	60-180	500**
	E	1-2	60-120	500**
	S	5	30-90	100
Mepivacaine	P	1-1.5	120-180	500**
	E	1-2	60-190	500**
Prilocaine	IV	0.25-0.5		600
	P	1.5-2	90-180	600
	E	1-3	60-150	600

*I = Infiltration, P = Peripheral Nerve Blocks, E = Epidural, S = Spinal,
T = Topical, IV = Intravenous
+General guide (for adults). Multiple factors influence this figure.
‡May cause methemoglobinemia when dose exceeds 600 mg.
**Plus epinephrine

Regional Anesthesia Techniques

A wide range of techniques are available for delivery of regional anesthesia but the techniques most commonly used are spinal and epidural anesthesia (also termed "central neural blockade" or "major regional" anesthesia), peripheral nerve blocks, and intravenous regional anesthesia.

Preparation for Regional Anesthesia

Well-conducted regional anesthesia is safe and efficacious. However, life-threatening events can occur, with disastrous complications, if preparation is inadequate. An intravenous line should be in place, and equipment must be immediately available and functional for full resuscitation from possible complications, including cardiopulmonary arrest. Patient monitoring should include electrocardiographic and blood pressure monitoring. Pulse oximetry is also highly recommended, particularly if intravenous sedation is administered. With increasing blood levels of local anesthetic, a continuum of patient responses occurs. Grand mal seizures and cardiac arrest are the most common serious side effects associated with toxic local anesthetic concentrations. Cardiac arrest caused by systemic local anesthetic toxicity may be extremely refractory to therapy (especially when bupivacaine is the anesthetic agent), and resuscitative efforts should be prolonged under these circumstances. Avoidance of catastrophic complications is aided by epinephrine-containing test doses, frequent aspiration as the needle is advanced, and incremental dosing. Maximum recommended doses should be known and must not be exceeded.

Spinal Anesthesia

Spinal anesthesia is induced by injecting local anesthetic into the cerebrospinal fluid in the subarachnoid space (usually in the lumbar area). Advantages include technical ease, profound anesthesia, avoidance of local anesthetic toxicity from systemic absorption because of low total dose of the drug, rapid onset, and a high rate of success. Spinal anesthesia may be performed as a single injection, or an intrathecal catheter may be used to facilitate a procedure of longer duration or allow titration of local anesthetic to the minimal dermatome required surgically. Narcotics may be introduced into the subarachnoid space as well, most often for postoperative pain management, but intrathecal catheters are usually not appropriate for extended postoperative use.

Complications of spinal anesthesia include hypotension, which is caused most commonly by vasodilation associated with sympathetic blockade; postdural puncture headache ("spinal" headache), which increases in likelihood with larger needles and younger patient age; and "high" or total spinal, which may have significant cardiopulmonary consequences. Back pain occurs with equal frequency after spinal or general anesthesia, and neurologic sequelae are extremely rare.

Epidural Anesthesia

Epidural anesthesia is induced by placing local anesthetic into the epidural space, usually in the lumbar area. Epidural anesthesia has certain advantages over spinal anesthesia. Unless the dura is punctured unintentionally, there is no risk of postdural puncture headache. The epidural space is well suited to catheter placement for continuous techniques, and the catheter may remain in place for several days to manage postsurgical pain. The hemodynamic effects are slower in onset and may be less profound. Compared with spinal anesthesia, disadvantages of epidural anesthesia include a greater risk of local anesthetic toxicity because of large volumes and/or intravascular injection, greater risk of "total" spinal resulting from inadvertent subarachnoid injection of a large volume, less profound anesthesia and relaxation, slower onset of anesthesia, and increased technical difficulty. Epidural anesthesia may be used in conjunction with general anesthesia; this technique is increasing in popularity, especially in high-risk patients.

Peripheral Nerve Blocks

Peripheral nerve blocks involve less physiologic trespass than commonly is associated with general anesthesia or central neural blockade. A variety of brachial plexus blocks are very useful for upper extremity anesthesia. Axillary blocks, which are most common, are performed by injecting local anesthetic into the fibrous sheath that surrounds the axillary artery. Numerous techniques have been described including seeking paresthesias, use of an electrical nerve stimulator, transarterial injection, and sheath techniques, whereby the neurovascular bundle is identified by a change in tissue consistency. The major risks associated with axillary blocks include neurologic injury, which can result in persistent paresthesias, and local anesthetic toxicity caused by an overly large dose or unintentional intravascular injection.

The brachial plexus also may be blocked by an interscalene or supraclavicular approach. Interscalene blocks are well suited for shoulder surgery. Spinal or epidural injection of local anesthetic is a risk as is local anesthetic toxicity, especially after inadvertent direct injection into the vertebral artery. Supraclavicular blocks are efficacious in providing anesthesia for elbow surgery. The most common complication of supraclavicular blocks is pneumothorax, with an incidence of approximately 1%, depending mostly on the experience of the practitioner. Interscalene and supraclavicular blocks often block the phrenic nerve as well, and the patient may report the sensation of dyspnea.

Lower extremity nerve blocks may also be performed although, except for ankle blocks, they are less common. This is partially because of the safety and efficacy of spinal and epidural anesthesia for lower extremity surgery.

Intravenous Regional Anesthesia

Intravenous regional anesthesia (Bier block) is simple and popular. It is accomplished by exsanguinating an extremity, inflating a tourniquet, and injecting relatively large volumes of local anesthetic intravenously. The major risk associated with the procedure is systemic anesthetic toxicity caused by inadequate function or early deflation of the tourniquet.

Management of the Patient With a Difficult Airway

Many candidates for orthopaedic surgery have an increased anesthetic risk because of the presence of a difficult anatomic airway. Congenital anomalies of the face and/or neck can be seen in children who will undergo extremity or back surgery. Orthopaedic trauma may be associated with injuries to the cervical spine and face. Patients with major traumatic injuries have a 1.5% to 3% risk of associated cervical spine trauma. Ankylosing spondylitis or rheumatoid arthritis can affect the cervical spine, jaw, and larynx. Unanticipated airway difficulty occurs with an incidence of 0.5% to 13%. Formulas proposed for preoperative prediction of this problem based on physical examination have proven to have poor sensitivity.

Patients with advanced ankylosing spondylitis may have complete ankylosis of the cervical spine and are at increased risk for cervical spine fractures that may result in significant neurologic dysfunction. These fractures can occur during routine intubation. Although regional anesthesia is not contraindicated in the patient with a difficult airway, it may be harder to accomplish because of difficulty in positioning the patient for the block or because of associated bony or cartilaginous changes associated with the underlying condition.

Prevention of complications in patients with airway abnormalities requires anticipation of the problem and a clear management plan for intubation, should it be necessary. When problems are anticipated, a fiber optic intubation, following appropriate upper airway anesthesia and sedation, is usually safe and successful. Other options include awake blind nasal intubation (contraindicated in patients with head trauma), retrograde wire placement, the use of intubating stylets and light wands, jet ventilation via a large bore needle inserted through the cricothyroid membrane, and, when other techniques fail, surgical cricothyrotomy or elective tracheostomy.

Spinal Surgery

Scoliosis

A thorough history and physical examination should be obtained, with particular attention given to the cardiac, respiratory, and neuromuscular systems, because the deformity may have a profound effect on the respiratory and cardiovascular systems. The thoracic cage and vertebral deformities of scoliosis may lead to reduced lung volumes, ventilation/perfusion abnormalities, reduced chest wall compliance, and increased pulmonary vascular resistance. Respiratory reserve is assessed by exercise tolerance, pulmonary function testing, and arterial blood gases. A history of hypercapnia, vital capacity less than 40% of predicted, or respiratory failure indicates poor respiratory reserve and increases the likelihood of a need for postoperative assisted ventilation.

Scoliosis also affects the cardiovascular system. Prolonged alveolar hypoxia resulting from the skeletal deformities eventually causes irreversible pulmonary vasoconstriction, pulmonary hypertension, and cor pulmonale. The echocardiogram is more sensitive than the electrocardiogram in detecting cardiopulmonary abnormalities. Echocardiography may also be used to determine the presence of mitral value prolapse, which is reported to be present in as many as 25% of patients with idiopathic scoliosis.

Anesthetic considerations in orthopaedic surgery for scoliosis include management of a patient in the prone position, hypothermia secondary to a long procedure with an extensive exposed surgical site, maintenance of spinal cord integrity, and replacement of blood and fluid losses. In addition to the usual anesthetic monitors, an arterial line is placed for direct blood pressure measurement and blood gas assessment. A central venous catheter (or a pulmonary artery catheter in patients with significant cardiopulmonary disease) may be useful in evaluating blood and fluid management and can be used to aspirate air should venous air embolism occur. Because the surgical incision is higher than the heart, a precardial Doppler may be used to detect venous air embolism.

A nitrous oxide-narcotic-relaxant technique is most commonly used for maintenance of anesthesia. Supplementation with low concentrations of volatile anesthetics will maintain normotension, reduce narcotic requirements, and allow satisfactory interpretation of somatosensory evoked potentials (SSEPs). Narcotics may be administered by either bolus or continuous infusion. A continuous narcotic infusion may reduce intraoperative narcotic requirements by 50% and results in a smoother and more rapidly achievable wake-up test. Neuromuscular blockade is monitored with a nerve stimulator. Supplemental doses of muscle relaxants are given, based on twitch height, to prevent overdosage and enable reversal during the wake-up test.

Blood loss during spinal instrumentation and fusion usually necessitates perioperative transfusions. The blood loss and subsequent transfusion requirements may be reduced through the use of positioning, intraoperative blood salvage, induced hypotension, and intraoperative hemodilution. Patient positioning should minimize epidural venous engorgement by freeing the abdomen. Subcutaneous infiltration of 1:500,000 epinephrine before skin incision reduces skin bleeding. Preoperative donation of autologous blood and infusion of crystalloid to reduce the hematocrit to 25% to 28% (normovolemic hemodilution) decreases blood viscosity and enhances organ blood flow.

Moderate induced hypotension (reduction of systolic pressure 20 mm Hg from baseline or lowering mean arterial pressure to 65 mm Hg in the normotensive patient) has been shown to decrease blood loss, reduce transfusion requirements by 50%, and shorten operating times. However, induced hypotension is not without risk and may cause spinal cord ischemia and neurologic deficits, particularly in the setting of preoperative hypertension, hypocapnia, anemia, rapid decrease in blood pressure, and intraoperative mean arterial pressure less than 60 mm Hg.

Hypotension should be induced before surgical incision and should be achieved gradually. The various agents used to induce hypotension include trimethaphan, nitroglycerine, sodium nitroprusside, halothane, enflurane, and isoflurane. The volatile agents provide anesthesia as well as hypotension. Enflurane and isoflurane have fewer myocardial depressant effects, decrease systemic vascular resistance to a greater extent, and are less arrhythmogenic than halothane. However, all volatile anesthetics produce a dose-dependent deterioration of somatosensory evoked potential (SSEP) waveforms. Sodium nitroprusside produces a reliable decrease in blood pressure and, at least initially, increases spinal cord blood flow, but it may be associated with tolerance, tachyphylaxis, toxicity, and rebound hypertension. Nitroglycerin maintains or increases spinal cord blood flow, but it may be ineffective in achieving target blood pressure. Pretreatment with a β-blocker such as propranol (0.06 mg/kg) or an angiotensin-converting enzyme inhibitor can prevent rebound hypertension and reflex tachycardia and reduce dose requirements and toxicity for intravenous hypotensive agents. Blood pressure is allowed to recover gradually at the end of the procedure to prevent reactionary hemorrhage.

Paraplegia is one of the most feared complications of spinal surgery. It is, therefore, essential that intraoperative compromise of spinal cord function be detected and reversed as early as possible. The two methods used to detect spinal cord compromise are the wake-up test and SSEP monitoring.

The wake-up test consists of the intraoperative awakening of patients after completion of spinal instrumentation. Ideally, the surgeon should notify the anesthesiologist 30 to 45 minutes in advance. During this period of time, the volatile anesthetic is discontinued and the patient is gradually allowed to awaken. No bolus of narcotic or muscle relaxant should be given during this time. Awakening is accomplished by withdrawing the nitrous oxide. The patient is then asked to move both hands, and after a positive response, both feet. Patients will usually respond within five minutes. If there is satisfactory movement of the hands, but not the feet, distraction on the rod is released one notch, and the wake-up test is repeated.

To date, there have been no false-negative wake-up results; no patient who was neurologically intact when awakened intraoperatively had a neurologic deficit on completion of the procedure. However, certain hazards of the wake-up test do exist, including recall, pain, rod dislocation, and accidental extubation or removal of intravenous or arterial lines. In addition, because the wake-up test requires patient cooperation, it may be difficult to perform on young children or mentally deficient individuals.

An adjunct or alternative to the wake-up test is the monitoring of SSEPs. Spinal cord function is continuously monitored by measuring the cortical or subcortical response to a peripheral sensory stimulus. Somatosensory stimulation of peripheral nerves follows the dorsal column pathways of vibration and proprioception. These sensory pathways are supplied by the posterior spinal artery, leaving the motor pathway, which is supplied by the anterior spinal artery, unmonitored. Because of this, some potential exists for postoperative paraplegia in a patient with preserved intraoperative SSEP monitoring.

A number of variables are known to alter the amplitude and latency of SSEP waveforms, including hypercarbia, hypoxia, hypotension, and hypothermia. All of the volatile anesthetic agents produce a dose-related decrease in the amplitude and an increase in the latency of cortical SSEPs. However, effective SSEP recording and interpretation can usually be accomplished if the concentration of the volatile anesthetics is limited to 0.5% to 1.0% expired concentration.

Acute alterations in SSEP amplitude or latency signify spinal cord compromise and may be the result of direct trauma, ischemia, compression, or hematoma. Should changes occur, it is recommended that surgery stop, blood pressure be returned to normal, and volatile agents be decreased. Arterial blood gases may be drawn to rule out a metabolic derangement. A wake-up test is often performed at this time to corroborate the high incidence of false-positive SSEPs or to definitely exclude neurologic deficits.

Most spinal fusion patients can be extubated immediately after the operation if preoperative pulmonary function tests and neurologic status were acceptable. Aggressive postoperative pulmonary care, including incentive spirometry, is necessary to avoid atelectasis and pneumonia. Careful monitoring of systemic and central venous pressures, urine output, and wound drainage is essential. Neurologic status must also be monitored closely for deterioration.

Degenerative Vertebral Column Disease

Although thoracolumbar laminectomy is usually performed prone, cervical laminectomy is performed in the prone, lateral, or sitting position. Patients undergoing this procedure should be assessed preoperatively for cervical range of motion and for the presence of neurologic symptoms during flexion, extension, or rotation. Only positions that do not produce pain or paresthesias should be used during induction, intubation, and surgery. Awake fiberoptic intubation may be necessary in patients with severely limited cervical movement.

Both general and regional anesthesia can be safely administered for lower thoracic and lumbar surgery. Some anesthesiologists and surgeons prefer to use spinal anesthesia; typically, a hypobaric solution is used. If the myelogram is done just before surgery, the spinal anesthetic may be administered through the same needle after the contrast medium is removed. Advocates of regional anesthesia maintain that this type of anesthesia reduced blood loss and improves operating conditions by shrinking epidural veins. If a regional technique is used, a local anesthetic of sufficient duration must be selected. Should surgery last longer than the regional block, conversion to general anesthesia is difficult. The majority of spine surgery, however, is performed under general endotracheal anesthesia. General anesthesia is preferred for essentially all thoracic and cervical procedures because of the high spinal level that would be required with a regional technique. In addition, general anesthesia ensures airway access, is associated with greater patient acceptance, and can be used for lengthy operations.

Pediatric Considerations

The pediatric population undergoing orthopaedic surgery presents many challenges to the orthopaedic anesthesiologist. In many instances, these patients have concomitant medical problems. Congenital abnormalities are often multiple, and trauma may be multisystem and require special consideration regarding anesthetic management.

Precise calculation of drug dosages, fluid replacement, and ventilator settings are of particular importance in treating children, and these generally are calculated on a weight basis. For this reason, it is imperative that all children be accurately weighed preoperatively. In addition, many pediatric procedures are done on an outpatient basis and need special preoperative and postoperative instructions and care.

Perioperative fluid management is extremely important in the pediatric age group. Recent data regarding the length of preoperative fasting have shown that children who receive no oral fluids for many hours can develop hypoglycemia. Current recommendations are as follows: on the night before surgery, no solid food, formula, or milk is given after midnight. Breast feeding and the ingestion of clear fluids, including water, apple juice, clear broth, and ice popsicles, may be continued up to two to three hours preoperatively.

Hourly maintenance fluid requirements are calculated as described in Table 3. Fluid deficits are calculated and administered as in Outline 2. The blood volume also should be estimated. In neonates this varies, but a general figure of about 80 ml/kg is accepted. It is important in assessing the need to transfuse blood. An ongoing blood loss of greater than 10% of the estimated blood volume should alert the anesthesiologist to consider transfusion. Any other operative blood losses (for example, from insensible loss if an abdomen is open) can be replaced by infusion of a colloid (such as albumin) or by infusion of a greater volume of a crystalloid solution.

Fluid overload is a complication that can occur, especially postoperatively. The use of an appropriate hourly fluid schedule, mini drippers, or infusion pumps may help avoid hypervolemia.

Regional Techniques

Regional anesthesia, once rarely used in the pediatric age group, is increasingly popular. Children often tolerate regional anesthesia well, especially with appropriate sedation. Regional anesthesia may also be used as an adjunct to general anesthesia (permitting, for example, avoidance of narcotics and thereby reducing the incidence of postoperative vomiting) and to provide postoperative analgesia. Any appropriate block may be used, but the most common are caudal anesthesia (using local anesthetics) for procedures below the umbilicus, and epidural anesthesia with narcotics and/or local anesthetics for other surgery, especially if continuous analgesia is

Table 3. Calculation of maintenance intravenous fluids

Weight	Calculated Hourly Requirements*
Up to 10 kg	4 ml/kg/hr
10-20 kg	40 ml + 2 ml/kg/hr above 10 kg
>20 kg	60 ml + 1 ml/kg/hr above 20 kg

*For a 13-kg child (40 + 3 kg x 2 ml/kg/hr = 6) = 46 ml/hr

Outline 2. Fluid deficit

The fluid deficit is calculated as follows: hours since nothing by mouth x hourly maintenance

Replace one-half the calculated deficit + maintenance in first hour

Replace one-fourth deficit + maintenance in each of the next two hours

required. Axillary blocks also provide good postoperative analgesia for upper-limb surgery.

Upper Respiratory Infections

A frequent dilemma in pediatric anesthesia involves the child who comes in for surgery with a possible upper respiratory infection. The history of the illness is important in the differentiation between an infectious or allergic cause of the "runny" nose. Studies show that the incidence of complications after anesthesia in children with upper respiratory infections is minimal for short procedures that do not require endotracheal intubation, but there may be an increased incidence of perioperative morbidity if endotracheal anesthesia is administered (for example, oxygen desaturation and more serious infections). Thus, it may be appropriate to cancel an elective case if an upper respiratory infection is present and endotracheal intubation is required.

Temperature Maintenance

Children lose heat quickly, especially from the head. Operating rooms should be warmed prior to pediatric surgery and measures should be taken to reduce heat loss during the procedure (for example, the head should be covered, anesthetic gases humidified, blood and fluids warmed, etc).

Postoperative Apnea in Premature Infants

All infants aged less than 44 weeks postconceptual age and premature infants (born less than 37 weeks gestation and at surgery aged less than 50 weeks postconceptual age) require admission for overnight observation for apnea after both general and regional anesthesia.

Outpatient Anesthesia

Outpatient procedures represent a large and increasing percentage of all orthopaedic surgical cases. A variety of anesthetic techniques may be used alone or in combination to provide the rapid, smooth emergence from anesthesia that is necessary for surgery in this setting.

Local and regional anesthesia, often with light intravenous sedation, offer several advantages in outpatient surgery, including shorter discharge times and excellent postoperative analgesia. For upper extremity procedures, a brachial plexus block, using the axillary approach, is performed simply and avoids the potential complications of interscalene and supraclavicular blocks, which include phrenic nerve block and pneumothorax. For lower extremity surgery, central neural blockade, including subarachnoid (spinal) and epidural techniques are used most commonly. Ankle blocks and a variety of individual peripheral nerve blocks (femoral, lateral femoral, cutaneous, sciatic) may also be used. Intravenous regional anesthesia is useful for short procedures, such as upper extremity fracture reduction, especially in children.

Short and intermediate acting local anesthetics are most appropriate for outpatient surgery, as prolonged motor block is usually undesirable. Lidocaine, mepivacaine, and chloroprocaine are commonly used for epidural and peripheral nerve blocks. Lidocaine is the preferred agent for outpatient subarachnoid (spinal) block, and it is also the most popular intravenous regional agent. Back pain in association with epidural chloroprocaine has been reported and has led to reduction in its use.

Many outpatient orthopaedic procedures are performed under general anesthesia as well. Drugs that are rapidly redistributed and metabolized, allowing rapid return of cognitive function, are optimal. Of the intravenous agents, short-acting barbiturates such as thiopental and methohexital are useful induction agents. Nonbarbiturates, such as propofol and the short acting benzodiazepine midazolam, can be used both as induction agents and as adjuvants in anesthetic maintenance. The narcotics fentanyl and alfentanil have short half lives and are well suited for outpatient surgery. Short-acting muscle relaxants, such as succinylcholine and newly available mivacurium, as well as intermediate acting relaxants, such as vecuronium and atracurium, may facilitate endotracheal intubation and provide surgical relaxation. Finally, relatively insoluble inhalational anesthetics such as nitrous oxide and isoflurane allow rapid awakening. The newer volatile anesthetic agents sevoflurane and desflurane are less soluble than isoflurane (their solubility is comparable to that of nitrous oxide) and may prove advantageous in the outpatient setting.

Criteria for safe discharge from the outpatient surgical unit have been described (Outline 3). In a large study of outpatient orthopaedic procedures, the most common reason for hospital admission was postoperative pain. Narcotics are useful for pain control but can cause nausea and vomiting. Local anesthetics can provide profound anesthesia with minimal side effects. For knee arthroscopy, intra-articular bupivacaine is effective in reducing postoperative pain. Instillation of local anesthetics directly into the surgical wound has also proven useful in some situations.

Susceptibility to Malignant Hyperthermia

Malignant hyperthermia (MH) is a rare clinical syndrome characterized by hypermetabolism and is triggered by specific anesthetic agents. This abnormal reaction is caused by uncontrolled calcium flux in the skeletal muscles, which results in a variable clinical syndrome of muscle rigidity, respiratory and metabolic acidosis, and elevation of temperature. The specific genetic defect underlying this condition has not been identified in humans, although in susceptible swine, a mutation of the gene for the ryanodine receptor, a large protein that comprises the calcium channel in the sarcoplasmic reticulum, recently has been identified. Inheritance in humans appears to be autosomal dominant with variable penetrance. Patients with MH rarely have physical or laboratory signs of muscle disease. However, scattered case reports and investigations of individuals with known myopathies and other muscle-related problems, such as acute rhabdomyolysis or idiopathic persistently elevated creatine kinase, suggest a possible association of MH with a variety of neuromuscular diseases and stress syndromes. This association is very strong in the case of central core disease (CCD), where it is supported by clinical and laboratory evidence, including the proximity of the CCD gene to the ryanodine receptor gene on chromosome 19. A variety of other diseases have been implicated and can be classified as possibly associated (King-Denborough syndrome, Duchenne muscular dystrophy) or unlikely to be associated (myotonia congenita, sudden infant death syndrome, limb girdle dystrophy, neuroleptic malignant syndrome). The purported increased incidence of MH in the population undergoing orthopaedic surgery is probably coincidental. A suggested association of susceptibility in children with scoliosis or clubbed feet has not been supported by careful epidemiologic studies.

The clinical syndrome is triggered by exposure to the potent volatile anesthetic gases (halothane, isoflurane, enflurane) and the depolarizing muscle relaxant, succinylcholine. It is characterized by marked variability in presentation and severity of symptoms. The classic fulminant case is rapid in onset following anesthetic induction with early evidence of severe acidosis, hypermetabolism, and elevation of temperature. Improved intraoperative monitoring has resulted in earlier diagnosis of MH episodes, sometimes at a stage when symptoms are mild and no temperature elevation has occurred. Although a family history of MH can be elicited preoperatively in some affected individuals, many patients with MH give no family history and have had previous triggering anesthetics without problems. Surgical patients with known MH are managed with nontriggering anesthetics and careful monitoring in the intraoperative and postoperative periods. Local anesthetics and a variety of nontriggering general anesthetic agents are safe for affected individuals. An acute MH episode is treated symptomatically with cooling and reversal of the acidosis. However, the cornerstone of therapy is the early administration of intravenous dantrolene sodium at doses of 2 to 10 mg/kg.

MH susceptibility can be diagnosed in centers that perform contracture testing with halothane and caffeine on fresh muscle strips from a vastus lateralis or rectus muscle biopsy. Other noninvasive or blood tests do not reliably predict susceptibility at this time.

Postoperative Pain Management

Over the past several years, it has become increasingly apparent that postoperative pain management plays an important role in duration of hospitalization and associated costs, patient satisfaction, and, ultimately, morbidity and mortality. The neurohumeral response to surgical stress and postoperative pain serves no useful purpose and can significantly contribute to increases in myocardial work, respiratory compromise, decreased gastrointestinal and genitourinary function, and a host of hormonal changes that result in altered metabolism and fluid disturbances.

Traditionally delivered intramuscular narcotics, given every three to four hours, produce wide swings in blood levels of these drugs, and the patient alternates between somnolence and respiratory depression and significant pain. In addition, interpatient variation in minimum effective blood levels varies up to sevenfold, making standard doses of parenteral narcotics near-toxic for some and totally ineffective in relieving the pain of others.

Efforts to improve postoperative pain management have centered on methods to minimize these cyclical variations by providing continuous delivery or intermittent patient-controlled doses based on need. New microprocessor-controlled delivery systems allow the patient to take some responsibility for administering the medications when needed, and also allow the physician to set limits on the frequency and the total dose available. The most frequently encountered problems with these patient-controlled analgesia (PCA) systems involve inadequate prescribing practices by physicians. It is necessary to achieve an adequate blood level of the narcotics to provide pain relief. If an initial bolus is omitted or if dosage intervals are too long, the patient may be uncomfortable for a longer period of time than is acceptable until this blood level is reached. In general, concerns about patients becoming drug addicts when given "free access" to narcotics in this manner are unfounded. Many patients will actually use less medication when using a PCA system than with the traditional IM delivery, and most patients will wean themselves within a few days.

A large number of patients undergoing orthopaedic surgery will have regional anesthetics. Many of these anesthetics are given using continuous infusion techniques that also can be used in the postoperative period and may be ideal for those patients for whom narcotics may not be advisable. Typically, the goal is to provide somatic pain relief, but limit the degree of motor block by adjusting the concentration and dose of the anesthetic adminis-

tered. With epidural infusions, the inclusion of a small amount of narcotic in the local anesthetic solution provides pain relief superior to that provided by either drug alone and has been shown to result in significantly less motor block (from the local anesthetic) and respiratory depression (from the narcotic) than occur with infusions of single drugs. Urinary retention may occur with either drug, and can be effectively treated by placing an indwelling bladder catheter for the two to three days that these infusions are maintained.

Continuous brachial plexus blocks can be administered by placing an indwelling catheter into the fibrous sheath surrounding the neurovascular bundle. These blocks are used to provide pain relief for patients requiring continuous passive motion devices and to provide sympathetic blockade to patients having replantation or revascularization of digits.

Ketoralac, a nonsteroidal anti-inflammatory agent given intramuscularly, has had great success in the treatment of postoperative pain. Studies have shown 30 to 90 mg intramuscular doses of ketoralac to be as effective as 6 to 12 mg of morphine in an acute pain setting, and ketoralac causes less nausea, vomiting, and drowsiness.

Annotated Bibliography

Preoperative Evaluation

Roizen MF: Preoperative evaluation, in Miller RD (ed): *Anesthesia*, ed 3. New York, Churchill Livingstone, 1990, pp 743-772.

The author presents a comprehensive review of the subject, including factors influencing risk, laboratory screening, medicolegal matters, and the implementation of change for improvement.

Positioning

Martin JT: *Positioning in Anesthesia and Surgery*, ed 2. Philadelphia, WB Saunders, 1987.

A comprehensive review of positioning for surgery with contributions from both anesthesiologists and surgeons. This volume includes a discussion of the physiologic alterations associated with posture changes as well as a number of excellent illustrations.

Regional Versus General Anesthesia

Yeager MP, Glass DD, Neff RK, et al: Epidural anesthesia and analgesia in high-risk surgical patients. *Anesthesiology* 1987;66:729-736.

A sentinel study showing that a combination of regional and general anesthesia may lower morbidity, mortality, and cost in high-risk patients.

Regional Anesthesia Techniques

Brown DL, Wedel DJ: Spinal, epidural and caudal anesthesia, in Miller RD (ed): *Anesthesia*, ed 3. New York, Churchill Livingstone, 1990, pp 1377-1402.

An excellent review of central neural blockade, including clinically relevant information about the techniques, local anesthetic pharmacology, and contraindications.

Wedel DJ, Brown DL: Nerve blocks, in Miller RD (ed): *Anesthesia*, ed 3. New York, Churchill Livingstone, 1990, pp 1407-1436.

A similarly excellent review of pertinent information regarding a wide variety of nerve blocks, including those that are less commonly performed. Diagrams effectively show a variety of techniques.

Management of the Patient With a Difficult Airway

Benumof JL: Management of the difficult adult airway: With special emphasis on awake tracheal intubation. *Anesthesiology* 1991;75:1087-1110.

An exhaustive review of airway management techniques, including recognition of the difficult airway, patient preparation, choice of tracheal intubation technique, and management of the unanticipated difficult airway.

Hastings RH, Marks JD: Airway management for trauma patients with potential cervical spine injuries. *Anesth Analg* 1991;73:471-482.

Mechanisms of the traumatic spine injury including physical and radiologic examination and methods of stabilization are reviewed. The authors emphasize airway management techniques and propose a case-specific strategy for tracheal intubation.

Spinal Surgery

Patel NJ, Patel BS, Paskin S, et al: Induced moderate hypotensive anesthesia for spinal fusion and Harrington-rod instrumentation. *J Bone Joint Surg* 1985;67A:1384-1387.

Moderate hypotensive anesthesia (systolic blood pressure 20-30 mm Hg below baseline) induced with enflurane reduced the average blood loss by 40% and the need for transfusion by nearly 45% in patients undergoing Harrington-rod instrumentation. Average operating time was shortened by 10%. There were no complications attributable to anesthetic technique.

Pediatric Considerations

Coté CJ: NPO after midnight for children: A reappraisal, comment. *Anesthesiology* 1990;72:589-592.

This editorial reexamines the need for withholding fluids from midnight the night before surgery. The risks of hypoglycemia in children are discussed as well as risks of aspiration of stomach contents. The discussion leads to a more moderate approach to nothing by mouth (NPO) orders for children, allowing clear fluids up to three hours before surgery.

Outpatient Anesthesia

Kinnard P, Lirette R: Outpatient orthopedic surgery: A retrospective study of 1996 patients. *Can J Surg* 1991;34:363-366.

A large retrospective review of outpatient orthopaedic surgical procedures. The unanticipated hospital admission rate was 6.3% and the complication rate was 1.3% with no life-threatening complication. Preoperative evaluation and safe discharge criteria are discussed.

Wetchler BV (ed): *Anesthesia for Ambulatory Surgery*, ed 2. Philadelphia, JB Lippincott, 1991.

This book is a reference book for anesthesia and ambulatory surgery. It contains detailed sections on patient selection, local and regional anesthesia, complications, and discharge criteria.

Susceptibility to Malignant Hyperthermia

Brownell AK: Malignant hyperthermia: Relationship to other diseases. *Br J Anaesth* 1988;60:303-308.

A review of malignant hyperthermia and its possible association with other neuromuscular diseases. The author classifies the relationship as likely or unlikely, based on a review of the literature.

Larach MG: Standardization of the caffeine halothane muscle contracture test. North American Hyperthermia Group. *Anesth Analg* 1989;69:511-515.

A description of the North American protocol for muscle contracture testing for malignant hyperthermia. A list of testing centers is included.

Postoperative Pain Management

Benumof JL, Oden RV (eds): *Management of Postoperative Pain, Anesthesiology Clinics of North America.* Philadelphia, WB Saunders, March 1989, vol 7, no 1.

A fairly comprehensive review of pain mechanisms, current pain practice, organization of an acute pain service, psychological factors, and outcome.

Bridenbaugh PO: Post-op pain relief: Does the technique matter? *Anesth Analg* 1992;74(suppl):35-38.

A general review of a wide variety of techniques for postoperative pain management with a practical bent. The author discusses techniques of pain management, factors that go into the choice, and potential side effects.

Yeager MP, Glass DD, Neff RK, et al: Epidural anesthesia and analgesia in high-risk surgical patients. *Anesthesiology* 1987;66:729-736.

A landmark study demonstrating the significant benefits of effective postoperative pain management in a high-risk surgical population.

18

Blood Transfusion Medicine: 1993

Blood transfusion continues its evolution as a rapidly changing treatment form of considerable importance to the orthopaedic surgeon.

Historic Perspective

The Past 50 Years

The era of modern transfusion medicine began immediately after World War II, with the advent of centers in which volunteer donors contributed blood. The product was tested, processed, and distributed to an entire community or surrounding area. These regional donor units were under the central control of the Food and Drug Administration (FDA) and either the American Association of Blood Banks (AABB) or the American Red Cross. Citrated whole blood was used almost exclusively during the first two decades. In the 1960s, the development of plastic containers, automated cell separators, and other sophisticated, ancillary technology allowed whole blood to be separated and processed into various types of red cells, plasma, platelets, cryoprecipitate, albumin, factor VIII or IX concentrate, and other derivatives. The era of component therapy started. It permitted more effective use of the blood donated by the 5% of the general population who, at that time, constituted the volunteer donor group.

The ready availability of such homologous blood components fostered the growth of much medical technology considered commonplace today: radical cancer surgery and chemotherapy; improved management of massively traumatized patients; cardiopulmonary bypass with definitive cardiovascular or thoracic procedures; and transplantation of kidney, heart, liver, and other organs. In the past decade, while overall transfusion needs increased 100%, blood collection rose a mere 30%. Meanwhile, problems with the national blood supply surfaced.

The Decade of the 1980s

As transfusion medicine grew dynamically, the education of physician users failed to keep pace. The inordinate or even inappropriate use of certain products, especially fresh frozen plasma and platelets, was obvious. In addition, the donor base had declined because of several factors. The aging of Americans had a decided negative impact on their roles as blood donors. Widespread changes in the economy included the loss of many manufacturing jobs and conversion of others to service-oriented ones. The volunteer donors had come chiefly from the manufacturing sector. Moreover, tests on donated blood for infectious disease transmissibility were added, with further loss of acceptable donors.

Most importantly of all, the discovery that the lethal retrovirus HIV-1, the causative agent of acquired immunodeficiency syndrome (AIDS), had penetrated the national blood supply brought to an end the period of seemingly inexhaustible amounts of safe, relatively inexpensive homologous blood. The public began to question seriously the safety of existing transfusion practices, putting medicine on the defensive. Through July 1990, in the United States, 140,822 cases of AIDS in adults and adolescents had been reported. Although the majority of infection occurred through sexual or drug usage routes, 4,609 individuals (3%) acquired the infection through exposure to blood products. These persons included 1,258 with hemophilia or other coagulation problems, some of whom received blood concentrates from multiple donors.

Since April 1985, when screening donors for antibody to HIV-1 became standard, transfusion-transmitted HIV-1 infection has become rare. It is estimated that the risk for contracting the virus by transfusion is now lower than one in 150,000 units transfused. Nevertheless, concern remains, because infection rates vary according to geographic locales of the donor, the "window" or period between exposure and antibody positivity is not certain, and conversion to positivity in recipients of antibody-positive blood transfusion has been shown in a recent study to be 90%. The rate of progression to AIDS within the 38 months after infection was similar to that reported for homosexual men and hemophiliacs. Lastly, AIDS has emerged as a leading cause of death among young adults in the United States in the period from 1981 to 1990.

In recent years, there has been increasing litigation stemming from adverse effects of transfusion therapy. Awards against physicians, hospitals, and blood banks have been considerable. Despite all safeguards applied from the national level downward it is apparent that significant risks may result from treatment with transfusion. For this reason, some accrediting agencies, such as the AABB, have recommended informed consent be obtained from the patient before administering blood products or derivatives. An informed-consent form would include a brief but detailed discussion of overall benefits, risks, and specific alternatives to conventional transfusion. It could even prove helpful in the management of the rare individual who refuses blood on the basis of religious convictions.

Benefits of Homologous Blood Transfusion

Benefits vary according to the blood product and are directly related to the appropriate use of each component. Criteria for proper usage have been established (Table 1). Peer reviews of the practice of transfusion medicine by each hospital medical staff are demanded by the Joint Commission on Accreditation of Healthcare Organizations as an integral part of its inspection process, which occurs every two years. In 1989, an alert, summarizing positive and negative points about the use of blood components, was issued by the National Institutes of Health in concurrence with the FDA.

Components

Homologous blood is best studied by analyzing each of the important components derived from whole blood, which is rarely used in current therapy. The most commonly transfused product is packed red blood cells. Packed red cells are usually available in a 225- to 300-ml unit, which contains most of the erythrocytes and, usually, many of the leukocytes and platelets of the original whole blood, suspended in about 60 ml of plasma. Often, 100 ml of normal saline with extra adenine has been added to increase the shelf life to 42 days. Other types of red cells that are seldom used are whole blood and frozen or washed red cells. The sole reason for transfusing red cells is to increase the oxygen-carrying capacity in a patient seriously compromised by anemia, a red cell deficit. When intravascular volume is adequate for perfusion, a hemoglobin of 7 g/dl or even less may meet the body's needs. Indeed, the new "transfusion trigger" has been decreased from the previous 10 g/dl to 7 g /dl.

The decision to transfuse red cells, even in an acute situation, depends not only on the degree and etiology of the anemia, but also on the patient's age, hemodynamic stability, and any coexisting cardiovascular or pulmonary problems. Red cells must never be transfused as volume expanders, hematinics, or enhancers of wound healing. Each type of red cell product confers on the recipient exposure to one donor. Because donor and recipient blood must be compatible, especially in the ABO system, crossmatching must be done before transfusion of any red cell components. This is done by mixing blood from the donor and the recipient and observing for compatibility in vitro.

Fresh frozen plasma contains all of the constituents of the citrated plasma derived from the original whole blood donation. The plasma is separated from the whole blood and is frozen. Usually, it is relatively cell free. All hemostatic factors are present, including procoagulant factors I through XIII; naturally occurring anticoagulants, AT III and proteins C and S; plasminogen; activators and inhibitors of coagulation and fibrinolysis; immunoglobulins; complement factors; and albumin. Fresh frozen plasma is appropriately used to correct either a discreet deficit in a hemostatic factor, like factor XI or AT III, or a global deficiency of many hemostatic factors

Table 1. Indicators for transfusion of most frequently used blood components or products

Component	Indication
Red blood cells	Increase oxygen delivery to tissues
Fresh frozen plasma (FFP)	Correct deficit in hemostasis:
	Discrete coagulation problem (Factor XI deficiency, for example)
	"Global" problem
	Systemic coagulation (DIC)
	Systemic fibrinolysis
	Miscellaneous
	AT III deficiency
	Protein C/protein S deficiency
	Plasminogen deficiency
	Coumarinized patient
	Other
Cryoprecipitate	Treat:
	Fibrinogen depletion
	Factor VIII C deficiency (Hemophilia A)
	Factor III R deficiency (Von Willebrand's disorder)
	Factor XIII deficiency
Platelets	Platelet deficiency or platelet dysfunction severe enough to be causing or contributing to significant bleeding
Albumin or purified protein factor (PPF)	Increase oncotic pressure of plasma/ increase intravascular blood volume

such as occurs in uncompensated disseminated intravascular coagulation. Its use should be monitored by proper laboratory testing, which will be dictated, in turn, by the individual case.

Each unit of fresh frozen plasma confers on the recipient one-donor exposure. Because ABO compatibility between the donor and recipient must be maintained, some variation of crossmatching usually is performed before transfusion. Fresh frozen plasma must never be used solely for volume expansion or simply as prophylaxis following multiple transfusions or cardiopulmonary bypass.

Platelets are available as random-donor or single-donor platelets. Random donor platelets contain most of the platelets and many of the leukocytes, especially lymphocytes, of the original whole blood unit, suspended in about 50 to 60 ml of citrated plasma. Small numbers of red cells are often present. Because it is often impossible to find adequate random donor platelets to maintain ABO compatibility, no crossmatching is attempted. Apheresis or one-donor product contains, in about 200 ml of donor plasma, platelets equivalent to 8 to 10 units of random donor product. All of this material is derived from one donor and confers on the recipient one-donor exposure. It often contains many of the leukocytes and some red cells from the donor. ABO compatibility must be maintained and appropriate pretransfusion testing is performed.

Platelets are administered to control or prevent clinically significant bleeding secondary to either severe thrombocytopenia or platelet dysfunction. Various factors, besides the platelet count, should be considered before platelets are administered. Platelets should never be used as pure prophylaxis following cardiopulmonary bypass or massive transfusion. It is important to note that when any product containing RhD-positive erythrocytes, even small amounts as in platelets, is administered to an RhD-negative recipient, a proper dose of Rh immune globulin must be administered within 72 hours of the transfusion to prevent allosensitization of the recipient.

Cryoprecipitate contains in a small volume (approximately 10 ml) concentrates of factors I, VIII C (antihemophiliac factor), VIII R (Von Willebrand factor), and XIII. It is used whenever there is a proven deficiency of any of these factors and small volume is needed. Each unit confers on the recipient one donor exposure. Except for small children, it is not absolutely necessary to maintain ABO compatibility.

Serum albumin and plasma protein fraction are used to increase the osmotic pressure of plasma and thereby restore decreased intravascular volume. Serum albumin contains 95% albumin; plasma protein fraction contains 83% albumin. In each product, the remainder is made up of immunoglobulins, complement factors, etc. Both are derived from multiple pooled plasmas; but, because they are pasteurized, no transfer of donor disease to the recipient has been reported.

Factor VIII (antihemophiliac factor) and factor IX (Christmas disease factor) concentrates are used to treat the congenital deficiencies of hemophilia A and B, respectively. Each is derived from multiple pooled donors and each unit confers on the recipient an incalculable number of donor exposures. Additionally, many of the pooled concentrates are manufactured using blood from donors who are paid for their plasma donations. In spite of the fact that such plasma is tested for infectious disease in the same way as is that from volunteer donors, and new modifications like heat treatment and monoclonal antibody processing are added as safety measures, the multiple-donor exposure derived from these sources has resulted in some increased disease transmission, especially in patients treated before 1985. In some series, hemophiliacs thus exposed show HIV-1 antibody positivity of 50% to 75%. Recombinant DNA factor VIII C, available at present for investigational use, should circumvent this problem, although all of the newer concentrates have added greatly to the cost of treatment of these disorders and recombinant product will probably be restricted to use in newly diagnosed cases.

Risks of Homologous Blood Transfusion

Risks of transfusion therapy are significant. The most common adverse effect, which occurs in 5% or more of all transfusions, is the febrile response, caused most often by antibodies against donor leukocytes received in previous transfusions or pregnancies. Resulting chills and fever can be severe. The patient may experience significant discomfort. The reaction can be avoided, or at least ameliorated, by the use of the newer leucocyte filters that remove 99% of donor white cells. In any patient in whom repeated transfusion will be a mainstay of treatment, the use of such special filters for red cell or platelet products is unquestionably indicated.

Although the occurrence is uncommon, an individual may sustain a nonspecific allergic reaction to one or more components in donor blood. This also produces chills, fever, and, usually, urticaria. Very rarely, especially in an IgA-deficient recipient, the allergic reaction may progress to anaphylaxis.

Because conventional pretransfusion blood typing is confined to that of the red cell antigens of ABO and RhD groups, alloimmunization to other important erythrocyte antigen systems may occur as a result of prior transfusions or of pregnancy. Compatibility testing, involving screening of donor and recipient for significant alloantibodies or autoantibodies directed against red cell antigens, and the traditional crossmatching in several phases, ensures that the donor and recipient blood are compatible at the laboratory level. In spite of all the sophisticated technology applied, however, incompatibility may occur with the actual transfusion and result in immune based hemolysis, which can be either delayed or immediate. Delayed hemolytic reactions usually happen after the patient's discharge. Although they can be severe enough to render the patient symptomatic, they are usually mild in nature and often go undetected. It has been found, however, that they often will compromise future transfusions.

Conversely, immediate hemolysis, often from small amounts of transfused blood, always elicits a serious symptom/sign complex in the patient. In one in 100,000 transfusions, such reactions are fatal. Usually, these involve ABO incompatibility generated by misidentification of the recipient or the donor. These reactions always require emergency care on the part of the transfusionist, nurse, or physician, cooperating closely with the medical director of the blood bank or transfusion service. Signs and symptoms may include chills, fever, tachycardia, pain in the chest and/or flank, dyspnea, nausea, vomiting, and, finally, bloody urine and shock. Management of a suspected hemolytic reaction should be directed at stopping the transfusion immediately; maintaining vascular access with normal saline infusion; notifying the attending physician and blood bank director; collecting posttransfusion blood and urine samples, which are sent along with intact transfusion tubing, filters, and the blood bag containing the remaining blood to the blood bank for comprehensive testing; instituting proper diuretic therapy to maintain renal output; and immediate treatment of shock and the frequent sequelae of disseminated intravascular coagulation, with compatible blood components, vasopressors, corticosteroids, etc. Such appropriate aggressive management may save the patient's life.

In recent years, the most feared adverse result of transfusion has been the transmission of an infectious disease,

Table 2. Transfusion transmitted diseases for which all blood is routinely screened

Test	Disease
Syphilis "Ab"	Syphilis
Hepatitis B Ag	Hepatitis B
Hepatitis B core Ab	Non-A, non-B hepatitis
Serum ALT (SGPT)	Non-A, non-B hepatitis
Hepatitis C Ab	Non-A, non-B hepatitis
HIV-1	AIDS
HIV-2*	AIDS
HTLV-1	Adult T-cell leukemia-lymphoma or HTLV-1 associated myelopathy (HAM)

*Started July 1992

especially AIDS. Donor blood is now routinely screened by eight infectious disease markers for the diseases listed in Table 2.

Transfusion-transmitted hepatitis is a major public health problem, worldwide. With increasingly sensitive tests for hepatitis B surface antigen, infection with this serious organism is rarely encountered in the United States. This is not true with non-A, non-B hepatitis, which by 1989 was estimated to occur with a frequency of one case per 100 units transfused. Since the mid 1980s, two screening tests for this disease in donor blood have been in place. They are the "surrogate" markers of elevated SGPT (serum ALT) and core antibody to hepatitis B. In May 1990, the more definitive antibody against hepatitis C, considered the chief, but not sole, cause of non-A, non-B hepatitis, was added. Although this infection often appears mild and may go undetected for months after transfusion, 30% of patients infected may develop chronic active hepatitis. A small but significant number of these may acquire cirrhosis leading to total hepatic failure. Liver transplantation may eventually be the only effective therapy.

Transmission of the potentially lethal retrovirus HIV-1, the causative agent of AIDS, has been considered earlier. Published current estimates of risk of acquiring this infection via transfusion are between 1:40,000 and 1:250,000 units transfused, depending on location of donation. A second etiologic agent of AIDS, HIV-2, has now been reported to have penetrated the United States blood supply. By July 31, 1991, 31 confirmed cases of HIV-2, including four in one state, had been reported to the Centers for Disease Control. Although there is some cross-reactivity of HIV-2 antibody positive blood with the exceedingly sensitive test used for antibody to HIV-1, a specific test for HIV-2 was scheduled for use on donor blood by July 1992.

Another serious retrovirus, human T-cell lymphotrophic virus type I (HTLV-1) is efficiently transmitted via blood from an infected donor. It has been linked to adult T-cell leukemia/lymphoma and to a degenerative neurologic disorder, HTLV-1 associated myelopathy (HAM) or tropical spastic paraparesis. In Japan, where the organism was endemic, there has been a strong association between HAM and prior blood transfusion. In

the United States, testing of donor blood for antibody to this organism started in January 1989. There is evidence that prevalence of antibody to HTLV-1 in donors may be as high as that of HIV-1, with which it is not related, although it is a retrovirus and can be spread by blood and sexual contacts. The first case report that directly linked blood transfusion and HAM appeared in an orthopaedic journal in November 1990.

"Look-back" procedures are those in which donors who are positive for HIV-1, HTLV-1, or hepatitis C antibody at a current donation are studied to see if they gave units before being tested. If so, previous donation records are sent to the hospital to which the blood was distributed, and attending physicians of any recipient are notified and asked to have the recipient tested for the disorder. Anonymity of both donor and recipient is maintained, but information is disseminated by the attending physician to either party as needed.

Donor blood is not routinely screened for other diseases that are easily transmitted by transfusion. These include parasitic infections, such as malaria and cytomegalovirus (CMV). Parasitic infections, in general, are an uncommon complication of transfusion in the United States. Malaria, the most frequently encountered, has been estimated to occur in the order of one infection per million transfusions. Undoubtedly, the policy of deferring blood donations from asymptomatic individuals who have been in endemic malarial areas has helped in lowering this risk. When veterans who had served in Vietnam became blood donors after their return to the United States, the incidence of transfusion-transmitted malaria rose. Anticipating a similar experience, the AABB, American Red Cross, and Council of Community Blood Centers have issued a joint statement concerning the donor status of military personnel with Persian Gulf area experience. This should avert the transmission of other rare blood parasites endemic to that area.

Babesia, toxoplasmosis, and Chagas disease are even rarer complications of transfusion in the United States. However, the incidence of Chagas' disease may be rising with the recent immigration of many Central and South Americans and Mexicans to the United States. A recent author questions whether special policies are in order to prevent contamination of the blood supply by this trypanosome. Cytomegalovirus (CMV) can be a devastating infection, especially in the frankly immunosuppressed patient or in the individual who is immunocompromised by medication, age, malignant disease, or other factors. It is good practice to give such patients, especially newborns and young children, who show no serologic evidence of previous exposure to the virus, CMV serologically negative blood.

Lastly, a less well-defined hazard, that of immunomodulation, exists for the recipient of homologous blood. In renal transplantation, the immunosuppressive effect of prior blood transfusion, which allowed better tolerance of cadaver kidneys, has been known for several years. Some increased susceptibility to severe infections in patients who have received massive blood transfusions following trauma has also been suggested. In the past seven years, moreover, comparison studies have appeared in the literature that described the survivorship of cancer patients matched for type of malignancy staging, treatment, age, sex, etc, and differing only by the presence or absence of blood transfusion in the perioperative period. Incontrovertible evidence emerges from these retrospective investigations that transfusion with homologous blood, regardless of the component used, can exert an adverse effect on survival of the cancer patient. Prospective studies to elucidate the cause of this immunomodulating effect are awaited. Another related post-transfusion event is the unlikely complication of the graft-versus-host reaction in which homologous blood T-lymphocytes literally reject the recipient and evoke a reaction that can be fatal. Most such reactions occur in the recipient who is compromised by premature birth, the posttransplant state, malignancy, or immunosuppressive drugs. These reactions also can occur in the situation in which the donor is a first-degree relative. The hazard can be obviated by appropriate irradiation of the blood before use.

Homologous blood transfusion can decrease morbidity and even save lives, but significant hazards exist. The physician user should be aware not only of the appropriate use of each product but also of the donor exposure provided by each. The term donor "dose" has been coined to convey such risk (Table 3).

Changes in the Practice of Transfusion Medicine

In recent years, the Joint Commission on Accreditation of Healthcare Organizations has demanded, as part of its accreditation process, a detailed review of appropriateness of transfusion of all blood products or derivatives in each institution. Blood banking processes are no longer scrutinized under laboratory activities, but are considered the practice of medicine with all responsibilities attendant thereon.

Reference has been made to an informed consent dedicated to blood transfusion becoming standard in the hospital practice of the near future. A recent study showed the physician user to be in need of additional education. A face-to-face survey of 122 general and orthopaedic surgeons and anesthesiologists was conducted regarding the influence of clinical knowledge, organizational context, and practice style on transfusion decision making. Widespread deficiencies were found. These involved, chiefly, a failure to appreciate transfusion risks and indications. Of the physicians surveyed, less than 50% understood risks and only 31% were knowledgeable about indications for transfusion. Attending physicians scored lower than residents. Indeed, there was a negative association between knowledge and years of practice. While the frequently used red blood cell product is of the utmost importance, the inappropriate transfusion of other compo-

Table 3. Donor "dose" or exposure risk per unit of homologous blood

Product	Donor Dose per Unit
Red blood cells	
Whole blood	1
Packed cells	1
Washed cells	1
Deglyc'ed cells	1
Platelets, random donor	1
Platelets, one donor "apheresis"	1
Fresh frozen plasma	1
Cryoprecipitate	1
Factor VIII or IX concentrate	Multiple

nents, especially platelets and fresh frozen plasma, appears to be increasing.

That the practice of transfusion medicine had already changed significantly in the past decade is suggested by a special article, published in 1990, which describes a national survey on the collection and transfusion of blood in the United States, 1982-1988. It chronicles that transfusions of various kinds of red cells peaked at 12.2 million units in 1986, declined to 11.6 million units in 1987, and continued to decline in 1988. Plasma used declined from a peak of 2.3 millions units in 1984 to 2.1 million in 1987. Growth of overall platelet use slowed somewhat after rising to 6.4 units in 1987, but the use of single-donor platelets rose from 11% in 1980 to 25% in 1987.

Growth in collection of homologous blood in general slowed after 1982. The total supply crested at 13.4 million units in 1986, but did not grow between 1986 and 1988. Autologous predeposit donations soared from fewer than 30,000 units in 1982 to 397,000 units in 1987, equivalent to 3% of homologous donations. It was concluded that the preoccupation of both the patient and physician with the AIDS epidemic had exerted widespread effects on the national blood supply, which was judged adequate throughout the period.

Alternatives

Multiple forces, then, are at play to alter even more the practice of transfusion medicine in the 1990s. Alternatives to the conventional use of homologous blood have been developed. They include directed donations in which a donor, considered safe by a prospective recipient or his family, contributes blood at the Red Cross or other licensed installation for a specific patient. At both the drawing center and hospital, such blood is handled in a manner identical to that from volunteer donors, including being tested for infectious disease transmissibility. If not distributed to the individual for whom it is intended, it is incorporated into the general blood supply. Directed donor blood is considered as safe as, but not safer than, that of volunteer donors. Indeed, some transfusion specialists believe safety is compromised somewhat by the vested interest of the prospective donor. Even though the practice does offer psychological support to the patient, it may indirectly increase the cost of blood and diminishes the blood supply by diverting donors from the general group who donate for the anonymous recipient. Directed donations remain controversial. There are fervent proponents and equally ardent antagonists. Often requests are based on emotion, rather than scientific principle. The exception is in infants and children, in whom there is a decided need to reduce the degree of donor exposure.

Another alternative being explored in some community drawing centers is that involving "pedigreed" donors. In this setting, individuals, with safety of their blood having been proven through a long period of previous donations, are chosen to give repeatedly, by automated apheresis methods, such products as platelets, fresh frozen plasma, and, rarely, granulocytes. This requires considerable dedication on the part of the donor. It includes some increased donor discomfort and time expenditure and results in a more costly product.

In general, more frugal use of all homologous blood has been emphasized. Another possibility is the use of no blood at all, especially in some clinical settings of elective surgery. For years, patients whose religious beliefs prohibit transfusion have chosen this alternative, often successfully. Pharmacologic agents such as desmopressin have also been used in some hemostatic disorders; for example, some varieties of Von Willebrand's disease or very mild hemophilia A. Certain anemias respond well to various hematinics, such as iron, folic acid, cyanocobalamins, or the recently offered recombinant erythropoietin.

The search for an effective synthetic blood substitute continues. To date, no fully satisfactory product has been obtained.

In a recent national seminar sponsored by the AABB, the inevitability of some type of informed consent dedicated to blood transfusion was discussed in detail by many professionals, including various medical disciplines, hospital administrators, and attorneys. Of all the alternatives to conventional homologous blood usage, autologous transfusion (autotransfusion) was cited as the most desirable. Indeed, the statement was made that if autotransfusion is not available in the hospital in which surgery is to be performed, but is possible in another institution in the community, the patient should probably be offered this information. In autotransfusion, the recipient and the donor are identical; many advantages follow.

Autologous blood is the only perfectly compatible blood; therefore, the possibility of immunization to foreign donor antigens, allergic reaction, graft-versus-host responses, and the other immunomodulating effects of homologous blood are avoided. It is readily available for salvage in an emergency. In addition, autologous blood conserves the stores of homologous products for the community. Most important of all, it will not transmit infectious disease from the donor to the recipient. When collected and reinfused perioperatively, it abolishes the need for compatibility testing and averts identification errors. On the disadvantage side, autologous blood may be more expensive than homologous, but this factor depends on the situation. In addition, there is a relative contraindication to the perioperative collection of autologous blood from the site of cancer surgery or overwhelming, obvious bacterial wound contamination.

Currently, comprehensive autotransfusion includes four facets—preoperative deposit plus the three types of perioperative salvage, preoperative, intraoperative, and postoperative. In the first preoperative deposit, the donor patient gives blood at a regional center preparatory to an anticipated surgical or obstetrical need. Such donations are handled exactly as are those of the volunteer donors, including testing of the blood for infectious disease, grouping, typing, etc. After processing, the blood component is sent to the hospital for later use. It is intended for the autologous patient only and, if not used, is discarded, because it is considered not strictly volunteer in origin. Such blood is usually crossmatched with the recipient before use. The indications for appropriate transfusion of predeposit autologous product are exactly the same as those for analogous homologous components. With careful planning on the part of the surgeon and patient, the blood needs of each individual can be carefully tailored and fully satisfied.

Several problems exist with predeposit. Economic ones center on the surcharge usually added to each unit at the drawing center and to the tremendous wastage of autologous blood that is not used. Under pressure from the patient, surgeons are ordering more predeposit units than would normally be requested if homologous blood were involved. Costs are consequently rising significantly. In addition, the volunteer donor base is eroded further by patients conserving their donations for their own future use. Regardless of the problems, the public's concern with safety issues is driving the growth of predeposit. It has been predicted by those knowledgeable in donor dynamics that this phase of autotransfusion will continue to expand, exceeding the growth of autologous donations of 30,000 in 1982 to 397,000 five years later. Indeed, donors with special risks of age, pregnancy, or preexisting medical conditions will be accepted for such contributions.

A recently published prospective, randomized study of elderly patients undergoing hip arthroplasty compared a predonation group of 45 individuals with 15 nondonating controls. Although the average age was 71 years, no major complications with either phlebotomy or anemia were encountered in the donor group. Moreover, perioperative blood needs were totally met by the autologous route. It was concluded that use of predeposit autologous blood in elective orthopaedics, regardless of the patient's age, is feasible, cost effective, and avoids risks associated with conventional transfusion.

It is usually recommended that special-risk donors should be monitored during and immediately after the donation, preferably in a hospital setting. Conversely, recent analysis of 5,660 preoperative autologous donations at 25 different nonhospital blood centers documented the infrequency of severe reactions even though 16% of the donors did not meet the usual criteria for safe donation. Most common variances were for cardiovascular disease. It was stressed, however, that donor patients should fully understand beforehand both the risks and benefits.

While the predeposit phase is flourishing, the major growth of autotransfusion resides in the three perioperative salvage areas. State-of-the-art technology, involving instrumentation and disposables, allows the automated recovery, processing, and reinfusion of various autologous components throughout the preoperative, intraoperative, and postoperative periods. Moreover, because this blood remains with the patient and is given immediately or within the prescribed six hours after collection, there are no rigid restrictions on its reinfusion as there are for the predeposit blood. Identification errors in this kind of transfusion are virtually nonexistent.

Autotransfusion in the immediate preoperative phase consists most commonly of platelet-rich-plasma collection. Here, the product is reserved in the operating room and given back when the patient is most in need of it, usually early in the postoperative phase. It is commonly reserved for cases in which blood losses are considerable, as in cardiovascular procedures, especially after completion of cardiopulmonary bypass.

Automated intraoperative or intratrauma salvage of autologous blood, with almost immediate reinfusion of washed red cells, has become a standard of therapy in most surgeries with significant blood loss. In the late 1970s it was confined to cardiovascular procedures and massive trauma. It has now become conventional in most cases in which homologous blood might be employed, including arthroplasties and spinal procedures.

In some situations where exsanguinating type bleeding occurs, both autologous and homologous transfusions can be used simultaneously. Such procedures may not only be life saving, they decrease the amount of donor exposure.

The remaining facet of perioperative autotransfusion occurs with postoperative salvage, especially in the two situations in which bleeding after surgery can be significant, namely after some cardiovascular operations and after joint surgery, particularly that involving the knee and hip. Several techniques are available whereby the blood drainage from the operated joint or mediastinum is collected at the bedside, processed, usually by anticoagulation and filtering, and returned to the patient. Considerable controversy about the safety of this product has been raised, especially in the orthopaedic sector where it is most commonly used. Various relatively undesirable substances, such as free hemoglobin and fibrin/fibrinogen degradation products, are present in the blood drained from a joint cavity. Some techniques of washing the red cells to provide a safer product have been reported. To date, washed red cells are not used as frequently as the unwashed. But the debate continues.

Autotransfusion in the past decade has grown almost exponentially. Special problems with cost, quality assurance, safety issues, and indications for usage remain troublesome. As one recent editorial suggests, the time is right for a national effort directed toward defining the role of autologous blood in the overall schema of transfusion medicine.

Administration of Blood Products

Several aspects of homologous blood usage in the clinical site should be considered. The quality of such transfusion depends to a large extent on meticulously establishing the identification of the recipient and on careful selection and monitoring of ancillary equipment, such as various blood filters, warmers, rapid infusion devices, and so forth.

Normal saline is the parenteral fluid of choice in the vessel in which blood products are infused. When multiple sites of vascular access are present, one dedicated to blood transfusion should be maintained with normal saline. Especially to be avoided is the use of crystalloid that contains calcium (for example, Ringer's lactate) with any blood product in which there is citrated plasma. Such practice could enhance localized coagulation in the recipient with possible development of a serious coagulopathy.

Washing homologous packed red cells before transfusion may rarely be indicated to remove excessive free hemoglobin, potassium, or other unwanted substances from the supernatant plasma of the donor. It is not an effective means of ridding the product of platelets or leukocytes and adds considerably to the cost of the component.

Special problems can arise in the treatment of the seriously traumatized patient. The inappropriate use of group O blood as "universal donor" type is common. With rare exception, as in those individuals treated on the spot or in transport by helicopter to the hospital, the prospective recipient can be rapidly blood grouped and administered compatible ABO-specific products with a definitive crossmatch to follow. Such practice conserves group O blood for the true group O patient, who can accept no other type.

Disseminated intravascular coagulation of a florid, uncompensated type often complicates massive trauma, especially when blood loss demands large volumes of replacement products. Automated autologous salvage and appropriate use of fresh frozen plasma to correct the underlying global deficits in hemostasis should be considered complementary to traditional transfusion. Thereby, the degree of donor exposure can be considerably lessened.

Future Trends

Throughout the past decade, the growth of transfusion medicine has been brisk. Continued progress is predicted, especially in the areas of reducing the degree of exposure to homologous donors. Fostering this drive toward greater safety will be computerized tracking to derive several components from one donor, when multiple types of products are used in the same recipient; procurement of certain derivatives, such as platelet concentrates and fresh frozen plasma, by apheresis techniques from frequently studied volunteer donors with an established track record or "pedigree"; adaptation of new methodologies geared especially to the pediatric patient; and increasingly sophisticated testing of all donor blood for its potential of infectious disease transmissibility.

Spearheading the drive toward quality will be the more widespread use of autotransfusion. The net result will be increased costs, but the benefits to the patient from improved transfusion practices will more than compensate.

Annotated Bibliography

Historical Perspective

Centers for Disease Control: Mortality attributable to HIV infections/AIDS: United States, 1981-1990. *JAMA* 1991;265:848-849.

These data from CDC show recent emergence of AIDS as a leading cause of death among young adults, male and female, in the United States.

Donegan E, Stuart M, Niland JC, et al: Infection with human immunodeficiency virus type I (HIV-1) among recipients of antibody-positive blood donations. *Ann Intern Med* 1990;113:733-739.

A true "look-back" multicenter study details the 90% infection transmission capability of anti-HIV positive blood transfusion in recipients, restricted to those with no known exposure to HIV other than the index transfusion. The rate of progression to AIDS within the first 38 months after infection was similar to that reported for homosexual men and hemophiliacs.

Klein RS, Friedland GH: Transmission of human immunodeficiency virus type I (HIV-1) by exposure to blood: Defining the risk. *Ann Intern Med* 1990;113:729-730.

The marked efficiency of HIV transmission to recipients of virus infected blood transfusion (89.5%) is contrasted with the relatively low risk associated with accidental occupational exposure of health-care workers to body fluids of infected patients (<1%).

Simonds RJ, Holmberg SD, Hurwitz RL, et al: Transmission of human immunodeficiency virus type I from a seronegative organ and tissue donor. *N Engl J Med* 1992;326:726-732.

The authors reemphasize that HIV-1 can be transmitted by a donor who is serologically negative but infectious.

Surgenor DM, Wallace EL, Hao SH, et al: Collection and transfusion of blood in the United States, 1982-1988. *N Engl J Med* 1990;322:1646-1651.

A national survey examines the significant trends in recent blood collection and transfusion practices in the United States.

Widmann FK: Informed consent for blood transfusion: Brief historical survey and summary of a conference. *Transfusion* 1990;30:460-470.

Salient topics presented at an American Association of Blood Banks sponsored conference are summarized. The article focuses on the relationship between patient and health-care provider; clinical and legal aspects of obtaining consent; and risks and benefits of, and alternatives to, traditional homologous transfusion.

Benefits of Homologous Blood Transfusion

Fontanarosa PB, Giorgio GT: Managing Jehovah's Witnesses: Medical, legal, and ethical challenges. *Ann Emerg Med* 1991;20:1148-1149.

The various challenges inherent in the management of the emergency patient who needs, but refuses, transfusion are discussed.

Welch HG, Meehan KR, Goodnough LT: Prudent strategies for elective red blood cell transfusion. *Ann Intern Med* 1992;116:393-402.

While concerns about transfusion-transmitted infections, especially HIV, have recently caused a decline in the use of homologous red cells, current practice remains variable because of differing physician attitudes toward appropriateness indicators.

Young FE, Benson JS, Nightingale SL (ed bd): Use of blood components. *FDA Drug Bulletin* 1989;19:14-15.

This report shows concurrence of the FDA with an alert issued by the National Institutes of Health on recently derived indications and contraindications for the use of red blood cells, platelets, and fresh frozen plasma.

Risk of Homologous Blood Transfusion

Aach RD, Stevens CE, Hollinger FB, et al: Hepatitic C virus infection in post-transfusion hepatitis: An analysis with first- and second-generation assays. *N Engl J Med* 1991;325:1325-1329.

Nearly all cases of non-A, non-B posttransfusion hepatitis are caused by hepatitis C virus.

Anderson KC, Weinstein HJ: Transfusion-associated graft-versus-host disease. *N Engl J Med* 1990;323:315-321.

Reports of transfusion-associated graft-versus-host disease persist, both in recipients with known predisposing risk factors and in those with no overt immunocompromise. Appropriate prophylactic gamma irradiation of blood products is discussed.

Blumberg N, Triulzi DJ, Heal JM: Transfusion-induced immunomodulation and its clinical consequences. *Transfus Med Rev* 1990;IV:24-35.

Although the best characterized effect of transfusion-induced immunomodulation remains the beneficial one of increased survival of renal allografts, homologous blood may also compromise host defenses against solid tumors, bacteria, and viruses.

Delamarter RB, Carr J, Saxton EH: HTLV-I viral-associated myelopathy after blood transfusion in a multiple trauma patient. *Clin Orthop* 1990;260:191-194.

This is the first report of this sequelae in American literature.

Greenbaum BH: Transfusion-associated graft-versus-host disease: Historical perspectives, incidence, and current use of irradiated blood products. *J Clin Oncol* 1991;9:1889-1902.

This problem is assuming increasing importance as a serious complication of modern therapy, especially that directed against malignant tumors. Its symptomatology, diagnosis, mortality potential, and treatment are extensively reviewed.

Manns A, Blattner WA: The epidemiology of the human T-cell lymphotrophic virus type I and type II: Etiologic role in human disease. *Transfusion* 1991;31:67-75.

General epidemiology of the two retroviruses is presented with special attention to the HTLV-1 associated diseases of adult T-cell leukemia lymphoma (ATLL) and HTLV-1 associated myelopathy tropical spastic paraparesis (HAM/TSP).

Quinn TC, Zacarias FR, St. John RK: HIV and HTLV-1 infections in the Americas: A regional perspective. *Medicine* 1989;68:189-209.

This is a detailed review of the entire disease spectrum produced by infection with the retroviruses, HIV-1, HIV-2, and HTLV-1, in North and South America.

Shulman IA: Parasitic infections, an uncommon risk of blood transfusion in the United States. *Transfusion* 1991;31:479-480.

Although it represents an unusual complication of blood transfusion in the United States, transmission of some serious parasitic infections is a distinct possibility.

Sullivan MT, Williams AE, Fang CT, et al: Transmission of human T-lymphotrophic virus types I and II by blood transfusion: A retrospective study of recipients of blood components (1983 through 1988). *Arch Intern Med* 1991;151:2043-2048.

This retrospective study of recipients of blood components from 1983 through 1988 concludes that HTLV-1/2 transmission occurred in approximately 700 patients per year before routine donor testing.

Tremolada F, Casarin C, Tagger A, et al: Antibody to hepatitis C virus in post-transfusion hepatitis. *Ann Intern Med* 1991;114:277-281.

This is the study in which hepatitis C virus is proven the major case of non-A, non-B posttransfusion hepatitis in 63 Italian patients. Time to seroconversion varies widely after hepatitis onset and bears no relation to acute illness or eventual outcome.

Changes in the Practice of Transfusion Medicine

AuBuchon JP, Popovsky MA: The safety of preoperative autologous blood donation in the nonhospital setting. *Transfusion* 1991;31:513-517.

A multicenter study documents the infrequency of severe reactions in this increasingly popular mode of autotransfusion. In 5,660 donations, only four reactions were regarded as severe: one transient ischemic attack and three anginal episodes.

Audet AM, Goodnough LT: Practice strategies for elective red blood cell transfusion. *Ann Intern Med* 1992;116:403-406.

A practical guideline for the use of red cell transfusion by the clinician in elective situations is presented.

Elawad AA, Jonsson S, Laurell M, et al: Predonation autologous blood in hip arthroplasty. *Acta Orthop Scand* 1991;62:218-222.

Use of predeposited autologous blood in elective orthopaedic surgery, even in the elderly, is supported as a practical, cost effective means of avoiding the risks of homologous blood transfusion.

Salem-Schatz SR, Avorn J, Soumerai SB: Influence of clinical knowledge, organizational context, and practice style on transfusion decision making: Implications for practice change strategies. *JAMA* 1990;264:476-483.

Several important reasons for inappropriate use of blood products provide insights into the development of improved transfusion practices that address problems of quality of care and cost containment.

Thomson A, Contreras M, Knowles S: Blood component treatment: A retrospective audit in five major London hospitals. *J Clin Pathol* 1991;44:734-737.

A study of the transfusion of platelets and fresh frozen plasma performed in London hospitals echoes the inappropriate use of these same components in American institutions.

Williamson KR, Taswell HF: Intraoperative blood salvage: A review. *Transfusion* 1991;31:662-675.

Intraoperative autotransfusion as a standard of modern therapy is extensively reviewed.

19

Microvascular Surgery

Introduction

Although the size of needles and suture materials and the degree of magnification that can be used limit the microsurgeon's ability to reliably repair structures with lumenal diameters of less than 0.3 mm, this limitation is not of great practical importance, because the smallest structures that require repair are in the 0.5 to 1.0 mm range. Vein grafting techniques are well established in microsurgery. Vein grafts are used to augment the length of the vascular pedicle in a free-tissue transfer, to reconstruct a damaged vessel (as in replantation of an avulsed digit), and to bypass a traumatized vascular bundle during extremity reconstruction. The reliability of a reversed vein graft in these situations can be brought to a high level by measures that decrease the reactive spasm of the graft. These measures include atraumatic dissection techniques, pharmacologic manipulation with agents such as papaverine, and gentle hydrostatic distention. Previous studies of the microsurgical treatment of ulnar artery thrombosis at the wrist have produced disappointing results. Greatly improved patency rates have now been obtained with use of interposition vein grafts. In eight cases at a minimum one year followup, 88% patency was found. Best results were in nonsmokers after a single, distinctly recalled history of trauma to the palm and were associated with preoperative symptoms of less than five months' duration before treatment.

Microsurgeons who treat trauma patients have observed a "zone of injury" that surrounds the traumatized area. Within this zone the vascular structures have absorbed energy and undergone irreversible intimal damage that will lead to high rates of thrombosis. A recent animal study in which arterial trauma was combined with island flap creation using the rat groin flap system provided evidence to support this observation. In animals who underwent this trauma arterial patency was 31%. Patency was improved to 71% with heparin administration. If the traumatized vessels were immediately completely resected and replaced with vein grafts, patency without heparinization improved to 92%. This study supports the aggressive use of vein grafts in traumatized regions.

Anastomotic Techniques

Traditional anastomotic suture techniques have a high degree of success. New methods that allow anastomoses to be completed in less time and on smaller vessels are being evaluated. The mechanical coupling device now in clinical use shows great promise. One difficulty encountered in suturing small, thin-walled vessels, such as veins or lymphatics, is that the vessel wall can easily be torn by the needle pass. One can also catch the back wall of the vessel during the needle pass, which leads to certain occlusion. The coupler acts as a stent to hold the anastomosis site open and eliminates lacerations of the vessel wall. Other experimental techniques, such as those using a thermal weld or the carbon dioxide laser, have not found clinical applications. An experimental study has shown that laser-assisted microsurgical anastomosis may have patency rates in traumatized blood vessels superior to those of conventional suture techniques. A CO_2 laser was used, and patency rates in traumatized rat femoral vessels that were crushed and avulsed were 25% to 40% better in the early postoperative period. The elimination of sutures probably improved rates because of the inherent thrombogenicity of the suture material within the lumen of the vessel. An innovative approach to anastomosing extremely small, thin-walled vessels is to use an absorbable stent to maintain the lumen during anastomosis. Experiments using this technique in rat femoral arteries showed faster repair, less dilatation at the anastomosis site (a problem commonly seen in experimental studies of couplers with late aneurysm formation), and less narrowing in distal segments with increased distal blood flow.

Pharmacology

Pharmacologic treatments that effectively reduce vessel spasm are used to prevent and treat thrombosis. Topical lidocaine and papaverine, which act to reduce tonicity in the smooth muscle of the vessel media, have both been shown to increase patency rates. Topical thorazine, which inhibits muscle contraction by blocking the formation of the calcium-calmodulin complex, is also effective. Heparin infusion in experimental models has been shown to increase patency, perhaps through a direct effect on vasospasm. The use of low doses of aspirin has been shown to decrease thromboxane levels in the platelets while not inhibiting the antiplatelet prostacyclin produced in the intimal cells of the vessel walls. Higher doses of aspirin inhibit prostacyclin and may negate the beneficial effect on the platelets. Topical prostacyclin, studied in an experimental model as an antithrombotic agent, was found to decrease vessel tone, interfere with blood flow, and promote thrombus formation. Streptokinase converts the inactive plasminogen to active plasmin and has been used to initiate thrombolysis and salvage a failing anastomosis. Adverse reactions can be severe and include fever, hypersensitivity reaction, and hemorrhage. Streptokinase should be used only as a last resort. To lessen the complication of excessive and potentially life-threatening bleeding associated with streptokinase and urokinase the flap can be perfused directly with these drugs and the venous effluent collected, which keeps it from entering the corporal circulation. After this initial cleanout, the systemic intake of these thrombolytic agents can be restricted. This method successfully reversed the "no reflow" phenomenon in four out of five failing free flaps.

A new approach to pharmacology in microsurgery has been provided by the use of the medicinal leech, *Hirudo medicinalis*. The leech secretes a heparin-like enzyme, hirudin, from its salivary glands. Because heparinization takes place only in the region where the leech is applied, the patient avoids the considerable risks of systemic heparinization. The leech remains attached for about 15 minutes and ingests 5 to 10 cc of blood. It then falls off, and the attachment site continues to bleed slowly for about 12 hours. The rate of bleeding is evidently well matched to the venous congestion. A report of salvaging seven replants without venous drainage showed success in all cases, and no patient needed a blood transfusion. In earlier techniques, in which the nail was removed and free bleeding, augmented by heparinized pledgets, was used to relieve venous congestion, patients often required transfusion. One potential disadvantage is that the leech harbors *Aeromonas hydrophila* in its gut instead of digestive enzymes for heme and could possibly infect the replanted digit. To date, no infection has been reported, but all patients should receive appropriate antibiotic coverage for this organism. In addition, leeches should not be used in cases where arterial inflow is compromised.

Monitoring

Clinical examination, with the observation of skin color, capillary refill time, and bleeding after laceration, remains the most common method of assessing the replanted part or free-tissue transfer. However, such examinations are subjective, and they must be repeated. Investigators have sought to develop instrumented methods that will constantly assess the tissue, are completely objective (without observer error), will reflect early changes in tissue vascularity, will indicate whether vascular compromise is venous or arterial, and are completely noninvasive. No method has been developed that satisfies all of these criteria. Measurement of tissue pH can differentiate between venous and arterial occlusion, because pH decreases rapidly with arterial problems and more slowly with venous blockage. The laser Doppler, which measures the movement of erythrocytes beneath the skin, has not been found to be reliable in the clinical setting.

Peripheral Nerve Repair

Various methods have been employed to improve fascicular matching during peripheral nerve repairs. Sensory and motor fascicles can be identified in the proximal and distal stumps with electrical stimulation or histochemical methods. Electrical stimulation is most useful in the acute phases after injury, before the distal motor fascicles have undergone degeneration, while they can still be identified. The most common histochemical technique identifies the enzyme acetylcholinesterase in the motor nerve fascicles. This technically demanding method is only used in few centers at this time, but results are promising. Knowledge of the anatomy of the nerve fascicles remains the most commonly used technique to improve matching. At the level of the wrist, a common site of laceration, the volar-radial location of the motor fascicles in the median nerve and dorsal-ulnar location of the motor fascicles of the ulnar nerve helps to match these structures during repair. Vascularized nerve grafting, most commonly using the sural nerve as a graft, has not been shown to be more effective than nonvascularized techniques.

The results of previous studies of nerve grafting and neurorrhaphy of the posterior tibial nerve have been discouraging. A series of eight patients with numbness of the foot so severe that they were possible candidates for amputation showed improved results with interfascicular interposition nerve grafting of the posterior tibial nerve at the ankle. The sural nerve was used as a donor in all cases, and sensory recovery was seen in all patients. There were no cases of foot ulcerations. This procedure appears to be worthwhile as an alternative to amputation.

The repair of partial lacerations of major peripheral nerves results in good recovery of function. In a study of 12 patients with partial, sharp, distal lacerations of the ulnar and median nerves treated within two weeks of the injury by end-to-end repair of the lacerated fascicles, there was no degeneration of the intact fascicles and sensory and motor recovery were good. Meticulous microsurgical repair of partially lacerated fascicular groups appears to be a reliable treatment method that does not harm adjacent intact fascicular groups. The results of primary microsurgical nerve repair in the upper extremity using an epineural or perineural technique show that in digital nerve repair static two-point discrimination was regained in 71% of cases. In median nerve repair the figure was 50%, and in ulnar nerve repair it was 70%. Results in moving two-point discrimination tests were similar. The age of the patient was the most critical factor. Associated injuries were also important. Good to excellent recovery was achieved in only 58% of patients with associated injuries, compared with 70% in those with nerve injury only.

Replantation

As experience with replantation increases, data are emerging that will refine the techniques used. It is now clear that survival rates for digital replantations can be enhanced by repairing both digital arteries and at least two veins. A study of 153 patients showed a survival rate of 86% when both arteries were repaired, compared with 79% when a single artery was anastomosed. Repairing two veins was associated with a 91% success rate versus 71% for single vein repairs. Recovery of digital sensibility and joint motion were most frequent with sharp amputations and were worse with crushing and avulsion injuries. The return of intrinsic muscle function was poor after hand replantation. Ischemic time was a factor only in amputated parts that underwent warm preservation for a period longer than 12 hours. Older patients did as well as younger ones. Because digital replantation in patients older than 65 can be accomplished with success rates comparable to those seen in younger patients, age by itself should not be the sole decisive factor.

Because of the thumb's unique role in the function of the hand, it is critical to replant this digit whenever feasible. The socioeconomic consequences of thumb amputation are significant. In a study of 25 patients with thumb amputations, the final outcome was good in eight patients, fair in 12, and poor in five. Only patients with amputations at or distal to the interphalangeal joint had normal key and pinch grip. The median time away from work was 114 days. Because the success of thumb replantation cannot be predicted from the initial severity of the injury, replantation should be attempted in all cases. A study of 42 complete thumb amputations that underwent replantation had a 38% failure rate. Thumbs with poor intraoperative blood flow had a 20% survival rate; 50% of those with no venous return survived. Even these cases, formerly thought to be hopeless, should not be amputated primarily. Total active motion (TAM) averaged 68 degrees for these patients and static two-point discrimination averaged 11 mm. Of avulsed thumbs, 46% survived.

Various methods are used to reconstruct thumbs that cannot be replanted. Toe-to-thumb transfer has been shown to be effective, although it is a technically demanding procedure. The transferred toe can be quite bulky on the hand. Anatomic studies have shown that the transverse diameter of the toe skeleton is greater at all levels than that of the thumb. A trimmed-toe technique has been used which involves reduction of both the bony and soft-tissue elements. A longitudinal osteotomy removes a 4 to 6 mm width of the medial joint prominence and 2 to 4 mm from the phalangeal shaft. A major drawback of this procedure is that because these osteotomies are intra-articular, they reduce motion.

Ring avulsion injuries represent one of the greatest replantation challenges. In a recent study of 55 of these injuries, the overall amputation rate was 20.5%. Using the Urbaniak classification system, the success rate was 86% for class 2 avulsions and 73% for class 3. Of class 3 patients, 69% had cold intolerance, compared with 26% of the class 2 patients. Digits with skeletal injury had a lower success rate.

Free Tissue Transfer

The advent of microvascular free tissue transfer has allowed the surgeon great flexibility in timing the reconstruction of both soft-tissue and bony defects. Microsurgical techniques allow early single-stage coverage and vascularized bone grafting after debridement. The risks of secondary infection and wound desiccation are thus decreased. Early range of motion of gliding structures and joints can thus be instituted. This is especially important in the hand. Obtaining wound coverage within the first 72 hours has the advantages of not allowing the vessels adjacent to the wound to become fibrotic, decreasing granulation tissue and infection, preventing desiccation, and preventing progressive bone and tendon necrosis. In trauma patients, free flap coverage within 72 hours has been shown to result in low infection rates and increased bone healing.

Free tissue transfer has been proven useful in the treatment of soft-tissue defects in patents with peripheral vascular disease. In diabetics microsurgical endarterectomy has prevented flap failures. The use of free gracilis muscle flaps to treat diabetic foot ulcers proved effective in a series of nine patients with ten infected foot ulcers. Although this flap is denervated and insensate, there was no recurrence of ulceration or of infection.

As microsurgical expertise has developed over the years, more complete single stage reconstructions have become possible. In a large series of patients who required complex reconstructive procedures using multiple flaps, it was found that several flaps could be transferred successfully at one time, with clear advantages over sequential procedures. Success rates were equivalent, the patients were spared repeated anesthesia, and the overall time of reconstruction was decreased. Microvascular surgery in children is safe and can be performed with a high success rate. A study of 43 procedures in 38 children (average age 5.4 years) had a success rate of 93%. The postoperative course was comparable to that seen in adults except that extra attention was paid to psychosocial care. Vessel size was not a problem, because external diameters generally exceeded 0.8 mm.

The latissimus dorsi flap, based on the thoracodorsal artery, is widely used in microsurgical reconstruction. It is easily harvested, provides a large amount of flat muscle for coverage, and leaves an acceptable donor defect. The flap can be tailored for improved coverage. There has now been a long experience with fibular bone graft for treatment of bone defects. This flap leaves a minimal donor site defect and can be tailored to produce two parallel struts. The proximal strut maintains both the periosteal and the endosteal blood supply; the distal survives on periosteal supply alone. The temporoparietal flap, one of the first fascial flaps used, has the distinct advantages of begin thin and pliable and providing an excellent gliding surface, which makes it well suited for use in the hand. However, it is difficult to harvest and may leave a significant cosmetic donor defect, especially if the patient later suffers hair loss. Newer techniques have found other sources for vascularized fascial tissue that are easier to harvest and have more acceptable donor sites. The dorsal thoracic fascia, a variant of the scapular flap, is based on the circumflex scapular vessels. More fascia is available with this flap than with the temporoparietal flap and the donor scar can be hidden in the axilla. Another new fascial flap is the free fascial forearm flap based on the radial artery. This fascia is very thin and is well suited for reconstruction of the hand and foot. The donor site morbidity is minimized compared to the radial artery based cutaneous forearm (Chinese) flap, because

skin closure is accomplished easily. As in the Chinese flap, the vascular pedicle is long and of reliable dimensions. This fascia can also be used with a distal pedicle as a reversed rotation flap.

The treatment of soft-tissue defects of the hand, especially of the palm, is a difficult problem. Palmar resurfacing requires a flap that is thick enough to provide padding and durable enough to survive repeated grips. It also must be stable or adherent to the underlying tissue. The inferior three slips of the serratus anterior muscle have been effective in this application. This flap is easily harvested and the donor site morbidity is minimal. If only the inferior three slips are harvested and the remaining muscle is not denervated, scapular winging will not occur. The muscle can be tailored because of the separate slips and can be transferred as an innervated active muscle. It can be used in this manner to replace the thenar muscles and assist in opposition of the thumb.

Annotated Bibliography

Cooley BC, Groner JP, Hoer SR, et al: Experimental study of the influence of arterial trauma on dependent distal tissue survival. *Microsurgery* 1991;12:86-88.

An experimental model in which arterial trauma was combined with island flap creation using the rat groin flap system has provided experimental evidence to support this. In animals who underwent this trauma, arterial patency was 31%. Patency was improved to 71% with heparin administration. If the traumatized vessels were immediately completely resected and replaced with vein grafts, patency without heparinization improved to 92%. This study supports the aggressive use of vein grafts in traumatized regions.

Mehlhoff TL, Wood MB: Ulnar artery thrombosis and the role of interposition vein grafting: Patency with microsurgical technique. *J Hand Surg* 1991;16:274-278.

Eight consecutive cases of chronic ulnar artery thrombosis at the wrist managed with microsurgical interposition vein grafting were evaluated for long-term patency. At minimum one year followup an 88% patency rate was found. Functional results in patent grafts were excellent in 57% and good in the remainder. Interposition vein grafts can effectively restore blood flow to painful digits.

Anastomotic Techniques

Ruiz-Razura A, Branfman GS: Laser-assisted microsurgical anastomoses in traumatized blood vessels. *J Reconstr Microsurg* 1990;6:55-59.

In this experimental model based on rat femoral artery anastomoses, laser anastomosis had an 80% patency rate in crushed vessels compared to a 65% patency rate for conventional suture anastomosis. The patency rates at two days postinjury in avulsed vessels were 85% for the laser and 45% for the suture technique.

Zhong C, Tang NX, Zheng CF, et al: Experimental study on microvascular anastomosis using dissolvable stent support in the lumen. *Microsurgery* 1991;12:67-71.

This is an experimental study of a new technique in the rat femoral artery in which an absorbable stent is placed in the lumen. It has shown faster repair, less dilatation at the anastomosis site (a problem commonly seen in experimental studies of couplers with late aneurysm formation), and less narrowing in distal segments with increased distal blood flow.

Pharmacology

Brody GA, Maloney WJ, Hentz VR: Digit replantation applying the leech *Hirudo medicinalis. Clin Orthop* 1989;245:133-137.

Four patients without a suitable vein for anastomosis and three in whom venous congestion developed postoperatively were treated with leeches. The incision bled for 12 hours after the leech dropped off. The average time of treatment was 4.7 days and all replanted digits survived. Patient acceptance was universal.

Goldberg J, Pederson W, Barwick W: Salvage of free tissue transfers using thrombolytic agents. *J Reconstr Microsurg* 1989;5:351-356.

Four of five failing free flaps with "no-reflow" phenomena were salvaged with a technique in which the flap circulation is washed out with urokinase/streptokinase and the venous effluent prevented from entering the general circulation. A restricted dose of these agents can then be used systemically to eliminate bleeding complications.

Salemark L, Wieslander JB, Dougan P, et al: Adverse effects of topical prostacyclin application in microvascular surgery: An experimental study. *J Reconstr Microsurg* 1991;7:27-30.

The efficacy of topical prostacyclin as an antithrombotic agent was tested in a rabbit ear arterial model. Patency was lower following prostacyclin administration with five of 15 occluding, as opposed to one of 12 in the control group. While these results were not significant they did suggest increased thrombus formation.

Peripheral Nerve Repair

Dellon AL, Mackinnon SE: Results of posterior tibial nerve grafting at the ankle. *J Reconstr Microsurg* 1991;7:81-83.

The results of interfascicular interposition nerve grafting for posterior tibial nerve deficit at the ankle are reported for eight patients. The sural nerve was used as a donor and the indication for surgery was numbness so severe as to consider amputation. Sensory recovery was to S4 level in two, to S3+ in four, and to S3 in two. There were no cases of foot ulceration. Grafting of the posterior tibial nerve is indicated for the treatment of pain and recovery of sensation in carefully selected patients and is capable of predictably restoring at least some touch sensibility.

Hurst LC, Dowd A, Sampson SP, et al: Partial lacerations of median and ulnar nerves. *J Hand Surg* 1991;16:207-210.

Twelve patients with sharp distal partial median and ulnar nerve lacerations were treated within two weeks of injury with fascicular repair. At an average followup of 21 months the results, based on the British Medical Research Council Rating Scale, were S = 3.81 (Normal = 4.0), and M = 4.0 (Normal = 5.0).

Mailänder P, Berger A, Schaller E, et al: Results of primary nerve repair in the upper extremity. *Microsurgery* 1989;10:147-150.

The results of primary microsurgical nerve repair in 147 patients from a single center showed good recovery of sensation. Age was an important factor as were associated injuries. This study provides a basis for reasonable expectations for nerve repair.

Replantation

Hovgaard C, Dalsgaard S, Gebuhr P: The social and economic consequences of failure to replant amputated thumbs. *J Hand Surg* 1989;14B:307-308.

Thumb amputation results in significant social and economic consequences. In a study of 25 patients with thumb amputations the final outcome was good in eight patients, fair in 12, and poor in five. Only patients with amputations at or distal to the interphalangeal joint had normal key and pinch grip. The median time away from work was 114 days.

Kay S, Werntz J, Wolff TW: Ring avulsion injuries: Classification and prognosis. *J Hand Surg* 1989;14A:204-213.

In this study of 55 ring avulsion injuries, an overall amputation rate of 20.5% for the entire series was found. Using the Urbaniak classification system there was a 86% success rate for class 2 avulsions and 73% for class 3. Of the class 3 patients, 69% had cold intolerance compared with 26% of the class 2 patients. Digits with skeletal injury had a lower success rate.

Okada T, Ishikura N, Tsukada S: Digital replantation in the aged patient. *J Reconstr Microsurg* 1988;4:351-357.

Seven men and one woman aged 65 to 74 underwent nine replantation procedures. Postoperative joint mobilization was the most difficult problem and was worse than that seen in a younger population. The final decision to carry out replantation should be based on the patient's health status and preference, and not on age.

Tark KC, Kim YW, Lee YH, et al: Replantation and revascularization of hands: Clinical analysis and functional results of 261 cases. *J Hand Surg* 1989;14A:17-27.

This study of 176 replantations and 85 revascularizations indicates that the results are best in bilateral restoration of digital arteries and repair of multiple veins, sharp amputations in zone III, and when the parts undergo cold preservation. Age was not a factor.

Ward WA, Tsai TM, Breidenbach W: Per primam thumb replantation for all patients with traumatic amputations. *Clin Orthop* 1991;266:90-95.

A study of 42 complete thumb amputations that underwent replantation had a 38% failure rate. Thumbs with poor intraoperative blood flow had a 20% survival rate and those with no venous return survived 50% of the time. Even these cases, formerly thought to be hopeless, should not be amputated primarily. Total active motion (TAM) averaged 68 degrees for these patients and static two-point discrimination averaged 11 mm. Avulsed thumbs survived 46% of the time. Replantation should be attempted in all cases of thumb amputation, because success cannot be predicted by mechanism or severity of the injury.

Wei FC, Chen HC, Chuang CC, et al: Reconstruction of the thumb with a trimmed-toe transfer technique. *Plast Reconstr Surg* 1988;82:506-515.

This article outlines the anatomic aspects of free toe-to-thumb transfer. A new technique involving a longitudinal osteotomy was used on 26 patients. While the cosmetic results are superior, there is decreased range of motion of the transfers because of the intra-articular nature of the osteotomy.

Free Tissue Transfer

Brody GA, Buncke HJ, Alpert BS, et al: Serratus anterior muscle transplantation for treatment of soft tissue defects in the hand. *J Hand Surg* 1990;15A:322-327.

The inferior three slips of the serratus anterior muscle were used to reconstruct palmar and dorsal defects in the hands of 18 patients. All flaps survived and there were no cases of scapular winging. The palmar reconstructions were stable and durable with no flap breakdown. There is minimal donor site morbidity and the scar is well concealed. The separate slips can be divided easily and the flap contoured.

Colen LB: Limb salvage in the patient with severe peripheral vascular disease: The role of microsurgical free-tissue transfer. *Plast Reconstr Surg* 1987;79:389-395.

Microsurgical free tissue transfer may allow limb salvage in carefully selected diabetics with peripheral vascular disease. The technique is particularly valuable in patients who have undergone amputation of the other leg.

Devaraj VS, Kay SP, Batchelor AG, et al: Microvascular surgery in children. *Br J Plast Surg* 1991;44:276-280.

Describes 43 procedures carried out in young children, with a 93% success rate.

Godina M: Early microsurgical reconstruction of complex trauma of the extremities. *Plast Reconstr Surg* 1986;78:285-292.

Free flap coverage of extremity wounds within 72 hours resulted in a decreased flap failure and infection rates and diminished bone healing times when compared with cases in which coverage was obtained after 72 hours. Radical debridement of devitalized tissues is the essential part of this technique.

Ismail T: The free fascial forearm flap. *Microsurgery* 1989;10:155-160.

This paper describes a modification of the well-known radial artery-based cutaneous forearm flap (Chinese flap). Only the fascia is taken. This flap can have particular application as a reversed rotation flap for hand coverage.

Jones NF, Swartz WM, Mears DC, et al: The "double-barrel" free vascularized fibular bone graft. *Plast Reconstr Surg* 1988;81:378-385.

The fibular shaft is bisected transversely, preserving the peroneal blood supply to the distal half. This creates two vascularized struts that can be placed parallel to one another to provide increased mechanical stability.

Kim PS, Gottlieb JR, Harris GD, et al: The dorsal thoracic fascia: Anatomic significance with clinical applications in reconstructive microsurgery. *Plast Reconstr Surg* 1987;79:72-80.

The circumflex scapular artery lies within the dorsal thoracic fascia and communicates with the myocutaneous perforators of the latissimus dorsi. The dorsal thoracic fascia can be transferred as a free flap or used to extend the latissimus dorsi myocutaneous flap.

Lai CS, Lin SD, Yang CC, et al: Limb salvage of infected diabetic foot ulcers with microsurgical free-muscle transfer. *Ann Plast Surg* 1991;26:212-220.

Nine diabetic patients with ten infected foot ulcers, four with osteomyelitis, and three with gangrene were successfully treated with free gracilis muscle transfers. There were no recurrences of the ulcers or infections.

Whitney TM, Buncke HJ, Lineaweaver WC, et al: Multiple microvascular transplants: A preliminary report of simultaneous versus sequential reconstruction. *Ann Plast Surg* 1989;22:391-404.

Two parallel series of patients, one undergoing sequential multiple free flaps and the other undergoing simultaneous free-flaps, were compared. There was no difference in the success rate and the patients undergoing simultaneous free tissue transfers had shorter hospitalizations with fewer anesthesias. The complication rates for the two groups showed no statistical difference.

20

Lasers in Orthopaedics

Introduction

The use of lasers in orthopaedics has lagged behind their use in other fields of surgery. The limited success of CO_2 lasers and free beam Nd:YAG lasers in the early 1980s for arthroscopic surgery led many leaders in the field to conclude that lasers were not likely to play a role in arthroscopic surgery. However, recent basic science studies and technologic advances have rekindled interests in lasers, and many researchers see exciting possibilities for their use both in diagnosing and in treating orthopaedic disorders.

Laser Principles

The term LASER is an acronym for **L**ight **A**mplification by **S**timulated **E**mission of **R**adiation. Albert Einstein first hypothesized the formation of laser light in 1917, in his *Quantitative Theory of Radiation*, but it was not until 1960 that Theodore Maiman developed the first working laser using a ruby crystal. The laser is an electro-optical device that transmits energy in the form of an intense beam of light.

Atoms can exist in several discrete energy states. When atoms are in an excited state, they are said to be in a higher energy level than when they are in a resting state. When atoms drop from a high-energy state to a low-energy state, they release energy in the form of photons; these photons are emitted as an intense beam of light known as a laser beam. Because the wavelength of this beam of light is a function of the difference between the two energy levels, it differs from one atom to another. The principle of laser operation involves pumping large amounts of energy into a substance to create a population inversion, in which more atoms are raised to a high-energy state. Ultimately, one of the high-energy atoms will spontaneously emit a photon. When this photon strikes another high-energy atom, a photon of identical wavelength and traveling in the same direction is emitted. As these two photons move in phase with each other, a light wave of double the original intensity is produced. This light wave can be transformed into heat energy that can simultaneously cut and coagulate tissues, and, thus, it is able to provide the surgeon with the means of making a precise and bloodless incision.

There are three basic components to all lasers: (1) a lasing medium, which can be a gas, a liquid, or a solid; (2) an excitation source that will pump high energy into the medium; and (3) a resonator, which is a chamber

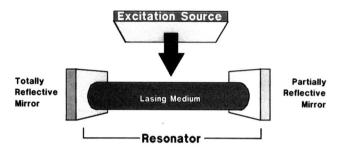

Fig. 1 The three basic components to all lasers are a lasing medium, an excitation source, and a resonator.

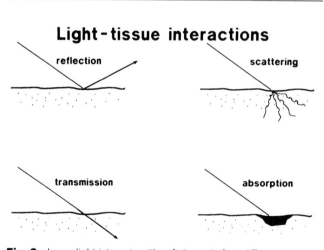

Fig. 2 Laser light interacts with soft tissue in four different ways: reflection, scattering, transmission, or absorption.

consisting of two parallel mirrors, one totally reflective, and the other partially reflective to allow egress of the laser light (Fig. 1).

A variety of factors determine the effect that a particular laser beam has on tissue. These include: (1) the power density or energy density, (2) the spot size, and (3) the nature of the light interaction with tissue. Light can be reflected from, transmitted through, scattered within, or absorbed by tissue (Fig. 2). Only when the light energy is absorbed by tissue is it transformed into effective thermal energy that can be used to cut, coagulate, or ablate target tissues. The ability of a laser beam to be absorbed by a tissue is determined by the wavelength of the laser light and the optical properties of the target tissue, that is, its absorption characteristics. In general, target tissues tend to absorb light at wavelengths that are similar to or near to their own. Through the adjustment of several variables, including manipulation of the laser's wavelength, it is possible to obtain the desired surgical effect of cutting, coagulation, vaporization, interstitial irradiation, or, possibly, tissue welding. The principal biologic advantage of laser energy over other thermal energies, such as electrocautery, is that the energy is focused at a point, instead of being dispersed in all directions from a particular point, as happens with electrocautery.

Types of Lasers

Laser light is a part of the electromagnetic spectrum, as are television and radio waves. Certain wavelengths are visible; others are not. All lasers are named for their medium.

Several laser systems are commercially available for orthopaedic use. The ones that have been used most frequently in orthopaedic surgery are the CO_2 laser (10.6 μm wavelength), the Nd:YAG laser (1.06 μm), the Ho:YAG laser (2.1 μm), the Excimer laser (308 nm), and the KTP laser, which is actually a YAG laser (1.06 μm) focused through KTP crystals that double the frequency. All of these laser systems, with the exception of the CO_2 laser system, are fiberoptically compatible and can be used in a saline medium. The need for a gaseous medium with the CO_2 laser and the attendant risks (subcutaneous emphysema and embolism) have limited the widespread acceptance of the CO_2 laser in arthroscopy and orthopaedics in general.

The contact Nd:YAG laser is particularly attractive for arthroscopic use because it provides tactile feedback that arthroscopic surgeons are most familiar with. Other advantages include its effects on articular cartilage in the knee. Experiments using rabbits as an animal model have shown that defects created by an Nd:YAG laser in knee articular cartilage have significantly enhanced healing compared with similar lesions created by a scalpel or electrocautery. Furthermore, both basic science and clinical studies using the contact Nd:YAG laser in arthroscopic meniscectomy have shown the laser to be a safe and effective tool for arthroscopic use.

Excimer lasers, like the Nd:YAG, are contact lasers that can be delivered fiberoptically and can be used in a saline medium. The excimer laser does not cut tissue by a thermal effect, but rather works by separating the molecules of the tissue. This process is known as photo-ablation or molecular dissociation. The Ho:YAG laser is also capable of being delivered fiberoptically and can be used in a saline medium. The Ho:YAG laser, however, is classified as a near contact pulsed laser system; it works by "blasting" away at a target tissue through microsecond pulses.

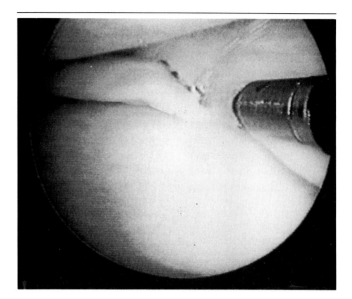

Fig. 3 Arthroscopic view of an Nd:YAG contact laser meniscectomy.

The KTP laser is similar to the Argon laser with respect to wavelength, power range, and tissue absorption characteristics. Unfortunately, a relatively weak output power may limit the use of these laser systems in orthopaedic surgery.

Laser Arthroscopy

Arthroscopic surgery with lasers offers a number of potential advantages. Because it has the ability to cut and coagulate simultaneously, use of the laser obviates the need for a tourniquet in the upper and lower extremities (Fig. 3). It also avoids the need to ground the patient. For most arthroscopic procedures, only a laser and arthroscopic shaver are necessary to perform surgery. The laser's small size allows the surgeon access to areas that are difficult to reach with standard instrumentation. The laser allows for either precise incising of meniscal tissue or ablation of larger areas of synovial tissue. The development of office arthroscopy with needle arthroscopes will make the laser even more valuable, because a surgeon will be able to introduce the laser percutaneously either to cut or to coagulate.

Certain lasers may play a role in articular cartilage stimulation (Figs. 4 and 5). However, because this capability has yet to be shown with human cell culture studies, it remains experimental at present.

Current arthroscopic surgical procedures that use lasers in the knee joint include meniscal excision, plica resection, lateral release, excision of scar tissue, and synovectomy. Lasers have been used in the shoulder for soft-tissue release with adhesive capsulitis, labral resection, synovectomy, arthroscopic acromioplasty (for coagula-

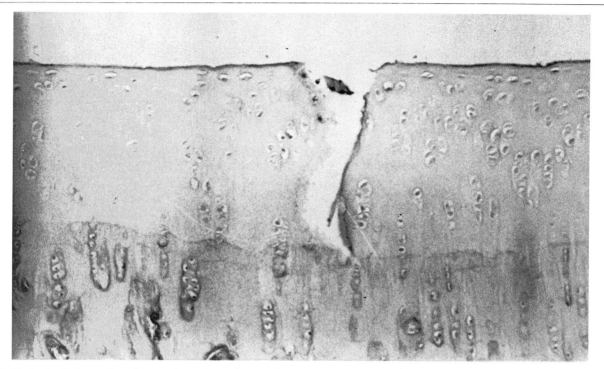

Fig. 4 Scalpel articular cartilage lesions showed no evidence of healing but exhibited no degeneration over time. (Reproduced with permission from O'Brien SJ, Miller MD: The contact neodymium-yttrium aluminum garnet laser. *Clin Orthop* 1990;252:98.)

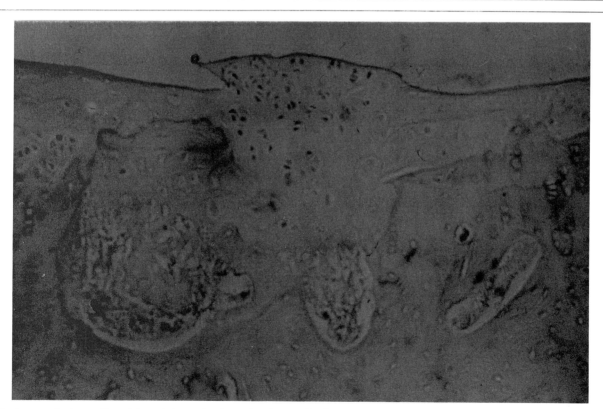

Fig. 5 Laser articular cartilage injury at six weeks showed a vigorous healing response, with increased vascularity, chondrocyte proliferation, and fibrocartilaginous repair.

tion), and arthroscopic rotator cuff repair (for coagulation).

Clinical evaluation studies show the laser to be both safe and effective, although further instrumentation advances as well as cost containment measures are needed before the use of lasers becomes widespread.

Other Orthopaedic Uses of Lasers

Lasers have been used in other types of orthopaedic surgery including excision of musculoskeletal tumors, spine surgery (diskectomy), revision arthroplasty (cement removal), amputation, tissue welding (peripheral nerve), and the treatment of selected foot (nail bed surgery) and hand disorders (arthroscopic carpal tunnel release). However, large clinical series with controls are still lacking at this time.

Future Directions

The basic science foundations and clinical applications for the use of lasers in orthopaedics are steadily growing. Lasers are being used for selective cutting of certain tissues (such as nerve and tumor), and new improved laser delivery systems continue to be devised. In addition to their use in arthroscopic surgery, laser systems for open surgery will be a subject for new research programs.

Annotated Bibliography

Lasers in Orthopaedic Surgery—An Overview

Metcalf RW: Lasers in orthopaedic surgery, in Dixon JA (ed): *Surgical Application of Lasers*, ed 2. Chicago, Yearbook Medical Publishers, 1987, pp 275-286.

The author provides a thorough discussion of the history, development, implementation, and subsequent use of lasers in orthopaedic surgery. Complications and shortcomings of initial protocols, trials, and laser systems are clearly pointed out. Initial studies using CO_2 and Nd:YAG systems are explained. Constructive critiques of these systems and their shortcomings are made, and plausible alternatives to correct these flaws and advance the use of lasers in orthopaedics are offered.

O'Brien SJ, Miller DV: The contact neodymium-yttrium aluminum garnet laser: A new approach to arthroscopic laser surgery. *Clin Orthop* 1990;252:95-100.

Reviews the physics of laser light emission and includes a detailed discussion of the contact Nd:YAG laser. Results from basic science and preliminary clinical trials using the contact Nd:YAG laser showed the laser to be a safe and effective alternative to conventional cutting instruments. Histologic examination at six weeks following articular cartilage stimulation with the contact Nd:YAG laser showed a vigorous healing response of articular cartilage, with increased vascularity, chondrocyte proliferation, and fibrocartilaginous repair. Scalpel- and laser-induced meniscal tears demonstrated evidence of regeneration upon histologic examination at six weeks.

O'Brien SJ, Miller DV, Fealy SV, et al: Lasers in the meniscus, in Mow VC, Arnoczky SP, Jackson DW (eds): *Knee Meniscus*. New York, Raven Press, 1992, pp 153-164.

This article reviews laser physics and current laser systems that are applicable for use in orthopaedic surgery. Contact Nd:YAG, CO_2, Excimer, KTP, and Ho:YAG laser systems are discussed. It provides information on future directions, including the study of the optical properties of human tissues.

Basic Science and Clinical Foundations

Miller DV, O'Brien SJ, Arnoczky SP, et al: The use of the contact Nd:YAG laser in arthroscopic surgery: Effects on articular cartilage and meniscal tissue. *Arthroscopy* 1989;5:245-253.

A two-pronged study using New Zealand white rabbits showed the contact Nd:YAG laser to produce effective results in both articular cartilage and meniscal studies when compared to similar lesions produced by electrocautery and scalpel. Articular cartilage lesions produced by the contact Nd:YAG laser seemed to heal significantly better than similar lesions created by scalpel or electrocautery. Rabbits undergoing meniscectomies with the contact Nd:YAG laser exhibited at six weeks a regeneration pattern similar to that produced by scalpel resection, and meniscal regeneration was not precluded. Scalpel meniscectomies at six weeks showed a loosely woven matrix populated by fibrocytes that "capped" the meniscus at the site of the lesion. Similar lesions produced by electrocautery failed to show meniscal regeneration, but instead demonstrated a wide band of cellular necrosis that increased with time.

Trauner K, Nishioka N, Patel D: Pulsed holmium:yttrium-aluminum-garnet (Ho:YAG) laser ablation of fibrocartilage and articular cartilage. *Am J Sports Med* 1990;18:316-320.

A new orthopaedic laser system, the Ho:YAG laser, was used to ablate bovine articular cartilage and meniscal fibrocartilage. The Ho:YAG laser has a 2.1 μm wavelength, and it was used in pulsed mode. Histologic examination revealed zones of thermal damage extending 550 μm from ablation sites. Tissue ablation rates were found to be proportional to laser radiant exposure when delivered above threshold. The Ho:YAG was found to be effective in a saline environment in direct contact with tissues. The laser was found to resect cartilaginous tissues with only limited tissue necrosis. The fact that Ho:YAG laser light can be delivered fiberoptically is a useful clinical advantage.

Waldow SM, Morrison PR, Grossweiner LI: Nd:YAG laser-induced hyperthermia in a mouse tumor model. *Lasers Surg Med* 1988;8:510-514.

An Nd:YAG laser was used in female mice with the SMT-F mammary carcinoma to induce a hyperthermic tumor response. Using 1 W of power, hyperthermic temperatures were found to be achieved at depths ranging from 3 to 8 mm in tumors. Positive responses in greater than 50% of the population were found in small tumors; control of large tumors was not achieved.

Whipple TL, Caspari RB, Meyers JF: Arthroscopic meniscectomy by CO_2 laser vaporization in a gas medium. *Arthroscopy* 1985;1:2-7.

Preliminary basic science studies using the CO_2 laser to perform subtotal meniscectomies on New Zealand white rabbits are described. The authors performed some of the earliest studies that evaluated CO_2 laser energy as a potential tool for arthroscopic meniscectomy. Postoperatively, they observed an excellent healing potential along the peripheral rim of the meniscus; complete healing was noted at ten weeks postoperatively. Healing was characterized by chondrocyte proliferation.

Procedures Using Lasers in Orthopaedic Surgery

Almquist EE: Nerve repair by laser. *Orthop Clin North Am* 1988;19:201-208.

Laser physics and medical applications of lasers are discussed. Argon, CO_2, Nd:YAG, and KTP laser systems are described briefly. Specific applications of several types of lasers in repairing damaged nerves are discussed and explained. Lasers can repair damaged nerves through the production of a minicuff of blood or a heat-induced fusion of epineural tissue. Both of these techniques work toward sealing gaps in tubular structures. Gaps in tubular structures secondary to nerve damage would lessen normal nerve function by allowing the entrance of scar tissue and the exit of axon sprouts.

Sherk HH, Kollmer C: Revision arthroplasty using a CO_2 laser, in Sherk HH (ed): *Lasers in Orthopaedics*. Philadelphia, JB Lippincott, 1990, pp 75-103.

The use of a CO_2 laser to remove polymethylmethacrylate (PMMA) in revision arthroplasty is discussed. CO_2 laser energy quickly changes solid PMMA found in the joint to a gaseous form. The laser's effects are studied with regard to heat transfer from PMMA to bone, comparative absorptive capacities of CO_2 laser energy, gaseous products of vaporization of PMMA, and histologic changes in bone following cement removal with the CO_2 laser. Initial clinical trials using the laser to remove PMMA during revision arthroplasty demonstrated no clear advantage over conventional mechanical instrumentation including reamers and burrs. Upon further experience and development of new techniques that refined the procedure using the laser, the authors report that they found use of the laser preferable. The CO_2 laser was used in 38 joint revisions, and it was found to be an effective alternative to mechanical instruments. Laser energy was found to remove PMMA without the inherent risks encountered during mechanical removal of this cement.

21
Bone Grafts

Skeletal deficits, whether congenital or acquired in any of numerous circumstances, present a spectrum of reconstructive challenges. Bone grafts, synthetic biomaterials, and manufactured implants provide enormous options and opportunities for repairing these various clinical disorders, and no single type of graft or implant is ideally suited to address the reparative needs of all bony defects. Increasing knowledge concerning the biology, immunology, and biomechanics of bone grafts; improvements in surgical implantation techniques; and advances in bone banking methodology, as well as a better definition of the relation between the graft and its host environment, have appeared in recent years. This information serves as the basis for choosing the most appropriate approach to specific patients, including selection of bone graft material, operative strategies, and postoperative management.

Terminology

Bone grafts are generally classified according to their tissue composition (cortical, cancellous), anatomic features (site of origin, size, shape), nature of their blood supply (nonvascularized, revascularized), preservation method (fresh, frozen, freeze-dried), additional chemical manipulations or exposures (demineralization, irradiation), and the degree of genetic disparity between the donor and the recipient (Table 1). Changes in any of these factors can influence the physiologic or structural properties of the graft; this, in turn, may affect its clinical efficacy in specific circumstances (Table 2).

Bone graft terminology and clinical applications belie the unique capacity of the skeleton to regenerate osseous tissue. Unlike solid organs, which require transplanted

cells to survive and function, transferred bone—even if devoid of viable donor cells—can participate in the process of regeneration. This newly formed bone is of host

Table 1. Transplantation terminology reflecting genetic relationships

Autograft	Transferred from elsewhere in the same individual (obtained from the iliac crest and used around a fracture in that same person)
Syngraft (or isograft)	Transplanted between genetically identical members of the same species (inbred strains of animals, human identical twins)
Allograft	Transplanted from one member of a species to a genetically dissimilar member of the same species (BALB/c mouse to A/He mouse; human to human)
Xenograft	Transplanted from one species to another species (dog to cow, cow to human)

Table 2. Advantages and disadvantages of available bone graft materials

Materials	Advantages	Disadvantages
Autografts		
Fresh	Optimal biologic behavior; no transfer of disease; histocompatible; best choice when donor site morbidity is acceptable and supply is sufficient	Limited availability; donor site morbidity; sacrifice of normal structures
Revascularized	Little dependence on host bed; rapid healing	Limited availability of donor sites; technically difficult; sacrifice of normal structures; donor site morbidity
Allografts		
Fresh	No preservation required; articular cartilage viable; well suited to joint resurfacing alone	Most intense immune response; need and availability may not coincide; little time to test for sterility or disease
Frozen	Simple; permits cartilage cryopreservation; decreased immunogenicity; no change in biomechanical properties; well suited to massive osteoarticular and segmental deficits	Requires careful screening of donors; expensive over the long term; cannot be sterilized secondarily; transit over long distances requires freezing temperature to be maintained; cartilage viability is limited
Freeze-dried	Can be stored indefinitely at room temperature; easy to transport; can be recovered clean and sterilized secondarily; compatible with demineralization; well suited to intercalary segmental loss or cystic defects	Storage and preservation techniques expensive and complicated; biomechanical changes; lengthy and perhaps less reliable incorporation; incompatible with cartilage cryopreservation
Demineralized	Potent osteoinducer; well suited to cystic defects and small or irregular bony gaps for supplementing stable fusions	Little intrinsic strength; complex processing; radiolucent

(recipient) rather than graft origins, the antithesis of the process achieved through solid organ transplantation. Thus, while there is some rationale for designating viable osseous tissues "grafts" and nonviable biologic preparations "implants" (transplanted versus implanted), common usage has tended to lump both categories together as "grafts" with appropriate descriptive adjectives appended: fresh revascularized segmental fibular autografts, freeze-dried irradiated cancellous wafer allografts, frozen distal femoral osteochondral allograft with cryopreserved articular cartilage, and the like.

Biology

Autografts

The process of bone graft incorporation has been well described histologically and represents a predictable sequence of events reflecting a partnership between graft-derived and host-derived factors. After implantation, the graft becomes enveloped in a hematoma. Unless the blood supply is immediately reestablished by vascular anastomosis, only those superficial cellular elements able to survive with the support of diffusion will persist. Most graft-derived cells will die within a few days, and this necrosis is responsible for inciting an inflammatory response. The host-tissue reaction is transformed into a fibrovascular stroma over the one to two weeks following placement of the graft. Blood vessels, accompanied by populations of host cells inducible or dedicated to the purposes of bone resorption and formation, converge at the graft. Because of its more open physical structure, cancellous tissue permits more rapid permeation of this new blood supply within its substance than does cortical bone. In cortex, the vascular response must find, transverse, and widen existing Volkmann and haversian canals to reestablish the blood flow (Figs. 1 and 2). Consequently, most of the remodeling of cortical autografts is confined to the osteonal rather than the interstitial lamellae.

The initial host-cell activity at the periphery and within bone grafts is resorptive and is mediated by osteoclasts derived from circulating monocytes of hematopoietic origin (Fig. 3). Osteoblasts, likewise arising from bone marrow precursors, subsequently synthesize and deposit osteoid on preexisting bony surfaces, particularly at sites of resorptive activity. While the normally stable net results of resorption and formation reflect their usually synchronous natures, the rates of these activities in individual cells differ substantially. Individual osteoclasts are capable of resorbing as much as 50 μm of bone matrix per day, while osteoblasts add new bone at a daily rate of 1.0 to 1.7 μm. The temporal sequence of these cellular events (resorption followed by formation) and their localization to the same or nearly the same sites on the surface of existing bone matrix suggest the expression of humeral signals or exposure of protein messengers at points of previous osteoclastic resorption. Furthermore,

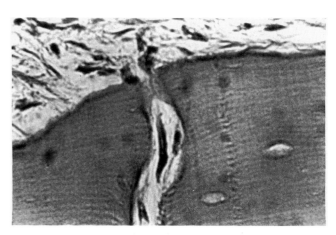

Fig. 1   The graft is initially surrounded by a hematoma that changes to fibrovascular tissue. From this response, blood vessels find their way into the avascular and acellular graft substance through preexisting Volkmann or haversian canals.

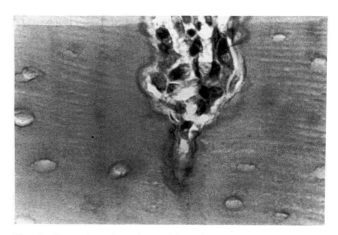

Fig. 2   Osteoclasts from the recipient site are conveyed into the graft, along with the new blood supply, and widen previous canals by resorbing matrix. This resorption substantially increases internal porosity, a state that persists until sufficient new bone has been formed.

the repair and remodeling observed during graft incorporation at a cellular (or physiologic) level is analogous to intact bone homeostasis (and fracture repair) and presumably relies on a cascade of circulating systemic factors and locally derived molecular signals.

The most notable group of molecules associated with bone induction and osteogenesis are the bone morphogenetic proteins (BMPs). Originally thought to be a single molecule with a molecular weight between 17,000 and 22,000, the BMP "family" is now known to include at least seven glycoproteins, four of which induce bone formation. These molecules have been isolated, purified,

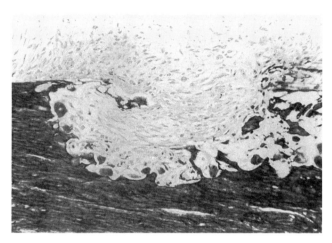

Fig. 3 In addition to performing internal resorption, osteoclasts vigorously remove existing matrix at the periphery of the graft.

synthesized, and, to various degrees, characterized and appear to exist as dimers of similar or identical protein chains of approximately 15,000 d each (30,000 d per dimer). Based on the significant homology of amino acid sequences, the BMPs appear related to the large group of molecules termed the "transforming growth factor-beta" (TGF-β) superfamily. Growing evidence suggests that a variety of different BMPs and other TGF-β molecules collaboratively and sequentially influence the recruitment, differentiation, maturation, and synthetic activities of the cells and events collectively producing bone graft incorporation.

It is important to recognize that incorporation is a collaborative effort between the graft and the host. The host contributes all the blood vessels and most, if not all, of the cells required for incorporation. Consequently, the regenerated bone is of recipient origin, an important issue when considering the fate of allogeneic and xenogeneic bone grafts. The primary functions of the graft are its passive service as a template or scaffold for the vascular and cellular events of incorporation (osteoconduction) or the active phenomenon whereby the graft matrix, and perhaps residual surviving cells, provide molecular signals to the host that are responsible for recruiting and sustaining the required cellular activity (osteoinduction). Although few, the graft-derived cells surviving transplantation clearly participate in the early phase of osteogenesis.

Variations in the sequence and intensity of these cellular events of graft incorporation are seen when autografts are immediately revascularized, when autogenous tissues are compared with allogeneic alternatives, and when allografts are treated before implantation.

Revascularized Autografts

Autografts transferred on a vascular pedicle or reanastomosed immediately to a blood supply do not undergo

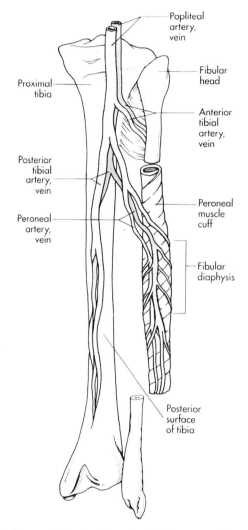

Fig. 4 Revascularized grafts are isolated on a vascular pedicle suitable for microvascular reanastomosis at the recipient site. The fibula is the most common donor site. Because of immunologic considerations, this approach is limited to autogenous tissues. (Reproduced with permission from Friedlander G, Tomford W, Galloway M, et al: Tissue transplantation, in Starzl TE, Shapiro R, Simmons RL (eds): *Atlas of Organ Transplantation*. New York, Raven Press, 1992, p 105.)

extensive cell necrosis and do not require the lengthy repair process characteristic of conventional graft incorporation (Fig. 4). Indeed, these grafts remain viable and heal at their osteosynthesis sites (graft-host bone junction) by events analogous to those of fracture repair.

The blood supply for revascularized grafts, usually the fibula, is based in part on the nutrient vessel(s) that penetrate into the medullary canal and then ascend and descend the internal diaphysis, as well as on the periosteal circulation emanating from the adjacent musculature. The relative contributions of these two sources remain controversial. Attempts to monitor the repair process of revascularized autografts noninvasively in canine models have been problematic. In particular, technetium bone scans are reliable indicators of blood flow to the graft only during the first postoperative week: thereafter, the results may be misleading.

The principal advantages of the revascularized bone graft are the relative speed of repair and the absence of dependence on the host site either for neovascularization (other than direct access to the peripheral circulation) or as a source of osteogenic cell populations. This absence of host dependence makes these grafts particularly useful when the local environment is compromised, such as by local irradiation or infection; when the orthotopic site is sufficiently abnormal to preclude a reliable source of osteoprogenitor cells, such as in pseudarthrosis of the tibia; or when a more rapid repair of a lengthy segmental defect is desirable than is possible with nonvascularized grafts.

The limitations of revascularized bone grafts reflect their technically demanding nature, the few available donor sites (fibula, rib, iliac crest), and, for practical purposes, the exclusive use of autogenous rather than allogeneic sources. Substantial immunosuppression in animal models has permitted the successful application of allografts, but clinically, the potential complications associated with altered immunocompetence have outweighed the benefits. There also remains controversy as to the degree of hypertrophy and the biomechanical properties of revascularized autografts. Recent studies in a canine model indicated that revascularized fibulae, with an intact medullary blood supply, are larger, stiffer, and stronger and possess greater bone mass than do nonvascularized alternatives.

Allografts

The histologic sequence of events associated with bone allograft repair is qualitatively similar, if not identical, to that seen in autografts. The biologic fate of allogeneic bone, however, is relatively inferior to that of autogenous bone, regardless of preservation techniques. These differences reflect the slower and less extensive incorporation associated with allografts in a variety of animal models. On the other hand, the extent of repair associated with allogeneic bone is often sufficient for the graft to respond to the physiologic stresses it will experience, making allograft use a reasonable alternative in many clinical circumstances.

As is true of bone autografts, allografts elicit a nonspecific inflammatory reaction based on cell necrosis. Unlike autografts, allogeneic bone evokes specific immune responses reflecting the degree of genetic disparity between the donor and the recipient. As the graft revascularizes, the new blood supply invades the allogeneic matrix and exposes the host to foreign antigens. Studies in rats have demonstrated the impaired ingrowth of blood vessels to fresh allogeneic bone in comparison with histocompatible tissue and suggest that this lack of vascularity was responsible for the lesser rates of both bone re-

sorption and formation observed in syngeneic versus allogeneic tissue. In dogs, the degree to which revascularization and remodeling (resorption and formation) are impaired directly parallels the extent of histocompatibility differences.

In a rat knee joint model, fresh revascularized allografts transferred against a strong histocompatibility mismatch demonstrate rapid cell death. The initial immunologic response probably targets the vascular endothelial cells of donor origin, causing disruption of the blood supply. Graft osteogenic cells probably are a secondary target of the immune response. Indeed, if the histocompatibility differences are minor, the intensity of the cellular response is weaker and more gradual in its evolution. In this case, the blood vessels remain patent, and the earliest cell necrosis occurs in osteoblasts, with osteoclasts succumbing later. Of additional note, physeal chondrocytes appear to survive transplantation across weak histocompatibility barriers.

Most bone allografts used clinically are subjected to some form of preservation, most commonly deep freezing, freeze-drying, demineralization, or combinations of these approaches. In animal models, studies of allograft incorporation have been confusing, because preservation techniques are known to diminish immune responses by reducing antigenicity on one hand but may also influence the osteogenic capacity of the graft independent of immunogenicity. Most studies focusing on differences in preservation techniques (fresh, frozen, freeze-dried) demonstrate all allografts to be biologically inferior to fresh autografts, and usually, the differences between variously preserved allografts are minor. For example, when the variables of immunogenicity are evaluated, closely matched frozen allografts—those that have only minor mismatches of major histocompatibility complex (MHC) antigens—are associated with significantly greater new bone formation than markedly disparate (major MHC mismatches) frozen allografts. The rates of revascularization, mineralization, and bone resorption are all greater in syngeneic animal grafts than in allografts.

Despite the biologic limitations of allografts compared with autografts, allogeneic bone has been associated with the successful repair of fracture nonunions, promotion of arthrodeses, and reliable segmental replacements of long bone and spinal segments (including the intervertebral disk) in a variety of animal models. There has been insufficient opportunity to evaluate these same biologic issues fully in humans, but there is reason to believe that bone graft repair in man is qualitatively similar to that observed in numerous animal models.

Demineralized Bone Matrix

Demineralized allogeneic bone matrix (DABM) has been studied extensively in many animal models and shown to be osteoinductive in nonskeletal sites in rats as well as in segmental long-bone defects in rats, rabbits, and dogs. Similarly, autolyzed antigen-extracted demineralized allogeneic bone has been effective in these same circumstances. However, DABM has not been useful in the repair of canine cranial defects, perhaps reflecting differences in the skull as a recipient site rather than inadequacies of this preserved bone. Of note, DABM from adult monkeys is osteoinductive in athymic rats but not when implanted in muscular sites in other adult monkeys. A well-recognized limitation of demineralized tissue has been its intrinsic biomechanical weakness prior to incorporation. One recent study suggested that less extensive demineralization can retain the osteogenic advantages of processing in this manner while preserving significant mechanical strength.

Allogeneic preparations of BMP have been successful in promoting the repair of segmental long-bone defects in dogs when combined with a suitable carrier such as polylactic acid polymer. Combinations of BMP and demineralized bone matrix have not proved efficacious in canine models.

Bone Marrow Aspirates

Recognizing the central importance of osteogenic cell populations in bone repair and graft incorporation, investigators have used bone marrow aspirates to provide the activity usually sought from conventional bone grafts but with a far less invasive procedure than is required to obtain the traditional iliac crest autograft. Unfractionated marrow cell populations have demonstrated osteogenic activity in rabbit segmental radius defects, and this response was enhanced by concentration, but not by fractionation, of the marrow if the separation was accomplished entirely on the basis of the weight characteristics of the heterogeneous cells in the aspirate. In rats, the combination of porous ceramics (hydroxyapatite) and syngeneic marrow cells (or allogeneic bone marrow implanted in nude mice) has been effective in repairing segmental bone defects. Furthermore, the combination of syngeneic marrow and xenogeneic bone grafts has proved efficacious in children.

Synthetic Substitutes

Synthetic alternatives to bone grafts, particularly hydroxyapatite and tricalcium phosphate, have attracted significant attention. Both materials can be found or manufactured with a physiologic range of pore sizes, 50 to 600 μm, and have been evaluated in animal models, usually dog or rabbit, either as single materials, mixed together, or supplemented with autograft or other sources of cells or BMP. Hydroxyapatite and tricalcium phosphate in cancellous skeletal sites are invaded by blood vessels and osteogenic cell populations from the host. Tricalcium phosphate is biodegradable, being replaced by new bone, whereas hydroxyapatite is nonbiodegradable but serves as an effective osteoconductive material. Neither hydroxyapatite nor tricalcium phosphate is significantly inductive, nor are their activities substantially enhanced by a pulsed electromagnetic field. These structurally weak materials appear suitable for filling cystic defects, where the intrinsic mechanical strength of the graft is less important.

Influence of Drugs and Irradiation

Many drugs, including cancer chemotherapy and nonsteroidal anti-inflammatory agents, adversely influence new bone formation in the intact skeleton and, to some degree, the repair associated with fractures in animal models. Similar findings follow irradiation. Although these effects have not yet been studied in bone grafts, it is reasonable to assume that some drugs and physical modalities will influence graft incorporation. Preliminary data suggest a higher incidence of nonunions in human recipients of osteochondral allografts who are simultaneously treated with chemotherapy. Physical barriers such as polymethylmethacrylate placed between the graft and its host bed also interfere with the ability of a graft to incorporate successfully by interfering with the ingress of blood vessels and the recruitment of osteogenic cells.

Immunology

Allogeneic and xenogeneic bone grafts are immunogenic. Over the past 40 years, numerous investigators have used the available methodology to confirm that fresh allografts evoke immune responses. These conclusions were based on the histologic nature of the associated inflammatory cells, nodal weight gain and blast transformation of small lymphocytes in regional lymph nodes, skin graft rejection patterns, and, more recently, the appearance of humoral antibodies and cell-mediated cytotoxicity in objective in vitro assays. Bone is a composite tissue, but the most immunogenic components of grafts clearly are the various cells, and, more specifically, their surface glycoproteins expressed under the control of the MHC. These are the HLA antigens in humans, referred to as class I when related to the HLA-A, -B, or -C loci (historically identified by serologic techniques) or the lymphocyte-defined class II antigens, reflecting the HLA-D (or -DR) locus. Using sensitive in vitro approaches and mice of selected recombinant strains with well-defined genetic maps, it has been determined that allogeneic bone in culture activates T lymphocytes, that this proliferation reflects the presence of both class I and class II MHC determinants, that stimulation does not depend on the presence of marrow, and that the alloreactive T lymphocytes are of the killer/suppressor phenotype.

Immune responses to fresh bone allografts have been detected in a number of animal models as well as in humans. These responses are reduced if the allograft is frozen prior to implantation, and the immunogenicity is further diminished by freeze-drying. What remains controversial is the influence of these immune responses on the biology of graft incorporation. There is growing evidence that these responses do alter graft biology in animals. In a well-studied canine model, the metabolic, histologic, and gross appearances of articular cartilage suffered most when osteochondral allografts were transplanted fresh across histocompatibility mismatches. Closely matched allografts maintained substantially more normal cartilage function than did the mismatched group. This same spectrum of biologic activity was documented in bone, with fresh autografts undergoing more rapid and more extensive new-bone formation than fresh mismatched allografts. Frozen allogeneic bone and matched fresh allografts were intermediate in their biologic activity.

Another approach to defining the influence of immunogenicity on allograft biology has focused on the use of immunosuppression. Cyclosporin A has improved the results of fresh allografts in rats and dogs. This same immunosuppressant improves the metabolic, histologic, and biomechanical fate of mismatched, immediately revascularized fibular allografts in dogs, again suggesting that the immune responses associated with osteochondral allografts are detrimental to bone incorporation.

Human recipients of allogeneic bone appear to develop immune responses similar in pattern to those observed in animals: fresh allografts are strongly immunogenic, deep freezing reduces this response, and freeze drying provides the most profound reduction in responsiveness. However, it has not been possible to evaluate allograft biology systematically in humans by invasive techniques. Failed frozen allografts available for study generally appear indolent in their internal repair, and the incorporation activity that does occur is a result of osteoconduction rather than osteoinduction. However, it is unclear whether these same patterns hold true in radiographically and clinically successful allografts, which represent 70% to 80% of most series. Consequently, bone allografts continue to be chosen for their anatomic sizes and shapes, mechanical strength, and intrinsic osteogenic potential rather than on the basis of blood or tissue types.

Bone Banking

In order to utilize the many innovative and efficacious approaches to reconstructing skeletal deficits, a program of bone banking is required to provide safe and appropriate grafts in a timely fashion. This banking requires attention to consent laws, donor selection criteria, laboratory (including microbiologic) testing, recovery techniques, and record keeping.

Consent Laws

As is true of other transplantable tissues and organs, permission of the donor or authorization by the appropriate next of kin is required in the United States before bone can be removed for transplantation. Some countries operate under "presumed consent" doctrines, whereby society expects that individuals will be donors if they meet selection criteria unless they or their next of kin object. Our traditional approach of "voluntary donation" was based on interested health-care workers voluntarily initiating requests for donation followed by the voluntary participation of donors, but legislation throughout the United States now requires health-care institutions to identify and ask all potential organ and tissue donors (or their next of kin) whether they wish to participate. The option remains completely voluntary. This approach is termed "required request" or "routine inquiry." It was designed to increase the frequency of organ and tissue donation, given the substantial unmet needs for all of these transplantable resources. There is evidence that this mechanism has been much more useful for increasing the supply of tissues than is the case for organs.

Donor Selection Criteria

In order to minimize, if not eliminate, transmission of potentially serious disease from donor to recipient, careful review of the patient's medical history and selected laboratory testing is required. Donors are screened carefully to avoid those individuals with infections of a bacterial, viral, or fungal origin (including hepatitis, venereal disease, slow virus disorders, and AIDS), either of a systemic nature or involving the tissues to be collected. Malignancies, with the exception of basal-cell carcinoma of the skin and some tumors confined to the central nervous system, diseases of unknown origin, disorders affecting the biologic or biomechanical nature of the skeleton (systemic collagen or metabolic bone diseases), and the presence of significant amounts of toxic substances (poisons, radioactivity) are all contraindications to tissue donation. The U.S. Public Health Service has also developed criteria for the exclusion of high-risk donors, focusing on HIV infection and circumstances that increase the chance of exposure to this virus (male homosexuality, intravenous drug abuse, hemophilia and other disorders managed with concentrates of clotting factors, immigration from high-prevalence regions, prostitution).

Laboratory Testing

Hepatitis has been transmitted by bone graft material, and it is important to utilize available screens for hepatitis B (core and surface antigens) and hepatitis C (C-100, C-33, and C-22 proteins). There are now four individuals in the United States who have contracted HIV infection through allogeneic bone grafts. These cases can be traced to two donors in 1985, both of whom would have been detected as HIV infected by today's screening methodology, including assays targeting the virus core antigen or DNA based on polymerase chain reaction (PCR) analysis. In the most recent report documenting HIV transmission from an organ and tissue (bone) donor, all four recipients of solid vascularized organs became infected, and three of the 41 tested recipients of tissue (bone, fascia, tendon, ligament, cornea, dura) were positive for the virus. All three of these individuals received frozen bone. The only other recipient of frozen bone, but with the marrow washed out, has no evidence of HIV infection; the other tissues were all lyophilized (freeze-dried), and some were additionally irradiated or exposed to ethanol.

The risk of contracting HIV infection from bone grafts is clearly present, but if donors are screened by the methods required for bank accreditation by the American Association of Tissue Banks, the incidence of infection has been estimated to be less than one in 1 million and certainly no more than the one in 40,000 associated with blood transfusions. Given the fact that one in 100 males and one in 800 females in the United States are estimated to be infected with HIV, it is clearly important to screen potential donors for this virus and other vectors of potentially harmful transmissible disease.

Banking Methods

There are two general approaches to the recovery of bone for transplantation. Tissues can be removed in a clean but nonsterile environment or in an operating room using standard aseptic technique. In the former case, the tissue needs to be secondarily sterilized, and this is usually accomplished by exposure to ethylene oxide, high-dose irradiation (10 to 30 x 10³ Gy), or strong acids (hydrochloric acid). Grafts sterilized in such a manner are usually freeze-dried for long-term storage. Tissues acquired in a sterile fashion can be preserved by any of a variety of techniques, including deep freezing to -70 to -80 C, the only long-term storage approach compatible with cryopreservation of articular cartilage. The other advantages of deep freezing are the retention of biomechanical properties, low cost, and ease of application. Freeze-drying permits storage for indefinite periods of time at room temperature, but the strength of the bone is reduced (often, this is of no relevance to its clinical application). Demineralization of bone prior to implantation enhances osteoinduction but at the expense of markedly reduced mechanical strength. In rabbits, lipid extraction of frozen grafts with chloroform-methanol also increases new bone formation.

Clinical Applications

Autografts

Fresh bone autografts continue to be used frequently and successfully for a wide variety of clinical indications such as acute comminuted fractures, nonunions, arthrodeses, and cystic or short segmental defects of traumatic, degenerative, or neoplastic origin and to supplement inadequate bone stock in the course of total joint arthroplasty. Indeed, fresh autogenous bone represents the maximum available and most reliable source of osteogenic activity. This type of graft is particularly useful in the presence of satisfactory soft-tissue coverage and in the absence of infection.

Recent reports emphasize the clinical efficacy of dual fibular autografts with substantial internal and external fixation for segmental defects as long as 24 cm and the usefulness of autogenous bone for repair of tibial non-

unions by posterolateral grafting (97% success rate), in combination with decompression to facilitate the healing of avascular necrosis of the femoral head, and to promote spine fusions. Autografts have been used extensively to augment acetabular defects or deficiencies and to enhance the osteointegration of porous-coated implants in conjunction with total joint replacement. However, long-term studies suggest loosening of as many as 46% of the acetabular components between 2.9 and 12.7 years in circumstances that necessitated use of supplemental bone stock at the time of the original procedure.

Vascularized Autografts

Vascularized autografts, especially based on the fibula or iliac crest, have been useful for reconstructing segmental deficits associated with a compromised local environment. By immediate reestablishment of the blood supply to the graft through microvascular reanastomosis, these grafts are effective in situations with inadequate soft-tissue coverage, in the presence of infection, or when local bone is biologically deficient in repair potential (congenital pseudarthrosis of the tibia). Revascularized fibulae heal rapidly and can be expected to unite and hypertrophy over time in at least 80% of cases. Such grafts have been effective in recalcitrant nonunions of the humerus and have been associated with successful repair of 95% of congenital tibial pseudarthroses. Vascularized grafts from the ilium have proved useful in the treatment of scaphoid nonunions, and vascularized portions of the iliac crest have been used to reconstruct the proximal humerus after resection of aggressive giant-cell tumors. This method also has been used to supplement large segmental allografts. Magnetic resonance imaging is the least morbid approach to the necessary preoperative assessment of donor site vascularity and is an alternative to angiography.

While autografts provide the optimum available biologic potential and avoid the issue of transfer of disease from donor to recipient, these tissues are associated with some morbidity and potential limitations. Autografts require sacrifice of a normal bony structure, usually at a second operative site, with a potential for longer operative time, additional blood loss, wound infection, and greater postoperative discomfort. Of more significance, autogenous bone grafts are limited in their available size, shape, and quantity.

Allografts

Bone allografts circumvent the disadvantages of autogenous tissues but present their own concerns, especially in the areas of biologic activity, transfer of disease, and consequences of immunogenicity. Decades of clinical experience have confirmed the efficacy of bone allografts preserved by a variety of methods but most notably deep freezing, freeze-drying, and demineralization. Seventy percent or more of frozen osteoarticular (including a joint surface) or intercalary (segments without an articular surface) allografts used after limb-sparing tumor re-

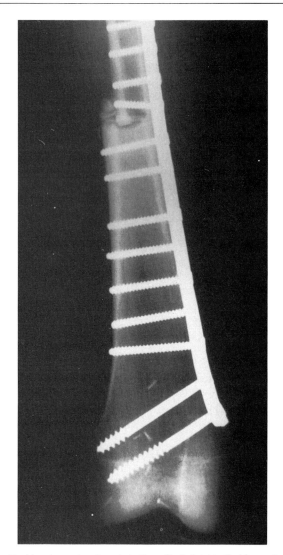

Fig. 5 Massive osteochondral allograft of distal half of femur in 12-year-old patient after resection of osteosarcoma. The graft was deep frozen, the cartilage was cryopreserved with exposure to dimethylsulfoxide, and the junction between the graft and the host was held by internal fixation and supplemented by autograft.

sections have been associated with satisfactory clinical function (Fig. 5). Complications, particularly during the first two postoperative years, include infection, fracture, or nonunion at the osteosynthesis site(s), each occurring in 5% to 15% of patients. Infection is the most devastating, usually necessitating removal of the graft, although an exchange of bone after eradication of the infection is

sometimes feasible. Massive allografts are particularly useful in limb reconstruction after tumor ablation. They allow for reattachment of soft tissues, avoid the long-term fixation problems associated with large custom implants, and are compatible with cemented endoprosthetics for joint surface replacement.

Preserved bone allografts also have been used with satisfactory success rates to reconstruct deficits of the proximal femur or acetabulum at the time of hip arthroplasty, including revision surgery prompted by aseptic loosening. Frozen allografts of femoral-head origin have behaved indistinguishably from fresh autografts in scoliosis fusions, and preserved allogeneic bone used to fill benign cystic lesions in children has been of similar efficacy in small defects although less impressive in larger lesions when compared with autografts. The operative time in these procedures was reduced significantly by the use of allogeneic bone. The incidence of nonunions in single-level anterior cervical spine fusions was identical (5%) whether autografts or freeze-dried allografts were used, although the time to fusion was longer with allografts. Allogeneic bone behaved less well than autogenous tissues in multilevel fusions.

The issue of transferring disease from donor to recipient remains important but can be addressed satisfactorily by rigorous attention to donor selection criteria and laboratory testing. The influence of allograft immunogenicity on bone incorporation in humans remains unresolved but clearly does not preclude a satisfactory clinical result in the majority of graft recipients. Consequently, preserved bone allografts have a clear role in reconstructive surgery and represent a safe and reliable alternative to autografts. However, autografts remain the superior choice when donor site morbidity is acceptable and can provide a sufficient quantity and the desired shape of tissue for the intended purposes.

Synthetic Substitutes

Biosynthetics have yet to be evaluated extensively in humans. Early information supports the osteoconductive nature of hydroxyapatite or tricalcium phosphate preparations in cystic defects. Similar ceramic coatings on metal femoral prostheses have likewise demonstrated osteointegration of the ingrowing bony response with the surface-bound hydroxyapatite material. Trials are now underway of combinations of ceramics, collagen, and marrow as alternatives to autogenous bone grafts, and there is reason to believe these approaches will prove useful in the future.

Annotated Bibliography

General Considerations

Friedlaender GE: Bone grafts: The basic science rationale for clinical applications. *J Bone Joint Surg* 1987;69A:786-790.

This is a concise summary of the cellular events characteristic of bone graft incorporation, stressing the relation between graft- and host-derived contributions and their clinical implications.

Friedlaender GE, Goldberg VM (eds): *Bone and Cartilage Allografts: Biology and Clinical Applications*. Park Ridge, IL, American Academy of Orthopaedic Surgeons, 1991.

This book reviews a wide spectrum of basic knowledge pertaining to the biology of bone autografts and allografts. Biomechanical and immunologic considerations are also reviewed. Clinical issues are explored; both bone banking practices and the use of conventional autografts, revascularized autografts, and preserved osteochondral allografts in a variety of disorders.

Biology

Aspenberg P, Lohmander LS, Thorngren KG: Monkey bone matrix induces bone formation in the athymic rat, but not in adult monkeys. *J Orthop Res* 1991;9:20-25.

Demineralized bone matrix from young and adult monkeys was evaluated after intramuscular implantation in athymic rats and adult monkeys. These preparations were osteoinductive in the immunocompromised rats but not in the monkeys. This finding is in contrast to the inductive properties of demineralized matrix often demonstrated in animal models lower than the nonhuman primates evaluated in this study, and raises doubt about the clinical behavior of human-derived implants.

Goldberg VM, Stevenson S, Shaffer JW, et al: Biological and physical properties of autogenous vascularized fibular grafts in dogs. *J Bone Joint Surg* 1990;72A:801-810.

The biologic and biomechanical properties of intact, nonvascularized, and revascularized autogenous fibulae were assessed in dogs three months after transplantation. Metabolic turnover, as assessed by preoperative isotope labeling of mineral and collagen, was similar for sham and revascularized grafts, as were biomechanical characteristics. In contrast, nonvascularized grafts were smaller, weaker, less stiff, and more porotic and exhibited faster turnover than the other types. This article confirms the biologic and biomechanical advantages of revascularized autografts.

Heckman JD, Boyan BD, Aufdemorte TB, et al: The use of bone morphogenetic protein in the treatment of non-union in a canine model. *J Bone Joint Surg* 1991;73A:750-764.

Using a canine segmental defect model, the investigators evaluated species-specific versus xenogeneic sources of BMP with and without a polylactic acid carrier. The best reparative response occurred with canine BMP combined with a resorbable carrier substance.

Kirkeby OJ: Revascularisation of bone grafts in rats. *J Bone Joint Surg* 1991;73B:501-505.

The rates of bone formation and resorption were substantially lower in rat allografts compared with syngeneic grafts. This difference appears related to impaired revascularization in allografts, demonstrated by a radioactive microsphere technique.

Kirkeby OJ, Larsen TB, Lereim P: Bone grafts in T-cell deficient rats. *Acta Orthop Scand* 1991;62:459-462.

The impaired revascularization of allografts noted in a normal rat model was improved in athymic rats, suggesting that T-cell responses are important in producing the less successful incorporation associated with allogeneic as opposed to syngeneic bone graft repair.

Köhler P, Ehrnberg A, Kreicbergs A: Osteogenic enhancement of diaphyseal reconstruction: Comparison of bone grafts in the rabbit. *Acta Orthop Scand* 1990;61:42-45.

The use of allogeneic demineralized bone matrix improved the incorporation of autoclaved autografts and frozen allografts in a rabbit segmental defect model.

Pelker RR, McKay J Jr, Troiano N, et al: Allograft incorporation: A biomechanical evaluation in a rat model. *J Orthop Res* 1989;7:585-589.

Segmental allografts in rats healed with similar mechanical strength in torsion regardless of whether the grafts were fresh or reduced in immunogenicity by deep freezing or irradiation. The influence of immune responses directed against bone graft-related antigens on the biology of repair remains unclear.

Bone Marrow Grafting

Connolly J, Guse R, Lippiello L, et al: Development of an osteogenic bone-marrow preparation. *J Bone Joint Surg* 1989;71A:684-691.

Osteogenesis was significantly increased when bone marrow was concentrated by simple centrifugation compared with equal volumes of nonprocessed marrow in ectopic or orthotopic sites in rabbits. These observations support the use of bone marrow aspirates to promote bony repair. While certain subpopulations of marrow may be most responsible for favorable outcomes, simple concentration appears particularly efficacious.

Weintraub S, Goodwin D, Khermosh O, et al: The clinical use of autologous marrow to improve osteogenic potential of bone grafts in pediatric orthopaedics. *J Pediatr Orthop* 1989;9:186-190.

Autologous bone marrow added to xenogeneic (Kiel) bone was associated with successful resolution of a variety of benign bone cysts and defects in 22 of 23 patients. The investigators speculate that the combination of autologous bone marrow and a variety of allogeneic, xenogeneic, and synthetic bone graft materials will prove clinically useful.

Immunology

Horowitz MC, Friedlaender GE: Induction of specific T-cell responsiveness to allogeneic bone. *J Bone Joint Surg* 1991;73A:1157-1168.

Using sensitive in vitro techniques and recombinant inbred strains of mice, the nature of bone allograft immunogenicity was explored. Both class I and class II cell-surface histocompatibility antigens appearing on osteogenic cells caused the activation and proliferation of T cells of the killer/suppressor phenotype. This response occurred even when marrow cells were removed from the stimulating bone cell population.

Rodrigo JJ, Schnaser AM, Reynolds HM Jr, et al: Inhibition of the immune response to experimental fresh osteoarticular allografts. *Clin Orthop* 1989;243:235-253.

A variety of approaches to immunosuppression were evaluated in rat and canine osteochondral allograft models, including systemic drugs, preadministration of blood, and coating the donor bone with biodegradable cement. Cyclosporin A was most effective both in decreasing the antibody response associated with this allograft and in enhancing articular cartilage function but also caused undesirable systemic toxicity.

Stevenson S, Li XQ, Martin B: The fate of cancellous and cortical bone after transplantation of fresh and frozen tissue-antigen-matched and mismatched osteochondral allografts in dogs. *J Bone Joint Surg* 1991;73A:1143-1156.

Fresh and frozen tissue-antigen-matched or -mismatched canine osteochondral allografts were evaluated 11 months after transplantation and compared with autografts. Fresh mismatched grafts, the most immunogenic combination, demonstrated the least fluorochrome uptake and new bone formation, the slowest revascularization, and the most fibrous connective tissue formation within the substance of the graft. This study suggests a direct correlation between successful graft biology and decreased immunogenicity in allograft transplantation.

Bone Banking

Buck BE, Malinin TI, Brown MD: Bone transplantation and human immunodeficiency virus: An estimate of risk of acquired immunodeficiency syndrome (AIDS). *Clin Orthop* 1989;240:129-136.

This article stresses the need to screen potential bone donors rigorously for the presence of harmful infectious organisms, including the human immunodeficiency virus (HIV). When the recommended methodology is used, the chance of receiving bone from an HIV-infected donor is estimated to be less than one in one million. Without proper screening the risk is unacceptably high.

Eggen BM, Nordbo SA: Transmission of HCV by organ transplantation: Letter to the editor. *N Engl J Med* 1992;326:411.

The authors document the transmission of hepatitis C virus in 1990 to the recipient of a frozen femoral-head allograft from a donor later found to be anti-HCV positive.

Simonds RJ, Homberg SD, Hurwitz RL, et al: Transmission of human immunodeficiency virus type 1 from a seronegative organ and tissue donor. *N Engl J Med* 1992;326:726-732.

The authors describe the transmission of HIV-1 from a donor to multiple organ and tissue recipients in 1985. Of 48 identified recipients, 41 were tested for HIV-1 antibody. All four organ recipients and three recipients of frozen, but otherwise unprocessed, bone were infected. Thirty-four recipients of other tissues (primarily freeze-dried bone) have remained seronegative. Using more sensitive present techniques for the detection of HIV infection, not available in 1985, this donor would have been identified as a carrier and excluded. The risk of HIV infection from an organ or tissue donor exists but appears exceedingly low if current screening techniques are used.

Tomford WW, Thongphasuk J, Mankin HJ, et al: Frozen musculoskeletal allografts: A study of the clinical

incidence and causes of infection associated with their use. *J Bone Joint Surg* 1990;72A:1137-1143.

A retrospective study of the incidence of clinically apparent infection was carried out in 324 patients having a variety of frozen musculoskeletal allografts distributed from this established tissue bank adhering to rigorous standards. Of patients receiving large grafts after tumor resection or revision arthroplasty, 4% to 5% became infected. In most cases, this was unlikely to have been secondary to contamination of the allografts. The infection rate with smaller grafts, including femoral heads, was negligible.

Clinical Experience
Autografts

Clarke HJ, Jinnah RH, Lennox D: Osteointegration of bone graft in porous-coated total hip arthroplasty. *Clin Orthop* 1990;258:160-167.

This clinical series of 19 patients followed radiographically since 1983 demonstrated the usefulness of bone grafting in association with porous-coated acetabular components. The average time needed to achieve incorporation of the graft was 12 months.

Mulroy RD Jr, Harris WH: Failure of acetabular autogenous grafts in total hip arthroplasty: Increasing incidence: A follow-up note. *J Bone Joint Surg* 1990;72A:1536-1540.

Forty-six hips in 37 patients were reevaluated nearly 12 years after autogenous femoral head grafting to address acetabular bone stock insufficiency at the time of total hip arthroplasty. Forty-six percent of the acetabula demonstrated loosening radiographically or at the time of revision.

Simpson JM, Ebraheim NA, An HS, et al: Posterolateral bone graft of the tibia. *Clin Orthop* 1990;251:200-206.

A total of 30 high-energy open and often comminuted fractures of the tibial diaphyses were treated by posterolateral bone autografts, 19 within six months of injury and the remainder after nonunion was established. Twenty-nine (97%) of the fractures went on to union an average of 4.7 months after the graft procedure, emphasizing the efficacy of this approach.

Steinberg ME, Brighton CT, Corces A, et al: Osteonecrosis of the femoral head: Results of core decompression and grafting with and without electrical stimulation. *Clin Orthop* 1989;249:199-208.

Core decompression and bone grafting of hips with avascular necrosis with or without direct-current stimulation were compared with each other and with nonoperative treatment. Both surgically treated groups had less radiographic progression and required fewer arthroplasties than patients treated without surgery. The addition of direct-current stimulation seemed to improve the results even more so than decompression and grafting without electrical stimulation.

Yadav SS: Dual-fibular grafting for massive bone gaps in the lower extremity. *J Bone Joint Surg* 1990;72A:486-494.

Fifty-two patients with segmental deficits in lower extremity long bones after tumor resection were reconstructed with dual-fibular autografts. The gaps ranged from 9 to 24 cm. Eight patients required subsequent corticocancellous bone grafts for nonunion and three for stress fracture. Adequate internal fixation was considered critical to the high success rate of this approach.

Vascularized Autografts

Jupiter JB: Complex non-union of the humeral diaphysis: Treatment with a medial approach, an anterior plate, and a vascularized fibular graft. *J Bone Joint Surg* 1990;72A:701-707.

Internal fixation and use of a vascularized fibular autograft led to union of all four atrophic synovial nonunions of the humeral shaft in this series. The average duration of the nonunion prior to this procedure was 33.5 months.

Manaster BJ, Coleman DA, Bell DA: Magnetic resonance imaging of vascular anatomy before vascularized fibular grafting. *J Bone Joint Surg* 1990;72A:409-414.

This study demonstrated the ability of MRI to delineate the vascular anatomy of the fibula and the remainder of the leg in preparation for use of the fibula on a vascular pedicle. This approach is more cost-effective and less morbid than traditional arteriography.

Nusbickel FR, Dell PC, McAndrew MP, et al: Vascularized autografts for reconstruction of skeletal defects following lower extremity trauma: A review. *Clin Orthop* 1989;243:65-70.

The applications of vascularized fibular autografts are reviewed, emphasizing the advantages of this approach over conventional grafting methods. Vascularized grafts are not dependent on an uninfected, well-vascularized host bed. They are associated with hypertrophy over time and reconstruct large segmental deficits successfully in approximately 80% of cases.

Weiland AJ, Weiss A-P, Moore JR, et al: Vascularized fibular grafts in the treatment of congenital pseudarthrosis of the tibia. *J Bone Joint Surg* 1990;72A:654-662.

Free vascularized fibulae were successful in repairing congenital pseudarthrosis of the tibia in 18 of 19 cases. Morbidity at the donor site was minimal.

Allografts

Berrey BH Jr, Lord CF, Gebhardt MC, et al: Fractures of allografts: Frequency, treatment, and end-results. *J Bone Joint Surg* 1990;72A:825-833.

Forty-three patients were identified who sustained a fracture through a massive osteochondral allograft; this represented a 16% incidence. Most patients were treated by operative reduction, fixation, and application of autogenous bone graft. The end results for this subgroup were similar to those of the entire patient population; that is, 75% achieved a good or excellent result. Thus, fracture of the allograft, which occurred an average of 28.6 months after transplantation, did not lead to a worse end result in most cases.

Gebhardt MC, Flugstad DI, Springfield DS, et al: The use of bone allografts for limb-salvage in high-grade extremity osteosarcoma. *Clin Orthop* 1991;270:181-196.

Massive frozen osteochondral allografts were used to reconstruct large deficits after resection of osteosarcomas in patients receiving adjuvant chemotherapy. While complication rates (infection, fracture, nonunion) were high, the overall results were satisfactory in 73% of the 53 patients.

Gitelis S, Piasecki P: Allograft prosthetic composite arthroplasty for osteosarcoma and other aggressive bone tumors. *Clin Orthop* 1991;270:197-201.

This study demonstrated the usefulness of combining frozen allografts with standard prosthetic components to address reconstructive needs after limb-sparing tumor resections, particularly those involving the hip or knee.

Clancy GL, Brugioni DJ, Eilert RE, et al: Autograft versus allograft for benign lesions in children. *Clin Orthop* 1991;262:28-33.

Autografts and allografts were compared in small- and large-volume benign bone lesions in children. Time to incorporation and success rates were similar for small lesions. Autografts were superior to allografts in larger defects (more than 60 cc) in terms of rate and completeness of repair. Nonetheless, allografts performed well enough to represent a satisfactory alternative when the availability of autograft or its associated morbidity is considered problematic.

Zdeblick TA, Ducker TB: The use of freeze-dried allograft bone for anterior cervical fusions. *Spine* 1991;16:726-729.

Tricortical iliac crest autograft and allografts were compared in 87 Smith-Robinson anterior cervical fusions. Symptomatic relief was similar regardless of the graft source. Autografts healed more rapidly and with less collapse and were substantially more reliable when more than one segment was fused. The nonunion rate for a single level was 5% with both autografts and allografts.

Synthetic Substitutes

Hardy DC, Frayssinet P, Guilhem A, et al: Bonding of hydroxyapatite-coated femoral prostheses: Histopathology of specimens from four cases. *J Bone Joint Surg* 1991;73B:732-740.

Specimens were examined from four patients with hydroxyapatite-coated femoral prostheses who died within nine months of their procedure. Biologic osteointegration was occurring in each case.

22

Prostheses: Materials, Fixation, and Design

Introduction

Orthopaedic prostheses are exposed to mechanical loading and environmental conditions that lead to fracture, wear, and corrosion of the materials of fabrication. Despite these ongoing processes of biomaterial failure, most prosthesis systems are able to function adequately for periods of ten to 20 years. Studies reported during the past three years indicate that the host response to wear-related particulate debris is the primary factor that limits the longevity of total joint replacement prostheses. The biologic reaction to wear particles causes resorption of bone surrounding the prosthesis, which leads to loosening and pain.

Many of the biomaterials issues reported in *Orthopaedic Knowledge Update 3* (*OKU 3*) related to the surface modification of existing orthopaedic materials, for example, ion implantation, and to the development of new substances, such as carbon fiber-reinforced polymer composites, to improve the performance of total joint replacement prostheses. More recent investigations have focused on obtaining a better understanding of the performance of existing orthopaedic biomaterials, particularly with respect to their wear and corrosion properties. Studies have added to our understanding of the mechanisms underlying the wear of polyethylene. Moreover, the increasing use of modular prostheses components has necessitated studies addressing fretting wear and corrosion, issues that previously were addressed in the context of the screw-plate junction of fracture fixation devices. Coupled with longer term clinical follow-up of devices, recent wear investigations have provided information about the longevity to be expected of total joint replacement prosthesis.

Studies of the wear of polyethylene have been complemented by continuing investigations of the biologic response to particles of this material. Closer examination of periprosthesis tissue, using polarized light microscopy, has suggested that there might be exceedingly large numbers of submicron polyethylene particles within the constituent macrophages and multinucleated foreign body giant cells. However, these light microscopy studies are limited by the resolution of the optical microscope (approximately 0.2 m). Other recent studies suggest that there may be an immune component to the host response to certain biomaterials. Several years ago the term "metal allergy" was used to describe the hypersensitivity response of certain patients who displayed an allergic response to nickel. Employing monoclonal antibodies to inflammatory cells and immunohistochemical techniques, recent publications have demonstrated the presence of immune cells, such as T-lymphocytes, around loose titanium alloy devices that have generated particulate debris.

An update of the strategies employed for implant fixation was provided in *OKU 3*. Studies reported during the past few years have focused primarily on the performance of hydroxyapatite coatings. Histologic investigations of hydroxyapatite-coated femoral stems obtained at autopsy have been particularly valuable in demonstrating the biologic response to and ultimate fate of the coatings. These findings have led to a reassessment of the process by which calcium phosphate coatings can improve the performance of a total joint replacement prosthesis.

Issues related to the design of total hip and knee replacement prostheses continue to be investigated. While there is a consensus that the devices should have inherent mechanical stability resulting from suitable filling of the medullary canal, questions remain as to the need for customizing the prosthesis for individual patients. The increased use of modular prosthetic systems has led to findings of fretting wear and corrosion of the components. However, because of the short-term clinical follow-up currently available, it is not yet possible to determine the long-term clinical sequelae of these processes.

The composition and molecular structure of orthopaedic biomaterials was presented in *OKU 1* and *OKU 2*. In addition, information about the mechanical properties of these materials relative to their performance for the fabrication of orthopaedic implants was also provided. Current materials-related problems with orthopaedic prostheses are associated with the wear and corrosion of materials, and these processes are described in this chapter. The previous *OKU* chapters have presented selected issues relating to the biocompatibility of orthopaedic materials. Continuing investigations of biological response to materials have deepened our understanding of the processes that comprise the host response to orthopaedic prostheses.

Wear

Conditions for Wear

Wear is generally defined as the loss of material from solid surfaces as a result of mechanical action. Several mechanisms can contribute to wear. In each case, fracture through the substance—loss of cohesive bonding—must occur for a fragment of the material to be removed from the surface. The three main mechanisms of wear are adhesive wear, abrasive wear, and fatigue wear. Adhesive wear occurs when the force of adhesion between contacting surfaces exceeds the cohesive force within one of the materials. When two surfaces come into contact, atomic bonding can occur between the materials (Fig. 1). Generally, when the surfaces separate, this bond is broken. However, in some cases this bond strength exceeds the strength of the atomic bonding in one of the two contacting materials. When the two surfaces separate, fracture occurs within the material, leading to loss of a transferred fragment. In adhesive wear, the amount of material lost is generally directly proportional to the applied load and to the distance slid. In many material systems, the amount of wear is inversely proportional to the hardness of the surface being worn away. These relationships are incorporated in the following equation, $V_{adh} = kWL/H$; where V_{adh} is the volume of adhesive wear, W is the load perpendicular to the surface, L is the indention hardness of the softer material, and H is the distance through which the surfaces slid. The dimensionless coefficient, k, is the fraction of adhesive junctions that eventually produces a wear particle and is generally less than 0.1 (ie, only one of ten adhesive junctions results in a wear particle)

Abrasive wear results when asperites on one material plow material from a softer contacting surface (Fig. 2). The loss of material that occurs as two surfaces contact can be referred to as two-body wear. When a third substance is interposed between the two surfaces, the process of abrasive wear is referred to as three-body wear (Fig. 3). The equation that evaluates the volume of material lost in abrasive wear is $V_{abr} = WL/H \pi \tan\theta$; where V_{abr} is the volume of abrasive wear and π is half the included angle of the asperite of the harder material plowing through the softer material. $\tan\theta$ is very small for sharp asperites, leading to high wear volume.

Fatigue wear results from repeated loading of contacting surfaces. The cyclic stresses initiate and/or propagate surface or subsurface cracks (Fig. 4). The fatigue wear process eventually leads to the loss of relatively large fragments of material.

The term fretting wear is used to describe the loss of material from contacting surfaces as they undergo oscillatory tangential displacement of small magnitude (ie, micrometers). The loss of material caused by fretting wear is the result of adhesion and/or abrasive wear.

During the past few years, much of the attention of orthopaedic biomaterials research has focused on the wear of the metal-polyethylene articulation surfaces and the fretting wear that occurs with modular prosthesis components. Analyses of the head-neck junction of modular components retrieved at revision arthroplasty have led to studies of the corrosion mechanisms that might be occurring at that site. In attempts to better understand the biologic mechanisms associated with prosthesis loosening, studies have continued to investigate the role of particulate debris in causing bone resorption. These studies have led to findings that suggest that there might

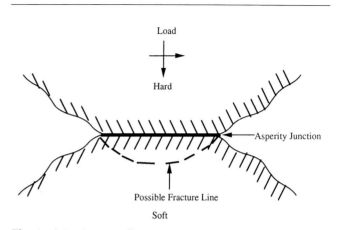

Fig. 1 Adhesive wear. The adhesive bond that develops between the hard and soft materials exceeds the cohesive strength of the soft material.

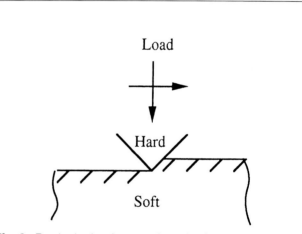

Fig. 2 Two-body abrasive wear due to hard asperites.

be an immune component to the biologic response to certain types of materials.

Wear of Orthopaedic Biomaterials

Wear can be found on the articulating surfaces, on portions of the device rubbing against surrounding bone cement or bone, and on the mated surfaces of modular components. A consensus has now developed that it is the wear of ultrahigh molecular weight polyethylene that limits the life of total joint replacement prostheses. However, metallic wear debris acting alone or with polyethylene can promote inflammatory processes that stimulate bone resorption.

Polyethylene Wear Characteristics of polyethylene wear were reviewed in the corresponding chapter in *OKU 3*. It is generally considered that acetabular cups undergo adhesive and abrasive wear and that tibial components undergo fatigue and abrasive wear. No new mechanisms of

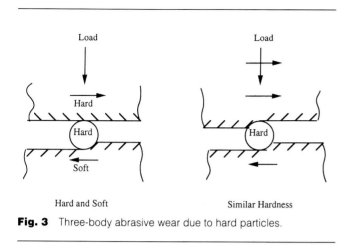

Fig. 3 Three-body abrasive wear due to hard particles.

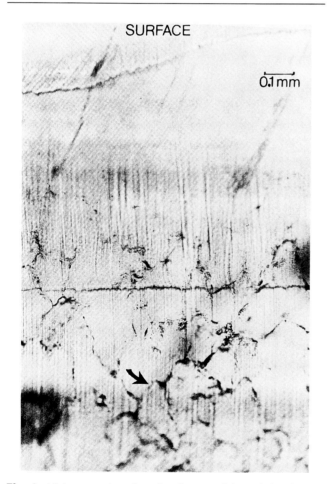

Fig. 4 High-power view of a subsurface crack (arrow) developing along planes of intergranular cracking. (Reproduced with permission from Landy MJ, Walker PS: Wear of ultra-high-molecular-weight polyethylene components of 90 retrieved knee prostheses. *J Arthroplasty* 1988;suppl:S73-S85.)

of wear of the ultrahigh molecular weight polyethylene components of total hip and knee replacement prostheses have increased in recent years. These increases result from the longer term performance of components before revision and the fact that heightened awareness of the untoward clinical sequelae has led to an increase in reporting of the problem. Recent reports of wear of cemented acetabular components have demonstrated a correlation between implantation time and penetration rate of the metallic head into the polyethylene cup. While bone cement particles continue to be the most likely cause of the accelerated wear, there is a suggestion that bone particles often can facilitate three-body abrasive wear that leads to higher penetration rates (when coupled with adhesive wear). Penetration rates have been found to range from 0.005 mm to 0.6 mm per year. Three factors that continue to be recognized as important influences on polyethylene performance are component thickness, conformity, and physical properties, such as density, of the polyethylene substance.

Particularly high incidences of wear of a specific type have been reported for certain types of tibial plateau inserts. Relatively thin (less than 6 mm) tibial plateau components of a relatively nonconforming design are susceptible to a delamination type of wear. In this wear process, subsurface cracks caused by fatigue failure of the polyethylene, as a result of the cyclic loading, led to removal of a lamina of polyethylene approximately 1 mm thick from large portions of the articulating surface. The cracks that caused these delaminations propagated parallel to the articulating surface at a depth of 1 mm (Fig. 5). Analysis of the variations in the density of polyethylene with depth below the surface of the tibial component revealed an increase in density at approximately 1 mm below the surface. This finding supports the hypothesis that fatigue fracture of the polyethylene at this site below the surface is related to the physical properties of the substance. It has been suggested that the process of heat-pressing tibial components during manufacture makes them more susceptible to fatigue wear. However, there are no remarkable differences between the depth profiles of density of heat-pressed polyethylene and nonheat-pressed components. Nevertheless, it is generally believed that the heat-pressing procedure alters the physical properties of polyethylene near the surface of the component and makes the device more susceptible for fracture at the subsurface juncture of the heat-press material and the bulk polyethylene. These recent studies continue to evidence the importance of polyethylene thickness and the conforming design of the components. Thinner components result in higher stresses that lead to the surface deformation. Recent laboratory wear testing has demonstrated that it is the sliding component of articulation that leads to the delamination type of wear seen in retrieved tibial components of total knee replacement prostheses.

Studies performed during the past few years have demonstrated that the physical properties of a block of ul-

wear have been revealed in studies performed during the past several years. However, the incidence and severity

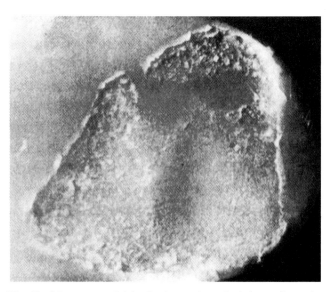

Fig. 5 A large area of delamination on the articulating surface of a polyethylene tibial component that had been implanted for seven years. (Reproduced with permission from Wright TM, Bartel DL: The problem of surface damage in polyethylene total knee components. *Clin Orthop* 1986;205:67-74)

trahigh molecular weight polyethylene from which a component is machined are not uniform throughout the block. Moreover, these properties are affected by the gamma radiation used for sterilization. Changes in the physical properties can also be found with time of exposure to ambient conditions; polyethylene components can undergo important changes in their density with time on the shelf. Additionally, environmental conditions and loading that occur with implantation can also change the physical characteristics and, therefore, the wear performance of polyethylene components. Predictions of the serviceable life of polyethylene components are confounded by the complex relationships between physical properties (and wear) and factors such as gamma irradiation, shelf life, and environmental factors that occur in vivo.

Wear of Metallic Articulating Surfaces Intuitively, the focus on wear occurring with metal-on-polyethylene articulations is on the polymer component. While the passivation oxide layer on the metallic surface is considerably harder than the polymer, the shear strength of the oxide-metal interface is relatively low. Shearing forces accompanying metal-polyethylene articulation lead to failure at the oxide-metal interface and release of titanium oxide particles. Areas of the titanium from which oxide has been lost reform an oxide layer spontaneously (in nanoseconds), drawing oxygen from the environment. Titanium oxide is more susceptible to this type of shear failure than the chromium oxide on cobalt-chromium alloy and stainless steel.

The release of the metallic oxide passivation layer can adversely affect the wear performance of the metal-polyethylene articulation in three ways. Firstly, loss of the oxide layer allows the very reactive metallic surface to interact with the opposing polyethylene during the period that the oxide is being reformed. This can facilitate polymer transfer from the polyethylene component to the metal surface thus accelerating adhesive wear of the polyethylene. Secondly, the instantaneous passivation in vivo of areas from which the oxide has been lost can result in a more irregular metallic surface that can eventually serve to facilitate abrasive wear of the polyethylene. Thirdly, the release of metallic oxide can contribute to three-body abrasive wear of the metallic and polyethylene surfaces. While the oxide particles are relatively thin (10 nm) they agglomerate to form larger aggregates that display the hardness of titanium oxide. The aggregates can serve to facilitate abrasive wear of the polyethylene and the metallic surface. The metallic surface roughened by this abrasive wear acts subsequently to abrade the polyethylene surface.

It is not yet clear to what extent the release of oxide caused by shear failure at the oxide-metal interface contributes to the wear of the metal-polyethylene articulation. Should concern be heightened about this issue, attention would have to turn to ceramic components for articulation against polyethylene. Because the oxide surface on ceramics such as aluminum oxide (alumina) and zirconium oxide (zirconia) is an integral part of the chemistry of the ceramic, there is no tendency for release of oxide surface layers from the ceramic as there is with metallic materials.

Wear of Modular Titanium Stems The requirement that noncemented femoral stems be canal-filling in order to have inherent mechanical stability and the economic constraints encouraging reductions in inventory have led to the implementation of modular proximal and distal sleeves. In order to reduce the amount of stress shielding and in order to take advantage of its biocompatibility, titanium alloy has been employed as the material of fabrication for these modular devices. However, the poor wear properties of titanium limit its usefulness for the fabrication of such devices. Care must be taken to use designs and machining techniques that minimize the fretting wear of the components.

Laboratory testing of a commercially available modular device with a proximal sleeve has demonstrated variable amounts of wear debris depending on the loading and stem constraint conditions. These test methods have yielded particulate debris in a size range comparable to that found in tissue retrieved with a variety of titanium alloy stem designs. The interpretation of the wear results is still in question because of the uncertainty about the amount of particulate debris necessary to initiate osteolytic responses. Despite this question about the interpretation of results the importance of laboratory testing of modular titanium stem designs prior to clinical trials is clear.

Another form of wear involves the process of corrosion. The oxide passivation layer on metals can be lost as a result of a wear process. The removal of this film can accelerate the corrosion process and lead to alterations in the oxide layer. These alterations can include an increase in rugosity (surface roughness) that leads to further abrasive wear of the opposing surface.

Corrosion

Whereas wear is the loss of solid fragments from surfaces as a result of mechanical action, corrosion is release of ions and compounds as a result of chemical action. Relatively little is known about the mechanisms underlying the corrosion of nonmetallic substances. The following paragraphs deal with corrosion of metallic substances.

Even relatively inert metals are soluble in aqueous solutions. Metal leaves the solid metallic state to form aqueous cations in electrolyte solutions. Passivation is the formation of an insoluble salt, such as oxide, on pure metals and metal alloys. The oxide layer inhibits metal egress and thus inhibits corrosion. This layer serves to protect the metal by insulating it from the electrolyte solution. A chromium oxide passivation layer forms on stainless steel and cobalt-chromium alloy. A titanium oxide layer forms on titanium and titanium alloys.

The electrochemical (Galvanic) series of metals rates the relative tendencies of metal ions to go into solution (Table 1). However, it is important to note that this classification of metals does not take into consideration the effect of an oxide layer on the surface of the metal. The electrochemical series shows that metallic elements such as gold are relatively insoluble while substances such as titanium and aluminum, when present in pure elemental form, are relatively soluble (and active). However, when these same reactive metallic elements are covered by their oxide layers, their tendency to go into aqueous solution is greatly reduced.

Titanium is a more active element than chromium; titanium and its alloys form oxide passivation layers more rapidly than do substances that contain chromium, such as cobalt-chromium alloy and stainless steel. However, while an active metal like titanium forms its oxide passivation layer spontaneously in any environment that contains oxygen, the strength of adhesion of the oxide layer to the underlying titanium metal is not as great as that of the chromium oxide layer to its metal substrate. In addition, the chromium oxide passivation film is more dense than the titanium oxide layer.

When a metal is immersed in an electrolyte solution, electrons, freed as the metal ions, enter the solution from one region of the specimen (the anode) and travel to other regions of the same specimen, making those areas cathodic. If the metallic sample is connected to (that is, if it touches) another metal specimen with less of a ten-

Table 1. The electrochemical series of metals. Normal electrode potentials measured in volts at 25 C, referred to hydrogen as zero.

Noble End	
Gold	+1.45
Platinum	+1.20
Silver	+0.80
Copper	+0.34
Hydrogen	0.00
Molybdenum	-0.20
Nickel	-0.25
Cobalt	-0.28
Iron	-0.44
Chromium	-0.73
Titanium	-1.63
Aluminum	-1.66
Magnesium	-2.37
Lithium	-3.05
Active End	

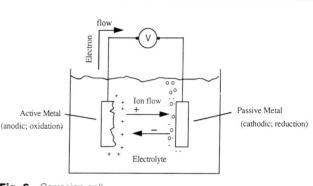

Fig. 6   Corrosion cell.

dency for corrosion, then the second metallic specimen becomes the cathode (Fig. 6). Corrosion of the anode can be accelerated by increasing the rate of reaction at the cathode. The anodic reaction is defined as $M > M^{n+}_{aqu} + ne^-_{met}$. There are two cathodic reactions. The reduction of dissolved oxygen is stated as $n/2(1/2O_2) + n/2H_2O + ne^-_{met} > nOH^-_{aqu}$ and the reduction of hydrogen ions is expressed as $nH^+ + ne^- > n/2H_2$.

The mechanisms that control corrosion relate to factors that favor either the anodic or cathodic reactions. Factors that facilitate electron transfer from the metal facilitate the anodic reaction; changes in oxygen concentration at sites along the metallic surface facilitate the cathodic reaction. The mechanisms of corrosion—pitting, crevice, and depletion—refer to situations in which there is relative depletion of oxygen at certain sites on a metal implant (Fig. 7). These sites take on an anodic character, favoring metal ion release. Salts can accumulate at sites of scratches (produced by instruments at the time of insertion). The depletion of oxygen at these sites can lead to corrosion, resulting in pitting of the surface. The low oxygen concentration at the bottom of the pits favors continuing corrosion. Crevices formed at the sites at which components are jointed (eg, in modular components of prostheses or at screw-plate junctions) are also

CREVICE

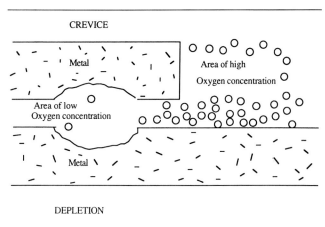

DEPLETION

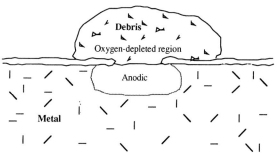

Fig. 7   Conditions predisposing metal implants to crevice (**top**) and depletion (**bottom**) corrosion.

microenvironments that can favor corrosion as a result of depleted oxygen. The depletion of oxygen can also occur under plaques of biological debris on the surface of devices, thus also favoring a so-called "concentration cell corrosion mechanism."

Another basic mechanism of corrosion can occur when dissimilar metals touch. The electrons tend to move from the more noble metal, which causes the former to become anodic, producing conditions that favor accelerated corrosion. This mechanism of corrosion has been referred to as Galvanic, two-metal, mixed-metal, or couple corrosion. The degree of Galvanic corrosion depends on the electrochemical nature of the two metals and the relative areas of contact and surfaces exposed to the solution. The term Galvanic corrosion is derived from an observation made by Galvani in 1791 as he was investigating the susceptibility of nerves to irritation. He found that if a rod of brass contacted the frog's foot while a silver rod contacted the spinal cord, the leg muscles would contract when the free ends of the rods touched. In 1800 Volta confirmed that the force that provoked the contraction was electrical in nature. The electric current generated by contact of dissimilar metals in an electrolyte solution has come to be referred to as Galvanic current.

In some situations the breakdown of material is caused by mechanical and chemical processes acting in concert. These mechanochemical processes include fretting cor-

rosion, stress corrosion, and metallic transfer (with subsequent Galvanic corrosion).

Fretting corrosion is a process in which abrasive wear is accompanied by corrosion. The protective oxide layer on the metal is removed by the abrasion wear process. Because the new passivation layer that forms after abrasion is neither as durable nor as chemically inert as the original layer, the metal is more susceptible to corrosion. Stainless steel and cobalt-chromium alloys are susceptible to fretting corrosion. This form of corrosion often occurs between screw heads and bone plates.

Stress corrosion is the process by which the presence of an electrolyte decreases the strength of the metal. Microcracks developed at anodic areas of the metallic device as the result of corrosion processes. These cracks propagate under applied stress. The tips of these microcracks are at a more highly strained condition than surrounding metal and are more susceptible to corrosion, which contributes to crack propagation.

As dissimilar metals contact one another there can be metallic transfer of small fragments of the softer metal to the harder one. These two metals then remain in contact, and Galvanic corrosion processes can occur. This is why it is suggested that implants be handled with instruments made of the same metal as the device.

Several methods are used to assess the liability of metals to corrosion. One can simply weigh the specimen after exposure to corrosive environments, or the bathing electrolyte solution can be assayed for corrosion products. An electrochemical method that has been valuable in characterizing the potential of metals to corrode is referred to as anodic polarization. In this experimental procedure, the test metal is made the anode of an electrolytic cell. An increasing voltage is applied between it and a reference cathode (usually platinum). The current density (current divided by cross-sectional areas of the anode) is a measure of the corrosion rate of the anodic metal in the particular electrolyte used. Table 2 shows the electrochemical potentials and tendency for corrosion, or current density, for the orthopaedic alloys. Because the current density for titanium alloy is significantly less than that of cobalt-chromium alloy and stainless steel, there is much less of a tendency for corrosion of titanium and its alloys. Because the release of metal is surface area dependent, a greater amount of metal is released from porous metal specimens. This remains an important issue when considering the use of porous metallic devices.

The Head-Neck Junction

In recent years there has been an increase in the number of reports of corrosion at the head-neck junction of modular hip prostheses. This corrosion has been evidence by discoloration of the metal, accumulation of debris, and pitting of the mated surfaces. A question remains as to the relative contributions of fretting wear and fretting corrosion, in addition to crevice corrosion, to breakdown of the metal at the head-neck junction. Moreover, for

Table 2. Electrochemical potentials and current densities for orthopaedic alloys

	Current density ($\mu_A m^2$)	Ec
Titanium alloy	0.003	-50
Cobalt-chromium alloy	0.011	-10
Stainless steel	0.028	-100

cases of mixed metals (ie, cobalt-chromium alloy heads on titanium alloy stems) there has been a suggestion that Galvanic as well as crevice corrosion might play a role. One consequence of corrosion at the head-neck junction is predisposition of the prosthesis for fracture at this site. In addition, the corrosion products can result in untoward histologic responses, including necrosis.

Factors that can contribute to the corrosion of the head-neck junction include metallurgy of the components, surface finish, and fit. Inferior metallic preparations resulting in inclusions of contaminants or porosity facilitate corrosion. Improperly prepared surfaces and inadequate designs can result in poorly mated components predisposed to crevice corrosion and to fretting processes associated with wear as well as corrosion.

Biologic Response

The biologic response to prostheses includes the local tissue response related to molecular and cellular interactions with the implant, stress-induced adaptive remodeling of surrounding tissue associated with alterations in the strain distribution in the tissue due to the presence of the prosthesis, and systemic effects due to substances released from the device. The following paragraphs provide a basis for understanding issues related to the local tissue response to biomaterials.

The local tissue response to the implant is determined initially by the effect of the prosthesis on the normal wound healing response to the surgical trauma of implantation (Fig. 8). Because of its capability for regeneration, bone should be expected to fill the surgically prepared cavity into which the implant was placed, and thereby, appose the prosthesis. If the prosthesis contains fenestrations or is coated with the porous material, new bone could be expected to fill these voids. The term osseointegration has been employed to describe the situation in which bone apposes the prosthesis, with no intervening fibrous tissue identifiable by light microscopy. The potential for osseointegration of a prosthesis is related to the capability of bone to regenerate and, therefore, does not necessitate a particular surface chemistry on the implant. This assumes that the surface chemistry does not interfere with bone regeneration. Osseointegration of prostheses implies that bone is contacting the surface of the implant; it does not require chemical bonding of bone to the prosthesis. In most cases it is the mechanical bond produced by the interdigitation of bone with surface features of the implant that provides the interfa-

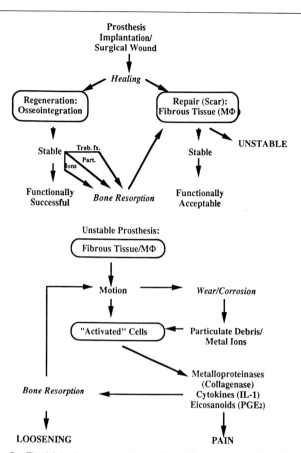

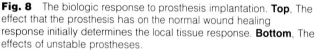

Fig. 8 The biologic response to prosthesis implantation. **Top,** The effect that the prosthesis has on the normal wound healing response initially determines the local tissue response. **Bottom,** The effects of unstable prostheses.

cial strength in compression and shear to provide for a stable implant. However, there is experimental evidence that bone can bond chemically to certain calcium phosphate substances, such as hydroxyapatite. This evidence is from mechanical testing and transmission electron microscopy studies. Push-out and pull-out tests of certain calcium phosphate-coated implants in bone yield relatively high interfacial shear strengths that cannot be explained on the basis of mechanical bonding alone. In addition, ultrastructural study of the interface by transmission electron microscopy displayed continuity of calcium phosphate crystallites from the bulk of the implant into the surrounding bone matrix. The mechanisms by which bone bonds to these calcium phosphate substances involves the initial precipitation of biologic apatites onto the surface of the implant within the first days of implantation. It is likely that adhesion proteins subsequently adsorb to this biologic apatite layer, facilitating subsequent attachment of bone cells.

The regeneration of bone in the process of healing following surgical trauma requires an intact stroma. Excessive motion of the prosthesis relative to the surrounding bone can destroy this framework for regeneration and lead to the production of scar (in the process of healing classically referred to as repair). During the process of fibrous tissue formation around the prosthesis macrophages gravitate to the prosthesis-tissue interface. Macrophages are attracted to and maintained at the surface of the implant by the microenvironment. The dead space caused by the presence of the implant results in an interface that has a low oxygen concentration, elevated lactate, and low pH.

Prostheses that are osseointegrated are generally functionally successful in that the patients are asymptomatic. However, it is possible that factors relating to the stiffness of the device so alter the strain distribution in surrounding bone that a redistribution of bone mass or net loss of bone places the device or bone at risk of fracture and jeopardizes revision procedures because of the loss of bone stock.

The bone around osseointegrated prostheses can be adversely affected by device-related factors acting over a period of years. For example, excessive mechanical loading of the device resulting from increased physical activities or trauma can lead to fracture of trabeculae comprising the bone supporting the prostheses. These fractured trabeculae can undergo regeneration to restore the osseointegrated stability of the device. In other circumstances, however, the regeneration process might be impaired by the continuing loading of the prosthesis, thus leading to the formation of fibrous tissue (scar) at the site of trabecular fracture. This loss of osseous support can place other regions of the bony interface at risk of fracture, eventually leading to replacement of bone by fibrous tissue at the interface along the entire perimeter of the device. In other circumstances, particulate debris generated within the joint space can migrate through the marrow spaces or interfacial fibrous tissue and elicit a response that can also result in a net loss of bone. Finally, ions released from the device can have an adverse effect on the osseous tissue, leading to bone loss. The effects of particulate debris and metallic ions on bone formation and resorption can be indirect, mediated by regulatory cells such as macrophages (or tissue-resident histiocytes) that release and produce factors that stimulate osteoclastic activity (eg, interleukin-1, formerly referred to as osteoclastic activating factor) or inhibit osteoblast function, and/or direct, activating osteoclasts or inhibiting osteoblasts.

In many cases, patients with fibrous-encapsulated prostheses are asymptomatic, which has led to the clinical impression that such tissue interfaces are functionally acceptable. However, the consensus is that fibrous tissue, which offers less mechanical support than bone, allows for a greater degree of micromotion of the prosthesis. This is believed to explain the higher incidence of pain in noncemented prostheses that are encapsulated in fibrous tissue.

The macrophages and fibroblasts that comprise the tissue around prostheses display the characteristics of synovium. Numerous studies of the periprosthetic tissue obtained at revision arthroplasty have demonstrated the elevated levels of such mediators of inflammation as prostaglandin E_2 and interleukin-1, which are known to be potent stimulators of bone resorption. The fact that the tissue around a loose prosthesis has characteristics of inflamed synovium has led to the use of the terms "prosthesis synovitis" and "implant bursitis" to describe this condition.

The tissue surrounding prostheses is affected by movement of the device, particulate debris generated by the prosthesis, and metallic ions released from the device. As the prosthesis moves relative to surrounding bone, conditions are produced that favor wear and corrosion and that lead to the generation of particulate debris and metallic ions. These conditions can increase the amount of bone resorption, which further reduces the stability of the device and leads to increased micromotion and more wear particles and corrosion products.

Relatively few studies have directly addressed the effects of motion and metal ions on the type of tissue that might be expected to form around a prosthesis. In a few studies, fibroblasts grown on flexible substrates were found to release prostaglandin E_2 when exposed to various strained conditions. In other studies, synovial cells were found to release prostaglandin when treated with cobalt ions.

Many studies have investigated the effects of particulate debris on cells in culture and in animal models. Generally, these studies have demonstrated that particulates of a wide variety of orthopaedic biomaterials are capable of provoking macrophages and fibroblasts to release proinflammatory agents, including interleukin-1 and prostaglandin E_2, known stimulators of bone resorption. However, it has not yet been possible to determine the role of chemistry, particle size distribution, concentration, shape, and topography on the inflammatory response.

Elements of the Biological Response to Particulate Debris

Issues related to the biocompatibility of orthopaedic biomaterials and the biologic response to particulate debris from these materials have been reviewed in the first three editions of *OKU*. Studies performed in recent years have added to our understanding of the mechanisms underlying the inflammation and bone resorption stimulated by particles released from orthopaedic prostheses.

Recent clinical findings of great concern are those that demonstrate focal osteolytic lesions at sites around asymptomatic femoral stems that radiographically appear to be well fixed. One hypothesis is that polyethylene wear debris from the joint space has migrated through fibrous tissue layers surrounding proximal regions of the device to reach distal sites along the stem, eliciting an inflammatory reaction and consequent bone resorption. The supposition is that this "lysis without loosening" has been caused by an extensive "effective joint space" facilitated by fibrous tissue interposed between the implant and surrounding bone. It is proposed that less fibrous tissue occurs with bone cement sheaths interdigitated with surrounding bone and with bone ingrowth into circumferentially porous-coated prostheses. However, if polyethylene particle migration alone is the cause of distal lytic lesions, then migration of particles through narrow spaces in bone and through pores of the coating in which bone has not formed could be expected eventually to cause a similar problem with all types of prostheses. Although there is some disagreement as to the role that polyethylene particles plays in various types of osteolytic conditions around prostheses, there is general agreement that an effort should be made to reduce the amount of polyethylene wear debris.

Analysis of Particles   Despite the repeated findings in vivo and in vitro of inflammation and bone resorption associated with particulate debris, it still has not been possible to rank orthopaedic biomaterials according to virulence of the response elicited by the substances in particulate form. This is because of the inability to obtain particles of biomaterials with the same size range and morphology. Ironically, despite its wear in vivo, the very nature of ultrahigh molecular weight polyethylene precludes the production of large numbers of particles in the laboratory for study. Therefore, most investigations of polyethylene have employed particles of the high density form of the polymer, from which particles in the 1 micrometer size range can be made more easily. It would not appear that the difference in molecular weight between high density (several hundred thousand) and ultrahigh molecular weight (several million) polyethylene would have a significant effect on the biologic response. However, this issue must be addressed before studies performed on high density polyethylene can be used to reach conclusions about ultrahigh molecular weight polymers.

Another problem encountered in performing studies of particles relates to the method of quantifying particle size, distribution, and number. Automated methods are available that determine particle size based on the dielectric property of the particle or its light scattering behavior. However, important assumptions need to be made relative to shape and other characteristics of the particles in order for particle size to be calculated. Moreover, there are uncertainties about the results of these techniques if particles of more than one material are present. Currently, the best method for quantifying particle size relies on measurements of individual particles made with a scanning electron microscope. While computerized image analysis apparatus can facilitate this procedure, it requires care in preparing specimens for analysis and assuring repeatable operating conditions with the microscope. An advantage of this method is that an energy dispersive x-ray (EDX) analysis accessory to the microscope can be used to obtain the elemental composition of the particle being viewed. A limitation of EDX is that only elements

with an atomic number greater than fluorine (atomic number 9) can be detected. Despite the promise of certain methods for providing reliable particle size information, no standards for these procedures have been developed.

The analysis of particles is greatly complicated if they are dispersed in tissue, as in the case of peri-implant specimens retrieved at revision arthroplasty. Reports are only now being published describing procedures to extract the particles from tissue. However, studies have yet to address the issue of whether the extraction process alters the chemistry of the particles.

The Cause of Bone Resorption   Studies of the cellular make-up and biochemistry of periprosthesis tissue recovered at revision arthroplasty continue to reveal the presence of macrophages and mediators of inflammation, such as PGE_2 and IL-1, that are known to be potent stimulators of bone resorption. It is generally assumed that these mediators lead to the recruitment and activation of osteoclasts in surrounding bone. This paradigm has been confirmed by recent in vitro studies that have shown that, in the process of phagocytosing particles, macrophages release agents that stimulate bone resorption, assayed in vitro. Particles of polyethylene and polymethylmethacrylate elicit a greater response in this system than do latex particles employed as "negative controls." However, it has not yet been possible to definitely rank orthopaedic biomaterials in order of the severity of the response that they elicit.

A canine model for the aseptic loose, cemented femoral stem was developed in order to investigate the biologic mechanisms that underly loosening and to evaluate the effects of treatment with a nonsteroidal anti-inflammatory drug (naproxen). The pseudomembrane around the loose canine stem was found by radiography, radionuclide imaging, histology, and biochemistry to be similar to the peri-implant tissue around loose prostheses in human subjects. In vitro treatment of cells obtained from the canine pseudomembrane led to a reduction in the production and release of PGE_2. There was a trend toward lower levels of PGE_2 in the pseudomembranes of animals treated with naproxen. However, because of the small number of animals in each group it was not possible to conclude that treatment with this drug led to a retardation or a reversal, or both, of the loosening process. The study demonstrated that cells comprising inflammatory tissue around loose prostheses are responsive to anti-inflammatory agents administered systemically. Additional studies are required before a rational treatment modality can be established for patients with prostheses that display signs of loosening.

The Role of the Immune System   Previous histologic investigations of the periprosthesis tissue removed at revision arthroplasty generally did not reveal the presence of lymphocytes and plasma cells, which are cellular elements of the immune system. Occasionally, infiltrates of acute inflammatory cells including lymphocytes were reported within the "pseudomembrane" removed with the prosthesis. In one study that distinguished the histological characteristics of pseudomembranes retrieved from joint replacement patients with rheumatoid arthritis and osteoarthritis, greater numbers of lymphocytes were found with the periprosthesis tissue of patients with rheumatoid arthritis. In a more recent investigation of the peri-implant tissue laden with titanium particulate debris, a lymphoplasmacytic response was noted. The lymphocytes and plasma cells comprising the infiltrate suggested an ongoing immune component to the response. In order to determine more definitively the presence of immune cells in periprosthesis tissue recovered at revision arthroplasty, investigators have recently employed panels of monoclonal antibodies to label specific cells. In one investigation, tissue obtained from patients in whom titanium screws were used to stabilized acetabular cups was analyzed using immunohistochemistry. The monoclonal antibody markers revealed large numbers of T-lymphocytes and many macrophages. Few, if any, B-lymphocytes were detected in the sections. Few granulocytes and mast cells were found. In an attempt to correlate the T cell response with an allergic reaction, patients were skin tested with titanium compounds. However, none of the patients showed a positive reaction. Although the hip replacement prostheses in the patients in this study comprised ultrahigh molecular weight polyethylene and cobalt-chromium alloy as well as titanium alloy, the supposition was that the black particulate debris was from the titanium alloy screws (and in one case a titanium alloy femoral head). The investigators concluded that the presence of the T-lymphocytes and the absence of the accompanying B-lymphocytes or plasma cells suggested a cell-mediated hypersensitivity response to titanium alloy. The absence of a positive skin test in response to challenges of titanium compounds could not be explained.

In another investigation of the cell type comprising the granulomatous response to loose prostheses, relatively few immunostaining T-lymphocytes were found around cemented cobalt-chromium alloy and stainless steel hip replacement prostheses. No B-lymphocytes or plasma cells were detected. The majority of the cells were macrophages. The T cells found in the periprosthesis tissue did not stain with monoclonal antibodies for certain receptors, which would have indicated that they were in an active state.

There continues to be a consensus that the macrophage is the predominant cell type in aggressive granulomatous lesions around loose prostheses. Multinucleated foreign body giant cells, the product of macrophage fusion, can also be found in this tissue, which might be characterized as being in a state of very active chronic inflammation. When lymphocytic infiltrates are found, they are composed of T-lymphocytes. A question remains as to the active nature of these cells and whether they are indicative of an ongoing immune response to the biomaterial.

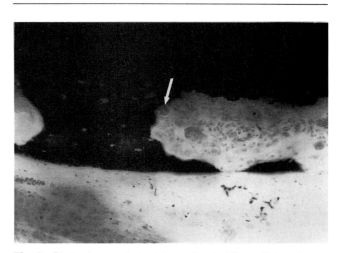

Fig. 9   Photomicrograph depicting osteoclast-like cells investing a hydroxyapatite-coated femoral stem of a prosthesis.

Strategies for Implant Fixation: Hydroxyapatite Coatings

Clinical investigations of the performance of hydroxyapatite-coated femoral stems continue to yield encouraging results. However, recent histologic studies of retrieved devices indicate that the coatings are susceptible to resorption by osteoclast-like cells (Fig. 9). As much as 20% of the coating might be removed within two years. While there is some indication that bone can become opposed to the exposed titanium substrate, there has been no evidence to demonstrate that osseous tissue can bond in chemical-like fashion to the titanium surface as it does to the original hydroxyapatite coating. Because of the uncertainty about the fate of hydroxyapatite coatings, no predictions can be made about the serviceable clinical performance to be expected from hydroxyapatite-coated devices.

Uncertainty about the permanence of hydroxyapatite coating has turned attention to the use of porous-coated prostheses as the substrate for hydroxyapatite coating. The rationale is that even if the hydroxyapatite coating is bioabsorbed in the body, the bone ingrowth into porous coating can serve as an attachment vehicle for the prosthesis. The benefit of the hydroxyapatite coating is the provision of higher attachment strengths within the first few weeks after implantation.

Initial animal studies comparing the strength of attachment of noncoated and hydroxyapatite-coated porous implants revealed a marginal, but significant, increase in the strength of attachment only at one time period (two weeks) postoperatively. Before and after two weeks, there was no difference in attachment strength of the specimens between the hydroxyapatite- and nonhydroxyapatite-coated groups. These studies were performed using specimens implanted into the medullary canal of dogs.

A more recent investigation comparing the strength of attachment of noncoated and hydroxyapatite-coated porous specimens implanted transcortically in dogs has reported high attachment strengths of the hydroxyapatite-coated specimens at all postoperative time periods. As noted in *OKU 3*, previous investigations have also shown the benefit of hydroxyapatite coatings in facilitating stabilization of specimens implanted into osteopenic bone or into sites where there are relatively large gaps between the implant surface and surrounding bone. A recent canine study compared the strength of hydroxyapatite-coated and noncoated titanium alloy implants designed to be unstable. The authors found that both types of implants, when exposed to loading that caused movement of the devices relative to surrounding bone, were surrounded by fibrous tissue. However, the interfacial shear strength of the hydroxyapatite-coated specimen was greater than the unstable noncoated titanium device and also the stable noncoated titanium control; stable hydroxyapatite-coated devices (those with no micromotion) had the highest strength of attachment to surrounding bone. The authors speculated that a denser fibrocollagenous material that formed around the unstable hydroxyapatite-coated device gave it a higher interfacial shear strength than was found with nonhydroxyapatite-coated implants. Despite these favorable results from animal investigations, additional studies are required to more clearly identify the clinical indications that require hydroxyapatite coatings.

Design Considerations: The Effect of Prosthesis Stiffness

Results of investigations of the bone remodeling around femoral stems in human subjects and canine models continue to demonstrate the stress-induced adaptive remodeling of bone around femoral stems. Findings during the past few years point to the importance of the influence of stem stiffness on remodeling. Several canine studies have demonstrated that more flexible femoral stems produced by reducing the cross-section moment of inertia (eg, using hollow titanium stems) or by decreasing the modulus of elasticity (eg, by using carbon fiber-reinforced polymer composite substances) reduce the bone loss associated with stress shielding. However, other recent studies comparing smooth-surfaced, noncemented, collarless, canal-filling titanium alloy and composite stems have not found the amount of bone loss observed in other investigations of the titanium stems in dogs. Moreover, these recent studies showed that there is a redistribution of bone mass within transverse sections of the femur. Examination of the original cortical area reveal a net loss of bone. However, examination of the entire cross section often showed a net increase in bone mass caused by the redistribution of bone. It is not yet clear how this redistribution of bone affects the mechanical properties of the femur. These findings demonstrate the importance of such design features as size and shape of the prosthesis and its degree of canal filling on the stresses transmitted to surrounding bone.

Issues related to stress shielding of bone around stiff metallic orthopaedic prostheses do not apply only to femoral stems. A recent study has demonstrated a loss of bone in a distal femur underlying metallic femoral components of total knee replacement prostheses. Bone loss occurred in the distal anterior femur in 68% of the cemented and noncemented femoral components reviewed. The prevalence of bone loss was independent of the mode of fixation and the implant design. By qualitative observation, radiographically detectable bone loss occurred within the first postoperative year and did not progress further. The apparent lack of progression may reflect the development of a new remodeling equilibrium under the altered stress conditions. The bone loss in the distal anterior femur underlying knee replacement prostheses has not been indicated as a source of failure. However, because the bone strength in the femoral region is compromised as it becomes osteopenic, bone failure might occur with longer periods of cyclic loading. Furthermore, as a result of bone loss, revision arthroplasty may be more difficult. Longer term clinical follow-up investigations will be required to determine if the stress shielding of bone under knee replacement prostheses contributes in any meaningful way to the failure of total knee arthroplasty.

Annotated Bibliography

Polyethylene Wear

Blunn GW, Walker PS, Joshi A, et al: The dominance of cyclic sliding in producing wear in total knee replacements. *Clin Orthop* 1991;273:253-260.

Laboratory wear testing of metal-on-polyethylene was performed in an attempt to simulate conditions producing wear of polyethylene knee replacement components. The results demonstrated that oscillatory sliding motion produces the type of severe surface and subsurface cracking and high wear seen in retrieved tibial components. The authors noted that low-conformity components inserted with high ligamentous laxity are susceptible to anteroposterior sliding and high wear.

Collier JP, Mayor MB, McNamara JL, et al: Analysis of the failure of 122 polyethylene inserts from uncemented tibial knee components. *Clin Orthop* 1991;273:232-242.

This analysis of polyethylene tibial inserts retrieved at revision arthroplasty revealed a correlation between the presence of unconsolidated polymer granules and the severity of wear of the articulating surface. Moreover, there was a positive correlation between the intensity of wear and the level of contact stress, with noncongruent designs having greater wear than fully congruent geometries. In the noncongruent designs, thinner polyethylene components showed greater wear than thicker polyethylene inserts of the same design.

Isaac GH, Wroblewski BM, Atkinson JR, et al: A tribological study of retrieved hip prostheses. *Clin Orthop* 1992;276:115-125.

The damaged condition of the polyethylene surface of cemented acetabular cups obtained at revision arthroplasty was classified according to the type of damage. The mean penetration of the metallic head into the cup was 1.69 mm and the mean penetration rate was 0.21 mm per year with a range from less than 0.005 mm to 0.6 mm per year. Roughening of the metallic femoral head was also noted, and attributed to abrasive wear produced by contrast medium debris resulting from fragmentation of the cement. The authors were unable to determine whether loosening and fragmentation of the cement led to wear at the articulating surface or if wear debris produced by articulation led to conditions predisposed to bone resorption and loosening of the cement.

Wright TM, Rimnac CM, Stulberg SD, et al: Wear of polyethylene in total joint replacement: Observations from retrieved PCA knee implants. *Clin Orthop* 1992;276:126-134.

Heat-pressed polyethylene tibial components obtained at revision arthroplasty were analyzed. Evaluation of wear and the physical characteristics of the polyethylene confirmed previous conclusions that nonconforming articulating surfaces on thin polyethylene components are at higher risk of damage than more confirming surfaces on thicker components. The density of polyethylene was found to vary with depth into the component. Well-defined peaks in density occurred at a depth of about 1 mm, corresponding to the level at which extensive cracking (parallel to the surface) occurred within the component. Comparison of the density profiles from the articulating surface of these heat-pressed components with profiles from specimens taken from the interior (nonheat-pressed surface) of these components and from specimens taken from other tibial designs (nonheat-pressed) indicated that the thermal treatments did not affect the shape of the density profile. The authors concluded that the predominant influence on alterations of the density of the polyethylene was the mechanical loading that occurred during function in vivo.

Wear of Metallic Articulating Surfaces

Davidson JA: Characteristics of metal and ceramic total hip bearing surfaces and the effect on long-term UHMWPE wear. *Clin Orthop*, in press.

This paper provides a scientific basis for understanding the changes in metallic surfaces as a result of articulation with polyethylene. Damage to or removal of the metal oxide film as a result of wear processes can contribute to metal ion release and a gradual increase in the surface roughness of the metal surface, which can subsequently result in accelerated abrasive wear of the opposing UHMWPE component.

Corrosion

Collier JP, Surprenant VA, Jensen RE, et al: Corrosion at the interface of cobalt-alloy heads on titanium-alloy stems. *Clin Orthop* 1991;271:305-312.

Examination of modular femoral stem components with cobalt-chromium alloy heads on titanium alloy stems, retrieved at revision arthroplasty, revealed that over 50% of the tapered connections had undergone some degree of crevice corrosion. These findings raised concerns about metal ion release from these sites and the potential failure of head-to-stem fixation.

Collier JP, Suprenant VA, Jensen RE, et al: Corrosion between the components of modular femoral hip prostheses. *J Bone Joint Surg* 1992;74B:511-517.

A total of 139 modular femoral components retrieved at revision arthroplasty were analyzed for corrosion at the femoral head-neck junction. There was no evidence of corrosion in the 91 prostheses fabricated using the same alloy for the head and stem. In contrast, definite corrosion was found in 25 of the 48 prostheses in which the stem was fabricated from titanium alloy and the head made of cobalt-chromium alloy. The corrosion that was found was time-dependent with no corrosion found in implants functioning for less than nine months; corrosion damage was found in all of the mixed-metal prostheses that were implanted for more than 40 months. These findings and other factors led the authors to conclude that the damage to the head-neck junction was due to galvanically accelerated crevice corrosion. This remains a controversial issue because this type of corrosion was not detected in previous laboratory testing of this type of mixed-metal prosthesis.

Mathiesen EB, Lindgren JU, Blomgren GG, et al: Corrosion of modular hip prostheses. *J Bone Joint Surg* 1991;73B:569-575.

Crevice corrosion was found at the head-neck junction of several modular femoral stems retrieved at revision arthroplasty. The devices studied in this paper were made of cast cobalt-chromium alloy with cobalt-chromium heads on cobalt-chromium alloy stems. The suboptimal metallurgy of the cast cobalt-chromium alloy used in these stems could have predisposed the head-neck junction to corrosion. However, another factor that could have contributed to corrosion is the nature of the mechanical fit of the components at the head-neck junction.

Biologic Response

Amstutz HC, Campbell P, Kossovsky N, et al: Mechanism and clinical significance of wear debris-induced osteolysis. *Clin Orthop* 1992;276:7-18.

This paper reviewed the issues related to wear particle-induced osteolysis. Macrophages, activated by the phagocytosis of particulate debris, are the key cells in this process, which can potentially occur in any implant system regardless of implant design or fixation mode.

Galante JP, Lemons J, Spector M, et al: The biologic effects of implant materials. *J Orthop Res* 1991;9:760-775.

This review addressed issues related to the biodegradation of orthopaedic biomaterials, paradigms for prosthesis loosening, the local and systemic responses to materials (including carcinogenicity), and the remodeling of bone around femoral stems.

Lalor PA, Revell PA, Gray AB, et al: Sensitivity to titanium: A cause of implant failure? *J Bone Joint Surg* 1991;73B:25-28.

Monoclonal antibody labeling was employed to determine the identity of cells in titanium particle-laden peri-implant tissue obtained at revision arthroplasty. In four cases the metallic debris resulted from titanium alloy screws used to fix the acetabular component; in the fifth case the debris might have also originated from a titanium alloy femoral head. Immunohistochemistry revealed abundant macrophages and T-lymphocytes that, in the absence of B-lymphocytes, suggested that the patients might be mounting a hypersensitivity response to titanium. However, skin patch testing with titanium compounds yielded negative results in all of the five patients. These findings were contradictory in that a T-lymphocyte mediated hypersensitivity reaction to the metallic prosthesis would be expected to yield positive results with conventional skin patch testing. The definitive finding of the T-lymphocytes, however, remains cause for concern that an immune component to the biologic response could be related to the presence of this commonly used metal.

Murray DW, Rushton N: Macrophages stimulate bone resorption when they phagocytose particles. *J Bone Joint Surg* 1990;72B:988-992.

This in vitro study investigated the response of macrophages to particles of bone cement and polyethylene. Particles of latex and zymosan served as negative and positive controls, respectively. Macrophages that phagocytosed these particles became activated, releasing agents that stimulated 15 times as much bone resorption, in an in vitro assay, as did control macrophages (with no particles). For activation to occur, 100 times more latex than zymosan had to be phagocytosed. The results obtained with the bone cement and polyethylene particles were intermediate between those of the negative and positive control particles. It was not possible in this study to rate the relative virulence of bone cement and polyethylene particles.

Santavirta S, Hoikka V, Eskola A, et al: Aggressive granulomatous lesions in cementless total hip arthroplasty. *J Bone Joint Surg* 1990;72B:980-984.

An attempt was made to distinguish the local immuno-pathologic response in patients who had an aggressive granulomatous lesion around a cemented hip prostheses from the response associated with common loosening of a cemented device. The granulomatous lesions were found to be highly vascularized, with well-organized connective tissue containing histiocytic-monocytic fibroblastic reactive zones. In contrast, the tissue around loose cemented stems with no granulomas comprised dense connective tissue. Immunohistologic methods revealed that most of the cells in the aggressive granulomatous tissue were multinucleated foreign body giant cells and macrophages.

Spector M, Shortkroff S, Hsu H-P, et al: Tissue changes around loose prostheses: A canine model to investigate the effects of an antiinflammatory agent. *Clin Orthop* 1990;261:140-152.

A canine model of the aseptic, loose, cemented femoral stem was employed to evaluate the effects of treatment with a nonsteroidal anti-inflammatory drug (naproxen), known to inhibit prostaglandin E$_2$ production/release.The results showed that cells in the pseudomembrane around the loose prostheses decreased production/release of PGE$_2$ when treated with naproxen in vitro. There was a trend toward lower levels of PGE$_2$ in the membranes of animals treated with this NSAID. However, it was not possible to determine if the process of loosening had been retarded or reversed by treatment with this drug.

Spector M, Shortkroff S, Sledge CB, et al: Advances in our understanding of the implant-bone interface: Factors effecting formation and degeneration, in Tullos HS (ed): *Instructional Course Lectures XL*. Park Ridge, IL,

American Academy of Orthopaedic Surgeons, 1991, pp 101-113.

This paper reviewed the factors influencing the formation and degeneration of tissue around prostheses. The effects of motion, particulate debris, and metal ions on the cells in the peri-implant tissue were presented.

Metallic Wear Debris

Betts F, Wright T, Salvati EA, et al: Cobalt-alloy metal debris in periarticular tissues from total hip revision arthroplasties: Metal contents and associated histologic findings. *Clin Orthop* 1992;276:75-82.

The concentration of metal ions in peri-implant tissue obtained during the revision of cobalt-chromium alloy hip replacement prostheses was determined. The metal content of the tissue did not correlate with the histologic findings, demographic variables, or duration of the implant. The highest amount of metal was found in cases revised for infection. The relative amounts of metal ions indicated that the metallic debris was present predominantly as wear particles. The findings suggested that much of the metallic debris was generated during the short period of time after significant loosening occurred.

Brien WW, Salvati EA, Betts F, et al: Metal levels in cemented total hip arthroplasty: A comparison of well-fixed and loose implants. *Clin Orthop* 1992;276:66-74.

In this prospective study the concentration of metal within the synovial fluid of patients receiving stainless steel, cobalt-chromium alloy, and titanium alloy cemented total hip implants was measured. The amount of metal in the synovial fluid of patients with loose stainless steel implants was five times greater than that found in patients with well-fixed stainless steel devices. There was a seven-fold increase in metal levels of loose compared with well-fixed cobalt-chromium alloy prostheses, and a 21-fold increase in metal levels of loose compared with well-fixed titanium alloy implants.

Huo MH, Salvati EA, Lieberman JR, et al: Metallic debris in femoral endosteolysis in failed cement total hip arthroplasties. *Clin Orthop* 1992;276:157-168.

Higher metal and barium levels were found in tissue obtained from the sites at which femoral endosteolysis was occurring than at other sites around cemented total hip prosthesis removed at revision arthroplasty because of aseptic loosening. Polyethylene and cement debris were noted in most cases. The authors concluded that cement, polyethylene, and metallic particulate wear debris may contribute to the pathogenesis and progression of osteolytic lesions at sites around cemented total hip arthroplasties.

Fretting Wear of Modular Components

Cook SD, Manley MT, Kester MA, et al: Evaluation of wear in a modular sleeve/stem hip system. Transactions of the combined meeting of the Orthopaedic Research Society of the USA, Japan and Canada, 1991, pp 229.

Laboratory testing was performed to determine the effect of cyclic loading on the fretting wear occurring with a modular sleeve/stem hip prosthesis system. The authors found that axial and torsional fatigue testing resulted in the generation and accumulation of a significant amount of wear debris. The particle size ranged from approximately 0.09 to 4 micrometers.

Krygier JJ, Bobyn JD, Dujovne AR, et al: Strength, stability, and wear analysis of a modular titanium femoral hip prosthesis tested in fatigue. Combined meeting of

Orthopaedic Research Society, Banff, Alberta, 1991, pp 194.

Laboratory fatigue testing of a modular sleeve/stem femoral component revealed metallic transfer between stem and sleeve surfaces at sites of high contact stress. The amount of wear debris produced by fretting varied with the magnitude of the applied loads and environmental conditions (wet versus dry).

Hydroxyapatite Coatings

Bauer TW, Geesink RCT, Zimmerman R, et al: Hydroxyapatite-coated femoral stems: Histological analysis of components retrieved at autopsy. *J Bone Joint Surg* 1991;73A:1439-1452.

Five hydroxyapatite-coated femoral stems, implanted for a mean duration of 12 months, were obtained at autopsy and evaluated histologically. Osteoclast-like cells could be found resorbing areas of the coating. Approximately 20% of the hydroxyapatite coating had been resorbed in the prostheses that were obtained at five to 25 months after implantation. The location from which the coating had resorbed varied in each of the five prostheses studied. The percentage of the stems apposed by bone varied from approximately 35% to 75%. These findings demonstrate that plasma-sprayed hydroxyapatite coatings might undergo cell-mediated resorption.

Søballe K, Hansen ES, Rasmussen HB, et al: Tissue ingrowth into titanium and hydroxyapatite-coated implants during stable and unstable mechanical conditions. *J Orthop Res* 1992;10:285-299.

The effect of micromotion on the bone apposition to hydroxyapatite-coated titanium alloy implants and noncoated devices in dogs was evaluated. Implants were inserted into the weightbearing regions of all four femoral condyles in each of seven dogs. The devices were designed to be either unstable, undergoing micromotion, or stable. Specimens subjected to micromovement were surrounded by fibrous tissue. However, the interfacial shear strength of unstable hydroxyapatite-coated implants was significantly greater than that of unstable titanium implants and comparable to the shear strength of stable titanium implants. Mechanically stable implants with hydroxyapatite coatings had the highest attachment strength to bone. The authors speculated that the presence of fibrocartilage in a higher collagen concentration in the fibrous membrane around the unstable hydroxyapatite implants might be responsible for their higher shear strength.

Effect of Prosthesis Stiffness

Cheal EJ, Grierson AE, Hsu H-P, et al: Comparable bone remodeling around composite and titanium alloy femoral stems in dogs as determined by QCT. *Trans Orthop Res Soc* 1992;17:386.

This study employed quantitative computed tomography to evaluate the distribution of bone mass in transverse sections of canine femurs containing titanium and carbon-fiber reinforced polymer composite femoral stem after six and 12 months. The carbon-fiber reinforced polyetheretherketone stem had approximately one half the stiffness of the metallic control. The results demonstrated a net increase in the amount of bone at proximal and distal sections around both types of stems. While the amount of bone at the site of the original cortex might have been reduced, there was a net increase in the amount of bone in the transverse section indicating a redistribution of bone mass. The fact that the titanium stems in this study did not yield the same type of proximal bone loss found in previous canine studies might have been due to the smooth surfaced, collarless, canal-filling design that yielded higher stresses in surrounding bone than titanium stem designs previously evaluated in dogs.

Mintzer CM, Robertson DD, Rackemann S, et al: Bone loss in the distal anterior femur after total knee arthroplasty. *Clin Orthop* 1990;260:135-143.

This investigation determined the prevalence of bone loss, detected radiographically, in areas underlying femoral and tibial components of cemented and noncemented total knee replacement prostheses of three designs. Bone loss occurred in the distal anterior femur in the majority of cases (68%); this bone loss was independent of mode of fixation and implant design. Radiographically detectable bone loss occurred within the first postoperative year and did not progress. It was proposed that this osteopenic condition resulted from stress shielding. This loss of bone occurred in asymptomatic patients, and has not been implicated as a source of failure. However, this osteopenic condition could place the bone at risk for failure with longer periods of cyclic loading. Moreover, as the result of bone loss, revision arthroplasty might be more difficult.

Sumner DR, Turner TM, Urban RM, et al: Remodeling and ingrowth of bone at two years in a canine cementless total hip arthroplasty model. *J Bone Joint Surg* 1992;74A:239-250.

Titanium alloy canine femoral stems with various types of porous coatings were evaluated for the amount and distribution of bone ingrowth into the coatings and the stress-induced adaptive remodeling around the prostheses. In general, about 15% to 18% of the cortical bone was loss adjacent to the levels of the stem that were covered with the porous coatings. The amount of loss of the cortical bone was similar to that observed in a previous six-month study, suggesting that a steady state had been achieved after that time period. The redistribution of bone in transverse sections was caused by a loss of subperiosteal bone proximally and endosteal resorption at the middle and distal levels of the stem. The amount of medullary bone increased proximally and distally.

23
Amputations and Prosthetics

Amputations are usually performed to remove diseased, mangled, or functionally useless parts. Although medical advances in antibiotics, peripheral and microvascular surgery, and the treatment of neoplasms have improved limb salvage, unwise or prolonged attempts to save a limb that should be amputated can cause excessive morbidity and even death. To adequately counsel patients contemplating amputation versus limb salvage, the surgeon must understand the entire surgical and rehabilitative process, as well as a realistic prognosis for achieving function. Limb salvage is not always in the patient's best interest.

The decision to amputate is an emotional process that often is accompanied by an attitude of unsurmountable disability or failure. The value of approaching amputation with a positive and reconstructive approach cannot be overemphasized. To achieve maximal function, the prospective amputee needs a clear understanding of amputation surgery, early postoperative prosthetic fitting, amputee rehabilitation, and the prosthetic prescription. The team approach, including input by nurses, prosthetists, and amputee support groups, can be invaluable in providing the psychological, emotional, and educational support needed for an amputee to return to a full and active life.

Pediatric Considerations

Pediatric amputations are typically the result of congenital limb deficiencies, trauma, or tumors. Congenital limb deficiencies are commonly described using the Burtch revision of the Frantz and O'Rahilly classification system: Amelia is the complete absence of a limb; hemimelia is the absence of a major portion of a limb; and phocomelia is the attachment of the terminal limb at or near the trunk. Hemimelias can be terminal, involving a complete transverse deficit; or they can be intercalary, involving an internal segmental deficit with variable distal formation. Preaxial refers to the radial or tibial side of a limb, and postaxial to the ulnar or fibular side. Amputation is rarely indicated in the case of a congenital upper limb deficiency; even rudimentary appendages can be functionally useful. In the lower limb, surgery may be indicated in proximal femoral focal deficiency and congenital absence of the fibula or tibia to produce a more functional residual limb and improve prosthetic replacement.

In the growing child, two major considerations are the proportional change in residual limb length and terminal overgrowth. A diaphyseal amputation removes one of the epiphyseal growth centers, and the bone involved does not continue to grow in proportion with the rest of the body. What initially appears to be a very long above-knee amputation in a small child can result in a very short limb that is difficult to fit with a prosthesis at skeletal maturity. All attempts should be made to save the distalmost epiphysis by disarticulation or, if this is not possible, to save as much bone length as possible.

Terminal overgrowth occurs when the appositional growth of bone in pediatric diaphyseal amputations exceeds the growth of the surrounding soft tissues. If untreated, the appositional bone often penetrates through the skin. Terminal overgrowth occurs most commonly in the humerus, fibula, tibia, and femur, in that order; and 8% to 12% occurrence has been reported in acquired pediatric amputations. Numerous surgical procedures have been described to manage this problem, but the best methods are stump revision with adequate resection of bone or autogenous osteochondral stump capping as described by Marquardt (Fig. 1). Although techniques using nonautologous material have been described, significant complications have been reported with this technique.

Fitting prosthetics for the growing child can be challenging, and frequent adjustments are required. Where available, specialty pediatric amputee clinics can ease this process, provide family support, and make care more cost efficient. Prosthetic fitting should be initiated to closely coincide with normal motor skill development. In the upper limb, this begins at the time of sitting balance, usually at 4 to 6 months of age. Initially, a passive terminal device with blunt rounded edges is used. Active cable control and a voluntary opening terminal device are added when the child exhibits initiative in placing objects in the terminal device, usually in the second or third year of life. Myoelectric devices are usually not prescribed until the child has mastered traditional body-powered devices. Because the physical demands placed on prosthetic devices by children can often exceed the durability of current myoelectric devices, maintenance and repair costs must be considered.

Prosthetic fitting for the lower extremity pediatric amputee usually coincides with crawling and pulling to stand at 8 to 12 months of age. For the above-knee amputee, control of a knee unit is not expected immediately. A locking knee unit should be used until the child is walking and demonstrates proficient use of the prosthesis. Initial gait pattern is not the normal heel-strike, midstance, toe-off pattern and this pattern should not be expected. For-

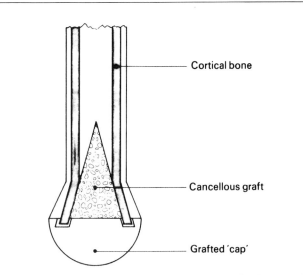

Cortical bone

Cancellous graft

Grafted 'cap'

Fig. 1 Diagram of the stump capping procedure. The bone end has been split longitudinally. (Reproduced with permission from Bernd L, Bläsius K, Lukoschek M, et al: The autologous stump plasty: Treatment for bony overgrowth in juvenile amputees. *J Bone Joint Surg* 1991;73B:203-206.)

mal gait training is seldom warranted until the child reaches 5 or 6 years of age. Attempts to force gait training too early can be frustrating for all involved, and children are surprisingly adept at developing efficient gait patterns as they develop the necessary motor coordination.

Preoperative Evaluation and Decision Making

The decision to amputate a limb and the choice of amputation level can be difficult and subject to differences in opinion. Advances in the treatment of infection, peripheral vascular disease, replantation, and limb salvage complicate the decision-making process. The goal is to optimize a patient's function and reduce morbidity.

Vascular Disease and Diabetes

Ischemia from peripheral vascular disease remains the most frequent reason for amputation in our society. Approximately half of these patients also have diabetes. The preoperative evaluation of these patients includes the clinical examination and evaluation of perfusion, nutrition, and immunocompetence. Preoperative screening tests can be helpful and predictive of successful healing, but no single test is 100% accurate, and all tests have false negative rates. Doppler ultrasound is the most readily available objective measurement of limb blood flow, but arterial wall calcification increases the pressure needed to compress these vessels. Low pressures are indicative of poor perfusion; however, normal and high values can be confusing because of vessel-wall calcification, and are not predictive of normal perfusion or of

wound healing. Toe blood pressure appears to be more predictive of healing than ankle-level pressures. Transcutaneous PO_2 and PCO_2 are noninvasive and becoming more readily available in many vascular laboratories. Both have been shown to be statistically accurate in predicting amputation healing, but false negatives still exist. Xenon 133 skin clearance has been used successfully to predict healing of amputations, but the preparation of the xenon 133 gas/saline solution and the application of this test are highly technician-dependent, expensive, and time consuming. After conducting a prospective trial, one previously enthusiastic author is no longer convinced of xenon 133's predictive value, and believes that $TcPO_2$ and $TcPCO_2$ are more predictive.

Nutrition and immunocompetence have been shown to correlate directly with amputation wound healing. Many laboratory tests are available to assess nutrition and immunocompetence; however, some are quite expensive. Scrum albumin and total lymphocyte count are readily available and inexpensive screening parameters. Several studies have shown increased healing of amputations in patients with impaired circulation who had an albumin of greater than 3.0 or 3.5 g/dl and a total lymphocyte count of over 1,500 cells/mm³. Preoperative nutritional screening is recommended to improve nutrition before surgery. If nutritional improvement is not possible, a higher level amputation should be considered.

The patient's activity level, ambulatory potential, cognitive skills, and overall medical condition must be evaluated to determine if amputation at the most distal level is really appropriate. In ambulatory patients, the goal is to achieve healing at the most distal level that can be fit with a prosthesis and to successfully rehabilitate the patient. In recent series of patients with impaired circulation and diabetes, 70% to 80% healed at the below-knee or more distal amputation levels. This is in sharp contrast to 25 years ago when 80% of all successful amputations were done at the above-knee level. For nonambulatory patients, the goal is to obtain wound healing, minimize complications, and improve sitting balance, transfers, and nursing care. For example, a bedridden patient with a knee flexion contracture might be better served with a knee disarticulation than a below-knee amputation. Preoperative assessment of the patient's potential to be a prosthetic user can contribute to wise selection of amputation level and to postoperative rehabilitation.

Trauma

The absolute indication for amputation in trauma remains an ischemic limb with unreconstructable vascular injury. With improvement in vascular reconstruction surgery, many limbs were salvaged initially, only to be amputated after multiple surgical procedures and substantial investment of time, money, and emotional energy. Recent studies show the value of early amputation in preventing the emotional, marital, financial, and addictive disasters that can follow unwise and desperate attempts at limb salvage.

Guidelines for immediate or early amputation of mangled limbs should differ for upper and lower extremities. An upper limb with severely diminished function usually serves better than a currently available upper extremity prosthesis as an assistive limb. However, a dysfunctional lower limb that cannot bear weight or is not durable because of pain, deformity, or sensory loss is often less functional than a prosthetic leg, especially if amputation is at the below-knee, Syme's, or partial foot level. Recently, grading scales for mangled lower limbs have been developed. These scoring systems are not absolute predictors of outcome or function, but should serve as guidelines to help the surgeon realize the gravity of the injury and the subsequent risks of salvage.

Tumors

Patients who have musculoskeletal neoplasms face new decisions about treatment with the development of limb salvage techniques and adjuvant chemotherapy and radiation therapy. The energy cost during gait after tumor surgery has been determined. A comparison of free-walking velocity, oxygen consumption per meter traveled, and the percent of maximum aerobic capacity used during walking indicated that patients with en bloc resection and knee replacement had a lower energy cost during gait than those with an above-knee amputation. Another comparison, of energy cost and functional outcome after above-knee amputation, resection arthrodesis, or replacement arthroplasty for malignant tumors adjacent to the knee, indicated there was no difference in self-selected walking velocity or oxygen consumption. The functional outcome analysis revealed that the patients with amputations were very active, and were the least worried about damaging the affected limb, but that they had difficulty walking on steep, rough, or slippery surfaces. The patients with arthrodeses had a more stable limb and performed the most demanding physical work and activities, but had difficulty sitting. The patients with arthroplasties led sedentary lives and were the most protective of the limb, but they were the least self-conscious about the limb.

In tumor patients, the amputation level must be carefully planned to achieve the appropriate surgical margin. If the surgical incision enters the lesion, the margin is intralesional; if the surgical incision enters the inflammatory zone but not the lesion, the margin is called marginal; if the surgical incision enters the same compartment, but is outside of the inflammatory zone, the margin is wide; and if the surgical incision is outside of the involved compartment, the margin is radical. All of these surgical margins are possible outcomes of a poorly or carefully planned amputation.

Surgical Techniques and Definitions

Surgical techniques, especially soft tissue handling, are more critical to wound healing and functional outcome in amputation surgery than in many other surgical procedures. The tissues often have impaired circulation or are traumatized, and the risk of wound failure, especially without close attention to soft tissue technique, is high. Flaps should be kept thick, avoiding unnecessary dissection between the skin, subcutaneous, fascial, and muscle planes. In adults, periosteum should not be stripped proximal to the level of transection. In children, removing 0.5 cm of the distal periosteum may help prevent terminal overgrowth. All bone edges should be rounded smooth.

Muscle loses its contractile function when the skeletal attachments are divided during amputation. Stabilizing the distal insertion of muscle can improve residual limb function by preventing atrophy, providing counterbalance to the deforming forces resulting from the amputation, and providing stable padding over the end of the bone. Myodesis, the direct suturing of muscle or tendon to bone, is most effective in above-knee and above-elbow amputations and knee and elbow disarticulations. Myoplasty involves suturing of muscles to periosteum or distally to each other. Stabilizing the muscle mass prevents distal formation of a mobile sling of muscle, which can result in a painful bursa.

All transected nerves result in the formation of neuromas. Surgical attempts to diminish neuromas include clean transection, ligation, crushing, cauterization, capping, and perineural closures and end loop anastomoses. None has proven more effective than careful retraction and clean resection of the nerve, allowing the cut end to retract into the soft tissues, away from the scar and prosthetic pressure points. Ligature of the nerve is indicated to control bleeding from the blood vessels contained within larger nerves.

Split-thickness skin grafts are generally discouraged except as a means to save a knee or elbow joint that has stable bone and good muscle coverage. Skin grafts do best with adequate soft-tissue support, and are least durable when closely adherent to bone. New prosthetic interfaces, such as the silicon-based liners, can help reduce the shear at the interface and improve durability in skin-grafted residual limbs.

Postoperative Care

The terminal amputation allows the unique opportunity to manipulate the physical environment of the wound during healing. Rigid dressings, controlled environment chambers, air splints, soft dressings, and skin traction are all described methods. The use of a rigid dressing controls edema, protects the limb from trauma, decreases postoperative pain, and allows early mobilization and rehabilitation. The use of the Immediate Post-Operative Prosthesis (IPOP) is proven to decrease the time to limb maturation and the time to definitive prosthetic fitting. Most surgeons will start partial weightbearing after the first cast change on day five to ten, if the wound appears stable. Immediate postoperative weightbearing can be initiated safely in select patients. Rigid dressings and

IPOP must be applied carefully, but their application is easily learned and well within the scope of interested orthopaedic surgeons. IPOP is also possible for upper extremity amputations, and early prosthetic training with these devices is believed to increase the long-term prosthetic use.

Complications

Pain   Phantom sensation, the feeling that all or a part of the amputated limb is still present, occurs in nearly all acquired amputees, but it is not always bothersome. Phantom sensation usually diminishes over time, and telescoping, the sensation that the phantom foot or hand has moved proximally toward the stump, commonly occurs. Phantom pain is a very bothersome, burning, painful sensation in the phantom limb that occurs in 1% to 10% of acquired amputees. Surgical intervention has not been very successful. Noninvasive treatments such as massage, intermittent compression, increased prosthetic use, or transcutaneous electrical stimulation can occasionally help. Often the symptoms are similar to those of reflex sympathetic dystrophy. Reflex sympathetic dystrophy can occur in amputated limbs and should be treated aggressively if present. Although it is rare, pain unrelated to the amputation is easy to overlook. The differential diagnosis includes radicular nerve pain from proximal entrapment or disc herniation, arthritis of proximal joints, ischemic pain, or referred visceral pain. Phantom pain has been prevented or decreased by perioperative epidural anesthesia or by postoperative intraneural anesthesia applied directly into the transected nerves.

Edema   Postoperative edema is common following amputation. Rigid dressings can help reduce this problem. If soft dressings are used, they should be combined with stump wrapping to control edema, especially if the patient is a candidate for a prosthesis. The major complication from stump wrapping is applying the elastic wrap too tightly at the proximal end, which can cause congestion, worsening edema, and a dumbbell-shaped residual limb. Another common mistake is not wrapping above-knee amputations in a waist high soft spica to fully include the the groin. If the stump is wrapped incorrectly, a narrow limb with a large adductor roll can result. The ideal shape of a residual limb is cylindrical, not conical.

A poor fitting prosthesis can lead to problems with the stump. Stump edema syndrome is commonly caused by proximal constriction. Its symptoms include edema, pain, blood in the skin, and increased pigmentation. This condition usually responds to temporarily not wearing the prosthesis, elevation, and compression. Verrucous hyperplasia is a wart-like overgrowth of skin, caused by a lack of distal contact and failure to remove normal keratin. A thick mass of keratin with fissuring and oozing develops at the distal end of the stump, and it often is infected. The infection should be addressed first, then the limb should be treated by soaking it and softening the keratin with salicylic acid paste. Occasionally, topical hydrocortisone can help resistant cases. Prosthetic modifications to improve distal contact must be made to prevent recurrences. Because the distal limb is often tender, and these prosthetic modifications uncomfortable, an aggressive prosthetic and physical therapy approach is warranted.

Joint Contractures   Joint contractures usually occur in the time between amputation and prosthetic fitting. Preoperative contractures seldom can be corrected postoperatively. In the above-knee amputee, the deforming forces are to flexion and abduction. Adductor and hamstring stabilization can oppose these deforming forces. Postoperatively, patients should avoid propping the leg up on a pillow, and they should be started on active and passive motion early, including lying prone to stretch the hip. In below-knee amputees, knee flexion contractures greater than 15 degrees can cause major prosthetic problems and failure. Long leg rigid dressings, early postoperative prosthetic fitting, quadriceps strengthening exercises, and hamstring stretching can prevent this complication. Prevention is best, because the very short lever arm makes established knee contractures difficult or impossible to correct. Elbow contractures often follow below-elbow amputation, especially when the residual limb is short. Efforts should be directed at prevention, but if a contracture occurs, step-up hinges can convert a limited range of motion into a greater arc of prosthetic motion.

Wound Failure   Wound failure is not uncommon, especially in diabetic and ischemic limbs. Most surgeons prefer open wound care for wounds less than 1 cm wide and revision surgery for more gapping wounds. There are reports of some success with rigid dressing and IPOP use in spite of local areas of wound failure.

Dermatologic Problems   Good general hygiene includes keeping the leg and prosthetic socket clean, rinsed well to remove all residual soap, and thoroughly dry. Patients should avoid the application of foreign materials and be encouraged not to shave the residual limb. Reactive hyperemia is the early onset of redness and tenderness after amputation. It is usually pressure related, and resolves spontaneously.

Epidermoid cysts commonly occur at the prosthetic socket brim, especially posteriorly. Epidermal cysts are very difficult to treat and commonly recur, even after excision. The best initial approach is to modify the socket and relieve pressure over the cyst.

Contact dermatitis can be confused with infection. Primary irritation contact dermatitis is caused by acids, bases, and caustics. Detergents and soaps commonly are to blame; usually the irritant is not washed out of prosthetic socks. Patients with this problem should use mild soap and rinse extremely well. Allergic contact dermatitis commonly is caused by the nickel and chrome in metal, antioxidants in rubber, carbon in neoprene, chromium salts used to treat leather, and unpolymerized epoxy and polyester resins in plastic laminated sockets. After ruling out infection, the treatment of contact dermatitis includes removal of the irritant, soaking the limb, application of topical steroid creams, and compression with Ace wraps or shrinkers.

Superficial skin infections are common in amputees. Folliculitis occurs in hairy areas, often soon after the amputee starts to wear a prosthesis. Pustules surround the hair follicles at the eccrine sweat glands. Folliculitis is often worse if the patient shaves. Hidradenitis, which occurs in apocrine glands in the groin and axilla, tends to be chronic and responds poorly to treatment. Socket modification to relieve any pressure in these areas can be helpful. Candidiasis and other dermatophytes cause scaly, itchy skin, often with vesicles at the border and clearing centrally. Fungal infections are diagnosed with a potassium hydroxide preparation and treated with topical antifungal agents.

Prosthetics

Major advances in lower limb prosthetics include the use of new lightweight structural materials, the incorporation of elastic response "energy storing" designs, and the use of computer-assisted design and computer-assisted manufacturing (CAD-CAM) technology in socket design. New electronic technology has increased the success and durability of myoelectric prostheses for the upper limb. The surgeon who prescribes prosthetic limbs should have a basic understanding of the general features available to obtain an optimal match of the components with the patient's specific needs. A good prosthetic prescription specifies the socket type, suspension, shank construction, specific joints, and terminal device.

The socket can be a hard socket with no or minimal interface, or it can incorporate a liner. For the above-knee amputee, a wide variety of socket shapes are available, from the traditional quadrilateral design to the newer narrow medial-lateral design. The prosthesis is suspended from the body by straps, belts, socket contour, suction, friction, or physiologic muscle control. Shank construction can be an exoskeletal shell or an endoskeletal rigid inner pylon with a cosmetic foam cover. Traditionally, exoskeletal systems were more durable, but as materials technology has improved, so have the durability and cosmetic appearance of endoskeletal systems. A large variety of elbow, wrist, knee, and ankle joints are available, as well as a multitude of terminal devices, including hands, hooks, feet, and special adaptive devices for sports and work. Without sensation, vision is mandatory to substitute for upper extremity proprioception. Often, cosmetic-appearing hands will block vision and make dexterous use of the terminal device difficult and clumsy. The simple hook provides better vision of objects and, usually, superior function. The

physician must individualize the prescription to present the most efficient system for a particular patient.

Nearly all prostheses are fabricated by forming a thermoplastic or laminate socket over a plaster mold. This mold is not an exact replica of the residual limb, but is modified to relieve the socket over areas that cannot tolerate pressure and to indent the socket over areas that can tolerate pressure. Test sockets of clear plastic commonly are made to visualize the blanching of the skin at troublesome areas. AFMA (Automated Fabrication of Mobility Aids) technology uses computer-assisted design and manufacturing to assist the prosthetist by digitizing the residual limb, adding the standard modifications usually applied to a mold, and allowing additional fine manipulation of the shape on the computer screen. The computer can direct the carving of the mold or fabrication of the socket. AFMA technology can decrease the prosthetist's hands-on fabrication time and allow more time for patient evaluation, prosthesis alignment, and gait training.

Myoelectric components are exciting, but generally should not be prescribed for patients until they have mastered traditional body-powered devices, and the residual limb volume is stable. Myoelectric devices have been used most successfully in the midlength, below-elbow amputee. Although a long below-elbow limb has better rotation, it leaves less room to contain the electronics for such a limb. The need is greater in the more proximal level upper-extremity amputee, but the weight and speed of myoelectric components have been a deterrent. Hybrid devices that use body power and myoelectric components can be effective. Muscles that were stabilized by myodesis or myoplasty techniques seem to generate a better signal for myoelectric use.

Amputation Levels and Prosthetic Principles

Upper Extremity

Hand Amputations Although microsurgical replantation techniques have reduced the incidence of these amputations, there are still many patients for whom replantation is not feasible or results in failure. Reconstruction to obtain prehension can be accomplished with pollicization, ray transposition, or toe-to-hand transfer. Functional partial hand prostheses attempt to provide a stable post against which to oppose the remaining digits or the palm. Function is limited. The hand is very visible and is an important part of our body image. Many patients with partial hand amputations can benefit tremendously from cosmetic partial hand prostheses.

Wrist Disarticulation The wrist disarticulation has two advantages over the shorter, below-elbow amputation: Retaining the distal radio-ulnar joint preserves more forearm rotation, and retaining the distal radial flare dramatically improves prosthetic suspension. There is no benefit to retaining the carpal bones. Tenodesis of the major forearm motors stabilizes the muscle units, improving physiologic and myoelectric performance. Prosthetic substitution for the wrist disarticulation is slightly more complicated than for a standard below-elbow amputation. Conventional wrist units generally are not used because of the additional length these add to the prosthetic arm, and, occasionally, the terminal device must be modified because of length. A wrist disarticulation is also harder to fit with a myoelectric prosthesis because less space is available in which to conceal the electronics and power supply. In spite of these prosthetic concerns, wrist disarticulation patients are often excellent upper extremity prosthetic users. Some patients with an unsatisfactory hand can gain improved function by undergoing a wrist disarticulation and using a standard prosthesis. This decision must be individualized and is based on such contributory factors as severity of tissue loss, pain, appearance, functional requirements, and the patient's body image.

Below-Elbow Amputation   The below-elbow amputation is extremely functional, and successful prosthetic rehabilitation and sustained use are achieved in 70% to 80% of patients. Forearm rotation and strength are proportional to the length retained. Myoplastic closure should be performed to prevent a painful bursa, to facilitate physiologic muscular suspension, and to facilitate myoelectric prosthetic use. A short below-elbow amputation needs the added suspension of a Münster socket, or side hinges and a humeral cuff. This type of suspension preserves elbow flexion and extension but further limits rotation. The value of preserving the elbow joint cannot be overemphasized. Skin grafts and even composite grafts should be considered to salvage the tremendous functional benefit of an elbow with some active motion. Step-up hinges can convert a limited active range of elbow motion to an improved prosthetic range of elbow motion. Although body-powered prostheses are extremely functional at this level, this has also been the most successful level at which myoelectric devices have been used.

Krukenberg's Amputation   Krukenberg's kineplastic operation transforms the below-elbow amputation stump into radial and ulnar pincers capable of strong prehension and excellent manipulative ability because of retained sensation on the "fingers" of the forearm. It may be performed as a secondary procedure in below-elbow amputees with residual limbs at least 10 cm from the tip of the olecranon, elbow flexion contracture of less than 70 degrees, and good psychological preparation and acceptance. It should not be performed as a primary amputation. Krukenberg amputees can become completely independent in their daily activities because of the retained sensory ability of the pincers, as well as the quality of the grasping mechanism (Fig. 2). Traditionally, this procedure has been indicated for the blind bilateral below-elbow amputee, but it may be indicated, at least uni-

laterally, in the bilateral below-elbow amputee with vision, or in patients with very limited access to prosthetic facilities. A conventional prosthesis can be worn over the Krukenberg forearm, and myoelectric devices could be adapted to use this unique forearm motion. The major disadvantage is the unique appearance of the arm, which many people consider grotesque and will not accept. As society is becoming more understanding and accepting of disabled and handicapped individuals, this concern may lessen. Intensive preoperative preparation and counseling are mandatory.

Elbow Disarticulation   The elbow disarticulation has the advantages of the condylar flair to improve prosthetic suspension and transfer of humeral rotation to the prosthesis. The longer lever arm improves strength. The disadvantage is in designing the elbow hinge. Outside hinges are bulky and hard on clothing. Conventional elbow units result in a disproportionately long upper arm and short forearm. Whether the advantages outweigh the disadvantages remains controversial.

Above-Elbow Amputation   All possible length that has suitable soft tissue coverage should be saved in performing an above-elbow amputation. Even if only the humeral head remains, and no functional length is salvageable, shoulder contour and cosmetic appearance are improved. Myodesis helps preserve biceps and triceps strength, prosthetic control, and myoelectric signals. Immediate postoperative rigid dressings and prosthetic fitting can be successfully applied to nearly all upper extremity amputations. Postamputation physical therapy for upper extremity amputees should emphasize proximal joint and muscle function. Because the terminal device is usually controlled by active shoulder girdle motion, early prosthetic use and therapy can prevent contracture and maintain strength.

Prosthetic suspension has traditionally been incorporated into the body-powered harness, but this can be somewhat uncomfortable. Newer techniques include suction suspension or, rarely, humeral angulation osteotomy. Many prosthetic options are available for the above-elbow amputee, including all body powered or hybrid prostheses that use myoelectric control of the elbow or terminal device and body power for the other. Many unilateral above-elbow amputees prefer not to wear a prosthesis or, only occasionally, to wear a light-weight cosmetic prosthesis.

Occasionally above-elbow amputation is elected to manage a dysfunctional arm following a severe brachial plexus injury. The advantages are unloading the weight from the shoulder and scapulothoracic joints, and removing a paralyzed arm that hinders function by getting in the way. The necessity for shoulder arthrodesis is controversial and should be individualized. One clinical series found somewhat better return to work in the group of patients with above-elbow amputation alone. Prosthetic expectations in these patients should be limited, because

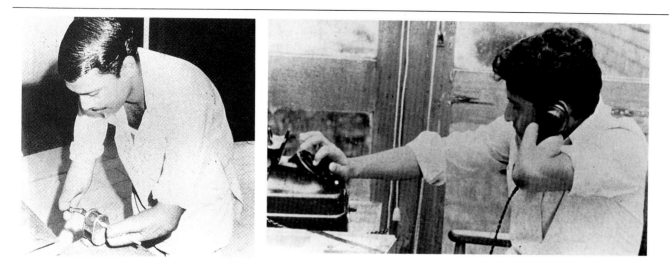

Fig. 2   **Left,** A patient with bilateral Krukenberg hands demonstrates bimanual dexterity in sharpening a pencil. **Right,** A blind patient with unilateral Krukenberg hand is employed as a telephone operator. (Reproduced with permission from Garst RJ: The Krukenberg hand. *J Bone Joint Surg* 1991;73B:385-388.)

attempting to use a prosthesis adds weight to a dysfunctional shoulder girdle, often defeating one of the original goals of the amputation.

Shoulder Disarticulation and Forequarter Amputation

These rare, mutilating amputations usually are performed only for malignancy or severe trauma. Elaborate myoelectric prostheses are available, but are very expensive and require intensive maintenance. Body-powered prostheses are very heavy, hard to suspend comfortably, and difficult to use. Most patients with these proximal amputations request prosthetic help for improved cosmesis and fitting of clothes. Often, a simple soft mold to fill out the shoulder meets these expectations and is an alternative to a full-arm cosmetic prosthesis.

Lower Extremity

Foot Amputations   Toe amputations can be performed with side-to-side or plantar-to-dorsal flaps to use the best available soft tissue. The bone should be shortened to a level that allows adequate soft tissue closure without tension, either disarticulated or metaphyseal. In great toe amputations, the sesamoids can be stabilized in position for weightbearing by leaving the base of the proximal phalanx intact or by tenodesis of the flexor hallucis brevis tendon. Beware of isolated second toe amputations, because a severe hallux valgus deformity of the first toe commonly results. This deformity may be prevented either by second ray amputation or by first metatarsal phalangeal fusion. In metatarsal phalangeal amputations, transferring the extensor tendon to the capsule may help to elevate the metatarsal head. Prosthetic replacement is not typically required after toe amputations.

A ray amputation removes the toe and all or some of the corresponding metatarsal. Isolated ray amputations can be durable, however multiple ray amputations, especially in patients with impaired circulation, can narrow the foot excessively and lead to uneven weightbearing and new areas of increased pressure, calluses, and ulceration. Prosthetic requirements include extra depth shoes with custom-molded insoles.

The transmetatarsal and Lisfranc amputations are reliable and durable. A long plantar flap is preferable, but equal dorsal and plantar flaps will work. Because a healthy, durable soft tissue envelope is more important than a specific anatomic level, bone should be shortened to allow soft tissue closure without tension, rather than shortened to a specific anatomic level. Muscle balance around the foot should be evaluated carefully preoperatively, with specific attention given to heelcord tightness, anterior tibialis, posterior tibialis, and peroneal muscle strength. Midfoot amputations significantly shorten the lever arm of the foot; therefore, Achilles tendon lengthening should be done if necessary. Tibial or peroneal muscle insertions should be reattached if they are released during bone resection. For example, if the base of the fifth metatarsal is resected, the peroneus-brevis insertion should be reinserted into the cuboid. In patients with impaired circulation, reinsertion can be done with minimal dissection to prevent further compromise of the tissues. Postoperative casting can help prevent deformities, control edema, and speed rehabilitation. Prosthetic requirements vary widely. Many patients benefit initially from an ankle-foot orthosis with a long foot plate and a toe filler. Later, a simple toe filler combined with a stiff-soled shoe can be adequate. Cosmetic partial foot prostheses are also available.

A Chopart amputation removes the forefoot and midfoot, saving only the talus and calcaneus. Rebalancing is required to prevent equinus and varus deformities, and can be accomplished by Achilles tenotomy, anterior tibialis or extensor digitorum transfer to the talus, and postoperative casting. If deformity can be prevented, patients with both a Chopart and a Syme's amputation prefer the Chopart level. The Boyd hindfoot amputation is a talectomy and calcaneal-tibial arthrodesis after forward translation of the calcaneus. The Pirogoff hindfoot amputation is a talectomy with calcaneal-tibial arthrodesis after vertical transection of the calcaneus through the midbody, and a forward rotation of the posterior process of the calcaneus under the tibia. These latter two amputations are done mostly in children to preserve length and growth centers, prevent heel pad migration, and improve socket suspension. Studies of children have shown improved function of hindfoot amputations compared to the Syme's amputation, provided that the hindfoot is balanced and no equinus deformity has developed. The hindfoot prosthesis requires more secure stabilization than a midfoot prosthesis to keep the heel from pistoning during gait. An anterior shell can be added to an ankle-foot orthotic type prosthesis, or a posterior opening prosthesis can be used.

Syme's Amputation   Syme's amputation is an ankle disarticulation in which the calcaneus and talus are removed by carefully dissecting bone to preserve the heel skin and fat pad to cover the distal tibia. The malleoli must be removed and contoured. Controversy exists on whether to remove the malleoli initially or at a second-stage operation six to eight weeks later. An advantage of two stages might be improved healing in patients with impaired circulation. Disadvantages include a delay in rehabilitation because of the inability to bear weight until after the second stage, and a second surgical procedure. No prospective, randomized studies have been done. A late complication of Syme's amputation is the posterior and medial migration of the fat pad. Options for stabilizing the fat pad include: tenodesis of the Achilles tendon to the posterior margin of the tibia through drill holes; transferring the anterior tibialis and extensor digitorum tendons to the anterior aspect of the fat pad; or removing the cartilage and subchondral bone to allow scarring of the fat pad to bone, with or without pin fixation. Careful casting postoperatively can also help keep the fat pad centered under the tibia during healing.

Syme's amputation is an end-bearing level. Retaining the smooth, broad surface of the distal tibia and the heel pad allows direct transfer of weight. The below-knee or above-knee amputations do not allow this direct transfer of weight. Because of this, the amputee occasionally can ambulate without a prosthesis in emergencies or bathroom activities.

The prosthesis for Syme's amputations is wider at the ankle level than a below-knee prosthesis. This cosmetic concern is occasionally bothersome. Newer materials and surgical narrowing of the malleolar flair have lessened this concern. Because of the low profile of some newer elastic-response feet, the Syme's amputee can now benefit from energy storing technology. Sockets do not need the high contour of a patellar-tendon bearing design because of the end-bearing quality of the residual limb. The socket can be windowed either posteriorly or medially if the limb is bulbous, or a flexible socket within a socket design can be used if the limb is less bulbous. Because of the tibial flare, the Syme's amputation socket is usually self suspending.

Below-Knee Amputation   The below-knee amputation is the most commonly performed major limb amputation. The long posterior flap technique has become standard, and good results can be expected even in most patients with impaired circulation. Anteroposterior, sagittal, and skewed flaps have all been described and can be useful in specific patients. The level of tibial transection should be as long as possible between the tibial tubercle and the junction of the middle and distal thirds of the tibia, based on the available, healthy soft tissues. Amputations in the distal third of the tibia have poor soft tissue padding and are more difficult to fit comfortably with a prosthesis. The goal is a cylindrically shaped residual limb with muscle stabilization, distal tibial padding, and a scar that is neither tender nor adherent (Fig. 3). The below-knee amputation is especially well suited to rigid dressings and immediate postoperative prosthetic management.

Distal tibiofibular synostosis, the Ertl procedure, is not commonly performed. The principle was to create a broad bone mass terminally to improve the distal-end bearing property of the limb, but this is rarely achieved. The complication of a painful nonunion can be difficult to treat. Distal tibiofibular synostosis may be indicated in a wide traumatic diastasis to improve stabilization of the bone and soft tissues, but it is rarely indicated in patients with impaired circulation.

A large variety of prosthetic designs are available for the below-knee amputee. Sockets can be designed to incorporate a liner to increase comfort and accommodate minor changes in residual limb volume. These liners also increase perspiration, and they can be uncomfortable and less sanitary in hot and humid climates. Hard sockets are designed to have cotton or wool stump socks of certain ply or thickness as the interface between the leg and the socket. Hard sockets are easier to clean and are more durable than the liners. The ISNY (Icelandic-Sweden-New York) socket uses a flexible socket material with more rigid outer supports. The flexible socket changes shape to accommodate underlying muscle contraction. This socket style also can be useful for scarred and difficult to fit limbs.

Open-ended sockets with side joints and thigh corset are not used much today except in patients who have worn them successfully in the past, or in patients with very limited access to prosthetic care. The patellar tendon bearing shape is most commonly used for the below-

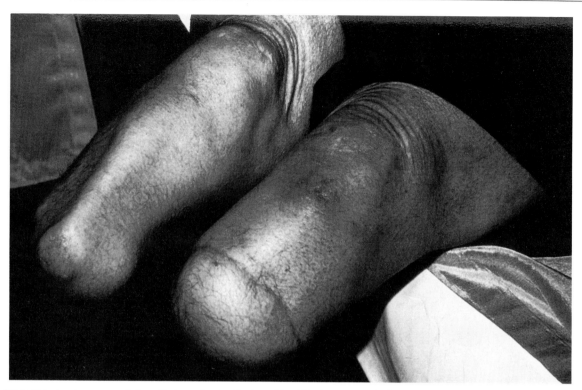

Fig. 3 Bilateral below-knee amputations that emphasize the benefits of the long posterior flap technique. The right limb, amputated by using equal anterior and posterior flaps, is conically shaped and atrophic. The left limb, amputated by using the long posterior flap technique, is cylindrical and well padded. (Reproduced with permission from McCollough NC III, Harris AR, Hampton FL: The bilateral lower limb amputee, in American Academy of Orthopaedic Surgeons *Atlas of Limb Prosthetics: Surgical and Prosthetic Principles.* St. Louis, CV Mosby, 1981, chap 28, p 418.)

knee amputee. In spite of its name, in this prosthesis the majority of the weight is borne on the medial tibial flare and, laterally, on the interosseus space, then to a lesser amount on the patellar tendon area.

Suspension of the below-knee prosthesis can vary extensively. The simplest and most common suspension is a suprapatellar strap, which wraps above the femoral condyles and patella. Sockets can be designed to incorporate a supracondylar mold or wedge to grip above the femoral condyles, but this higher profile is bulkier and less cosmetic in sitting. A waist belt and fork strap suspension is helpful for very short below-knee amputees to decrease pistoning in the socket, or for patients whose activities require very secure suspension. For the limb with poor soft tissue or intrinsic knee pain, side hinges and thigh corset can help unload the lower leg and transfer some weight to the thigh. Suspension sleeves made of latex or neoprene are being used more commonly. The latex is more cosmetic, but is less durable and can be constricting. The neoprene is more durable and not as constricting, but patients can occasionally get a contact dermatitis. The newest suspension uses a silicon-based liner that is rolled on over the residual leg, having an intimate friction fit. A small metal post on the distal end of the liner then locks into a catch in the prosthetic socket to securely

suspend the socket to the liner. Many patients like the secure suspension and feeling of improved control of this prosthesis. These silicon-based liners are less durable and commonly need frequent replacement. Many prosthetic feet now are available, from the original solid-ankle cushion heel, to the newer energy-storing or elastic-response technology with a variety of heel, ankle, and pylon designs. Cost and function can vary widely, and care should be used in prescribing an appropriate prosthetic foot for an individual patient (Table 1).

Through-Knee Amputation Disarticulation through the knee joint is indicated in ambulatory patients when a below-knee amputation is not possible, but suitable soft tissue is present for a knee disarticulation. This occurs most commonly in trauma. In patients with impaired circulation, the blood supply is such that for most patients in whom a knee disarticulation would heal, a short below-knee amputation will also heal. The knee disarticulation is indicated in circulation-impaired patients who are not ambulatory, especially if knee flexion contractures are present. Sagittal flaps appear to heal more readily than the traditional anteroposterior flaps. The patella is retained, and the patellar tendon is sutured to the cruciate stumps to stabilize the quadriceps complex. The biceps

Table 1. A comparison of prosthetic feet

Component	Cost/Weight	Indication	Advantages	Disadvantages	Typical Sports Applications	Ankle Mechanism	Permits Forefoot Pro/Supination	Permits Hindfoot in/ Eversion/Rotation
Sach	Low/medium	General use	Reliable, inexpensive, accommodates numerous shoe styles	Fairly rigid, limited range of motion	Sprinting	Fixed	No	No
Single axis	Mod/heavy	To enhance knee stability	Adds stability to prosthetic knees	Slightly increased cost, weight, maintenance	Limited	Articulated	No	No
Greissinger	Mod/heavy	Accommodate uneven surfaces, absorb rotary torques	Multi-directional motion	Slightly increased cost, weight, maintenance less ML stability	General, to absorb stresses	Articulated	Yes	Yes
Safe	Mod/heavy	Accommodate uneven surfaces, absorb rotary torques, smooth rollover	Multi-directional motion, moisture & grit resistant	Slightly increased cost, weight, less ML stability	General, to absorb stresses		Yes	Yes
Sten-Foot	Mod/medium	Smooth rollover	Moderate cost & weight; accommodates numerous shoe styles; ML stability similar to Sach	Slightly increased cost, weight	General, for smoother rollover	Fixed	Yes	No
Seattle Foot™	High/heavy	Jogging, general sports, "conserve energy"	"energy storing" smooth rollover	Increased cost, weight, difficult to fit in shoes	General, jogging		No	No
Carbon Copy II	High/light	Jogging, general sports, "conserve energy"	"Energy storing," smooth roll-over, very stable ML, highest solid ankle foot	Increased cost, difficult to fit in shoes	General, jogging		No	No
Flex-Foot™	Very high/ very light	Running, jumping, vigorous sports, "conserve energy"	Most "energy storing," most stable ML, lowest inertia, wide range of applications	High cost, complex fabrication & alignment, not feasible for very long residual limbs	Vigorous sports jumping, running	Flexible	No	No

(Reproduced from Michael JW: Energy storing feet: A clinical comparison. *Clin Prosthet Orthot* 1987;11:154-168.)

tendons can also be stabilized to the patellar tendon. A short section of gastrocnemius can be sutured to the anterior capsule to pad the distal end. Although many techniques have been described for trimming the condyles of the femur, this is rarely necessary, and radical trimming can decrease some of the advantages of the knee disarticulation.

For ambulatory patients, the advantages over an above-knee amputation include improved socket suspension by contouring above the femoral condyles, the added strength of a longer lever arm, the retained muscle balance of the thigh, and, most importantly, the end bearing potential to directly transfer weight to the prosthesis. In the past, the objections of a bulky prosthesis

and an asymmetric knee-joint level led many surgeons to abandon this level. New materials allow a less bulky prosthesis to be fabricated, and the four-bar linkage knee unit, which can fold under the socket, improves the appearance when the patient is sitting. The four-bar linkage knee is the prosthetic knee of choice for a knee disarticulation. It is low profile, has excellent stability, and can incorporate a hydraulic unit for swing-phase control.

For nonambulatory patients, a knee disarticulation will eliminate the problem of knee flexion contractures, provide a balanced thigh to decrease hip contractures, and provide a long lever arm for good sitting support and transfers.

In the Gritti-Stokes amputation, the patella is advanced distally and arthrodesed to the distal femur to accept weightbearing. This does not provide a physiologic weightbearing surface, because, even in normal kneeling, the weight is born on the pretibial and patellar tendon areas and not the patella. The added length complicates prosthetic fitting and the asymmetry of the knee joints. This amputation is not recommended. Transcondylar amputation can be performed, however the advantages of end bearing and suspension appear to be diminished by this technique, as compared to the knee disarticulation.

Above-Knee Amputation The above-knee amputation usually is performed with equal anterior and posterior fish-mouth flaps. A typical flap can and should be used to save all possible femoral length in cases of trauma, because increased function is directly proportional to the length of the residual limb. Muscle stabilization is more important in the above-knee amputation than in any other major limb amputation. The major deforming force is into abduction and flexion. Myodesis of the adductor muscles through drill holes in the femur can counteract the abductors, improve prosthetic control, and avoid a difficult adductor tissue roll in the groin (Fig. 4). Without muscle stabilization, the femur commonly migrates laterally through the soft tissue envelope to a subcutaneous location. Newer above-knee socket designs attempt to better control the position of the femur, but they are not as effective as muscle stabilization. Even in nonambulatory patients, muscle stabilization is helpful in creating a more durable, padded residual limb by preventing migration of the femur.

Immediate postoperative prosthetic rigid dressings for the above-knee amputee are more difficult to apply and keep positioned than in more distal amputations. IPOP techniques do offer the advantages of early rehabilitation and control of edema and pain; they are preferred if the expertise is available. Soft compressive dressings alone can be used. These dressings should be carried proximally as a spica to better suspend the dressing and to include the medial thigh, which will prevent the development of an adductor roll of tissue. Proper postoperative positioning and therapy are essential to prevent hip flexion contractures. The limb should not be elevated on a pillow, but should be flat on the bed, and hip extension exercises and prone positioning should be started early.

Suspension of the above-knee prosthesis is more complicated than suspension of prostheses for more distal amputations because of the short residual limb, lack of bony contours, and increased weight of the prosthesis. The prosthesis can be suspended by suction, Silesian bandage, or hip joint and pelvic band. Suction suspension works when the skin forms an airtight seal against the socket. Air is forced out a small one-way valve distally when the prosthesis is donned and, with each step during gait, maintains negative pressure distally in the socket. No prosthetic sock or other liner is used between

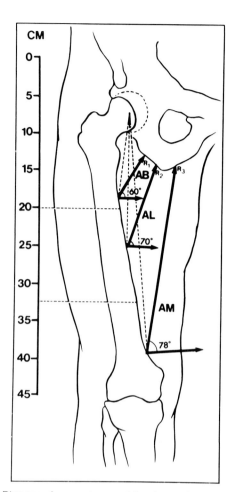

Fig. 4 Diagram of moment arms of the three adductor muscles. Loss of the distal attachment of the adductor magnus will result in a loss of 70% of the adductor pull. (Reproduced with permission from Gottschalk FA, Kourosh S, Stills M, et al: Does socket configuration influence the position of the femur in above-knee amputation? *J Prosthet Orthot* 1989;2:94-102.)

the hard socket and the limb, because air would leak out around the sock and prevent suction from developing. Donning a suction suspension prosthesis requires skill and exertion, and patients must have good coordination, upper extremity function, and balance to perform this task. Suction suspension works well for average to long above-knee amputations with good soft tissues, and stable shape and volume. It is usually very comfortable and the most cosmetic method of socket suspension.

A Silesian bandage is a flexible strap that attaches laterally to the prosthesis, wraps back around the waist and over the countralateral iliac crest, and then comes forward to attach to the anterior proximal socket. It provides good suspension and added rotational control of the prosthesis. A Silesian bandage commonly is used to augment suction suspension for shorter residual limbs or for patients whose activities require more secure suspension than suction alone.

The hip joint and pelvic band provides very secure suspension and control, but is also bulky and the least cosmetic method of suspension. It also is the least comfortable, especially during sitting. The pelvic band is made of metal or plastic and is thicker than a Silesian bandage. The pelvic band runs from the hip hinge around the waist between the contralateral iliac crest and trochanter back to the hip hinge. The hinge is located laterally, just anterior to the trochanter, over the anatomic axis of the hip joint. Hip joint and pelvic band suspension is indicated for very short above-knee limbs, geriatric patients who cannot don a suction suspension, and obese patients who cannot get adequate control with suction or Silesian band suspension.

Socket design for the above-knee amputee has undergone recent changes. The traditional quadrilateral socket has a narrow anteroposterior diameter to keep the ischium positioned back and up on top of the posterior brim of the socket for weightbearing. The anterior wall of the socket is 5 to 7 cm higher than the posterior wall to hold the leg back on the ischial seat. Anterior pain, a frequent complaint, should be addressed by very local relief, for example, over the anterior superior iliac spine. If the entire anterior wall is lowered or relieved, the ischium will slip inside the socket and totally alter the load transfer and pressure areas. Even though the lateral wall is contoured to hold the femur in adduction, the overall dimensions of the quadrilateral socket are not anatomic and provide poor femoral stability in the coronal plane. The ISNY (Icelandic-Swedish-New York) socket is a quadrilateral shaped socket of flexible material with reinforced posterior and medial walls. The flexible material allows socket wall expansion with underlying muscle contraction. Patients report improved comfort in walking and sitting, and possibly improved muscular efficiency. One drawback is that the flexible material is less durable, and cracks can result in the loss of suction suspension.

Narrow medial-lateral above-knee socket designs attempt to solve the problems of a traditional quadrilateral socket by contouring the posterior wall to set the ischium down inside the socket, not up on the brim. Weight is transferred through the gluteal muscle mass and lateral thigh instead of the ischium. This eliminates the need for anterior pressure from a high anterior wall. Attention is then focused on a narrow medial-lateral contour to attempt to better hold the femur in adduction, and to minimize the relative motion between the limb and the socket. The NSNA (Normal Shape, Normal Alignment) and the CAT-CAM (contoured adducted trochanteric-controlled alignment method) sockets are two of the narrow medial-lateral designs available.

Prosthetic knee joints are available in many designs to address specific patient needs. The traditional standard has been the single axis constant friction knee. The constant friction knee is simple, durable, lightweight, and inexpensive. The friction can be set at only one level to optimize function at one cadence, and patients must compensate when walking at different speeds. Outside hinges were the old standard for the knee disarticulation patient, to better approximate the center of motion of the knee. This unit is poor in cosmesis, and has been replaced by a polycentric four-bar knee unit except in patients who have used outside hinges successfully in the past and do not want to change. The safety knee has a weight-activated friction unit that increases friction, and, therefore, stability and resistance to buckling as more weight is applied. This unit is particularly useful in geriatric or insecure patients, and in those patients with very short residual limbs, poor hip extensors, or hip flexion contractures. The variable friction knee unit changes the friction according to the degree of knee flexion, thereby improving the swing phase. This unit is cheaper and requires less maintenance than a hydraulic unit, but is not as effective. A polycentric knee provides a changing center of rotation that is located more posterior than

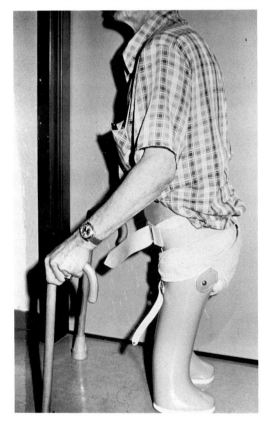

Fig. 5 A 72-year-old male with bilateral above-knee amputations ambulates daily with conventional stubbies, Silesian bandage suspension, and two canes for balance. (Reproduced with permission from Smith DG, Burgess EM, Zettl: Special considerations in fitting and training the bilateral lower-limb amputee, in Bowker JH, Michael JW (eds): *Atlas of Limb Prosthetics, Surgical, Prosthetics and Rehabilitation*, ed 2. St. Louis, Mosby-Year Book, 1992, p 618.)

other knee joints. The posterior center of rotation provides more stability in stance and in the first few degrees of flexion than is provided by other knee units. The four-bar knee is one of many polycentric knee units available.

A hydraulic unit can be added to most knee joints to provide superior control of the prosthesis in swing phase by using fluid hydraulics to vary the resistance according to the speed of gait. This option is very useful in active amputees who walk and run at different speeds. A manual locking option can also be added to most knee units to lock the knee in full extension. Locking is helpful in bilateral amputees, insecure or blind patients, and those patients with very short residual limbs.

The patient with bilateral above-knee amputations is a unique rehabilitation challenge. The use of stubbies as the initial prosthesis is recommended for all patients with bilateral knee disarticulation or above-knee amputation, regardless of age, who are candidates for walking and who lost both legs simultaneously. Stubbies consist of prosthetic sockets mounted directly over rocker-bottom platforms that serve as feet. The rocker-bottom platforms have a long posterior extension to prevent the tendency for the patient to fall backwards. The shortened anterior process allows smooth rollover into the push-off phase of gait. The use of stubbies results in a lowering of the center of gravity, and the rocker bottom provides a broad base of support that teaches trunk balance and provides stability and confidence to the patient during standing and walking (Fig. 5). As the patient's confi-

dence and skills improve, periodic lengthening of the stubbies is permitted until the height becomes nearly compatible with full-length prostheses, at which time the transition is attempted. Many patients reject full-length prostheses, and prefer the stability and balance afforded by the stubbies.

Hip Disarticulation or Hemipelvectomy Hip disarticulation is rarely performed. In the patient with impaired circulation, prosthetic replacement for a hip disarticulation generally is not indicated. A prosthesis can be successfully used, however, by healthier patients who required hip disarticulation because of trauma or malignancy. The prosthesis is heavy, difficult to use, and requires a lot of energy. The standard prosthesis is the Canadian hip disarticulation prosthesis. The socket contains the involved hemipelvis and suspends over the iliac crests. A lightweight hip joint with a locking option and lightweight endoskeletal components are used to keep the weight to a minimum. Many ambulatory patients will use crutches and no prosthesis because this is more comfortable and faster, but prosthetic use does allow freer use of the upper extremities.

Hemipelvectomy is even less frequently required, usually for trauma or malignancy about the pelvis. Prosthetic use is extremely rare after this procedure. Special considerations for seating are occasionally required after hemipelvectomy.

Annotated Bibliography

Pediatric Considerations

Bernd L, Bläsius K, Lukoschek M, et al: The autologous stump plasty: Treatment for bony overgrowth in juvenile amputees. *J Bone Joint Surg* 1991;73B:203-206.

The technique of autologous stump plasty is well described. Fifty procedures carried out on 41 children resulted in a failure rate of only 12% (six cases). The results were age related (six failures in 31 patients under ten years old, versus zero failures in ten patients over ten years old). All six failures were in the humerus, and there were no failures in the lower extremity.

Dysvascular Patients

Lind J, Kramhøft M, Bødtker S: The influence of smoking on complications after primary amputations of the lower extremity. *Clin Orthop* 1991; 267:211-217.

Retrospective review of 165 primary above-knee and below-knee amputations in 137 patients found the risk of infection and reamputation was 2.5 times higher in cigarette smokers. The effects of smoking on coagulation, hemoglobin, perfusion, and wound healing are reviewed.

Malone JM, Anderson GG, Lalka SG, et al: Prospective comparison of noninvasive techniques for amputation level selection. *Am J Surg* 1987;154:179-184.

Transcutaneous oxygen, transcutaneous carbon dioxide, transcutaneous oxygen to transcutaneous carbon dioxide, foot to chest transcutaneous oxygen, intradermal xenon 133, ankle/brachial index, and absolute popliteal artery Doppler systolic pressure were compared prospectively in 52 limbs of 48 patients for accuracy in predicting healing in major lower extremity amputations. The decision of amputation level was based only on xenon 133 skin blood flow data, and clinical judgment. Intradermal xenon 133 skin blood flow was not found to be statistically reliable. Because this group has previously reported a good correlation with xenon 133, this result was surprising. The investigators now believe that xenon's value in amputation level prediction is poor. Ankle/brachial index and popliteal Doppler pressure also were not statistically accurate in predicting successful healing. Transcutaneous measurements of oxygen and carbon dioxide were statistically reliable in prospectively predicting successful healing.

Trauma

Johansen K, Daines M, Howey T, et al: Objective criteria accurately predict amputation following lower extremity trauma. *J Trauma* 1990;30:568-573.

A simple rating scale for massive lower extremity trauma, the mangled extremity severity score (MESS), is detailed. The system scores four variables: skeletal/soft tissue damage, limb ischemia, shock, and age. Analysis of 25 limbs retrospectively, and of 26 limbs prospectively, demonstrated a significant difference in the scores of limbs that were salvaged and those that ultimately required amputation. In both series, a MESS value greater than or equal to seven predicted amputation with 100% accuracy.

Robertson PA: Prediction of amputation after severe lower limb trauma. *J Bone Joint Surg* 1991;73B:816-818.

The mangled extremity severity score (MESS) was applied retrospectively to 164 severely traumatized limbs in 152 patients. All cases with a score of seven or more required amputation. Of the 121 limbs that required amputation, 61 had a score of seven or greater, and 60 had a score of less than seven. Of the 43 salvaged limbs, all had a score of less than seven. Using a score of seven as predictive of amputation, the MESS resulted in no false-positive results indicating 100% specificity; but because many patients with a MESS of less than seven eventually underwent amputation, the method lacks sensitivity.

Tumors

Harris IE, Leff AR, Gitelis S, et al: Function after amputation, arthrodesis, or arthroplasty for tumors about the knee. *J Bone Joint Surg* 1990;72A:1477-1485.

The functional outcome of 22 patients who had a malignant tumor adjacent to the knee treated by above-knee amputation (seven patients), resection arthrodesis (nine patients), or replacement arthroplasty (six patients) revealed no difference in self-selected walking velocity or oxygen consumption. The patients with amputation were very active, and were the least worried about damaging the affected limb, but had difficulty walking on steep rough or slippery surfaces. The patients with arthrodeses had a more stable limb and performed the most demanding physical work and activities, but had difficulty sitting. The patients with arthroplasty led sedentary lives and were the most protective of the limb, but they were the least self-conscious about the limb.

Upper Extremity

Garst RJ: The Krukenberg hand. *J Bone Joint Surg* 1991;73B:385-388.

The author describes his personal experience with 35 Krukenberg procedures over 36 years, reviewing the operative indications, surgical technique, and functional results. Only two patients were blind. The author believes that with the excellent functional results obtained, our traditional indications of a blind patient with bilateral hand amputations may be too restrictive. Proposed indications are: (1) a well healed below-elbow residual limb of > 10 cm length, measured from the tip of the olecranon; (2) no flexion contracture, or less than 70 degrees; and (3) good psychological preparation and acceptance.

Lower Extremity

Gottschalk FA, Kourosh S, Stills M, et al: Does socket configuration influence the position of the femur in above-knee amputation? *J Prosthet Orthot* 1989;2:94-102.

Fifty above-knee amputees who wear a prosthesis every day were divided into two groups: 27 patients with quadrilateral socket design and 23 patients with a narrow medial-lateral socket design. Standing radiographs revealed no difference between the two socket designs in controlling the alignment of the femur. The importance of the adductor muscles and the role of adductor myodesis are discussed.

Unruh T, Fisher DF, Unruh TA, et al: Hip disarticulation: An 11-year experience. *Arch Surg* 1990;125:791-793.

A retrospective review of 38 hip disarticulations in 34 patients for atherosclerosis (17 cases), femoral osteomyelitis (10 cases), and trauma (11 cases) found an overall mortality of 44%. Mortality was statistically higher in atherosclerotic and trauma patients with active infection versus those without active infection. Complications were frequent, and only five of 34 patients had an uncomplicated course. Of the 19 surviving patients, four walked with crutches or a walker, no patient used a prosthesis, 12 patients used a wheelchair, and three were confined to bed.

Pain

Bach S, Noreng MF, Tjéllden NU: Phantom limb pain in amputees during the first 12 months following limb amputation, after preoperative lumbar epidural blockade. *Pain* 1988;33:297-301.

A prospective study of 25 patients with preoperative limb pain in which a study group of 11 patients received lumbar epidural bupivacaine and morphine for 72 hours before amputation, while a control group of 14 patients were treated preoperatively with their usual oral analgesics. All patients received epidural or spinal analgesia for surgery, and meperidine, paracetamol, or acetylsalicylic acid for postoperative pain. Phantom pain was reduced at seven days, at six months, and at one year in the study group compared to the controls.

Fisher A, Meller Y: Continuous postoperative regional analgesia by nerve sheath block for amputation surgery: A pilot study. *Anesth Analg* 1991;72:300-303.

A catheter was introduced into the sciatic or posterior tibial nerve sheath at the time of amputation in 11 patients. Effective postoperative analgesia was obtained with continuous infusion of 0.25% bupivacaine at a rate of 10ml/hr for 72 hours. The need for on-demand narcotic analgesics decreased significantly from 18.4 mg of morphine in the retrospective control group to 1.4 mg of morphine in the study group. One year follow-up showed no phantom pain despite the presence of preoperative limb pain in this small group. No complications related to this technique were seen.

Malawer MM, Buch R, Khurana JS, et al: Postoperative infusional continuous regional analgesia: A technique for relief of postoperative pain following major extremity surgery. *Clin Orthop* 1991;266:227-237.

Bupivacaine was delivered into peripheral nerve sheaths via catheters placed during surgery in 23 patients. Eleven of the 23 patients required no supplemental narcotic, and the remaining 12 patients required approximately one-third of the narcotic units when compared to 11 patients receiving epidural morphine, and an 80% reduction in narcotic units when compared to a group of historical controls. None of the 12 amputees reported phantom pain. No catheter-related complications were reported.

Melzack R: Phantom limbs. *Scientific American* 1992;266(4):120-126.

Originally known for his "gate control" theory of pain, Dr. Melzack discusses phantom sensation and phantom pain, the historic and new theories on this unique phenomenon, and the current treatment approaches. To better explain phantom limbs, he presents his theory that the brain itself generates the experience of the body, and that sensory inputs merely modulate that experience but do not directly cause it.

Prosthetics

Michael JW: Reflections on CAD/CAM in prosthetics and orthotics. *J Prosthet Orthot* 1988;1:116-121.

This editorial introduces an entire issue of the journal devoted to computer-assisted design and manufacturing in the field of prosthetics and orthotics. Principles of digitization of complex shapes, rectification maps, and computer-controlled carving and manufacturing are introduced and discussed throughout this issue.

Michael J: Energy storing feet: A clinical comparison. *Clin Prosthet Orthot* 1987;11:154-168.

This article is an excellent description and review of the physical characteristics of eight commonly used prosthetic feet. The indications, advantages, and disadvantages of the different feet are also discussed to help in appropriately prescribing these prosthetic components.

Torburn L, Perry J, Ayyappa E, et al: Below-knee amputee gait with dynamic elastic response prosthetic feet: A pilot study. *J Rehab Res Dev* 1990;27:369-384.

The gait of five below-knee amputees was investigated while they were wearing a standard SACH foot and four different dynamic energy response feet. Each subject used each foot for one month prior to testing. Compared to the other feet, the Flex-Foot resulted in significantly different gait kinematics at the "ankle" but did not show an increase in velocity or improvement in energy costs. The results of this small study indicated no clinically significant advantages of any of the feet used during free or fast-paced walking on level ground.

III

Upper Extremity

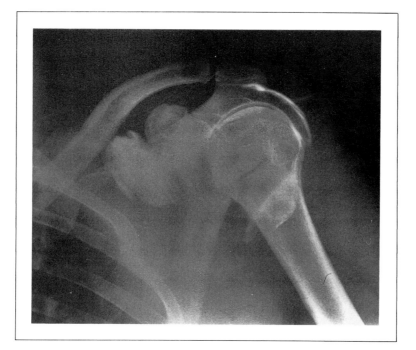

24
Shoulder: Pediatric

Embryology

The upper limb bud first becomes visible at 26 days of fetal life, and rapid development of the shoulder girdle occurs over the following four weeks. Caudal migration of the scapula from the lower cervical level to the upper thoracic level begins during the fifth fetal week and is completed by the eighth week. The three secondary ossification centers of the proximal humerus do not become visible until between four and six months. Separate secondary centers exist for the humeral head and for each of the tuberosities. These three epiphyses coalesce between the ages of 6 and 13 years. The primary center of ossification for the scapula is visible radiographically at birth. Secondary centers arise from the coracoid process and the acromion. These secondary centers do not unite with the body of the scapula until the second, sometimes the third, decade.

Congenital Abnormalities

Sprengel's Deformity

Sprengel's deformity is an uncommon congenital anomaly resulting from interruption of the normal caudal migration of the scapula. It is associated with a high incidence of congenital skeletal and soft-tissue deformities including scoliosis, cervical ribs, torticollis, renal abnormalities, segmentation anomalies of the spine, and muscular hypoplasia, especially involving the trapezius.

The deformity is characterized by elevation and medial rotation of the inferior scapula with resultant loss of shoulder abduction and forward flexion. The involved scapula is both smaller and more cephalad than normal. In 30% of patients, the scapula is attached to the cervical spine by an omovertebral bone, cartilage, or fibrous tissue, which, when present, can severely limit scapulothoracic motion. If an omovertebral bone is present, abduction of the shoulder is commonly limited to less than 90 degrees. Because pain is an unusual finding, many patients are not diagnosed until adolescence. Because of the scapular asymmetry, some children are referred to scoliosis clinics by school screening programs. Minor asymmetries commonly seen between the right and left scapula should not be designated Sprengel's deformity.

Because passive stretching exercises advocated in the past are not successful, treatment is primarily surgical. Surgery is indicated for children between 3 and 8 years of age with significant deformities, both functional and cosmetic. Patients older than 8 years of age are not good candidates for scapular displacement procedures.

Several different procedures have been described for detaching the medial and superior scapular muscles, repositioning the scapula caudad, and subsequently reattaching the muscles to the lowered scapula. The Woodward procedure involves resection of the omovertebral bone and division of the vertebral attachments of the trapezius, rhomboids, and levator scapula. The scapula is then rotated and translated caudally before the detached muscle origins are sutured to more inferior vertebral spinous processes. Three weeks of postoperative immobilization are necessary. Osteotomy or morcellation of the clavicle may be required to prevent compression of the neurovascular structures against the first rib by the straight clavicle.

Both the Green and Woodward procedures and their modifications continue to be performed with 80% satisfactory functional and cosmetic results. Increased shoulder abduction following surgery ranges from 34 to 60 degrees. The child's age at operation and differing methods of measurement play the largest role in accounting for these differences. Younger patients obtain better motion and postoperative correction. Caudad displacement of the scapula is reported to be 1.9 vertebra body heights in one series and 4 cm in another (Fig. 1). Postoperative improvement in shoulder abduction is maintained, although some loss of scapular translation can occur in the first four months postoperatively. One third of patients will have widening of their surgical scars, which can be cosmetically disturbing.

Congenital Pseudarthrosis of the Clavicle

Failure of union between the medial and lateral ossification centers of the clavicle is thought to be the source of this unusual congenital anomaly. Almost all cases involve the right clavicle. The diagnosis is usually made shortly after birth when painless, nontender ends of the ununited clavicle can be palpated. Pseudoparalysis and pain are distinctly unusual, suggesting that birth trauma does not play a role in the development of this condition. Radiographs show lack of callous formation, with a rounded appearance to the ends of the two fragments.

Even in older children, congenital pseudarthrosis of the clavicle causes little or no discomfort. Open reduction, internal fixation, and bone grafting can be performed if asymmetry and cosmetic considerations are unacceptable to the patient or if there are functional limitations. Surgical intervention is more successful than for the more familiar but unrelated congenital pseudarthrosis of the tibia.

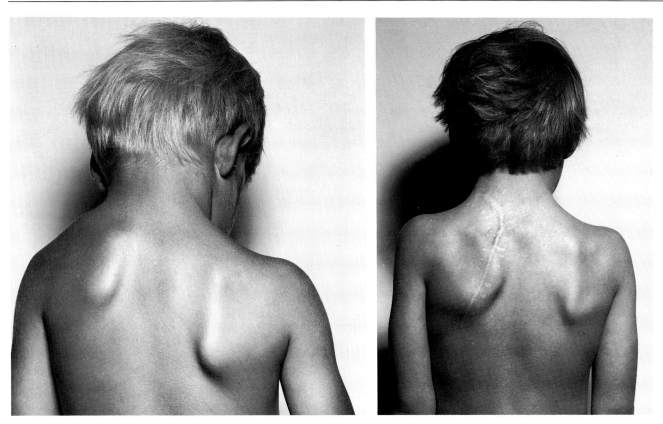

Fig. 1   Left, Preoperative photograph of child with Sprengel's deformity of the left shoulder. **Right**, Nine months following modified Green procedure for left Sprengel's deformity there has been correction of scapular elevation, medial rotation, and neck contour.

Congenital Amputations

Congenital amputations at the level of the shoulder are uncommon. Such amputations may be secondary to constriction or amnionic band syndromes, failure of formation, genetic deficiencies, or teratogens. Most children with shoulder level or above-elbow amputations function exceptionally well if they have a normal contralateral upper extremity. Early prosthetic fitting at 3 to 6 months of age reportedly improves prosthetic acceptance. Initially, a static terminal device is used, and, at approximately 2 years of age, a functional terminal device can be added. Patients with amelia often prefer to do without a prosthesis.

Infection

The shoulder and proximal humerus are common sites for osteomyelitis and septic arthritis in children. Trauma, illness, and malnutrition have been implicated as sources of these infections, but the etiology remains unknown. In the younger child, diagnosis is often delayed. A high clinical suspicion of infection is necessary to detect osteomyelitis in unusual sites such as the proximal humerus. In the acute stage, acute hematogenous osteomyelitis of the proximal humerus shows no radiographic changes. The white blood cell count is within normal limits in the majority of cases. An elevated erythrocyte sedimentation rate usually is present, but it cannot be used to reliably make or exclude the diagnosis, especially in the neonate. Technetium bone scans can localize the affected area, but also are not specific enough to make the diagnosis of osteomyelitis. Direct aspiration of the site for Gram stain, cultures, and sensitivities is required for the diagnosis to be made.

It has long been known that acute hematogenous osteomyelitis of the intra-articular proximal humeral metaphysis can lead to purulent septic arthritis. This may occur when a metaphyseal abscess ruptures into the joint. The intra-articular biceps tendon also provides a route for metaphyseal abscesses to communicate with the shoulder joint. Purulent osteomyelitis of the proximal humeral metaphysis has been shown to communicate with the shoulder joint by extension along the bicipital groove. Acute septic arthritis of the shoulder in children requires formal arthrotomy, irrigation, and appropriate antibiotic treatment. When acute hematogenous osteomyelitis in the proximal humerus is suspected, metaphyseal osteomyelitic foci should be debrided.

Trauma

Clavicle Fractures

The clavicle is the most commonly fractured bone in children. Displacement of the fracture is related directly to the energy absorbed at the time of injury. In infants, 95% of birth fractures involve the clavicle and are associated with breech deliveries. The accompanying pseudoparalysis can be distinguished from birth-related brachial plexus injury, because reflexes remain intact following isolated clavicle fractures. Clavicular birth fractures heal rapidly. Among toddlers and older children, 80% of clavicle fractures occur in the midshaft. Older children can be managed equally well with a figure-eight dressing or a simple arm sling. If significant growth remains, most of the resulting prominence will be incorporated by the growing clavicle. Older children and adolescents may be left with a small prominence. Surgical intervention is rarely indicated. Emergency operative reduction may be required for posteriorly displaced medial clavicle fractures with impingement of the mediastinal structures. Internal fixation is not necessary.

Significant displaced distal clavicle fractures occasionally require surgical reduction and fixation. These fractures usually involve the distal clavicular physis with periosteal stripping of the proximal clavicle (Fig. 2). Specifically, surgery is recommended for distal clavicle fractures with dorsal displacement of the proximal fragment into a subcutaneous position, and rare inferior dislocations of the clavicle beneath the coracoid. Finally, large intra-articular glenoid fractures with displacement, especially those involving the anterior rim, may require open reduction and internal fixation.

Proximal Humerus Fractures

Fractures of the humeral shaft are less common in children than in adults. Most are easily treated by closed reduction and immobilization with an arm sling, shoulder immobilizer, plaster splint, or hanging arm cast. Unicameral and aneurysmal bone cysts are quite common in the diaphysis and metaphysis of the proximal humerus. Most are discovered when pathologic fractures occur through the lesions. Such fractures should be immobilized and allowed to heal before any treatment of the lesion.

Fractures involving the proximal humeral physis are common between the ages of 11 and 15, and are three times more common in males than in females. Most such fractures are of the Salter-Harris I and II types. Because 80% of the growth of the humerus occurs at the proximal physis, tremendous remodeling potential exists, especially in children younger than 12 years of age. As a result, 20 to 40 degrees of angulation can be accepted. Most fractures can be immobilized with the arm at the side or in slight abduction. Closed reduction may be required for significantly displaced or angulated fractures in children near the end of growth.

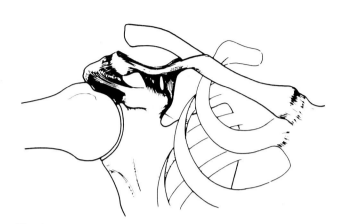

Fig. 2 Distal clavicle fracture with displacement of the clavicle from the periosteal sleeve. These childhood fractures mimic adult acromioclavicular separations. (Reprinted with permission from Havranek RH: Injuries of distal clavicular physis in children. *J Pediatr Orthop* 1989;9:213-215.)

A report of 64 proximal humerus fractures suggests that full remodeling of displaced fractures occurs in all cases. Ten percent of patients have slight sequelae such as transient pain, mild restricted range of motion, or mild weakness. Radiographic evidence of nonunion, malunion, or avascular necrosis of the humeral head is rare. The good prognosis associated with nonsurgical treatment of these fractures is due to the enormous remodeling potential of the proximal humeral physis and the great mobility of the glenohumeral joint (Fig. 3).

Although most fractures about the shoulder in children can be managed without surgery, several specific fractures are best managed surgically. In general, displaced fractures with intra-articular extension (Salter-Harris IV), fractures associated with neurovascular injuries, and open fractures demand surgical treatment (Fig. 4).

Other Fractures

Scapula fractures are uncommon in children and usually involve the body of the scapula. These are treated nonsurgically with immobilization.

Acromioclavicular injuries rarely occur in children. When acromioclavicular joint injuries do occur, they tend to be physeal injuries. Their classification and treatment is the same as for adults sustaining such injuries.

Sternoclavicular injuries are also uncommon in children. Most injuries are Salter-Harris type I or type II fractures. Treatment is nonsurgical in almost all cases. Because the physis at the sternal end of the clavicle does not close until 20 to 25 years of age, these injuries are also seen in adults.

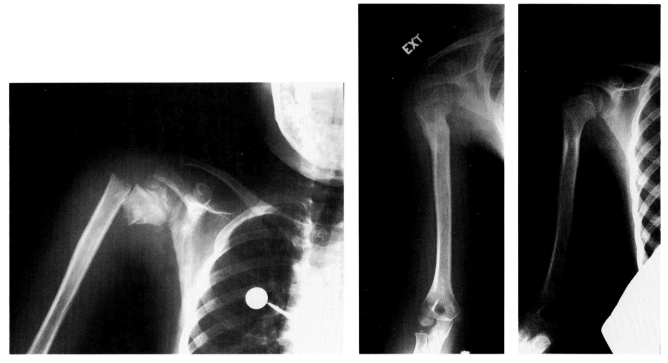

Fig. 3 **Left**, Left proximal humerus fracture in a 5-year-old boy who fell from a tree. Treatment was immobilization. **Center**, Radiographic appearance 12 weeks following fracture. **Right**, Six months after injury there has been complete remodeling of the proximal humerus fracture.

Paralytic Shoulder Injuries

Congenital Brachial Plexus Injury

The incidence of brachial plexus birth palsy is approximately two per 1,000 live births. The most common palsy involves the C-5 and C-6 roots (Erb's palsy). Total brachial plexus involvement and lower root (C-7 and C-8) palsies also occur but are less common and affect hand function. Pseudoparalysis resulting from clavicle and humerus fractures or osteomyelitis must be excluded when considering the differential diagnosis. Brachial plexus injuries can range from mild neuropraxia with early recovery to complete disruption with no potential for recovery. Fortunately, between 80% and 90% of children with such injuries will attain normal or near-normal function.

The natural history of obstetric brachial plexus injuries suggests that children so injured who show evidence of biceps function before 6 months of age have near-normal to excellent function. Therefore, treatment in this first six-month interval is directed specifically at prevention of fixed deformities. Gentle range of motion exercise is necessary to retain external rotation and abduction at the shoulder. Children who show no clinical or electromyographic evidence of biceps function by 6 months of age have a poor prognosis and can be considered for brachial plexus exploration, neurolysis, end-to-end repair, nerve grafting, or neurotization. Recent studies suggest a

better prognosis for patients who have surgical intervention soon after reaching 6 months of age.

Late deformities associated with the more common upper root lesions include internal rotation and adduction of the shoulder and flexion at the elbow. In time, these deformities can become fixed. For those children who have incomplete recovery or residual deformity, the modified L'Episcopo procedure can be most useful in improving shoulder function. This procedure involves lengthening of the pectoralis major and subscapularis tendons with transfer of the teres major and latissimus dorsi insertions into the posterior surface of the humerus to act as external rotators. Several different modifications have been described. For older children with fixed bony adaptive changes, proximal humeral external rotation osteotomy can be considered.

Obstetric Brachial Plexus Injury

Early microsurgical repair continues to gain acceptance for children having obstetric palsies. The concern is no longer whether early surgery is indicated, but rather how early those patients requiring surgery can be identified. Current studies suggest that children in whom biceps function is not clinically or electrically present by six months have a poor prognosis. This represents 10% to 20% of children with obstetric palsies. Early microsurgical repair, grafting, neurolysis, or neurotization can be of benefit in these cases.

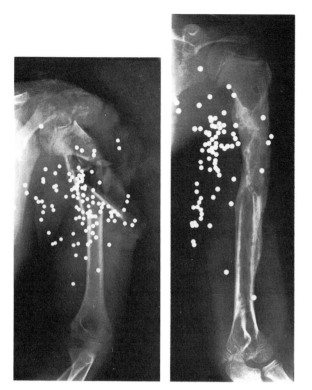

Fig. 4 **Left**, Open comminuted left proximal humerus fracture in a 7-year-old girl as a result of shotgun injury. Treatment involved debridement and application of an external fixator. **Right**, Five months after fracture, bony healing is complete. Humeral length and rotation have been restored.

Because complete nerve transections and root avulsions have a poor prognosis, methods are being explored to identify these lesions early. These methods include myelography, computed tomographic (CT) myelography, sensory evoked potentials, and magnetic resonance imaging (MRI). CT myelography appears to be more sensitive in the detection of traumatic meningoceles; however, nerve root avulsion is not always accompanied by the presence of a meningocele. Sensory evoked potentials cannot discriminate intact nerve roots from those that are incompletely avulsed. MRI allows for identification of distal as well as proximal lesions, but is troubled by occasional false-negative reports and has been used only intermittently to date. Although these different methods do supplement clinical examination, they still do not identify independently those patients who will benefit from early surgery.

Finally, it has been suggested that posterior dislocation of the shoulder can occur in association with obstetric brachial plexus palsies. Some controversy exists as to whether these dislocations are a direct result of a traumatic birth injury or are secondary to nerve injury and muscle imbalance. Indirect evidence exists that suggests that posterior dislocations can occur at birth. When associated with an obstetric brachial plexus palsy, dislocation

results in a considerable loss of function. Correction by open reduction results in marked improvement. External rotational osteotomy of the proximal humerus can be performed in older children who have secondary bony changes in the glenohumeral joint.

Traumatic Brachial Plexus Palsy in Children

Nonbirth-related brachial plexus injuries in children are rare. As a result, very little has been written about this topic. A recent study of 25 children with traumatic brachial plexus injuries suggests that these injuries have a less favorable prognosis than obstetric palsies and more closely resemble adult brachial plexus injuries. Nearly 70% of such injuries are sustained as a result of motor vehicle accidents. Over 50% have associated head injuries consistent with high-energy trauma. Supraclavicular nerve lesions predominate as in obstetric palsies. Root avulsion is common.

The natural history of such injuries suggests that between 22% and 66% of patients will show some spontaneous recovery. The prognosis is good if there is early, partial neurologic recovery before the third month, with continued recovery until the fifteenth month following injury. The prognosis is poor when there is a lack of clinical neurologic recovery by the third month following injury. In such cases, early surgical intervention is warranted. Surgery should be directed primarily at restoration of hand sensation and elbow flexion. Steps to improve shoulder and forearm function can be attempted later, if necessary. Nerve grafting, neurotization, tendon transfer, rotational osteotomy, and arthrodesis can all be used by surgeons skilled in these techniques. It is dangerous to perform simultaneous ipsilateral phrenic and intercostal neurotization, because to do so can lead to dyspnea and pneumonia in children.

Fascioscapulohumeral Muscular Dystrophy

Fascioscapulohumeral muscular dystrophy is a rare autosomal dominant atrophic myopathy that appears in the second decade of life. It is characterized by progressive atrophy of the face and shoulder girdle. Life expectancy is normal. Involvement of the serratus anterior, trapezius, and rhomboids leads to winging of the scapula. Without scapular stability, the spared deltoid is unable to abduct or flex the arm.

Several surgical methods have been described to stabilize the scapula. Scapulothoracic arthrodesis remains the treatment of choice; it is indicated when shoulder function and cosmesis are significantly affected by the disease process. Intact deltoid function is necessary for the procedure to be beneficial. Scapulothoracic arthrodesis increases abduction and flexion by an average of 25 to 30 degrees and eliminates scapular winging. This usually restores the patient's ability to perform most tasks requiring up to 100 degrees of abduction and flexion at the shoulder, including combing hair and dressing without assistance. Several techniques of scapulothoracic arthrodesis have been described.

Complications unfamiliar to orthopaedic surgeons can occur following scapulothoracic arthrodesis. These may include pneumothorax, pleural effusion, atelectasis, and rib fractures, as well as pseudarthrosis.

Shoulder Arthrodesis

Shoulder arthrodesis remains a reliable procedure for stabilization of the flail shoulder in children who have localized paralysis of shoulder-girdle muscles for which good tendon transfers often are not available. Controversy exists regarding the optimum age and angle for arthrodesis. A recent study of five children between 7 and 15 years of age undergoing arthrodesis in 30 degrees of abduction showed loss of 10 to 20 degrees of abduction during the first 12 postoperative months. Because it is difficult to predict the final position, some surgeons advocate delaying shoulder arthrodesis until skeletal maturity. A different study of ten children between 8 and 15 years of age who underwent shoulder arthrodesis showed no loss of abduction and good functional results when the shoulder was fused in 45 degrees of abduction, 25 degrees of flexion, and 25 degrees of internal rotation. The controversy over timing of surgical arthrodesis, therefore, persists.

Subjectively, patients are improved following arthrodesis, with an increased active shoulder abduction of between 20 and 60 degrees. The functional results are related most directly to the neurologic status of the distal arm and hand. Best results are obtained in those patients having isolated paralysis of the shoulder girdle with intact distal function. The possibility of tendon transfer rather than arthrodesis should be considered in this group of patients.

If arthrodesis is attempted in the immature child, the shoulder should be placed in 45 degrees of abduction, 25 degrees of flexion, and 25 degrees of internal rotation. Excessive abduction should be avoided, because excessive scapular winging can result. Similarly, less than 30 degrees of abduction can be associated with eventual loss of abduction. A solid fusion is technically difficult to achieve in children because of the cartilaginous makeup of the humeral head. Pseudarthrosis rates of up to 20% have been reported.

Childhood Disorders with Shoulder Manifestations

Arthrogryposis

This musculoskeletal disorder is characterized by congenital immobility of multiple joints. There may be as many as 10 to 20 specific arthrogrypotic disorders, all with similar joint manifestations. While the distal extremities are more severely affected than the proximal extremities, it is not uncommon for the shoulders to be fixed in adduction and internal rotation. The shoulders rarely require treatment. In selected individuals, severe internal rotation contractures can be corrected with proximal external rotational osteotomy of the humerus.

Juvenile Rheumatoid Arthritis

Fortunately, shoulder involvement is quite rare in this disorder. When it does occur, initial manifestations include radiographic cyst formation and erosions in the proximal humerus. Continued involvement can lead to flattening of the humeral head. Treatment, largely nonsurgical, includes use of medication and physiotherapy.

Shoulder pain with restricted range of motion is present in one third of children with juvenile rheumatoid arthritis, and incidence varies considerably with subtype. Specifically, shoulder involvement is present in 2% of children with pauciarticular onset, 50% with polyarticular onset, and 80% with systemic onset (Table 1). Internal rotation is the most common limited motion, followed by abduction. Children with systemic onset juvenile rheumatoid arthritis are more likely to have early shoulder involvement and more severely limited range of motion. Individuals with the systemic and polyarticular onset disease require more aggressive medical and rehabilitation management.

Table 1. Shoulder involvement in children with juvenile rheumatoid arthritis

Type of Onset	Patients	No. of Shoulders Involved (%)	Unilateral Involvement (%)	Bilateral Involvement (%)
Pauciarticular	45	1 (2.2%)	100	0
Polyarticular	40	20 (50%)	15	85
Systemic	15	12 (80%)	0	100

(Reproduced with permission from Libby AK, Sherry OD, Dudgeon BJ: Shoulder limitation in juvenile rheumatoid arthritis. *Arch Phys Med Rehab* 1991;72:382-384.)

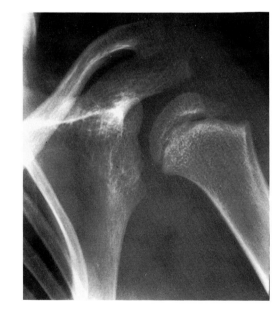

Fig. 5 Mild multiple epiphyseal dysplasia involving the shoulder in an 11-year-old boy. There is slight irregularity of the humeral head and glenoid with decreased height of the epiphysis.

Multiple Epiphyseal Dysplasia

Although hip and other lower extremity symptoms predominate in children with multiple epiphyseal dysplasia, up to one third can expect to have shoulder symptoms sometime during their lives. Patients with minor epiphyseal abnormalities, such as slight irregularity of the humeral head or decreased height of the proximal humeral epiphysis, retain a spherical head in a well-formed glenoid fossa (Fig. 5). Many such patients remain asymptomatic until middle age, when osteoarthritis causes bilateral symmetric pain with minimal loss of motion. Patients who have more marked involvement with early deformity of the humeral head and glenoid often have no pain, but they may have restricted range of motion during their adolescence and early adulthood. Like those individuals with minor epiphyseal involvement, the more severely involved patients experience increased shoulder pain with advancing age. Surgical intervention at an early age is not indicated. Total shoulder arthroplasty may be indicated for patients who become symptomatic as adults.

Conditions Requiring Humeral Lengthening

A variety of conditions, both congenital and acquired, can lead to unilateral or bilateral shortening of the humerus. These conditions include achondroplasia, infantile septic arthritis, obstetric brachial plexus palsy, fractures, congenital shortening, and neoplasms. Until recently, humeral lengthening has not been recommended for many such deformities, because the discrepancy was felt to be cosmetic rather than functional. Recent changes in limb lengthening technology suggest that significant lengthening of between 5 and 16 cm can be achieved with manageable risks. Surgery is indicated in patients with unilateral humeral discrepancies of more than 6 cm who have unsatisfactory appearance and function. Bilateral lengthenings have been performed in patients with dwarfing conditions such as achondroplasia. The indications for this procedure remain controversial.

Humeral lengthening, using corticotomy-distraction techniques, requires from four to 14 months of treatment. Complications include temporary neuropraxis, angular deformity, premature consolidation at the lengthening site, and fracture through new bone after the lengthening apparatus is removed. All of these complications can be managed but require meticulous attention to detail.

Overuse Syndromes

Epiphysiolysis of the Proximal Humerus

Repetitive upper extremity activities, especially throwing, can cause painful widening of the proximal humeral physis. This condition, which is uncommon, occurs most frequently in adolescent male baseball pitchers. Pain and tenderness are localized to the proximal humeral physis. Radiographs show widening of the physis. The condition is most analogous to epiphysiolysis of the distal radius seen in young gymnasts. Treatment involves rest and activity modifications. Most patients report symptomatic relief in one to two months. Radiographic improvement usually lags behind clinical improvement and may take up to six months or more.

Annotated Bibliography

Sprengel's Deformity

Griffin PP, Young R: Sprengel's deformity: A comparison of the Green and Woodward procedures. Presented at the Pediatric Orthopaedic Society of North America Annual Meeting, San Francisco, CA, May 6-9, 1990.

Fifty-eight Green and 17 Woodward procedures were performed for Sprengel's deformity. Eighty percent of patients were found to be improved in function and cosmesis at average follow-up of six years. Increased shoulder abduction was 34 degrees for the Green procedure and 52 degrees for the Woodward procedure.

Leibovic SJ, Ehrlich MG, Zaleske DJ: Sprengel deformity. *J Bone Joint Surg* 1990;72A:192-197.

Sixteen patients with Sprengel's deformity were treated using a modified Green procedure. Moderate or dramatic cosmetic improvement resulted postoperatively. Total shoulder abduction improved from an average of 91 to 148 degrees. Children older than 6 years of age are not good candidates for scapular displacement procedures.

Infection

Danielsson LG, Gupta RP: Four cases of purulent arthritis of the shoulder secondary to hematogenous osteomyelitis. *Acta Orthop Scand* 1989;60:591-592.

Acute hematogenous osteomyelitis of the proximal humerus can spread to the shoulder joint along the biceps tendon. Treatment must address both the osteomyelitic focus and the resultant purulent arthritis.

Trauma

Curtis RJ: Operative management of children's fractures of the shoulder region. *Orthop Clin North Am* 1990;21:315-324.

Fractures about the shoulder in children are reviewed with emphasis directed at those fractures requiring surgical intervention. Open reduction and internal fixation is recommended for open fractures, those with neurovascular compromise, and irreducible fractures. Specific clavicle and glenoid fractures requiring open reduction and internal fixation are also discussed.

Havranek P: Injuries of distal clavicular physis in children. *J Pediatr Orthop* 1989;9:213-215.

Ten patients with distal clavicular physeal injuries are reviewed. All fractures healed without functional deficits. A cosmetic prominence or shortening occurred in 70% of those fractures treated nonsurgically. Open reduction and internal fixation are recommended for distal clavicle fractures with significant displacement.

Ireland ML, Andrews JR: Shoulder and elbow injuries in the young athlete. *Clin Sports Med* 1988;7:473-494.

Common athletic injuries to the adolescent shoulder and elbow are reviewed. These are related to the type of sporting activity and age of the patient.

Larsen CF: Fractures of the proximal humerus in children. *Acta Orthop Scand* 1990;61:255-257.

Seventy-seven patients with proximal humerus fractures are reviewed retrospectively with nine-year follow-up. All but one were treated nonsurgically. All patients were subjectively satisfied with their treatment. Ten percent had slight pain or a minor loss of motion. Full remodeling occurred in all fractures left displaced at the time of treatment. Nonsurgical treatment for proximal humeral fractures in children is recommended.

Obstetric Brachial Plexus Injuries

Dunkerton MC: Posterior dislocation of the shoulder associated with obstetric brachial plexus palsy. *J Bone Joint Surg* 1989;71B:764-766.

Four cases of posterior dislocation of the shoulder in association with obstetrical brachial plexus palsies are presented.

Gupta RK, Mehta VS, Banerji AK, et al: MR evaluation of brachial plexus injuries. *Neuroradiology* 1989;31:377-381.

MRI was used in ten cases of brachial plexus injuries to identify the level and extent of nerve damage.

Hashimoto T, Mitomo M, Hrabuki N, et al: Nerve root avulsion of birth palsy: Comparison of myelography with CT myelography and somatosensory evoked potential. *Radiology* 1991;178:841-845.

Myelography, CT myelography, and somatosensory evoked potentials were compared in this study of 21 patients with obstetrical palsies.

Jackson ST, Hoffer MM, Parrish N: Brachial plexus palsy in the newborn. *J Bone Joint Surg* 1988;70A:1217-1220.

The incidence of congenital brachial plexus palsies in this group of 21 patients was 2.5 per 1,000 live births. Eighty percent of palsies showed full spontaneous recovery at an average of three months.

Traumatic Brachial Plexus Palsy in Children

Dumontier C, Gilbert A: Traumatic brachial plexus palsy in children. *Ann Hand Surg* 1990;9:351-357.

Twenty-five children with traumatic brachial plexus injuries are reviewed. Associated lesions were noted in 68%. Early surgical intervention is recommended for children who have no evidence of nerve recovery three months following injury.

Gao Z, Yu G, De C, et al: Root avulsion of brachial plexus in infants and children. *Chin Med J* 1990;103:424-427.

Twenty-one patients with traumatic brachial plexus injuries are reported. Simultaneous transfer of the ipsilateral phrenic and intercostal nerve leads to respiratory embarrassment.

Fascioscapulohumeral Muscular Dystrophy

Letournel E, Fardeau M, Lytle JO, et al: Scapulothoracic arthrodesis for patients who have fascioscapulohumeral muscular dystrophy. *J Bone Joint Surg* 1990;72A:78-84.

Nine patients with fascioscapulohumeral muscular dystrophy are reviewed. All were treated with scapulothoracic arthrodesis between the ages of 17 and 36 years. Shoulder abduction and flexion improved significantly. A new surgical technique is presented, which differs from those advanced by Copeland and Ketenjian. Both older techniques are referenced and should be reviewed by any surgeon planning to perform this procedure.

Shoulder Arthrodesis

Mah JY, Hall JE: Arthrodesis of the shoulder in children. *J Bone Joint Surg* 1990;72A:582-586.

Ten children with a shoulder arthrodesis are evaluated from five- to 27-year follow-up. The angle of arthrodesis was 45 degrees of abduction, 25 degrees of flexion, and 25 degrees of internal rotation. All patients were satisfied and none lost abduction postoperatively.

White JI, Hoffer MM, Lehman M: Arthrodesis of the paralytic shoulder. *J Pediatr Orthop* 1989;9:684-686.

Five children with paralytic conditions underwent shoulder arthrodesis. Progressive loss of fused abduction occurred with time. The authors recommend delaying such surgery until skeletal maturity.

Juvenile Rheumatoid Arthritis

Libby AK, Sherry DD, Dudgeon DJ: Shoulder limitation in juvenile rheumatoid arthritis. *Arch Phys Med Rehabil* 1991;72:382-384.

One hundred children with juvenile rheumatoid arthritis of all types are reviewed. Shoulder symptoms were virtually absent in children with pauciarticular onset disease. Polyarticular onset and systemic onset disease led to shoulder pain and decreased range of motion in 50% and 80% of patients, respectively. Internal rotation was the most commonly and severely affected motion.

Multiple Epiphyseal Dysplasia

Ingram RR: The shoulder in multiple epiphyseal dysplasia. *J Bone Joint Surg* 1991;73B:277-279.

One hundred shoulders are assessed in 50 patients with multiple epiphyseal dysplasia. Those that developed symptoms did so as a result of osteoarthritis in middle age. Symptoms were almost always bilateral.

Conditions Requiring Humeral Lengthening

Cattaneo R, Villa A, Catagni MA, et al: Lengthening of the humerus using the Ilizarov technique: Description of the method and report of 43 cases. *Clin Orthop* 1990;250:117-124.

Forty-three humeral lengthenings are reported using the Ilizarov technique. Preoperative diagnoses varied. The humerus was lengthened from 5 to 16 cm over a time period of 4 to 14 months. Functional results are reported as excellent or good. Complications are discussed.

25

Shoulder: Trauma

Proximal Humerus Fractures

Proximal humerus fractures are classified according to the presence or absence of displacement of each of the four major segments: the humeral head, the greater and lesser tuberosities, and the humeral shaft. A segment is considered displaced if it has greater than 1.0-cm displacement of 45-degree angulation. The Neer classification of proximal humerus fractures is the one most commonly used. However, the reliability among different observers has been assessed and was found to vary from 24% to 59%, a relatively low level of agreement. The degree of interobserver agreement was dependent on the observer's level of experience. However, this study used only anteroposterior and lateral radiographs; use of the standard trauma series (Fig. 1) might have improved the level of agreement.

Clinical evaluation should include a thorough neurologic examination because associated injuries to the axillary nerve and brachial plexus are common. It is essential to assess fracture stability and determine whether the fracture segments move as a unit. Radiographic evaluation should include scapular anteroposterior (Fig. 1, *top left*), scapular lateral (Fig. 1, *top right*), and axillary views (Fig. 1, *bottom left*). These radiographs are referred to as the trauma series. The computed tomographic scan has been suggested as an effective method for determining the amount of displacement or rotation of fragments, especially for fractures involving the lesser or greater tuberosities and impression or head splitting fractures. Computed tomography (CT) is helpful in determining the size of humeral head articular surface defects (Fig. 2).

General treatment considerations include the degree of segment displacement, bone quality, the age and functional demands of the patient, arm dominance, preexisting functional deficits, patient expectations, and anticipated compliance. Eighty percent of proximal humerus fractures are minimally displaced and can be treated with protective immobilization and early range of motion based on fracture stability. One study, which compared one week versus three weeks of immobilization, found that the shorter period brought improved results three months after fracture. However, by six months the results in both groups were essentially the same. By 12 months the degree of recovery was complete for both groups.

Displaced proximal humerus fractures generally require restoration of anatomic alignment. This can be accomplished by closed reduction or by open reduction and internal fixation; in some cases, prosthetic replacement is preferred. Methods of internal fixation include use of tension band wires, screws, percutaneous pins, plates, and screw devices; or intramedullary nailing.

The principles of treatment of displaced proximal humerus fractures have not changed significantly. However, additional experience with the use of specific internal fixation devices has been reported. Plate and screw devices, including the AO buttress plate and a modified semitubular plate, were used for three-part fractures and two- and three-part fracture-dislocations; satisfactory results were noted. Significant factors affecting outcome included the presence of adequate bone stock, performance of an acromioplasty to prevent impingement of the plate on the acromion, and the presence of a rotator cuff tear, particularly when optimal repair was not possible.

Two-part lesser tuberosity fractures are usually associated with a posterior glenohumeral dislocation. Small fragments can be treated without surgery; fragments require open reduction and internal fixation. Two-part greater tuberosity fractures displace superiorly or medially and result in a longitudinal rotator cuff tear. They require open reduction and internal fixation using tension band technique or screw fixation and repair of the rotator cuff tear. Two-part fractures involving the anatomic neck are very uncommon and carry a high risk of osteonecrosis. Closed reduction is very difficult; younger patients should have an open reduction and internal fixation and older patients, a hemiarthroplasty. Surgical management of two-part displaced greater tuberosity fractures was successful in a series of 12 patients treated with a specific protocol. Exposure was through a deltoid-splitting approach; the displaced fragment was sutured back to its bed using heavy, nonabsorbable sutures through drill holes in bone, and the longitudinal tear of the rotator cuff was repaired. The importance of a structured, supervised postoperative rehabilitation program was stressed.

Two-part surgical neck fractures are either impacted (stable but malaligned), or completely displaced and unstable. Treatment options include closed reduction, with or without percutaneous pinning, or open reduction and internal fixation. Closed reduction and percutaneous pin fixation of displaced fractures has been used to a limited extent with variable results. Satisfactory results were achieved using this technique in a large series of elderly patients with two-part surgical neck fractures. An acceptable reduction (less than 20-degrees angulation, 3-mm displacement, and 5-mm impaction) was achieved in all cases. The protocol included two to three weeks of im-

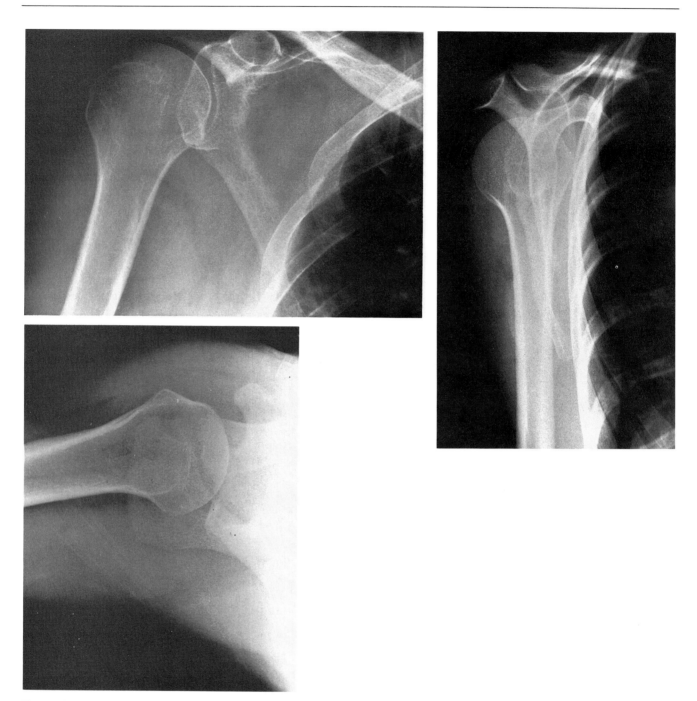

Fig. 1 Standard trauma series. **Top left**, Scapular anteroposterior radiograph. **Top right**, Scapular lateral (Y view) radiograph. **Bottom left**, Axillary radiograph.

mobilization after insertion, with pin removal six to seven weeks after insertion. The most common complications were upper extremity edema (17%) and pin site drainage (14%). However, less satisfactory results were reported in a smaller series that included three- and four-part fractures. Unsatisfactory outcomes occurred in patients older than 50 years of age and in those with an inadequate reduction. Because migration of smooth pins was also a significant problem, the recommendation was made that only threaded pins be used. Nonunion most often follows two-part surgical neck fractures. Various treatment approaches are available, including open reduction and internal fixation and proximal humeral replacement. In one series, open reduction and internal

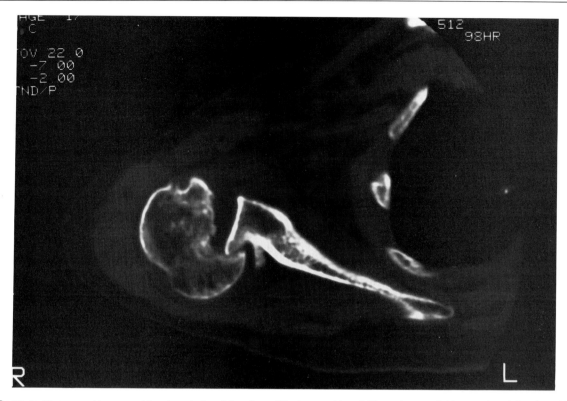

Fig. 2 Computed tomographic scan of fixed posterior dislocation of the humeral head. The anteromedial impression defect is evident.

fixation with a T-plate and tension band wire gave better results than use of intramedullary devices or proximal humeral replacement. Use of the tension band wire that fixed the rotator cuff and proximal humerus to the plate/shaft construct was stressed as an important method of enhancing fixation.

Three-part fractures (Fig. 3) usually require open reduction; closed reduction is difficult to obtain and maintain. Different techniques of internal fixation are available. A tension band wiring technique is often preferred because the rotator cuff can be used to enhance the security of fixation. Hemiarthroplasty with tuberosity/rotator cuff reconstruction may be indicated in elderly patients with severely osteoporotic or comminuted fractures.

In four-part fractures, the articular segment is devoid of soft-tissue attachment and has a high risk of osteonecrosis. Young patients or those with good bone quality can be considered for open reduction and internal fixation; however, in general, hemiarthroplasty is preferred. The technique of hemiarthroplasty must include meticulous reattachment of the tuberosities to the prosthesis and humeral shaft and repair of the rotator interval. In a specific type of displaced four-part fracture of the proximal humerus consisting of a valgus impaction of the humeral head with displacement of the tuberosities, the impaction of the articular segment (as opposed to wide displacement evident in the classic four-part pattern) re-

sults in a rate of osteonecrosis lower than that seen in other displaced four-part fractures. For a series of 19 fractures, all of which were treated by closed or open reduction and minimal internal fixation, 74% satisfactory results and an osteonecrosis rate of 26% were reported.

Fracture-dislocations are higher energy injuries. Proper radiographic evaluation is essential; posterior fracture-dislocations are often missed initially as a result of an inadequate radiographic assessment (Figs. 4-6). Two-part fracture-dislocations can be treated by closed reduction of the dislocation and internal fixation of displaced segments. Three-part fracture-dislocations require open reduction and internal fixation or prosthetic replacement as discussed. Four-part fracture-dislocations are best treated by hemiarthroplasty with tuberosity/rotator cuff reconstruction; in young patients with good quality bone, open reduction and internal fixation can be considered. Chronic fracture-dislocations are uncommon but difficult problems. Surgical treatment is indicated after careful patient selection and proper preoperative planning directed at accurate assessment of deformity/tuberosity position.

External fixation has been used for the treatment of a variety of displaced fractures and fracture-dislocations. Although the results have been generally satisfactory, specific indications for the use of external fixation have not been defined except in patients with significant asso-

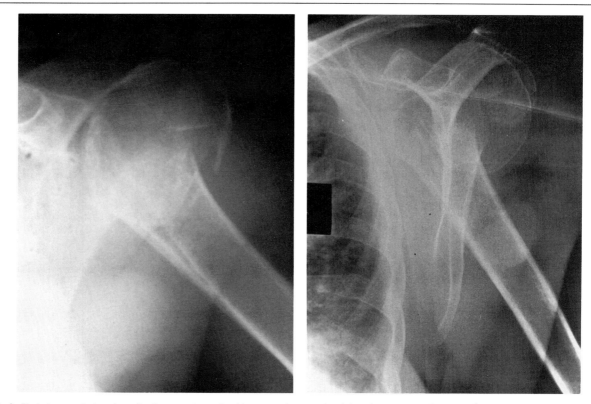

Fig. 3   **Left**, Anteroposterior view of a three-part proximal humerus fracture involving the greater tuberosity. **Right**, Scapular Y view.

ciated soft-tissue injury. In most of the series reported, external fixation was used for fractures that could have been treated by a variety of other methods. In a prospective randomized series comparing closed reduction with external fixation, the external fixation group had significantly better results, as indicated by achievement of a more anatomic reduction and improved functional results. However, the authors did caution about the problems of pin-tract infection, poor fixation of the pins in osteoporotic bone, and the need for patient compliance.

Head-splitting fractures are often associated with other injuries. It is essential to identify the degree of articular surface injury. Large fragments in young patients should be reduced and stabilized; comminuted fractures and fractures occurring in osteoporotic bone generally require hemiarthroplasty. Articular impression fractures of the humeral head are associated with chronic dislocations (Figs. 4-6). Treatment is based on the percentage of articular surface involvement and the duration of dislocation. In general, closed reduction can be considered in dislocations of less than six weeks' duration; after six weeks, open reduction is necessary. Articular surface defects of less than 20% will be stable following a period of immobilization; defects of 20% to 40% will usually require a subscapularis (posterior dislocations) or infraspinatus (anterior dislocations) transfer; defects of greater than 40% or with significant degenerative changes require hemiarthroplasty.

Complications following proximal humerus fractures include loss of motion, nonunion, malunion, and osteonecrosis. The degree of motion loss depends on the severity of injury, fracture pattern, length of immobilization, fracture reduction, and status of the rotator cuff. Nonunion most commonly occurs after two-part surgical neck fractures and may be related to soft-tissue interposition (deltoid, long head of triceps) or inadequate immobilization. Other factors associated with nonunion include the severity of the initial trauma, degree of displacement, distraction of the fragments, alcoholism, diabetes mellitus, or inadequate primary internal fixation. Surgery should be avoided when there is absence of function of the anterior deltoid. Malunion may be related either to inadequate initial reduction or to loss of reduction. Osteonecrosis is most common after four-part fractures and fracture-dislocations.

Fractures of the Clavicle

Fractures of the clavicle result from direct trauma or a fall onto an outstretched hand. Less than 3% of clavicle fractures have associated injuries. Clavicle fractures are classified by location into medial-third (6%), middle-third (82%), and lateral-third (12%) fractures. Only 6% of a large series of middle-third fractures could be attributed to a fall on the outstretched hand; 94% resulted

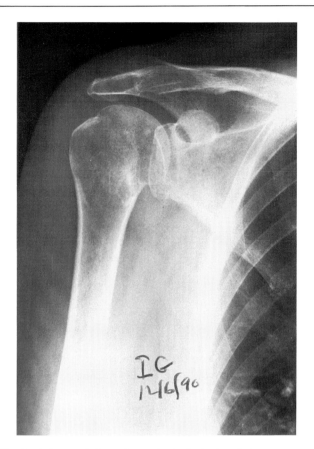

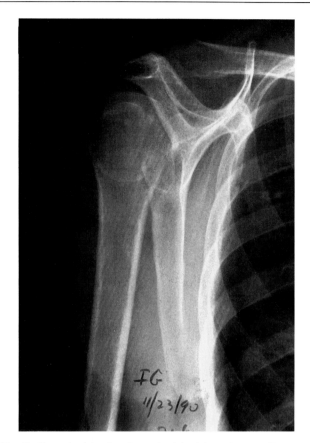

Fig. 4 Anteroposterior radiograph of a locked posterior dislocation in a 65-year-old woman. This dislocation was identified three months following a motor vehicle injury.

Fig. 5 Scapular lateral radiograph of the injury shown in Figure 4.

from a direct blow to the shoulder. Displaced middle-third fractures have a classic pattern in which the medial fragment is displaced upward by the sternocleidomastoid and trapezius muscles and the lateral fragment is displaced downward and medially by the weight of the arm and the pectoralis major, respectively. The attached ligaments may cause up to 40% rotation between two fragments. Lateral-third fractures are further classified according to the functional status of the coracoclavicular ligaments. Type I distal clavicle fractures are minimally displaced, and the coracoclavicular ligaments are functionally attached to the medial fragment. Type II fractures are displaced and the coracoclavicular ligaments are functionally detached from the medial fragment. Type III fractures involve the articular surface of the lateral clavicle.

Radiographic evaluation should include anteroposterior and 15-degree cephalic tilt radiographs to evaluate superoinferior and anteroposterior displacement, respectively. Weighted views may be helpful in lateral-third fractures to evaluate the status of the coracoclavicular ligaments. Computed tomographic scanning is useful in

the assessment of medial-third and lateral-third fractures involving the articular surface.

Treatment is dependent on fracture location, displacement, and associated injuries. The vast majority of middle-third fractures are treated nonsurgically, with either a figure-eight bandage or an arm sling. In a study comparing figure-eight and sling immobilization, no differences were found in the speed of recovery. Regardless of the type of immobilization, shortening and residual deformity result; however, an improperly positioned figure-eight might increase the deformity. In most cases this is painless and does not interfere with shoulder function. Indications for surgery for middle-third fractures include open fractures, displaced fractures with potential compromise of the overlying skin, and fractures with associated neurovascular injury. Internal fixation usually consists of either intramedullary devices or plate and screws. Bone grafting should be considered for comminuted fractures. One recent series described the use of external fixation in 20 cases of acute fracture and nonunion. All fractures and nonunions united and complications related to the pins were minimal, but the indications and advantages of this technique over more standard techniques remain unclear.

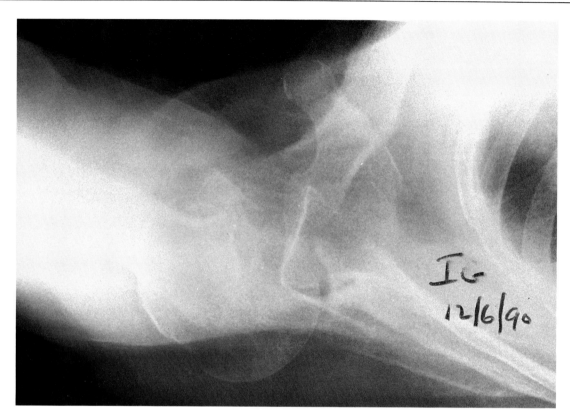

Fig. 6 Axillary radiograph of injury shown in Figures 4 and 5 showing the humeral head locked on the posterior portion of the glenoid with a moderate-sized articular impression defect present.

Types I and III lateral-third fractures are generally treated with sling support and early range of motion. The treatment of type II fractures is controversial. Because these fractures are associated with an increased incidence of nonunion, some authors advocate primary open reduction with either intramedullary or coracoclavicular stabilization. Displaced type II lateral clavicle fractures have generally been considered an indication for surgical management because of an increased risk of nonunion. In one series of 19 patients treated surgically, 17% had unsatisfactory results. Transacromial Kirschner wire fixation gave the poorest results: 46% nonunion, 38% infection. Based on these results, the authors recommended initial nonsurgical management unless the skin is at risk, and late reconstruction if significant disability is present.

Complications following clavicle fracture are uncommon and include nonunion, malunion, neurovascular compromise, and posttraumatic arthritis. Nonunion is probably more common than is generally appreciated. Predisposing factors for nonunion are inadequate immobilization, fracture location (lateral third), severity of trauma, soft-tissue interposition, refracture, and primary open reduction and internal fixation.

Malunion is common, though rarely symptomatic. Angulatory deformities are primarily a cosmetic problem, but significant shortening may lead to muscular dysfunction. Neurovascular complications may be acute secondary to fracture displacement, or delayed secondary to compromise by exuberant fracture callus or mobile nonunion. Posttraumatic arthritis can result from intra-articular fractures of either end of the clavicle.

Hypertrophic callus formation can result in neurovascular compromise by encroachment into the space between the first rib and clavicle. This usually required resection of the prominent callus. Nonunions are also uncommon and can be a cause of pain, dysfunction, or neurovascular compromise, although they may be asymptomatic. A series of 50 midshaft clavicle nonunions were reported, in which 16 were treated without surgery because the patients had minimal symptoms or general health that precluded surgery. Of the 34 patients treated surgically, 23 underwent intramedullary fixation with a modified Hagie pin combined with autogenous bone grafting. This technique resulted in healing in 95% of cases. Another series of 15 nonunions reported thoracic outlet symptoms or brachial plexus impingement in seven patients (four of whom had subclavian vessel compression). Treatment recommendations included intramedullary fixation for hypertrophic nonunion and plate and screw fixation with bone grafting for atrophic nonunions. The authors specifically stressed the importance of restoring clavicular length (with tricortical graft) in non-unions that result from midclavicle resections for subclavian vessel exposure.

Fractures of the Scapula

Fractures of the scapula are usually the result of high energy trauma. It is not surprising that 80% to 90% of scapula fractures have associated injuries. These injuries most commonly involve the thorax, ribs, or clavicle. Brachial plexus and vascular injuries are much less common. These associated injuries can be life-threatening, and their evaluation and treatment should take precedence over the scapula fracture. A fracture of the scapula with an associated underlying first rib fracture is particularly serious because of the potential for associated pulmonary and neurovascular injury.

In a series of 148 scapular fractures, 96% of patients had associated injuries. Rib fractures were the most common, followed by pulmonary injuries (hemopneumothorax, pulmonary contusion), head injury, ipsilateral clavicle fractures, and spinal cord injury. This study also reported on a follow-up group of 24 patients and found that significant disability was present following displaced scapular spine and neck fractures. The authors concluded that in addition to displaced intra-articular fracture, indications for surgical management should be extended to include some types of displaced scapular neck and spine fractures. However, these conclusions were based on a relatively small number of fractures. Additional studies will be necessary to determine specific indications or guidelines for surgical management of these fractures.

The combination of subtle clinical findings and the severity of the associated injuries often leads to delayed diagnosis of the scapula fracture. Radiographic evaluation should include a chest radiograph, scapula anteroposterior, scapular Y, and axillary view. A 45-degree cephalic tilt is useful for the evaluation of coracoid fractures; computed tomographic scanning can provide additional information and is particularly helpful in the evaluation of intra-articular glenoid fractures.

Scapula fractures are classified anatomically as either body, neck, glenoid, acromion, spine, or coracoid fractures. These fractures often represent a combination of these specific patterns. Glenoid fractures have been further classified based on the location and direction of the fracture line(s).

The treatment for the vast majority of scapula fractures is nonsurgical, consisting of ice, support with a sling, and early range of motion. Surgery is indicated only for (1) intra-articular glenoid fractures with subluxation and instability of the humeral head; (2) depressed acromion fractures that encroach on the subacromial space and interfere with rotator cuff function; (3) coracoid fractures with an associated acromioclavicular separation resulting in compromise of the overlying skin; and

(4) scapular neck fractures with severe angulation of the glenoid articular surface that predisposes to glenohumeral instability.

Complications related to scapula fracture include suprascapular nerve injury, nonunion, and malunion. Suprascapular nerve injury is associated with fractures of the coracoid and scapula body that involve the suprascapular notch. Nonunion is rare, because of the scapula's abundant soft-tissue cover and vascular supply. Malunion is rarely symptomatic.

Scapulothoracic Dissociation

Scapulothoracic dissociation is a rare, often fatal closed injury manifested by lateral displacement of the scapula with associated neurovascular injury and either acromioclavicular or sternoclavicular separation, or clavicle fracture. The mechanism of injury is a violent force applied to the anterolateral portion of the shoulder. The associated brachial plexus injury is usually complete; the vascular injury commonly occurs at the level of the subclavian vessels and can result in a pulseless extremity.

The possibility of scapulothoracic dissociation should be considered in any patient who has sustained massive trauma to the upper extremity associated with a neurovascular deficit. Diagnosis is made on an anteroposterior chest radiograph by comparing the locations of the two scapulae; the involved scapula is significantly displaced laterally. Immediate evaluation of the ipsilateral vascular structures by angiography is mandatory to avoid fatal internal hemorrhage.

After the level of vascular injury is determined, surgical exploration of the appropriate vessel is indicated to restore vascularity to the ischemic limb. Careful neurologic examination is necessary to assess the level and degree of injury. Complete brachial plexus injuries with root avulsions result in a flail limb with no potential for neurologic recovery; these injuries are probably best treated with a shoulder arthrodesis and above- or below-elbow amputation. Patients with partial root avulsions or postganglionic lesions may be candidates for exploratory surgery and nerve repair or grafting.

Humeral Shaft Fractures

Humeral shaft fractures are common injuries that usually result from a direct blow or a fall on the outstretched arm. Recently, a series of five fractures were reported that occurred during arm wrestling, probably as a result of the significant torsional and bending stresses. They occurred in young, healthy patients with nonpathologic bone.

Successful nonsurgical management of the vast majority of humeral shaft fractures continues to be supported by the literature. The more frequently used techniques include the hanging arm cast, coaptation splints, Velpeau immobilization, and functional bracing. The hanging cast requires patient cooperation and care must be taken to avoid distraction, especially with transverse or short oblique patterns. Functional braces are usually applied after initial splinting, usually within seven to ten days of injury; studies have demonstrated a high rate of union, early restoration of joint mobility, and minimal complications associated with functional bracing.

A prefabricated standardized humeral fracture brace was used in a series of 170 patients that included 43 open fractures. A 98% union rate was achieved in an average of 10.6 weeks (9.5 weeks for closed fractures; 13.6 for open fractures). A 96% union rate was reported in another series of 85 patients with distal shaft fractures using a similar brace.

Indications for surgical management of acute humeral shaft fractures include open fractures, unacceptable reduction after attempted closed reduction, segmental fractures, floating elbows, polytrauma, bilateral humeral fractures, vascular injury, intra-articular fracture extension, pathologic fracture, and radial nerve palsy following closed reduction. The specific problem of humeral shaft fractures in patients with ipsilateral brachial plexus injuries was studied in 21 patients. Nonsurgical management resulted in a 64% incidence of delayed union and nonunion, compared with 40% for the surgical group. The best results were obtained following compression plating. Primary surgical management is recommended to avoid healing complications and enhance rehabilitation.

The intramedullary fixation of humeral shaft fractures with Ender nails or Rush rods have been reported. More recently, locked nailing has been used and preliminary results have been reported. Nail insertion generally follows reaming and the nail can be inserted either antegrade or retrograde, using different types of locking mechanisms. Although the results have been satisfactory, the experience is limited. More experience will be necessary to determine the advantages these devices have over those used previously and the specific indications for use.

External fixation of humeral shaft fractures has an important place in the management of severe upper extremity injuries with extensive soft-tissue damage. Two studies have documented the difficulty of obtaining satisfactory results in these complex injuries. Specific protocols that include immediate external fixation, meticulous open wound management, delayed bone grafting, and, if necessary, late internal fixation (for delayed unions) have been most effective.

Up to 18% of humeral shaft fractures have an associated radial nerve palsy. It occurs most commonly with middle-third humeral fractures, although the Holstein-Lewis fracture (oblique, distal-third) is best known for its association with this neurologic injury. Most nerve injuries represent a neuropraxia or axonotmesis; 90% will resolve in three to four months. The primary indications for early nerve exploration are a radial nerve palsy associated with an open fracture or one that develops after closed reduction.

The management of radial nerve palsy in association with humeral shaft fractures continues to be an area of controversy. One study reported on 42 cases treated either without surgery or by early or late surgical exploration. Of the 14 cases treated nonsurgically, 86% recovered fully. All 18 cases treated by early exploration (within 30 days) recovered; however, only 33% were found to have a lesion that obviously required surgery (ie, nerve caught in the fracture site or nerve lacerated). In comparison, all ten of the late explorations (after four months) were found to have a lesion that required surgical correction (ie, compression, disruption) but functional recovery was noted in only 50%. The decision of early versus late exploratory surgery should be based upon four criteria: fracture site, degree of displacement, extent of exposure (open fractures), and degree of neurologic deficit.

Another study reported 37 cases of radial nerve palsy treated by late surgical exploration. Most radial nerve injuries occurred in association with middle-third fractures. Overall, there were 73% good or excellent results. Surgical exploration three or four months after injury was recommended for the following reasons: (1) enough time had passed for recovery from neuropraxia or axonotmesis; (2) precise evaluation of the nerve lesion is possible; (3) the associated fracture can be expected to be healed; and (4) secondary repair can be expected to be as efficacious as primary repair. Passive range of motion exercises and dynamic splinting should be performed. Monitoring for return of nerve function should include clinical and electrodiagnostic testing. If there has been no function recovery after three months, late exploratory surgery should be considered.

The nonunion rate following humeral shaft fractures ranges from zero to 15%. Factors associated with nonunion include transverse fracture, fracture distraction, soft-tissue interposition, and primary open reduction and internal fixation. Vascular injuries are uncommon and are associated primarily with open injuries.

Nonunions of humeral shaft fractures have been treated by a variety of techniques. However, compression plating combined with cancellous bone grafting has been the most effective. Two series of 32 and 25 cases of nonunion reported healing in 97% and 96%, respectively. Both series used protocols that included excision of all nonunion tissue, compression plating with a broad dynamic compression plate, and autogenous cancellous bone grafting. The Ilizarov method has also been used successfully in a small number of cases. The complex atrophic, synovial pseudarthrosis that has had multiple previous attempts at gaining union has been successfully treated using a medial approach for insertion of a vascularized fibula, anterior plating, and cancellous autogenous grafting.

Radiography

Different studies have investigated the specific radiographic views that are most helpful in the evaluation of acute shoulder injuries. Specifically, the apical oblique projection was compared to the transscapular and transthoracic views in two separate studies. One study found that 111 of 112 injuries could be identified with a trauma series consisting of the anteroposterior and apical oblique views; the transthoracic view was recommended only when the initial views indicated the presence of a proximal humerus or humeral shaft fracture. In another study, the apical oblique was compared to the transscapular (scapular Y) view in a series of 80 patients with acute shoulder injuries. The apical oblique was found by both orthopaedic surgeons and radiologists to permit more accurate diagnosis of fractures and dislocations. At present the standard trauma series usually consists of three views: anteroposterior, transscapular, and axillary (Fig. 1). The apical oblique is not routinely used. Additional study will be necessary to determine if the apical oblique should replace any of the views currently included in the trauma series.

Annotated Bibliography

Proximal Humerus

Cofield RH: Comminuted fractures of the proximal humerus. *Clin Orthop* 1988;230:49-57.

This review article addresses important aspects of the evaluation and management of comminuted fractures of the proximal humerus. A review of the relevant literature is also included.

Flatow EL, Cuomo F, Maday MG, et al: Open reduction and internal fixation of two-part displaced fractures of the greater tuberosity of the proximal part of the humerus. *J Bone Joint Surg* 1991;73A:1213-1218.

A series of 12 two-part greater tuberosity fractures were treated surgically by open reduction and internal fixation using heavy nonabsorbable sutures and careful repair of the rotator cuff. All fractures healed. Initiation of early passive range of motion resulted in good or excellent results in all patients.

Healy W, Jupiter J, Kristiansen T, et al: Nonunion of the proximal humerus. *J Orthop Trauma* 1990;4:424-431.

In this series of 25 nonunions, 11 patients underwent surgical management because of significant pain and disability. The best results were obtained after open reduction with internal fixation and bone grafting using a tension band construction that fixed the rotator cuff.

Jakob RP, Miniaci A, Anson PS, et al: Four-part valgus impacted fractures of the proximal humerus. *J Bone Joint Surg* 1991;73B:295-298.

The authors describe a specific type of displaced four-part fracture of the proximal humerus that consists of valgus impaction of the articular segment with outward displacement of the tuberosities. They recommend either closed reduction or limited open reduction and minimal internal fixation. In their series of 19 fractures, satisfactory results were achieved in 74%. The incidence of osteonecrosis was much lower than would be expected for "classic" four-part fracture patterns.

Jupiter JB: Complex non-union of the humeral diaphysis: Treatment with a medial approach, an anterior plate, and a vascularized fibular graft. *J Bone Joint Surg* 1990;72A:701-707.

The specific problem of an atrophic nonunion of the humeral diaphysis that has been recalcitrant to previous surgical attempts at achieving union was treated by a medial surgical approach, anterior plating, vascularized fibular bone graft, and autogenous cancellous bone grafting. Union was achieved in all four patients reported.

Kilcoyne RF, Shuman WP, Matsen FA III, et al: The Neer classification of displaced proximal humeral fractures: Spectrum of findings on plain radiographs and CT scans. *AJR* 1990;154:1029-1033.

Computed tomographic scans can be an important adjunct to plain radiographs in the evaluation of proximal humerus fractures. Determination of the degree of displacement or rotation of fragments and assessment of impression or head-splitting humeral head fractures can often be more easily evaluated.

Kowalkowski A, Wallace WA: Closed percutaneous K-wire stabilization for displaced fractures of the surgical neck of the humerus. *Injury* 1990;2:209-212.

This technique was used in a series of 22 displaced fractures. Significant problems were encountered, including difficulties obtaining an adequate reduction and migration of smooth Kirschner wires. Unsatisfactory results were much more common in the older age group (older than age 50 years) than in younger patients (82% versus zero).

Kristiansen B: Treatment of displaced fractures of the proximal humerus: Transcutaneous reduction and Hoffman's external fixation. *Injury* 1989;20:195-199.

Transcutaneous reduction combined with external fixation was used to treat a variety of two-, three-, and four-part proximal humerus fractures. The most satisfactory results were associated with obtaining a satisfactory reduction. Pin loosening was a problem and was most common in cases with severe osteoporosis, head-splitting fractures, or when reduction was unsatisfactory.

Kristiansen B, Angermann P, Larsen TK: Functional results following fractures of the proximal humerus: A controlled clinical study comparing two periods of immobilization. *Arch Orthop Trauma Surg* 1989;108:339-341.

This prospective, randomized study of proximal humerus fractures (approximately 80% minimally displaced) compared one and three weeks of sling immobilization before initiation of a physiotherapy program. Shorter duration of immobilization resulted in better functional results during the first three months. After six months, the results in both groups were essentially the same.

Kristiansen B, Kofoed H: Transcutaneous reduction and external fixation of displaced fractures of the proximal humerus: A controlled clinical trial. *J Bone Joint Surg* 1988;70B:821-824.

This prospective, randomized study compared closed reduction with transcutaneous reduction and external fixation in a series of 30 patients with a variety of displaced proximal humerus fractures. The external fixation method provided a better reduction, safer healing, and superior function than did the closed reduction approach.

Moda SK, Chadha NS, Sangwan SS, et al: Open reduction and fixation of proximal humeral fractures and fracture-dislocations. *J Bone Joint Surg* 1990;72B:1050-1052.

Satisfactory results were obtained in 21 of 25 fractures and fracture-dislocations treated by open reduction and insertion of either a T-plate or semitubular plate modified to a blade plate. Unsatisfactory results were associated with associated rotator cuff injury.

Savoie FH, Geissler WB, Van der Griend RA: Open reduction and internal fixation of three-part fractures of the proximal humerus. *Orthopaedics* 1989;12:65-70.

Open reduction and internal fixation with plate and screw devices gave satisfactory results in this series of 11 patients. Patients who underwent acromioplasty at the time of the initial surgery had slightly better function and range of motion than did the remaining patients.

Smith DK, Cooney WP: External fixation of high-energy upper extremity injuries. *J Orthop Trauma* 1990;4:7-18.

This series of 40 patients with complex open injuries of the upper extremity stressed the importance of immediate external fixation, management of open wounds, delayed bone grafting, and late internal fixation when necessary. Good or excellent results were obtained in 73%.

Clavicle

Boehme D, Curtis RJ Jr, DeHaan JT, et al: Non-unions of fractures of the mid-shaft of the clavicle: Treatment with a modified Hagie intramedullary pin and autogenous bone-grafting. *J Bone Joint Surg* 1991;73A:1219-1226.

In a series of 50 patients with a nonunion of a fracture of the clavicle, 16 were treated nonsurgically and 34 required surgical management. The authors describe their preferred approach using a modified Hagie intramedullary pin and autogenous bone grafting, which was successful in achieving union in 20 of 21 patients.

Connolly JF, Dehne R: Nonunion of the clavicle and thoracic outlet syndrome. *J Trauma* 1989;29:1127-1133.

In this series of 15 clavicular nonunions, symptoms consistent with thoracic outlet were identified in seven. This was most commonly found in association with hypertrophic nonunions that narrowed the costoclavicular space.

Kona J, Bosse MJ, Staeheli JW, et al: Type II distal clavicle fractures: A retrospective review of surgical treatment. *J Orthop Trauma* 1990;4:115-120.

The authors reported satisfactory results in only ten of 19 patients treated surgically. Transacromial Kirschner wire fixation was associated with the highest incidence of complications. They recommend nonsurgical management as the treatment of choice except in cases where the skin is at risk; and late reconstruction if significant symptoms persist.

Post M: Current concepts in the treatment of fractures of the clavicle. *Clin Orthop* 1989;245:89-101.

This review article addresses the important aspects of the evaluation and management of clavicle fractures. Nonsurgical and surgical management of lateral-, middle-, and medial-third fractures in adults and children are discussed.

Schuind F, Pay-pay E, Andrianne Y, et al: External fixation of the clavicle for fracture or non-union in adults. *J Bone Joint Surg* 1988;70A:692-695.

The authors utilized external fixation to treat a variety of clavicle fractures including open fractures, impending skin compromise, multiple trauma, delayed unions, and nonunions. The external fixation device remained in place an average of 51 days. Union was achieved in all 20 patients.

Stanley D, Norris S: Recovery following fractures of the clavicle treated conservatively. *Injury* 1988;19:162-164.

This study compared treatment of clavicle fractures with either a figure-eight bandage or a standard arm sling and found no significant difference in the speed of recovery.

Stanley D, Trowbridge EA, Norris SH: The mechanism of clavicular fracture: A clinical and biomechanical analysis. *J Bone Joint Surg* 1988;70B:461-464.

The mechanism of injury was carefully studied in a large series of clavicle fractures. Only 6% resulted from an indirect mechanism (fall on the outstretched arm) while 94% resulted from a direct mechanism (blow to the shoulder).

Scapula

Ada JR, Miller ME: Scapular fractures: Analysis of 113 cases. *Clin Orthop* 1991;269:174-180.

This series of 113 cases with follow-up on a smaller group of 24 patients identified significant long-term disability associated with displaced fractures of the scapular spine and neck. The authors concluded that the indications for surgical management of scapular fractures should be expanded to include these fracture patterns.

Scapulothoracic Dissociation

Ebraheim NA, An HS, Jackson WT, et al: Scapulothoracic dissociation. *J Bone Joint Surg* 1988;70A:428-432.

A series of 15 patients with scapulothoracic dissociation documents the devastating nature of this injury. All patients had a flail upper extremity secondary to complete brachial plexus injuries.

Humeral Shaft

Barquet A, Fernandez A, Luvizio J, et al: A combined therapeutic protocol for aseptic nonunion of the humeral shaft: A report of 25 cases. *J Trauma* 1989;29:95-98.

The authors used a standard treatment protocol—decortication, internal fixation with a broad, straight dynamic compression plate, and autogenous cancellous bone grafting—to achieve union in 24 of 25 cases of aseptic nonunion of the humeral shaft.

Brien WW, Gellman H, Becker V, et al: Management of fractures of the humerus in patients who have an injury of the ipsilateral brachial plexus. *J Bone Joint Surg* 1990;72A:1208-1210.

Surgical management of humeral shaft fractures in patients with ipsilateral brachial plexus injury resulted in a higher rate of union and improved rehabilitation than nonsurgical management. Compression plating was superior to intramedullary fixation.

Chiu K, Pun W, Chow S: Humeral shaft fracture and arm wrestling. *J R Coll Surg Edinb* 1990;35:264-265.

A series of five cases are reported in which spiral, displaced humeral shaft fractures resulted from arm wrestling.

Postacchini F, Morace G: Fractures of the humerus associated with paralysis of the radial nerve. *Ital J Orthop Traumatol* 1988;14:455-464.

The results of nonsurgical and surgical management of radial nerve injuries associated with humeral shaft fractures was reported in a series of 42 cases. The authors concluded that the choice of treatment (nonsurgical versus surgical) should be based on careful assessment of each individual case, particularly with respect to the location of the fracture, degree of displacement, associated soft-tissue injury, and the degree of neurologic deficit.

Rosen H: The treatment of nonunions and pseudarthrosis of the humeral shaft. *Orthop Clin North Am* 1990;21:725-742.

This article reviews the principles of the evaluation and management of nonunions of humeral shaft fractures. The author also reports personal experience with 32 nonunions in which healing was obtained after one surgical procedure in 31 cases (97%).

Sarmiento A, Horowitch A, Aboulafia A, et al: Functional bracing for comminuted extra-articular fractures of the distal third of the humerus. *J Bone Joint Surg* 1990;72B:283-287.

In this series of 85 extra-articular comminuted distal-third humerus fractures, 96% union was achieved using a prefabricated plastic orthosis. At union, varus deformity averaged 9 degrees in 81% of the patients, but this did not appear to affect functional outcomes.

Zagorski JB, Latta LL, Zych GA, et al: Diaphyseal fractures of the humerus: Treatment with prefabricated braces. *J Bone Joint Surg* 1988;70A:607-610.

The authors report a large series in which humeral shaft fractures were treated with a prefabricated fracture brace. Union was achieved in 98% of cases with an average time to union of 10.6 weeks. Good or excellent functional outcomes were obtained in 98%.

Radiography

Brems-Dalgaard E, Davidsen E, Sloth C: Radiographic examination of the acute shoulder. *Eur J Radiol* 1990;11:10-14.

This study compared two lateral radiographs of the shoulder—transthoracic and apical oblique—to determine which projection, when used in combination with an anteroposterior view, provided more diagnostic information. They found that the apical oblique and anteroposterior views were the most effective combination. The transthoracic view was helpful only when a humerus fracture was present.

Richardson JB, Ramsay A, Davidson JK, et al: Radiographs in shoulder trauma. *J Bone Joint Surg* 1988;70B:457-460.

This study compared two lateral radiographs of the shoulder—Neer transscapular (Y view) and apical oblique—with respect to the ability to establish a diagnosis following a shoulder injury. Both views were combined with an anteroposterior view. The apical oblique view permitted a more accurate diagnosis of fractures and dislocation by all examiners.

26

Shoulder: Instability

In order to properly treat shoulder instability, the type of instability must be known. A classification of shoulder instability is presented in Outline 1. Before commencing surgery, it is of critical importance to determine the direction, degree, and volition of the instability.

Examination and Radiologic Evaluation

Careful examination of the patient with shoulder instability will usually determine the direction and degree of instability. The apprehension and sulcus signs are very useful. The apprehension sign is manifested by guarding and apprehension when the arm is placed and stressed in a provocative position. The provocative position for anterior instability is one of abduction and external rotation. The provocative position for posterior instability is in adduction, flexion, and internal rotation. The sulcus sign—a gap between the humeral head and undersurface of the acromion—appears when longitudinal traction is placed on the humeral shaft with the arm at the side while in a seated position. The sulcus sign is felt to be pathognomonic of multidirectional instability.

For acute dislocations, a trauma series (see Shoulder: Trauma), including true anteroposterior, axillary lateral, and Y-lateral views, is mandatory to determine the presence and direction of a dislocation. Chronic missed dislocations are usually the result of a failure to obtain such a series at the time of the initial injury.

A Bankart lesion can be defined as an avulsion of the anteroinferior glenoid labrum at its attachment to the inferior glenohumeral ligament complex. This is rarely seen on plain radiographs, but recent studies have demonstrated that the lesion is usually well visualized on double contrast computed tomographic arthrography.

Magnetic resonance imaging is currently being explored as a means of imaging shoulder problems. However, to date, its primary use has been in evaluating the rotator cuff. Large-scale studies of imaging the glenoid labrum in suspected instability have been done but the results are preliminary.

In cases where examination is difficult without anesthesia because of patient apprehension, examination of the shoulder under anesthesia is used to evaluate and determine the precise directions of instability.

Diagnostic arthroscopy is now used more frequently to determine the etiology of shoulder problems. Arthroscopic examination begins with an examination under anesthesia and possible fluoroscopic confirmation of the findings. The arthroscopy itself is useful in determining

Outline 1. Classification of Shoulder Instability

I. Frequency
   a. Acute
   b. Recurrent
   c. Fixed
II. Direction
   a. Anterior
   b. Posterior
   c. Multidirectional
III. Onset
   a. Traumatic
   b. Atraumatic
   c. Overuse
IV. Volition
   a. Voluntary
   b. Involuntary
V. Degree
   a. Dislocation
   b. Subluxation

(Adapted with permission from Hawkins RJ, Mohtadi NGH: Clinical evaluation of shoulder instability. *Clin J Sports Med* 1991;1:59-64.)

directions of instability by examining the integrity of the anteroinferior and posteroinferior margins of the glenoid labrum. Tears seen at arthroscopy will increase the clinician's suspicion that the shoulder problem is one of instability in the direction of the labral tear.

Anterior Instability

Anterior instability is by far the most common instability seen. The most important determining factor in whether a patient with an acute dislocation will have recurrent dislocations is the patient's age. Older studies showed that a primary dislocation in a 20-year-old carried a 90% chance of becoming a recurrent problem. More recent studies have supported the age hypothesis, but the chance of recurrence in the highest risk group (15-25) is now felt to be in the range of 50% to 70%.

Other factors important in prognosis are the presence of an associated fracture and the degree of trauma required to cause the initial dislocation. Patients who sustain a fracture at the time of their initial dislocation (usually of the greater tuberosity) have a relatively low rate of recurrence. Severe trauma causing the dislocation is also associated with lower rates of recurrence.

Treatment of a primary dislocation usually involves a period of immobilization, rehabilitation of the muscles around the shoulder girdle, and restriction from sports activities. The length of immobilization has varied in different studies, but it has never been shown that immobilization for a fixed length of time will decrease the chance of a patient becoming a recurrent dislocator.

The use of exercise and rehabilitation to prevent recurrence is also controversial. A study at the U.S. Naval Academy was relatively successful; 15 of 20 midshipmen followed for three years did not have a recurrence. However, the patients were required to have a very high compliance with the program and the follow-up should be considered short for this problem.

Repairs for recurrent anterior instability now favor attempting to fix the anatomic lesion responsible for the problem. This is usually felt to be a Bankart lesion. The Bankart repair, which repairs the defect in the anterior glenoid labrum and reattaches the inferior glenohumeral ligaments, is currently favored by most shoulder surgeons. The most common complication after all methods of repair has been loss of motion, with loss of external rotation being an almost universal complication of the procedures.

A recent study has shown the need to be very careful when placing any hardware about the shoulder joint. Repairs for anterior instability that place hardware within the shoulder capsule should be carefully considered, because high rates of complications are associated with such procedures.

Current research into the problem of recurrent anterior instability has focused on: (1) improving our understanding of the exact anatomy and biomechanics of the glenohumeral joint, (2) decreasing the incidence of recurrence after a primary dislocation, (3) defining the exact cause ("the essential lesion") of recurrent anterior instability, (4) attempting arthroscopic reconstruction of recurrent instability, and (5) finding the "best" method of reconstructing the shoulder with recurrent anterior instability.

In a recent, more precise definition of the anatomy of the inferior glenohumeral ligament, it was shown that the ligament should be considered a complex, referred to as the inferior glenohumeral ligament complex (IGHLC). The complex (Fig. 1) consists of fibrous thickenings of the ligament both anteriorly and posteriorly, termed the anterior and posterior bands. Between the bands lies a very thin, fibrous axillary pouch. The strength of the complex rests primarily in the anterior and posterior bands.

The relationship of the musculocutaneous nerve to the inferior border of the glenohumeral joint capsule has also been studied recently. This relationship is important in open repairs because of the proximity of the nerve to the capsule. We now know that the nerve enters the coracobrachialis at a point much closer to the coracoid process than was previously believed (averaging 31 mm, minimum studied 17 mm). The importance of this was shown in a study of nerve injury after surgical repair of recurrent instability. Of eight patients with nerve injury after anterior shoulder repair, six had injury to the musculocutaneous nerve.

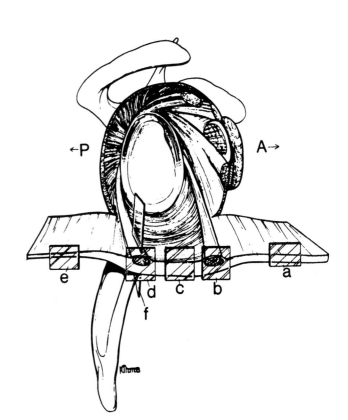

Fig. 1 Schematic drawing of a shoulder specimen showing the location and orientation of the histologic sections. A, anterior; P, posterior; a, sagittal section through anterior joint capsule; b, sagittal section through anterior band of the IGHLC; c, sagittal section through axillary pouch of IGHLC; d, sagittal section through posterior band of the IGHLC; e, sagittal section through posterior joint capsule; f, coronal section through posterior band of the IGHLC. (Reproduced with permission from O'Brien SJ, Neves MC, Arnoczky SP: The anatomy and histology of the interior glenohumeral ligament complex of the shoulder. *Am J Sports Med* 1990;18:449-456.)

Attempts to decrease the incidence of recurrence after a primary dislocation usually focus on immobilization and rehabilitation, but the efficacy of this treatment is debatable. In a recent study of arthroscopic evaluation after a primary dislocation, treatment consisted of debridement of the anterior glenoid rim near the labral tear. Although this treatment dramatically reduced the rate of recurrent dislocation, the follow-up period was short, and other reports confirming this finding are still awaited.

The exact nature of the "essential lesion" of recurrent instability is still not well understood. The current focus is on the Bankart lesion, or avulsion of the inferior glenohumeral ligament complex at its insertion to the glenoid labrum. Other possible causes of recurrent instability include abnormal glenoid version, abnormal humeral version, Hill-Sachs lesion, and subscapularis laxity.

Several recent studies evaluating the version of the glenoid and humeral head and their relationship to recurrent anterior instability have had contradictory results. However, it appears that glenoid or humeral version contributes to recurrent anterior instability only in extreme cases.

In earlier studies, the Hill-Sachs defect and subscapularis laxity were thought to be possible causes of recurrent instability. Although recent studies have not supported these conclusions, a recent arthroscopic study of first-time dislocators did show that almost all sustain some degree of Hill-Sachs injury. Subscapularis laxity has not to date been demonstrated to occur in these patients.

Arthroscopy to reconstruct recurrent anterior instability is an attractive option because it decreases trauma to the shoulder joint and reduces the risk of losing motion, specifically external rotation, after the repair. Several studies have evaluated various arthroscopic methods of repair. To date, none of these have had the success of open repair with respect to eliminating further recurrence.

Recently, open methods of repair have focused primarily on finding ways to eliminate anterior instability while retaining motion, specifically external rotation. In addition, because these injuries occur in a young population who are often athletic, return to sport after the surgery is often an important consideration.

Evaluation of loss of external rotation after the Bankart, Putti-Platt, Magnuson-Stack, Bristow, Eden-Hybinnette, and Weber procedures showed, when combining the results of multiple studies, that there were no significant differences among the procedures in loss of motion.

Previously, the Bristow procedure or variants (transfer of the coracoid with the conjoint tendon to the anteroinferior glenoid neck) were thought to be associated with less loss of motion and higher rates of return to sport. However, one study showed that, after a Bristow procedure, athletic individuals with involvement of the dominant shoulder were not capable of returning to high performance levels of overhead sports activity.

The Bankart procedure and its variants, although technically difficult, are currently favored by many surgeons. One recent variant that has attractive possibilities entails dividing the subscapularis in line with its fibers, rather than transversely near its insertion. This variant, which is thought to allow closure with less shortening of the subscapularis and possibly decrease loss of external rotation, may allow higher rates of return to sport. Long-term studies are not yet available.

Another variant of the Bankart procedure, developed because of the technical difficulty of the original operation, involves using metallic suture anchors placed in the anterior glenoid neck and using the attached sutures to repair the glenoid capsuloligamentous defect. Although this involves the risk of placing hardware within the shoulder capsule, one preliminary study of 32 patients showed no complications from the hardware at one-year follow-up.

Other recent studies have looked at complication rates after surgical repairs. Of eight cases of nerve injury after surgical repair for anterior instability, the musculocutaneous nerve was injured in six patients and the axillary nerve in two patients. All cases of nerve injury occurred after a Putti-Platt or Bristow procedure. Because of the high rates of laceration or suture entrapment of nerves, early exploration is recommended if nerve injury occurs after surgical repair for anterior instability.

Another series of patients developed osteoarthritis of the glenohumeral joint after Putti-Platt repairs. This was felt to have been caused by a technical error, in which the imbrication of the subscapularis was made excessively tight.

Posterior Instability

Posterior dislocations comprise less than 5% of all shoulder dislocations. Because of their rarity and the often subtle findings on a plain anteroposterior radiograph, it is felt that an initial posterior dislocation is not diagnosed in as many as 50% to 75% of occurrences. However, the diagnosis should not be missed if a complete trauma series is obtained at the time of injury. Examination of the patient with a posterior dislocation will also often reveal the problem. A patient with a posterior dislocation will be unable to externally rotate the arm to neutral while at the side.

Recurrent posterior instability is difficult to treat. The initial treatment is conservative and emphasizes muscle strengthening of the shoulder girdle, especially the external rotators and shoulder extensors. Education and lifestyle modification are also emphasized to help the patient avoid provocative positions.

Because of its rarity, large series of surgical repairs for posterior instability are not common. All series discussing the various repairs have had high recurrence rates (often greater than 50%) and high rates of complications. Thus, selection of patients for surgical reconstruction must be done with great care, and should be limited to patients who remain disabled by the problem despite completion of an adequate rehabilitation protocol.

Multidirectional Instability

Neer pointed out the importance of multidirectional instability in diagnosis. Diagnosis is made by demonstrating instability in at least two planes. A sulcus sign, representing inferior laxity, should also be present. This difficult problem should always be treated initially by physical therapy, concentrating on strengthening all the muscles about the shoulder girdle. Neer presented a preliminary study of an inferior capsular shift for this problem. The operation can be performed from an anterior

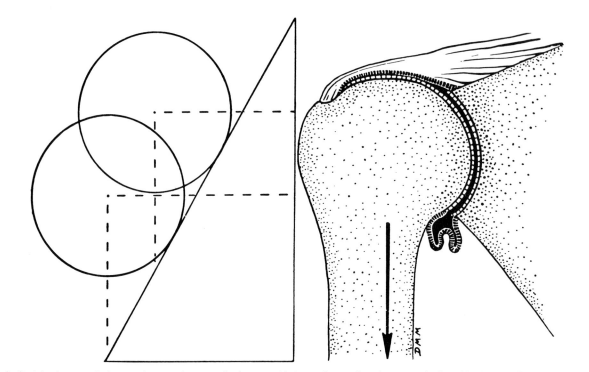

Fig. 2 **Left**, A body moved along a slope undergoes displacement in two primary directions—vertical and horizontal. Restricting the movement in one primary direction acts as a lock, preventing movement in the other direction. **Right**, The superior part of the capsule of the joint and the associated supraspinatus tighten when the humeral head is pulled downward on the slope of the glenoid fossa. (Reproduced with permission from Basmajian JV, Bazant FJ, Kingston CM: Factors preventing downward dislocation of the adducted shoulder joint. *J Bone Joint Surg* 1959;41A;1182-1186.)

or posterior approach, depending on the direction of most of the instability.

Because multidirectional instability (MDI) is a difficult problem which has not responded well to operative treatment, surgical repair of this problem should be considered only for patients who are disabled by it and who fail intensive rehabilitation. Recent studies have shed some light on the reasons for the difficulty in treating MDI. Hawkins and Tsutsui, who both studied the collagen of patient's shoulders with MDI, revealed abnormalities in the rate of formation and the amount of cross-links formed in the collagen from these shoulders.

The importance of the superior structures of the glenohumeral in the etiology and treatment of multidirectional instability has achieved a recent renaissance. It was shown in 1959 by Basmajian and Bazant that the superior capsule and supraspinatus were the primary structures responsible for preventing inferior subluxation of the humeral head (Fig. 2). More recently, a cadaveric study showed that sectioning of the coracohumeral ligament produced inferior instability, primarily anteroinferior instability. Another similar study showed that the rotator interval between the supraspinatus and subscapularis provided resistance to posterior and inferior displacement of the humeral head. It has also been postulated that imbrication and tightening of the rotator interval

may help prevent inferior instability. This may have future importance in the design of repairs for multidirectional instability.

Inferior Instability

Inferior glenohumeral dislocation, "luxatio erecta," is a very uncommon lesion. The dislocation, which usually is reduced easily by overhead traction, rarely becomes a recurrent problem. However, the dislocation is far from innocuous, and a recent evaluation of the literature has stressed the high incidence of associated injuries. In a review of 83 cases, 80% of the patients sustained a greater tuberosity fracture or rotator cuff tear, 60% of the patients sustained transient neurologic compromise with variable rates of recovery, and 3.3% of patients demonstrated vascular compromise to some degree.

Chronic Unreduced Dislocations

Most chronic dislocations occur after a missed posterior dislocation. Treatment options in these patients depend on how much time has passed since the original dislocation and the degree of destruction of the articular surfaces. The consensus is that dislocations less than six weeks old can be treated by reduction, usually open. Closed reduction may be attempted under anesthesia.

Dislocations between six weeks and six months old usually require surgical stabilization to maintain a reduction obtained by an open procedure. Posterior dislocations are usually reduced using a McLaughlin procedure (or Neer modification), in which the subscapularis tendon is moved into the reverse Hill-Sachs defect to render the defect an extra-articular problem. Untreated anterior dislocations, though rare, can be treated by the analogous Connolly procedure, in which the infraspinatus is moved into the Hill-Sachs defect.

Chronic unreduced dislocations of greater than six months duration usually involve massive destruction of the humeral head from large Hill-Sachs or reverse Hill-Sachs defects. These usually require a humeral head replacement. Concurrent degenerative arthritis of the glenoid may necessitate use of a total shoulder replacement. In this surgery, the humeral component is placed either in 60 to 75 degrees of retroversion (chronic posterior) or near neutral version (chronic anterior).

Annotated Bibliography

Flatow EL, Bigliani LU, April EW: An anatomic study of the musculocutaneous nerve and its relationship to the coracoid process. *Clin Orthop* 1989;244:166-171.

This study of cadaver shoulders demonstrated the close proximity of the musculocutaneous nerve to the coracoid process. The researchers found branches of the nerve entering the coracobrachialis as close as 17 mm to the coracoid and averaging 31 mm. They concluded that the frequently cited range of 5 to 8 cm below the coracoid for the level of penetration of the nerve cannot be relied on and great care should be taken when dissecting below the coracoid because of this.

Harryman DT II, Sidles JA, Harris SL, et al: The role of the rotator interval capsule in passive motion and stability of the shoulder. *J Bone Joint Surg* 1992;74A:53-66.

Harryman and associates studied the rotator interval in eight fresh-frozen cadavers. They concluded that release of this portion of the superior glenohumeral capsule may improve range of motion in shoulders with limited flexion and external rotation and, conversely, that imbrication of the rotator interval may help control posteroinferior instability of the glenohumeral joint.

Hawkins RJ, Angelo RL: Glenohumeral osteoarthrosis: A late complication of the Putti-Platt repair. *J Bone Joint Surg* 1990;72A:1193-1197.

Hawkins demonstrated that glenohumeral osteoarthrosis can result after the Putti-Platt repair if the repair is initially made too tight. This study evaluated ten referral cases, of which seven were unsuccessfully treated with an anterior Z-lengthening of the subscapularis.

Hawkins RJ, Mohtadi NG: Clinical evaluation of shoulder instability. *Clin J Sports Med* 1991;1:59-64.

This is an excellent review of classification, history of injury review, and physical examination of the patient with shoulder instability.

Helming P, Søjbjerg JO, Kjærsgaard-Andersen P, et al: Distal humeral migration as a component of multidirectional shoulder instability: An anatomical study in autopsy specimens. *Clin Orthop* 1990;252:139-143.

This cadaveric study looked at the importance of the coracohumeral ligament in preventing inferior and especially anteroinferior instability of the humeral head.

Mallon WJ, Bassett FH III, Goldner RD: Luxatio erecta: The inferior glenohumeral dislocation. *J Orthop Trauma* 1990;4:19-24.

The literature of 83 luxatio erecta is studied. Associated injuries were common as 80% of patients sustained a greater tuberosity fracture or rotator cuff tear, 60% of patients sustained transient neurologic compromise, and 3.3% of patients demonstrated vascular compromise.

O'Brien SJ, Neves MC, Arnoczky SP, et al: The anatomy and histology of the inferior glenohumeral ligament complex of the shoulder. *Am J Sports Med* 1990;18:449-456.

The study of cadaver shoulder demonstrated that the inferior glenohumeral ligament was more complicated than previously described. The authors found an anterior band, a posterior band and axillary pouch as distinct structures in all specimens. The possible clinical correlates are also discussed.

Richards RR, Hudson AR, Bertoia JT, et al: Injury to the brachial plexus during Putti-Platt and Bristow procedures. *Am J Sports Med* 1987;15:374-380.

Eight patients were studied with nerve injury after anterior shoulder repair. Early exploration was performed with satisfactory motor recovery in seven cases. The musculocutaneous nerve (6) was most frequently injured.

Richmond JC, Donaldson WR, Fu F, et al: Modification of the Bankart reconstruction with a suture anchor: Report of a new technique. *Am J Sports Med* 1991;19:343-346.

This preliminary article discusses the results of using a suture anchor to help perform a Bankart repair in 32 patients. At one-year average follow-up, 94% of the patients were considered to have good or excellent results. There were no complications from the technique or from use of hardware within the shoulder joint. Only one patient, a football player who sustained another severe trauma, had a recurrent dislocation after the surgery.

Rowe CR: Prognosis in dislocations of the shoulder. *J Bone Joint Surg* 1956;38A:957-977.

Though now slightly dated, this article remains the absolute classic in the field. More recent work does dispute somewhat the high rates of recurrence (around 90%) among primary dislocators in the 15 to 25 age group.

Snyder SJ, Karzel RP, Del Pizzo W, et al: SLAP lesions of the shoulder. *J Arthroscopy Rel Surg* 1990;6:274-279.

This was the first comprehensive description of the SLAP (Superior Labrum, Anterior and Posterior) lesion. Twenty-seven cases were studied with avulsions of the superior glenoid labrum near the origin of the biceps tendon.

Tsutsui H, Yamamoto R, Kuroki Y, et al: Biochemical study on collagen from the loose shoulder joint capsules, in Post M, Morrey BF, Hawkins RJ (eds): *Surgery of the Shoulder*. St. Louis, CV Mosby, 1991, p 108.

Tsutsui studied the collagen obtained from biopsies of eight shoulders with multidirectional instability. This was compared to collagen obtained from fresh cadaveric shoulders. These showed that collagen from the unstable patients formed fewer reducible crosslinks than that of normal shoulders.

Zuckerman JD, Matsen FA III: Complications about the glenohumeral joint related to the use of screws and staples. *J Bone Joint Surg* 1984;66A:175-180.

This study evaluated 37 patients with complications related to the implantation of screws or staples near the glenohumeral joints. They noted that such hardware can cause complications requiring reoperation and permanent loss of joint function. Great care must be exercised when placing such devices near the glenohumeral joint.

27

Shoulder: Reconstruction

Reconstructive shoulder surgery has continued to be an active area of basic and clinical research. Advances in the basic sciences have improved our knowledge of anatomy and function, while clinical research has helped refine patient selection and surgical techniques. Much of this work has concentrated on the diagnosis and treatment of rotator cuff disease as well as on prosthetic arthroplasty. As our understanding of shoulder pathology expands and our surgical techniques improve, a vast array of clinical pathology involving the shoulder girdle can be successfully managed through both rehabilitation and operative intervention.

Glenohumeral Joint

Anatomy

The glenohumeral geometry allows a wide range of movement but affords little intrinsic joint stability. The glenoid usually has a slightly greater radius of curvature than the humeral head and has about one fourth the surface area of the proximal humerus. The glenoid cartilage is thinner at the center than at the periphery. The densely fibrous labrum adds approximately 1 cm to the glenoid diameter, but little or no additional joint stability is attributable to the labrum itself. However, the labrum is an important attachment site for the joint capsule and the glenohumeral ligaments. The proximal humerus is retroverted 12 to 36 degrees with a neck-shaft angle of 115 to 129 degrees.

Static Stabilizers

Within the circumferential joint capsule are variable thickenings defined as the superior, middle, and inferior glenohumeral ligaments, which represent the primary components of static restraint in the glenohumeral joint. The inferior glenohumeral ligament has been established as the primary restraint to anterior and anteroinferior instability. Arthroscopic and histologic study of cadaver shoulders has shown that the inferior glenohumeral ligament consists of anterior and posterior bands that are connected to the proximal humerus in a collar-like or "V" attachment.

Together, the three glenohumeral ligaments limit the extremes of motion and help control the center of joint rotation, as demonstrated by instrumented strain gauge evaluation of these ligaments during joint movement. During motion, there is reciprocal tension sharing among the glenohumeral ligaments and transference of tension between themselves and the joint capsule. Cadaver studies also have demonstrated variations in the strain on these ligaments as a function of shoulder position. At zero degrees abduction, the superior and middle glenohumeral ligaments developed the most strain. At 45 degrees, the inferior and middle glenohumeral ligaments developed the greatest strain. At 90 degrees abduction, the inferior glenohumeral ligament developed the most strain. With the body upright and the arm in a dependent position, the coracohumeral and middle glenohumeral ligaments play important roles in resisting inferior translation. The rotator interval capsule (coracohumeral ligament and underlying joint capsule) acts to limit flexion and external rotation. In cadaver experiments, imbrication of the interval capsule helped to eliminate posterior and inferior instability. Thus, the three glenohumeral ligaments and coracohumeral ligaments, together with the joint capsule, are positioned in a finely tuned interrelated pattern to achieve static joint stability.

Dynamic Stabilizers

Dynamic stability is provided by the rotator cuff and should girdle musculature and is determined by arm position. Electromyographic studies show that the deltoid muscle is the primary force causing displacement (movement) and that the supraspinatus exerts a constant force that stabilizes the joint's center of rotation during movement. The infraspinatus is the primary muscle force responsible for external rotation. When the arm is in a position of anterior instability (90 degrees abduction and 90 degrees external rotation), the role of the dynamic stabilizers changes. In this position, the primary flexors that resist anterior dislocation are the pectoral, short head of the biceps, coracobrachial, anterior deltoid, and subscapular muscles.

Many individual components combine to form a given line of action in a single muscle. In the rotator cuff, for example, a histomorphometric study showed that the anterior portion of the supraspinatus is stronger and may contain contractile tissue and that the posterior part is entirely tendinous and passive. Biomechanical analyses show that the long head of the biceps tendon plays a major role in resisting upward migration of the humerus. The attachment site of the biceps long head has been found to be at the superior glenoid labrum in the majority of cadaveric specimens; only 25% had attachments into the supraglenoid tubercle.

Exercise programs have developed to isolate muscle groups in an effort to improve athletic performance or compensate for deficiencies. External rotation strength appears to be significantly greater when rotation is at the zero position of Saha than when it is in the frontal plane, implying that isokinetic strengthening and testing should be done in the scapular plane. It has become popular to perform strength testing on isokinetic equipment. One study has shown excellent correlation of tests with isokinetic testing and tests with hand-held office dynamometers, suggesting reliable information can be obtained with less costly equipment.

Blood Supply

A detailed cadaver study of 29 specimens confirmed that the humeral head is consistently perfused by an anterolateral branch of the anterior humeral circumflex artery. This vessel continues lateral to the long head of the biceps and forms the so-called arcuate artery, which perfuses the entire epiphysis of the humeral head. The posterior circumflex artery perfused only a small area in the posteroinferior aspect of the humeral head.

Rotator Cuff Disease

Etiology

The pathogenesis of rotator cuff disease appears to be multifactorial. Earlier theories focused on extrinsic factors leading to impingement with attendant reduction of available subacromial space and subsequent mechanical wear and degeneration in the supraspinatus tendon. More recent studies are focusing on intrinsic etiologic factors. The supraspinatus tendon receives its blood supply from the anterior humeral circumflex and suprascapular arteries, and it has an avascular zone characterized by a very sparse capillary web at the supraspinatus insertion site. A separate study of 18 cadaveric specimens showed this hypovascular area to involve only the articular side of the insertion site, which may account for the majority of partial thickness tears seen in this location. Another study corroborates previous work and suggests that once these intrinsic changes occur, imbalance and subtle upward humerus migration may result, leading to a decreased subacromial space and secondary acromial degenerative changes. In this study of 76 autopsy specimens, rotator cuff tearing correlated with increasing age but acromial degenerative changes did not. Thus, primary intrinsic degenerative tendonopathy may be the initiating factor in older patients with rotator cuff disease (Fig. 1).

The actual incidence of rotator cuff tearing has been studied as well. In 122 autopsy dissections with an average age of 79, the prevalence of partial tears was 28.7% and of complete tears, 30.3%. Under the age of 70, the prevalence of tears was 30%; for ages 71 to 80, it was 57.5%; and for over 80 years, it was 69.4%. In this study, unlike previous studies, prevalence of rupture was higher in women than in men.

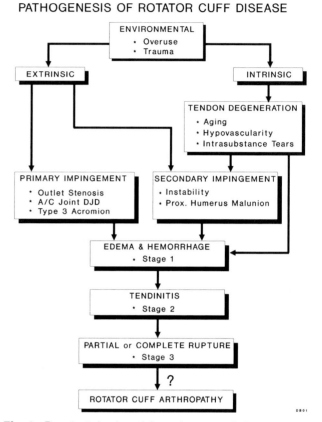

Fig. 1 Flowchart showing etiology of rotator cuff disease.

Physical Examination

The patient should be examined for abnormal masses, bone prominences (particularly the acromioclavicular joint), and muscle atrophy. In addition to measuring active range of motion, the fluidity and positions of pain are recorded. Particular attention should be paid to external rotation at 0 and 90 degrees abduction; loss of a small amount of external rotation can result in subacromial impingement, and this impingement prevents the greater tuberosity from rotating clear of the acromion during arm elevation.

As passive motion is recorded, impingement signs can be documented. The presence of pain in maximum forward elevation with the examiner stabilizing the scapula is known as the primary impingement sign. Pain during abduction of the arm to 80 degrees and internal rotation is a secondary impingement sign. Areas of tenderness are localized, particularly around the acromioclavicular joint and the supraspinatus insertion at the greater tuberosity. The joint is then examined for stability, particularly in younger, more active patients. Active muscle testing quantifies strength as well as eliciting pain. The supraspinatus muscle is tested with the shoulder abducted 90 degrees, flexed 30 degrees, and then maximally internally rotated. Downward pressure is resisted primarily by the supraspinatus. The infraspinatus and teres minor are tested with the shoulder adducted and the elbows flexed 90 degrees. Finally, the neurologic and vascular status of the upper extremities is documented.

Imaging

Routine radiographs in patients suspected of having rotator cuff disease should include an anteroposterior view in internal and external rotation and an axillary view. Patients without rotator cuff tears or with small to medium size tears may have normal appearing plain radiographs with an acromiohumeral interval of 1 to 1.5 cm. In chronic rotator cuff disease, with or without tearing, there may be evidence of greater tuberosity sclerosis and spurring with cyst formation and subacromial spurring. When the acromiohumeral interval measures 5 mm or less, a significant tear of the rotator cuff should be suspected. The active abduction view described in a recent study may allow use of plain radiographs for detection of patients with complete rotator cuff tears. In seven of 16 shoulders for which plain radiographs were normal and full thickness tears were seen on arthrography, the active abduction view showed narrowing of the acromiohumeral space to 2 mm or less. This view is obtained by having the patient actively abduct the shoulder to 90 degrees and repeating an anteroposterior radiograph. This supports a previous study of this view showing similar results when the arm is abducted to 30 degrees while holding a 2-kg weight or pushing up out of a chair.

Single- and double-contrast arthrography have shown over 85% sensitivity and specificity in the diagnosis of complete rotator cuff tears and are cost effective when trying to establish the absence or presence of complete rotator cuff disruption (Fig. 2). Arthrography is not as accurate in the diagnosis of partial rotator cuff tears and does not diagnose intrasubstance and bursal side tearing.

Ultrasonography is used to confirm the presence of significant rotator cuff disruption; it has a positive predictive value approaching 85% in that setting. However, it is extremely operator dependent. In a prospective study comparing it with arthrography, ultrasonography was found, on surgical confirmation, to be diagnostic in only seven (35%) of 20 patients with full thickness tears and diagnostic in only two of seven (29%) with partial tearing.

Magnetic resonance imaging (MRI) has emerged as the most sensitive and comprehensive noninvasive diagnostic tool in the evaluation of rotator cuff disease (Fig. 3). It remains costly, however, and is still thought by many to be most applicable when the diagnostic methods mentioned above would not suffice. In a large study of 106 patients undergoing MRI with operative confirmation, this test had a specificity of 100% with a sensitivity of 95% in the diagnosis of complete rotator cuff tears. In differentiating rotator cuff tendinitis from degeneration and partial tearing, the values were 82% and 85%, respectively. Currently, it is still difficult to differentiate between severe tendinitis, partial tearing, or an ex-

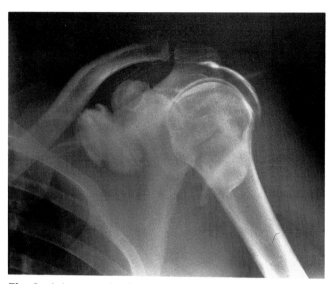

Fig. 2 Arthrogram showing a complete rotator cuff tear.

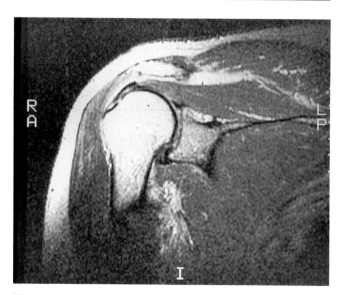

Fig. 3 Magnetic resonance T2-weighted image showing a partial rotator cuff tear.

tremely small complete rotator cuff tear on MRI. As technology improves, enhanced specificity should allow this differentiation.

Diagnostic arthroscopy for rotator cuff disease has had an increasingly limited role as MRI continues to improve. Although direct visualization of articular as well as bursal side tearing is possible, intratendinous degeneration cannot be visualized.

Treatment

Earlier methods of treatment consisted of complete acromionectomy but results were unsatisfactory. Since 1972, open acromioplasty has consisted of resection of only the anterior inferior aspect of the acromion and has shown satisfactory results in approximately 80% of properly selected patients when performed for refractory rotator cuff tendinitis. Acromioplasty is the usual treatment for stage II impingement with encroachment of the subacromial space by an abnormally shaped or sloped acromion, inferior acromioclavicular joint osteophytes, or greater tuberosity malunion. Arthroscopic or conventional open techniques are both successful. The management of complete thickness tears of the rotator cuff also remains controversial, but the weight of evidence favors repair through conventional open techniques.

Surgical Technique   Certain general principles apply to the management of the tissues about the shoulder. The deltoid may be elevated subperiosteally and, therefore, not detached from the acromion, or it may be detached. If detached, the fascial origin should be preserved. A secure, anatomic reattachment of the deltoid origin to bone using nonabsorbable sutures is mandatory. Effective clearance for the rotator cuff to pass within the subacromial space is required. To achieve this goal, an inferior acromioplasty most often is required. Partial anterior acromionectomy may also be required if an acromial protuberance is projecting anterior to the front of the acromioclavicular joint.

Resection of the coracoacromial ligament rather than division is preferable. Resection of the distal clavicle is less common today than in the past. The main indication for distal clavicle resection is pain localized by palpation to the acromioclavicular joint. Radiographic changes without that clinical finding are not an indication. Inferiorly directed acromioclavicular joint osteophytes can be removed at the time of surgery without formal resection of the distal clavicle. Resection of the subacromial bursa is necessary when that structure is chronically thickened and acting as a space-occupying lesion or if the bursa is adherent to the rotator cuff and prevents complete tendon visualization. Additional principles of surgery depend on whether the tear is a complete tear or a partial thickness tear or if the tendon is merely thickened and fibrotic.

Postoperative Rehabilitation   Passive range of motion in elevation and external rotation is started as soon as the surgeon feels secure that the newly sutured rotator cuff attachment will take the stresses. At six weeks, the tendon attachment should be strong enough to allow active motion. Passive range of motion exercises also are continued until fluid, full passive motion is achieved. Grip strengthening and gentle deltoid isometrics also are started. Three months after surgery, rotator cuff fixation is secure enough to allow rotator cuff muscle strengthening. Work and sports rehabilitation programs can be initiated on an individual basis.

Special Problems   Perhaps the greatest current area of controversy involves the management of irreparable rotator cuff tears. The options include: open or arthroscopic wide debridement and decompression without repair, local tendon transfers, latissimus dorsi transfer, primary repair with the arm in abduction, and the use of synthetic graft materials.

Arthroscopic acromioplasty and subacromial decompression do not require deltoid detachment and are associated with cost savings and more rapid rehabilitation. However, the basic principles described above should be realized. It is performed as an outpatient procedure and patients begin shoulder rehabilitation immediately, without immobilization (Fig. 4). In a comparative study of ten open versus ten arthroscopic decompression procedures, range of motion returned more rapidly and overall recovery occurred four months earlier in the arthroscopic group. Arthroscopic results have paralleled open surgery results. A report of 89 arthroscopic decompressions in patients who had stage II impingement syndrome without rotator cuff tears showed marked improvement in 81 (91%) at a 2.5-year average follow-up. Significant improvement was seen in patients with partial rotator cuff tears who underwent arthroscopic acromioplasty, but occurred less often than in those without tears. Of 40 patients, 33 (82%) had successful outcomes. In complete rotator cuff tears, only 14 of 25 patients (56%) had satisfactory results, and seven later underwent open rotator cuff repair. Arthroscopic decompression has been successful in patients with stage II impingement syndrome and in those with partial rotator cuff tears, but it has not been shown to be successful in patients with complete rotator cuff tears. An analysis of 31 patients with partial rotator cuff tears showed that results of debriding articular-side partial tears without performing an acromioplasty were equal to results with acromioplasty at short-term follow-up. It was concluded that an acromioplasty should be performed primarily for bursal-side partial tears.

Intra-articular glenohumeral examination is a routine part of evaluation in patients undergoing arthroscopic rotator cuff debridement or decompression. The reported risks of fluid extravasation, bleeding, articular damage, nerve injury, and infection are quite low. A recent study reported four cases of competitive athletes with persistent symptomatic rotator cuff tears requiring open repair. The tears had apparently occurred as a result of arthroscope placement through the posterior portal site. Patients with persistent pain should undergo thorough reevaluation to rule out an incorrect initial diagnosis (such as secondary impingement from an instability problem) or possible iatrogenic rotator cuff tearing. In a study of 67 failed acromioplasties performed for stage II impingement syndrome without tearing, 27 (40%) were felt to be secondary to an incorrect initial diagnosis and 28 (42%) resulted from operative errors. Revision or secondary surgeries in nonworkers' compensation cases showed a 75% success rate.

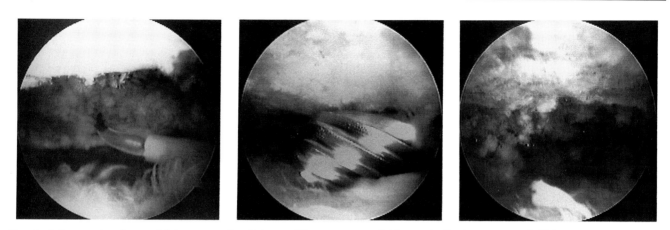

Fig. 4 Arthroscopic subacromial decompression: Release of the coracoacromial ligament with electrocautery (**left**), insertion of burr beneath the anterior acromion (**center**), and completed acromioplasty (**right**).

Rotator Cuff Repair

The vast majority of patients with partial rotator cuff tears can be managed successfully without surgery. Most symptomatic complete rotator cuff tears are chronic in nature or represent an acute extension of a preexisting tear in a degenerative tendon. In spite of long-standing symptoms, approximately 50% of these patients can successfully be managed without surgery, depending on the patient's age, activity level, and expectations. Patients who fail to respond to conservative measures may be candidates for open surgical tendon repair combined with subtotal bursectomy, anterior acromioplasty, coracoacromial ligament excision, and distal clavicle excision if symptomatic acromioclavicular joint arthritis coexists. While some studies have shown satisfactory pain relief following debridement and acromioplasty alone, the best long-term pain relief and return of function are seen following tendon repair. Small and medium size tears are managed by debridement of diseased tendon and direct repair into a bone trough or side-to-side with heavy absorbable or nonabsorbable sutures. A water-tight anatomic repair, which provides maximum restoration of dynamic rotator cuff power and contains synovial fluid within the joint for adequate cartilage nutrition, is best.

Large and massive rotator cuff tears are a complex reconstructive challenge. Less complicated repair techniques are used whenever possible. It is necessary to release the remaining scarred and retracted rotator cuff by mobilizing both the articular and bursal sides of the tendons. This includes a circumferential capsular release at the glenoid rim and release of the rotator interval capsule and cuff with the coracohumeral ligament. The extent to which the tendons can be mobilized is limited, however. A cadaver study of 18 shoulders indicated that more than 1 cm of lateral advancement of the supraspinatus or infraspinatus tendons might jeopardize function of the suprascapular nerve and should be avoided. If anatomic repair is not possible after mobilization, a McLaughlin V-Y

repair is used. Occasionally, the long head of the biceps tendon is incorporated into the repair. If adequate closure still is not possible, transposition of the upper half of the subscapularis tendon is performed. Postoperative immobilization with an abduction brace relieves tension on the repair during healing.

Fascial grafts, muscle transfers, and synthetic materials have been described for the repair of massive rotator cuff defects, but the results have not been predictable and follow-up has been short. One recent study of 16 patients with massive rotator cuff tears undergoing latissimus dorsi muscle transfers did show encouraging results at an average of 33 months follow-up. Of those patients with an intact subscapularis tendon preoperatively, 94% achieved satisfactory pain relief and had an average improvement of 67 degrees active flexion. Another study reported 11 of 14 patients had satisfactory results at four-year average follow-up when a synthetic carbon fiber was used to augment the repair in medium to massive rotator cuff tears. These procedures should still be considered experimental.

Using direct repair and local tendon transposition techniques, surgery has yielded satisfactory results in 85% to 90% of patients with follow-up for as long as 14 years. Successful pain relief is not affected by tear size, but return of function is less dramatic in patients with massive tears. Most reports indicate that the results in terms of pain relief do not deteriorate with time but the integrity of the repair may. One published study of 105 patients who underwent rotator cuff repairs, at five year average follow-up, showed recurrent defect in 20% of patients with only supraspinatus involvement and 50% of patients with tears involving more than just the supraspinatus. Although recurrent tearing did not seem to affect pain relief, it was associated with deterioration in shoulder function.

Revision rotator cuff repair surgery is less successful than primary surgery and depends on the quality and mobility of the remaining rotator cuff tendons. Pain can be reduced, but improved function is rare, so surgery is directed primarily at pain relief. Surgery to repair deltoid retraction is difficult and rarely improves function.

Update of Rotator Cuff Disease

Currently, rotator cuff disease is thought to arise from two distinct, though not mutually exclusive causes, grouped as structural and functional. Those who favor a structural etiology focus on those factors that change the size of the subacromial space, either by increasing the thickness of the soft tissue contents or by bony changes that result in a decreased volume through which the soft tissue structures must pass.

Those who favor functional cause focus more on dynamic abnormalities that allow symptoms to develop without true or permanent alterations in the bone or soft tissues.

Structural Causes These can be divided into bone and soft tissue changes. Variations in acromial shape have been described, and significant correlations between that bone shape and the extent of rotator cuff disease have been documented. The acromial shape has been classified as type I (flat), type II (gently curving), or type III (hook shaped) (Fig. 5). The type III acromion allows minimal rotator cuff clearance and is associated with a higher incidence of significant rotator cuff disease. The presence of an os acromionale also is significant. This failure of ossification in the acromion can displace with minimal trauma, which causes the acromion to tilt inferiorly and compromise the subacromial space. If an acromioplasty is required in the presence of an os acromionale, open reduction, internal fixation, and bone grafting can be performed.

Acromioclavicular arthritis or inferior acromioclavicular joint osteophytes can result in impingement and mechanical irritation to the rotator cuff tendons. A similar phenomenon can occur after displaced acromioclavicular separations. More rarely, an elongated or more laterally directed coracoid process can impinge on the rotator cuff tendons when the arm is adducted. Greater tuberosity fractures can cause impingement if the fragment migrates superiorly. In a similar phenomenon, humeral neck fractures heal in a varus position and cause the greater tuberosity to tilt more superiorly.

Soft tissue structural causes include bursal abnormalities, as a result of inflammation, trauma, or aging. The rotator cuff can become thickened as a result of repetitive microtrauma or, less commonly, a single isolated traumatic event. Calcium deposits may be present, and inflammation can result in fibrosis and scarring. Partial tears with flaps of soft tissue can cause irritation to the remaining tendon and bursa and result in an increased soft tissue volume within the subacromial space.

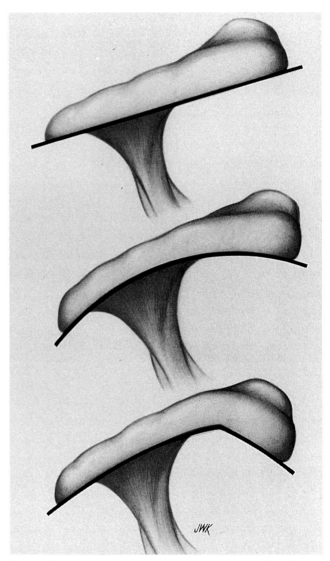

Fig. 5 Three acromial types: Type I (**top**) is flat; type II (**middle**) is curved; type III (**bottom**) is hooked.

Functional Causes Loss of normal humeral head depression by the rotator cuff can result from rotator cuff tear or weakness, a C5-6 lesion, suprascapular nerve palsy, or biceps tendon rupture. Each of these conditions allows excessive superior movement of the humeral head.

Loss of the humeral head fulcrum through humeral head resection, rheumatoid arthritis, sepsis, or avascular necrosis will cause abnormalities in rotator cuff function. Abnormal scapular motion may be seen with trapezius fatigue in the competitive swimmer. Lower extremity functional loss, as seen in paraplegics, amputees, and multijoint arthritis, can cause a "weightbearing upper extremity" as the individual places increased reliance on the arms to support body weight. More recently, attention has been focused on the interplay of the capsule and movements of the humeral head. It has been shown that a tight posterior capsule can lead to an obligatory anterosuperior migration of the humeral head.

Another etiology of rotator cuff disease is the overlapping of glenohumeral instability and rotator cuff injuries. Repetitive overhead throwing results in the gradual stretching and laxity of the anteroinferior glenohumeral ligament, anteroinferior subluxation, and traction tendinitis of the rotator cuff. The individual has classic symptoms of "impingement." Treatment of what appears to be the obvious source of pain, the rotator cuff, without addressing the true abnormality, instability, will result in clinical failure. The reverse may also be true. An individual may have subclinical asymptomatic subluxation that is well controlled through properly coordinated rotator cuff function. With rotator cuff injury, rotator cuff weakness develops and increased humeral head translation becomes symptomatic instability.

In addition to the more chronic etiologies of rotator cuff disease, acute trauma may produce significant rotator cuff pathology. The younger individual with major shoulder trauma can sustain a full-thickness rotator cuff tear. The individual over 45 years of age who sustains a dislocation must be examined carefully for an accompanying rotator cuff tear. Failure of normal arm elevation or rotator cuff strength should alert the examiner to the possibility of a full-thickness tear of the rotator cuff.

Prosthetic Arthroplasty

Before the advent of prosthetic shoulder arthroplasty, the options for reconstruction of the glenohumeral joint were joint debridement, synovectomy, resectional arthroplasty, arthrodesis, or osteotomy. Synovectomy still has a limited role in the treatment of early rheumatoid disease of the shoulder, but resection arthroplasty is now used as a salvage procedure only. Arthrodesis can be considered in young, active individuals with degenerative arthritis, uncontrollable joint sepsis, loss of both rotator cuff and deltoid function, or as a salvage procedure following failed total joint arthroplasty. Procedures such as the Benjamin double osteotomy carry significant risks of nonunion and/or osteonecrosis and cannot be recommended.

Design

Prosthetic arthroplasty of the shoulder initially centered on the use of constrained implant designs but their usefulness has been limited by high mechanical failure rates resulting from periarticular fractures and glenoid loosening. Since 1952, glenohumeral joint arthroplasty has focused on the use of an unconstrained proximal humeral component with or without glenoid resurfacing as dictated by the disease process. Unconstrained implants are characterized by a near anatomic design that depends on

an intact or repairable rotator cuff to maintain stability and center of joint rotation, as well as an intact deltoid. The humeral component is designed to preserve metaphyseal bone stock for adequate fixation and to maintain the integrity of the rotator cuff attachment site at the anatomic neck. The glenoid component preserves subchondral bone and achieves fixation in the glenoid metaphysis. Most patients who are candidates for total shoulder arthroplasty have intact or repairable rotator cuff tendons, making any intrinsic glenoid component stability unnecessary and undesirable.

Some systems are semiconstrained, having a superior polyethylene hood built into the glenoid component to help prevent superior humeral head migration, but this is accomplished at the cost of increased glenoid keel stresses. Early finite element analysis studies showed improved cortical bone stress transfer with metal backing, but more recent finite element analyses suggest that an all-polyethylene component may transfer stress in a more physiologic manner.

Technique

Proper preoperative planning is essential. All patients should have radiographs, including an anteroposterior radiograph in internal and external rotation as well as an axillary view to assess glenoid deficiencies. The deltopectoral approach provides excellent exposure without requiring release of the anterior deltoid. Many patients with osteoarthritis have posterior glenoid bone loss, and patients with rheumatoid arthritis often have central (medial) erosion. If significant posterior bone loss is present, it may be necessary to alter the amount of humeral retroversion from the normal 35 degrees to a less retroverted position to prevent postoperative posterior instability and eccentric glenoid component loading. In severe cases of glenoid bone deficiency, it may be necessary to consider the use of an angled keel component or use of a bone graft, which has been shown to successfully reconstruct and reorient the glenoid to a near anatomic position. In most patients, the glenoid component is cemented in place, although younger individuals with adequate bone quality may be candidates for an uncemented prosthesis designed to promote tissue ingrowth (Fig. 6).

The humeral component can be press fit in place in most patients. Cement augmentation should be used if bone quality is poor or if metaphyseal bone deficiency is present. Hemiarthroplasty can be considered in a young patient with osteoarthritis, posttraumatic conditions without glenoid involvement, osteonecrosis, or rotator cuff arthropathy. Glenoid resurfacing in patients with osteoarthritis or rheumatoid arthritis has yielded a higher percentage of patients with satisfactory pain relief than has hemiarthroplasty. Glenoid loosening rates, which, in part, result from eccentric loading and excessive glenoid wear debris, are significantly higher in patients with rotator cuff arthropathy than they are in patients with osteoarthritis (Fig. 7).

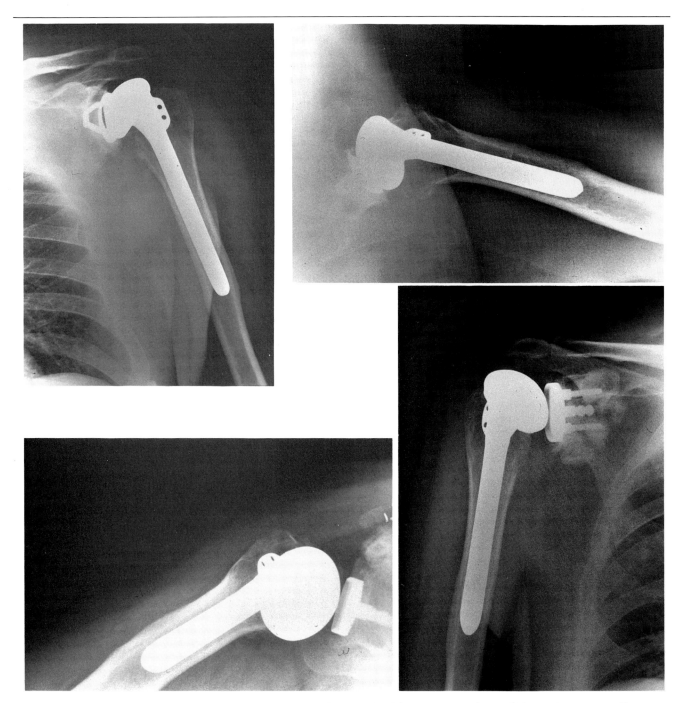

Fig. 6 Total shoulder arthroplasty. **Top,** Use of a cemented metal-backed glenoid component and press-fit humeral component. **Bottom,** Use of an ingrowth glenoid component in a patient with severe glenohumeral degenerative joint disease and synovial chondromatosis.

The postoperative rehabilitation program varies with disease process and patient motivation and must be individualized. Most patients wear a shoulder immobilizer at night and a sling during the day for four to six weeks. Passive shoulder range of motion begins the day after surgery, and active motion begins at three to six weeks. At eight weeks, patients may begin a gentle stretching and strengthening program.

Results

Long-term follow-up studies are now available for hemiarthroplasty and for total shoulder arthroplasty using a cemented glenoid component for a variety of glenohumeral disease processes. Pain relief has been excellent in all groups, but return of function depends on the integrity of the rotator cuff. Surveillance for as long as 15 years with an average of eight years in osteoarthritis pa-

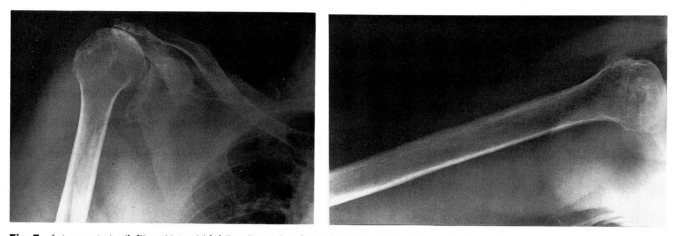

Fig. 7   Anteroposterior (**left**) and lateral (**right**) radiographs of a patient with severe rotator cuff arthropathy.

tients has shown satisfactory pain relief in 90% to 95%. Hemiarthroplasty in this same group yields 85% to 90% satisfactory pain relief, although one study suggests that long-term pain relief may be less. Although most diagnostic categories show a gain in function, patients with osteoarthritis and osteonecrosis obtain the best functional results, followed by patients with rheumatoid arthritis. Patients with posttraumatic arthritis usually have significant associated rotator cuff scarring and achieve less dramatic functional gains.

Implant longevity has compared favorably with total hip and total knee arthroplasty. Most studies indicate a revision rate of approximately 11% at 10 years. A 27% failure rate at 11 years postoperatively has been predicted based on survivorship analysis, where failure is defined as the surgeon's recommendation of revision based on intractable pain or radiographic evidence of loosening.

Radiolucent lines in the glenoid have not correlated directly with symptoms or the need for revision surgery. Glenoid keel lucencies present the greatest concern, especially if they are greater than 1.5 cm and complete. An analysis of 33 total shoulder arthroplasties using a cemented Neer glenoid component, followed up for an average of five years, showed 49% of glenoid components developed 1 to 2 mm of circumferential lucent lines, but only one showed migration and loosening. Whatever the reported prevalence of glenoid lucent lines, these figures are undoubtedly underestimated because of the difficulty in orienting the x-ray beam perpendicular to the bone-cement interfaces. Fluoroscopic spot films may help to better define the incidence of lucent lines, but it seems clear that their correlation with clinical loosening is not linear. The presence of lucent lines may be as high as 60%, but their presence usually is not associated with clinical symptoms.

Patients with rheumatoid arthritis in general show lesser gains in function, which correlate with their preoperative disease severity. However, a recent series of 24 arthroplasties performed in patients with severe rheumatoid arthritis showed satisfactory pain relief in 92% at 4.5 years average follow-up. Seventy-five percent of patients reported no significant functional limitations.

Complications

Proximal migration of the humeral component in total shoulder arthroplasty is not an infrequent finding (Fig. 8). In a study of 131 unconstrained total shoulder arthroplasties followed an average of 55 months, 22% showed significant proximal migration. This migration was not associated with pain relief, range of motion, or glenoid loosening rates. Also, it was not directly related to preoperative rotator cuff integrity. Twenty-one percent of those without migration and 24% of those with proximal migration had rotator cuff tears preoperatively. These data support the use of an unconstrained prosthesis, even in the presence of irreparable rotator cuff tears. Proximal migration appears to be multifactorial and includes factors such as late rotator cuff thinning or tearing or deltoid and rotator cuff imbalance.

Currently, the need for revision total shoulder arthroplasty appears to be low and can result from a variety of factors. The most common causes are glenoid loosening, instability, late rotator cuff tearing, humeral component loosening, and infection.

Less Common Causes of Glenohumeral Arthroplasty

The true incidence of glenohumeral joint involvement in hemophilic arthropathy is unknown, but it is thought to be uncommon. Shoulder involvement produces intra-articular degenerative changes as well as rotator cuff disease. A report of adult hemophiliacs suggests a 37% incidence of shoulder involvement and, of those, eight of 12 (66%) had rotator cuff tears.

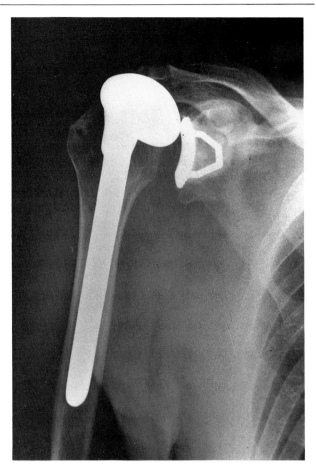

Fig. 8 Anteroposterior radiograph of proximal humeral component migration following total shoulder arthroplasty in a patient with rotator cuff arthropathy.

Multiple epiphyseal dysplasia most commonly affects the hip and knee, but shoulder involvement is not unusual. In a study of 50 patients with multiple epiphyseal dysplasia, one third had bilateral shoulder symptoms and most developed painful osteoarthritis in middle age. Patients with a "hatchet head" deformity usually have significant stiffness from an early age, but remain relatively pain free until middle age.

Septic glenohumeral arthritis is uncommon, but there is often a delay in appropriate diagnosis and treatment. Some underlying cause is common. An analysis of 18 patients with shoulder septic arthritis showed all but one had a significant associated disease; eight had an intra-articular injection or aspirating before developing infection. Open debridement yielded better results than repeated joint aspiration.

Acromioclavicular Joint

Acromioclavicular joint arthritis and posttraumatic osteolysis can occur as isolated symptomatic entities or can coexist with glenohumeral arthritis and rotator cuff disease. It is important to isolate the acromioclavicular joint in the history and physical examination. Anteroposterior and axillary shoulder radiographs should be inspected for acromioclavicular joint narrowing, osteolysis, and inferiorly projecting osteophytes. Additional information can be gained through bone scanning and MRI. Selective lidocaine injection may be useful to isolate acromioclavicular joint symptoms from other causes of shoulder pain. In general, the treatment is similar to that for rotator cuff disease. If symptoms are refractory, surgical intervention may be considered.

Arthritis of the acromioclavicular joint or osteolysis of the distal clavicle can be managed by distal clavicle excision as an isolated procedure or as part of a larger shoulder reconstructive procedure, such as total shoulder arthroplasty, acromioplasty, or rotator cuff repair. Ten millimeters of the distal clavicle and 5 mm of the medial acromion can also be resected arthroscopically. An analysis of ten cadaver shoulders showed that arthroscopic resection could be performed with precision comparable to open resection.

Biceps Tendon

Inflammation of the long head of the biceps tendon and its synovial lining usually is associated with rotator cuff inflammation, although it may be a predominant source of symptoms. The long head of the biceps tendon has an important contribution as a humeral head depressor, and tenodesis can lead to aggravation of rotator cuff inflammation and impingement symptoms. Isolated biceps tenodesis has not produced satisfactory long-term results and now usually is performed only if significant degeneration or rupture of the tendon is found as part of a shoulder reconstructive procedure.

Posttraumatic degenerative changes can be seen in the superior labrum, posteriorly and anteriorly involving the biceps long head anchor point (SLAP lesion). Satisfactory short-term results were reported after arthroscopic debridement in a study of 26 patients who had this lesion. However, the natural history of this lesion is unknown, and prolonged nonoperative management should precede surgical intervention.

Calcific Tendinitis

Symptomatic calcific tendinitis of the shoulder can be divided into acute and chronic phases, but the composition of calcium deposits in rotator cuff tendons is the same. The deposit is composed of H_2O, CO_3, and PO_4 in addition to organic molecules. Its dissolution and disintegration probably depend on a change in the binding capacity of these organic molecules. For unknown reasons, diabetic patients are more likely to develop asymptomatic rotator cuff calcium deposits. In one radiographic study, 31.8% of insulin-dependent diabetics had tendon calcification while only 10.3% of nondiabetics had the calcific lesion. Most cases of calcific tendinitis of the shoulder resolve spontaneously, but refractory cases can be managed by cortisone injection, needling, or arthroscopic calcium excision.

Suprascapular Nerve Entrapment

Suprascapular neuropathy is uncommon but is a clinical entity that can cause pain and weakness primarily when the arm is in external rotation and less commonly in abduction. Entrapment can occur at the suprascapular notch or spinoglenoid notch. If it occurs at the suprascapular notch, both the supraspinatus and infraspinatus can be affected, whereas spinoglenoid entrapment produces weakness solely in the infraspinatus muscle. Electromyography, ultrasonography, computed tomographic scanning, and MRI be helpful in establishing the etiology. In addition to trauma, tumor, and fracture, entrapment of the suprascapular nerve in the spinoglenoid notch may be caused by ganglia. Of three reported cases, all were successfully treated by ganglia excision and decompression of the suprascapular nerve.

Frozen Shoulder

The etiology of frozen shoulder (adhesive capsulitis) is multifactorial. Associated diseases include insulin-dependent diabetes mellitus, Parkinsonism, thyroid disorders, and cardiovascular disease. Frozen shoulder syndrome can occur secondary to other shoulder pathology. A study of 150 patients with glenohumeral stiffness showed that 37 had primary frozen shoulder syndrome, while the remaining patients had associated rotator cuff tears or impingement syndrome. Arthroscopic findings in the 37 patients with primary frozen shoulder disclosed an absence of intra-articular adhesions. However, a vascular reaction was identified around the biceps long-head tendon as it opened into the subscapularis bursa. Contractures also have been described in the joint capsule associated with intra-articular synovitis. A study of 17 recalcitrant cases treated surgically also showed significant contracture of the coracohumeral ligament and rotator interval. Resection of these structures led to reduction of pain and return of motion.

In most cases, the symptoms of pain and stiffness begin insidiously. The majority of patients show gradual reduction of pain and return of motion over a period of eight to 18 months. Treatment consists of gentle physical therapy, anti-inflammatory medication, and judicious use of subacromial and intra-articular cortisone injections. Patients who fail to show improvement may be candidates for manipulation under anesthesia. Arthroscopic distention and debridement may occasionally be helpful. Open releases are rarely indicated and can accentuate permanent residual stiffness.

Annotated Bibliography

Basic Science

Bassett RW, Browne AO, Morrey BF, et al: Glenohumeral muscle force and movement mechanics in a position of shoulder instability. *J Biomech* 1990;23:405-415.

With the arm in a position of anterior instability of 90 degrees abduction and 90 degrees external rotation in five cadaver specimens examined using computer assisted cross-sectional analysis, the most effective flexors of the shoulder that appeared to resist anterior dislocation were the pectoral, short head of the biceps, coracobrachialis, anterior deltoid, and the subscapularis.

Ferrari DA: Capsular ligaments of the shoulder: Anatomical and functional study of the anterior superior capsule. *Am J Sports Med* 1990;18:20-24.

In a study of 100 cadaver shoulder specimens, the coracohumeral ligament was found to be a consistent structure and worked in conjunction with the middle glenohumeral ligament to support the arm in a dependent position.

Gagey N, Gagey O, Bastian G, et al: The fibrous frame of the supraspinatus muscle: Correlations between anatomy and MRI findings. *Surg Radiol Anat* 1990;12:291-292.

Data from 30 patients who underwent MRI examination of the shoulder were compared with data from 20 cadaver shoulders that were carefully dissected. This histomorphometric study showed the anterior part of the supraspinatus muscle to have a longer and stronger fibrous frame than the posterior aspect, implying that it may function as contractile tendon.

Gerber C, Schneeberger AG, Vinh TS: The arterial vascularization of the humeral head: An anatomical study. *J Bone Joint Surg* 1990;72A:1486-1494.

All 29 cadaver specimens were shown to have the humeral head perfused by the anterolateral ascending branch of the anterior humeral circumflex artery, which then became the so-called arcuate artery. The posterior humeral circumflex artery perfused a small portion of the posteroinferior part of the humeral head.

Greenfield BH, Donatelli R, Wooden MJ, et al: Isokinetic evaluation of shoulder rotational strength between the plane of scapula and the frontal plane. *Am J Sports Med* 1990;18:124-128.

Isokinetic shoulder girdle strength testing in 20 subjects demonstrated that external rotational strength values were significantly higher in the plane of the scapula than in the frontal plane.

Harryman DT II, Sidles JA, Harris SL, et al: The role of the rotator interval capsule in passive motion and stability of the shoulder. *J Bone Joint Surg* 1992;74A:53-66.

In a cadaver study using position sensors and torque transducers to determine glenohumeral motion, translation, and stability, the rotator interval capsule (coracohumeral ligament and underlying joint capsule) acted to limit flexion and external rotation. Imbrication of the interval helped to eliminate posterior and inferior instability.

Magnusson SP, Gleim GW, Nicholas JA: Subject variability of shoulder abduction strength testing. *Am J Sports Med* 1990;18:349-353.

In nine test subjects, isokinetic equipment was compared to an office hand-held dynamometer and showed excellent correlation between these two methods of evaluation.

O'Brien SJ, Neves MC, Arnoczky SP, et al: The anatomy and histology of the inferior glenohumeral ligament complex of the shoulder. *Am J Sports Med* 1990;18:449-456.

An arthroscopic and histologic study of the inferior glenohumeral ligament in 11 cadaver specimens showed it to be complex structure consisting of an anterior and posterior band. The proximal humerus attachment site was collar-like or in a "V" arrangement adjacent to the articular edge of the humeral head.

O'Connell PW, Nuber GW, Mileski RA, et al: The contribution of the glenohumeral ligaments to anterior stability of the shoulder joint. *Am J Sports Med* 1990;18:579-584.

In a cadaver study of six specimens, strain-gauge instrumentation was applied to the glenohumeral ligaments. The superior and middle glenohumeral ligaments developed most strain at 0 degrees abduction. At 45 degrees abduction, the inferior and middle glenohumeral ligaments developed the greatest strain. At 90 degrees abduction, the inferior glenohumeral ligament developed the greatest strain with a lesser amount of strain developing in the middle glenohumeral ligament.

Pal GP, Bhatt RH, Patel VS: Relationship between the tendon of the long head of biceps brachii and the glenoidal labrum in humans. *Anat Rec* 1991;229:278-280.

A study of 24 cadaver specimens showed that the long head of the biceps tendon inserts into the superior labrum. The major portion of the tendon attached to the supraglenoid tubercle in only 25% of specimens.

Terry GC, Hammond D, France P, et al: The stabilizing function of passive shoulder restraints. *Am J Sports Med* 1991;19:26-34.

Four of 11 fresh frozen shoulder specimens underwent motion analysis and seven were instrumented with glenohumeral ligament strain gauges. The results demonstrated a reciprocal tension-sharing relationship among all ligament components and a transference of tension among these components when changes in joint position were compared.

Rotator Cuff Disease

Etiology

Jerosch J, Müller T, Castro WM: The incidence of rotator cuff rupture: An anatomic study. *Acta Orthop Belg* 1991;57:124-129.

In 122 autopsy dissections with an average age of 79 years, the incidence of partial rotator cuff tears was 28.7%, and of complete tears was 30.3%. The incidence of tearing in patients under the age of 70 years was 30%, at age 71 to 80 was 57.5%, and over 80 was 69.4%. Women showed a higher incidence of rupture (66.7%); men had ruptures in 43.9%.

Ling SC, Chen CF, Wan RX: A study on the vascular supply of the supraspinatus tendon. *Surg Radiol Anat* 1990;12:161-165.

Twenty-two cadaver specimens were injected with gelatin and India ink and were evaluated by scanning electron microscopy. This showed that the primary blood supply to the supraspinatus tendon came from the anterior humeral circumflex and suprascapular arteries. An avascular zone at the supraspinatus insertion site showed a very sparse capillary web.

Lohr JF, Uhthoff HK: The microvascular pattern of the supraspinatus tendon. *Clin Orthop* 1990;254:35-38.

Eighteen cadaver specimens underwent selective silicone rubber vascular injection and histologic examination. The articular side of the supraspinatus tendon insertion site showed consistent hypovascularity; the bursal side was well perfused.

Ogata S, Uhthoff HK: Acromial enthesopathy and rotator cuff tear: A radiologic and histologic postmortem investigation of the coracoacromial arch. *Clin Orthop* 1990;254:39-48.

Seventy-six autopsy specimens were dissected, and a positive correlation was found between the incidence of rotator cuff tears and increasing age. No such correlation was found between acromial degenerative changes and age. This implies that rotator cuff tearing occurs as a result of an intrinsic tendinopathy, and acromial changes occur secondarily.

Imaging

Bloom RA: The active abduction view: A new maneuver in the diagnosis of rotator cuff tears. *Skeletal Radiol* 1991;20:255-258.

Active abduction radiographs were obtained in 48 patients. Normal routine radiographs of the shoulder showed that 16 of the 48 had arthrographic evidence of complete rotator cuff tears. In seven of these 16 patients (44%) the acromiohumeral interval narrowed to 2 mm or less during active abduction.

Iannotti JP, Zlatkin MB, Esterhai JL, et al: Magnetic resonance imaging of the shoulder: Sensitivity, specificity, and predictive value. *J Bone Joint Surg* 1991;73A:17-29.

One hundred and six patients underwent magnetic resonance shoulder imaging with surgical confirmation. In complete tears, the sensitivity was 100% and the specificity was 95%. In differentiating tendinitis from tendon degeneration, the values were 82% and 85%, respectively.

Misamore GW, Woodward C: Evaluation of degenerative lesions of the rotator cuff: A comparison of arthrography and ultrasonography. *J Bone Joint Surg* 1991;73A:704-706.

In a prospective study of 32 patients with suspected rotator cuff disease, the results of ultrasonography were compared to arthrography with surgical confirmation. Ultrasonography was accurate in detecting 37% of partial and complete rotator cuff tears; arthrography was diagnostic in 87%.

Acromioplasty

Altchek DW, Warren RF, Wickiewicz TL, et al: Arthroscopic acromioplasty: Technique and results. *J Bone Joint Surg* 1990;72A:1198-1207.

Arthroscopic acromioplasty was performed in 40 patients (average age, 43.2) after at least six months of nonoperative therapy. The mean follow-up was 17 months. Satisfactory results were seen in 20 of 24 (83%) patients with intact rotator cuffs and stage 2 impingement syndrome, four of six patients with partial tears, and six of ten with complete tears.

Bosley RC: Total acromionectomy: A twenty-year review. *J Bone Joint Surg* 1991;73A:961-968.

At an average of 5.6 years following total acromionectomy for impingement syndrome, 29 of 34 shoulders (85%) achieved a satisfactory result. Secure deltoid repair was felt to be essential to the success of this operation.

Burkhart SS: Arthroscopic treatment of massive rotator cuff tears. *Clin Orthop* 1991;267:45-56.

Ten patients with painful, massive (>5 cm) complete rotator cuff tears were treated with arthroscopic acromioplasty and rotator cuff debridement. All ten obtained pain relief and normal motion and strength.

Gartsman GM: Arthroscopic acromioplasty for lesions of the rotator cuff. *J Bone Joint Surg* 1990;72A:169-180.

Patients who underwent arthroscopic acromioplasty had satisfactory results at an average of 31.2 months follow-up in 81 of 86 (94%) shoulders with stage 2 impingement syndrome, 33 of 40 (82%) with partial tears, and 14 of 25 (56%) with complete tears.

Norlin R: Arthroscopic subacromial decompression versus open acromioplasty. *Arthroscopy* 1989;5:321-323.

In a random prospective study, ten patients each were treated with either open or arthroscopic subacromial decompression. At short-term follow-up, range of motion returned more rapidly and recovery time was decreased in the arthroscopic surgery group.

Norwood LA, Fowler HL: Rotator cuff tears: A shoulder arthroscopy complication. *Am J Sports Med* 1989;17:837-841.

Four patients who had undergone shoulder arthroscopic surgery returned with persistent pain and had open rotator cuff repair surgery for iatrogenic partial tears in the supraspinatus tendon. This appeared to be a result of tendon damage caused by arthroscope insertion through a posterior portal site.

Ogilvie-Harris DJ, Wiley AM, Sattarian J: Failed acromioplasty for impingement syndrome. *J Bone Joint Surg* 1990;72B:1070-1072.

Sixty-seven patients with persistent symptoms for two or more years following open anterior acromioplasty were evaluated and treated. The cause of failure was felt to be secondary to diagnostic errors in 27 (40%) and operative errors in 28 (41%). Revision surgery yielded a success rate of 75% in patients not receiving worker's compensation.

Paulos LE, Franklin JL: Arthroscopic shoulder decompression development and application: A five year experience. *Am J Sports Med* 1990;18:235-244.

Eighty shoulders with refractory rotator cuff tendinitis were treated by arthroscopic decompression and achieved 80% satisfactory results at 32 month average follow-up. Additional pathology, including significant labral tears, biceps fraying, or loose bodies, was detected in 18 of 80 shoulders at the time of the intra-articular examination.

Snyder SJ, Pachelli AF, Del Pizzo W, et al: Partial thickness rotator cuff tears: Results of arthroscopic treatment. *Arthroscopy* 1991;7:1-7.

Thirty-one patients underwent arthroscopic debridement with or without arthroscopic decompression for partial thickness rotator cuff tears. Satisfactory results were achieved in 84% and extent of the partial tear did not influence the results. Subacromial decompression is recommended if bursal side tearing is present.

Rotator Cuff Repair

Gerber C: Latissimus dorsi transfer for the treatment of irreparable tears of the rotator cuff. *Clin Orthop* 1992;275:152-160.

Sixteen patients underwent latissimus dorsi transfers for massive rotator cuff tears, with an average follow-up of 33 months. Of patients with an intact subscapularis tendon preoperatively, 94% achieved satisfactory pain relief and had an average increase in active flexion of 67 degrees.

Harryman DT II, Mack LA, Wang KY, et al: Repairs of the rotator cuff: Correlation of functional results with integrity of the cuff. *J Bone Joint Surg* 1991;73A:982-989.

At an average of five years following rotator cuff repair surgery, 105 patients were evaluated with ultrasonography. Of repairs characterized as small or medium sized, 80% were intact at follow-up while less than 50% were intact if the tear involved more than the supraspinatus tendon. Pain relief remained satisfactory and was unrelated to the presence of retearing, but function deteriorated if retearing was present.

Visuri T, Kiviluoto O, Eskelin M: Carbon fiber for repair of the rotator cuff: A 4-year follow-up of 14 cases. *Acta Orthop Scand* 1991;62:356-359.

Four year median follow-up of 14 patients with medium to massive sized rotator cuff tears treated with a carbon fiber implant showed satisfactory results in 11 of 14 (78%).

Warner JP, Krushell RJ, Masquelet A, et al: Anatomy and relationships of the suprascapular nerve: Anatomical constraints to mobilization of the supraspinatus and infraspinatus muscles in the management of massive rotator-cuff tears. *J Bone Joint Surg* 1992;74A:36-45.

In 18 cadaver shoulders, mobilizing the supraspinatus or infraspinatus muscles more than 1 cm jeopardized the suprascapular nerve.

Update of Rotator Cuff Disease

Harryman DT II, Sidles JA, Clark JM, et al: Translation of the humeral head on the glenoid with passive glenohumeral motion. *J Bone Joint Surg* 1990;72A:1334-1343.

Posterior capsule contracture produces an obligatory anterosuperior translation of the humeral head.

Jobe FW, Tibone JE, Jobe CW, et al: The shoulder in sports, in Rockwood CA Jr, Matsen FA III (eds): *The Shoulder.* Philadelphia, WB Saunders, 1990, pp 961-989.

Biomechanics of the throwing motion and the relationship between impingement and instability are presented.

Neviaser RJ, Neviaser TJ, Neviaser JS: Concurrent rupture of the rotator cuff and anterior dislocation of the shoulder in the older patient. *J Bone Joint Surg* 1988;70A:1308-1311.

Thirty-one patents who were unable to abduct the involved arm after reduction of a primary anterior dislocation of the glenohumeral joint were found to have a ruptured rotator cuff. All of the patients were more than 35 years old. The incidence of axillary nerve injury was 7.8%.

Prosthetic Arthroplasty

Boyd AD Jr, Aliabadi P, Thornhill TS: Postoperative proximal migration in total shoulder arthroplasty: Incidence and significance. *J Arthroplasty* 1991;6:31-37.

One hundred and thirty-one total shoulder arthroplasties followed an average of 55 months showed proximal humeral component migration in 22% but were not associated with increased pain, loss of motion, or glenoid loosening. Proximal migration was not directly related to preoperative rotator cuff pathology.

Boyd AD Jr, Thomas WH, Scott RD, et al: Total shoulder arthroplasty versus hemiarthroplasty: Indications for glenoid resurfacing. *J Arthroplasty* 1990;5:329-336.

Sixty-four Neer hemiarthroplasties were compared with 59 total shoulder arthroplasties at 44 month follow-up. Functional improvement was similar. Pain relief was better after total shoulder arthroplasty in patients with rheumatoid arthritis. Although early pain relief was similar, patients with osteoarthritis experienced increasing discomfort following hemiarthroplasty with longer follow-up.

Brenner BC, Ferlic DC, Clayton ML, et al: Survivorship of unconstrained total shoulder arthroplasty. *J Bone Joint Surg* 1989;71A:1289-1296.

Fifty-three total shoulder arthroplasties were followed for an average of 67 months. After 11 years, 73% did not have revision surgery recommended to correct loosening or to relieve intractable pain. At follow-up, 82% continued to experience satisfactory pain relief.

Friedman RJ, Thornhill TS, Thomas WH, et al: Non-constrained total shoulder replacement in patients who have rheumatoid arthritis and class-IV function. *J Bone Joint Surg* 1989;71A:494-498.

Twenty-four unconstrained total shoulder arthroplasties were evaluated in patients with severe class IV functional capacity rheumatoid arthritis at 4.5-year average follow-up. Satisfactory pain relief was achieved in 92%, and 75% reported no significant functional limitations. Active elevation improved 88%.

Friedman RT, Laberge M, Dooley RL: Finite element modeling of the glenoid component: An effect of design parameter on stress distribution. *J Shoulder Elbow*, in press.

Finite element analysis showed that the stresses in surrounding bone are more physiologic with an all polyethylene glenoid component than with a metal-backed component.

Weiss AP, Adams MA, Moore JR, et al: Unconstrained shoulder arthroplasty: A five-year average follow-up study. *Clin Orthop* 1990;257:86-90.

Forty-two total shoulder arthroplasties with five-year average follow-up showed pain improvement in 94% and an average gain in active flexion of 47 degrees. Patients with preoperative rotator cuff tears experienced less improvement in function. Of glenoid components, 36% showed lucent lines. Superior migration was noted in 28%, all with preoperative rotator cuff tears.

Glenohumeral Arthropathy

Ingram RR: The shoulder in multiple epiphyseal dysplasia. *J Bone Joint Surg* 1991;73B:277-279.

In a study of 50 patients with multiple epiphyseal dysplasia, patients with minor epiphyseal abnormalities developed painful osteoarthritis and loss of motion in middle age, whereas patients with a "hatchet head" appearance developed loss of motion at an early age.

Leslie BM, Harris JM III, Driscoll D: Septic arthritis of the shoulder in adults. *J Bone Joint Surg* 1989;71A:1516-1522.

In a study of 18 patients with septic arthritis of the shoulder, all but one had a significant associated disease and eight had either a joint aspiration or intra-articular cortisone injection prior to the onset of symptoms. Open debridement yielded better results than repeated aspiration, but functional results remained poor.

MacDonald PB, Locht RC, Lindsay D, et al: Haemophilic arthropathy of the shoulder. *J Bone Joint Surg* 1990;72B:470-471.

In a study of 41 adult hemophiliac patients, 15 suffered shoulder symptoms. Eight of 12 studied with ultrasonography showed rotator cuff tears.

Acromioclavicular Joint

Gartsman GM, Combs AH, Davis PF, et al: Arthroscopic acromioclavicular joint resection: An anatomical study. *Am J Sports Med* 1991;19:2-5.

In ten cadaver shoulders, five each underwent either open or arthroscopic distal clavicle and medial acromion resection. Arthroscopic resection showed comparable accuracy to open resection.

Biceps

Snyder SJ, Karzel RP, Del Pizzo W, et al: SLAP lesions of the shoulder. *Arthroscopy* 1990;6:274-279.

Twenty-six patients underwent arthroscopic debridement for SLAP (superior labral anterior and posterior) lesions of the shoulder with satisfactory short-term follow-up.

Calcific Tendinitis

Gartner J, Simons B: Analysis of calcific deposits in calcifying tendinitis. *Clin Orthop* 1990; 254:111-120.

Twenty-five patients with calcific rotator cuff tendinitis had analysis of calcium deposits in the acute and chronic phases of disease. Little difference was found in the two phases. The deposits contained H_2O, CO_3, PO_4, and organic molecules, which were responsible for the deposit's binding properties.

Mavrikakis ME, Drimis S, Kontoyannis DA, et al: Calcific shoulder periarthritis (tendinitis) in adult onset diabetes mellitus: A controlled study. *Ann Rheum Dis* 1989;48:211-214.

Radiographic evidence of rotator cuff calcific tendinitis was found in 31.8% of 824 adult insulin-dependent diabetics; 320 nondiabetics had an incidence of 10.3%.

Suprascapular Neuropathy

Ogino T, Minami A, Kato H, et al: Entrapment neuropathy of the suprascapular nerve by a ganglion: A report of three cases. *J Bone Joint Surg* 1991;73A:141-147.

Three cases of suprascapular nerve entrapment are reported. All were caused by ganglia compression at the spinoglenoid notch and were successfully treated by decompression and ganglia excision.

Frozen Shoulder

Ozaki J, Nakagawa Y, Sakurai G, et al: Recalcitrant chronic adhesive capsulitis of the shoulder: Role of contracture of the coracohumeral ligament and rotator interval in pathogenesis and treatment. *J Bone Joint Surg* 1989;71A:1511-1515.

Seventeen surgically treated patients with recalcitrant adhesive capsulitis were shown to have significant contracture of the coracohumeral ligament and rotator interval. Resection of these structures relieved pain and restored motion.

Wiley AM: Arthroscopic appearance of frozen shoulder. *Arthroscopy* 1991;7:138-143.

In 150 patients with glenohumeral stiffness, 75% showed rotator cuff tears or impingement syndrome. Arthroscopic findings in the remaining 37 patients with primary frozen shoulder syndrome showed no intra-articular adhesions with vascular reaction around the biceps long-head tendon and opening into the subscapularis bursa.

28
Elbow and Forearm: Trauma

Anatomy and Biomechanics

The elbow is a hinged-pivotal joint with three articulations to allow 0 to 150 degrees of flexion through the ulnohumeral joint, as well as 75 degrees of pronation and 85 degrees of supination through the radiocapitellar and proximal radioulnar joints. Most activities of daily living are performed through a 100-degree functional arc of motion from 30 to 130 degrees of flexion for the elbow, as well as a 100-degree arc of motion for the forearm from 50 degrees of supination to 50 degrees of pronation. Pronation is favored by the dominant extremity for most activities of daily living, while supination is favored by the nondominant extremity. Arthrodesis of the elbow or the forearm severely impairs the ability to position the hand; hence, there is no one best position for arthrodesis.

Elbow

The stability of the elbow is determined by its congruous osseous anatomy and its ligament support.

The medial collateral ligament is the primary stabilizer of the elbow joint, consisting of the anterior oblique ligament, posterior oblique ligament, and small transverse ligament (Fig. 1). The anterior oblique ligament is strong and well-defined, arising from the inferior surface of the medial epicondyle to insert at a tubercle on the coronoid of the ulna. The humeral origin of the medial collateral ligament (MCL) lies posterior to the axis of elbow flexion, creating a cam effect, so that the anterior fibers are stressed in extension and the posterior fibers are stressed in flexion. The posterior oblique ligament, a weak fan-shaped thickening of the capsule, is absent in primates. The small transverse ligament is nonfunctional.

The lateral collateral ligament complex is primarily a thickening of the capsule consisting of the radial collateral ligament, the lateral ulnar collateral ligament, and the accessory collateral ligament (Fig. 2). The radial collateral ligament proper arises from the lateral epicondyle and inserts onto the annular ligament. The lateral ulnar collateral ligament passes over the annular ligament to insert onto the supinator tubercle of the ulna. The flexion axis of the elbow passes through the origin of the lateral collateral ligament so the length of the structure does not change during elbow flexion.

In vitro cadaveric studies have defined the ligamentous and osseous contributions to valgus stability for the elbow. The MCL, specifically the anterior oblique ligament, is the primary stabilizer of the elbow for the functional range of motion from 20 to 120 degrees of flexion. In flexion, the medial collateral ligament provides 54%

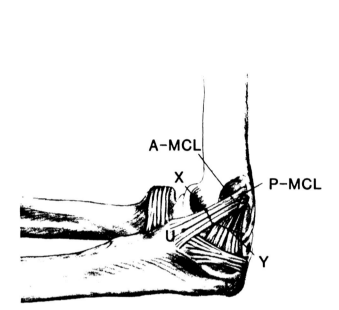

Fig. 1 Classic representation of the medial collateral ligament complex. (Reproduced with permission from Mayo Foundation.)

of the valgus stability, while the osseous articulation provides 33% of the stability, and the capsule 10% of the stability (Table 1). The radial head is the most important secondary stabilizer to valgus stress. The flexor pronator mass is a dynamic contributor to valgus stability.

In a recent cadaveric model simulating active elbow motion and muscle activity, serial release of the MCL and excision of the radial head was performed to define the primary and secondary constraints of valgus stability. When the MCL was intact, the radial head could be resected with no significant effect on valgus stability. When the MCL was released, some joint instability was observed, but abduction rotation measured only 6 to 8 degrees in the model with an intact radial head. However, resection of both the MCL and radial head resulted in gross instability of the elbow, observing elbow subluxation and dislocation with applied muscle stress.

Insufficiency of the medial collateral ligament can be inferred from gravity stress radiography. With the patient supine, the shoulder is externally rotated and the elbow flexed to 30 degrees to clear the olecranon fossa. If the elbow is unstable, the weight of the forearm will open the medial ulnohumeral joint with gravity stress, implying rupture of the MCL and flexor pronator mass. With

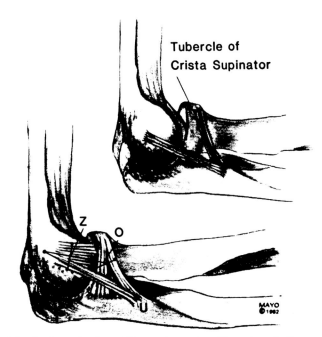

Fig. 2 Lateral collateral ligament complex. (Reproduced with permission from Mayo Foundation.)

Table 1. Contribution to resist applied valgus stress*

| | Valgus Stress, 3 Degrees Position | |
	Extended	90 Degrees
Medial collateral ligament	31	54
Soft tissue, capsule	38	10
Osseous, articulation	31	33

*Mean percent, four specimens
(Reproduced with permission from Morrey BF, An KN: Articular and ligamentous contributions to the stability of the elbow joint. *Am J Sports Med* 1983;11:315-319.)

Table 2. Contribution to resist applied varus stress*

| | Valgus Stress, 3 Degrees Position | |
	Extended	90 Degrees
Lateral collateral ligament	14	9
Soft tissue, capsule	32	13
Osseous, articulation	55	75

*Mean percent, four specimens
(Reproduced with permission from Morrey BF, An KN: Articular and ligamentous contributions to the stability of the elbow joint. *Am J Sports Med* 1983;11:315-319.)

regard to varus stability, the lateral collateral ligament accounts for 9% of stability to varus stress, while the osseous ulnohumeral articulation accounts for 75% of stability, and the capsule for 13% of stability (Table 2). The anconeus is a dynamic contributor to varus stability.

Laxity of the lateral collateral ligament complex can be demonstrated by a lateral pivot-shift test of the proxi-

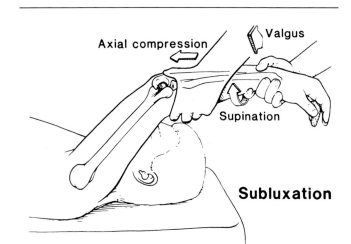

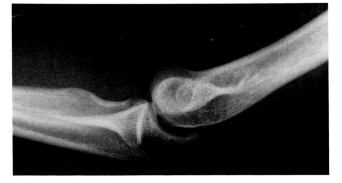

Fig. 3 **Top**, Lateral pivot-shift test. The same procedure is performed much more easily with the arm over the patient's head. Full external rotation of the shoulder provides a counterforce for the supination of the forearm and leaves one hand of the examiner free to control valgus moments. **Bottom**, In the lateral radiograph the radiohumeral joint is dislocated posterolaterally, and there is rotatory subluxation of the ulnohumeral joint. The semilunar notch of the ulna is rotated away from the trochlea. (Reproduced with permission from O'Driscoll SW, Bell DF, Morrey BF: Posterolateral rotatory instability of the elbow. *J Bone Joint Surg* 1991;73A:441-443.)

mal ulna on the humerus, indicating posterolateral rotatory instability (Fig. 3). Supination of the forearm with a valgus moment and axial compression while the elbow is flexed 40 degrees from full extension will produce a sudden reduction of subluxation if instability is present.

Anterior and posterior stability of the elbow is highly dependent on the osseous articulations. The trochlea is spool-shaped and firmly seated into the olecranon under usual compressive loads. Insufficiency or absence of the coronoid will result in posterior instability.

Forearm

Malalignment of the radius or ulna in the forearm will impair range of motion of the forearm. With simulated fractures of both bones in cadavers, a 10-degree angulatory deformity resulted in an 18% loss of pronation-supination, and a 15-degree angulatory deformity resulted in a 27% loss of forearm rotation. Angulation greater than 20 degrees, or any rotational deformity, significantly impaired forearm rotation. Deformity at the mid-shaft was more limiting than deformity distal in the forearm.

Recent studies have also demonstrated the importance of the interosseous membrane to axial stability of the forearm, particularly after radial head excision. One cadaveric study reported the central band of the interosseous membrane contributed 71% of the longitudinal stiffness of the forearm, while the triangular fibrocartilage complex (TFCC) contributes 8%. Another study emphasized the importance of both the interosseous membrane (IOM) (50%) and the TFCC (50%) to forearm stability. Sectioning either the IOM or the TFCC with the radial head fracture resulted in 3 to 7 mm of proximal migration under axial load across the forearm. Sectioning both of these structures resulted in 12 to 23 mm of proximal migration of the radius, which remained displaced after removal of the stress.

The potential for proximal migration of the radius can be identified with stress testing for axial instability. A stress anteroposterior radiograph performed with the forearm under axial compression is compared to an anteroposterior radiograph with the forearm under axial distraction. A change in ulnar variance exceeding 10 mm suggests insufficiency of the interosseous membrane, or axial instability of the forearm.

Adult Fractures and Dislocations

Simple Elbow Dislocations

Dislocations of the elbow usually result from a fall onto the outstretched extended elbow. In fact, the anatomic morphology of the semilunar notch may predispose to elbow dislocation. The central angle of the semilunar notch was found to be significantly large in a group of patients who had dislocation of the elbow compared to normals.

Elbow dislocations without fracture are termed "simple." These dislocations are classified according to the direction of dislocation, namely posterior, posterolateral, posteromedial, lateral, medial, or divergent.

The pathoanatomy of the simple elbow dislocation includes rupture of the capsule, rupture of the medial collateral ligament, rupture of the flexor pronator mass to a variable extent, injury to the brachialis muscle, and perhaps even chondral damage. Rupture of the brachial artery has been reported and requires an index of suspicion, confirmed by arteriography. Neuropraxia is reported in 20% of cases, usually involving the ulnar or median nerves. Most neurologic deficits are transient and will resolve. Entrapment of the medial nerve within the elbow joint after manipulation is more common in children.

Gentle closed reduction of the elbow is recommended, usually under general anesthesia, with early return to

protected motion. Repeated manipulations should be avoided. Longitudinal traction followed by flexion of the elbow usually succeeds in obtaining a congruent reduction. Passive range of motion to within 20 degrees of full extension without subluxation implies a stable reduction, and best results are obtained with early protected motion begun before two weeks. Inherent stability of the osseous articulation will allow for early flexion and extension if exacerbating valgus stress is prevented after reduction. No enhancement from open repair of the medial collateral ligament over closed management has been documented for simple elbow dislocations.

The final clinical outcome for simple dislocations of the elbow is dramatically affected by the duration of immobilization. While mild loss of extension is a common sequela, prolonged immobilization over two weeks is associated with greater flexion contracture and more pain at follow-up, and does not decrease symptoms of instability. Recurrent dislocation is unusual. Redislocation of an elbow with passive range of motion or redislocation in plaster implies severe valgus instability with rupture of both the MCL and flexor forearm muscles. Under these circumstances, repair of the medial collateral ligament is mandatory.

Neglected or unrecognized chronic dislocation of the elbow may benefit from open reduction for salvage. A series reported 70% recovery of flexion-extension movement and 40% recovery of forearm rotation, even when open reduction was performed at six weeks or later.

Complex Elbow Dislocations

Dislocations of the elbow associated with fracture are termed "complex," and comprise 49% of elbow dislocations. Complex dislocations are the exception to closed management, since most are inherently unstable, and usually require surgery. Again, prolonged elbow immobilization produces poor results. Operative intervention must achieve sufficient stability to allow early range of motion. Fractures associated with elbow dislocation may include the medial epicondyle, coronoid process, or the radial head.

Dislocations With Medial Epicondyle Fracture Following closed reduction, the medial epicondyle fracture is classified with regard to displacement. If it is displaced less than 5 mm and does not move with gentle valgus stress test, then continued closed treatment is indicated. Open reduction and internal fixation of the fracture is indicated for displacement exceeding 10 mm, severe valgus instability (suggested by a positive gravity stress test), associated ulnar nerve symptoms, or incarceration of the fragment within the ulnohumeral joint.

Dislocations With Coronoid Process Fracture These fractures have recently been classified. Type I is an avulsion of the tip of the coronoid process, type II is a fragment involving less than 50% of the process, and type III is a fragment involving more than 50% of the process

(Fig. 4). Closed reduction and early motion within three weeks of injury is recommended for type I or type II fractures. Type III coronoid fractures are unstable and associated with a high redislocation rate. These fractures require open reduction and internal fixation to restore anteroposterior stability, as well as valgus stability since the MCL inserts onto the fracture fragment.

Dislocations With Radial Head Fracture   The treatment of elbow dislocations associated with radial head fractures remains controversial. The radial head is an important secondary stabilizer, and open reduction and internal fixation of the radial head is preferable to excision if the fracture is salvageable. If radial head excision is dictated by severe comminution, then use of a Silastic or metallic radial head prosthesis may be necessary as a temporary spacer. The prosthesis will serve as a secondary stabilizer to valgus stress during healing of the medial collateral ligament. Furthermore, open repair of the medial collateral ligament and flexor pronator mass may be required in these cases as well. Intraoperative use of valgus stress with the spacer in place will help with surgical decision-making.

Most of these Silastic prostheses may later fracture at the head-stem junction, but associated synovitis is usually mild and will respond to removal of the implant. The long-term clinical and radiographic results of 46 High-Performance Silastic radial head prostheses in 39 patients were assessed at follow-up of 7.2 years. Radiographic failure was demonstrated in 41 of 46 cases, or 89%. The spacer effect was maintained in 52%, but compromised in 48%. Reoperation was needed in 20%, usually removal.

Supracondylar and T-Y Fractures

Supracondylar fractures   These fractures are classified by the displacement of the distal fragment. The most common type of supracondylar fracture is a posteriorly displaced fracture, usually due to an extension injury. Nondisplaced fractures can be treated with splinting or even percutaneous pinning. However, most supracondylar fractures in adults are displaced or have intra-articular extension of the fracture, and will require open reduction and internal fixation in order to begin early motion.

Transcondylar fractures   These fractures are supracondylar fractures that occur within the capsule of the elbow joint. They are most commonly encountered in elderly patients with osteoporotic bone. Treatment alternatives include percutaneous K-wire fixation, overhead olecranon pin traction, or anatomic restoration with open reduction and internal fixation. Poor bone quality makes fixation difficult, and total elbow arthroplasty may be

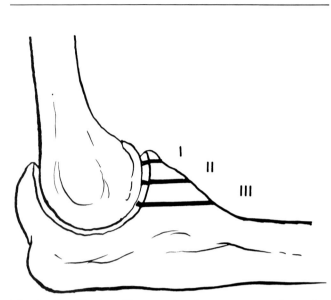

Fig. 4   Classification of fractures into three types according to the degree of involvement of the coronoid process. (Reproduced with permission from Regan W, Morrey B: Fractures of the coronoid process of the ulna. *J Bone Joint Surg* 1989;71A:1348-1354.)

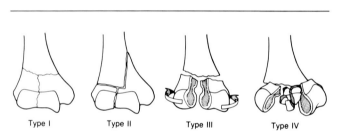

Type I   Type II   Type III   Type IV

Fig. 5   Riseborough and Radin's classification of intercondylar fractures. (Reproduced with permission from Henley MB, Bone LB, Parker B: Operative management of displaced intraarticular fractures of the distal humerus. *J Orthop Trauma* 1987;1:24-35.)

indicated primarily or as a salvage procedure for elderly patients.

Intercondylar fractures   These fractures of the distal humerus are the result of an additional wedging force transmitted by the ulna into the trochlea between the condyles. The condyles will split with various degrees of displacement, rotation, and comminution (Fig. 5). Type I nondisplaced fractures are very rare, and can be treated with cast immobilization. Displaced type II or type III fractures are best treated with accurate open reduction and rigid internal fixation. Surgical exposure of the fracture can be obtained with a triceps-sparing approach or olecranon osteotomy. The articular surface is restored using interfragmentary lag screw reconstruction of the condyles. The condyles are then stabilized to the humeral shaft with medial and lateral plates. The coronoid and olecranon fossa must not be violated with fixation.

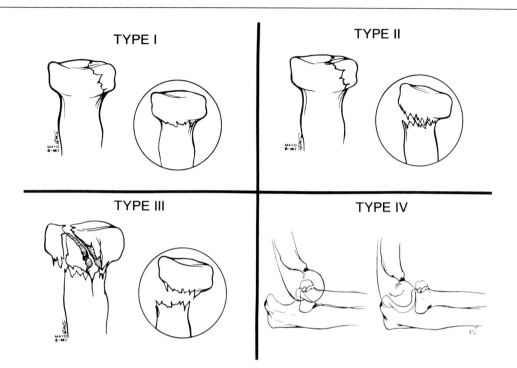

Fig. 6 Mason classification of radial head fractures. (Reproduced with permission from Broberg MA, Morrey BF: Results of treatment of fracture dislocations of the elbow. *Clin Orthop* 1987;216:109-119.)

Ulnar nerve transposition may be required. Successful outcome requires meticulous surgical technique, stable internal skeletal fixation, and early controlled postoperative mobilization within two weeks. In type IV fractures with comminution, it is more difficult to obtain stable internal fixation. Even so, open reduction and internal fixation to obtain adequate reduction of the articular surface is still recommended, despite being technically demanding. Care should be taken not to narrow the width of the trochlea spool by overcompressing the condyles, and bone grafting may be necessary.

Nonunion of fractures of the distal humerus usually occurs when stable internal fixation has not been achieved and is a difficult problem. While radiographic union was obtained in 17 of 18 cases with repeat open reduction and internal fixation and bone grafting, patients continued to have long-term disability secondary to limited motion. In a mobile elbow, the plate should be positioned posteriorly or laterally. In a stiff elbow, the plate should be positioned anteriorly on the humerus. Some nonunions of the supracondylar humerus in elderly patients can be salvaged with semiconstrained total elbow arthroplasty.

Capitellum Fractures

The type I, or Hahn-Steinthal, fracture is a fracture of the capitellum in the coronal plane. The fracture hinges anteriorly between the radial head and radial fossa, producing a block to flexion. If closed reduction can be ob-

tained, then the reduction is usually stable with elbow flexion. Open reduction and internal fixation of the fracture with Herbert screw fixation, followed by early range of motion, has been reported to give excellent results. The advantages of Herbert screw fixation are several, namely the jig maintains the reduction and compresses the fracture, the screw is buried beneath the cartilage and does not need to be removed, and fixation does not require detachment of the lateral collateral ligament. If the fracture is comminuted, then excision is recommended.

The type II, or Kocher-Lorenz, fracture is a sleeve fracture of the articular surface with little osseous bone. Healing potential is minimal and excision is recommended for these injuries.

Radial Head Fractures

Mason's classification is the most widely accepted and is useful for treatment (Fig. 6). Radial head fractures can be "isolated," but might also be associated with fracture of the capitellum, rupture of the triceps tendon, valgus instability of the elbow due to rupture of the medial collateral ligament, or axial instability of the forearm due to tearing of the interosseous membrane and distal radial ulnar joint ligaments. These associated injuries will have important therapeutic implications.

Type I fractures are nondisplaced and may be missed on routine radiographic views. A posterior fat pad sign should suggest further oblique views, including the radial head-capitellum (RHC) view. Mason type I fractures are adequately treated with brief splinting, followed by early mobilization to minimize posttraumatic stiffness.

Type II fractures are marginal radial head fractures with displacement, depression, or angulation. Treatment options include brief protection and early motion, open reduction and internal fixation, or excision of displaced radial head fragments. Because the results of late excision of the radial head have been shown to be as good as those for early excision, conservation management is usually indicated initially. Open reduction and internal fixation of large fragments may be accomplished with small mini-fragmentary screws or Herbert screws. Excellent results were obtained for Mason type II fractures in recent series, with less than 4 degrees flexion contracture. The fixation must be subarticular so as to not impinge on the proximal radioulnar joint during forearm rotation. If stable anatomic reduction cannot be obtained, then the fracture fragment should be excised.

Comminuted fractures of the entire head are classified as type III fractures. These fractures require excision. The long-term result for excision of the "isolated" radial head fracture with competent MCL and interosseous membrane are good. However, if the fracture is associated with valgus instability of the elbow due to medial collateral ligament insufficiency, replacement with a Silastic or metallic radial head prosthesis may be necessary to serve as a temporary spacer following repair of the MCL and flexor-pronator mass. Similarly, if the radial head fracture is associated with axial instability of the forearm due to interosseous membrane insufficiency, use of the radial head prosthesis may be necessary to minimize proximal migration of the radius. To this end, stress radiography is mandatory to assess the potential for valgus instability of the elbow, or for proximal migration of the radius in the forearm, when deciding to use a radial head implant.

Essex-Lopresti Lesion

A violent longitudinal force across the forearm, usually a fall from a height, may result in fracture of the radial head associated with disruption of the distal radioulnar joint ligaments and the interosseous membrane in the forearm (Fig. 7). Excision of the radial head will lead to disastrous proximal migration of the radius, resulting in pain at the wrist due to ulnacarpal impingement, and pain at the elbow due to radiocapitellar impingement. Late reconstruction of the instability is poor. Suboptimal results are reported for cases where definitive management was delayed four to ten weeks. The lesion must be recognized early. Open reduction and internal fixation of the radial head is recommended, or use of the Silastic radial head prosthesis if excision is unavoidable. Restoration of radial length and stabilization of the distal radioulnar joint with pinning for six weeks is necessary to allow for anatomic healing of the interosseous membrane. The radial head spacer alone does not restore satisfactory axial stability without pinning the distal radioulnar joint.

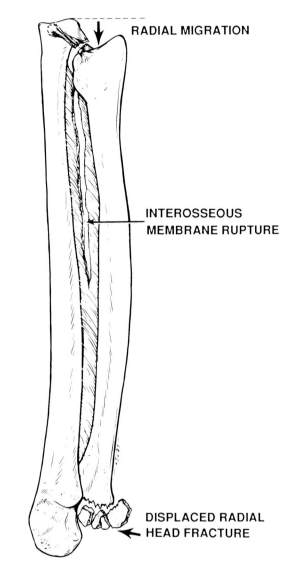

Fig. 7 Essex-Lopresti lesion. (Reproduced with permission from Edwards GS Jr, Jupiter JB: Radial head fractures with acute radioulnar dislocation: Essex-Lopresti revisited. *Clin Orthop* 1988;234:61-69.)

Olecranon Fractures

Olecranon fractures usually result from a direct blow to the olecranon with the elbow in flexion, or occasionally from indirect trauma onto the outstretched arm with sudden contraction of the triceps. Nondisplaced olecranon fractures can be treated with elbow immobilization in 40 degrees of flexion for three weeks, followed by a protected range of motion. Displaced fractures of the proximal olecranon will require open reduction and internal fixation of the fracture to restore triceps tendon function and minimize posttraumatic arthritis of the ulnohumeral joint secondary to joint incongruity. Tension band wiring with intramedullary 6.5-mm cancellous screws or parallel K-wires is generally recommended. Intramedullary fixation without the tension banding is not reliable. However, long oblique fractures of the proximal olecranon may be internally fixed with bicortical screw fixation. The triceps tendon expansions are also repaired at the time of surgery. Articular surface incongruity greater than 2 mm was associated with poor results in one study, although presence of gaps in the intra-articular surface of the semilunar notch of the ulna produced no ill effects and was compatible with excellent results. Symptomatic metal prominence is particularly common after AO tension band wiring, as frequent as 80% in one series. Minor loss of terminal elbow extension is common, but not functionally significant.

In elderly patients with comminution, excision of up to 50% of the olecranon with repair of the triceps tendon to the subarticular surface has been recommended. A postoperative regimen of three weeks immobilization followed by protected range of motion resulted in a range of motion from 10 to 120 degrees flexion, with no complaints of pain and no clinical evidence of instability.

Fractures of the Radius and Ulna

In the adult, displaced diaphyseal fractures of the radius and ulna should be treated with open reduction and internal fixation, utilizing the 3.5-mm AO dynamic compression plate. A recent large series confirmed union in 98% of fractures, with 92% of patients achieving excellent or satisfactory functional results. Rigid adherence to AO principles is necessary for success. Axial and rotational alignment must be achieved, and the radial bow must be maintained. Rigid internal fixation with compression technique should utilize at least a five-hole plate with interfragmentary screw compression if possible. Comminution involving more than one third of the circumference of the shaft may necessitate bone grafting. The bone grafting should be away from the interosseous membrane to decrease the risk for synostosis. Both bone fractures of the forearm should be approached through two separate incisions to minimize the risk for cross-union. Segmental defects of the diaphysis can be managed with interposed tricortical iliac crest bone graft incorporated into the fixation. By affixing the iliac crest graft to the plate with one or two screws, early postoperative range of motion can be permitted. If necessary, one of the bones can be shortened as much as 5 cm.

Cross-union complicating fracture of the forearm has been classified. Type I cross-union is between the distal intra-articular part of the radius and ulna. Type II cross-union involves the middle third or nonarticular distal third of the radius and ulna, and type III cross-union involves the proximal third of the radius and ulna. Type I cross-union was rare and occurred after fractures of the intra-articular distal radius that were managed with closed reduction. These cross-unions frequently recurred

after excision. Type II and III cross-unions were associated with delayed open reduction, presence of bone fragments in the interosseous space between the radius and ulna, use of inappropriately long screws that protruded through the opposite cortex, and severe trauma or head injury. Results of excision for type II cross-unions were better than for type III.

Debate still continues over the need for removal of internal fixation from the forearm. Refracture may occur through an unhealed fracture site if the plate is removed prematurely, through a screw hole if the forearm is not protected following plate removal, or even through a screw hole of a still implanted plate. Studies with single photon absorptiometry suggest that plates should be retained for at least 21 months to allow bone density to return to its prefracture level before removal of the plates. The forearm should be protected for six weeks following removal. Fractures with greater initial displacement or comminution, plating with the 4.5-mm DCP, early plate removal, and lack of post-removal protection are associated with increased risk for refracture.

Monteggia Fractures

Fracture of the ulnar shaft associated with dislocation of the radial head has been classified as type I through IV by Bado (Fig. 8). Monteggia fractures in adults usually require anatomic and rigid open reduction and internal fixation of the ulna, with complete and usually closed reduction of the radial head. Early range of motion is necessary to avoid limited elbow or forearm motion.

Galeazzi Fractures

Fracture of the distal third of the radius associated with dislocation of the distal radial ulnar joint is referred to as Galeazzi's fracture, the reverse Monteggia's fracture, the Piedmont fracture, or the "fracture of necessity." Open reduction and internal fixation of the radius with compression plating on the volar surface of the radius is recommended, with closed reduction of the distal radioulnar joint. Reduction of the distal radioulnar joint is maintained with immobilization of the forearm in supination, or stabilization with K-wire fixation for six weeks.

"Night Stick" Fractures

Isolated fractures of the ulnar shaft with minimal displacement can be successfully treated with functional bracing. Displaced ulnar shaft fractures will require open reduction and internal fixation.

Pediatric Fractures and Dislocations

Elbow Dislocations

Elbow dislocations are a relatively uncommon injury in

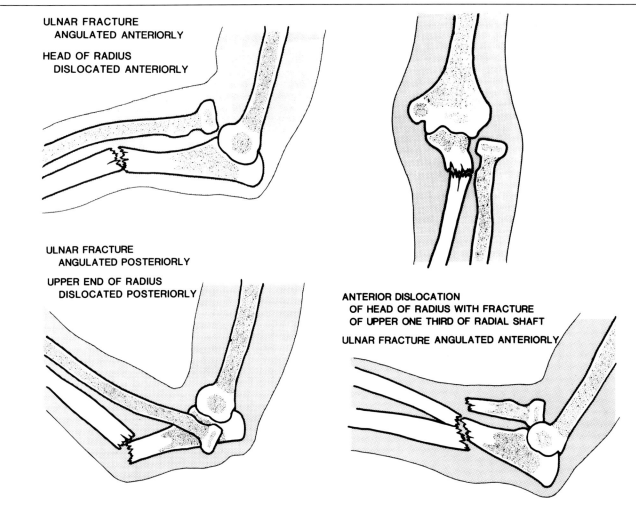

ULNAR FRACTURE
ANGULATED ANTERIORLY

HEAD OF RADIUS
DISLOCATED ANTERIORLY

ULNAR FRACTURE
ANGULATED POSTERIORLY

UPPER END OF RADIUS
DISLOCATED POSTERIORLY

ANTERIOR DISLOCATION
OF HEAD OF RADIUS WITH FRACTURE
OF UPPER ONE THIRD OF RADIAL SHAFT

ULNAR FRACTURE ANGULATED ANTERIORLY

Fig. 8 Monteggia lesions. **Top left**, Type 1 Monteggia lesion. **Top right**, Type 2 Monteggia lesion. **Bottom left**, Type 3 Monteggia lesion. **Bottom right**, Type 4 Monteggia lesion. (Reproduced with permission from Olney BW, Menelaus MB: Monteggia and equivalent lesions in childhood. *J Pediatr Orthop* 1989;9:219-223.)

children; the incidence being 3% to 6% of all elbow injuries depending on the series quoted. The peak incidence occurs in adolescence between the ages of 13 and 14 years.

Posterior dislocations of the elbow in children must be carefully assessed for associated fractures or neurovascular injury. Since ossification of the medial epicondyle can be delayed until age 5 years, associated displacement of the apophysis of the medial epicondyle may be missed. An entrapped medial epicondyle may be mistaken for a trochlear ossification center. Furthermore, distal humerus epiphyseal separation injuries may be confused with elbow dislocations, especially since these injuries are most common in children under 2 years of age. A recent review of 12 cases of fracture separation of the distal humeral epiphysis noted four cases to be initially misdiagnosed.

Postreduction radiographs are necessary and should be scrutinized for possible soft or bony tissue interposition in the joint space. Careful postoperative neurovascular examination must be performed. The patient should be monitored for 12 to 24 hours after reduction for any late neurovascular compromise.

Intra-articular entrapment of the median nerve may follow close reduction of elbow dislocations in children. The diagnosis of median nerve entrapment is often delayed. A proximal median nerve deficit, limited passive elbow motion, or an associated medial epicondyle avulsion after reduction should alert the surgeon to the possibility of a nerve entrapment. Management consists of early surgical exploration. Prolonged entrapment of the median nerve may result in a depression on the posterior surface of the medial epicondylar ridge, known as Matev's sign.

In a series of 58 traumatic dislocations, closed reduction failed in 10% of cases. Failure to achieve closed reduction should suggest an entrapped medial epicondyle, an inverted cartilaginous flap, or an osteochondral fragment.

Late posttraumatic sequelae following simple dislocation in children are rare, with better outcomes than in adults. A 24-year follow-up of 28 pediatric dislocations demonstrated few residual symptoms and a flexion contracture averaging 4 degrees.

Management of untreated posterior dislocations of the elbow three or more weeks after injury may require open reduction. A posterior approach with lengthening of the triceps, removal of fibrous tissue, and possible K-wire stabilization has been recommended.

Supracondylar Fractures

Supracondylar fractures in children may be nondisplaced or displaced. Nondisplaced supracondylar fractures (Gartland type I) can be managed with careful splinting with the elbow in 110 to 120 degrees of flexion, followed by protected range of motion at three weeks.

Most displaced supracondylar fractures (Gartland type III) are of the extension type (97%). Fractures of the extension type are associated with the most serious complications and the highest rate of residual cosmetic deformity. A medial spike may tether the median nerve or the brachial artery. A lateral spike may tether the radial nerve. Anterior interosseous nerve injury is frequently missed because of the lack of sensory changes. The diagnosis is made by discreet functional deficit of the flexor pollicis longus and the flexor digitorum longus to the index finger. All suspected extension-type supracondylar fractures should be initially splinted in 20 degrees of elbow flexion pending evaluation and treatment. Vascular injury is the most serious complication. If the radial pulse is absent, but the hand is well profused without evidence of ischemia, there is no need for immediate arteriography. In 17 cases with vascular impairment, 14 cases were managed successfully with rapid reduction and K-wire stabilization, indicating the correct way to proceed. If the pulse has not returned within 24 hours of close observation, arteriography followed by exploration and repair of the problem is probably indicated. If the hand is not profused, then immediate exploration of the artery at the fracture site is indicated. A radial pulse present before reduction and absent after reduction should suggest the possibility of arterial entrapment in the fracture site.

A large review of displaced supracondylar fractures of the humerus in children with several different treatments demonstrated best results with traction techniques or well-performed Kirschner pin transfixion. The worst results occurred with manipulation and splint immobilization alone. Displaced fractures are usually best managed with closed reduction followed by percutaneous pinning. Fluoroscopic C-arm control under general anesthesia is used to inspect the reduction in extension. The pinning allows maintenance of the reduction with the elbow at 90 degrees of flexion to allow for swelling.

To obtain closed reduction, length is first restored by using countertraction, followed by realignment of the distal fragment to the humeral shaft. Then medial or lateral displacement of the distal fragment is corrected, as well as rotation. The elbow is flexed while pushing the distal fragment anterior to reduce it. Flexion is maintained to hold the reduction while the pins are placed. If the initial displacement of the distal fragment was medial, the forearm is then pronated to tighten the medial periosteal hinge. If the initial displacement of the distal fragment was lateral, the forearm is then supinated to tighten the lateral periosteal hinge. Anatomic reduction should be confirmed with multiple fluoroscopic views, including oblique views. Repetitive manipulation should be avoided in the treatment of these injuries.

Either two lateral pins, or one lateral and one medial pin may be used and both should penetrate the cortex. Biomechanics studies have showed that the latter technique provides better stabilization. Baumann's angle, the angle between the long axis of the humeral shaft and the growth plate of the capitellum, will reliably predict the final carrying angle after reduction. This method of treatment is especially useful in management of cases with severe swelling that prohibits flexion of the elbow due to vascular compromise, and in cases with other concomitant fractures in the same extremity. Skin or skeletal traction are also treatment options for severe swelling, severe displacement, or a late presentation of the injury.

Cubitus varus deformity, the most common complication following supracondylar fracture, results from malrotation of the fragments, which then permits the distal fragment to tilt into varus. Thus, a small amount of medial or lateral displacement or a small amount of anterior or posterior angulation may be tolerated, but any malrotation should not be accepted. Rotation is verified radiographically with the anteroposterior view, the lateral view, and both oblique views, which profile the medial and lateral condyles and can demonstrate which one is not completely reduced. If reduction cannot be obtained, there may be soft-tissue interposition and open reduction is indicated.

Nerve and vessel injuries are the most serious complications associated with the supracondylar fracture. Nerve injuries occur in 7.7% of the fractures with the radial nerve being the most commonly injured. It is generally injured by the anterior spike of the proximal fragment of the humerus in the supracondylar fracture with posterior medial displacement.

The next most common neural injury is to the median nerve. This is typically seen injured in the posterior laterally displaced supracondylar fracture and is frequently associated with vascular injuries.

The most dreaded complication, Volkmann's ischemic contracture, is rarely seen today. Its occurrence is not necessarily associated with an absent radial pulse, but is best thought of in terms of the pathophysiology and diagnosis of a compartment syndrome of the forearm. This fact underlines the importance of eliminating venous obstruction at the elbow to avoid this complication.

Humeral Physeal Fractures

Distal humeral physeal fractures are classified according to the degree of ossification of the lateral condyle. The first is in infants where the lateral condyle is totally unossified. A second type of distal humeral physeal fracture is characterized by the appearance of an ossified lateral condyle. A third type has an ossified lateral condyle, accompanied by a large metaphyseal fragment. These occur mainly in older children and can be confused with lateral condyle fractures.

A significantly displaced distal humeral physeal fracture can be reduced in a method similar to that of the supracondylar fracture. Utilizing image intensification, longitudinal traction is applied after the distal fragment has been aligned with the more proximal fragment. The traction is initiated with the elbow held at approximately 20 to 30 degrees of flexion with pressure being applied along the proximal forearm in line with the long axis of the humerus. This allows the distal fragment to be distracted past the end of the more proximal fragment. Once this is accomplished, the elbow is flexed, which allows the distal fragment to ride anteriorly and lock onto the more proximal fragment.

Lateral Condyle Fractures

The most common injury to the distal humeral physis is the fracture of the lateral condyle. This injury comprises almost 17% of all distal humeral fractures and 54% of all distal humeral physeal injuries. This fracture has been classically described as being a Salter-Harris type IV physeal fracture. Treatment of this fracture depends again on the amount of displacement. Less severe displacement may also have a translational component. There is a significant step-off of the lateral cortex, which, despite a narrow fracture line, indicates that there is significant articular discontinuity. An oblique radiograph of the distal humerus with the arm internally rotated will best demonstrate the amount of displacement and rotation of the lateral condyle fragment.

If treated closed, the patient returns for radiographic examination between two and three weeks later. The cast is removed and radiographs are taken in the anteroposterior and oblique positions to demonstrate the lateral condyle. If the fracture is not displaced, it is not likely to displace and the cast treatment is continued. If the fracture has displaced, proceed with surgical reduction.

An open reduction is indicated in those fractures with displacement of the fracture fragment. It is generally performed through a Kocher incision placed over the lateral aspect of the elbow. The posterior aspect of the fracture fragment should be left unmolested because that is the source of the blood supply to the capitellum and the adjacent cartilaginous structures.

Once a congruent reduction is obtained it can be held in place by applying two K-wires in a divergent or parallel fashion through puncture wounds in the skin posterior and lateral to the initial skin incision.

Fractures of the lateral condyle are associated with several complications. The classic deformity associated with a lateral condyle fracture is that of cubitus valgus. This may occur with or without union of the condylar fragment. Treatment involves establishing a union of the lateral condylar fragment with or without a varus-producing osteotomy to realign the valgus deformity, depending on its severity. Reduction of the fragment is difficult in late cases and should be attempted only when the fragment is severely displaced.

A tardy ulnar nerve palsy appears as a late complication. This is generally associated with a nonunion and subsequent cubitus valgus formation. The symptoms are gradual in onset with motor loss occurring prior to sensory changes. It is generally felt that the best treatment for this problem is anterior transposition of the ulnar nerve.

Medial Condyle Fractures

Fracture of this condyle is rare and comprises only approximately 0.3% of distal humeral physeal fractures. Treatment is based on the degree of displacement. Less displaced fractures can be treated easily with elbow flexion and neutral forearm rotation. More extensive displacement requires open reduction and internal fixation by a posterior medial approach. Due to its predominantly cartilaginous nature, this portion of the fracture fragment is healed in about three to four weeks and the pins can be safely removed and range of motion begun.

Avascular necrosis of the trochlea is an uncommon but interesting result of trauma to the distal humeral physis. It occurs because of damage to one of the multiple sources of blood supply to the distal humeral physis. This has been observed after both medial and lateral condyle fractures, as well as supracondylar fractures.

Radial Neck Fractures

In children, fractures of the proximal radius involve the physis or the neck in 90% of instances and are usually Salter-Harris type II fractures. This may result in angulation or lateral translation of the radial head to a varying degree (Jeffrey type I). Total displacement, especially in a posterior direction, may occur following spontaneous relocation of an elbow dislocation (Jeffrey type II).

In a younger child, up to 10 degrees of residual neck angulation will correct spontaneously with growth, and up to 30 degrees of residual angulation can be accepted. If the angulation is greater than 30 degrees, closed manipulative reduction, as advocated by Patterson, is recommended, or use of a percutaneous pin to manipulate the fracture. Poor results are associated with age greater than 10 years, residual angulation greater than 30 degrees, or translocation greater than 3 mm. Inability to reduce angulation less than 45 degrees, or to reduce severe displacement, may require open reduction and internal fixation. Crossed K-wire fixation of the proximal radius is preferred. Radiocapitellar transfixion with K-wires should be avoided, because the wire usually breaks. Excision of the radial head in children is disastrous, with uniformly poor results due to cubitus valgus, proximal migration of the radius, and synostosis. More than half of radial neck fractures are associated with other injuries in the elbow, particularly fractures of the olecranon process, which should be treated on their own merits. Before age 4, lateral sloping of the radial neck is a vagary of the proximal radius and may be misinterpreted as representing an injury. Also, a notch at the lateral aspect of the proximal radial metaphysis may be seen in older children and should not be confused with injury.

Olecranon Fractures

Nondisplaced fractures of the olecranon in children can be treated closed, but displaced fractures will require open reduction and internal fixation with tension band wiring. Articular surface must be reduced to within 2 mm.

Vagaries of the physis of the proximal olecranon may also be confused with fracture. Identifying the normal sclerotic margins of the physis and noting that it is wider in the posterior portion will distinguish a normal physis from a fracture.

Medial Epicondyle Fractures

Fractures involving the medial epicondylar apophysis are most common between the ages of 9 and 14 years. Minimally displaced fractures can be treated conservatively with casting until fibrous union is complete. If the fracture fragment is incarcerated within the joint, if there is dysfunction of the ulnar nerve, or if there is severe displacement of a large fragment with associated valgus instability of the elbow, open reduction and internal fixation of the medial epicondyle should be considered. A recent study examining surgical treatment of the medial epicondyle fractures in these cases gave consistently good results with good range of motion, good stability, no ulnar nerve symptoms, and no deformity. Unless the fracture is severely displaced, conservative treatment is generally recommended with good results as well.

Shaft Fractures of the Radius and Ulna

Unlike adults, most forearm fractures in children are managed with closed reduction and cast immobilization. In children less than 6 years of age, up to 15 degrees of angulation, and even 5 degrees of rotation, can be tolerated because remodeling will improve alignment with growth. Between the ages of 6 and 10 years, 10 degrees of angulation should remodel. For children older than 12 years of age, a more aggressive treatment may be required, including open reduction and compression plating since no angulatory or rotational deformity is considered acceptable.

Recent studies reconfirm the importance of follow-up radiographs at one- and two-week intervals after the initial reduction. A review of 90 pediatric forearm fractures concluded 7% were subject to reangulation or displace-

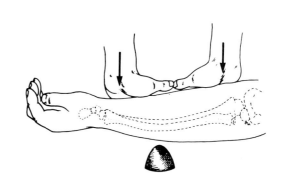

Fig. 9 Demonstration of reduction technique for plastic deformation. The apex of the plastically deformed bone is placed over a fulcrum and pressure is applied to each limb of the curve as shown. (Reproduced with permission from Sanders WE, Heckman JD: Traumatic plastic deformation of the radius and ulna. *Clin Orthop* 1984;188:58-67.)

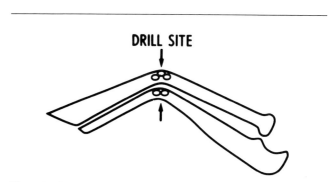

Fig. 10 Drill osteoclasis for malunion of the forearm. This line drawing of the technique indicates the drill sites. (Reproduced with permission from Sanders WE, Heckman JD: Traumatic plastic deformation of the radius and ulna. *Clin Orthop* 1984;188:58-67.)

ment. The authors recommend that a loss of acceptable alignment should be treated by remanipulation. Nonepiphyseal fractures were safely manipulated up to 24 days postfracture. Bayonet apposition may be acceptable, particularly for those children less than 10 years of age, although end to end apposition is preferred. Greenstick fractures in the mid-forearm have both an angulatory and a rotational component, both of which must be corrected with manipulation. Plastic deformation may occur to either the ulna or radius. Children less than age 4 have sufficient remodeling potential to recover full function, but older children may require manipulation of the plastic deformation under general anesthesia if forearm rotation is limited. A reduction technique (Fig. 9) using a fulcrum under general anesthesia may improve deformity by an average correction of 85%. Malunion of the forearm can be corrected with open osteotomy or, preferably, drill osteoclasis using a semiclosed technique (Fig. 10). Cross-union of the forearm is uncommon in children, but may follow high-energy trauma or operative intervention of a forearm fracture through one incision. In a recent series of ten cross-unions in children, four were type II and six were type III. The results after excision of the cross-union were not as good in children as in adults.

Monteggia Fractures

All four Bado types of the Monteggia fracture dislocation are pertinent to children, including Monteggia equivalents. Type I with the head anterior is the most common lesion comprising approximately 75% in most series. The type III Monteggia fracture has a lateral dislocation of the radial head with an ulnar metaphyseal fracture, usually a greenstick type of fracture. This is most commonly associated with radial nerve injuries and is the second most common type of Monteggia fracture comprising approximately 24% of the lesions. The fracture of the ulna may be a complete fracture, a greenstick fracture, or a bowing of the ulna due to plastic deformation. In contrast to adults, most of these injuries are treated closed by manipulation. Reduction of the radial head must be confirmed. For type I, III, and IV Monteggia injuries, immobilization of the elbow in 100 degrees of flexion with the forearm fully supinated for six weeks is recommended. For type II injuries, immobilization with the elbow extended for four weeks is recommended.

Open reduction is usually indicated only if it is necessary to reduce the radial head. If the reduction of the radial head cannot be maintained, intramedullary fixation of the ulna fracture may be necessary, or even more rarely, open reconstruction of the annular ligament with use of a transcapitellar pin to stabilize the radius. In a recent review, the type I equivalent lesion required operative treatment in ten of 14 children. Late presentation of a Monteggia injury with malunion of the ulna may be corrected by osteotomy.

Complications

Radial nerve injury is most commonly observed after type III fractures. Fortunately, as with the adult, this usually resolves completely with time. Occasionally there is persistent ulnar bowing, occurring most commonly in type III lesions. This can produce subluxation of the radial head with subsequent symptoms of pain. An opening wedge osteotomy of the ulna will generally reduce both the ulnar deformity and the subluxation of the radial head. Delayed reduction of a dislocated radial head is performed by open reduction, and the orbicular ligament, which must be excised, is reconstructed with a strip of triceps fascia.

Annotated Bibliography

Anatomy and Biomechanics

Hotchkiss RN, An KN, Sowa DT, et al: An anatomic and mechanical study of the interosseous membrane of the forearm: Pathomechanics of proximal migration of the radius. *J Hand Surg* 1989;14A:256-261.

Cadaveric study of the IOM revealed the central band to contribute 71% of the longitudinal stiffness to the forearm, with the TFCC contributing 8%. Silicone radial head implants are less stiff than the intact IOM.

Morrey BF, Tanaka S, An KN: Valgus stability of the elbow: A definition of primary and secondary constraints. *Clin Orthop* 1991;265:187-195.

The radial head is an important secondary constraint to valgus stability. While the radial head can be excised if the MCL is intact, gross instability resulted with release of the MCL and excision of the radial head.

O'Driscoll SW, Bell DF, Morrey BF: Posterolateral rotatory instability of the elbow. *J Bone Joint Surg* 1991;73A:440-446.

The clinical stress test to assess for posterolateral rotatory instability of the elbow due to laxity of the LCL is described. Operative repair is reported in patients.

Søjbjerg JO, Ovesen J, Nielsen S: Experimental elbow instability after transection of the medial collateral ligament. *Clin Orthop* 1987;218:186-190.

This study clearly identifies the MCL to be the primary stabilizer of the elbow from 20 to 120 degrees of flexion.

Adult Fractures and Dislocations

Broberg MA, Morrey BF: Results of treatment of fracture dislocations of the elbow. *Clin Orthop* 1987;216:109-119.

Prolonged immobilization (greater than four weeks) is associated with poor results.

Josefsson PO, Gentz CF, Johnell O, et al: Surgical versus nonsurgical treatment of ligamentous injuries following dislocation of the elbow joint. *Clin Orthop* 1987;214:165-169.

With random assignment to treatment group, no clear difference was demonstrated for surgical repair of the ligaments in simple elbow dislocations. A greater degree of injury to the flexor-pronator mass was associated with greater instability of the elbow under anesthesia.

Josefsson PO, Gentz CF, Johnell O, et al: Dislocations of the elbow and intraarticular fractures. *Clin Orthop* 1989;246:126-130.

In a series of 23 complex elbow dislocations, 19 underwent excision of the radial head with poor results. The authors recommend preserving the radial head if possible. If the radial head is resected, repair of the ligaments and muscles at the epicondyles is stressed.

Mehlhoff TL, Noble PC, Bennett JB, et al: Simple dislocation of the elbow in the adult: Results after closed treatment. *J Bone Joint Surg* 1988;70A:244-249.

Long-term results in 52 adult simple elbow dislocations revealed flexion contracture exceeding 30 degrees in 15%, residual pain in 45%, and pain on valgus stress in 35%. Early active motion is key to successful rehabilitation after dislocation.

Regan W, Morrey BF: Fractures of the coronoid process of the ulna. *J Bone Joint Surg* 1989;71A:1348-1354.

Fractures of the coronoid process are classified. Type III coronoid fractures are unstable and require open reduction and internal fixation (ORIF) to allow early motion.

Supracondylar and Intercondylar Fractures

Ackerman G, Jupiter JB: Non-union of fractures of the distal end of the humerus. *J Bone Joint Surg* 1988;70A:75-83.

In a series of 20 patients, 17 of 18 nonunions ultimately united with repeat ORIF and bone grafting, but continued to have significantly impaired motion.

Figgie MP, Inglis AE, Mow CS, et al: Salvage of non-union of supracondylar fracture of the humerus by total elbow arthroplasty. *J Bone Joint Surg* 1989;71A:1058-1065.

Salvage of symptomatic nonunions of the supracondylar humerus in elderly patients with the semiconstrained total elbow arthroplasty is reported in 14 patients, with good to excellent results in eight, and poor results in three, patients.

Henley MB, Bone LB, Parker B: Operative management of displaced intraarticular fractures of the distal humerus. *J Orthop Trauma* 1987;1:24-35.

The operative management of displaced intra-articular fractures of the distal humerus in 33 patients is reviewed. The authors stress the importance of rigid fixation and early range of motion. A high rate of complication with the transolecranon osteotomy is reported.

Richards RR, Khoury GW, Burke FD, et al: Internal fixation of capitellar fractures using Herbert screws: A report of four cases. *Can J Surg* 1987;30:188-191.

The advantages of Herbert screw fixation for these capitellar fractures is discussed.

Radial Head Fractures

Edwards GS Jr, Jupiter JB: Radial head fractures with acute distal radioulnar dislocation: Essex-Lopresti revisited. *Clin Orthop* 1988;234:61-69.

The authors stress the importance of early recognition and management for the Essix-Lopresti lesion. Suboptimal results occurred in four patients when definitive surgery was delayed four to ten weeks.

King GJ, Evans DC, Kellam JF: Open reduction and internal fixation of radial head fractures. *J Orthop Trauma* 1991;5:21-28.

Excellent results for ORIF of Mason type II fractures can be obtained with anatomical reduction, stable fixation, and early range of motion. Comminuted type III injuries require alternative treatment methods.

Olecranon Fractures

Murphy DF, Greene WB, Dameron TB Jr: Displaced olecranon fractures in adults: Clinical evaluation. *Clin Orthop* 1987;224:215-223.

Displaced fractures of the olecranon were reviewed in 38 cases. Malreduction of the articular surface >2 mm was associated with poor results, as was articular surface involvement ≥60%. Excision of >60% of the olecranon led to instability in one case. Symptomatic metal prominence occurred in 80%.

Wolfgang G, Burke F, Bush D, et al: Surgical treatment of displaced olecranon fractures by tension band wiring technique. *Clin Orthop* 1987;224:192-204.

While some loss of terminal extension was noted in 59% of cases, tension-band wiring of isolated olecranon fractures gave good to excellent results in 29 of 30 cases over a 13-year period.

Forearm Fractures

Chapman MW, Gordon JE, Zissimos AG: Compression-plate fixation of acute fractures of the diaphyses of the radius and ulna. *J Bone Joint Surg* 1989;71A:159-169.

A retrospective review of 129 diaphyseal fractures in 87 patients treated with AO DC plates obtained union in 98% of fractures. No refracture occurred following removal of 3.5-mm plates, but two refractures occurred following removal of 4.5-mm plates. Immediate fixation of open fractures had a low rate of complications.

Rosson JW, Petley GW, Shearer JR: Bone structure after removal of internal fixation plates. *J Bone Joint Surg* 1991;73B:65-67.

Using single-photon absorptiometry, these investigators determined bone density to return to its prefracture level at 21 months after plating.

Rumball K, Finnegan M: Refractures after forearm plate removal. *J Orthop Trauma* 1990;4:124-129.

In a review of 63 patients undergoing forearm plate removal, refracture occurred in four, for an incidence of 6%.

Vince KG, Miller JE: Cross-union complicating fracture of the forearm. Part I: Adults. *J Bone Joint Surg* 1987;69A:640-653.

Twenty-eight adults with cross-union of the forearm were classified. Seventeen cross-unions were excised. While none of ten type II recurred, three of four type I and two of three type III cross-unions recurred.

Pediatric Fractures and Dislocations

Beaty JH: Fractures and dislocations about the elbow in children, in Eilert RE (ed): American Academy of Orthopaedic Surgeons *Instructional Course Lectures, XLI.* Park Ridge, IL, American Academy of Orthopaedic Surgeons 1992, pp 373-384.

The authors present the description, classification, and treatment of lateral humeral condyle, medial epicondyle, T-condylar, olecranon, and radial head and neck fractures; Monteggia fracture-dislocations; and elbow dislocations.

Elbow Dislocations

De Jager LT, Hoffman EB: Fracture-separation of the distal humeral epiphysis. *J Bone Joint Surg* 1991;73B:143-146.

The diagnosis of fracture-separation of the distal humerus epiphysis is difficult, especially in children under age 2 who usually have Salter-Harris I injuries. Arthrography may be needed. Closed reduction and pinning is recommended by the authors to assess carrying angle in children under 2 years of age.

Dias JJ, Lamont AC, Jones JM: Ultrasonic diagnosis of neonatal separation of the distal humeral epiphysis. *J Bone Joint Surg* 1988;70B:825-828.

This review article on this separation demonstrates the difficulty in making a diagnosis between this injury and an elbow dislocation. The article demonstrated that sonography was helpful on its own merits and even more helpful when associated with an arthrogram.

Floyd WE III, Gebhardt MC, Emans JB: Intra-articular entrapment of the medial nerve after elbow dislocation in children. *J Hand Surg* 1987;12A:704-707.

Intra-articular entrapment of the median nerve after closed reduction of elbow dislocation in children is described, with a report of two cases. Early recognition and surgical exploration is advised.

Gerardi JA, Houkom JA, Mack GR: Pediatric update #10: Treatment of displaced supracondylar fractures of the humerus in children by closed reduction and percutaneous pinning. *Orthop Rev* 1989;18:1089-1095.

This retrospective review studies 25 displaced supracondylar fractures treated by closed reduction and percutaneous pin fixation. The average follow-up was 16 months. Only one fracture demonstrated less than excellent or good results.

Kurer MH, Regan MW: Completely displaced supracondylar fracture of the humerus in children: A review of 1708 comparable cases. *Clin Orthop* 1990;256:205-214.

A large review of 1,708 comparable cases in the literature determined the best results in cases managed with traction or wheel-performed K-wire techniques. The worst results occurred with manipulation and splint immobilization alone.

Pirone AM, Graham HK, Krajbich JI: Management of displaced extension-type supracondylar fractures of the humerus in children. *J Bone Joint Surg* 1988;70A:641-650.

A very large series of 230 patients with type III supracondylar fractures treated with closed reduction and cast immobilization was reviewed. This series demonstrated a significantly lower percentage of excellent results with a higher percentage of complications than a series treated with closed reduction and percutaneous pinning. It was concluded that closed reduction with percutaneous pinning was the procedure of choice. Certain patients with significant soft-tissue swelling were, however, treated with skeletal traction with apparently acceptable results.

Shaw BA, Kasser JR, Emans JB, et al: Management of vascular injuries in displaced supracondylar humerus fractures without arteriography. *J Orthop Trauma* 1990;4:25-29.

Rapid reduction and K-wire stabilization for displaced supracondylar humerus fractures with signs of vascular impairment successfully restored circulation in 14 of 17 cases without need for prereduction arteriography.

Yates C, Sullivan JA: Arthrographic diagnosis of elbow injuries in children. *J Pediatr Orthop* 1987;7:54-60.

This is a prospective study reviewing 36 arthrograms. There was a 19% incidence of changed diagnosis secondary to the arthrogram. The authors found this very helpful in differentiating the diagnosis between the medial epicondyle and the medial condylar fractures.

Lateral Condyle Fractures

Badelon O, Bensahel H, Mazoa K, et al: Lateral humeral condylar fractures in children: A report of 47 cases. *J Pediatr Orthop* 1988;8:31-34.

This is a retrospective review including 47 children. Four were treated after a five-month delay. A classification was presented including four types. The best results were those treated with an open reduction and internal fixation. The authors pointed out that a fracture, though minimally displaced laterally, that is, less than 2 mm, is potentially an unstable fracture and needs to be opened and stabilized.

Dhillon KS, Sengupta S, Singh BJ: Delayed management of fracture of the lateral humeral condyle in children. *Acta Orthop Scand* 1988;59:419-424.

This article reviewed 39 displaced fractures, with an average follow up of five years. Fractures treated at less than two weeks did well; after a six-week delay they did poorly with variable results in the intervening interval. There is approximately a 10% incidence of avascular necrosis.

Flynn JC: Nonunion of slightly displaced fractures of the lateral humeral condyle in children: An update. *J Pediatr Orthop* 1989;9:691-696.

This author has a strong background of treatment of fractures of the lateral humeral condyle. He suggests that the best treatment for the established nonunion is early stabilization and bone grafting, provided that the position of the fragment is acceptable and the physis is not closed.

Thönell S, Mortensson W, Thomasson B: Prediction of the stability of minimally displaced fractures of the lateral humeral condyle. *Acta Radiol* 1988;29:367-370.

In this retrospective study of 159 children, fractures were classified into three groups based on the fracture pattern. It showed that late instability is predictable and can be as high as 44% in one type of fracture pattern. This classification is helpful in dealing with fractures that are minimally displaced and in determining a fracture management program.

Medial Condyle Fractures

Papavasiliou V, Nenopoulos S, Venturis T: Fracture of the medial condyle of the humerus in childhood. *J Pediatr Orthop* 1987;7:421-423.

These authors reviewed their series of medial condylar fractures and classified them into three types according to Kilfoyle. Their recommendation for treatment was cast immobilization for type I fractures and open reduction and internal fixation with K-wires for types II and III. They utilized a supracondylar closing wedge osteotomy for reconstruction for a cubitus varus deformity secondary to this fracture.

Radial Neck Fractures

Fowles JV, Kassab MT: Observations concerning radial neck fractures in children. *J Pediatr Orthop* 1986;6:51-57.

Angulation >60 degrees was treated with open reduction and internal fixation. Oblique K-wire fixation that avoids the humerus is recommended.

Silberstein MJ, Brodeur AE, Graviss ER: Some vagaries of the radial head and neck. *J Bone Joint Surg* 1982;64A:1153-1157.

The normal appearance of the developing radial head and neck are prone to misinterpretation as being due to trauma.

Steinberg EL, Golomb D, Salama R, et al: Radial head and neck fractures in children. *J Pediatr Orthop* 1988; 8:35-40.

In a review of 42 consecutive fractures of the radial neck in children, primary angulation was the most important factor affecting the results. Complications included periarticular ossification, avascular necrosis, and enlargement of the radial head.

Medial Epicondyle Fractures

Hines RF, Herndon WA, Evans JP: Operative treatment of medial epicondyle fractures in children. *Clin Orthop* 1987;223:170-174.

The operative management of displaced medial epicondyle fractures in 31 patients is reviewed at four years follow-up, with good results.

Silberstein MJ, Brodeur AE, Graviss ER, et al: Some vagaries of the medial epicondyle. *J Bone Joint Surg* 1981;63A:524-528.

This article reviews the radiographic variations of the medial epicondyle. It points out that the medial epicondyle usually appears at 4 years of age, and the fracture represents the third most common fracture of the elbow.

Forearm Fractures

Kramhøft M, Solgaard S: Displaced diaphyseal forearm fractures in children: Classification and evaluation of the early radiographic prognosis. *J Pediatr Orthop* 1989;9:586-589.

All displaced diaphyseal forearm fractures in children should be radiographed after one week and after two weeks postfracture.

Olney BW, Menelaus MB: Monteggia and equivalent lesions in childhood. *J Pediatr Orthop* 1989;9:219-223.

Most Monteggia fracture-dislocations in 102 children could be treated closed with good results, except type I equivalent lesions, which required operative treatment in 10 of 14 children.

Vince KG, Miller JE: Cross-union complicating fracture of the forearm. Part II: Children. *J Bone Joint Surg* 1987;69A:654-661.

Ten cross-unions in children's forearm fractures are reported. The results for excision in children were less favorable than in adults.

Vittas D, Larsen E, Torp-Pederson S: Angular remodeling of midshaft forearm fractures in children. *Clin Orthop* 1991;265:261-264.

For children younger than age 11 years, there was a significant correlation between angular remodeling of the midshaft forearm and change in epiphyseal plate angulation, with the highest degree of correction being 13 degrees.

Voto SJ, Weiner DS, Leighley B: Redisplacement after closed reduction of forearm fractures in children. *J Pediatr Orthop* 1990;10:79-84.

A review of 90 pediatric forearm fractures concluded 7% were subject to angulation or displacement. Nonepiphyseal fractures were safely remanipulated up to 24 days postfracture.

29

Elbow: Reconstruction

A patient with an elbow problem may complain of any of the following five problems: pain, stiffness, weakness, instability, or cosmetic deformity. Much information and clinical experience have been accumulated recently regarding arthroscopy, treatment of instability, stiffness, arthritis, and the flail elbow. New diagnostic methods include magnetic resonance imaging (MRI) but its role remains to be determined.

Diagnostic Studies

A careful history and physical examination combined with plain radiographs, special views, and tomograms yield adequate information to proceed with treatment in at least 90% of cases. Electrodiagnostic studies and bone scans are also contributory. With the exception of patients with suspected tumorous conditions, the roles of computed tomography and MRI have not assumed significant importance. The value of elbow arthroscopy is in the process of being defined.

Biomechanics and Kinematics

The elbow behaves as a loose hinge with respect to flexion and extension. There is a slight degree of varus/valgus and rotational laxity (3 to 5 degrees) throughout the flexion-extension arc, which is almost perfectly centered on a single axis. The anterior band of the medial collateral ligament is the primary constraint to valgus instability, and the radial head is of secondary importance. Replacement of the radial head with a Silastic implant does not restore biomechanical stability to normal. It does, however, act as a spacer, and it is capable of maintaining stability provided that the forces and moments applied to the elbow are small. In fact, the radial head assumes importance only when the medial collateral ligament (MCL) is dysfunctional. The remaining portions of the MCL, the posterior and transverse bands, do not appear to play important roles. The capsule is an important constraint to instability only in full extension.

Functional Anatomy

The bony and soft-tissue anatomy in the region of the elbow has been the source of ongoing anatomic studies. The cubital tunnel begins where the ulnar nerve passes beneath the cubital tunnel retinaculum, a fibrous band about 4-mm wide that extends from the medial epicon-

dyle to the olecranon. Together with the aponeurosis of the flexor carpi ulnaris, the cubital tunnel retinaculum forms the roof of the cubital tunnel. The floor of the cubital tunnel is formed by the elbow joint capsule as well as the posterior and transverse components of the MCL. The anterior band of the medial collateral ligament (AMCL) is anterior to the ulnar nerve, which does not cross it. This important relationship is valuable to know when operating in this area. The cubital tunnel retinaculum can be absent, permitting ulnar nerve subluxation. When present, it is normally tight in full flexion, but if pathologically thick or shortened, the cubital tunnel retinaculum will be tight in 90 to 120 degrees of flexion, thereby potentially causing dynamic nerve compression with elbow flexion. It may also be represented by a muscle, the anconeus epitrochlearis, from which it is a remnant.

The MCL consists of three bands, the anterior, posterior and transverse. The AMCL is the primary constraint to valgus instability; its precise origin is relevant to medial epicondylectomy, medial epicondyle transfer (Steindler transfer), or fractures. The AMCL originates exclusively from the middle two thirds of the anteroinferior surface of medial epicondyle, but does not attach to the trochlea (Fig. 1). Only 20% of the width of the epicondyle can be removed without violating part of the origin of the AMCL. Excision of the entire epicondyle as ini-

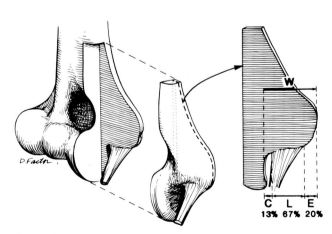

Fig. 1 The anterior band of the medial collateral ligament originates exclusively from the middle two-thirds of the anteroinferior surface of the epicondyle. (Reproduced with permission from O'Driscoll SW, Jaloszynski R, Morrey BF, et al: Origin of the medial collateral ligament. *J Hand Surg* 1992;17A:164-168.)

tially recommended for ulnar neuropathy will therefore completely detach this ligament and can potentiate instability. More bone can be removed posteriorly than anteriorly and, therefore, the ideal plane of osteotomy lies between the sagittal and coronal planes.

Further studies have also been conducted to clarify the anatomy of the lateral collateral ligament (LCL). The ulnar part of the LCL, previously described as the lateral ulnar collateral ligament, plays an important role in rotatory instability. This structure has been identified as part of the lateral capsuloligamentous complex (Fig. 2). At its origin on the lateral epicondyle, the ulnar part of the LCL blends with the fibers of the lateral collateral complex from which it is indistinguishable. As it courses superficially over the annular ligament, it blends with that ligament and then curves posteriorly and medially to insert on the tubercle of the supinator crest of the ulna. Its fibers are distinct at its insertion, which is beneath the fascia that covers the supinator and the extensor carpi ulnaris muscles. It can be palpated by applying a varus or supination moment to the elbow. The paucity of anatomic descriptions of this ligament may be related to the fact that it lies beneath a fascial layer and, therefore, is not routinely exposed. Its function is to prevent varus and posterolateral rotatory instability of the elbow.

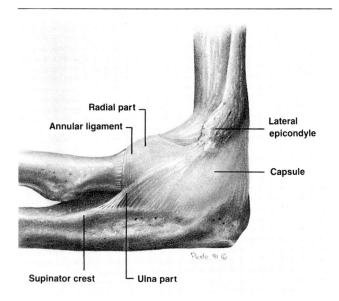

Fig. 2 The lateral collateral ligament is part of a capsuloligamentous complex. The ligament consists of an ulnar part, which is about 4 mm wide and extends from the lateral epicondyle down over the annular ligament (with which it blends) to insert onto the tubercle of the supinator crest on the ulna. It is homologous with the anterior band of the medial collateral ligament and is the primary constraint to both varus and posterolateral rotatory instability of the elbow. The other parts are the radial part and the annular ligament. The lateral collateral ligament complex is isometric at its origin on the lateral epicondyle. (Reproduced with permission from O'Driscoll SW, Horii E, Morrey BF, et al: Anatomy of the ulnar part of the lateral collateral ligament of the elbow. *Clin Anat* 1992;5:1-8.)

Surgical Exposures

It has been said that the front door to the elbow is at the back. Although there are many different surgical approaches to the elbow, each with its own specific advantages and disadvantages, fewer and fewer of the specific approaches are being used as a result of the versatility of the posterior approach. A posteriorly placed skin incision, which can be slightly medial or slightly lateral, permits posteromedial or posterolateral arthrotomies as well as access to the ulnar nerve and to the anterior elbow via the deep portion of the Kocher approach, and is the most useful approach for the elbow. The incision should not cross the tip of the olecranon, especially in patients with olecranon bursitis or rheumatoid arthritis in whom the soft tissues are more susceptible to wound infection or breakdown. This incision is analogous to the straight anterior approach to the knee. Access to the elbow joint for internal fixation of comminuted distal humeral fractures or for total elbow replacement can be attained by reflecting the triceps and anconeus as a flap with or without a piece of bone at the insertion of the triceps. If an olecranon osteotomy is performed, the ulna is cut only part way through and then fractured with an osteotome the remainder of the way to permit precise articular realignment. The anconeus muscle must not be denervated by transecting it, because it is innervated in an axial direction by a terminal branch of the radial nerve passing through the triceps. Therefore, it is raised as a flap with the olecranon that has been osteotomized. This muscle serves as a dynamic stabilizer, preventing varus or posterolateral rotatory subluxation, and provides the majority of soft tissue bulk over the posterolateral aspect of the elbow.

Arthroscopy

Arthroscopy is assuming a greater role in diagnosis and management of elbow problems, as it is in other joints, with definite indications beginning to emerge (Fig. 3). Whether it is performed for diagnosis only, for treatment only, or for diagnosis and treatment, approximately two-thirds to three-quarters of the patients who undergo elbow arthroscopy benefit in the sense that their outcomes are positively influenced by the findings or treatment of the arthroscopy.

Diagnostic Arthroscopy

Those patients with pain and objective abnormal clinical or radiographic findings but without a confirmed diagnosis can be diagnosed definitely in the majority of cases. Also, those patients with suspected loose bodies, snapping, and idiopathic contractures of spontaneous onset usually have recognizable intra-articular pathology that permits a diagnosis to be established. Patients who have pain without objective findings on examination and standard investigations typically remain undiagnosed after arthroscopy. Thus, diagnostic arthroscopy does not sub-

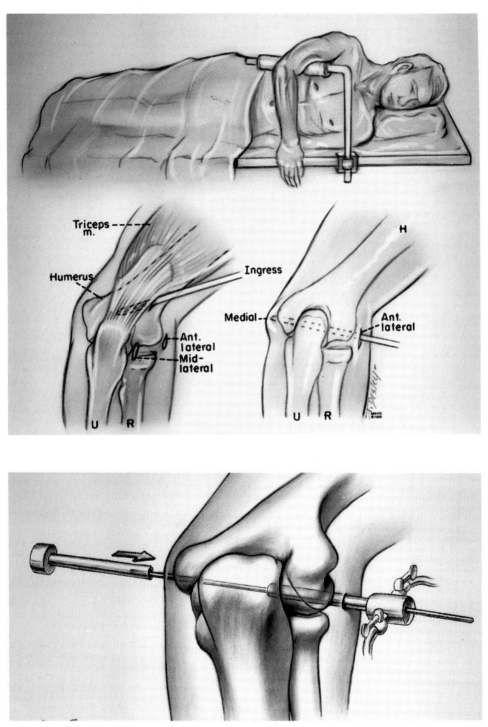

Fig. 3 **Top**, The position of the patient for arthroscopy is the lateral decubitus position with the involved limb supported by a padded bolster and the elbow flexed to 90 degrees. The midlateral and anterolateral portals are shown. **Bottom**, To establish the anterior portals, a sharp Steinmann pin is passed through the scope and out the other side. A cannula is then passed back into the joint over this pin, the pin removed, and the scope reinserted. (Reproduced by permission of Mayo Foundation.)

stitute for a careful history and physical examination or routine investigations.

Therapeutic Arthroscopy

The ideal patient for operative arthroscopy is one with isolated loose bodies or loose bodies associated with osteochondritis dissecans. It must be emphasized, however, that patients with posttraumatic or primary degenerative arthritis associated with loose bodies do not benefit from simple removal of the loose body. The same is true for those with contractures. Other indications for operative arthroscopy include debridement and localized synovectomy in patients with posttraumatic arthritis, and removal of osteophytes from the olecranon and coronoid as well as from the olecranon and coronoid fossae in patients who have primary degenerative arthrosis in the early stages. Synovectomy is practical and efficacious for the management of inflammatory or septic arthritis, although it is technically highly demanding. The surgeon must constantly be aware that the neurovascular structures may be within 2 mm of the operating instruments in the anterior part of the elbow.

Minor complications occur in 10% to 20% of patients and usually are not permanent. The frequency of serious complications such as injury to a nerve is not yet known. It would be considered essential that substantial experience with arthroscopy in general and a thorough knowledge of both the normal and the abnormal anatomy of the elbow are prerequisites to the safe and successful use of this procedure.

Elbow Instability: Current Concepts

The pathoanatomy, mechanism of injury, kinematics, and clinical aspects of elbow instability are now better understood. This has led to the new concept that elbow subluxation and dislocation are part of a spectrum of instability (Figs. 4 and 5). Instability of the elbow can be classified anatomically into ulnohumeral instability, chronic valgus overload, and radio-ulnar instability.

The pathoanatomy can be thought of as a circle of soft tissue disruption from lateral to medial in three stages (Fig. 4). In stage 1 the ulnar part of the LCL is disrupted, resulting in posterolateral rotatory subluxation of the elbow, which reduces spontaneously (Fig. 5). With further disruption anteriorly and posteriorly, the elbow in stage 2 instability is capable of an incomplete posterolateral dislocation. When this occurs, the concave medial edge of the ulna rests on the trochlea in such a way that on a lateral radiograph the coronoid appears to be perched on the trochlea (Fig. 6). This can be reduced with minimal force or by the patient manipulating the elbow him/herself. Stage 3 is subdivided into 2 parts. In stage 3-A, all the soft tissues are disrupted around to and including the posterior part of the MCL, leaving the important anterior band intact. This permits posterior dislocation by the previously described posterolateral rotatory

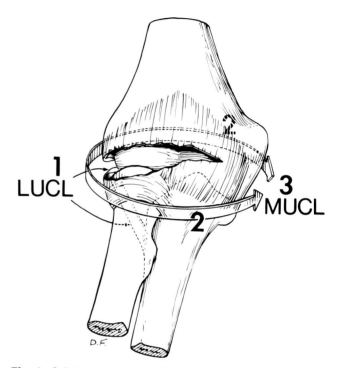

Fig. 4 Soft-tissue disruption with elbow subluxation or dislocation progresses in a circle from lateral to medial in three stages that correlate with the stages of instability in Figure 5. The first stage is disruption of the lateral ulnar collateral ligament; second, the anterior and posterior capsule and remaining lateral structures; and third, the medial ulnar collateral ligament starting with the posterior band and then finally the anterior band of the medial collateral ligament. (Reproduced with permission from O'Driscoll SW, Morrey BF, Korinek S, et al: Elbow subluxation and dislocation: A spectrum of instability. *Clin Orthop* 1992;280:17-28.)

mechanism. The elbow pivots around on the intact AMCL. Reduction is accomplished by gentle manipulation of the elbow in supination and valgus, temporarily recreating the deformity. The intact AMCL provides valgus stability, provided that the elbow is kept in pronation to prevent posterolateral rotatory subluxation during valgus testing. In stage 3-B the entire MCL complex is disrupted. Gross varus and valgus as well as rotatory instability are present following reduction because all ligaments and the capsule are disrupted. The role of the flexor/pronator muscle origin is not known, but its integrity could be relevant.

Treatment recommendations following acute injuries correspond to the stages outlined in the spectrum of instability. Valgus stability following reduction is present with the forearm fully pronated in stages 1 to 3-A. These are treated by immediate unlimited flexion and extension in a cast brace which is applied with the forearm in full pronation. In stage 3-B, the elbow is unstable in extension and a cast brace (usually in neutral rotation) is applied with an extension block incorporated to prevent

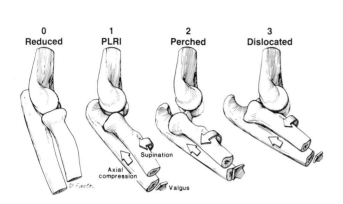

Fig. 5 The three stages of clinical instability that correlate with the pathoanatomic stages of capsuloligamentous disruption in Figure 4 are illustrated. PLRI refers to posterior lateral rotatory instability. The forces and moments responsible for displacements are illustrated by the arrows. (Reproduced with permission from O'Driscoll SW, Morrey BF, Korinek S, et al: Elbow subluxation and dislocation: A spectrum of instability. *Clin Orthop* 1992;280:17-28.)

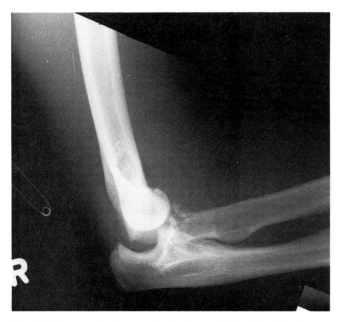

Fig. 6 An example of a perched, or incomplete, dislocation. In this case, there are associated fractures of the coronoid and radial head. This second stage of instability is actually more common than one might think.

extension beyond the point of instability. This is gradually extended during the healing phase.

Recurrent instability of the elbow involves a common pathway of posterolateral rotatory subluxation, and in virtually all of these unstable elbows, the ulnar part of the LCL is detached or attenuated. The MCL may or may not be intact. Posterolateral rotatory instability is being diagnosed with increasing frequency since its discovery, probably as a result of increased awareness of the condition. Patients typically indicate a history of recurrent painful clicking, snapping, clunking, or locking of the elbow, and careful interrogation reveals that this occurs in the extension half of the arc with the forearm in supination. A history of preceding trauma or surgery is always present, and this history might include a previous dislocation or an injury as subtle as a sprain resulting from a fall on the outstretched hand. Surgical causes include radial head excision and lateral release for tennis elbow (caused by violation of the ulnar part of the LCL). The physical examination is typically unremarkable except for a positive lateral pivot shift apprehension test or posterolateral rotatory apprehension test (Figs. 7 and 8). With the patient in the supine position and the affected extremity overhead, the wrist and elbow are grasped in the same way as the ankle and knee when examining the leg for anterior cruciate insufficiency of the knee. The elbow is supinated with a mild force at the wrist, and a valgus moment is applied to the elbow during flexion. This results in a typical apprehension response with reproduction of the patient's symptoms and a sense that the elbow is about to dislocate. Reproducing the actual subluxation and the clunk that occurs with reduction usually can be accomplished only with the patient under general anesthetic or, occasionally, after injecting local anesthetic into the elbow joint. The lateral pivot shift test performed in that manner results in subluxation of the radius and ulna off the humerus, causing a prominence posterolaterally over the radial head and a dimple between the radial head and the capitellum (Fig. 7, *right*). As the elbow is flexed to approximately 40 to 60 degrees or more, reduction of the ulna and radius together on the humerus occurs suddenly with a palpable visible clunk. It is the reduction that is apparent. A lateral stress radiograph taken before the clunk may show the rotatory subluxation.

Surgical correction is performed by reattaching the avulsed lateral ulnar collateral ligament or reconstructing it with a tendon graft (for example, the palmaris longus or the semitendinosus (Fig. 9). The current reconstruction technique involves isometric placement of the origin on the lateral epicondyle and fixation to bone at either end. Surgery is performed in young patients so as to prevent violation of the epiphyseal plate on the lateral side of the humerus. Clinical outcomes have been successful in patients from 4 to 46 years of age with diagnoses including recurrent subluxations and/or dislocations. Patients with valgus as well as posterolateral rotatory instability must have the anterior band of the MCL reconstructed as well. Motion in a cast brace is initiated immediately following surgery, with the forearm in full pronation (unless the AMCL was also reconstructed) and, usually, with no extension block.

Experimental data indicate that the only requirement for valgus, varus, and rotatory stability of the elbow is the presence of a normal articular surface, the anterior

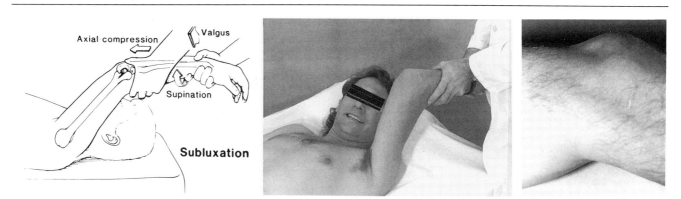

Fig. 7 **Left,** The lateral pivot shift test of the elbow for the posterolateral rotatory instability is most easily performed with the arm in the overhead position. While flexing the elbow from the extended position, a combination of axial compression as well as valgus and supination moments are applied to the elbow to cause it to subluxate. When the elbow is flexed past a certain position (typically 30 to 60 degrees of flexion) the subluxation reduces with a palpable visible clunk. (Reproduced with permission from O'Driscoll SW, Bell DF, Morrey BF: Posterolateral rotatory instability of the elbow. *J Bone Joint Surg* 1991;73A:440-446.) **Center,** A patient with posterolateral rotatory instability of the elbow demonstrating a positive apprehension sign during the lateral pivot shift test. This is highly sensitive sign and, in fact, the most important one in the awake patient, because most patients are not able to relax adequately to permit subluxation of the elbow during the lateral pivot shift test. **Right,** A close up lateral view of the elbow with the arm in the same position as shown in Figure 7, *center* (overhead, so that the head of the patient is to the left and the hand is to the right). At the point of maximum subluxation during the lateral pivot shift test, the elbow can be seen to be subluxated (once again, only under general anesthesia, or occasionally with local or no anesthesia if the patient is able to relax adequately). Subluxation is marked by a prominence over the posterolateral aspect of the elbow and a dimple behind the radial head where the skin is "sucked into" the space between the ulna and the humerus as the elbow opens up.

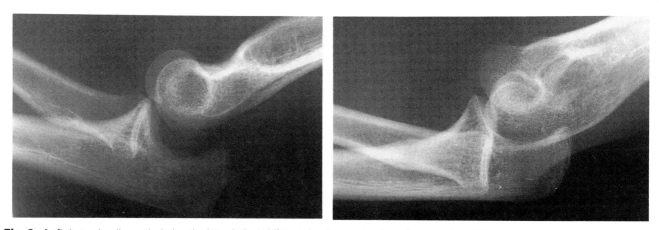

Fig. 8 **Left,** Lateral radiograph during the lateral pivot shift test showing posterolateral rotatory instability of the elbow, the features of which are ulnohumeral rotatory subluxation with the ulna supinating away from the humerus and creating a gap there. The radial head moves with the ulna so that the radiohumeral joint is also subluxated. **Right,** An oblique radiograph of the same elbow. This is what is typically seen and is responsible for the confusion in diagnosis. Here the ulnohumeral subluxation is not as obvious because of overlying bone shadows. Also, the radial head appears to be subluxated posteriorly. This combination of features is responsible for this condition being mistakenly diagnosed as posterior dislocation of the radial head when, in fact, the proximal radioulnar joint is reduced and the annular ligament is intact.

band of the MCL, the ulnar part of the LCL, and the annular ligament. Thus, there appears to be no need for unusual, nonanatomic procedures for ligament reconstruction in recurrent or chronic instability. Also, transarticular pinning of the elbow for subluxation is no longer indicated. Early clinical results from aggressive ligament reconstruction in complex fracture dislocations of the elbow have been very promising. Immediate motion is possible, and stability has been maintained. The

current approach is to start immediate motion in all injured and operated elbows; those that are unstable are reconstructed to permit such early motion. Future studies will be necessary to validate these observations.

The AMCL has been shown to be the primary constraint to valgus instability. The radial head is a secondary constraint. The radial head can be excised without significant valgus instability if the AMCL is intact; it becomes very important if the AMCL is cut. Replacement

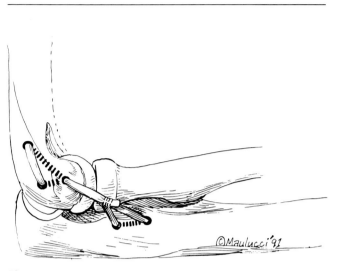

Fig. 9 Reconstruction of the ulnar part of the lateral collateral ligament (lateral ulnar collateral ligament), for the treatment of posterolateral rotatory instability of the elbow, is performed using the palmaris longus tendon graft attached to the ulna on either side of the tubercle of the supinator crest and to the humerus at the isometric point of origin on the lateral epicondyle. (Reproduced with permission from Gino Maulucci.)

of the radial head is not indicated following excision for a fracture unless there is medial collateral laxity and valgus instability or damage to the articulation (such as a coronoid fracture) that also compromises stability. What appears clinically to be valgus instability is often posterolateral rotatory instability, and the two are distinguished by testing for valgus with the forearm fully pronated (to prevent the ulna subluxating off the humerus).

Chronic valgus overload in throwers and athletes who constantly stress the elbow in a throwing motion can result in attenuation or detachment of the AMCL and is successfully treated by reconstruction using a palmaris longus tendon graft. Ulnar nerve symptoms frequently accompany this condition. The role of ulnar nerve transposition is not clear, because in a small percentage of operations ulnar nerve irritation or deficit occurs following routine submuscular transposition.

Isolated chronic posterior subluxation and dislocation of the radial head has been classified into three types, according to whether the anterior margin of the radial head is above (I) or below (II) a horizontal line through the middle of the capitellum, or (III) is posterior to a vertical line through the middle of the capitellum. Type I is the most likely and type III the least likely to go on to early painful degenerative changes, analogous to what occurs in congenital displacement of the hips comparing subluxated incongruent hips to those with high posterior dislocations. This very useful classification system can be applied directly to clinical practices. Early radial head excision did not cause distal radioulnar problems.

Stiffness and Ankylosis

It has been a generally held impression that the elbow is more prone to stiffness than most other joints in the body, and that it has a specific predilection for the development of heterotopic ossification. Whether this is true or is dependent on the treatment methods used is not known. Soft-tissue contractures are prevented largely by early (preferably immediate) movement through a relatively full arc of motion in flexion/extension as well as supination and pronation, but physiotherapy tends to be unsuccessful in the treatment of established contractures. In these patients, nonsurgical treatment of elbow stiffness caused by soft-tissue contractures begins with patient-adjusted static splints (Fig. 10). This method is highly effective for regaining range of motion, especially in the early period following injury or surgery. Clinically important improvements can occur even after six months, but the likelihood of such improvement decreases up to a year following injury or surgery. After one year virtually no improvement can be expected.

The indications for surgery include impairment of function with limitation in the activities of daily living or of occupation. Because the functional arc of motion of the elbow is from 30 to 130 degrees of flexion, it is rare to offer surgery for contractures less than 45 degrees. Preoperative evaluation includes a careful history, physical examination, and standard radiographs. Contractures can be classified into extrinsic and intrinsic. Intrinsic contractures involve adhesions between the articular surfaces and/or disruption of the normal articular congruity. Extrinsic contractures involve the periarticular soft tissues and may be associated with heterotopic ossification or extra-articular malunion. Lateral tomograms are recommended to make the distinction. All intrinsic contractures also have extrinsic soft-tissue contractures.

The surgical approach includes access to the anterior and posterior aspects of the elbow. The surgeon must be prepared to identify all neurovascular structures in order to protect them. A posterior approach is the most versatile. With this approach, raising flaps permits identification of the ulnar nerve, as well as access to the front of the joint from the lateral side for anterior capsulectomy. A lateral approach is highly versatile, although it sometimes requires a separate medial incision to ensure safety of the ulnar nerve. The anterior approach is indicated only in the presence of an isolated flexion contracture, with normal full flexion of the elbow and no evidence on the preoperative tomograms of bony abnormalities at the olecranon or in the olecranon fossa. The use of this exposure in the presence of an extension contracture (loss of full flexion) is contraindicated, because it will not permit improvement in flexion and its use has been associated with loss of flexion. Both flexion contractures and extension contractures should be released at the same time if they are present.

Further details of the surgical approach have been described along with the anticipated results. The typical

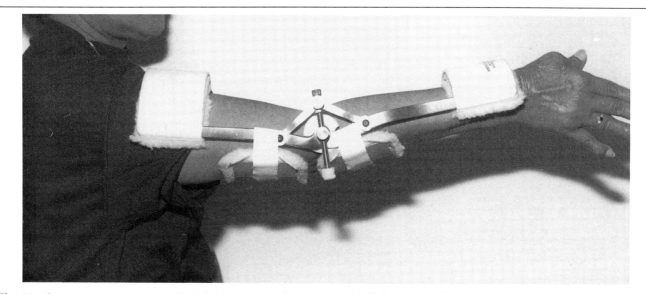

Fig. 10 Contracture braces are used both for the nonoperative treatment of stiff elbows as well as for postoperative management of elbows following surgery for trauma or reconstruction. This patient had undergone total elbow arthroplasty and was slow to regain her extension.

outcome from this surgery is a functional arc of motion from about 30 to about 130 degrees. Results are similar for more complex procedures, including distraction arthroplasty using fascia lata. This surgery is highly demanding and requires significant experience.

Radioulnar Synostosis

Radioulnar synostosis can occur whenever subperiosteal stripping is performed and the radius and ulna are exposed through the same incision. Examples include such surgery as open reduction and internal fixation of both bones of the forearm or repair of a ruptured distal biceps tendon by the two-incision technique. Treatment of a radioulnar synostosis depends to a certain extent on the level of the cross union, but overall a functional or nearly functional range of motion is achieved in approximately half of the cases. Rarely is it possible to achieve a nearly full arc of pronation-supination, probably because of soft-tissue contracture.

Osteoarthrosis

Degenerative joint disease of the elbow is a clinical entity which, although not frequently recognized, is characteristic in its clinical and radiographic presentations. The patient, who requests treatment in the third to eighth decade, has a characteristic history of mechanical impingement pain at the end of motion, which typically is greater in extension than in flexion. A history of significant overuse or repetitive trauma is often present. Carrying heavy objects, such as a suitcase, briefcase, or heavy bag of groceries, is possible only for short periods of time. Pain in the mid arc of motion is present only in the late stage. A flexion contracture of approximately 30 degrees is typical and often is associated with some loss of flexion as well. There may be crepitus in the elbow, but the characteristic finding is pain on forced extension or flexion at the end point. The anteroposterior and lateral radiographs reveal characteristic changes (Fig 11). In the advanced stages, the radioulnar joint and, finally, the radiohumeral joint may become involved.

Treatment consists of decompressing the impinging areas. One recently popularized procedure, termed ulnohumeral (Outerbridge-Kashiwagi) arthroplasty, involves a short posterior incision to split the triceps, excision of the olecranon osteophyte, and use of the Cloward drill to remove a core of bone from the olecranon fossa through to the coronoid fossa. This is followed by removal of the coronoid osteophyte (Figs. 12-14). The procedure characteristically relieves impingement pain and frequently permits some improvement in range of motion, provided that the patient undergoes a postoperative rehabilitation program involving the use of a patient-adjusted static brace.

Flail Elbow

A flail elbow typically results in significant functional impairment, because the patient does not have control of the hand and cannot place it in space. It is not necessarily a painful condition. Treatment options are few, and bracing is not particularly successful. If the elbow is flail because of periarticular or intra-articular nonunions and the patient is young, treatment by open reduction and internal fixation with bone grafting is appropriate. Satisfactory results also are being achieved with aggressive re-

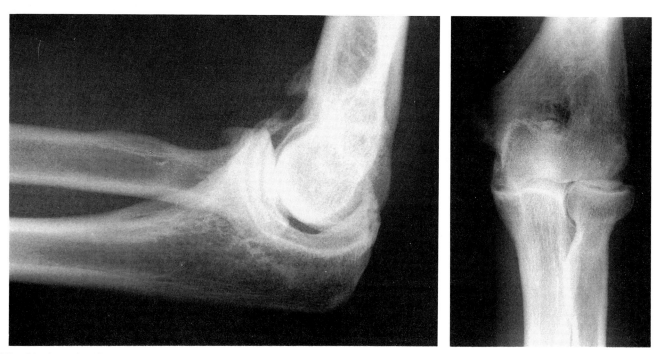

Fig. 11 Lateral and anteroposterior radiographs showing the characteristic findings of osteoarthritis of the elbow with osteophytes on the tips of the olecranon and coronoid as well as in the coronoid fossa and olecranon fossa, as indicated by filling in of the fossae. A small loose body can be seen there as well.

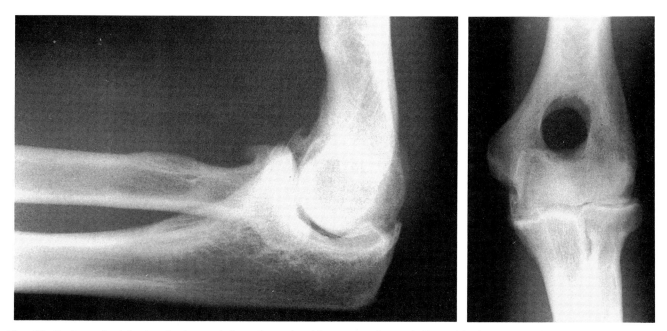

Fig. 12 Postoperative lateral and anteroposterior radiographs of the same patient as in Figure 14, after removal of the osteophytes from the olecranon and coronoid processes, as well as those around the olecranon and coronoid fossae, by removing a core of bone through the distal humerus. The significant stress riser is not a serious concern, because the bone in the region of this hole is normally very thin, and sometimes absent.

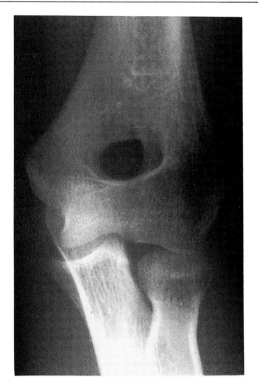

Fig. 13 Anteroposterior radiograph of a patient with congenital absence of bone in the region of the olecranon and coronoid fossae, which is similar to that created surgically by the Outerbridge-Kashiwagi arthroplasty. (Reproduced with permission from O'Driscoll S: Surgery of elbow arthritis, in McCarty D (ed): *Arthritis and Allied Conditions*, ed 12. Malvern, PA, Lea & Febiger, 1992, vol 1, chap 51, pp 951-962.)

lease of contractures and rigid internal fixation. Replacement of the elbow with a semiconstrained total elbow arthroplasty has also been shown to have good success. In the older patient in whom an arthroplasty is not a contraindication, this is the operation of choice (Figs. 15 and 16).

Total Elbow Arthroplasty

Two problems have thwarted early progress in total elbow replacement: mechanical loosening of constrained (hinged) designs and dislocation of nonconstrained designs. The early hinged design was a fully constrained prosthesis that directly linked the ulnar and humeral components. The failure rate was unacceptably high, so that there is no longer any indication for a fully constrained elbow prosthesis. The elbow has been erroneously referred to as a nonweightbearing joint, but the forces across it can exceed three times body weight. The principal moments (rotational forces or torques) about the humeral component are posteriorly and rotational.

Two types of elbow arthroplasties are in current use: semiconstrained (loose-hinge or sloppy-hinge) and non-

constrained, which would better be termed minimally constrained, because articulation itself affords a degree of constraint. Nonconstrained elbow arthroplasties have been in use since 1972. There was an initial trend to simply replace the articular surfaces of the distal humerus and proximal ulna, but without intramedullary stems these components had a tendency to loosen and displace. The majority of components now available have intramedullary stems, and loosening is no longer a common problem. Instability (dislocation, subluxation, or maltracking) has been a problem in 5% to 20% of nonconstrained total elbow arthroplasties. This problem can be overcome using the single-axis linked semiconstrained prostheses, which are in common use currently. These differ from snap-fit semiconstrained prostheses, which can become disengaged and dislocate. In both types of semiconstrained designs, the linkage between the ulna and humerus allows for a degree of laxity that permits the soft tissues to absorb some of the stresses that would normally be applied to the prosthesis-bone interface. Its indications include all cases of elbow replacement in which bone stock or soft tissue integrity is not adequate for a minimally constrained design to be used. Although in theory it might be more likely to loosen than a minimally constrained design, it has not done so in clinical experience. Thus, some consider a semiconstrained arthroplasty to be indicated in any patient requiring elbow replacement surgery. Others reserve minimally constrained types for young patients.

The indication for elbow arthroplasty is the same as for replacement of the hip, knee, or shoulder—improvement in the quality of life by restoration of pain-free function (motion, stability, and strength) in a joint that is causing functional impairment. Elbow arthroplasty is indicated when such a goal cannot be met by nonsurgical means or other less invasive surgical options. Other indications include the treatment of supracondylar/intercondylar nonunions of the distal humerus, severely comminuted acute supracondylar/intercondylar fractures of the distal humerus in elderly patients with osteoporotic bone that cannot be reduced and fixed adequately, and flail elbow caused by posttraumatic loss of bone or structural integrity. The only contraindication to total elbow arthroplasty is active infection of the joint. Although most authorities recommend reserving total elbow arthroplasty for patients over the age of 60, youth is not an absolute contraindication, just as it is not in the shoulder, knee, or hip. Loss of, or destruction of bone or soft tissue is not a contraindication to total elbow arthroplasty, for these problems can be dealt with surgically. With appropriate implant selection, custom components are rarely required and usually are reserved for revisions or patients with juvenile rheumatoid arthritis (Fig. 17).

Patients with rheumatoid arthritis who require total elbow arthroplasty may have advanced involvement of the ipsilateral shoulder as well. Although there has been considerable discussion regarding which joint should be replaced first, the joint that is most disabling is generally

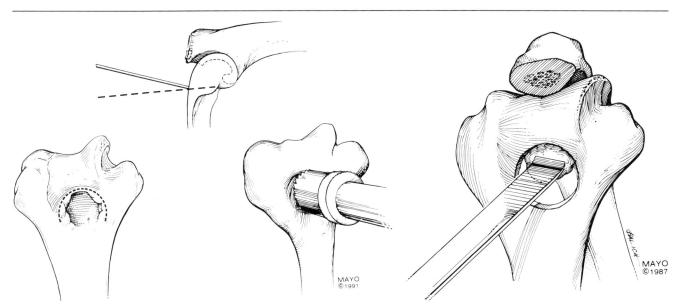

Fig. 14 The Outerbridge-Kashiwagi arthroplasty is performed through a split in the triceps tendon. It involves excision of the osteophytes from the tip of the olecranon by osteotomy. The Cloward drill is used to remove a core of bone from the olecranon fossa to the coronoid fossa, which takes with it the rim osteophytes around each fossa. This is drilled at a 30-degree angle, so that it does not penetrate the articular surface anteriorly. It is performed with the elbow fully flexed. The osteophytes on the coronoid can be removed through the hole in the distal humerus. (Reproduced by permission of Mayo Foundation.)

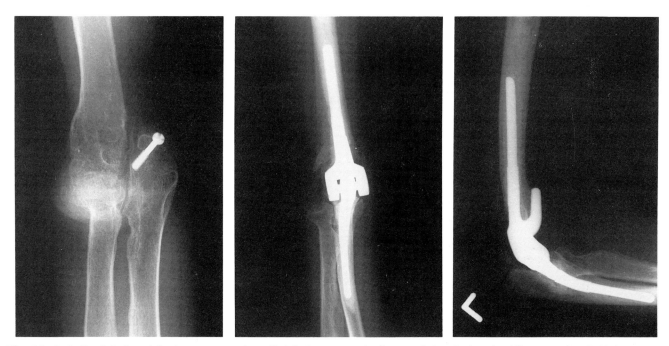

Fig. 15 **Left**, The flail elbow following trauma and usually failed surgery typically severely impairs function. When associated with bone loss, it is best treated by semiconstrained total elbow arthroplasty. Anteroposterior (**center**) and lateral (**right**) radiographs of the same patient following a Morrey-Coonrad semiconstrained total elbow arthroplasty, showing incorporation of a bone graft beneath the anterior flange over the distal humerus at the site of porous ingrowth on the prosthesis.

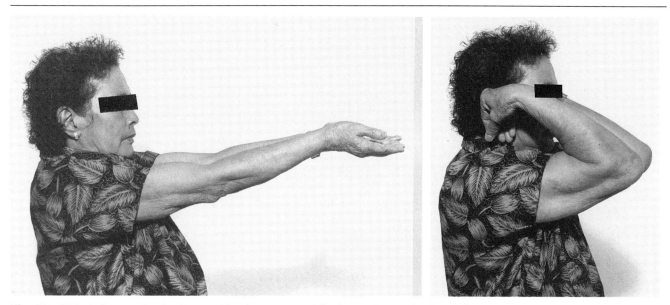

Fig. 16   Clinical photographs of a 64-year-old patient, one year following semiconstrained total elbow arthroplasty for a flail elbow, illustrated in Figure 15. Her arm previously had been completely functionless with less than half of normal range of motion. After reconstruction, function was virtually normal.

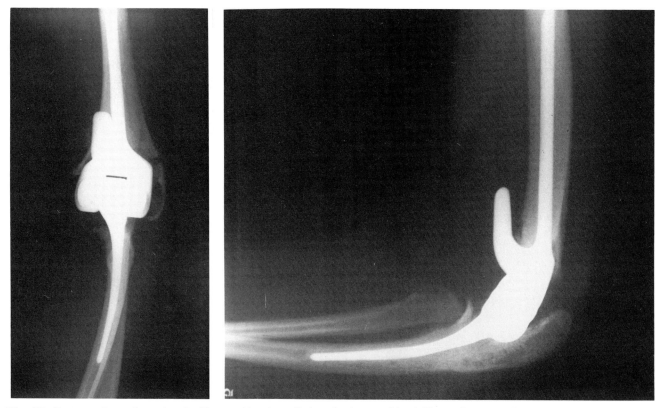

Fig. 17   Postoperative radiographs of a 30-year-old patient with juvenile rheumatoid arthritis causing severe incapacity because of elbow involvement. She previously had had replacement arthroplasties in both lower extremities. The small deformed bones frequently require custom arthroplasty. The soft brittle nature of the bone predisposes to the intraoperative fracture as seen with the fractured epicondyle. This healed in six weeks.

operated on first. The results of either arthroplasty are similar to those seen following replacement of a single joint. The results are not compromised by the presence of severe involvement or contracture. The results of bilateral elbow arthroplasties in patients with rheumatoid arthritis are as good as single joint replacements. The elbow, like the shoulder, becomes a true weightbearing joint in many patients with rheumatoid arthritis because of arthritis in the lower extremities. The need for subsequent lower extremity surgery, resulting in the requirement for walking aids, is not a contraindication for elbow replacement.

A posterior approach is used, as has been discussed. Careful handling of the skin and soft tissues is important, and the skin incision must not devascularize a compromised region of skin created by previous incisions. The ulnar nerve is explored and retracted gently; it usually is transposed anteriorly as part of the procedure. The triceps mechanism is reflected, unless there is significant laxity resulting from bone loss or soft tissue laxity, in which case it can be left intact. If a nonconstrained prosthesis is used, alignment of the components and proper soft-tissue balancing are critical for stability. The ulnar part of the lateral collateral ligament must be properly repaired to prevent posterolateral ulnohumeral rotatory subluxation.

The limb is kept elevated by suspending it for two days. The drain is removed after 24 to 36 hours, and the bulky compressive dressing is removed the next day. The patient is encouraged simply to use the hand for activities of daily living, which gradually results in attainment of a functional arc of motion. A motivated patient requires no physiotherapy, because he or she is able to perform activities that had been impossible or very painful. Exceptions to this rule include patients with significant preoperative contractures. Such patients are sometimes treated with contracture braces to prevent postoperative recurrence of their contractures (Fig. 10).

Results of elbow replacement have improved dramatically in the last 10 years. At least 90% of patients are highly satisfied with pain relief. Functional improvement is predictable following total elbow arthroplasty. Results of a prospective study showed that strength increased 90% in flexion and 60% to 70% in pronation/supination. Extension strength remains relatively unchanged, which might be explained on the basis of surgical approach (detachment and reattachment of the triceps) and offset of the axis of rotation of the prosthesis. The average postoperative arcs of motion are 100 degrees of flexion-extension and 130 degrees of pronation-supination. These ranges include the functional arcs of motion requirement for activities of daily living. Excellent range of motion is also possible in patients with complete preoperative ankylosis of the elbow.

The minimally constrained total elbow arthroplasties have been used with satisfactory long-term success since 1974, with reported average follow-ups of from 6 to 7 years, with a maximum of up to 15 years. Revisions are required in 5% to 10% of the cases. Survivorship analyses suggest a 10% to 20% failure rate by five to ten years. The problem of instability (recurrent dislocation or subluxation) of a nonconstrained elbow prosthesis might at least partially be overcome with improved understanding of the mechanism of elbow instability. The important ulnar part of the lateral collateral ligament complex is violated during a total elbow replacement, and it must be reconstructed.

Loosening of the constrained hinge type of prostheses and dislocation of the nonconstrained designs have been largely overcome by the semiconstrained design. Semiconstrained implants have been in use since 1976, and surveillance averaging up to nine years has been reported, with mechanical (nonseptic) loosening rates of less than 5% and satisfactory results in 90% to 95% of patients. Range of motion, strength, and function are predictably improved. Biomechanical studies have shown that a semiconstrained design can mimic normal elbow kinematics. Loading of the muscles across the elbow permits reproduction of a nearly normal kinematic pattern and limits the varus or valgus deflections. These data are thought to explain at least partially the low clinical rates of loosening observed in the past decade.

Excisional Arthroplasty

Excisional arthroplasty remains an option, particularly following failed total elbow arthroplasty. Its success (relatively pain-free satisfactory range of active motion with reasonable stability) is more likely if the medial and lateral columns of the distal humerus remain present. If the elbow becomes flail or grossly unstable it is usually nonfunctional, as outlined previously in the discussion of flail elbow.

Arthrodesis

Arthrodesis of the elbow is incompatible with satisfactory function because range of motion of the elbow is essential for use of the hand. It is, therefore, rarely indicated as a primary procedure. Its indications are for intractable sepsis or for patients in whom there is no possibility of reconstruction by total elbow revision. There might be an indication in a young man who performs heavy labor. Unfortunately there is no single optimum position.

Tendonopathies and Tendon Injuries

Tennis Elbow

Cortisone injection is used less commonly in current nonoperative treatment of tennis elbow. Furthermore, the concurrent existence of posterior interosseous entrapment at the arcade of Frohse is recognized in approximately 5% of patients.

If surgery is performed, the pathologic findings have been shown to include hyaline degeneration and vascular proliferation in the region of the origin of the extensor carpi radialis brevis tendon, without any evidence of chronic or acute inflammatory changes. The area of pathology is distinguished from a normal tendon by its gray amorphous appearance. It is typically found at the extensor carpi radialis brevis tendon. It is excised and the defect repaired. If posterior interosseous nerve compression coexists with this condition, the two can be treated through one incision that is slightly more anterior and distal.

Fortunately most patients do not require surgery. Conservative treatment includes rest and avoidance of overuse, physical therapy with stretching and strengthening by graduated resisted wrist extension (but never exceeding the patient's pain threshold), and a forearm band. Steroid injections still may be used occasionally, but must not be abused. Manipulation (forced elbow extension with the forearm pronated and the wrist and fingers flexed) has been found by some authors to be effective. There is no role for arthroscopic treatment of this condition, because it is not an intra-articular condition. Complete tenotomy also is inappropriate, because it will violate the lateral collateral ligament. Posterolateral rotatory instability of the elbow is a recognized complication of lateral release, and the lateral pivot shift test should be used at the end of surgery to test for such instability.

Medial epicondylitis is similar to lateral epicondylitis, and involves the common flexor pronator origin. As with lateral epicondylitis, conservative treatment is usually successful. The principles of surgery also are similar.

Rupture of the biceps insertion characteristically occurs in the dominant extremity of muscular men whose age averages about 50 years. A single traumatic event involving flexion against a resistance, with the elbow at a right angle results in a sudden sharp tearing sensation. Weakness of flexion and supination results. A small percentage of these patients may have radiographic irregularities at the bicipital tuberosity on the radius. This condition is treated surgically by reattachment through the two-technique incision discussed above. All patients treated nonsurgically remain weak, especially in supination. Decrease in endurance strength averages 40%. Following surgical repair, most patients achieve nearly normal isometric strength, and many are capable of relatively normal endurance. Rerupture is uncommon. Surgery should be performed early rather than late, because of the ease of the procedure and because with excessive delay it is no longer possible to reattach the tendon into the radius. In such cases, it must be attached to the brachialis instead, which does not improve supination strength.

The two-incision technique of Boyd and Anderson for reattaching the avulsed tendon of the distal biceps can result in radioulnar synostosis because of subperiosteal stripping of the ulna during exposure of the radius. Four such cases have been reported with a discussion of the rationale for a modified approach. A curved blunt instrument is passed down the biceps sheath onto the tuberosity on the radius, which it passes, and tents the skin posteriorly. A limited muscle-splitting approach is made directly down onto the instrument without exposing the ulna. This technique, which is easy, safe, and theoretically should not cause a synostosis, is to be recommended. Avulsion of the triceps occurs with a flake of bone that is seen in about 80% of radiographs. As with the biceps tendon, surgical repair is indicated.

Annotated Bibliography

Biomechanics and Kinetics

Morrey BF, An KN, Stormont TJ: Force transmission through the radial head. *J Bone Joint Surg* 1988;70A:250-256.

The force across the radiohumeral joint is maximal with the elbow extended and the forearm pronated. This corresponds to the position of loading of the radial head with radial head fractures.

Functional Anatomy

O'Driscoll SW, Horii E, Carmichael SW, et al: The cubital tunnel and ulnar neuropathy. *J Bone Joint Surg* 1991;73B:613-617.

The roof of the cubital tunnel is formed by a retinaculum, the cubital tunnel retinaculum (CTR), and the aponeurosis of the flexor carpi ulnaris. The four types of CTR, absent, normal, thick/tight, muscle (anconeus epitrochlearis), correspond to clinical causes of ulnar neuritis, neuropathy, and dislocation. The floor of the tunnel is formed by the medial capsule and the posterior and transverse bands of the MCL, but not the anterior band. The nerve lies just posterior to the anterior band, an important surgical relationship for procedures in this area.

O'Driscoll SW, Horii E, Morrey BF, et al: Anatomy of the ulnar part of the lateral collateral ligament of the elbow. *Clin Anat* 1992;5:1-8.

This anatomic study advances our knowledge and corrects our misunderstanding about the anatomy of the lateral collateral ligament (LCL). There is indeed a "true ligament" on the lateral side, the ulnar part of the LCL, which originates isometrically on the lateral epicondyle and inserts on the ulna at the tubercle of the supinator crest just distal to the annular ligament, over which it passes. This lateral ulnar collateral ligament is the primary constraint to posterolateral rotatory instability and is analogous to the anterior band of the medial collateral ligament. It has been overlooked in previous studies and surgery because it lies beneath the fascia of the supinator.

O'Driscoll SW, Jaloszynski R, Morrey BF, et al: Origin of the medial ulnar collateral ligament. *J Hand Surg* 1992;17A:164-168.

The origin of the medial collateral ligament (MCL) has been variably described as the epicondyle alone or the epicondyle and trochlea. This study proves that the MCL originates from the middle half of the anterior inferior surface of the epicondyle only. Implications for epicondylectomy and Steindler transfer are discussed.

Surgical Exposures

Bryan RS, Morrey BF: Extensive posterior exposure of the elbow: A triceps-sparing approach. *Clin Orthop* 1982;166:188-192.

This is a classic article on the triceps reflecting approach to the elbow, which can be used for most reconstructive procedures as well as for trauma. Variations on this exposure make it virtually universal for elbow surgery.

Arthroscopy

Jackson DW, Silvino N, Reiman P: Osteochondritis in the female gymnast's elbow. *Arthroscopy* 1989;5:129-136.

Some authors have claimed that this condition can be satisfactorily treated arthroscopically by debridement and removal of loose bodies, sometimes with drilling of the defect. These authors found this treatment gave unsatisfactory results in high-performance gymnasts. It may be that the result is the same for all patients and that the extent to which the result is satisfactory is determined by the expectations and demands placed on the elbow by the patient. Valgus stress at the elbow is significant in gymnastics, which may explain why there was only a 10% satisfactory outcome in the patients treated in this series. These patients might benefit from some form of reconstruction of the articular surface itself with the newer methods of articular cartilage regeneration, but these are admittedly experimental.

O'Driscoll SW, Morrey BF: Arthroscopy of the elbow: Diagnostic and therapeutic benefits and hazards. *J Bone Joint Surg* 1992;74A:84-94.

This article details the risks and benefits of arthroscopy of the elbow from an overall viewpoint and describes the diagnostic and therapeutic roles of this procedure. The current techniques are described and illustrated, and a detailed statistical analysis of a large series of patients is provided.

O'Driscoll SW, Morrey BF, An KN: Intraarticular pressure and capacity of the elbow. *Arthroscopy* 1990;6:100-103.

The average capacity of the elbow capsule is about 20 ml, and rupture can occur at relatively low pressures (about 80 mm Hg). The capacity is maximum at 80 degree of flexion, which explains the position of comfort and also the typical position of a stiff elbow.

Vahvanen V, Eskola A, Peltonen J: Results of elbow synovectomy in rheumatoid arthritis. *Arch Orthop Trauma Surg* 1991;110:151-154.

Synovectomy of the elbow is certainly indicated in the early stages of rheumatoid arthritis. As the authors experienced in their review of 54 patients, satisfactory outcome was obtained in three quarters of patients followed an average of almost eight years. These results, similar to the findings of others, support the use of this more limited surgical intervention in the early stages of arthritis.

Elbow Instability: Current Concepts

Bell SN, Morrey BF, Bianco AJ Jr: Chronic posterior subluxation and dislocation of the radial head. *J Bone Joint Surg* 1991;73A:392-396.

Isolated chronic posterior dislocation or subluxation of the radial head is not a common condition, and its treatment is somewhat uncertain. This condition has been clearly classified into three types based on anatomic, prognostic, and treatment implications. Long-term follow-up is available in a relatively large group of patients. Radial head excision in this condition does not necessarily lead to proximal or medial migration or significant growth disturbances.

Conway JE, Jobe FW, Glousman RE, et al: Medial instability of the elbow in throwing athletes: Treatment by repair or reconstruction of the ulnar collateral ligament. *J Bone Joint Surg* 1992;74A:67-83.

This is an extensive review of 68 patients followed for an average of over six years following medial collateral ligament (MCL) repair or reconstruction. Direct repair permitted half of the patients to return to sports, whereas two thirds returned to their same level of participation following reconstruction, typically with a palmaris longus tendon graft. This was performed primarily in throwers. Fifteen patients had postoperative ulnar neuropathy and nine of these required further surgery for this problem. The authors recommend reconstruction rather than repair.

Hotchkiss RN, An KN, Sowa DT, et al: An anatomic and mechanical study of the interosseous membrane of the forearm: Pathomechanics of proximal migration of the radius. *J Hand Surg* 1989;14A:256-261.

This article clearly demonstrates the importance of a central portion of the interosseous ligament to the prevention of proximal migration of the radius following radial head excision and to the transfer of load from the radius to the ulna. This structure contributes 70% to the overall load transfer. There was minimal restoration of this effect by silicone radial head replacement.

Hotchkiss RN, Weiland AJ: Valgus stability of the elbow. *J Orthop Res* 1987;5:372-377.

This is a detailed biomechanical study of the constraints to valgus instability in cadaver elbows. It shows that the anterior band of the medial collateral ligament is the primary constraint to valgus instability. The posterior portion is relatively insignificant. The radial head was found to contribute 30% of valgus stability, but this is probably artificially high because the radius and ulna were fixed with respect to each other. A subsequent study by Morrey did not confirm this. Replacement of the excised radial head with a Silastic prosthesis did not significantly improve biomechanical stability.

Jupiter JB, Goodman LJ: The management of complex distal humerus nonunion in the elderly by elbow capsulectomy, triple plating, and ulnar nerve neurolysis. *J Shoulder Elbow Surg* 1992;1:37-46.

Previously very discouraging results have been reported for supracondylar/intercondylar nonunion treated by open reduction/

internal fixation and bone grafting. However, this article reveals that with advanced surgical technique it may be possible to achieve satisfactory results in these patients. Six of six patients regained an adequate range of motion and function in the elbow following treatment for such conditions using triple plating and bone grafting. This probably will be the first of a series of papers reporting such experience.

Morrey BF, Tanaka S, An KN: Valgus stability of the elbow. A definition of primary and secondary constraints. *Clin Orthop* 1991;265:187-195.

Using sophisticated aerospace technology and a highly accurate electromagnetic tracking system to map the position and orientation of a body in three-dimensional space, the authors demonstrated with sequential cutting and resection that the anterior band of the medial collateral ligament is the primary constraint to valgus instability, and the radial head is a secondary constraint. Minimal instability occurs throughout the arc of motion following radial head excision if the medial collateral ligament (MCL) is intact. Based on the data in this paper, the indication for radial head replacement is valgus instability caused by combined MCL laxity and absence of the radial head due to excision. Of course, it is possible that adequate MCL repair might obviate the need for radial head replacement.

O'Driscoll SW, Bell DF, Morrey BF: Posterolateral rotatory instability of the elbow. *J Bone Joint Surg* 1991;73A:440-446.

Posterolateral rotatory instability of the elbow is a condition that previously has not been described. The clinical and radiographic characteristics of this condition are described in detail, and this report is the first of a series that describe the anatomy, pathology, kinematics, surgical technique, and results of surgery for this condition. Elbow instability is a spectrum from recurrent subluxation to dislocation, with this posterolateral rotatory pattern of instability being the common denominator.

O'Driscoll SW, Morrey BF, Korinek S, et al: Elbow subluxation and dislocation: A spectrum of instability. *Clin Orthop* 1992;280:17-28.

Elbow subluxation and dislocation are part of a spectrum of instability with a common mechanism of posterolateral rotatory displacement. This occurs by a combination of axial load and valgus and supination moments as the elbow flexes. Soft-tissue disruption starts on the lateral side and progresses in a circle anteriorly and posteriorly to the medial side in three stages that have anatomic, clinical (symptoms and signs), and radiographic correlations, which also predict treatment. This applies to acute, recurrent, and chronic instability.

Stiffness and Ankylosis

Bennett GB, Helm P, Purdue GF, et al: Serial casting: A method for treating burn contractures. *J Burn Care Rehabil* 1989;10:543-545.

This paper advocates the use of serial casting in the treatment of burn contractures of the elbow. This is certainly a viable option. The experience of some would indicate that more frequent adjustment of position than that made possible by application of a cast is desirable. The use of patient-adjusted static splints has been highly successful in the hands of some authors. We should remember that nonsurgical treatment is often successful in the management of patients with elbow contracture.

Duke JB, Tessler RH, Dell PC: Manipulation of the stiff elbow with patient under anesthesia. *J Hand Surg* 1991;16A:19-24.

We have traditionally thought that manipulation plays little role in the treatment of a stiff elbow. It is important to note that ten of the 11 patients in this series had had previous surgery. Half improved their motion, two lost motion, and three had no change. Only one patient had a functional arc of motion and only five of the 11 had close to a functional arc of motion. The authors recommend this treatment, but it would seem more appropriate to consider the use of contracture braces and, failing that, surgical intervention followed by appropriate postoperative management.

Husband JB, Hastings H II: The lateral approach for operative release of posttraumatic contracture of the elbow. *J Bone Joint Surg* 1990;72A:1353-1358.

The authors demonstrate that the lateral approach can be used safely and effectively to treat elbow contracture. All seven patients increased extension as well as their arcs of motion, and the average arc of motion was within the functional range. There is current interest in the nonsurgical and surgical treatment of elbow contractures, and this is one of several articles advocating this procedure. This approach is relatively extensile and has many of the advantages of the posterior approach, except one cannot safely expose the ulnar nerve. A separate medial incision can be used for that purpose when the lateral approach is used.

Morrey BF: Post-traumatic contracture of the elbow. Operative treatment, including distraction arthroplasty. *J Bone Joint Surg* 1990;72A:601-618.

This comprehensive article deals with elbow contracture and ankylosis, including all aspects from preoperative evaluation through postoperative rehabilitation. It clearly demonstrates that even for the most serious derangements of the elbow, a functional outcome is usually possible. The surgery is highly demanding, with significant risk of complications, although in experienced hands these should be minimized. The patient's satisfaction is extremely high, despite the potential for complications. The concept of distraction interposition arthroplasty as a salvage for the elbow with a completely destroyed joint surface brings new possibilities to reconstructive surgery.

Radioulnar Synostosis

Failla JM, Amadio PC, Morrey BF, et al: Proximal radioulnar synostosis after repair of distal biceps brachii rupture by the two-incision technique: Report of four cases. *Clin Orthop* 1990;253:133-136.

The two-incision technique of Boyd and Anderson with subperiosteal exposure of the ulna and radius can result in radioulnar synostosis. This risk can be avoided by a muscle-splitting technique for exposure of the tendon insertion of the radius.

Flail Elbow

Botte MJ, Wood MB: Flexorplasty of the elbow. *Clin Orthop* 1989;245:110-116.

This is an overview of different procedural options for restoration of elbow flexion power. A number of tendon transfers are available for restoration of elbow flexion power. The latissimus and pectoralis major transfers result in satisfactory flexion, range of motion, and strength, but the cosmetic deformity of this transfer is significant in female patients. The triceps to biceps transfer is excellent in flexion function, but active extension is sacrificed; therefore, this procedure is contraindicated in those requiring active extension, such as for the use of a cane, crutches, wheelchair, or for overhead function. As pointed out by the authors, the possibility of combined procedures can also be considered.

Total Elbow Arthroplasty

Figgie MP, Inglis AE, Mow CS, et al: Salvage of non-union of supracondylar fracture of the humerus by total elbow arthroplasty. *J Bone Joint Surg* 1989;71A:1058-1065.

Fourteen patients who had failed previous attempts at open reduction and internal fixation, with or without bone grafting, for supracondylar nonunions had satisfactory results following semiconstrained total elbow arthroplasty. This is one of the several indications for total elbow arthroplasty and, indeed, provides the surgeon with the opportunity for one of the most significant improvements in function of a patient. Frequently, these patients have a completely nonfunctional extremity and, following surgery, may well be capable of excellent or close to normal function, assuming normal neurovascular and soft-tissue integrity. A custom total elbow replacement was used in many cases, but this is not necessary with other designs that are commercially available.

Figgie MP, Inglis AE, Mow CS, et al: Total elbow arthroplasty for complete ankylosis of the elbow. *J Bone Joint Surg* 1989;71A:513-520.

Fifteen of 16 patients with ankylosis of the elbow had a good or excellent result with an average range of motion of 80 degrees of flexion and extension. A semi-constrained device was used, and removal of the prosthesis or revision was required in only one patient because of infection. Five required manipulation under anesthetic postoperatively. However, the ultimate range of motion was not significantly affected in those five elbows (average 60-degree range). Current experience indicates that ankylosis is not a contraindication to elbow replacement and that the results can be highly gratifying.

Kudo H, Iwano K: Total elbow arthroplasty with a non-constrained surface-replacement prosthesis in patients who have rheumatoid arthritis. *J Bone Joint Surg* 1990;72A:355-362.

The Kudo elbow, a nonconstrained surface replacement of the humerus and ulna without a radial head prosthesis, is probably the least constrained of the various devices in current use. This is a long-term follow-up of patients previously reported in the short-term follow-up. At the short-term, the results were excellent, but loosening of the nonstemmed humeral component was a major complication in this long-term series. This has also been true in other surface replacement devices. The humeral component tends to loosen because of the posteriorly directed joint resultant force factor as well as the torsional moment about the humeral component. This prosthesis was converted to a stemmed component when this complication was recognized. Loosening of the ulnar component was seen in only 5%.

Lindenfeld TN: Medial approach in elbow arthroplasty. *Am J Sports Med* 1990;18:413-417.

The major risks of arthroscopic instrumentation of the anterior aspect of the elbow are encountered during establishment of the anterolateral or anteromedial portals. In a study of six cadaver elbows, the author showed that the radial nerve was, on average, only 3 mm away from the arthroscope in the anterolateral portal, but the median nerve was, on average, at least 11 mm away from the scope in the anteromedial portal. A valid argument is presented for the routine use of the anteromedial portal as the first portal. However, if both portals are required, as is the case for anterior compartment procedures, we don't know if the risk to the radial nerve is lower with direct antegrade entry or with the use of the switch-stick technique.

Morrey BF, Adams RA, Bryan RS: Total replacement for post-traumatic arthritis of the elbow. *J Bone Joint Surg* 1991;73B:607-612.

This paper reports the authors' experience over a course of a decade and a half and three sequential designs of prosthesis, ranging from the fully constrained to the currently used semiconstrained device, in 53 patients with posttraumatic arthritis. These patients are generally younger than those treated for osteoarthritis and many have undergone multiple operations (as many as eight in these series). The success rate can be expected to be lower and the complication rate higher than in the treatment of rheumatoid or osteoarthritis. Nevertheless, the results are satisfactory in three quarters of cases with the current design, and this would be expected to be higher if replacement arthroplasty was performed only in patients over the age of 60 as recommended by the authors.

O'Driscoll SW, An K-N, Korinek S, et al: Kinematics of semi-constrained total elbow arthroplasty. *J Bone Joint Surg* 1992;74B:297-299.

This biomechanical study in human cadaver elbows is the first to demonstrate that a semiconstrained elbow arthroplasty can mimic the normal kinematics of the elbow during simulated active motion with the muscles loaded. Varus and valgus moments are absorbed, at least in part, by the muscles about the elbow rather than being transferred to the prosthesis-bone interface. This suggests an explanation for the low clinical rates of loosening of at least one of the semiconstrained designs in current use.

Pöll RG, Rozing PM: Use of the Souter-Strathclyde total elbow prosthesis in patients who have rheumatoid arthritis. *J Bone Joint Surg* 1991;73A:1227-1233.

This is a report of 33 patients with this unconstrained (minimally constrained) prosthesis, which is one of the more commonly used nonconstrained elbows. Dislocation occurred in 9%, which is compatible with the other nonconstrained elbows. This was the commonest cause for revision, although loosening of the humeral component because of a short intramedullary stem was another cause. The typical mode of failure, with posterior tilting of the articular surface and extrusion of the proximal stem anteriorly, was noted. Function and pain relief were excellent in the remaining patients. Ulnar nerve problems were seen in only 6% of patients.

Ruth JT, Wilde AH: Capitellocondylar total elbow replacement: A long-term follow-up study. *J Bone Joint Surg* 1992;74A:95-100.

This is a long-term follow-up of the capitellocondylar prosthesis. The early experience with this procedure was noted for its high complication rate, and this is reflected in the data. Pain relief was complete in 85% and partial in 15%. Six percent dislocated, and 31% experienced an ulnar neuropathy. With current techniques for exposure of the elbow, this complication relating to the ulnar nerve should be drastically reduced. There were three revisions and two with radiographic evidence of loosening. Survivorship analysis revealed 80% survival between five and six years. Survivorship was similar after just over a year, indicating that most of the failures occur early on.

Trepman E, Vella IM, Ewald FC: Radial head replacement in capitellocondylar total elbow arthroplasty: 2- to 6-year follow-up evaluation in rheumatoid arthritis. *J Arthroplasty* 1991;6:67-77.

This is a very limited review of six patients in whom a radial head replacement had been performed, associated with a capitellocondylar arthroplasty. The results were satisfactory, with only one case of loosening. The authors suggest that a radial head prosthesis may be indicated. This suggestion is in contrast to their early experience with the surface replacement in which they thought that the radial head replacement tended to predispose to humeral component loosening. The role of radial head replacement and surface arthroplasty of the elbow remains controversial.

Weiland AJ, Weiss AP, Wills RP, et al: Capitellocondylar total elbow replacement: A long-term follow-up study. *J Bone Joint Surg* 1989;71A:217-222.

This is a long-term study of one of the more commonly used prostheses. The function was significantly improved in terms of motion and pain relief, as reported by others. Instability occurred in 29% of patients and lucent lines in 25%. These were not associated with symptoms or loosening. As the lateral approach was used and the lateral collateral ligament complex disrupted, it would be likely that the mechanism of instability was at least in part due to posterolateral rotatory instability. This problem appears to have been reduced in more recent studies and might be further reduced now that we understand this mechanism as well as the treatment of it. Extension was not improved in these patients, which is in contrast to the experience with semi-constrained elbows.

Wolfe SW, Ranawat CS: The osteo-anconeus flap: An approach for total elbow arthroplasty. *J Bone Joint Surg* 1990;72A:684-688.

This variation on the posterior approach to the elbow is reported in this paper to have very good results and is theoretically appealing because it is faster than the traditional triceps-reflecting approach described by Bryan and Morrey. Our personal experience with this approach, however, has been disappointing in that there has been a substantial nonunion rate, although this was reported by the original authors to be a very unlikely complication.

Excisional Arthroplasty

Figgie MP, Inglis AE, Mow CS, et al: Results of reconstruction for failed total elbow arthroplasty. *Clin Orthop* 1990;253:123-132.

Failure of total elbow arthroplasty can be salvaged by resection arthroplasty. Results were satisfactory in three quarters of this series of 11 patients, and this depended on whether or not the epicondyles were present. These results provide a good argument for maintenance of bone stock with elbow reconstructive surgery. Fusion after failed total elbow is difficult, and resection arthroplasty appears to be the alternative of choice.

Tendonopathies and Tendon Injuries

Coonrad RW: Tendonopathies at the elbow, in Tullos HS (ed): American Academy of Orthopaedic Surgeons *Instructional Course Lecture XL*. Park Ridge, IL, American Academy of Orthopaedic Surgeons, 1991, pp 25-32.

Tennis elbow is something that is poorly understood by many. The pathology, clinical presentation, treatment, and prognosis are well delineated in this chapter. The conservative approach, including manipulation, is described in detail and is worthy of study.

Morrey M: Reoperation for failed surgical treatment of refractory lateral epicondylitis. *J Shoulder Elbow Surg* 1992;1:47-55.

Tennis elbow is a condition that remains a thorn in the side of physicians and surgeons in many ways. Failure of surgical treatment sometimes results in despair. This paper provides a logical and constructive approach to the failed tennis elbow surgery patient. If symptoms remained the same postoperatively, the cause was usually inadequate release or incorrect diagnosis. If the symptoms were different, the cause was usually ligamentous laxity. The real value of this paper is probably in the generic approach to failed surgery for any operation, and we would be well served by carefully studying the philosophy of this approach.

30

Wrist and Hand: Congenital Anomalies and Pediatric Reconstruction

The American and International Societies for the Surgery of the Hand have developed a classification that simplifies the previously confusing nomenclature for congenital anomalies of the upper extremity. *Failure of formation* results in transverse congenital amputations, radial or ulnar ray deficiencies of the bone or muscles, central ray deficiencies of the cleft hand, and intercalated deficiency of the humerus or forearm with an intact hand (phocomelia). *Failure of programmed cell death* results in syndactyly and synostoses. *Duplication* results in polydactyly. While *overgrowth* results in hemihypertrophy and macrodactyly, *undergrowth* results in short metacarpals and phalanges. Lastly, there is the *constriction band syndrome*.

Embryology

The limb bud develops from the lateral-plate mesoderm and ectoderm. The inner layer of the ectoderm, called the apical ectodermal ridge, directs the proximal-distal outgrowth and differentiation of the limb-bud mesoderm. Transverse deficiencies may result if this ectodermal influence is lost. Intercalary deficiencies may result from a more localized absence of the ectodermal inductive capacity or may be secondary to a later-stage failure of mesenchymal differentiation to cartilage or of cartilage to bone. Phocomelia, a complete intercalary deficiency, may result from a temporary loss of proliferation of the cells—the progress zone—that would have formed the missing humerus or forearm, with resumed proliferation and differentiation of the more distal hand structures. The limb bud rotates outward, then flattens and broadens to form a pentagonal hand plate. Programmed cell death, still in control of the apical ectodermal ridge, results in interdigital collapse and separation of the rays. Syndactyly occurs when these clefts form abnormally.

Although initially continuous without gaps, the mesenchymal skeleton differentiates to cartilage, and a three-layered interzone forms at the site of the future joints. Between the two chondrogenic layers that are destined to become articular cartilage is a less dense intermediate zone that gives rise to synovium and cavitates to form the joint at the time of joint motion. Distal interphalangeal and some carpal joints form by cavitation of adjacent cartilage without interzone formation. The hands move at 8 weeks' gestation, and creases will form at that time unless the fetus has restricted joint movement, which is seen with arthrogryposis or fusion of the interphalangeal (IP) joints.

Timing of Surgery

The proper timing of surgery remains debated. Most authorities would agree that surgery should wait until the anesthesiologist, who must consider cardiopulmonary, immunologic, or associated musculoskeletal factors, feels it is safe. Also, the body parts must have developed sufficiently that the anomaly has defined itself fully and disposable parts are identifiable. The parts must be able to be immobilized well enough to prevent loss of skin grafts, to preserve soft-tissue reconstructions, and to maintain the position of osteotomies. In the older child, flaps are more easily designed, and larger parts are easier to operate on. Although grasp develops early in infancy, three-digit prehension in hand-eye coordination does not develop until 2 to 3 years of age. Surgeons who believe hand function is encoded earlier perform early surgery. Certainly, surgery should be performed early if there is tethering by unequal growth of adjacent parts or a circulatory disturbance with constriction ring syndrome. Early surgery allows better bone remodeling, as seen with flaring of the distal ulna after centralization of a radial club hand, broadening of the proximal phalanx of the index finger to serve as a thumb metacarpal in pollicization, and improved incorporation of iliac crest bone graft with lengthening.

Most operations for radial club hands, central polysyndactylies, complex syndactylies, transverse phalanges, cleft hands, tight constriction bands, and thumb-index web release are done at 6 to 18 months of age. In other conditions, surgery should be done before school age to avoid teasing by peers and to improve use during the formative years.

Anomalies

Polydactyly

Polydactyly is the most common hand anomaly. Although patients function well, the deformity is unacceptable cosmetically in many cultures. These disorders of the small finger are often inherited or part of a syndrome. Thumb or radial polydactyly has been classified as types I through VII based on the level of duplication. Type IV, at the level of the metacarpophalangeal (MCP) joint of the thumb, is most common, where two proximal phalanges rest on a single broad metacarpal. When duplication is at the level of the joint, types II and IV, the collateral ligament of the digit to be discarded needs to be preserved and sewn to the remaining digit across the retained joint. Similarly, for polydactyly of the small finger, the abductor digiti minimi needs to be attached to the retained digit. Central polydactyly is often inherited and associated with syndactyly. The good web should be preserved and the digit removed.

Ulnar Dimelia

Duplication of all but the radial ray results in a hand with seven or eight fingers and no thumb, called "mirror hand." The ulna is duplicated, and the radius is absent. The humerus has two poorly developed trochlea and the olecranon fossae of the ulnas at the elbow face one another. The elbow is stiff in extension, pronation and supination are limited, the wrist is flexed, the hand is flat, and neither border can oppose. Reconstructive procedures are directed toward restoring elbow flexion, forearm supination, wrist extension, and pollicization to allow opposition.

Syndactyly

Syndactyly is most common in the middle and ring fingers. There is a shortage of skin; the combined circumference of the two digits is 1.4 times the circumference of two digits held side to side. Skin grafts, usually full thickness, are therefore needed at the base of the digit next to the web. The web is most commonly re-created using a dorsal flap or two triangular flaps, one volar and one dorsal. A Z-plasty is used to prevent scar contracture. The common digital artery division may limit the depth of the web. Digital nerves and arteries may be branched, entwined, or absent within the bridge, usually to the degree of associated bony fusions and hypoplasia in complex and complicated syndactyly. One side of a digit should be operated on at a time, and nerves should be teased apart using magnification. Once conjoined nails and the underlying bone or cartilaginous connections have been freed, palmar pulp is defatted and advanced dorsally to create a nail fold.

Failure of the procedure is most often attributable to loss of the skin graft and inadequate postoperative dressing. The fingers should be abducted with a fluff stent, and held with a cling wrap and long arm plaster with the elbow flexed.

The age at which a syndactyly should be released is controversial. Traditionally, the operation was postponed until age 3 or 4 years to obtain better patient cooperation, but many surgeons do the release at 9 months to 1 year of age or even earlier. Certainly, patients should be treated as young as possible if one digit is shorter and is tethering the growth of the other. Bilateral procedures are done in children less than 14 months of age and avoided in the older child.

When all digits are joined, as is common in the spoon hand of Apert's syndrome (acrocephalosyndactyly), it is important to release the border digits—thumb and small finger—first. The remaining three joined fingers can be managed by removing the middle digit, thus creating a three-fingered hand with a thumb and sufficient skin for closure. The thumb often has a delta phalanx, requiring osteotomy or excision.

More recently, there have been trials of release of syndactyly at birth. Newer methods have been used for re-creating nail folds, including flaps from the separated digit, composite grafts from the lateral great toe, or a thenar flap in complex syndactyly. Tissue expansion techniques have been applied to avoid the need for skin grafting. Greater attention has been paid to the arterial supply to the digits, and a preoperative arteriogram is recommended in many cases. One vessel intact to each digit is sufficient. If the common vessel is inadvertently damaged or is absent, both digits usually remain viable. However, if an artery is injured or divided and absence is known on the other side, reanastomosis of the artery under a microscope is indicated.

Constriction Band Syndrome

Normally programmed cell death progresses from distal to proximal in the web. In syndactyly that is associated with amniotic bands, the fingers separate and then reattach distally, often leaving a characteristic epidermal-lined sinus proximally, which can be probed from dorsal to palmar.

Constriction bands may be related to intrauterine fibrous sheets seen on ultrasound. They may encase the limb circumferentially, resulting in indentation, edema, vascular insufficiency, neurologic loss, or amputation. These amputations differ from other congenital amputations in that the proximal structures are normal and overgrowth is possible. Staged releases are performed on 50% of the digit at a time using Z-plasties with or without a shift of the surrounding fat to fill in the indentation (Fig. 1). Syndactyly is released, and any sinus is completely excised to prevent epidermal inclusion cysts.

Transverse Absences

Transverse absences of the forearm usually do not mandate excision of nubbins or the skin for prosthetic fit. Bilateral amputees may be candidates for the Krukenberg procedure, where the radius and ulna are separated to serve as prehensile pincers. This is the operation of choice for blind, bilateral upper-extremity amputees. Early fit of a passive mitten or hand at 6 months of age encourages integration of the prosthesis into daily activities and body image. Otherwise, children will prefer to use the deficient limb as a helper without the prosthesis. A hook and shoulder harness can be added at 2 years of age.

Myoelectric prostheses, where thumb-index pinch is triggered by skin electrodes over contracting muscles, are increasingly popular, and mechanical breakdown and need for surface repairs have become less common. When a wrist is present and mobile, a prosthesis with a palmar plate extending distally can be used as a post on which the flexed wrist can hold objects.

When metacarpal bones are present in a transverse deficiency, it may be possible to create a mobile radial ray and a post on which it can oppose. The presence of a

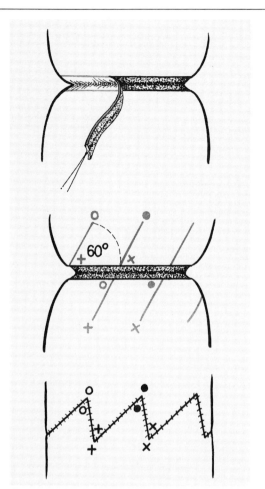

Fig. 1 Treatment of constriction ring. Excision of skin and deeper tissues is followed by multiple Z-plasties. (Reproduced with permission from Buck-Gramcko D: Congenital malformations, in Nigst H, Buck-Gramcko D, Millesi H, et al (eds): *Hand Surgery: General Aspects: Elective Surgery*. New York, Thieme Medical Publishers, 1988, vol 1, p 12.45.)

joint at the base of the thumb metacarpal and the presence of thenar muscles are important. Options include web deepening, transferring central metacarpals to lengthen a border ray, insertion of an autogenous bone graft, metacarpal distraction lengthening, or vascularized toe-to-hand transfer. Toe transfers are more difficult in the young and less predictable in the absence of muscle-tendon units in the forearm. Free, nonvascularized transfer of proximal phalanges of toes with open epiphyses will take and even grow if periosteum and collateral ligaments are left attached. These transplants can be added on top of existing metacarpals or phalanges of the thumb and index rays. Flexor and extensor tendons, which are usually looped over the bone end of the congenital defect, can be split and sutured to the base of the transplanted phalanx.

In the hand with no digits, transplantation of the proximal phalanx of the fourth toe from the ipsilateral foot can create a thumb when both sides of the thumb carpometacarpal joint are present. Microvascular transplantation of the second toe from the contralateral foot is then used to create a pincer on the ulnar side. Metacarpal distraction lengthening followed by grafting of iliac crest, fibula, allograft material, demineralized bone matrix, or nonfunctional skeletal elements in the hand has been used in adactylia. Distraction osteogenesis without the need for bone grafting has been successful using unilateral frames. Similar considerations are applicable for phalangeal-level terminal deficiencies, but function is usually excellent if the majority of the proximal phalanx is present.

Phocomelia

Intercalated loss of arm and forearm elements was seen in the 1960s when the sedative thalidomide was taken by women in the first trimester of pregnancy. The hand attaches directly to the shoulder or humerus. When the forearm is present with the hand, a radial or ulnar deficiency is often found. Surgery is rarely required unless to enhance prosthetic fit. Digits that function by intrinsic muscles can trigger a prosthetic terminal device.

Longitudinal Deficiencies

When one of two parallel bones normally present is missing, the remaining bone curves, often tethered by a fibrocartilaginous anlage. A short ulna may cause the longer radius to dislocate at the elbow. The ulna supports the elbow, and the radius supports the wrist. Thus, ulnar deficiencies more severely affect the elbow, whereas radial deficiencies affect the wrist. Radial absences have serious associated marrow and visceral abnormalities, whereas ulnar absence does not. Radial absence is bilateral in 50% of cases, whereas ulnar absence is rarely so.

Radial Deficiency

Radial deficiency includes shortened or absent radius, thenar muscle deficiencies, and absent thumb. Radial deficiencies are associated with cardiac abnormalities (Holt-Oram syndrome), thrombocytopenia (TAR syndrome), aplastic (Fanconi's) anemia, and a host of skeletal and visceral abnormalities (VATER syndrome).

Shortened or Absent Radius: Radial Club Hand

Serial plasters are used to stretch tight structures on the radial side. The distal ulna is squared off and inserted into a rectangular notch on the radial side of the carpus. A fibrous pseudarthrosis provides wrist stability, which can be enhanced by imbricating the ulnar capsule and extensor carpi ulnaris. Carpal bones need not be resected if the carpus is placed on the distal ulna at between 6 and 12 months of age (Fig. 2). Wrist motion is better preserved and alignment maintained by transfer of the flexor and extensor carpi radialis tendons to the ulnar side.

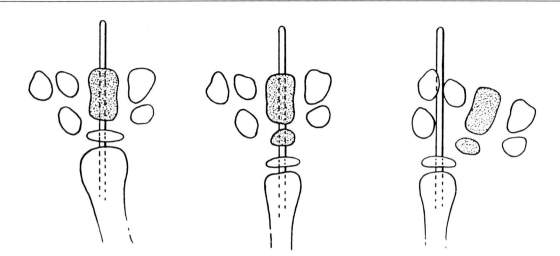

Fig. 2 Treatment of radial club hand. **Left**, Centralization by carpal resection and pinning. **Center**, Centralization by reduction on end of radius without carpal excision. **Right**, Radialization with reduction of carpus and pinning in ulnar deviation. (Reproduced with permission from Upton J: Congenital anomalies of the hand and forearm, in McCarthy JG (ed): *Plastic Surgery*. New York, WB Saunders, 1990, pp 5213-5399.)

The forearm is expected to be two thirds of the normal length, and further shortening is prevented by avoiding damage to the distal ulnar growth plate. After centralization, consideration may be given to ulnar lengthening. Bowing of the ulna is not progressive, but if it is severe, the bone can be osteotomized.

If all of the radius is present but the wrist deviates to the radial side, the contracted radial capsule is released. The radial tendons may be transferred to the extensor carpi ulnaris, which in turn can be advanced distally, shortened, or transferred to the third metacarpal. If the radius is present but short, the carpus may be supported radially without need for centralizing by serial lengthening of the radius with external fixation or by transfer of vascularized fibula and its epiphyseal plate, which will grow with the ulna.

Thenar Deficiency
Opposition can be restored by transfer of the abductor digiti minimi across the palm to the thumb. The ulnar collateral ligament of the metacarpophalangeal joint is always lax and therefore must be tightened. If the radial collateral ligament is lax, it should likewise be tightened; if the metacarpophalangeal joint is unstable, a fusion may be needed.

Absent Thumb
In order to grasp objects, one digit needs to be separated from the others. The index finger can be repositioned to the first metacarpal head. The proximal two thirds of the first metacarpal can be excised, and the preserved metacarpal head can be rotated to prevent hyperextension of the transferred digit. When the first metacarpal is absent, the head of the second metacarpal is used to create a new carpometacarpal joint. A thumb web space is created, and index muscles and tendons are rerouted to serve thumb function. More than 50% of patients need additional procedures, including tenolysis, shortening, fusion, or abductor digiti minimi opponensplasty. A transferred toe has no cortical representation and is not recommended for reconstruction of an absent thumb.

Ulnar Deficiency
Management of an ulnar deficiency depends on whether a fibrocartilaginous anlage results in a progressive deformity, whether pronation and supination are preserved, and whether the proximal radius is dislocated, fused to the humerus, or in normal relationship to the capitellum. In most cases of partial or complete absence of the ulna, a fibrocartilaginous anlage will tether the growth of the radius with dislocation of the radial head or bowing. If the anlage is excised within the first 6 months of life, the proximal radius probably will remain in normal relation to the capitellum, and pronation and supination will be maintained. As long as forearm rotation is preserved, there is no need to fuse the radius and ulna, even if the radial head is dislocated. One need merely excise the anlage if it is tethering the radius. However, if no pronation or supination is present, the dislocated radial head should be excised to create a one-bone forearm. Whenever a radial head is excised to improve cosmesis, the distal radius should be fused to the proximal ulna for forearm stability, but this procedure should be performed only if the patient will be better off without forearm rotation.

When the radius is fused to the humerus, the anlage is excised to prevent bowing of the radius and wedging of the distal radial epiphysis. If the elbows are fused bilaterally in extension, one elbow should be fused in flexion. A distal radial osteotomy may be necessary to prevent tilt.

The fourth and fifth rays are often absent, webbed, or fused to the other digits. In these patients, the forearms should be treated before the hands, but early surgery on the hand is needed if short ulnar rays are deforming the long finger.

Cleft Hand

The typical cleft hand has a V-shaped defect where the long ray is absent. The malformation is bilateral and familial, and the feet are also involved. The index ray may also be absent, and the border digits may be syndactylized, in which case, the thumb may be abducted. The ring ray is rarely absent.

The atypical cleft hand has a U-shaped defect between the remaining border digits, and more than one central ray is missing. This condition is unilateral, and the feet are not involved. The atypical form is really a symbrachydactyly because the metacarpals are present, and the phalanges are replaced by small nubbins. The thumb and small border rays remain, giving the hand a lobster-claw appearance. It has been suggested that damage to the hand plate centripetally suppresses the development of rays radialward and then ulnarward. Another theory, supporting the association between cleft hands and polydactyly, proposes that rays have been duplicated so numerously that they are no longer recognized as digits.

Patients with a cleft hand function well but are embarrassed by the appearance of the hand. Treatment of the typical cleft hand is to close the cleft, reapproximate the metacarpals by reconstruction of the intermetacarpal ligament, and form a new distal commissure using a diamond-shaped flap. Border digit syndactyly is released. If thumb mobility is limited by an adduction contracture, either a flap of dorsal skin can be rotated into the thumb web or the index ray can be transposed ulnarward to the base of the third metacarpal. The palmar side of the cleft is then used to deepen the web.

The type of surgery appropriate for a typical cleft hand depends on the function of the border digits. If apposition is possible, no surgery is necessary. If the cleft prevents grip of the border rays, the cleft may be deepened. Unstable border digits may be fused. If border digits are stable and have good passive motion, a graft of palmaris longus tendon can be attached to a wrist flexor or extensor to restore active motion to the digits.

Camptodactyly

The pathologic anatomy responsible for the fixed proximal interphalangeal flexion deformity is controversial, but this deformity is likely an imbalance caused by extensor hood insufficiency, a tight flexor digitorum superficialis, or abnormal intrinsic insertion volarward. Nonsurgical treatment—stretching and splinting—is preferred (Fig. 3). If required, the aberrant lumbrical muscle can be excised and the flexor superficialis transferred to the lateral band from a dorsal or combined dorsal and volar approach.

Symphalangia

Stiff fingers with absent joints are best left untreated. Arthroplasties have failed, resulting in unstable joints. An unossified epiphysis may be mistaken for the joint space. A well-segmented joint space in a young child may be freed by collateral and dorsal capsule release, but attempted resection of a cartilaginous bar will result in fusion. Associated syndactyly in Poland's or Apert's syndrome often necessitates separation of the digits and conversion to a functional three-fingered hand.

Radioulnar Synostosis

The radial and ulnar anlagen separate longitudinally by segmentation and cavitation from distal to proximal at a time when the embryologic forearm is in pronation. Thus, the proximal one third of the forearm is the most common site of bony union, and the forearm is pronated. Patients with a unilateral deformity or with a bilateral deformity and minimal pronation do not need surgery. Resection and interposition procedures fail. Derotational osteotomy through the area of synostosis is recommended, placing one side in 10 to 20 degrees of pronation and the other forearm in a neutral position or slight supination for function. In patients with severe bilateral hyperpronation, osteotomy of the nondominant extremity, to create supination, is indicated.

Clinodactyly

Incurving of a digit, usually the small finger, because of a trapezoidal middle phalanx is best left untreated. If, at skeletal maturity, the digits overlap with the making of a fist, a radial opening or ulnar closing wedge osteotomy can be performed. The middle phalanx of the small finger is the last bone in the hand to ossify.

Congenital Trigger Finger or Thumb

Congenital trigger digit is a fixed interphalangeal flexion deformity that is treated by division of the A_1 pulley if it does not resolve spontaneously by 12 months of age. Care must be taken to avoid injury to the radial digital nerve, which lies directly beneath the skin.

Delta Phalanx

Also called longitudinally bracketed epiphysis, delta phalanx is a condition in which the physeal plate with a proximal epiphysis curves around from its transverse orientation to a longitudinal one from proximal to distal along one side of the phalanx, thus forming a C. This results in a trapezoidal phalanx. Longitudinal growth is impossible and angulation inevitable. Treatment is designed to restore length, preserving the horizontal portion of the physis and destroying the longitudinally oriented portion. This is accomplished by an opening wedge osteotomy on the narrow side of the trapezoidal phalanx or by a reverse wedge osteotomy, in which the wedge is excised as a triangle and reinserted on the opposite side of the phalanx. Excision of the abnormal part of the

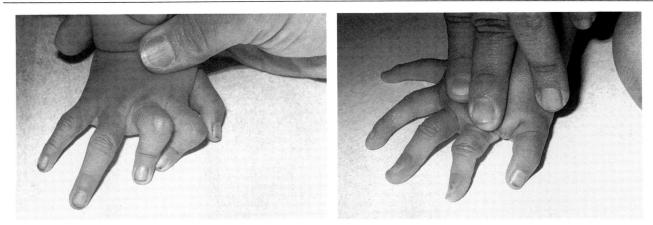

Fig. 3   **Left**, Camptodactyly of index and long fingers of left hand. **Right**, Improved with stretching and splinting.

physeal plate may result in resumption of more normal growth.

Kirner Deformity

The Kirner deformity is a dominantly inherited palmar and radialward deviation of the distal phalanx of the small finger usually seen at 8 to 12 years of age. Treatment is usually unnecessary. When it is, an osteotomy is performed through a midlateral incision and held with a Kirschner wire.

Gigantism

Macrodactyly is a hamartomatous enlargement of the soft tissue and underlying bone that can be static, growing commensurately with the hand, or progressive, growing faster than the rest of the hand. The term "nerve territory-oriented macrodactyly" relates the observed enlargement of the nerve supply to the affected digits that more commonly follow the distribution of the median nerve than that of the ulnar nerve. Children may complain of paresthesia, and, by adulthood, the enlarged median nerve can be compressed beneath the transverse carpal ligament. Macrodactyly is considered by many authorities to be a form of neurofibromatosis, as fat and fibrous tissue are found in the peripheral nerves of both conditions. Besides its association with nerve-oriented lipofibromatosis and neurofibromatosis, macrodactyly can be seen with osteochondral expansions of the phalanges or metacarpals and with hemihypertrophy. Treatment is by staged debulking, dealing with one side of the digit or hand at a time, because the blood supply to the skin of the enlarged digits is poor. Appropriately timed epiphysiodesis of the involved bones is performed during growth; alternatively, later bone resections and fusions can be carried out. Thumb reduction has been performed by excising the central third and attaching the two lateral portions of bone side to side.

Madelung's Deformity

Madelung's deformity (carpus curvus) is the result of an epiphyseal arrest on the ulnar and volar half of the distal radius, which causes the articular surface to be directed ulnarward and volarward (Fig. 4). A generalized dysplasia should be suspected if the condition is bilateral or if there is a positive family history, short stature, or mesomelia. Pain from radioulnar subluxation or radiolunate impingement usually becomes less severe at maturity. Pain and mild deformity can be treated with distal ulnar resection. The traditional treatment for severe deformity is distal radial osteotomy at maturity. Arthrodesis is considered if the carpus subluxates off the radius.

Multiple Hereditary Exostosis

Bowed radius with ulnar deviation and translocation of the wrist occurs in 50% of patients with multiple hereditary exostosis. The distal ulna contributes more to total bone length than does the distal radius, and the cross-sectional area of the ulnar growth plate is less than one quarter that of the distal radius. An exostosis of equal size will retard a greater proportion of the longitudinal growth of the ulna, and the faster-growing radius will either bend or dislocate at the radiohumeral joint. Excision of a distal osteochondroma unpredictably slows the shortening of the ulna and only occasionally improves forearm rotation. Ulnar lengthening may temporarily correct ulnar translocation at the wrist, but shortening recurs. Ulnar lengthening and correction of the radial angulation by distal radial osteotomy or stapling of the radial hemiepiphysis improves the angulation of the wrist as well as pronation and supination. The radial head should never by excised in a growing patient and is excised in the mature patient only to improve cosmesis.

Multiple Enchondromatosis

A deformity similar to that of multiple hereditary exostosis is multiple enchondromatosis. The condition results in a short ulna and dislocation of the radial head.

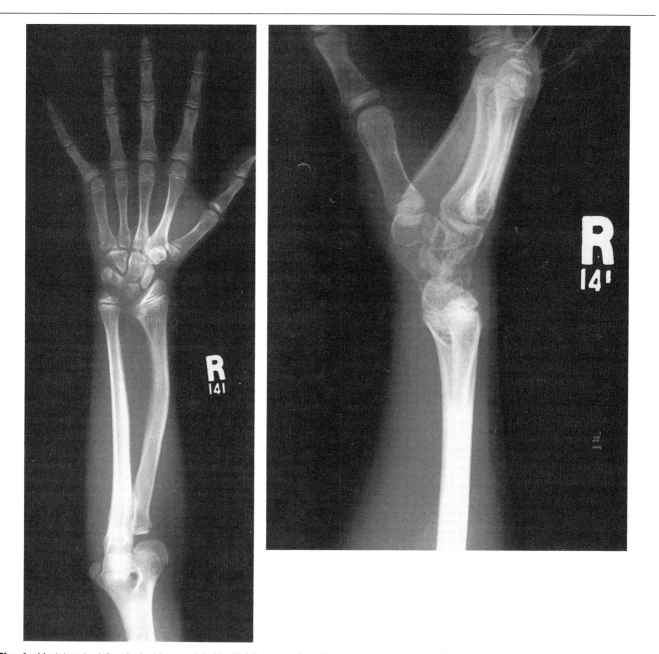

Fig. 4 Madelung's deformity in 11-year-old girl with bilateral deformity and short stature. **Left**, Anteroposterior view shows fusion of the ulnar part of the physis with ulnar tilt of the distal articular surface of radius. The carpus, shaped like a V, is driven like a wedge between the radius and ulna, the distal ulna is subluxated. **Right**, On lateral view, the dorsal tilt of distal radius is apparent.

Hand in Cerebral Palsy

Most patients with cerebral palsy have a functionless hand marked by spasticity, weakness, flexion deformity of the wrist and fingers, thumb-in-palm deformity, and loss of sensation and proprioception. Surgery will improve cosmesis but not function, and wrist fusion or tendon transfers may be offered to adolescents who are affected by the appearance of the hand. Procedures involving an inlay iliac-crest graft are most successful,

and the wrist should be held in the neutral position by a large Kirshner wire placed in the third metacarpal across the wrist and into the radius. If the finger and thumb flexors remain tight, the sublimis tendons are divided at the wrist, the profundus tendons are lengthened, and the thumb is released.

A few patients, usually those with hemiplegia, have a useful hand marked by a fair grasp and release, fair sensation, a flexed wrist, and thumb-in-palm. They may benefit from transfer of the flexor carpi ulnaris around the ulnar border of the wrist to the extensor carpi radialis brevis to restore active dorsiflexion of the wrist. Patients must have sufficient active finger extension to enable them to release objects in the absence of palmar flexion. The abductor pollicis longus and extensor pollicis brevis may be plicated, and the extensor pollicis longus may be rerouted to a more radial position with the addition of tendon transfer after fusion of the metacarpophalangeal joint of the thumb and release of the thumb adductor. The thumb-in-palm deformity can be overcome, but active abduction of the thumb is only partly achieved.

Hand in Arthrogryposis

The hands of patients with arthrogryposis are marked by weak motor muscles, stiff metacarpophalangeal and interphalangeal joints, an adducted thumb, and a flexed and ulnar-deviated wrist. In children who have learned to manage personal hygiene and feeding, surgery runs the risk of making their function worse. Restoration of flexion of one elbow is a primary consideration in the management of the upper extremity. The hand that has pinch and grasp is best left untreated. One of the few predictable procedures is sublimis release for flexion of the proximal interphalangeal joint. Fingers that are stiff in full extension may be improved by releasing the joints and allowing the fingers to stiffen in flexion. The adducted thumb requires web release, skin grafting, and tendon transfers to the extensor and abductors, most often using sublimis. Serial casting of a flexed wrist should precede proposed arthrodesis to confirm functional improvement. The flexed wrist is commonly of benefit to allow bent fingers to hook objects.

Juvenile Chronic Polyarthropathy

Children with seronegative arthritis usually present before age 5 years and have iridocyclitis if fewer than five joints are involved. The destruction of their joints is less severe than that of seropositive children, who present after age 10 and have adult-like disease progression. The inflammatory hyperemia results in osteopenia and early ossification of the carpal bones visible on radiographs. The distal ulnar physis matures early, and the short ulna contributes to ulnar translocation of the carpus along the incline of the articular surface of the distal radius. In the adult with rheumatoid arthritis, flexor and extensor tendons pull the fingers ulnarward at the metacarpophalangeal joint; via intercalary linkage, a zigzag radial deviation of the radiocarpal and carpometacarpal joints results. Forces of usage are contributory, accounting for the fact that children, with no work demands, have a lower incidence of ulnar drift than do adults.

Surgery is not often needed in childhood. Physical therapy, home exercises, and splinting may prevent the loss of wrist extension, ulnar translocation at the wrist, loss of flexion at the metacarpophalangeal joints, and hyperextension of the proximal interphalangeal joint. Children are not tolerant of the painful movement needed to preserve function. Severe swelling and pain

may necessitate synovectomy. Although the procedure is controversial, synovectomy performed early, before bony erosion, is of greater benefit and may retard the course of the disease.

The wrist is most commonly involved. Synovectomy after radiographic changes have occurred relieves pain in half the patients, but recurrent synovitis and persistent erosion and subluxation are likely. Surgical fusion or arthroplasty may be required. Metacarpophalangeal synovitis is more often seen in the seropositive child and, unlike the situation in adults, may affect only one or two joints. Synovectomy, repositioning of the extensor tendon over the metacarpophalangeal joint, and intrinsic release or transfer for tightness may be performed. Collateral ligament release has been used to improve metacarpophalangeal flexion. Swan neck deformity in children usually responds to use of a splint, preventing extension but allowing flexion. Landsmeer's ligament may need to be reconstructed using the radial intrinsic, leaving the ulnar intrinsic for transfer. Boutonnière deformity, a result of thinning of the central slip of the extensor tendon with forward subluxation of the lateral bands, is not predictably improved by reconstruction of the extensor mechanism. The boutonnière deformity may need to be converted to a mallet deformity by dividing the extensor mechanism just proximal to the distal interphalangeal joint. Injection of the tendon sheaths with corticosteroids often improves range of motion. Tendon ruptures are rare in children and, unlike those in adults, can be treated by primary repair rather than tendon transfer.

Bone and Soft-Tissue Tumors

Vascular Malformations

The most common soft-tissue lesions in children are vascular in origin. The term "hemangioma" is reserved by some authors for the superficial strawberry or deeper blue lesion that proliferates and grows faster than the child by 2 months of age but shows spontaneous involution by 4 to 5 years of age. Venous malformations, although present at birth, often are not noticed until 1 year of age. They engorge when dependent, decompress when elevated, and enlarge with trauma, puberty, pregnancy, or use of oral contraceptives. Lymphatic malformations contain catacomb-like spaces, may have associated skin blebs, can exude serous fluid, and have an increased incidence of β-streptococcus infections (Fig. 5).

Low-flow venous and lymphatic malformations can be treated either conservatively by compression garments or surgically by staged debulking, avoiding the need to return later to a previously scarred area. Surgery is complicated by bleeding or lymphatic leaks, hematoma or seroma, formation, skin necrosis, scarring, ulceration, contractures, and distention of channels in the same or adjacent areas. High-flow arteriovenous malformations are even more difficult to treat, and staged partial exci-

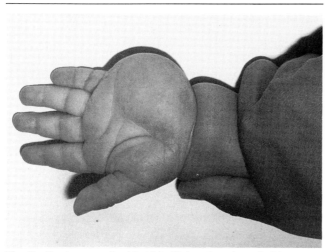

Fig. 5 Fourteen-month-old child with lymphangioma that has grown commensurate with child since birth.

sions are mostly palliative. Proximal ligation only increases collateralization, and embolization carries a high risk of digital ischemia. The YAG laser, used in direct contact with tissue for incision and thermal coagulation, has allowed subtotal excision of complicated hemangiomas of the hand previously thought to be untreatable. However, the laser will not stop bleeding from blood vessels with lumen diameters greater than 1 mm.

Benign Soft-Tissue and Bone Tumors of the Hand

Soft-tissue tumors of the hand in children are usually asymptomatic. They have a high rate of local recurrence, suggesting that greater attention should be paid to correct diagnosis and an adequate surgical margin. Ganglia occur much less commonly in children than in adults. Calcification in a lesion suggests a cavernous hemangioma, with phleboliths, tumoral calcinosis, soft-tissue chondroma, synovial chondromatosis, and calcification being seen with dermatomyositis, secondary hyperparathyroidism, hypervitaminosis D, idiopathic hypercalcemia, or milk alkali syndrome. A giant-cell tumor of a tendon sheath may erode the adjacent phalanx. Aggressive fibromatosis, with its tendency to invade locally and recur after excision, may require adjuvant radiother-

apy for control. Lipomatous tumors may involve the median nerve and are difficult to excise without risk of local recurrence.

The most common primary bone tumors, enchondromas and osteochondromas, are easily recognized when multiple but may cause confusion when single. Osteoid osteomas show an intense sclerotic reaction with periosteal thickening and a radiolucent nidus. Hematogenous osteomyelitis, which might be confused with the tumor, is extremely rare in the hands of children. Aneurysmal bone cysts may be expansile and resemble reparative granulomas. Cystic radiolucency in the distal phalanx is characteristic of epidermoid cyst. Glomus tumors are more common in adults. Benign bone tumors are treated by intralesional curettage and bone grafting or by resection if large or locally recurrent.

Malignant Soft-Tissue and Bone Tumors of the Hand

Malignant soft-tissue and bone tumors are extremely rare in children, accounting for only a case or two in any series. The few reported instances include a fibrosarcoma, a synovial sarcoma, a malignant fibrous histiocytoma, and a rhabdomyosarcoma. A series of 18 patients with primary malignant bone tumors seen at the Mayo Clinic from 1920 through 1985 including one 5-year-old child with a Ewing's sarcoma of the proximal phalanx that was irradiated before metastases developed. Three cases of Ewing's sarcoma were the only malignant lesions reported among 21 primary bone tumors of the hand collected from eight pediatric hospitals worldwide.

A precise definition of the anatomic extent of disease with magnetic resonance imaging and preoperative or postoperative adjuvant treatment has permitted limb salvage surgery even in the distal extremity. Preoperative radiotherapy is usually given for soft-tissue sarcomas, and chemotherapy is used for malignant bone tumors before wide excision. In general, lesions of the middle and distal phalanges are treated with cross-bone amputation or interphalangeal disarticulation. Proximal phalangeal or large metacarpal lesions often necessitate the resection of two or three rays to prevent marginal excisions, which have a high rate of local recurrence. Reconstruction with flap coverage, tendon transfer, and nerve and bone grafts can preserve function.

Annotated Bibliography

Timing of Surgery

Buck-Gramcko D: Progress in the treatment of congenital malformations of the hand. *World J Surg* 1990;14:715-724.

Microsurgery has allowed surgery in the first and second years of life, providing improved cosmesis, function, and bone and soft-tissue remodeling. Free second-toe transplantation and fourth-toe top to proximal-phalanx transplantation allows the surgeon to provide pincer function in hands with one or no digits.

After syndactyly separation, nail walls can be reconstructed using pulp tissue from the opposite digit. Good parts of a duplicated digit can be used to replace poor parts of digit to be retained. Radialization of a radial club hand may result in better motion than does ulnocarpal fusion when the central carpus is resected.

Polydactyly

Lister G: Pollex abductus in hypoplasia and duplication of the thumb. *J Hand Surg* 1991;16A:626-633.

An anomalous slip from the flexor to the extensor pollicis longus passes around the radial border of the thumb and results in abduction rather than flexion of the MP and IP joints in 20% of thumb duplications and 35% of hypoplastic thumbs. The abducted thumb is corrected by excision of the intertendinous slip, sometimes combined with rerouting and pulley reconstruction. Recognized by the absence of extensor and flexor creases of the IP joint and the absence of active with retained passive IP flexion, it is a likely cause of abduction at the IP joint after removal of a duplicate thumb.

Syndactyly

Colville J: Syndactyly correction. *Br J Plast Surg* 1989;42:12-16.

At 1 year of age, volar and dorsal rectangular flaps designed to allow closure on the important opposition ulnar side of the cleft and partial full-thickness grafting of the radial side of the cleft are carried out. The web is reconstructed using a kite-shaped dorsal island flap, which is moved on a VY principle. The defect created can be closed primarily or by split-skin graft. No web contracture has been seen.

Moss ALH, Foucher G: Syndactyly: Can web creep be avoided? *J Hand Surg* 1990;15B:193-200.

Web space creep is a partial recurrence of the syndactyly. Longitudinal scars on the lateral sides of the adjacent separated digits do not grow as fast as the remaining digit and pull the commissure distally. A technique using two triangular skin flaps on the palmar side of the proximal phalanges prevents this longitudinal scarring.

Ogawa Y, Kasai K, Doi H, et al: The preoperative use of extra-tissue expander for syndactyly. *Ann Plast Surg* 1989;23:552-559.

Skin grafts were avoided in four patients undergoing simple syndactyly release by stretching and compressing the volar and dorsal interdigital skin to form a hollow between the two mobile digits prior to separation.

Ostrowski DM, Feagin CA, Gould JS: A three-flap web-plasty for release of short congenital syndactyly and dorsal adduction contracture. *J Hand Surg* 1991;16A:634-641.

A rectangle is outlined on both the dorsal and the volar webbed skin. Opposite corners of the volar rectangle are connected in either direction to create two triangles, which are later sewn to the sides of the dorsal rectangular flap. The method is offered as an alternative to the butterfly flap for release of partial syndactyly proximal to the PIP joint.

Percival NJ, Sykes PJ: Syndactyly: A review of the factors which influence surgical treatment. *J Hand Surg* 1989;14B:196-200.

The incidence of web space creep, 22%, was similar for three techniques of web floor reconstruction: dorsal quadrilateral flap, interdigitating palmar and dorsal triangular flaps, and dorsal triangular or horseshoe flap. There was a higher incidence of flexion contracture, web creep, and need for revision surgery when split-thickness rather than full-thickness grafts were used and in complex rather than simple syndactyly.

Constriction Band Syndrome

Askins G, Ger E: Congenital constriction band syndrome. *J Pediatr Orthop* 1988;8:461-466.

Constriction band syndrome in 55 patients affected longer central fingers and multiple extremities asymmetrically, supporting an amniotic band theory of pathogenesis. The more proximal the involvement, the more likely is a neurodeficit. Staged half-circumferential excisions with Z-plasty are used for deep bands associated with edema or neurovascular compression.

Hill LM, Kislak S, Jones N: Prenatal ultrasound diagnosis of a forearm constriction band. *J Ultrasound Med* 1988;7:293-295.

Asymmetric extremity edema seen on prenatal ultrasound examination suggests blockage of venous and lymphatic drainage by an amniotic band. An indentation of subcutaneous and muscle tissue without edema may be seen at the site of a constriction band later in gestation.

Uchida Y, Sugioka Y: Peripheral nerve palsy associated with congenital constriction band syndrome. *J Hand Surg* 1991;16B:109-112.

Peripheral nerve palsy is common when a constriction band occurs above the wrist. On exploration, the nerves beneath the band were flattened and degenerated in two cases. Surgical decompression soon after birth, with or without nerve grafting, may improve function.

Upton J, Tan C: Correction of constriction rings. *J Hand Surg* 1991;16A:947-953.

Excision of the ring and part of the neighboring adipose tissue with mobilization of the remaining adipose tissue into the groove prevents the recurrent contour deformities that otherwise were seen in 29 patients with deep rings who were treated by simple Z-plasties alone. Staged corrections are recommended. A W-plasty or Z-plasty over the dorsum of the digit indents with time, and these flaps should be confined to the sides of the digit; dorsal skin should be closed in a straight line.

Transverse Absences

Koshima I, Moriguchi T, Soeda S, et al: Free second toe transfer for reconstruction of the distal phalanx of the fingers. *Br J Plast Surg* 1991;44:456-458.

Survival of a free microvascular transplantation of the second toe is improved by making as many vascular anastomoses as possible. Both plantar digital arteries and the dorsalis pedis artery may be anastomosed to both digital arteries in the hand and the radial artery in the snuff box. Two or more branches of the dorsal cutaneous vein of the foot should be left with the toe.

Phocomelia

Seitz WH Jr, Froimson AI: Callotasis lengthening in the upper extremity: Indications, techniques, and pitfalls. *J Hand Surg* 1991;16A:932-939.

Lengthening through fracture callus using half-frame configurations put one hand in phocomelia 13 cm farther away from the shoulder, increased the length of one ulna in radial agenesis and of two ulnas with short congenital amputations near the elbow, and lengthened seven phalanges with congenital amputations near the elbow, and lengthened seven phalanges with congenital amputation of fingers. Digital lengthenings improved chuck and key pinch; forearm and phocomelia lengthenings allowed the use of below-elbow instead of above-elbow prostheses. The circular frame for lengthening and angular adjustment is recommended for Madelung's deformity.

Radial Deficiency

Bayne LG, Klug MS: Long-term review of the surgical treatment of radial deficiencies. *J Hand Surg* 1987;12A:169-179.

A nontraditional goal of wrist motion of 20-degree dorsiflexion and 20-degree volar flexion was achieved in 21 to 51 centralizations without radiocarpal fusion or carpal bone resection. Recurrence was avoided by careful radial release followed by ulnocarpal capsular flap and flexor and extensor carpi ulnaris advancement. Postoperative bracing was mandatory after Kirschner wire removal at eight weeks. The best results were achieved when surgery was performed at 6 months of age after preliminary stretching.

Brons JT, van der Harten HJ, van Geijn HP, et al: Prenatal ultrasonographic diagnosis of radial-ray reduction malformations. *Prenat Diagn* 1990;10:279-288.

Prenatal diagnosis of skeletal abnormalities is a rapidly growing field. Ultrasound scanning may detect absent radius or thumb and hypoplasia during the second and third trimester of pregnancy. Because radial ray reduction malformations may be associated with lethal cardiac, urogenital, or central nervous system abnormalities, early detection can have profound implications for further evaluation and clinical management.

Kato H, Ogino T, Minami A, et al: Experimental study of radial ray deficiency. *J Hand Surg* 1990;15B:470-476.

Radial and ulnar ray deficiencies were induced in rats by maternal administration of Myleran, an alkylating agent that interferes with mitosis. The results suggest that the deficiencies may follow exposure to environmental factors at a critical period of embryogenesis.

Sawaizumi M, Maruyama Y, Okajima K, et al: Free vascularised epiphyseal transfer designed on the reverse anterior tibial artery. *Br J Plast Surg* 1991;44:57-59.

In a 29-month-old boy with an absent distal half radius, continued growth of the proximal fibular physis was observed after a vascularized transfer based on the anterior tibial artery.

Urban MA, Osterman AL: Management of radial dysplasia. *Hand Clin* 1990;6:589-605.

Associated with radial dysplasia are a multitude of hematologic, cardiac, and renal anomalies, as well as a thickened median nerve, absent radial artery, conjoined muscles, and absent carpal bones. Between 6 and 12 months of age, after preoperative splintage, the carpus may be reduced on the distal ulna with or without carpal resection and held in place with tendon transfers and Kirschner wire. Index pollicization for absent thumb is performed 6 months later. Alternatively, the radial side of the carpus can be supported either by lengthening the shortened radius or by a vascularized fibular epiphyseal plate transfer that grows with the patient. After centralization, a one-bone forearm can be osteotomized if the ulna is bowed severely or lengthened by Ilizarov methods if the ulna is short.

Shortened or Absent Radius: Radial Club Hand

Kessler I: Centralisation of the radial club hand by gradual distraction. *J Hand Surg* 1989;14B:37-42.

Gradual disengagement of the carpus at daily increments with an external fixator allows centralization of the carpus on top of the distal ulna for long-standing radial club hand with less risk to neurovascular structures.

Tetsworth K, Krome J, Paley D: Lengthening and deformity correction of the upper extremity by the Ilizarov technique. *Orthop Clin North Am* 1991;22:689-713.

Techniques of frame construction, corticotomy, and prevention of complications are outlined for lengthening in the five types of forearm deformity.

Villa A, Paley D, Catagni MA, et al: Lengthening of the forearm by the Ilizarov technique. *Clin Orthop* 1990;250:125-137.

Functional, cosmetic, and psychological benefits were obtained from 2 to 13 cm increases in forearm length with the Ilizarov method for a difference in length between the radius and the ulna or short one-bone forearm. Eleven complications occurred in 12 patients; three radial nerve palsies resolved, but three patients had persistent limited motion.

Absent Thumb

Lister G: Microsurgical transfer of the second toe for congenital deficiency of the thumb. *Plast Reconstr Surg* 1988;82:658-665.

Good use was made of 11 of 12 second-toe transplantations for reconstruction of the congenitally deficient thumb. Absence of tissue in all three cases of symbrachydactyly and all six cases of transverse absences necessitated connection of the transferred nerves, tendons, and vessels to the most appropriate remaining structures. Interphalangeal motion was achieved in only three patients.

Cleft Hand

Ogino T: Teratogenic relationship between polydactyly, syndactyly and cleft hand. *J Hand Surg* 1990;15B:201-209.

Advanced central polydactyly of the middle finger and osseous syndactyly of the middle and ring fingers where the fusion extends proximally to the proximal phalanx or metacarpal appear identical to typical cleft hand. The clinical features of these anomalies induced in rats by the administration of Myleran are the same as those in clinical cases. The findings suggest that polydactyly, syndactyly, and cleft hand have the same teratogenic mechanism by which induction of the finger rays fails.

Camptodactyly

Hori M, Nakamura R, Inoue G, et al: Nonoperative treatment of camptodactyly. *J Hand Surg* 1987;12A:1061-1065.

Use of a dynamic splint for stretching 24 hours a day achieved near-full extension in 20 of 34 fingers in 22 of 24 patients with proximal IP joint-flexion deformities of the small finger. Recurrences may be prevented by continued splinting for 8 hours daily perhaps until the growth plates close.

Koman LA, Toby EB, Poehling GG: Congenital flexion deformities of the proximal interphalangeal joint in children: A subgroup of camptodactyly. *J Hand Surg* 1990;15A:582-586.

Little improvement was seen when only the contracted palmar structures were released and the flexor digitorum superficialis tendon was lengthened. Improvement in active and passive extension was seen only when the palmarly subluxated lateral bands were realigned by releasing the transverse retinacular ligament, augmented by transfer of the flexor digitorum superficialis through the lumbrical canal to reinforce the central slip.

Siegert JJ, Cooney WP, Dobyns JH: Management of simple camptodactyly. *J Hand Surg* 1990;15B:181-189.

The authors conclude that an extensor abnormality is not of significance. Operative treatment should include a palmar release of the tight flexor digitorum superficialis without complicated transfers to the extensor mechanism. Loss of flexion is common postoperatively, so stretching and splinting are recommended, and operative treatment is avoided unless the flexion deformity is greater than 60 degrees.

Congenital Trigger Finger

Ger E, Kupcha P, Ger D: The management of trigger thumb in children. *J Hand Surg* 1991;16A:944-947.

Trigger thumb failed to improve spontaneously, as widely accepted, despite an average of 40 months' observation in 17 thumbs diagnosed before 6 months of age and in 28 patients whose condition was diagnosed before 6 months of age and in 28 patients whose condition was diagnosed after 6 months of age. Contracture may persist if surgical release of the A_1 pulley is performed after 3 years of age.

Eyres KS, McLaren MI: Trigger thumb in children: Results of surgical correction. *J R Coll Surg Edinb* 1991;36:197-198.

Three of 15 cases reportedly occurred after direct trauma to the thumb. In the differential diagnosis is the congenital flexion-adduction deformity of the clasped thumb that can be passively abducted and extended.

Delta Phalanx

Burgess RC: Use of an H-graft in the treatment of a delta phalanx. *J Hand Surg* 1988;13A:297-298.

The magnitude of the opening wedge osteotomy in a delta phalanx makes insertion of wedge-shaped graft difficult, and displacement can occur. An H-shaped graft from the distal radius with an oblique Kirschner wire is used for secure fixation.

Madelung's Deformity

White GM, Weiland AJ: Madelung's deformity: Treatment by osteotomy of the radius and Lauenstein procedure. *J Hand Surg* 1987;12A:202-204.

Osteotomy of the distal radius in conjunction with arthrodesis of the distal radioulnar joint and creation of a pseudarthrosis in the ulna proximal to the fusion (Lauenstein procedure) can relieve pain and limited motion attributable to radioulnar incongruity. The procedure provides pain-free wrist and forearm motion and correction of the angular deformity of the distal radius and prevents the ulnar translocation of the carpus sometimes seen when a Darrach procedure alone is performed.

Hand in Cerebral Palsy

Goldner JL, Koman LA, Gelberman R, et al: Arthrodesis of the metacarpophalangeal joint of the thumb in children and adults: Adjunctive treatment of thumb-in-palm deformity in cerebral palsy. *Clin Orthop* 1990:253:75-89.

Chondrodesis or arthrodesis of the thumb MCP joint alone or in combination with release of the adductor and first dorsal interosseous muscles, or extrinsic tendon transfer functionally improved thumb-in-palm deformity when the MCP joint

hyperflexed or hyperextended. No significant disturbance in longitudinal or circumferential growth occurred.

Hoffer MM, Lehman M, Mitani M: Surgical indications in children with cerebral palsy. *Hand Clin* 1989;5:69-74.

Quadriplegics and diplegics usually do not require hand surgery. Athetoids with movement disorders rather than increased tone should not have surgery. Patients need reasonable cognition, sensibility, and proprioception. Spasticity and contractures are treated with lengthening, while abnormal patterns of muscle use are treated by tendon transfer. Postoperative management is emphasized; tendon transfers are gradually lengthened using serial splints, nonresistive activity, and gradually longer unprotected periods.

Koman LA, Gelberman RH, Toby EB, et al: Cerebral palsy: Management of the upper extremity. *Clin Orthop* 1990;253:62-74.

Only a few patients with cerebral palsy, mainly hemiplegics, require surgery for the hand. The authors feel that most patients have a problem with release and need augmentation of finger extension. Wrist and finger flexion deformities are treated with flexor carpi ulnaris transfer to the extensor digitorum communis with Z lengthenings of the contracted flexor digitorum superficialis. The profundus almost never needs release. Adduction deformity of the thumb is treated with division of the adductor pollicis and first dorsal interosseous release from the first and second metacarpals.

Strecker WB, Emanuel JP, Dailey L, et al: Comparison of pronator tenotomy and pronator rerouting in children with spastic cerebral palsy. *J Hand Surg* 1988;13A:540-543.

Pronator rerouting through the interosseous membrane into a hole in the radius restores more active supination for debilitating pronation deformity than does pronator tenotomy alone.

Thometz JG, Tachdjian M: Long-term follow-up of the flexor carpi ulnaris transfer in spastic hemiplegic children. *J Pediatr Orthop* 1988;8:407-412.

Flexor carpi ulnaris transfer to both extensor carpi radialis tendons improved dorsiflexion of the wrist to an average of 44 degrees with concomitant loss of palmar flexion to an average of 19 degrees. Patients must, therefore, not require palmar flexion for release of grasp and should be able to extend the fingers actively with the wrist in 20 degrees of dorsiflexion. Function was improved more in those patients with stereognosis and ability to cooperate with the therapist.

Wenner SM, Johnson KA: Transfer of the flexor carpi ulnaris to the radial wrist extensors in cerebral palsy. *J Hand Surg* 1988;13A:231-233.

Flexor carpi ulnaris transfer to the radial wrist extensors resulted in a gain of an average of 18 degrees of active wrist extension. Grasp and release is improved if the fingers can be extended in any position of the wrist but not if active extension is absent.

Juvenile Chronic Polyarthropathy

Gedalia A, Gewanter H, Baum J: Dark skin discoloration of finger joints in juvenile arthritis. *J Rheumatol* 1989;16:797-799.

Hyperpigmentation of the skin over the PIP joints in juvenile rheumatoid arthritis reflects the chronicity of joint inflammation. It is not seen in other connective tissue diseases.

Hanff G, Sollerman C, Elborgh R, et al: Wrist synovectomy in juvenile chronic arthritis (JCA). *Scand J Rheumatol* 1990;19:280-284.

Wrist synovectomy for pain and radiographic changes in 20 patients with juvenile rheumatoid arthritis gave results comparable to those of wrist synovectomy in adults. Half the patients had less pain, although half had continued radiographic deterioration. Although the range of motion was more limited, the average grip strength doubled. Nine patients developed recurrent synovitis, four required arthrodesis for continued pain, and one had spontaneous fusion.

Vascular Malformations

Apfelberg DB, Maser MR, Lash H, et al: YAG laser resection of complicated hemangiomas of the hand and upper extremity. *J Hand Surg* 1990;15A:765-773.

The YAG laser offers advantages over Ar and CO_2 lasers by allowing direct tissue contact for excision of hemangiomas while controlling hemorrhage. Surgical excision for very diffuse and infiltrating hemangiomas is unlikely to be curative because of their extensive nature. Hemangiomas present at birth may resolve spontaneously and should be observed six to eight years before excision. Ligation of afferent vessels and arteriography with selective embolization may still be necessary for control of hemorrhage. The laser coagulates only vessels less than 1 mm in diameter.

Malignant Soft-Tissue and Bone Tumors of the Hand

Azouz EM, Kozlowski K, Masel J: Soft-tissue tumors of the hand and wrist in children. *J Can Assoc Radiol* 1989;40:251-255.

Second to ganglia, tumors of blood- and lymph-vessel origin were the most common soft-tissue tumors of the hand in this series. Plain films remain the most important examination and may show calcifications, leading to the diagnosis of cavernous hemangioma with pheboliths, soft-tissue chondroma, myositis ossificans, extra-articular synovial chondromatosis, periosteal chondroma, tumoral calcinosis, and disorders producing metastatic calcification.

Frassica FJ, Amadio PC, Wold LE, et al: Primary malignant bone tumors of the hand. *J Hand Surg* 1989;14A:1022-1028.

Malignant bone tumors of the hand are rare, especially in children. Even with adjuvant treatment, wide surgical margin is needed to prevent local recurrence.

Kozlowski K, Azouz EM, Campbell J, et al: Primary bone tumours of the hand: Report of 21 cases. *Pediatr Radiol* 1988;18:140-148.

Twenty-one primary bone tumors, excluding osteochondromas and enchondromas, were collected from eight pediatric hospitals. Common tumors, including osteoid osteoma (six cases), aneurysmal bone cyst (five cases), and epidermoid cysts (two cases), have characteristic appearances, but uncommon tumors were more difficult to identify. Destruction of cortex with a soft-tissue mass was seen in three cases of Ewing's sarcoma.

Angiography in Congenital Hand Deformity

Hadidi AT, Kaddah NT, Zaki MS, et al: Congenital malformations of the hand: A study of the vascular pattern. *J Hand Surg* 1990;15B:171-180.

Angiography by direct exposure and catheterization of the brachial artery is safe and shows that each type of congenital hand deformity is associated with specific vascular alterations.

Mantero R, Rossello MI, Grandis C: Digital subtraction angiography in preoperative examination of congenital hand malformations. *J Hand Surg* 1989;14A:351-352.

Evaluation of blood supply is important to select the correct surgical procedure. Distal subtraction angiography is useful to detect distal arterial forks, agenesis of one or both palmar arches, a single digital artery, and supply from the radial or ulnar artery alone.

31

Wrist and Hand: Trauma

Wrist Injuries

Distal Radius Fractures

The optimum treatment of distal radius fractures continues to be controversial. The alternatives include closed reduction and casting, pins and plaster, external fixation with or without bone grafting, and open reduction with internal fixation. To diminish the development of post-traumatic arthritis, anatomic reduction and fixation are emphasized in treating intra-articular fractures. In Colles' fracture, restoration of volar tilt, radial inclination, and proper length are stressed, especially in young patients. If closed reduction is performed and residual displacement is uncorrected, the resultant malunion can produce a weak, deformed, stiff, and often painful wrist.

In addition to distal radial joint incongruity, the most significant factors leading to a poor result are the degree of carpal malalignment as measured by the radial tilt and the radiolunate, lunocapitate, and scapholunate angles. Because of these problems, attention continues to focus on alternative treatments. One approach taken with comminuted distal radius fractures is treatment by distraction, application of an external fixator, and autogenous cancellous iliac crest bone grafting, followed by functional bracing (Fig. 1). Fifteen to 20 months after treatment, the results are reported as generally excellent, although a small number of patients report mild wrist pain or residual pain over the ulnar aspect of the joint. With this treatment, the retained range of motion was 70% to 80% of normal, and grip strength was 85% of

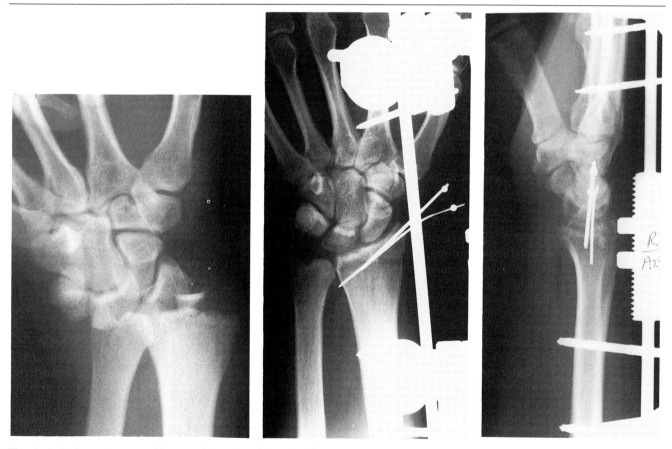

Fig. 1 **Left**, Severe intercarpal fracture dislocation of the wrist. **Center**, External fixator was used to provide ligamentotaxis and to stabilize the wrist. A volar approach was used to anatomically reduce the articular surface, which was then stabilized with wires. Currently less bulky fixators are used. **Right**, Lateral view showing satisfactory carpal alignment and distal radial tilt.

the unaffected side. Radiographs reveal that radiopalmar tilt and radial articular angles are maintained. However, complications do exist, including second metacarpal fracture, superficial pin tract infection, reflex sympathetic dystrophy, transient radial and/or median nerve sensory impairment, and bone graft donor site hematoma.

The preceding results are comparable to the outcome reported in 75 consecutive patients with Frykman type VIII fractures of the distal radius who were treated by primary external fixation. A comparison group of 32 patients were treated by closed reduction and cast immobilization. All fractures treated with external fixation remained well reduced, while 88% of those treated with casts had unsatisfactory alignment despite the fact that 30% had a second attempt at reduction. Most patients treated with external fixation had good or excellent functional outcome, although half of the cast group had fair and poor results. Wrist motion was significantly better in the group treated by external fixation. Residual grip strength was 90% in the operatively treated group and 65% in the casted group. Complications noted among patients treated with external fixation included ulnar nerve palsy, reflex sympathetic dystrophy, extensor pollicis longus tendon rupture, radial nerve irritation, pin infection, and loose fixator pins.

Not all studies have achieved this level of success. In a prospective, randomized study of patients greater than 60 years of age, there was no advantage in using an external fixator when compared with use of closed reduction and plaster cast immobilization. In the cast group, there were no complications, no cases of reflex sympathetic dystrophy, and no remanipulations necessary during the course of treatment. In the external fixator group, 21% of patients experienced problems with the pin sites, and 26% reported symptoms suggesting radial nerve irritation. Complications of external fixation (pin loosening, fracture through pin sites, intrinsic contracture) can be decreased by using a limited open surgical approach for predrilling and central placement of fixator pins and by using 4-mm half pins. Compared to 3-mm pins, these 4-mm self-tapping half pins demonstrate a significantly higher pull-out strength, and there is only a small decrease in torsional strength of the bone. Proximal pins are placed in the radius. Distal pins should be through six cortices of the bases of the second and third metacarpals. If two pins are used at the metacarpal level, six cortices are obtained by the distal pin capturing two cortices of the second metacarpal and the more proximal pin capturing two cortices of the second and two cortices of the third metacarpal at the base.

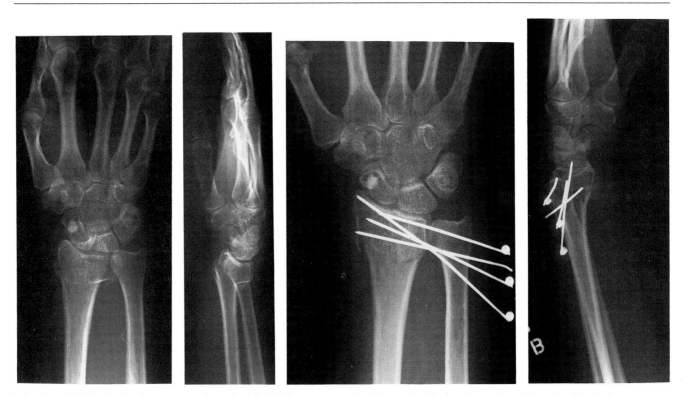

Fig. 2 **Left**, Distal radial fracture with shortening. **Center left**, The dorsal tilt is noted on the lateral radiograph. **Center right**, The posteroanterior view showing reduction of the distal radial fracture with fixation using transulnar percutaneous pins. Radial length is maintained. **Right**, Lateral view demonstrating satisfactory reduction of the distal radius.

This method does not violate the interosseous muscles of the second intrinsic compartment. An alternative to external fixation is transulnar percutaneous pinning of displaced, unstable distal radius fractures (Fig. 2). Four or five 0.045-in. Kirschner pins are placed percutaneously from the ulna through the radius. In small cohorts of patients, excellent or good results have been reported. The proponents of this technique note that radial sensory nerves are avoided, the use of a lightweight splint at three weeks promotes patient comfort and facilitates finger range-of-motion exercises, percutaneous pins are removed easily without anesthesia in the office, and pin sites are barely perceptible at follow-up in the majority of patients. Eight weeks of pinning of the distal radioulnar joint has not been detrimental to ultimate pronation and supination in these patients.

Another alternative is open reduction and internal fixation. One study analyzed younger patients (average age 40), whose comminuted, intra-articular distal radius fractures were treated with open reduction and internal fixation. When closed reduction failed to achieve or maintain congruity, the surgery was performed at an average of 6.5 days after the injury. Fractures were reduced under direct vision and were internally stabilized with Kirschner wires (K-wires) or plates and screws. By the criteria of Gartland and Worley, 81% had an excellent or good result. By a modified system of Green and O'Brien, 56% had an excellent or good result, but none was judged poor. All patients were able to return to domestic duties or to their occupations. The worst results tended to be in patients who had high-energy trauma resulting in severely comminuted fractures. The prognosis was directly related to the amount of intra-articular incongruity that was present when the fracture united, and all fractures that healed with a step-off of 2 mm or more had later degenerative changes.

In another review, patients who underwent open reduction and internal fixation of comminuted intra-articular fractures of the distal radius were followed for an average of 3.25 years. The early complication rate was 15%; the late complication rate was 35%. However, patient satisfaction was very high, and 89% returned to their previous occupations. Function was excellent, and radiographic results revealed that articular congruity was restored in 88% of patients. Suggested indications for this procedure are the presence of residual articular incongruency of greater than 2 mm after closed reduction, as assessed by plain radiographs, computed tomography (CT) scan, or tomograms.

A prospective, randomized study sought to determine if repairing the triangular ligament and stabilizing the ulnar styloid would improve results from Colles' fractures. Of 41 patients with closed, extra-articular fracture-dislocation of the distal radius, 19 were randomly allocated to a group treated by closed reduction of the radius with subsequent suture of the triangular ligament and stabilization of the ulnar styloid. The other 22 patients were treated by closed reduction and above-elbow casts.

Radiographic examination immediately after treatment in both groups revealed that all fractures were reduced, and alignment was maintained one week later. Later arthrograms of the radio-carpal joint showed that all patients had a complete rupture of the triangular ligament. Examination two years after injury demonstrated no differences in distal radial fragment deterioration or ulnar styloid union. Contrast medium leaked into the distal radial joint from the radiocarpal joint equally in both groups. In addition, four of 19 patients treated surgically and seven of 22 patients who were not operated on complained of painful or restricted forearm rotation. These findings indicate that surgical repair of the ruptured triangular ligament in Colles' fractures is no better than nonsurgical treatment. Unless there is gross instability of the wrist or dislocation of the distal radioulnar joint, acute repair of the triangular fibrocartilage and the ulnar styloid does not appear to be indicated.

Scaphoid Fractures

It is generally recommended for the wrist to be immobilized in a thumb spica splint or cast when an individual sustains a wrist injury, has tenderness in the anatomic snuffbox, and has radiographs negative for fracture. The radiographs are repeated seven to ten days later. If the tenderness persists and the new radiographs are negative, immobilization is continued or additional imaging, such as bone scan, trispiral tomography, or CT, is obtained. The reported rationale for the prophylactic immobilization is to reduce the frequency of delayed union and nonunion.

To determine the relationship between delay before immobilization and development of nonunion or delayed union, 285 fractures of the scaphoid were analyzed. Thirty-two fractures (11%) were not detected at the first radiographic examination. Ten to 14 days later, 28 of the 32 fractures were apparent in the new radiographs. A third radiographic examination identified four more fractures. Treatment for the diagnosed scaphoid fracture was above-elbow plaster cast until radiographic union.

Sixteen of the 285 (6%) developed nonunion, and 27 (11%) had delayed union. The common denominator for delayed union and nonunion was an adult who had a fracture involving the proximal pole or waist. The frequency of nonunion was definitely increased by a delay in treatment of longer than four weeks, but nonunion was not associated with delay of immobilization between one and 28 days. In fractures of the proximal two thirds of the scaphoid, nonunion was found in only 5% when immobilization began within the first day after injury, but 45% had nonunion when the delay exceeded four weeks.

Another important issue deals with the optimum cast technique in treating scaphoid fractures. Many physicians feel that a short arm thumb spica cast produces satisfactory results, while others favor a long arm cast. A prospective study of 51 patients with nondisplaced scaphoid fractures compared treatment with long (28 patients) and short (23 patients) thumb spica casts, neither of which included the interphalangeal (IP) joint of the thumb. Those initially treated with a long cast were placed in a short cast after six weeks. The fractures treated with a long thumb spica cast united in an average of 9.5 weeks; those treated with a short thumb spica cast healed in an average of 12.7 weeks. There were no non-unions and two delayed unions in the long cast group, compared with two nonunions and six delayed unions in the short cast group. The improved results seen with elbow immobilization are thought to be caused by the diminished sheer stresses across the fracture site. Time to union was significantly shorter for fractures of the proximal and middle third of the scaphoid that were treated initially in a long thumb spica cast. Fractures of the distal third did well regardless of the type of immobilization. The development of aseptic necrosis, while associated with a delay in union, was not related to the type of immobilization, but rather to the level of the fracture.

Even when a scaphoid fracture unites, subsequent arthritis is not necessarily prevented. Five percent of patients with primary healing of scaphoid waist fractures have had radiographic evidence of radiocarpal arthrosis at a minimum follow-up of seven or more years after their fracture. Alteration of carpal dynamics due to malunion, with deformation and shortening of the scaphoid, is thought to be the most likely cause.

Anatomic reduction and internal fixation of scaphoid fractures is recommended if the fracture fragments are displaced by 1 mm or more, if the radiolunate angle is greater than 15 degrees, or if the scapholunate angle is greater than 60 degrees. Smooth K-wires, cancellous bone screws, and Herbert screws (Fig. 3) are alternative fixation devices. Excellent results have been achieved with the Herbert screw although compressive force is greater with the ASIF 4-mm cancellous screw. Cannulated screws are available for insertion over an accurately placed K-wire. The position of the K-wire must be confirmed by intraoperative radiographs before the screw is inserted. Technical precision is mandatory when using any of these methods, and incorrect screw length or inaccurate or eccentric screw placement can decrease the rate of union.

Dorsal Transscaphoid Perilunate Dislocations

The results of treatment continue to be reported in small groups of patients. For example, 13 patients with 14 dorsal transscaphoid perilunate dislocations were treated with open reduction and internal fixation of the scaphoid using the Herbert screw. The perilunate dislocations were transscaphoid in 10, transradial styloid and transscaphoid in three, and transscaphoid transcapitate in one. The results, based on Cooney's clinical scoring system, were two, excellent; six, good; five, fair; and one, poor. Somewhat better results have been reported for other small series when dorsal transscaphoid perilunate dislocations are treated with the Herbert screw.

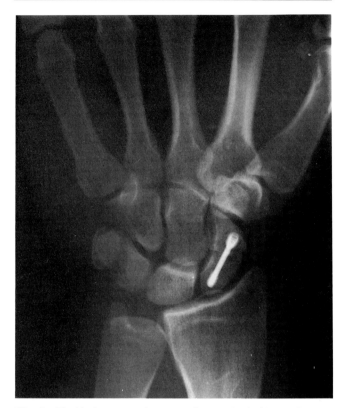

Fig. 3   The Herbert screw is an excellent method of internally fixing scaphoid fractures. Technical expertise is required for optimal results.

Scaphoid Fractures with Scapholunate Ligament Disruption

A cadaveric biomechanical analysis of scaphoid fractures associated with scapholunate ligament disruption suggests the ligament rupture occurs first, followed by continued deformation until the scaphoid fractures. It seems unlikely that sufficient loads can be generated to cause ligament disruption after the scaphoid has fractured. The presence of a widened scapholunate gap, in addition to an acute scaphoid fracture, is an indication of ligamentous instability. The objective of treatment must be to produce scaphoid union and correct rotary subluxation (Fig. 4). Failure to correct the ligamentous instability can lead to radioscaphoid and intercarpal arthritis.

Scapholunate Dissociation

Scapholunate dissociation alters wrist mechanics and can lead to degenerative arthritis at the radioscaphoid and the intercarpal joints (Fig. 5). The exact contribution of the various supporting ligaments is still being clarified in scapholunate diastasis with rotary subluxation of the scaphoid (stage I perilunar instability by Mayfield's Classification). The scapholunate stabilizing ligaments (radioscapholunate, palmar scapholunate interosseous, dorsal scapholunate interosseous, and radiocapitate) were se-

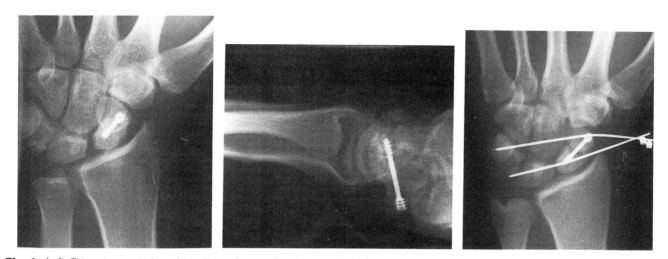

Fig. 4 **Left**, This anteroposterior wrist radiograph was taken after scaphoid fracture was stabilized using a Herbert screw. Volar flexion of the scaphoid and widened scapholunate gap are noted. **Center**, Radiograph of the same patient showing increased scapholunate angle on lateral view. **Right**, This wrist was approached through dorsal and palmar incisions, the scapholunate ligaments were repaired, and C-wires were placed to maintain adequate alignment of the carpus. The wires do not cross the radial carpal joint.

quentially sectioned to simulate a progressive wrist injury caused by extension, intercarpal supination, and ulnar deviation forces. After each ligament was sectioned, standard and stress radiographs were obtained using the radiographic limits of carpal instability, which are a scapholunate gap of 3 mm and a lateral scapholunate angle of 70 degrees. These radiographic limits were not exceeded until the radioscapholunate, the scapholunate interosseous ligament, and the radiocapitate ligaments were completely disrupted. The lateral scapholunate angle most closely reflected the progressive nature of injury. However, it was possible to have complete disruption of the radioscapholunate and scapholunate interosseous ligaments and a normal scapholunate gap and lateral scapholunate angle. These experimental results would imply the need for further studies such as arthrograms or arthroscopy, where clinically indicated, in patients with normal radiographs. The carpal height ratio, ulnar carpal distance ratio, and lateral radiolunate and capitolunate angles appear to be of little clinical significance in assessing ligament damage incurred with mild hyperextension injuries.

Lunotriquetral Instability

Progressive ligament disruption at the lunotriquetral joint results in increasingly severe ulnar-sided perilunate disability that causes dynamic and, subsequently, static volar intercalated segment instability. Cadaver dissections and load studies have been performed to develop a staging system for ulnar-sided perilunate instability. Stage I includes partial or complete disruption of the lunotriquetral interosseous ligament, which, by itself, does not produce clinical and/or radiographic evidence of dynamic or static volar intercalated segment instability.

Stage II includes disruption of both the lunotriquetral interosseous and the palmar lunotriquetral ligaments. With compressive loads on the wrist, this disruption produces clinical and/or radiographic evidence of dynamic volar intercalated segment instability. Stage III includes complete disruption of the lunotriquetral interosseous and palmar lunotriquetral ligaments, and attenuation or disruption of the dorsal radiocarpal ligament, and it produces clinical and/or radiographic evidence of static volar intercalated segment instability. Others have shown the essential lesion in producing a static volar intercalated segment instability is division of the dorsal radiotriquetral and scaphotriquetral ligaments in association with sectioning of the lunotriquetral and interosseous ligaments.

Complete lunotriquetral ligament tears frequently result from hyperextension of the wrist. Ulnar wrist pain, limited motion, and tenderness over the lunotriquetral joint are present. Standard radiographs are normal, but arthrography is reported to reliably demonstrate the ligament tear. Operative treatment of acute injuries appears warranted if static irreducible instability is present radiographically. Limited studies indicate that ligament reconstruction is not a durable procedure. Lunotriquetral arthrodesis appears to be the treatment of choice for chronic, complete lunotriquetral injuries. In a report of 11 patients, fusion was achieved between two and five months in all cases, although three patients had persistent pain. Postoperative reductions are observed in wrist flexion, extension, ulnar deviation, and maximum grip strength.

Hamate Fracture

Most isolated fractures of the hook of the hamate are the result of athletic activity (swinging a racket, golf club, or

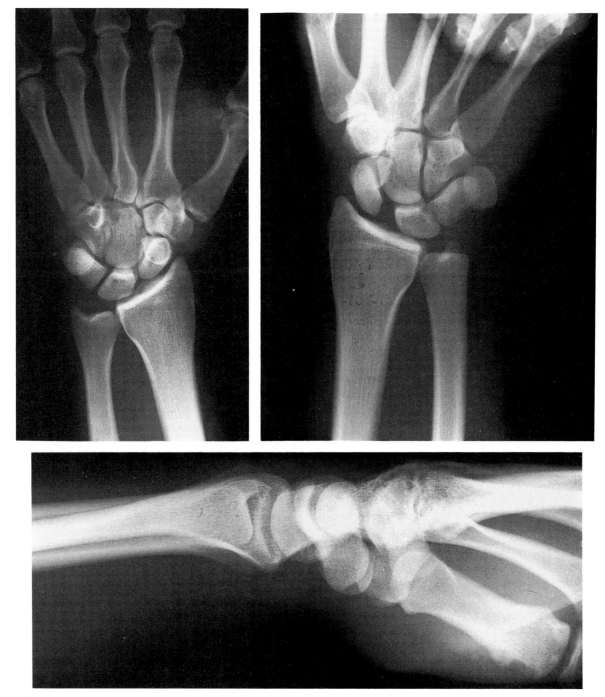

Fig. 5 **Top left**, Posteroanterior view of the left wrist, demonstrating widening of scapholunate joint and excessive volar flexion of the scaphoid as seen with scapholunate dissociation. **Top right**, Anteroposterior clinched fist view demonstrated widened scapholunate gap. This "Terry Thomas" sign seen with scapholunate dissociation is often less obvious. **Bottom**, Lateral radiograph revealing increased scapholunate angle as seen with static scapholunate dissociation (dorsal intercalated segment instability).

baseball bat), but some are caused by striking the palm on a solid object, by falling on the palm, or by a crush injury to the hand. Almost all patients complain of pain and tenderness on the ulnar side of the palm or on the dorsoulnar aspect of the wrist. However, the most common symptom is pain in the palm aggravated by grasp. Diminished grip strength, dorsal wrist pain, ulnar nerve paresthesias or weakness, and mild carpal tunnel syndrome are frequent. Tenosynovitis, tendon fraying, or tendon rupture may be demonstrated in 25% of the cases and is unrelated to the use of steroids. Most of the fractures can be diagnosed conclusively on a carpal tunnel radiograph or on a special oblique radiograph with the wrist supinated; however, CT scan is the definitive imaging technique for demonstrating this fracture. Immediate immobilization of acute fractures may promote fracture healing and obviate operative intervention. A nonathletic injury or the presence of crush injury adversely affects the outcome. Open reduction and internal fixation is feasible but offers little advantage over excision, which generally produces excellent results.

When a symptomatic nonunion occurs, excision is the treatment of choice. The complication rate associated with excision, reported as 3%, includes injury to the ulnar nerve or the superficial palmar arch, and median nerve paresthesias. These complications are attributed to surgical exposure and retraction rather than to the actual excision.

Carpometacarpal Dislocations

Transcarpal carpometacarpal fracture dislocations are often unrecognized. In one study, early diagnosis was made in only eight of 13 patients. Posteroanterior views demonstrate abnormal overlapping of the articular surfaces in some instances, lateral views are helpful in other instances, and pronation oblique views may be useful in delineating injuries to the fourth and fifth rays. However, lateral trispiral tomography or CT scan is by far the most effective method of diagnosis. When the diagnosis is early, recommended treatment has been open reduction, pin or screw fixation, and immobilization for four to six weeks. Complications are minimal and excellent functional recovery is reported.

Often the diagnosis is not immediate, but is suspected because patients have continued pain, loss of grip strength, and mild limitation of finger motion. Acute carpal tunnel syndrome can be observed a few days after an injury. Results were variable in a small series of patients treated with open reduction, bone grafting, fixation with multiple pins, and immobilization until fracture consolidation. A larger study reported 20 patients with dislocation of one or all of the medial four carpometacarpal joints and an average follow-up of 6.5 years. Fifteen patients were treated with open reduction and internal fixation during the first two weeks after injury, and the long-term results were excellent in 13. Three of the four unsatisfactory results were in patients who had injuries to the normally rigid second and third carpometacarpal joints or who had a concomitant ulnar nerve injury.

Others who treated patients with closed multiple carpometacarpal dislocations found that closed manipulation can be performed successfully within two days of the injury. After closed reduction, percutaneous K-wire fixation supplemented by plaster cast immobilization is reported to give excellent results.

Bennett's Fracture

Alternative treatments for Bennett's fracture include closed reduction and plaster immobilization (infrequent), percutaneous K-wire fixation, and open reduction. The main determinant of an excellent long-term result is the accuracy of reduction. Residual displacement is often associated with symptoms, although most are mild. Radiographic signs of arthritis are more common when there is residual displacement.

Hand Injuries

Metacarpophalangeal Joint

Closed crush injuries from direct blows to the dorsum of the hand can produce significant metacarpophalangeal joint symptoms or dysfunction. Only two of 11 patients who had chronic metacarpophalangeal joint pain and swelling without extensor tendon subluxations responded to nonsurgical measures. All nine who were treated surgically had an anatomic lesion that consisted of a partial, arcuate tear of the sagittal fibers. Intra-articular pathology was seen in 25% of these patients. All patients improved postoperatively.

Cadaver dissections of the dorsal metacarpophalangeal tendon mechanism demonstrate that neither partial nor complete transection of the ulnar sagittal fibers produces radial dislocation of the extensor tendons. However, radial sagittal fiber transections frequently produce ulnar tendon dislocation. Patients who have closed, impacted injuries to the metacarpophalangeal joints and who have long-standing pain, swelling, and limited motion, without extensor tendon migration, may have sustained unrecognized partial ulnar sagittal fiber disruption. Repair of the partial sagittal fiber tear and exploration of the metacarpophalangeal joint is indicated.

Metacarpal Fractures

Functional casting appears to have advantages over traditional plaster casting. One hundred subcapital or diaphyseal fractures of the second through fifth metacarpals were randomized to either a dorsoulnar plaster cast, which immobilized the wrist and the joints of the involved digits, or to a functional cast, which allowed the wrist and digits a free range of motion. Both types of casts were removed at three weeks. Compared with plaster cast immobilization, functional casting reduced volar angulation by two thirds in metacarpal shaft fractures and by one third in metacarpal neck fractures. Restriction of wrist, metacarpophalangeal, and interphalangeal joint movement was more frequent in the cast group, but did not influence overall function three months after injury. When compared with the plaster cast group, sick leave was reduced by two thirds after functional casting.

In another study, 40 patients with isolated closed fractures of the fifth metacarpal neck were treated conservatively (25) and surgically (15). Both groups were statistically comparable. The conservative group was treated with buddy taping, bulky dressing, and plaster splint for no longer than three weeks. In the surgical group, ten patients were treated with closed reduction and percutaneous intramedullary K-wire fixation and the other five underwent open reduction, three with intramedullary K-wire fixation and two with interosseous crossed K-wire fixation.

All patients obtained good results. Subjectively, no patient had long-term pain or dissatisfaction with the functional or cosmetic result. Objectively, all patients regained normal grip strength and full joint motion, but the conservative group had less extension lag. Mild rotary malalignment was present in both groups. The main difference was considerably less residual dorsal angulation in the surgical group. This dorsal angulation was not associated with functional disability.

A variety of alternative internal fixation techniques have been evaluated, including composite wiring techniques using various configurations of K-wires and stainless steel wire sutures. Contraindications to this technique are bone loss, osteoporosis, or comminution preventing firm cortical apposition. When the composite technique was used, no malunion, nonunion, infection, loss of reduction, or tendon rupture was observed in a series of 33 fractures. However, 50% had pin loosening and protrusion, which necessitated pin removal after fracture healing. Extensor tenolysis was performed in ten digits.

Others have used internal fixation with AO minifragment screws and plates to treat displaced or rotated metacarpal fractures. Fractures consistently united without deformity or infection; the mean time off work was six weeks. No patient had persistent symptoms that caused difficulty with work or sport. Movement was restricted in patients with open fractures, divided extensor tendons, or intra-articular fractures of the metacarpal heads.

Ulnar Collateral Ligament Injury of the Thumb Metacarpophalangeal Joint

Early operative repair has been favored for complete rupture of the ulnar collateral ligament of the thumb if a Stener lesion is present, but incomplete rupture can be treated adequately without surgery. In patients with posttraumatic instability of the metacarpophalangeal joint of the thumb, clinical examination included instability test and palpation of the injured ulnar collateral ligament. These clinical techniques have been used to separate patients into two groups: nondisplaced and displaced ruptures. In one series of 24 patients, palpable displaced ruptures were treated surgically, while nonpalpable lesions were interpreted as nondisplaced and were treated with plaster, irrespective of the instability. At follow-up one year later, both groups had similar results with respect to strength, stability, and function. The results indicate that a clinical examination with palpation of torn ligament ends identifies displaced ruptures

of the collateral ligament (those cases needing surgery) and that nondisplaced ruptures may be treated successfully without surgery.

In another study, patients with acute metacarpophalangeal joint injuries were assessed by stress radiography, arthrography, and clinical examination. Arthrograms served to assess tissue injury by the extent and location of dye leaks, including the differentiation of displaced tears (Stener lesions) from undisplaced tears of the ulnar collateral ligament. Patients were treated for a minimum of six weeks with a custom removable splint and daily range-of-motion exercises. In the 32 patients available for examination at least one year after injury, mean relative instability improved from 17 degrees (at injury) to 2.3 degrees. Subjective and functional outcomes were good or satisfactory in more than 90% of patients; outcomes for all patients with Stener lesions were satisfactory, although joint stability was less than for the group as a whole.

Analysis of 34 of 42 patients who had undergone surgical repair of collateral ligament injuries of the thumb metacarpophalangeal joint indicated that, at a mean of 38.7 months later, 23 had symptoms that were minor in all but one patient, and 43% had less than 80% of the pinch strength of the opposite side. Findings were not related to the presence of symptoms or to demonstrable instability of the joint; however, the prevalence of weakness increased when surgery had been delayed by more than three weeks.

Collateral Ligament Injury of the Metacarpophalangeal Joint of the Fingers

In acute and chronic collateral ligament injuries, arthrographic findings correlate with the degree of joint stability. Although good results can be obtained after conservative treatment of this injury, severely unstable joint injuries should be treated surgically. Local repair is usually an effective treatment method, but tendon graft is recommended if an insufficient amount of ligament remains for reconstruction. In elderly patients, intrinsic transfer is an adequate method for controlling lateral instability.

Conservative treatment is indicated for an acute injury unless there is gross instability at the joint. Gross instability is present if there is no firm endpoint when a lateral force is applied to the digit. In this situation, the collateral ligament is completely ruptured and surgery is advisable. The most common reported site of rupture is the radial collateral ligament of the little finger. Patients have pain, swelling, and instability. When examined under local nerve block with the metacarpophalangeal joint flexed 90 degrees, radial force produces deviation of more than 40 degrees with no firm endpoint. The pathology is rupture of the ligament at its distal insertion, often associated with small avulsion fragments or flecks of bone attached to the torn ligament. In surgical treatment, the ligament and bone are reapproximated with a pull-out suture through a drill hole in the proximal phalanx.

Fractures of the Sesamoid Bones of the Thumb

The sesamoids of the metacarpophalangeal joint of the thumb are embedded within the fibrous substance of the palmar plate at the origin of the fibrous tunnel of the flexor pollicis longus. The accessory collateral ligaments insert into the lateral margins of the sesamoids. The tendon of the adductor pollicis inserts on the ulnar sesamoid, and the tendon of the flexor pollicis brevis inserts on the radial sesamoid. Fracture of one or both of the sesamoids may be associated with complete or partial rupture of the palmar plate or accessory collateral ligaments. Fractures of the thumb metacarpophalangeal joint may be classified as type I, with palmar plate intact, or type II, with palmar plate ruptured. In type I, the patient maintains normal flexion posture of the metacarpophalangeal joint, as well as the ability to flex it and the interphalangeal joint. In type II injuries, the metacarpophalangeal joint assumes a hyperextension posture, and the patient is unable to flex it.

The patient describes hyperextension injury to the metacarpophalangeal joint of the thumb, ecchymosis on the flexor side of the joint extending to the thenar eminence, and tenderness over one or both sesamoid bones. The joint should be examined for palmar plate and collateral ligament injuries by stressing these structures appropriately. Radial and ulnar oblique views of the metacarpophalangeal joint should be obtained, and comparative views of the opposite thumb are helpful to exclude the possibility of bipartite sesamoids.

In closed sesamoid fractures of the thumb, surgical repair of the palmar plate is not essential unless hyperextension instability of the metacarpophalangeal joint can be demonstrated clinically. The palmar plate is fibrous and not fibrocartilaginous, and it has an excellent chance of healing if the edges are approximated by immobilizing the metacarpophalangeal joint in comfortable flexion. In open fractures of the sesamoids, the fracture fragments are approximated to reinforce the palmar plate repair. This prevents a hyperextension deformity of the metacarpophalangeal joint of the thumb. Angulation or displacement of the fracture fragments has not been shown to cause painful arthritis.

Digit Fractures

Controversy remains as to which hand fractures are treated best with screws, plates, pins, external fixation, or splinting. Often the outcome of the fracture depends on the amount of bone or soft-tissue trauma sustained at the initial injury. Factors important in the selection of treatment method are acceptable alignment, functional stability, and associated significant soft-tissue injuries. The definition of acceptable alignment in one series was 10 degrees of angulation in both sagittal and coronal planes except in the metaphyseal region, in which a 20-degree angulation in the sagittal plane was acceptable. In

fractures of the fifth metacarpal neck, 45 degrees of angulation in the sagittal plan was acceptable. Fifty percent overlap of the fracture site was considered necessary for rapid bone healing, and no rotational deformity was accepted. A fracture that was markedly displaced before reduction did not necessarily require internal fixation after adequate reduction. In this series, 26 (15%) of 171 markedly displaced fractures that were functionally stable after closed reduction were treated successfully by mobilization. Results were comparable in displaced and undisplaced fractures.

Regardless of the anatomic site of the fracture, treatment of unstable fractures by splints or K-wire fixation produced unsatisfactory results. Unfavorable prognostic factors are open fracture, comminuted fracture, and associated significant soft-tissue injury. Interfragmentary fixation with mini screws is useful in selected phalangeal fractures (Fig. 6).

Nonsalvageable, open intra-articular metacarpophalangeal and proximal interphalangeal joint injuries have been treated with immediate Swanson Silastic arthroplasty. The results are variable, but nonamputated digits seem to have better results than those that were completely amputated. Unlike arthrodesis, Silastic arthroplasty maintains length and mobility. In selected cases, emergency implant arthroplasty can be useful treatment. Adequate soft-tissue coverage is mandatory, and using a prosthesis in a border digit is discouraged.

Mallet Fracture

In most instances, closed treatment of a mallet fracture provides a satisfactory functional outcome, but a dorsal bump is common and posttraumatic arthritis is usually present radiographically. Possible candidates for open reduction and internal fixation are individuals whose fracture involves more than one third of the articular surface, who have fracture subluxation that cannot be reduced by closed means, or who are younger and work at occupations that require normal or near-normal distal interphalangeal joint extension.

One operative treatment is a dorsal "H" shaped incision with elevation of a flap of the extensor tendon. The fracture fragment is left attached to the extensor tendon and is immobilized, with care taken to avoid the germinal matrix of the nail bed. Temporary fixation is provided by a 0.28-mm K-wire through the fracture and driven in a retrograde fashion out the distal phalanx. The distal interphalangeal joint is held with the same K-wire guided proximally. In most cases, a second 0.28-mm K-wire is driven dorsally across the fracture site to hold the dorsal fragment to the distal phalanx. Comparison of this technique to nonoperative treatment has shown less dorsal prominence, less extensor lag, and somewhat improved range of flexion.

Open Fractures

Retrospective series continue to define the optimum management of open fractures. For example, analysis of

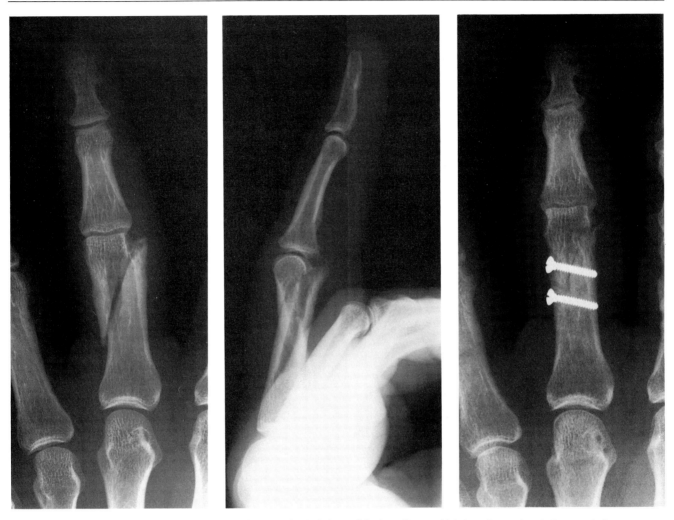

Fig. 6 **Left**, Two-week-old long oblique fracture of the proximal phalanx of the long finger which is malrotated and shortened. **Center**, Lateral view demonstrating volar angulation and dorsal displacement of the proximal phalanx fracture. **Right**, In view of the length of time since injury, closed reduction and percutaneous pinning was not an option. This fracture was amenable to open reduction and internal fixation using two cortical mini fragment screws.

200 open fractures distal to the carpus in 121 patients indicated that the infection rate increased in the presence of wound contamination (grass, dirt, or debris; human or animal bite; warm lake or river injury; barnyard injury), when treatment had been delayed for a period longer than 24 hours, or in those patients who had some significant systemic illness. When any of these conditions are present, delayed closure should be considered. When risk factors are absent, infection is not increased by the presence of internal fixation, immediate wound closure, or large wound size; by tendon, nerve, or vascular injury; or by high-energy mechanism of injury.

The infection rate was 20% in contaminated fractures and 1.2% in noncontaminated fractures. These results generally have been replicated in other studies. *Staphylococcus aureus* is the most commonly reported organism isolated from infected hand wounds, but polymicrobial agents are reported as causative in more than one third of the infections.

To prevent these infections, the role of antibiotics has been investigated in prospective studies of open finger fractures, distal to the metacarpophalangeal joint. In one study, antibiotics were administered to alternate patients; all patients were treated with aggressive surgical irrigation and debridement. In each group, 4% of patients developed clinical signs of infection. However, osteomyelitis did not develop, and no secondary surgical procedures were required in either group. These data suggest vigorous irrigation and debridement is adequate primary treatment for open fractures in fingers with intact digital arteries. Early antibiotic treatment may play a role in helping prevent infections in fingers of patients who have significant amounts of devitalized tissue or who are noncompliant in follow-up care.

In another study, the use of cephalosporin antibiotics was analyzed to determine their effectiveness in preventing infections and encouraging wound healing in open hand wounds treated on an outpatient basis. Eighty-seven patients with acute, open hand trauma participated in a prospective, double-blind trial. Severity ranged from single nail bed injuries with open fractures to moderately contaminated wounds involving tendon, bone, joint, and neurovascular structures. Human bite wounds, outpatient replantation procedures, and superficial skin wounds without injury to deeper structures and without severe contamination were excluded. All wounds were treated in the operating room, where they were irrigated and debrided under tourniquet control with good visualization.

The antibiotic regimen included intravenous cephamandol and oral cephalexin or intravenous and orally administered placebo. The overall infection rate was 1.1%. There were no infections in the antibiotic group; 2.1% of the placebo group developed an infection. Preventive antibiotics are not necessary in the treatment of selected wounds when accompanied by debridement, irrigation, and rapid primary repair in an operating room environment.

Flexor Tendons

The weakness of flexor tendon sutures remains a limiting factor in the postoperative rehabilitation of the hand. The core suture is currently believed to be the most important element for a strong repair. Biomechanical studies of cadaver finger tendons have compared the strengths of a core suture alone, a core suture with a simple running surface suture, and a core suture with a new modification involving a running peripheral Halsted horizontal mattress technique using 5-0 suture. The horizontal mattress configuration results in the suture grasping the epitenon and tendon fiber bundles with its multiple transverse passes across the axially running tendon fibers. The multiple passes share the load evenly and, thus, multiply the strength of the relatively weak suture material. If a bulky tendon repair does not result from this technique, the improved maximum strength could lead to better tendon gliding and decreased rates of tendon rupture.

After tendon repair, early motion is initiated to decrease tendon adhesions that can limit digit motion. The best means of achieving controlled passive motion, however, has not been determined conclusively. The Kleinert splint combines a dorsal extension block with rubber-band traction proximal to the wrist. This passively flexes the fingers, and the patient actively extends within the limits of the splint. The Brooke Army Hospital splint uses rubber-band traction to passively flex the fingers, but the traction is through a pulley at the distal palmar crease, which increases passive flexion at the interphalangeal joints.

Prospective randomized studies have been carried out to determine whether improved tendon gliding can be achieved with greater durations of daily passive motion rehabilitation (eight to 12 hours per day) after flexor tendon repair. A continuous passive motion device was compared with the traditional early passive motion protocol (rubber band traction). The duration of daily controlled motion significantly and favorably affected the function of repaired flexor tendons. However, difficulties encountered with the use of the continuous passive motion device included power failures, mechanical breakages, and lack of patient compliance. These problems require spending more time in patient education, both initially and at intervals throughout the rehabilitation program.

Other studies have analyzed the rehabilitation of flexor tendon repair and grafting using controlled active extension against passive rubber band flexion combined with the use of controlled passive extension and flexion. During active extension exercises, the patient is instructed to hold the metacarpophalangeal joint in the flexed position and then to extend fully the interphalangeal joints. In this way, full excursion of the interphalangeal joint is obtained while the tendon repair is protected. Of 66 patients (78 fingers) with complete lacerations of the profundus and superficialis in "no man's land," 80% were rated excellent; 18%, good; and 2%, fair, based on the Strickland formula. None was rated as poor.

A comparison of 51 patients with isolated flexor pollicis longus tendon repairs was undertaken to determine the value of postoperative splinting. Of the patients treated by immobilization postoperatively, 44% achieved good to excellent results compared with 60% treated by dynamic traction, but this difference was not statistically significant. However, for repairs between the A1 pulley at the metacarpophalangeal joint and the A2 pulley at the interphalangeal joint, the results of mobilization were significantly better than those for fixed splinting.

Nerve Repair

Efforts are underway to improve results of nerve repair by improvement of alignment and repair techniques. Nerves are commonly repaired using an operating microscope and a perineurial or epineurial repair. The age of the patient is the single most critical factor in sensory recovery after nerve repair, and results are adversely affected by associated injuries to muscle, tendon, and bone. Sensory recovery also correlates with the experience of the surgeon. Vein conduits 1 to 3 cm long may improve early digital nerve repair, but delayed repair with vein conduits has had poor results.

The anterior branch of the medial antebrachial cutaneous nerve is a useful adjunct to digital nerve repair. There are several advantages to using this graft source: the nerve is subcutaneous and easy to isolate, the incision is confined to the upper extremity, and sensibility is not lost anywhere in the hand.

When simultaneous laceration of both median and ulnar nerves occurs with flexor tendon laceration at the wrist, restoration of hand mobility and strength of tendon repair are good, but the results of nerve repair are less reliable. The majority of patients have diminished protective sensation, and the recovery of two-point discrimination is almost uniformly poor. However, these patients compensate well for their impairment and usually return to full employment. Despite significantly reduced dexterity and impaired tactile gnosis, both therapist and patients often believe they function well.

Fingertip Injuries

A conservative method of treating fingertip injuries was prescribed for 71 patients with 89 fingertip injuries. The injured finger is soaked in betadine solution, followed by hydrogen peroxide solution. The tip of the finger of a surgical glove is filled with silver sulfadiazine cream and is pulled over the injured digit. The resulting occlusion dressing is taped at the base to prevent leakage and is changed every other day for ten days, but less frequently thereafter. Of the 71 patients, 15 returned to work one week after injury. By one year none of the fingers was hypersensitive, all had full motion, and 86 had good appearance.

When the fingertip is amputated, one technique is to fillet the severed tip and replace it as a "cap" over the skeletonized distal phalanx of the stump. A 2-mm remnant of germinal matrix is preserved for nail regrowth. Although the reconstructed fingers are shortened by an average of 6 mm, the illusion is that of a normal finger. The "cap" technique of nonmicrosurgical reattachment is a simple, reliable means of achieving both functional preservation of pulp tissue and acceptable appearance of the nail complex in amputations at the level of the lunula when replantation is inappropriate or impossible.

Replantation

Indications for replantation are being refined, and results of replantation of various types of amputations are being scrutinized. Disadvantages to replantation of single digit amputations at the distal interphalangeal joint or distal phalanx are that initial operating time is longer, the procedure requires microsurgical training, and it is more expensive. Advantages are that it is a one-stage procedure that gives good soft-tissue coverage, adequate sensibility without painful neuroma, and good metacarpophalangeal and proximal interphalangeal joint motion; it preserves the nail, maintains digit length, and is cosmetically pleasing.

Forty-two complete thumb replantations were attempted for amputations, regardless of the mechanism or severity of injury. Sixteen (38%) failed intraoperatively or postoperatively. Thumbs with narrow zones of injury had significantly higher survival rates than those with wide zones of injury. Of those with poor arterial flow intraoperatively, 80% ultimately failed despite pharmacologic treatment and multiple vein grafts. Survival rate of avulsed thumbs was 46%. Reexploration for loss of perfusion succeeded in 60% of cases. Cold intolerance was seldom a problem beyond one year postoperatively.

It is recommended that replantation be attempted for all thumb amputations, because success cannot be predicted, either by mechanism or severity of injury.

Another article reviewed the results that followed rotating shaft avulsion amputations of the thumb. Survival rate was 82% in 23 patients at a mean of 20.5 months after injury, grip strength was 95% of the unaffected side, and key pinch was 77%. It is concluded this aggressive surgical approach produces better function than that obtained with other reconstructive methods.

Of 25 patients whose thumb amputations were not replanted, 13 amputations were at the distal phalanx and 12 were more proximal. The final outcome was good in eight patients, fair in 12, and poor in five. Only patients with amputations at or distal to the interphalangeal joint had normal key grip and pinch grip. Six patients never returned to work, and two carpenters worked at a lower capacity. The median time out of work was 114 days. The most frequent complaints were hypersensitivity, difficulty in picking up small objects, cold intolerance, and pain when using the remaining part of the digit.

Other investigators have evaluated patients with complete thumb amputations treated by replantation or revision. Ninety percent of the replantations were between the metacarpophalangeal joint and the proximal third of the distal phalanx. Eighty percent of both groups were able to perform activities of daily living at 80% of their uninjured side. Grip strength was approximately 84% that of the uninjured hand in each group. Work simulator assessment of lateral and three-point pinch was better in the revision group.

In this group of patients, it was not possible to demonstrate uniform superiority of replantation over revision. Median time for return to work for replant patients was 11 weeks compared with eight weeks for revisions, but the range was large. In the replant group, 87% returned to their preinjury job, compared with 70% (12 of 17) of the revision group. Among those patients who had complaints, the most frequent was that of poor sensibility. Patients with replanted thumbs with good sensibility tend to perform better in tasks requiring fine dexterity than do those with revision. Patients with isolated thumb revision usually have stronger pinch but they have more difficulty holding certain tools and large objects. Most patients with isolated thumb amputation distal to the metacarpophalangeal joint, whether replanted or revised, adapt to their injury and resume activities of daily living and their jobs.

Infections

Mycobacterium marinum

Unusual hand infections, in themselves seen infrequently, are encountered frequently enough when taken as a group that the orthopaedist should be cognizant of them. The key to the diagnosis of *Mycobacterium marinum* is a high index of suspicion, a thorough history with emphasis on possible exposure to *M marinum* sources, awareness that inoculation can occur as a result of seemingly trivial trauma, and use of tissue for culture and for histologic examination. The reported sources of *M marinum* include contaminated swimming pools, fishing tanks, boat piers, brackish water, fish bites or injuries caused by fins or spines, and even laboratory accidents. The most common complaint is painful swelling in the hand, either a subcutaneous mass or tenosynovitis, which involves the extensors more frequently than the flexors (Fig. 7). *M marinum* organisms require Lowenstein-Jensen media and incubation at 30 C, because routine tuberculosis cultures incubated at 35 C to 37 C frequently failed to show this organism. Ethambutol and rifampin have been used successfully in treatment.

Sporotrichosis

Subcutaneous inoculation with the ubiquitous fungus *Sporothrix schenckii* leads to chronic granulomatous infection that involves skin and subcutaneous tissues. Less commonly, deeper structures such as joints, muscles, and bone are involved. The majority of infected patients handled plants or soil at work or recreationally; others recall a specific injury, such as a thorn puncture. Delay in diagnosis is common, averaging four months for the lymphocutaneous form and 25 months for deep infection. The risk for infection is greater in the immunocompromised patient. Lymphocutaneous disease generally can be treated orally with saturated potassium iodine solution, while those with pulmonary or deep infection require amphotericin or ketoconazole. Most patients become free of lymphocutaneous disease, but most of those with joint involvement have residual functional impairment. Sporotrichosis should be considered in the differential diagnosis of chronic inflammatory monoarticular arthritis and tenosynovitis, especially where there is a risk of inoculation with spores.

Vibrio vulnificus

Vibrio vulnificus, a gram-negative facultative coccobacillus, is a rare cause of hand infection. In the United States these infections occur mainly on the Gulf Coast and Southern Atlantic Seaboard. These ubiquitous organisms tend to proliferate in the warm months from May through October, in waters of moderate salinity and alkaline pH. The two known sources of infection are direct inoculation and enteric involvement from ingestion of raw seafood. This infection spreads rapidly, especially if antibiotic therapy and radical debridement of all infected and necrotic tissue are delayed. Gram-negative septicemia and septic shock may begin within hours of onset, and cardiovascular collapse may occur rapidly. Infection accompanied by septicemia is most common in immunocompromised hosts, including those who have diabetes mellitus. Once the organism invades the tissue, destruction may be extensive and may be accompanied by bulli, vasculitis, arterial and venous thrombosis, massive necrosis to the deep fascia, and septic myositis.

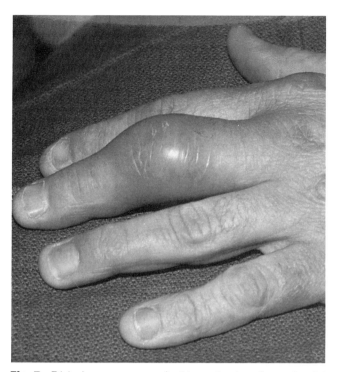

Fig. 7 Etiologies are numerous for this swollen long finger. Careful history revealed that four months earlier this patient sustained a puncture wound from a seashell fragment. Culture of the debrided tissue revealed *Mycobacterium marinum*, which responded to ethambutol and refampin.

The organism is sensitive to a variety of broad-spectrum antibiotics, including doxycycline (perhaps the antibiotic of choice), tetracycline, ampicillin, most cephalosporins, and gentamicin. Nonetheless, in patients with severe, advanced infection, radical operative debridement down to the level of uninvolved tissues is mandatory, in addition to administration of antibiotics. When a gram-negative bacillus is evident on a smear of an infected wound that was incurred through a scratch or puncture contaminated by warm sea water, the diagnosis should be suspected.

Pyoderma Gangrenosum

Pyoderma gangrenosum is a poorly understood but well described papulovesicular skin disorder that presents problems in both diagnosis and management. It usually occurs in the hand and is very rare in other sites. The appearance of progressive, painful bulli following injury is noted. The initial symptoms of this disease mimic several infectious processes; however, surgical treatment of the lesion rarely is curative. An underlying systemic disease is present in up to 78% of cases, and ulcerative colitis is reported in 36% to 60% of infected patients. Infection, while probably not a direct cause, may play a secondary role in the development of lesions. No relation has been shown between this and AIDS.

The lesions characteristically have acute, rapid, painful development, usually beginning as red or black papules. Within hours they become pustular, spreading rapidly and undergoing central necrosis. The border, purple and shaggy with an erythematous halo, advances centrifugally at the rate of 1 to 2 mm a day. Once the lesion develops, the consistent symptom is pain. If the disease remains untreated, enlargement slows and the ulcer becomes indolent. Nonpathognomonic histologic findings are seen on biopsy. Except in cases of secondary infection, staining and cultures for microorganisms are negative. The diagnosis is made on clinical grounds and by process of exclusion.

Management consists of local treatment of the lesions, systemic treatment of the skin disease, and search for any associated systemic diseases. Minimal superficial debridement is done so as not to incite the pathergic response. Appropriate cultures are taken to exclude atypical or secondary infections. Gentle serial whirlpools, the application of topical sulphone compound, and enteral or parenteral administration of high-dose steroids, 60 to 80 mg of prednisone per day in divided doses, are recommended. The dose is tapered with time and response. If contraindications to the above routes of administration exist, intralesional corticosteroid instillation may be beneficial.

Self-Inflicted Hand Injuries

The physical manifestations of self-inflicted hand injuries include factitious lymphedema of the hand, usually caused by a tourniquet from some type of self-applied circular bandage; hard edema of the dorsum of the hand, usually caused by repeated self-inflicted blows to the back of the hand; clinched fist syndrome; various skin disorders, mostly infections; and a passive form of Munchausen syndrome.

Prolonged healing and failure of wounds to heal are usually ascribed to physiologic conditions such as infection, immune deficiency, or trauma, without considering the possibility that the patient may be causing the lesion. Ulceration and local skin infections are frequently the patient's complaint. The wounds do not progress gradually but instead appear fully developed, often overnight in previously normal skin. Close observation of the patient or use of an occlusive dressing typically interrupts the development of further lesions. The common finding is the patient's denial of any responsibility for his/her illness. However, there is no characteristic psychological profile of a patient with self-inflicted disease; diagnosis is usually made by exclusion, often after prolonged hospitalization.

Treatment of such injuries is a major problem. The physician must give the patient an opportunity to save face without depriving him/her of defenses that maintain emotional integrity. The patient should not be confronted with evidence of self mutilation until a plan for social and psychiatric care is arranged. Although psycho-therapy is the main treatment, the physician should not neglect a coexisting medical illness.

Burns

Acute thermal hand burns require a systematic approach to obtain optimal results. Although controversy exists concerning the most appropriate treatment of the second-degree hand burn, an algorithm for treatment of the burned hand clarifies the treatment options available to the surgeon (Fig. 8).

Flaps

A variety of flaps (free, axial, fasciocutaneous) are being used immediately after injury and within several days after injury to cover soft-tissue defects in the hand. Flap coverage of damaged palmar and dorsal hand soft tissue should provide a durable surface, cosmetic contour, appropriate bulk, suitable bed for tendon gliding or grafting, and an acceptable donor site. The inferior three slips of the serratus anterior muscle have been used for free tissue transfer for the reconstruction of dorsal and palmar defects in the hand. This flap has low donor site morbidity, has three separate slips that are easily divisible for contouring, is durable, and adheres to provide a stable surface for grasp.

Although the Chinese fasciocutaneous radial forearm flap has gained popularity, donor site appearance has prevented its widespread acceptance. The standard forearm flap is vascularized by a pedicle that consists of the radial artery and two vena comitantes that are ligated proximally and turned distally toward the defect in the hand. The donor defect is resurfaced with split-thickness skin graft. To minimize donor site morbidity, the fascial component of the forearm flap can be used to reconstruct hand defects. Split-thickness skin is placed over the flap, and the donor site is closed primarily. This flap requires a pulsatile ulnar artery and positive Allen test. It provides a thin, vascularized wound cover and a vascular bed for skin grafting. The disadvantages are that skin graft of fascia is not as ideal as that of full-thickness skin, and that the radial artery is sacrificed, although this is not necessarily a problem if the ulnar artery is intact.

The free scapular fascial flap resurfaced with skin graft provides less bulk than the cutaneous scapular flap. It is supplied by the circumflex scapular artery, which emerges at the lateral border of the scapula and divides into cutaneous scapular and periscapular arteries. It has the advantage of a constant vascular pedicle and a well-hidden donor site, although the scar does spread.

The dorsal metacarpal vessels contribute to the fascial plexus, which supplies the skin of the dorsum of the hand. The reverse dorsal metacarpal flap, based on the dorsal metacarpal arteries, can cover small soft-tissue defects in the hand. The axis of this flap parallels the dorsal interosseous muscles. Subcutaneous fat, fascia, and dor-

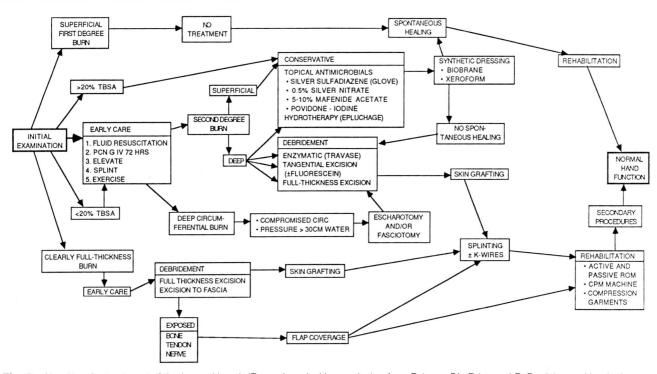

Fig. 8 Algorithm for treatment of the burned hand. (Reproduced with permission from Falcone PA, Edstrom LE: Decision making in the acute thermal hand burn: An algorithm for treatment. *Hand Clin* 1990;6:233-238.)

sal metacarpal vessels are included in the flap and divided proximally. The proximal end of the flap is elevated and dissection of the flap and its pedicle is continued distally to the web space. Because the fourth and fifth metacarpal arteries are absent in one third of cases, this flap might not be dependable on the ulnar side.

The second dorsal metacarpal artery neurovascular island flap can be used after release of first web contractures and to resurface radiopalmar and thumb defects. It is proximally based, and if it is extended beyond the proximal interphalangeal joint, distal flap necrosis and donor-site difficulties can result. The point at which the extensor tendon to the index and long fingers separates is the pivot point for the flap pedicle. The dorsal interosseous fascia must be included with the pedicle over the full width of the muscle to safeguard the artery. The flap is dissected from distal to proximal. The communication with the palmar metacarpal artery is identified and ligated when the second web is reached. The flap is passed through a subcutaneous tunnel and the donor site closed with split thickness or full thickness skin graft.

The homodigital neurovascular island flap provides flap mobility, blood supply, and innervation. When the lost tissue is mainly volar, an advancement flap can maintain digit length and preserve sensibility. With loss of sensibility on the radial side of the index finger, an exchange island flap can be moved from the ulnar border to the radial border.

Arterialized venous skin flaps consist of subcutaneous vein along with the skin, and usually are taken from the flexor side of the distal forearm or the dorsal aspect of the foot. The vein is interposed between missing segments of the distal artery. This method restores circulation and covers the skin defect. There are several variations of the procedure: Both ends of the vein in the skin flap are anastomosed to a vein in the finger. One end of the vein in the flap is anastomosed to an artery in the finger and the other end of the vein flap is anastomosed to a vein in the finger. Both ends of the vein in the skin flap are anastomosed to an artery in the finger. When a skin defect is accompanied by injury to the digital artery, the venous skin flap is positioned between the two healthy segments of artery. Both microsurgical and conventional techniques continue to play an important role in hand reconstruction after trauma.

Annotated Bibliography

Wrist and Hand Trauma

Distal Radius Fractures

af Ekenstam F, Jakobsson OP, Wadin K: Repair of the triangular ligament in Colles' fracture: No effect in a prospective randomized study. *Acta Orthop Scand* 1989;60:393-396.

In a prospective, randomized study, the authors examine the importance of ulnar styloid injury and triangular fibrocartilage repair in Colles' fractures. Closed reduction of the fractured radius, followed by suturing the triangular ligament and stabilization of the ulnar styloid did not produce better results than closed reduction and application of an above-elbow plaster cast unless there was gross instability of the wrist or dislocation of the distal radioulnar joint.

Axelrod TS, McMurtry RY: Open reduction and internal fixation of comminuted intraarticular fractures of the distal radius. *J Hand Surg* 1990;15A:1-11.

This paper demonstrates the importance of accurate reduction for intra-articular distal radial fractures and also notes some of the problems associated with using open reduction and internal fixation to achieve this. The overall complication rate is 50%.

Bickerstaff DR, Bell MJ: Carpal malalignment in Colles' fractures. *J Hand Surg* 1989;14B:155-160.

A study of 32 patients demonstrates that abnormalities in carpal alignment contribute to a poor functional result after a Colles' fracture.

Bradway JK, Amadio PC, Cooney WP: Open reduction and internal fixation of displaced, comminuted intra-articular fractures of the distal end of the radius. *J Bone Joint Surg* 1989;71A;839-847.

This retrospective review of 16 patients with AO type C2 or C3 fracture of the distal radius demonstrated excellent or good results in the majority of the patents who underwent open reduction, internal fixation.

Horne JG, Devane P, Purdie G: A prospective randomized trial of external fixation and plaster cast immobilization in the treatment of distal radial fractures. *J Orthop Trauma* 1990;4:30-34.

Because of the significant complication rate and the failure to demonstrate superior end results, the use of external fixation in distal radial fractures in patients older than 60 years of age has been abandoned at the senior author's institution.

Kongsholm J, Olerud C: Plaster cast versus external fixation for unstable intra-articular Colles' fractures. *Clin Orthop* 1989;241:57-64.

External fixation to treat unstable intra-articular Colles' fractures revealed superior results with respect to functional outcome, range of motion, and grip strength when compared with plaster cast treatment of similar fractures.

Leung KS, Shen W, Tsang HK, et al: An effective treatment of comminuted fractures of the distal radius. *J Hand Surg* 1990;15A:11-17.

These authors used the combination of external fixation and bone grafting to treat 100 patients with comminuted distal radial fractures. Results were generally excellent in this series.

McQueen M, Caspers J: Colles Fracture: Does the anatomical result affect the final function? *J Bone Joint Surg* 1988;70B:649-651.

Thirty patients who had sustained a Colles' fracture at least four years earlier were examined functionally and radiographically. Seventeen had a good radiographic result and 13 were considered to have malunion. Function was significantly worse in the displaced group than in the undisplaced group.

Rayhack JM, Langworthy JN, Belsole RJ: Transulnar percutaneous pinning of displaced distal radial fractures: A preliminary report. *J Orthop Trauma* 1989;3:107-114.

Fourteen patients, averaging 48 years of age, were analyzed as to subjective patient responses, range of motion, grip strength, and radiographic appearance. At 15 months, two had excellent and 12 had good results.

Seitz WH Jr, Froimson AI, Brooks DB, et al: Biomechanical analysis of pin placement and pin size for external fixation of distal radius fractures. *Clin Orthop* 1990;251:207-212.

Biomechanical analysis of external fixator pin placement and pin size for fractures of the distal radius provides information that should help decrease the incidence of pin loosening, fracture through pin sites, collapse at the fracture site, and intrinsic contracture.

Scaphoid Fractures

Adams BD, Blair WF, Reagan DS, et al: Technical factors related to Herbert Screw Fixation. *J Hand Surg* 1988;13A:893-899.

Twenty-four patients with acute fractures or nonunion of the scaphoid were treated with Herbert screw fixation. Fracture healing correlated strongly with technical factors of the procedure, including poor scaphoid realignment, inaccurate gig placement, or improper screw length.

Gelberman RH, Wolock BS, Siegel DB: Fractures and nonunions of the carpal scaphoid. *J Bone Joint Surg* 1989;71A:1560-1565.

This comprehensive review includes vascular anatomy, biomechanics, imaging, and diagnosis and treatment of scaphoid fractures and nonunions.

Gellman H, Caputo RJ, Carter V, et al: Comparison of short and long thumb-spica casts for nondisplaced fractures of the carpal scaphoid. *J Bone Joint Surg* 1989;71A:354-357.

Fifty-one patients with nondisplaced scaphoid fractures were randomly assigned to treatment with either a long or short thumb spica cast. Based on these results, the authors recommended an initial period of six weeks of immobilization in a long thumb spica cast followed by a short thumb spica cast when treating proximal or middle fractures. Fracture of the distal third did well regardless of the type of immobilization.

Inoue G, Tanaka Y, Nakamura R: Treatment of trans-scaphoid perilunate dislocations by internal fixation with the Herbert screw. *J Hand Surg* 1990;15B:449-454.

This review of 13 patients with 14 dorsal transscaphoid perilunate dislocations suggests that satisfactory results can be obtained with Herbert screw fixation of the scaphoid. Ligamentous repair and restoration of carpal alignment by temporary K-wire fixation are sometimes indicated.

Langhoff O, Andersen JL: Consequences of late immobilization of scaphoid fractures. *J Hand Surg* 1988;13B:77-79.

Records and radiographs of 285 scaphoid fractures were reviewed to determine the relationship between delay before immobilization and the development of nonunion or delayed union. The authors felt that it was unnecessary to immobilize the wrist if there was clinical suspicion of a fracture but it was not demonstrable radiographically. If the scaphoid fat strip was abnormal or missing, a second radiograph and reexamination at about two weeks were recommended. They concluded that the frequency of nonunion would not increase if correct immobilization was commenced at that time.

Lindström G, Nyström A: Incidence of posttraumatic arthrosis after primary healing of scaphoid fractures: A clinical and radiological study. *J Hand Surg* 1990;15B:11-13.

This retrospective study of 229 patients with healed fractures of the waist of the scaphoid demonstrates relatively high incidence of radiocarpal arthrosis after primary healing of the scaphoid. This was attributed to malunion and recommendation was for open reduction and internal fixation of unstable, severely displaced, angulated, or compressed fractures.

Vender MI, Watson HK, Black DM, et al: Acute scaphoid fracture with scapholunate gap. *J Hand Surg* 1989;14A:1004-1007.

Two cases were presented to demonstrate the simultaneous occurrence of acute scaphoid fracture and scapholunate gap. The recommended treatment in acute cases is open reduction, internal fixation of the fracture, and open stabilization of the scaphoid.

Viegas SF, Bean JW, Schram RA: Transscaphoid fracture/dislocations treated with open reduction and Herbert screw internal fixation. *J Hand Surg* 1987;12A:992-999.

These authors reviewed six cases of dorsal and two cases of palmar transscaphoid perilunate fracture dislocation treated by open reduction and internal fixation of the scaphoid with Herbert screw. The results of the six dorsal injures were three excellent, one good, one fair, while both palmar injuries were poor.

Carpal Instability

Horii E, Garcia-Elias M, An KN, et al: A kinematic study of lunotriquetral dissociations. *J Hand Surg* 1991;16A:355-362.

Stereoradiographic methods were used to analyze carpal motion after sectioning of the ligamentous support of the lunotriquetral joint. A complete injury of the lunotriquetral ligament results in increased mobility of the triquetrum but does not show a static volar intercalated segment instability.

Meade TD, Schneider LH, Cherry K: Radiographic analysis of selective ligament sectioning at the carpal

scaphoid: A cadaver study. *J Hand Surg* 1990;15A:855-862.

This experimental study used six fresh frozen cadaver specimens to demonstrate the radiographic changes seen on standard and stress wrist radiographs that correlate with the sequential sectioning of the scapholunate stabilizing ligaments. Significant ligamentous injury must occur before commonly used radiographic limits are exceeded. The lateral scapholunate angle most closely reflected the progressive nature of this injury.

Pin PG, Young VL, Gilula LA, et al: Management of chronic lunotriquetral ligament tears. *J Hand Surg* 1989;14A:77-83.

Eleven patients treated by lunotriquetral fusion with use of a compression screw are reported. The mechanism of disruption of the lunotriquetral ligament, symptoms, signs, and imaging studies are discussed, as well as the results of arthrodesis.

Taleisnik J: Current concepts review: Carpal instability. *J Bone Joint Surg* 1988;70A:1262-1268.

This comprehensive review includes the anatomy, kinematics, mechanism of injury, diagnosis, and treatment of scapholunate dissociation, lunotriquetral instability, ulnar translocation, and dynamic volar and dorsal intercalated segment instability.

Viegas SF, Patterson RM, Peterson PD, et al: Ulnar sided perilunate instability: An anatomic and biomechanic study. *J Hand Surg* 1990;15A:268-278.

These authors stage ulnar-sided wrist instability and delineate the pathophysiology of lunotriquetral dissociation and subsequent volar intercalated segment instability.

Hamate Fractures

Bishop AT, Beckenbaugh RD: Fracture of the hamate hook. *J Hand Surg* 1988;13A:135-139.

These authors review the diagnosis and treatment of 21 hamate fractures. Although open reduction and internal fixation may be successful, these authors conclude that excision produces equal or better results.

Smith P III, Wright TW, Wallace PF, et al: Excision of the hook of the hamate: A retrospective survey and review of the literature. *J Hand Surg* 1988;13A:612-615.

A retrospective review of 133 cases of excision of the hook of the hamate to treat nonunion confirms that excision is the treatment of choice for fractures of the hook of the hamate.

Stark HH, Chao EK, Zemel NP, et al: Fracture of the hook of the hamate. *J Bone Joint Surg* 1989;71A:1202-1207.

Conclusion after reviewing 59 patients was that a fractured hook of the hamate, where it is acute, chronic, or even considered partially united, should be removed. This treatment reliably eliminates the symptoms and lessens the likelihood of subsequent rupture of nearby flexor tendons.

Carpometacarpal Dislocations

DeBeer JD, Maloon S, Anderson P, et al: Multiple carpo-metacarpal dislocations. *J Hand Surg* 1989;14B:105-108.

Closed manipulation was found to be successful in carpometacarpal dislocations if performed within two days of the injury. Plaster cast immobilization supplemented by percutaneous K-wire fixation is recommended in maintaining reduction because of the unstable nature of the dislocation.

Lawlis JF III, Gunther SF: Carpometacarpal dislocations. Long-term follow-up. *J Bone Joint Surg* 1991;73A:52-59.

After reviewing 20 patients who had a dislocation of one or all of the medial four carpometacarpal joints, recommendations were for open reduction and pinning. Closed reduction and percutaneous fixation with pins was not used as a method of treatment in these patients.

Bennett's Fractures

Kjaer-Petersen K, Langhoff O, Andersen K: Bennett's fracture. *J Hand Surg* 1990;15B:58-61.

This series of 41 Bennett's fractures included patients treated by closed reduction, percutaneous fixation, and open reduction. No patient had significant symptoms at follow-up after median 7.3 years. However, the authors found a positive association between the position in which the fracture healed and the occurrence of late symptoms in addition to an increased tendency toward the development of arthritic changes after less perfect reduction and a positive correlation between pain and arthritis.

Metacarpophalangeal Joint

Koniuch MP, Peimer CA, VanGorder T, et al: Closed crush injury of the metacarpophalangeal joint. *J Hand Surg* 1987;12A:750-757.

Patients with chronic symptoms after closed impact injuries to the metacarpophalangeal joint, without extensor tendon migration or positive radiographs, who are unresponsive to nonoperative treatment should have surgical exploration of the painful area. The sagittal fiber tear and any contiguous capsular lesion should be repaired and the metacarpophalangeal joint explored to exclude encompassing intra-articular pathology.

Metacarpal Fractures

Ford DJ, El-Hadidi S, Lunn PG, et al: Fractures of the metacarpals: Treatment by AO screw and plate fixation. *J Hand Surg* 1989;12B:34-37.

These authors used AO minifragment screws and plates to treat 22 patients with 26 metacarpal fractures that were multiple, unstable, displaced, or rotated. Fourteen patients regained full movement. Restricted movement was present in patients with open fractures, divided extensor tendons, or intra-articular fractures of the metacarpal head, but results were felt to be uniformly satisfactory.

Greene TL, Noellert RC, Belsole RJ, et al: Composite wiring of metacarpal and phalangeal fractures. *J Hand Surg* 1989;14A:665-669.

Sixty-three metacarpal and phalangeal fractures were treated by a combination of K-wires and stainless steel wire loupes, making a composite of bone, pin, and a wire. The K-wires (0.035 in) are used to secure the fragments, and monofilament stainless steel wire, 24, 26, or 28 gauge, is incorporated around the ends of the K-wires.

Konradsen L, Nielsen PT, Albrecht-Beste E: Functional treatment of metacarpal fractures: One hundred randomized cases with or without fixation. *Acta Orthop Scand* 1990;61:531-534.

These authors compare results of 100 subcapital or diaphyseal fractures of the second through fifth metacarpals, randomized to either a dorsal/ulnar plaster cast immobilizing the wrist and the joints of the involved digits, or a functional cast allowing the wrist and digits a free range of motion.

McKerrell J, Bowen V, Johnston G, et al: Boxer's fractures: Conservative or operative management. *J Trauma* 1987;27:486-490.

Of 63 consecutive patients with isolated closed fractures of the fifth metacarpal neck, 40 were divided into a conservative and an operative group. All patients obtained good results. The authors concluded that operative treatment should be reserved for patients demanding perfect cosmesis and willing to accept a longer period of disability.

Metacarpophalangeal Joint Collateral Ligament Injuries

Albrahamsson SO, Sollerman C, Lundborg G, et al: Diagnosis of displaced ulnar collateral ligament of the metacarpophalangeal joint of the thumb. *J Hand Surg* 1990;15A:457-460.

After prospectively studying 24 consecutive patients with posttraumatic instability of the metacarpophalangeal joint of the thumb, the authors conclude that palpation of the displaced collateral ligament combined with instability testing is an improved diagnostic method for detecting a Stenner lesion. They suggest that ligament ruptures of the thumb without ligament displacement can be treated successfully with immobilization, irrespective of the instability found, and that only cases with palpable ligament displacement and gross instability should be treated with surgery.

Helm RH: Hand function after injuries to the collateral ligaments of the metacarpophalangeal joint of the thumb. *J Hand Surg* 1989;12B:252-255.

Thirty-four patients who had undergone surgical repair of collateral ligament injuries of the metacarpophalangeal joint of the thumb were assessed as to symptoms, range of motion, pinch strength, and instability.

Ishizuki M: Injury to collateral ligament of the metacarpophalangeal joint of a finger. *J Hand Surg* 1988;13A:444-448.

Arthrography was performed in 22 patients with injury to the collateral ligament of the metacarpophalangeal joint of the finger and correlated with grade of joint stability. Severely unstable joints should be treated surgically.

Pichora DR, McMurtry RY, Bell MJ: Gamekeepers thumb: A prospective study of functional bracing. *J Hand Surg* 1989;14A:567-573.

Thirty-two patients had acute thumb metacarpophalangeal joint injuries assessed by stress radiography, arthrography, and clinical examination, and treated by splinting combined with daily active motion. The authors found this to be a simple, economical, noninvasive, and effective treatment for the majority of active metacarpophalangeal joint injuries routinely encountered in the clinic.

Schubiner JM, Mass DP: Operation for collateral ligament ruptures of the metacarpophalangeal joints of the fingers. *J Bone Joint Surg* 1989;71B:388-389.

Ten cases of complete rupture of the collateral ligaments of the metacarpophalangeal finger joints were reported. The nature of this injury, the preoperative morbidity, and the intraoperative pathology were analyzed. In all cases, surgery was performed with satisfactory results. Operations improved joint stability and grip and pinch strength, relieved pain, and led to early functional recovery.

Sesamoid Fractures

Patel MR, Pearlman HS, Bassini L, et al: Fractures of the sesamoid bones of the thumb. *J Hand Surg* 1990;15A:776-781.

A literature review of 25 patients with sesamoid fractures of the thumb and three additional cases were used to discuss classification and treatment of thumb sesamoid fractures.

Digit Fractures

Nagle DJ, af Ekenstam FW, Lister GD: Immediate silastic arthroplasty for nonsalvageable intraarticular phalangeal fractures. *Scand J Plast Reconstr Surg* 1989;23:47-50.

Fourteen patients with open nonsalvageable, intra-articular fractures of the proximal interphalangeal or metacarpophalangeal joint had immediate Silastic arthroplasty. Metacarpophalangeal joints averaged 60 degrees of motion and proximal interphalangeal joints averaged 30. No postoperative infections were noted. All joints with the exception of one proximal interphalangeal were stable. Three of the six that remained painful were replants. Six patients rated the joint as satisfactory, three had complaints, and five were dissatisfied.

Pun WK, Chow SP, So YC, et al: A prospective study of 284 digital fractures of the hand. *J Hand Surg* 1989;14A:474-481.

These authors report a prospective study of 284 digital fractures of the hand in 235 patients. It was important to distinguish stable and unstable fractures, because many stable fractures of the hand do well with early active mobilization treatment. The best method to manage unstable fractures was not determined, but splinting was not successful in patients with associated skin problems.

Mallet Fractures

Lubahn JD: Mallet finger fractures: A comparison of open and closed technique. *J Hand Surg* 1989;14A:394-396.

Thirty mallet fractures were treated closed in 19 cases and open in 11. In this series, open treatment with anatomic restoration of the joint provided a cosmetically and functionally better result than that seen in patients treated by the closed technique. Indications for open treatment included joint subluxation and fracture involving more than one third of the articular surface.

Warren RA, Kay NR, Ferguson DG: Mallet finger: Comparison between operative and conservative management in those cases failing to be cured by splintage. *J Hand Surg* 1988;13B:159-160.

Sixty-nine patients with mallet finger who failed to be cured by a period of splinting were offered either tenodermodesis or K-wire fixation of the distal interphalangeal joint. Eleven (16%) accepted the offer, and eight of these were significantly improved. Of those patients declining surgery, 30 were available for review after a minimum period of six months; of these 13 (43%) had undergone a significant spontaneous improvement.

Open Fractures

McLain RF, Steyers C, Stoddard M: Infections in open fractures of the hand. *J Hand Surg* 1991;16A:108-112.

This study of 46 consecutive patients with open hand fractures has identified several injury factors associated with increased risk of infection, as well as risk factors for poor outcome following

this type of injury. Hands with injuries characterized by significant soft-tissue damage, severe skeletal trauma, or gross wound contamination should be considered compromised and at a high risk for infection.

Peacock KC, Hanna DP, Kirkpatrick K, et al: Efficacy of perioperative cefamandole with postoperative cephalexin in the primary outpatient treatment of open wounds of the hand. *J Hand Surg* 1988;13A:960-964.

This prospective, double-blind study of 87 patients suggests that perioperative administration of antibiotics in treatment of common, open traumatic hand wounds is not of significant benefit when compared with placebo.

Suprock MD, Hood JM, Lubahn JD: Role of antibiotics in open fractures of the finger. *J Hand Surg* 1990;15A:761-764.

After investigating prospectively 91 open finger fractures, these authors conclude that the early use of antibiotics in fractures of the phalanges that have been aggressively irrigated and debrided is of no benefit in the prevention of infections, when compared with treatment via aggressive irrigation and debridement alone.

Swanson TV, Szabo RM, Anderson DD: Open hand fractures: Prognosis and classification. *J Hand Surg* 1991;16A:101-107.

Two hundred open hand fractures distal to the carpus were reviewed with attention to wound infection, malunion, delayed or nonunion, fixation problems, and amputations. A classification predictive of infection is suggested. Fracture stabilization is chosen on the basis of the mechanical needs of the fracture, regardless of the wound size, injury, or contamination. Wound closure was determined by the degree of contamination.

Flexor Tendons

Chow JA, Thomes LJ, Dovelle S, et al: Controlled motion rehabilitation after flexor tendon repair and grafting: A multi-centre study. *J Bone Joint Surg* 1988;70B:591-595.

This multicenter study incorporates the Brooke Army Hospital modification of the rubber band passive flexion splint, which provides increased range of passive flexion of the finger. It emphasizes active extension of the proximal interphalangeal and distal interphalangeal joints with the metacarpophalangeal joint blocked in the flexion position, and it incorporates full passive extension and flexion of the proximal interphalangeal and distal interphalangeal joints performed with the metacarpophalangeal joint flexed by the surgeon or hand therapist.

Gelberman RH, Nunley JA II, Osterman AL, et al: Influences of the protected passive mobilization interval on flexor tendon healing: A prospective randomized clinical study. *Clin Orthop* 1991;264:189-196.

In this prospective multicenter clinical study, 51 patients were randomly placed into two controlled passive motion protocols. Group I patients received greater intervals of passive motion using a continuous passive motion device. Group II patients were treated with a traditional early passive motion protocol (rubber-band traction) for tendon rehabilitation.

Percival NJ, Sykes PJ: Flexor pollicis longus tendon repair: A comparison between dynamic and static splintage. *J Hand Surg* 1989;14B:412-415.

This retrospective review of 51 patients with isolated flexor pollicis longus repairs documents that patients treated with dynamic traction had better results than those treated by fixed splinting.

Wade PJ, Wetherell RG, Amis AA: Flexor tendon repair: Significant gain in strength from the Halsted peripheral suture technique. *J Hand Surg* 1989;14B:232-235.

Tensile strength of tendon suture techniques were compared for Kessler, Kleinert, and Halsted repairs, the latter being tested with prolene, PDS, and ethibond.

Nerves

Mailänder P, Berger A, Schaller E, et al: Results of primary nerve repair in the upper extremity. *Microsurgery* 1989;10:147-150.

Primary nerve repair was performed on 143 peripheral nerve injuries in the upper extremities in 120 patients. Sensibility was tested using Weber static and Dellon's moving two-point discrimination test. Sensory reeducation was also assessed.

Nunley JA, Ugino MR, Goldner RD, et al: Use of the anterior branch of the medial antebrachial cutaneous nerve as a graft for the repair of defects of the digital nerve. *J Bone Joint Surg* 1989;71A:563-567.

In 21 digital nerves of 14 patients, all but one nerve graft restored the ability to distinguish between sharp and dull stimuli and all but three restored two-point discrimination between 5 and 15 mm with an average of 9 mm.

Rogers GD, Henshall AL, Sach RP, et al: Simultaneous laceration of the median and ulnar nerves with flexor tendons at the wrist. *J Hand Surg* 1990;15A:990-995.

Simultaneous laceration of the median and ulnar nerves with flexor tendons at the wrist was reviewed in 26 patients treated over a 10-year period. Mean age was 28.7 years. Grip in the affected hand varied from 17% to 86% of that in the normal hand, but five of eight patients had regained better than 70% of the normal grip strength. Key grip in all patients varied from 40% to 100% of that of the unaffected side (average 69%). Most of the patients performed below the population average on functional testing.

Walton RL, Brown RE, Matory WE Jr, et al: Autogenous vein graft repair of digital nerve defects in the finger: A retrospective clinical study. *Plast Reconstr Surg* 1989;84:944-952.

Fourteen patients who had 22 digital nerve defects repaired with autogenous vein grafts were reviewed retrospectively. In 11 acute digital nerve repairs using vein conduits 1 to 3 cm long, two-point discrimination averaged 4.6 mm.

Fingertip Injuries

Arbel R, Goodwin DRA, Otremski I: Treatment of fingertip injuries with silver sulphadiazine occlusion dressing. *Injury* 1989;20:161-163.

A conservative method of treatment of fingertip injuries was shown to be simple, with excellent functional and cosmetic results.

Rose EH, Norris MS, Kowalski TA, et al: The "cap" technique: Nonmicrosurgical reattachment of fingertip amputation. *J Hand Surg* 1989;14A:513-518.

The "cap" technique is a simple and reliable method of eponychial nonmicrosurgical reattachment that preserves the specialized pulp tissue of the tip. Salvaging the nail complex gives the illusion of a normal digit, although actually shortened in comparison with the adjacent fingers.

Replantation

Bowen CV, Beveridge J, Milliken RG, et al: Rotating shaft avulsion amputations of the thumb. *J Hand Surg* 1991;16A:117-121.

Twenty-three of 29 patients with rotating shaft avulsion of the thumb were considered suitable for replantation. Survival was achieved in 19 of 23 replantations. Grip, pinch, and sensibility were good enough to encourage an aggressive microsurgical approach to these injuries.

Goldner RD, Howson MP, Nunley JA, et al: One hundred eleven thumb amputations: Replantation versus revision. *Microsurgery* 1990;11:243-250.

Of patients sustaining isolated complete thumb amputations, 25 who underwent replantation and 18 who underwent revision of amputation underwent testing that consisted of interview and physical examination, test of activities of daily living, Jebson test of hand function, and both static and dynamic testing on the BTE work simulator.

Goldner RD, Stevanovic MV, Nunley JA, et al: Digital replantation at the level of the distal interphalangeal joint and distal phalanx. *J Hand Surg* 1989;14A:214-220.

Forty-two complete, single digital amputations at the distal interphalangeal joint or distal phalanx were reviewed. Success rate, return of sensibility, range of motion, time lost from work, and average total cost of treatment are discussed in comparing replantation with conventional procedures.

Hovgaard C, Dalsgaard S, Gebuhr P: The social and economic consequences of failure to replant amputated thumbs. *J Hand Surg* 1989;14B:307-308

Because replantation of the amputated thumb is not always possible, the effects of complete amputation at various levels were examined in 32 patients.

Ward WA, Tsai TM, Breidenbach W: Per primam thumb replantation for all patients with traumatic amputations. *Clin Orthop* 1991;266:90-95.

These authors review 42 patients with complete thumb amputations replanted between 1980 and 1984. Success rate, factors affecting survival, range of motion, sensibility, and results of reexploration are discussed.

Infections

Hurst LC, Amadio PC, Badalamente MA, et al: *Mycobacterium marinum* infections of the hand. *J Hand Surg* 1987;12A:428-435.

Fifteen patients with culture-proven *Mycobacterium marinum* were assessed with regard to laboratory and radiographic studies, histology and microbiology, skin testing, immunologic studies, surgical procedures, drug therapy, and results of treatment.

Kaye JJ: *Vibrio vulnificus* infection in the hand: Report of three patients. *J Bone Joint Surg* 1990;72A:283-285.

Although *Vibrio vulnificus* infection is rare, it is important because a few hours' delay in treatment can lead to septic shock, which usually can be avoided if diagnosis and treatment are begun early.

Papilion JD, Bergfield TG: Pyoderma gangrenosum complicating infection of the hand: A case report and review of the literature. *Clin Orthop* 1990;254:144-146.

This is an excellent review of pyoderma gangrenosum.

Rowe JG, Amadio PC, Edson RS: Sporotrichosis. *Orthopaedics* 1989;12:981-985.

This article reviews history, diagnosis, and treatment of 49 culture-proven cases of sporotrichosis involving the hand.

Self-Inflicted Hand Injuries

Friedman B, Yaffe B, Blankstein A, et al: Self-inflicted hand injuries: Diagnostic challenge and treatment. *Ann Plast Surg* 1988;20:345-350.

The aim of this article is to draw attention to factitious hand injuries and to alert the physician to this possible diagnosis, because early detection and proper psychotherapy may prevent irreversible damage.

Burns

Falcone PA, Edstrom LE: Decision making in the acute thermal hand burn: An algorithm for treatment. *Hand Clin* 1990;6:233-238.

This article summarizes significant studies that deal with the care of hand burns. Controversy remains regarding the most appropriate treatment of the second-degree burn. The algorithm presented by these authors covers the spectrum of care with the ultimate goal of returning normal hand function.

Flaps

Brody GA, Buncke HJ, Alpert BS, et al: Serratus anterior muscle transplantation for treatment of soft tissue defects in the hand. *J Hand Surg* 1990;15A;322-327.

These authors review their experience with the serratus anterior muscle free flap.

Earley MJ: The second dorsal metacarpal artery neurovascular island flap. *J Hand Surg* 1989;14B:434-440.

Eleven patients who had second dorsal metacarpal sensate island flaps to cover local skin defects are reviewed.

Foucher G, Smith D, Pempinello C, et al: Homodigital neurovascular island flaps for digital pulp loss. *J Hand Surg* 1989;14B:204-208.

Sixty-four homodigital monopedicle island flaps were used to replace soft-tissue loss of the digit. Success for this procedure requires a clear understanding of surgical indications and anatomic variations in addition to a technically skilled surgeon.

Ismail TIA: The free fascial forearm flap. *Microsurgery* 1989;10:155-160.

These authors describe their experience using the free fascial forearm flap in eight patients. Six of the overlying skin grafts survived entirely. In the other two flaps, marginal graft loss over the ulnar aspect of the flap healed spontaneously within three weeks.

Maruyama Y: The reverse dorsal metacarpal flap. *Br J Plast Surg* 1990;43:24-27.

The reversed dorsal metacarpal flap based on the dorsal metacarpal arteries was used in eight patients. Results were good in seven cases. One individual had distal partial necrosis.

Nishi G, Shibata Y, Kumabe Y, et al: Arterialized venous skin flaps for the injured finger. *J Reconstr Microsurg* 1989;5:357-365.

This procedure was used in seven patients. In two it was used to reconstruct skin defects and restore blood circulation in replanted amputated digits. In five patients, it was used to repair missing skin and an interdigital artery on one side of the finger. Flaps range in size from 1 x 1 to 4.5 x 3 cm. The dorsal aspect of the foot was the donor site in three patients and the flexor side of the distal forearm was the donor site in four.

Reyes FA, Burkhalter WE: The fascial radial flap. *J Hand Surg* 1988;13A:432-437.

Six patients with full-thickness skin loss complicating traumatic problems of the hand each had a retrograde forearm fascia flap transfer. Four patients had an uncomplicated one-stage flap transfer. Two patients had postoperative hematoma, but no further procedures were required. One patient had superficial necrosis of more than one fourth of the flap.

32

Wrist and Hand: Reconstruction

Hand and wrist reconstructions continue to be improved by an increasing knowledge of the biomechanics of the wrist. New studies are leading to better understanding of the different instability patterns secondary to ligamentous injuries in the wrist. The reported results of various intercarpal fusions are influencing our treatment choices. The new diagnostic techniques, including magnetic resonance imaging (MRI), computed tomographic (CT) scans, and wrist arthroscopy, have added significantly to the understanding of hand and wrist pathology. Arthroplasties and arthrodeses of the hand and wrist, as well as tendon reconstructions and nerve repairs, remain important in hand and wrist reconstruction. Treatment of Dupuytren's contracture, carpal tunnel syndrome, and arthritis continue to dominate the hand literature.

Biomechanics of the Wrist

In vitro analysis of wrist motion has established the relative contributions of the radiocarpal and midcarpal joints. In a cadaver study, 63% of wrist flexion and 53% of wrist extension occurred at the radiocarpal joint, and 44% of radial deviation and 45% of ulnar deviation occurred at the radiocarpal joint. The remaining motion in each position occurred at the midcarpal level. The use of pressure-sensitive film in a cadaver study led to the discovery that the scaphoid fossa bears an increased load with perilunate instability. Scaphotrapeziotrapezoid or scaphocapitate fusion did not alter this load transmission via the scaphoid fossa. However, scapholunate, scapholunate-capitate, or capitate-lunate fusions are better biomechanically, because they transmit the load proportionately through both the scaphoid and lunate fossae. The scaphoid contact area is 1.47 times that of the lunate, and each area of contact between the scaphoid and the lunate and the distal radius and triangular fibrocartilage complex is separate and distinct. The contact area is greatest with the scaphoid more horizontally oriented in ulnar deviation, and the contact area of the scaphoid and lunate with the distal radius and triangular fibrocartilage complex increases as the wrist moves from radial to ulnar deviation and/or from flexion to extension.

Diagnostic Imaging Evaluation of the Wrist

The etiology of wrist pain can be elusive. Bone scans are nonspecific, and when arthrograms are performed, injection of the radiocarpal, midcarpal, and radioulnar joints is necessary for a complete diagnostic evaluation. A recent report demonstrated the value of various imaging techniques in locating foreign bodies such as glass, gravel, and wood.

In certain conditions, MRI is superior to both standard radiography and CT for evaluating the wrist. Early studies supported its use in establishing the diagnosis of ganglia, rheumatoid arthritis, arteriovenous malformations, carpal fractures, and carpal tunnel syndrome. In patients suspected of having osteonecrosis of either the proximal fracture fragment of the scaphoid or the lunate in Kienböck's disease, the MRI findings correlate with later histologic findings. In fact, MRI may detect osteonecrosis even before the onset of carpal collapse. MRI also is more specific than routine radiographs or bone scans for the diagnosis of osteonecrosis of the lunate. Care should be taken, however, not to abuse this expensive imaging modality.

CT scans continue to be of superior value in many situations because of their increased bone detail. For specific problems, such as radioulnar subluxation and fractures of the hook of the hamate, transaxial images are superior to other techniques.

Arthroscopy of the Wrist

The primary indication for wrist arthroscopy is persistent symptoms with evidence of mechanical wrist derangement. Arthroscopy is useful to confirm a suspected diagnosis, and often reveals additional undiagnosed articular disorders.

The most commonly used radiocarpal portals are the 3-4 portal, the 4-5 portal, and 6R portal (Fig. 1).

The 3-4 portal is the initial viewing portal. Located between the extensor pollicis longus and extensor digitorum communis tendons, it offers excellent visualization of the scaphoid and lunate and of their respective radial articular facets. The extrinsic radioscaphocapitate, radiolunotriquetral, and radioscapholunate ligaments, and the intrinsic scapholunate ligament and triangular fibrocartilage complex also can be inspected through this portal (Fig. 2 A, B).

The 4-5 portal, which serves as the initial instrumentation portal, is established between the extensor digitorum communis and extensor digiti minimi tendons, approximately 1 cm ulnar to the 3-4 portal.

The 6R portal is used most commonly as an outflow pressure monitoring portal for a mechanical infusion sys-

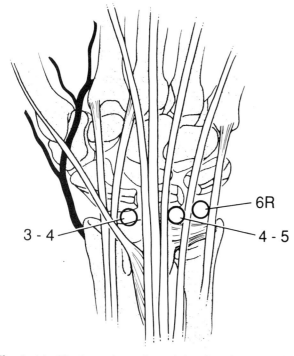

Fig. 1   Identification and use of portals in wrist arthroscopy: 3-4, Primary visualization portal, secondary instrumentation portal. 4-5, Primary instrumentation portal, secondary visualization portal. 6R, Primary outflow pressure monitor portal or inflow portal.

tem or as the inflow portal for a gravity flow system. However, it may also be used for visualization or instrumentation on the ulnar side of the wrist. This portal is established radial to the extensor carpi ulnaris tendon.

While wrist arthroscopy is emerging as an excellent diagnostic tool, there is wide disagreement on its effectiveness as a therapeutic measure. The most accepted application is debridement of central tears of the articular disk of the triangular fibrocartilage complex, a well-accepted procedure that used to be done through an arthrotomy. Visibility is improved by the bright arthroscopic illumination and magnification, allowing more precise resection and contouring of the triangular fibrocartilage. Good or excellent results can be expected in a high percentage of patients with isolated tears of the triangular fibrocartilage.

Articular cartilage debridement may be effective for early degenerative or traumatic lesions of the articular surface. The management of ligamentous instability of the wrist is highly controversial. The effectiveness of pinning the scapholunate joint or the lunotriquetral joint, or of debridement alone in partial tears of these ligaments, has not been verified in long-term studies.

Finally, some have attempted to reassemble the distal radius after fracture and to supplement percutaneous pinning and external fixation. No results have been reported that verify the effectiveness of this approach.

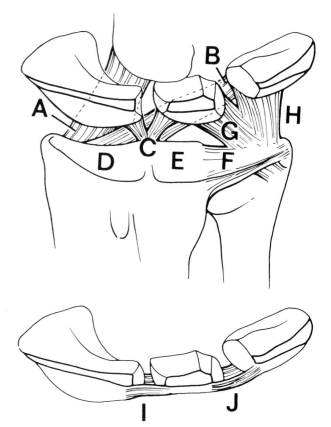

Fig. 2   Arthroscopic anatomy of the radiocarpal joint. (**A**), Radioscaphocapitate ligament: Scaphoid pivots on this ligament; first volar ligament on radial side. (**B**), Radiolunotriquetral ligament: Second volar ligament on radial side; forms the interosseous lunotriquetral ligament on the volar distal portion. (**C**), Radioscapholunate ligament: Excellent insertional landmark; Y-shaped with puff of fat; ligament of Testu. (**D**), Scaphoid facet: Home for the scaphoid. (**E**), Lunate facet: Home for the lunate. (**F**), Triangular fibrocartilage: Part of the triangular fibrocartilage complex which also includes the ulnocarpal ligaments; connection of radius to base of ulnar styloid; thick on the edges and thin in the center. (**G**), Ulnolunate ligament: Part of the triangular fibrocartilage complex—most radial; part of the volar sling—important in stabilizing the distal ulna. (**H**), Ulnotriquetral ligament: Part of the triangular fibrocartilage complex—most ulnar; part of the volar sling—important in stabilizing the distal ulna. (**I**), Scapholunate interosseous ligament: Partial and/or complete tears are present in scapholunate dissociation; ligament is distally placed; tears often lead to deformity from dorsal intercalated scaphoid instability and degeneration of most radial compartments (scaphoid facet). (**J** and **L**) lunotriquetral interosseous ligament: partial or complete tears constitute a lunotriquetral dissociation; ligament is distally placed; tears often lead to a deformity from volar intercalated scaphoid instability.

Posttraumatic Problems of the Wrist

Kienböck's Disease

Kienböck's disease continues to present problems in diagnosis and treatment. As noted above, MRI is the imaging technique of choice for osteonecrosis of the lunate and is more specific than a bone scan. In fact, a subclassification of Lichtman's stage II is now based on T1 and T2 patterns on MRI.

In early disease with a negative ulnar variance, radial shortening continues to be a popular surgical treatment. In ulnar neutral variance, a medial closing or lateral opening radial wedge osteotomy is recommended. Each of these three procedures unloads the lunate fossa and redistributes the load to the scaphoid fossa and the ulnar column. Scaphotrapeziotrapezoid fusion and scaphocapitate fusion unload the lunate fossa and transfer all the load to the scaphoid fossa, whereas capitohamate fusion does not unload the lunate fossa. The use of alternative treatments, such as silicone replacements, appears to be less favorable over the long term. A recent report of a series of ten silicone replacements followed for five years stated that only 50% had satisfactory results. Silicone synovitis was noted in three patients. The authors have modified their previous classification of stages of disease (Fig. 3). A previous report stated that patients with ad-

vanced collapse, stages III and IV, demonstrated progression of carpal collapse and osteoarthritis with either silicone implants or tendon arthroplasties.

Scaphoid Nonunion and Osteonecrosis

Untreated or persistent scaphoid nonunion results in a high prevalence of periscaphoid arthritis in the radioscaphoid and midcarpal joints. Russe bone grafting leads to a high rate of union (92%). Other satisfactory methods of fixation include the use of percutaneous pins or the Herbert screw. With percutaneous pinning, complication rates are low, and the reported union rate is 77%. A similarly high union rate is achieved with Herbert screw fixation. Reported advantages of this technique include decreased immobilization time and improved wrist motion, with an early return of wrist function. However, introduction of the screw is technically demanding. A modification of the technique to facilitate the introduction of the screw has been described in which a volar trough is made in the trapezium (Fig. 4), facilitating the placement of the jig. The Herbert screw has also been useful for fixation of the small proximal fragment. In these cases the screw is introduced retrograde without need of the jig.

A personal technique for the treatment of scaphoid nonunion was recently reported. To preserve surface cartilage, the scaphoid is prepared by drilling a hole from the distal tuberosity and then filling it with cancellous bone and a cortical bone peg that was obtained from a

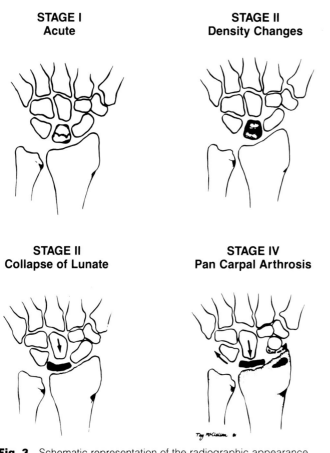

STAGE I
Acute

STAGE II
Density Changes

STAGE II
Collapse of Lunate

STAGE IV
Pan Carpal Arthrosis

Fig. 3 Schematic representation of the radiographic appearance of stages I to IV Kienböck's disease. We now subdivide stage III into IIIA (without fixed scaphoid rotation) and IIIB (with fixed scaphoid ["ring sign"] rotation). (Reproduced with permission from Alexander AH, Turner MA, Alexander CE, et al: Lunate silicone replacement arthroplasty in Keinböck's disease: A long-term follow-up. *J Hand Surg* 1990;15A:401-407.)

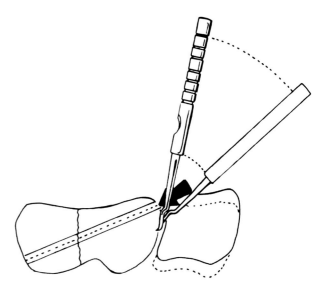

Fig. 4 The technique of elevation of distal pole after complete ligamentous mobilization. The bulk of the trapezium necessitates an anterior position of the barrel of the jig and thus oblique line of the screw across the scaphoid defect. (Reproduced with permission from Chun S, Wicks BP, Meyerdierks E, et al: Two modifications for insertion of the Herbert screw in the fractured scaphoid. *J Hand Surg* 1990;15A:669-671.)

radial styloidectomy. Radiographs showed consolidation in 50 of 52 cases reviewed.

Later complications associated with nonunion include carpal instability, carpal displacement, volar angulation, osteonecrosis, and fractures of the proximal third of the scaphoid. Patients in whom bone grafting has failed and who have early posttraumatic arthritic changes often remain symptomatic after additional procedures, even when union is achieved. Salvage procedures, such as the use of an allograft to replace the small proximal fragment, may be reasonable alternatives to continued attempts at bone grafting in such cases. The silicone scaphoid prosthesis has fallen into disfavor because of late particulate synovitis. The process appears to worsen with time and can be prevented by removing the implant, synovectomy, curettage of the lytic lesions, and bone grafting the defects if they are large enough. Because of this complication, patients with silicone implants should be monitored regularly. Titanium implants are now being introduced as an alternative treatment. Some authorities have advised scaphoid excision combined with intercarpal fusions. However, total wrist fusion remains the ultimate treatment to salvage failed surgical attempts to achieve scaphoid union. Two cases are reported in which a scaphoid osteotomy was performed for scaphoid malunions in patients with abnormal wrist alignment and pain. The author feels that this procedure may reduce the risk of late arthritis. Although recognizing the risks involved, the author feels that the improved internal fixation techniques make this approach feasible.

Arthritis of the Wrist

Total Joint Replacement

Although most patients who receive silicone rubber wrist implants obtain early relief of pain with a functional range of motion, there are later significant fracture rates accompanied by progressive radiographic collapse. Prosthetic fracture often leads to increasing pain, stability of deformity, and diminished function. Excessive wrist motion, overuse, and inadequate surgical technique appear to contribute to this high rate of failure. The use of titanium grommets and capsular tightening to restrict motion can minimize these complications. However, for severely deformed or unstable wrists, fusion is the procedure of choice. In patients with severe bilateral wrist involvement, arthrodesis on one side and a replacement on the opposite side may be the preferred approach.

Some authors favor arthroplasty. Other surgeons have been unable to duplicate the results obtained by Volz. His prosthesis is currently undergoing design changes, and future trials will be necessary to evaluate its success. A combination of radiocarpal fusion and condylar silicone implant to replace the capitate, which allows motion at the midcarpal level, has been suggested. In a study comparing 33 patients with rheumatoid arthritis who un-

derwent wrist fusion with 37 who underwent silicone wrist implant arthroplasty, results were good or excellent in 97% of the arthrodesis cases and 78% of the arthroplasty cases. Postoperative flexion averaged 32 degrees and extension averaged 29 degrees; most patients reported that dexterity and strength were adequate. Arthroplasties on dominant hands gave better results than those on the nondominant side. There were no pseudarthroses in the group, and the complication rate in the fusion group was 18%. In the arthroplasty group, 25% required revisions. Interestingly, bone resorption was noted about the implants in 14%, and subsidence was noted in 11%. Swanson has predicted that that the use of titanium grommets would lead to minimal resorption and settling. The grommets also theoretically protect the surface of the implant from debriding by bone that could result in the development of silicone synovitis. Arthroplasties may be inappropriate for young patients because of the progressive nature of the disease and the possibility that they may require ambulatory aids as they get older.

A recent report of results with the Trispherical total wrist arthroplasty in rheumatoid arthritis described 28 good or excellent results in 34 patients with an average follow up of nine years. Two patients required revisions (arthrodesis) for loosening and pain. The authors stress the need for adequate preoperative wrist extensor power. The pain was relieved in a small series of cases, and average postoperative range of motion was 42 degrees of extension and 23 degrees of flexion. These early results are encouraging. However, because rheumatoid arthritis involves all the joints of the carpus, progression of the disease process is still possible.

Arthroplasty results were not predictable in patients with class IV rheumatoid arthritis who had anterior wrist dislocations, in patients receiving long-term steroids, and in patients using ambulatory aids. Wrist fusion is recommended for patients with marked osseous destruction and in patients whose wrist extensor tendons are absent. Previous infection that has resolved is also an indication for fusion rather than arthroplasty.

Limited Arthrodesis

Limited arthrodesis of the wrist continues to be an area of interest and change. Studies to determine the amount of motion lost with various combinations of intercarpal fusions have been reported. In one study, it was noted that fusions that crossed the radiocarpal joint resulted in a loss of 55% of the arc of flexion and extension, while fusions that crossed only the intercarpal joint resulted in loss of 27% of this arc. Scaphotrapeziotrapezoid arthrodesis has been used to manage rotary instability of the scaphoid and to prevent carpal collapse in advanced osteonecrosis of the lunate. The operation usually is performed via a dorsal approach. A report by Essman describes a volar approach to STT fusion with Herbert screw fixation combined with a bone graft from the distal radius. He felt that this made the procedure easier than the dorsal approach. In a study of 93 scaphotrapeziotrapezoid fusions 33% radio-styloid impingement was noted and radial styloidectomy is recommended as part of the procedure. A report of 46 patients (47 wrists) undergoing scaphotrapeziotrapezoid fusion for dynamic scapholunate instability noted a significant (50%) complication rate, including radiostyloid impingement, persistent pain with incomplete scaphoid reduction, and failure of fusion. As an alternate treatment to scaphotrapeziotrapezoid arthrodesis, scaphocapitate arthrodesis has been performed for rotary subluxation of the scaphoid, scaphoid nonunion, or Kienböck's disease. This fusion leads to some loss of motion in several planes, especially radial deviation and flexion. However, some surgeons report fusion is technically easier to perform than scaphotrapeziotrapezoid fusion, and the results are comparable. Nonunion in a small series is reported as 12%. However, rates of nonunion are increased when there is gross instability. For example, successful scapholunate arthrodesis for scapholunate dissociation was found in only one of seven patients in a recent study. Three patients with a fibrous union achieved good clinical outcomes. This procedure was concluded to be unpredictable, and has been abandoned in favor of other alternatives.

Wrist Arthroplasty Versus Arthrodesis

Arthrodesis of the wrist is currently used in posttraumatic conditions, destruction of the wrist after infection, paralytic conditions, spastic cerebral palsy, certain tumors, degenerative arthritis, failed arthroplasty, and rheumatoid arthritis. In rheumatoid patients, freedom from pain, ability to function, and stability of the wrist are important. Initial enthusiasm for silicone implant arthroplasty of the wrist has waned because of an increased fracture rate, bone resorption with sinking of the prosthesis, and recurrent deformity. However, there are also disadvantages with arthrodesis.

Many activities of daily living require some wrist motion, and patients with arthrodeses who have rheumatoid involvement in other upper-extremity joints often find it difficult to write, dress, eat, and perform other activities around the house. Therefore, in cases of multiple joint involvement, preservation of some wrist motion can be a major benefit to the patient. In 20 consecutive patients who were treated with arthrodesis, average time to fusion was 11 weeks. The patients with solid fusion obtained relief of pain and had satisfactory functional results. In a later functional assessment in patients with bilateral wrist arthrodeses, the Jebsten-Taylor function test gave normal results 38% of the time and abnormal results 62% of the time. Of nine patients, two thought function remained unchanged and seven thought function had improved. Rayan and associates concluded that grip strength improved even in patients with rheumatoid arthritis, and that bilateral wrist arthrodeses did not adversely affect upper extremity function.

Proximal Row Carpectomy

Proximal row carpectomy is again coming into favor as a reconstructive procedure for severely involved wrists resulting from various causes. These include late scapholunate dissociation, dorsiflexion instability with secondary arthritis, carpal instability secondary to nonunion of the scaphoid, failed silicone lunate implant arthroplasty, and Kienböck's disease. In a recent study, pain relief was achieved in 26 of 27 patients. Almost all of the patients were able to return to their previous work. The grip strengths were found to be 80% of the opposite side. Proximal row carpectomy has also been used in patients with arthrogryposis multiplex congenita, but the results are less predictable. Biomechanical analyses of the capitate radius articulation after proximal row carpectomy shows a decrease in the radius curvature of the lunate fossa, suggesting wear deformation. This finding suggests that clinical results may deteriorate with further observation (Fig. 5). It has been suggested that proximal row carpectomy is contraindicated if there is evidence of arthritic change in the lunate fossa and/or distal involvement of the head of the capitate.

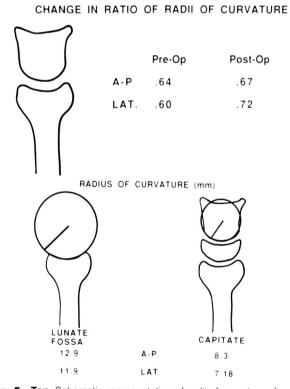

Fig. 5 Top, Schematic representation of radii of curvature of lunate fossa of radius and capitate. **Bottom**, Postoperative changes in radius of curvature for capitate and lunate fossa of radius. Curvatures more closely approximate each other with time. (Reproduced with permission from Imbriglia JE, Broudy AS, Hagberg WC, et al: Proximal row carpectomy: Clinical evaluation. *J Hand Surg* 1990;15A:426-430.)

Distal Radioulnar Joint Dysfunction

The Darrach procedure remains the classic treatment for distal radioulnar joint derangement. Careful minimal bone resection and soft-tissue reconstruction are essential for good results. In a recent study, the authors were unable to identify any radiographic differences between 20 patients with limited function and pain after the Darrach procedure and patients who had successful Darrach resections. They concluded that the Darrach procedure can lead to serious disability in young patients and in patients with lax ligaments. Others have supported this concept by stating that the triangular fibrocartilage complex is functionally disabled by the Darrach procedure. Obviously, excessive bone resection with the Darrach procedure leads to distal instability of the ulna with pain, prominence of the distal ulna, and mechanical impingement against the radius with rotation. A previously described technique called "hemi-section interposition arthroplasty" produced stable, painless motion in 85% of patients with rheumatoid arthritis and in 100% of those with degenerative or posttraumatic arthritis.

In a type of arthroplasty that preserves ulnar length, the styloid process, and the triangular fibrocartilage complex, the radial side of the distal ulna is resected to match the opposing surface of the radius throughout the arch of forearm rotation. After an average follow-up of six years, each of the 44 wrists had a stable distal ulna and painless rotation averaging 80 degrees of pronation and 88 degrees of supination. No patient required additional surgery.

A corrective osteotomy and reconstruction of the radioulnar ligament in a malunited distal radius in cases of derangement of the distal radioulnar joint yielded excellent results in 17 cases, good in 19, fair in two, and poor in one. There was a good correlation between the radiographic results and the functional results. Tears of the triangular fibrocartilage frequently cause pain on the ulnar side of the wrist. In a recent study of 13 patients with traumatic peripheral separation treated with repair, eight achieved normal painless function. The diagnosis of this type of triangular fibrocartilage complex tear was made by wrist arthroscopy.

Another procedure that maintains the function of the triangular fibrocartilage complex while restoring forearm rotation is the Sauve Kapandji (Lauenstein) procedure, which resects a portion of the distal ulna but preserves the distal ulna. Although the clinical results are limited, it has the advantage of preserving the triangular fibrocartilage complex as well as maintaining the normal anatomic configuration of the wrist. However, if excessive bone is resected, a distal portion of the proximal ulna may be unstable. If inadequate bone is resected, reactive bone may form at the osteotomy site, limiting motion.

Each of these procedures has its advocates, and the results vary in different clinical series. In elderly patients, a carefully performed Darrach procedure is recommended. In younger patients with distal radioulnar joint dysfunction, the treatment of choice appears to be resection arthroplasty of the distal radioulnar joint with preservation of ulnar length, the ulnar styloid, and the triangular fibrocartilage complex and, possibly, interposition of tissue between the distal radius and the ulna.

In cases of malunion of the distal radius with involvement of the ulnar joint, the recommended treatment is corrective osteotomy and soft-tissue reconstruction of the ligamentous support of the distal radioulnar joint. One should differentiate between radioulnar joint dysfunction and ulna impingement against the carpus. Ulna shortening has become a popular way to treat this latter condition. This procedure is thought to tighten the ulnar carpal ligaments and eliminate any impingement of the ulna against the carpus.

Posttraumatic Problems of the Hand

Soft-Tissue Defects

In recent years there has been an interest in pedicled axial flaps of the forearm to cover defects on the hand. A recent report describes the result of a retrograde posterior interosseous flap nourished by perforating vessels from the posterior interosseous artery. In this series, 36 patients underwent this surgery to cover soft-tissue defects resulting from trauma, infections, or burns. Although there was no loss of a flap in this series, there were significant complications with major partial necrosis in 12%. The flap requires careful preoperative assessment of the vascular anatomy and has distinct limitation of distal reach. It is an alternative to other standard methods of coverage including the Chinese forearm flap, the axial pedicle groin flap, or any free flap.

Tendon Transfers

In addition to traditional transfers, new techniques are being developed for selected conditions.

Camptodactyly Gupta and Burke consider the primary deformity in camptodactyly to be an imbalance between the flexors and the extensors, giving rise to an intrinsic-minus deformity. They have used the extensor indicis proprius as a transfer to the radial side of the extensor of the little finger to supplement the intrinsic action (Fig. 6). The early results are promising.

Extensor Pollicis Longus Ruptures As an alternative to tendon transfer for the treatment of traumatic extensor pollicis longus ruptures, Magnell reported 21 patients treated an average of six weeks after rupture with an intercalated tendon graft. Although there was a small loss of interphalangeal joint extension, all patients were able to extend the thumb to the palmar level.

Crossed intrinsic transfer of the ulnar lateral band to the radial lateral band has been modified by Blair to attach the transfer to the collateral ligament. The procedure appeared to prevent long-term recurrent deformity

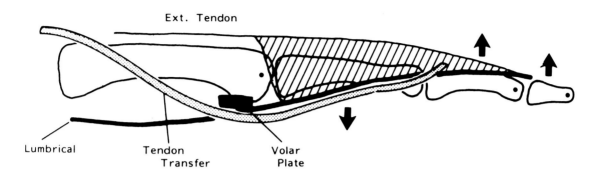

Fig. 6   Depiction of the transfer of the extensor indicis proprius to the radial side of the extensor of the little finger to resolve the primary deformity in camptodactyly. (Reproduced with permission from Gupta A, Burke FD: Correction of camptodactyly: Preliminary results of extensor indicis transfer. *J Hand Surg* 1990;15B:168-170.)

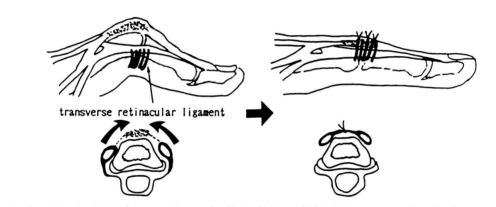

Fig. 7   Through a dorsal longitudinal incision over the proximal interphalangeal joint, the transverse retinacular ligaments are identified and are sharply separated from their insertion anteriorly. The ligaments are turned over onto the dorsal aspect of the proximal interphalangeal joint, thus lifting the lateral bands dorsally, and sutured to one another. (Reproduced with permission from Ohshio I, Ogino T, Minami A, et al: Reconstruction of the central slip by the transverse retinacular ligament for Boutonniere deformity. *J Hand Surg* 1990;15B:407-409.)

after the correction of ulnar drift, despite progression in the hand.

Nerve Injury   The value of the extensor indicis proprius opponensplasty first described by Durkwalter has been reported by G. A. Anderson and associates. They followed 39 patients with 40 transfers for high and low median nerve palsy as well as mixed median and ulnar nerve palsies. The results were generally successful and reeducation was uncomplicated. There were few complications.

Tendon Injuries or Ruptures

Boutonniere Deformity   A variety of methods have been advocated to restore extensor tendon force to the proximal interphalangeal joints in posttraumatic boutonniere deformities. For the treatment of boutonniere deformities with good passive correction, a modification of the Salvi procedure has been described in which the trans-

verse retinacular ligaments are freed from the palmar plate and then transferred dorsally to lift the lateral bands (Fig. 7). Two of six patients had limited distal interphalangeal joint flexion, but improved proximal interphalangeal extension was reduced from 69 to 21 degrees. In one technique, a swallow-tailed flap of fibrous tissue is excised, with care taken to assure anchoring of the proximal edge of the central slip (Fig. 8). A 3-mm portion of scar tissue is removed. Kirschner wire fixation obliquely across the joint is used for four weeks. Following pin removal, a dynamic digital splint is used for an additional two weeks to maintain extension. A review of 18 patients with chronic boutonniere deformity demonstrated 13 (72.2%) had excellent results. This technique also can be used in fixed deformities, preceded by a first stage soft-tissue release to obtain full passive extension.

Extensor Tendon   The results of extensor tendon repair do not now appear to be as good as previously thought.

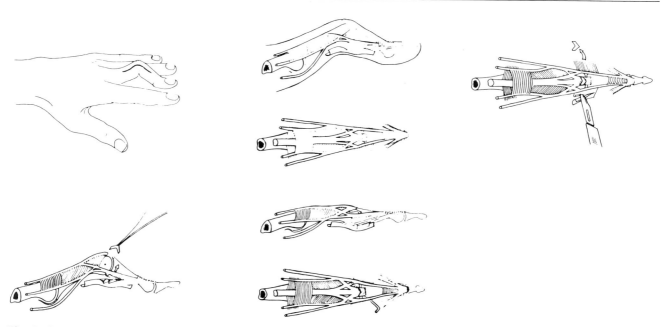

Fig. 8 Direct repair of the central tendon according to Caroli. **Top left,** Deformity and incision; **Top center,** Scar tissue assures the continuity of the central tendon; **Top right,** The swallow-tailed flap is designed over the scarred capsular tissue. The transverse retinacular ligament is often released; **Bottom left,** 3 mm excision of the scar tissue; **Bottom center,** Anchoring of the proximal end of the central slip. The proximal interphalangeal joint is fixed with a K-wire inserted obliquely. (Reproduced with permission from Caroli A, Zonasi S, Squarzina PB, et al: Operative treatment of the post-traumatic Boutonniere deformity: A modification of the direct anatomical repair technique. *J Hand Surg* 1990;15B:410-415.)

A study of the long-term results of extensor tendon repair was carried out in 62 patients with 101 digits having extensor tendon laceration. For injured fingers, excluding the thumb, the total active motion averaged 218 degrees. When the results were evaluated according to the zone in which the injury occurred, it was noted that the more distal injuries produced a higher percentage of poor results. In general, a higher percentage of fingers lost flexion than lost extension.

Fifty-two patients with extensor tendon ruptures between the wrist and the mid aspect of the proximal phalanx were treated with repair followed by the use of an extension splint allowing active flexion. They had no ruptures, and full flexion was achieved in all.

In a review of 115 flexor tendon ruptures in patients with rheumatoid arthritis, those ruptures distal to the wrist were caused by invasive tenosynovitis. Ruptures of the flexor pollicis longus were often the result of attrition of the scaphoid, which had eroded through the volar wrist capsule. Those ruptures within the flexor tendon sheath had the poorest prognosis. Flexor pollicis longus ruptures had the best prognosis and were treated by bridge grafts or tendon transfer. In a review of 116 patients with ruptures of the extensor pollicis longus after Colles' fracture and rheumatoid arthritis, the site of tendon rupture was categorized into three anatomical levels (Fig. 9 and Table 1), called proximal, intermediate, and distal in relationship to the extensor hood at the metacar-

pophalangeal joint level. The authors compared their results with direct suture, tendon transfer, and tendon grafts. They preferred the extensor carpus radialis longus when performing the transfer, but recently have found postoperative training easier with the bridge grafts.

Arthritis of the Hand

Joint Replacement

The role of joint replacement continues to be reassessed. In a study of 23 female patients undergoing 38 distal interphalangeal silicone interpositional arthroplasties for osteoarthritis there was an average extensor lag of 12.7 degrees with a range of motion of 33 degrees. An 89% patient satisfaction was noted. The use of arthroplasty was compared with fusion of the proximal interphalangeal joint in 24 patients undergoing 43 proximal interphalangeal procedures. Eighty-three percent of the patients had erosive arthritis. In this series, cemented implants frequently fractured at the hinge. Improved key pinch strength was noted with fusion of the proximal interphalangeal joint of the index finger, but silicone implants were advised for the ulnar digits. In that series, a flexion arc of 56 degrees with satisfactory pain relief was noted after two years.

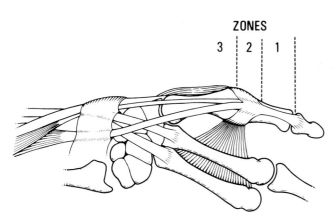

Fig. 9 Zones in which the extensor pollicis longus tendon may rupture or be cut. (Reproduced with permission from Mannerfelt L, Oetker R, Ostlund B, et al: Rupture of the extensor pollicis longus tendon after Colles fracture and by rheumatoid arthritis. *J Hand Surg* 1990;15B:49-50.)

Table 1. Operations performed

	Cuts	After Colles' Fracture	Rheumatoid Arthritis	Total
Suture	60	0	0	60
Tendon transfer	10	10	21	41
Free tendon graft	6	5	4	15
Total	76	15	25	116

(Adapted with permission from Mannerfelt L, Oetker R, Ostlund B, et al: Rupture of the extensor pollicis longus tendon after Colles fracture and by rheumatoid arthritis. *J Hand Surg* 1990;15B:49-50.)

Results were reported for Silastic replacement arthroplasties for posttraumatic arthritis of the metatarsophalangeal, proximal interphalangeal, and distal interphalangeal joints. Between 1981 and 1987, 59 joints were replaced and 49 reviewed. Six patients required revisions, but 80% were thought to have achieved good or fair results with an extensor lag of 12 to 25 degrees. Preservation of passive extension allows the hand to flatten, which is an advantage over fusions. The proximal interphalangeal joint of the index was deemed to give the least successful results, and fusions were the preferred treatment for this area.

In a study of 50 patients with 59 implants at the metatarsophalangeal joint of the rheumatoid thumb, all had reduced pain with an average range of motion of 25 degrees and 46 reported improvement in activities of daily living. Joint stability was deemed to be adequate and pinch strength averaged 4 lbs. Nalebuff reviewed the factors influencing the results of implant surgery in the rheumatoid hand. The implant design was deemed the least important factor. Important factors included the state of the hand (condition of adjacent joint, controlling tendons, stabilizing structure) and of the patient (motivation, pain threshold, and tissue elasticity) (Table 2). The surgical technique and hand therapy were also rated

Table 2. Implant surgery

Importance	Factor
****	**State of hand** Adjacent joints Controlling tendons Stabilizing structure
***	**Patient** Motivation Pain threshold Tissue elasticity
**	**Surgeon** Judgment Technical skill
**	**Therapist**
*	**Implant**

The number of stars indicates the importance of that factor.
(Adapted with permission from Nalebuff EA: Factors influencing the results of implant surgery in the rheumatoid hand. *J Hand Surg* 1990;15B:395-403.)

higher than the implant in importance. Indications for salvage surgery following implant surgery include limited motion, pain, infection, fracture, or dislocation of the implant. Again, the final result of surgery appears to depend on many factors, some of which are beyond the control of the surgeon.

Arthrodesis

Union has been reported in 170 of 171 arthrodeses of the small joints in the hand. To achieve this success, the joint surfaces are resected back to medullary bone, tightly coapted, and fixed with Kirschner wires. Bone grafting is used when necessary. Proximal interphalangeal joint arthrodesis using the Herbert screw for compression was successful in 50 of 51 joints. The joints fused within six weeks and required only minimal external protection. For arthrodesis of the digital joints in children, without interference with growth, the articular cartilage is removed down to the ossific nucleus. Subchondral bone is carefully removed to expose cancellous bone on each side of the joint. The surface is coapted and held with cross K-wires. This technique produced no detectable growth disturbance over an average three-year surveillance.

Fifty-three patients with rheumatoid boutonniere deformities of the thumb were classified according to passive metacarpophalangeal joint correction. In mild cases, synovectomy and extensor pollicis longus rerouting were performed, but the recurrence rate was high. Most of the patients advanced to more severe deformity in which metacarpophalangeal fusion was the procedure of choice.

The authors found that tenotomy of the extensor to correct interphalangeal extension was usually not successful. In advanced cases with fixed deformity at both the metacarpophalangeal and interphalangeal joints, they advised metacarpophalangeal arthroplasty with interphalangeal joint fusion.

Trapeziometacarpal Joint

Because silicone synovitis is becoming increasingly common, alternatives to the use of silicone have been sought as a replacement for the trapezium. A 25% failure rate is identified at an average of four years after silicone replacement, including subluxation and loss of implant height (nearly 50%), resulting in shortening of the thumb and silicone synovitis.

Tendon interposition arthroplasty is now the more accepted technique for surgical management of severe osteoarthritis of the trapeziometacarpal joint. Several techniques have been described, including one report that compared tendon interposition with silicone implant arthroplasty. In this series of 25 cases followed up for an average of two years, the initial arthroplasty space collapsed in only three cases, subluxation averaged 7% of the width of the metacarpal (compared with 35% with the silicone implant), and excellent results were obtained in 23 cases. No revisions were necessary. The technique is similar to that in which the distally based radial half of the flexor carpi radialis is used to reconstruct the ligamentous support for the metacarpal. Two additional steps are performed: (1) A supporting ligamentous sling is made by passing the tendon through the center of the base of the metacarpal and its ulnar cortex. This maintains length and prevents radial subluxation. (2) The remaining tendon is folded and placed into the area of the absent trapezium as a spacer. In one series of 89 cases, 65 patients were satisfied after resection arthroplasty that used the flexor carpi radialis tendon. A strip of tendon was wrapped around the main portion of the flexor carpi radialis and the abductor pollicis longus. Adduction contracture was relieved in only one half of the cases.

Carpal Tunnel Syndrome

Carpal tunnel syndrome continues to be the most common cause of hand pain. Studies have confirmed that intracarpal canal pressure is greater in patients with carpal tunnel syndrome than in normal control patients. This pressure increases further with exercise and persists for a longer period of time than in the control patients. While evidence indicates that carpal tunnel syndrome is an occupational disease, it cannot be determined whether or not an individual case of carpal tunnel is occupationally related.

The condition is often first noted during pregnancy. Carpal tunnel syndrome developed in 40 women during pregnancy and in 18 post partum. The latter group tended to be older, were primiparous and breast feeding, and showed little evidence of peripheral edema. Many of these patients have associated "trigger" fingers or other sites of tendinitis. In some patients, congenital abnormalities of the palmar muscles cause median nerve compression. The condition is often brought on after malunion of wrist fractures or carpal malalignment.

Splinting, steroid injections, and vitamin B6 are the conservative treatments most commonly used. The indications for carpal ligament release include persistent symptoms in spite of conservative treatment. Thenar muscle atrophy is an indication for surgery without a long trial of splinting or steroid injections. Patients with rheumatoid flexor tenosynovitis and carpal tunnel syndrome should have the nerve decompressed by flexor tenosynovectomy. A widening of the transverse carpal arch with decreased grip strength has been noted after carpal tunnel release. Carpal tunnel release also produces an increase in the anteroposterior volume of the carpal canal with palmar displacement of the carpal contents, as indicated by MRI studies. If the transverse ligament is reconstructed in a lengthening state, there is no decrease in grip strength. It is thus felt that the reconstructed ligament stabilizes the transverse carpal arch while protecting the median nerve and preventing bowstring of the flexor tendons. A recent report on a series of 30 patients who had simultaneous release of the carpal tunnel and fasciectomy for Dupuytren's contracture indicated that no great morbidity than after fasciectomy alone, in contrast to previous reports of frequent complications when the two procedures were simultaneously performed. The current interest in arthroscopically controlled carpal tunnel release is under assessment. It is too early to judge its effectiveness at this time.

Dupuytren's Contracture

A study of the relationship between cigarette smoking and Dupuytren's contracture suggests that cigarette smoking may produce microvascular occlusion and subsequent fibrosis and contracture. Dupuytren's contracture in women has been treated by a limited fasciectomy, that is, removal of the diseased fascia. Women are more than twice as likely as men to have a flare reaction after surgery. The report of this study of 83 women noted that finger flexion was diminished in 76% of patients who had a flare reaction and 35% of those without a flare reaction. Because women have a flare reaction if they undergo a carpal tunnel release when the palmar fascia is excised, it may be prudent to stage these procedures.

Segmental removal of diseased fascia thru multiple small curved incisions has been reported in 213 cases. It was shown that this procedure could achieve corrections that could not be achieved with fasciotomy, but had less complications than seen after limited fasciectomy. Others have shown that the procedure was fast and safe and could be done on an outpatient basis.

Annotated Bibliography

Biomechanics of the Wrist

Gellman H, Kauffman D, Lenihan M, et al: An in vitro analysis of wrist motion: The effect of limited intercarpal arthrodesis and the contributions of the radiocarpal and midcarpal joints. *J Hand Surg* 1988;13A:378-383.

The authors simulated radiocarpal and intercarpal fusions in fresh cadaver specimens to determine loss of motion of various types of fusions.

Viegas S, Patterson RM, Peterson PD, et al: Evaluation of the biomechanical efficacy of limited intercarpal fusions for the treatment of scapho-lunate dissociation. *J Hand Surg* 1990;15A:120-128.

The effects of ligament section producing instabilities and various intercarpal fusions were studied to determine the areas of increased load distribution in the wrist.

Diagnostic Evaluation

DeMaagd RL, Engber WD: Retrograde Herbert screw fixation for treatment of proximal pole scaphoid nonunions. *J Hand Surg* 1989;14A:996-1003.

The authors reviewed 12 patients with nonunion or fractures of the proximal pole of the scaphoid treated with Herbert screw fixation via the dorsal approach. Healing was achieved in 11 of the 12 cases.

Osterman AL: Arthroscopic debridement of triangular fibrocartilage complex tears. *Arthroscopy* 1990;6:120-124.

This prospective study involved 52 consecutive patients treated arthroscopically for triangular fibrocartilage complex tears. Both arthrography and arthroscopy were more diagnostic than stress films; arthroscopy had a 9% false-negative rate, arthrography a 9% false-positive rate. Repair often included removal of 2 to 3 mm of the ulnar head. Of 41 patients followed for 13 to 42 months, 88% considered the procedure worthwhile and 73% had complete relief of pain.

Palmer AK: Triangular fibrocartilage disorders: Injury patterns and treatment. *Arthroscopy* 1990;6:125-132.

This article reviews the anatomy and biomechanics of the triangular fibrocartilage complex, classifies patterns of triangular fibrocartilage complex injury, and suggests treatment for each pattern. Treatments include arthroscopic debridement of the horizontal portion of the triangular fibrocartilage complex for central perforations and arthroscopic removal of the distal 2 mm of the ulnar head for degenerative perforation of the horizontal portion of the triangular fibrocartilage complex with associated underlying ulnar head chondromalacia.

Roth JH, Poehling GG, Whipple TL: Arthroscopic surgery of the wrist, in Bassett FH III (ed): American Academy of Orthopaedic Surgeons *Instructional Course Lectures, XXXVII*. Park Ridge, IL, American Academy of Orthopaedic Surgeons, 1988, pp 183-194.

This article presents the techniques of wrist arthroscopy, reviews the principles and strategy of arthroscopy, describes wrist anatomy, compares arthroscopy and arthrography, and illustrates several cases of arthroscopic wrist surgery.

Russell RC, Williamson DA, Sullivan JW, et al: Detection of foreign bodies in the hand. *J Hand Surg* 1991;16A:2-11.

Using fresh cadaver, the authors compared the ability of routine radiographs, CT scans, and MRI studies to identify various types of foreign bodies. Wood particles were difficult to identify by standard radiograph but were readily identified by CT scan. Gravel, difficult to see by standard examinations, was readily found by MRI studies.

Sowa DT, Holder LE, Patt PG, et al: Application of magnetic resonance imaging to ischemic necrosis of the lunate. *J Hand Surg* 1989;14A:1008-1016.

The authors studied 20 patients with aseptic necrosis of the lunate and found that MRI is the definitive test in evaluating ischemic necrosis of the lunate. It can be used to follow the progress in both untreated and treated cases.

Trumble TE, Irving J: Histological and magnetic resonance imaging correlations in Kienböck's disease. *J Hand Surg* 1990;15A:879-884.

Nine patients were studied to evaluate midcarpal pain. Six patients had the diagnosis of Kienböck's disease made by this technique. In four of these patients the plain films were abnormal, but this technique confirmed the diagnosis in two patients.

Whipple TL, Cooney WP, Poehlng GG: Intraarticular fractures, in McGinty JB, Caspari RB, Jackson RW, et al (eds): *Operative Arthroscopy*. New York, Raven Press, 1991, pp 651-654.

This chapter on arthroscopic management of intra-articular fractures of the wrist discusses fracture patterns and common problems following open repair, the usefulness of arthroscopy in fracture repair, and the arthroscopic technique.

Whipple TL, Martin D: Triangular fibrocartilage complex, in McGinty JB, Caspari RB, Jackson RW, et al (eds): *Operative Arthroscopy*. New York, Raven Press, 1991, pp 655-657.

This very recent chapter discusses the rationale for and technique of arthroscopic repair of triangular fibrocartilage rupture.

Posttraumatic Problems of the Wrist

Kienböck's Disease

Alexander AH, Turner MA, Alexander CE, et al: Lunate silicone replacement arthroplasty in Kienböck's disease: A long-term follow-up. *J Hand Surg* 1990;15A:401-407.

Poor results were noted with the silicone lunate implant when used in stage III Kienböck's disease.

Kato H, Usui M, Minami A: Long-term results of Kienböck's disease treated by excisional arthroplasty with a silicone implant or coiled palmaris longus tendon. *J Hand Surg* 1986;11A:645-653.

Thirty-two patients with Kienböck's disease underwent 19 lunate implant replacement and 13 patients had palmaris longus tendon replacement. The silicone implants did not give good clinical results in advanced cases with collapse but were better than the tendon replacements in early cases.

Scaphoid Nonunion and Osteonecrosis

Birchard D, Pichora D: Experimental corrective scaphoid osteotomy for scaphoid malunion with abnormal wrist mechanics. *J Hand Surg* 1990;15A:863-868.

The use of a corrective osteotomy for the hump-back deformity in the healed scaphoid fracture is described in an attempt to reduce the risk of late wrist arthritis.

Brunelli GA, Brunelli GR: A personal technique for treatment of scaphoid non-union. *J Hand Surg* 1991;16B:148-152.

The authors describe a technique for the treatment of nonunion of the scaphoid consisting of a styloidectomy with axial perforation of the scaphoid, emptying of bone, and filling it with grafts from the styloid. A bone peg from the styloid is used to achieve fixation. A very high success rate was achieved.

Carter PR, Malinin TI, Abbey PA, et al: The scaphoid allograft: A new operation for treatment of the very proximal scaphoid nonunion or for the necrotic, fragmented scaphoid proximal pole. *J Hand Surg* 1989;14A:1-12.

This is a preliminary report of eight cases in which an allograft was used to replace the proximal one half of the scaphoid in cases of nonunion or necrosis of the proximal fragment.

Chun S, Wicks BP, Meyerdierks E, et al: Two modifications for insertion of the Herbert screw in the fractured scaphoid. *J Hand Surg* 1990;15A:669-671.

Two modifications of the technique to insert a Herbert screw using the jig are presented. A trough in the palmar aspect of the trapezium was thought to simplify the proper jig placement.

Arthritis of the Wrist

Limited Arthrodesis

Essman JA, Reilly TJ, Forshew FC: Palmar approach for treatment of scapho-trapezio-trapezoid arthrodesis. *J Hand Surg* 1990;15A:672-674.

A palmar approach to scaphotrapeziotrapezoid fusion is presented to minimize common complications seen following the dorsal radial approach to perform this intercarpal fusion.

Hom S, Ruby LK: Attempted scapholunate arthrodesis for chronic scapholunate dissociation. *J Hand Surg* 1991;16A;334-339.

The authors reviewed their experience with seven scapholunate fusions and found that fusion was seldom achieved. The authors felt that this was not a reliable procedure for scapholunate dissociation.

Kleinman WB, Carroll C IV: Scapho-trapezio-trapezoid arthrodesis for treatment of chronic static and dynamic scapho-lunate instability: A 10-year perspective on pitfalls and complications. *J Hand Surg* 1990;15A:408-414.

Complications of the scaphotrapeziotrapezoid fusion are common, and careful attention to detail in placement of the scaphoid is critical.

Pisano SM, Peimer CA, Wheeler DR, et al: Scaphocapitate intercarpal arthrodesis. *J Hand Surg* 1991;16A:328-333.

A review of 17 patient after scaphocapitate fusion showed a reduction in radial deviation and flexion. There were two nonunions in the series. The procedure maintained carpal bone relationships.

Rogers WD, Watson HK: Radial styloid impingement after triscaphi arthrodesis. *J Hand Surg* 1989;14A:297-301.

In a series of 93 triscaphi arthrodeses, 31 patients were found to have radial styloid impingement. On the basis of this study, the authors incorporate radial styloidectomy as part of the routine procedure during a triscaphi arthrodesis.

Wrist Arthroplasty Versus Arthrodesis

Figgie MP, Ranawat CS, Inglis AE, et al: Trispherical total wrist arthroplasty in rheumatoid arthritis. *J Hand Surg* 1990;15A:217-223.

Thirty-four patients with 35 trispherical total wrist arthroplasties are presented. Only two patents have required revisions. The best results were seen in patients with intact extensor tendons.

Rayan GM, Brentlinger A, Purnell D, et al: Functional assessment of bilateral wrist arthrodeses. *J Hand Surg* 1987;12A:1020-1024.

In this study of nine patients who had bilateral wrist fusions, the patients did not seem to be adversely affected in regard to function of the upper extremity.

Proximal Row Carpectomy

Hermansdorfer JD, Kleinman WB: Management of chronic peripheral tears of the triangular fibrocartilage complex. *J Hand Surg* 1991;16A:340-346.

Thirteen patients with traumatic separation of the triangular fibrocartilage from its peripheral origin had an anatomic reconstruction by surgical reattachment to the ulna. Eight patients regained normal, painless activity with a follow-up of one year.

Imbriglia JE, Broudy AS, Hagberg WC, et al: Proximal row carpectomy: Clinical evaluation. *J Hand Surg* 1990;15A:426-430.

This is a review of 27 patients undergoing proximal row carpectomy. Almost all patients returned to work. The authors feel that this procedure is an acceptable alternative to wrist fusion.

Posttraumatic Problems of the Hand

Soft-Tissue Defects

Buchler U, Frey HP: Retrograde posterior interosseous flap. *J Hand Surg* 1991;16A:283-292.

Thirty-six distally based posterior interosseous island flaps were reviewed. Donor morbidity was minimal but the flaps were slightly bulky in 30% of the cases.

Tendon Transfers

Anderson GA, Lee V, Sundararaj GD: Extensor indicis proprius opponensplasty. *J Hand Surg* 1991;16B:334-338.

This is an analysis of 39 patients (40 hands) that underwent an extensor indicis proprius opponensplasty. Excellent or good results were seen in 87.5%.

Gupta A, Burke FD: Correction of camptodactyly: Preliminary results of extensor indicis transfer. *J Hand Surg* 1990;15B:168-170.

The extensor indicis proprius tendon was used as a transfer to overcome passively correctable camptodactyly. The early results were encouraging.

Mannerfelt L, Oetker R, Ostlund B, et al: Rupture of the extensor pollicis longus tendon after Colles fracture and by rheumatoid arthritis. *J Hand Surg* 1990;15B:49-50.

One hundred and sixteen patients with rupture of the extensor pollicis longus tendon were operated on. The lesions were categorized into three anatomical levels. The results of tendon transfers and free tendon grafts were reviewed.

Oster LH Jr, Blair WF, Steyers CM: Crossed intrinsic transfer. *J Hand Surg* 1990;15A:811.

A crossed intrinsic transfer technique using the ulnar lateral band transferred to the radial collateral ligament is described.

Tendon Injuries

Browne EZ Jr, Ribik CA: Early dynamic splinting for extensor tendon injuries. *J Hand Surg* 1989;14A:72-76.

The authors used dynamic splinting following the treatment of extensor tendon repairs. They had no ruptures and noted full restoration of flexion in all patients.

Caroli A, Zonasi S, Squarzina PB, et al: Operative treatment of the post-traumatic Boutonniere deformity: A modification of the direct anatomical repair technique. *J Hand Surg* 1990;15B:410-415.

Twenty cases of posttraumatic boutonniere deformity treated by a modified direct anatomical repair are described. The authors excise a swallow-tailed flap from the fibrous tissue between the tendon ends. Excellent results were obtained in a high percentage of cases.

Ertel AN, Millender LH, Nalebuff E, et al: Flexor tendon ruptures in patients with rheumatoid arthritis. *J Hand Surg* 1988;13A:860-866.

The authors reviewed their combined experience with flexor tendon ruptures as the result of rheumatoid arthritis.

Gerbino PG II, Saldana MJ, Westerbeck P, et al: Complications experienced in the rehabilitation of zone I flexor tendon injuries with dynamic traction splinting. *J Hand Surg* 1991;16A:680-686.

This is a review of 163 flexor tendon lacerations in 83 patients. All patients were treated with passive motion exercises of the interphalangeal joints in the first two weeks. A high rate of complications with zone I patients prompted the authors to modify their postoperative technique.

Hagberg L, Selvik G: Tendon excursion and dehiscence during early controlled mobilization after flexor tendon repair in zone II: An x-ray stereophotogrammetric analysis. *J Hand Surg* 1991;16A:669-680.

The effect of different methods on early controlled mobilization of flexor profundus tendon excursion and dehiscence was examined during the treatment of 20 tendons in 18 patients. A new radiographic method to determine tendon excursion is presented.

Magnell TD, Pochron MD, Condit DP: The intercalated tendon graft for treatment of extensor pollicis longus tendon rupture. *J Hand Surg* 1988;13A:105-109.

Twenty-one patients with extensor pollicis longus rupture were treated with tendon grafts. There was near uniform satisfaction with the procedure, which the authors felt was simple, reliable, and effective.

Newport ML, Blair WF, Steyers CM Jr: Long term results of extensor tendon repair. *J Hand Surg* 1990;15A:961-966.

The results following extensor tendon injuries are most affected by the presence or absence of associated injuries. Only 64% achieved good/excellent results in simple cases while only 45% had good/excellent reults when associated injuries were present.

Ohshio I, Ogino T, Minami A, et al: Reconstruction of the central slip by the transverse retinacular ligament for Boutonniere deformity. *J Hand Surg* 1990;15B:407-409.

A new method of repair for the boutonniere deformity is described using the transverse retinacular ligament.

Arthritis of the Hand

Joint Replacement

Conolly WB, Roth S: Silastic implant arthroplasty for post traumatic stiffness of the finger joints. *J Hand Surg* 1991;16B:286-292.

Fifty patients undergoing 59 Silastic joint replacements for posttraumatic stiffness were reviewed. Most patients were satisfied with the procedure based on relief of pain, correction of deformity, stability, and overall finger function.

Figgie MP, Inglis AE, Sobel M, et al: Metacarpal-phalangeal joint arthroplasty of the rheumatoid thumb. *J Hand Surg* 1990;15A:210-216.

Fifty patients underwent metacarpophalangeal arthroplasties of the thumb in rheumatoid arthritis. The maintenance of motion was thought to improve hand function.

Nalebuff EA: Factors influencing the results of implant surgery in the rheumatoid hand. *J Hand Surg* 1990;15B:395-403.

The various factors thought to influence the results of arthroplasties are reviewed. The implant was thought to be the least important factor with the patient and the condition of the controlling tendons and adjacent joint to be of prime importance.

Pellegrini VD Jr, Burton RI: Osteoarthritis of the proximal interphalangeal joint of the hand: Arthroplasty or fusion? *J Hand Surg* 1990;15A:194-209.

The alternate treatments for osteoarthritis of the proximal interphalangeal joints are reviewed. Fusions were preferred for the radial digits to improve stability. Bone absorption was noted in long-term follow-up evaluation of the arthroplasties.

Arthrodesis

Rayan GM, Brentlinger A, Purnell D, et al: Functional assessment of bilateral wrist arthrodesis. *J Hand Surg* 1987;12A:1020-1024.

In this study of nine patients who had bilateral wrist fusions, the patients did not seem to be adversely affected in regard to function of the upper extremity.

Carpal Tunnel Syndrome

Fuchs PC, Nathan PA, Myers LD: Synovial histology in carpal tunnel syndrome. *J Hand Surg* 1991;16A:753-758.

This study investigated the relationship between idiopathic carpal tunnel syndrome and tenosynovial histology. It was concluded that tenosynovitis is uncommon in patients undergoing surgery.

Gonzalez F, Watson HK: Simultaneous carpal tunnel release and Dupuytren's fasciectomy. *J Hand Surg* 1991;16B:175-178.

The authors reviewed their experience with 30 patients undergoing simultaneous fasciectomy and carpal tunnel release. Their complication rate was low and their results better than in previous reports on this subject.

Jakab E, Ganos D, Cook FW: Transverse carpal ligament reconstruction in surgery for carpal tunnel syndrome: A new technique. *J Hand Surg* 1991;16A:202-206.

A two-year follow-up of a technique to reconstruct the transverse carpal ligament following carpal tunnel release surgery is reported. The results were excellent with 97% of patients returning to work within two months of surgery.

Richman JA, Gelberman RH, Rydevik BL, et al: Carpal tunnel syndrome: Morphologic changes after release of

the transverse carpal ligament. *J Hand Surg* 1989; 14A:852-857.

The morphologic changes that follow division of the transverse carpal ligament are described.

Wand JS: Carpal tunnel syndrome in pregnancy and lactation. *J Hand Surg* 1990;15B:93-95.

This is a retrospective study of 40 women with carpal tunnel syndrome developing in pregnancy. These patients were thought to react differently than those patients who developed the syndrome in the postpartum stage.

Dupuytren's Contracture

Andrew JG, Kay NRM: Segmental aponeurectomy for Dupuytren's disease: A prospective study. *J Hand Surg* 1991;16B:255-257.

In this prospective study of 46 patients, a segmental aponeurectomy was performed. The incidence of recurrence at one year was no higher than with other more extensive techniques. It was felt that this approach was particularly suited for elderly patients.

Moermans JP: Segmental aponeurectomy in Dupuytren's disease. *J Hand Surg* 1991;16B:243-254.

This is a report of 213 consecutive segmental aponeurectomies in 175 patients. No attempt was made to remove all of the diseased tissue. The authors feel that this technique has fewer complications than more standard surgical treatment.

IV
Spine

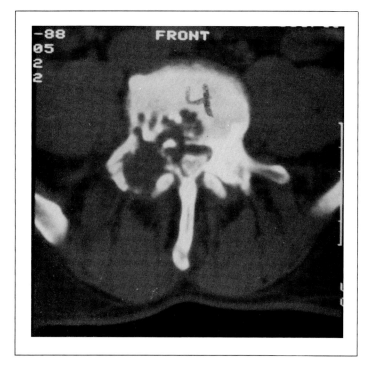

33
Cervical Spine: Pediatric

Anatomy and Embryology

The anatomy of the upper cervical spine differs significantly from that of the remainder of the spine, and its evaluation can be a source of confusion. Congenital anomalies may result either from a failure of segmentation, as occurs in the Klippel-Feil syndrome, or from failure of coalescence of secondary centers of ossification, as is seen in os odontoideum. The atlas (C-1) has ossification centers at both posterior neural arches with a posterior synchondrosis. A neurocentral synchondrosis forms on each side anteriorly and appears at 6 to 24 months of age. The anterior arch of the immature atlas occasionally has multiple ossification centers. At 4 to 6 years of age, the posterior and anterior centers fuse, and the space available for the spinal cord is defined. Posterior bifid arches of C-1 are found in 5% of the population; anterior bifid arches of C-1 are rare.

The dens forms from two primary centers of ossification that coalesce at 1 to 3 months of age. The centers are separated from the vertebral body by a basilar synchondrosis. At 8 to 10 years of age, the ossiculum terminale forms at the apex of the dens and then fuses to the dens at 10 to 13 years of age.

The orientation of the facet joints of the cervical spine changes with growth. In the young child, the angle of the upper cervical facets from C-2 to C-4 is nearly horizontal in the sagittal plane (30 to 35 degrees) permitting more translation in flexion and extension than is seen in the adult spine. In the preadolescent child, the facet angle becomes more vertical (75 to 80 degrees) and less mobile. The orientation of the lower cervical facets changes from 55 to 70 degrees during the same period of growth.

The cervical spine can be stretched considerably in the young child without permanent injury to the spinal column. The spinal cord, however, is not as elastic as the spinal column, and may be injured without bony injury to the cervical spine.

The combination of incomplete ossification, relative ligamentous laxity, and shallow facet joint angles results in greater translation motion of the immature cervical spine. The firm ligamentous fixation between the atlas, axis, and occiput and the relatively larger size and weight of the child's skull result in a higher cervical fulcrum at C2-C3 as compared to the eventual adult fulcrum at C5-C6.

The motion pattern of the cervical spine in children younger than 8 years of age differs considerably from that of the adult. Pseudosubluxation of C-2 on C-3 in flexion refers to the normal mobility in this area, which may be so pronounced as to be mistaken for pathologic motion. The application of adult standards of kinematics to the child's spine is not reliable. The straight-line relationship of the spinolaminar line of C-1, C-2, and C-3 in flexion is helpful in differentiating physiologic from pathologic anterior displacement of C-2 and C-3. In flexion, the posterior arch of C-2 will lie on or behind a straight line connecting the posterior arches of C-1 and C-3 in the normal immature spine (Fig. 1). The differentiation of these variants from congenital anomalies of the cervical spine is important to avoid misdiagnosis and inappropriate investigation or treatment.

Widening of the cervical canal is not a reliable indicator of pathology in children younger than 10 years of age because of normal variations in width throughout the entire cervical canal. The radiographic finding does not merit further investigation unless there are accompanying neurologic signs and symptoms.

Congenital Disorders

Basilar Impression

Basilar impression is a deformity of osseous structures that form the base of the skull and the foramen magnum.

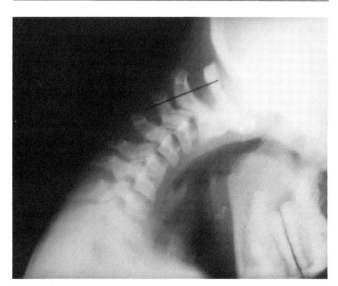

Fig. 1 Swischuk's spinolaminar line bridging from C-1 to C-3 lies anterior to the spinolaminar line of C-2 in patients presenting with pseudosubluxation.

Lateral radiographs of the skull and cervical spine will reveal indentation of the floor of the skull by the upper cervical spine. The tip of the odontoid may intrude into the foramen magnum, encroach on the brain stem, and interfere with the vascular supply of the spinal cord and with the flow of cerebrospinal fluid. Computed tomography (CT) and magnetic resonance imaging (MRI) have simplified the identification of this problem and allowed for detailed evaluation. Projection of the tip of the odontoid above McRae's line is associated with neurologic compromise. In those individuals in whom the odontoid tip remains caudal to the foramen magnum, neurologic compromise is unusual.

Primary basilar impression is congenital and is associated with such vertebral anomalies as atlantooccipital fusion, hypoplasia of the atlas, odontoid abnormalities, and the Klippel-Feil syndrome, as well as with such skeletal dysplasias as achondroplasia, spondyloepiphyseal dysplasia, and Morquio syndrome. Secondary basilar impression is a development condition resulting from softening of the osseous structures of the base of the skull and may be caused by severe osteoporosis, osteomalacia, rickets, renal osteodystrophy, Paget's disease, osteogenesis imperfecta, rheumatoid arthritis, neurofibromatosis, or trauma.

Basilar impression is usually inconsequential, but it may be clinically important because of its association with treatable neurologic problems such as syringomyelia, cerebellar herniation (Arnold-Chiari syndrome), atlantoaxial instability, and spinal cord compression at the foramen magnum. If instability exists, the odontoid may encroach on the medulla oblongata and increase intracranial pressure with blockade of the aqueduct of Sylvius resulting in hydrocephalus. In addition, instability may produce compression of the cerebellum, herniation of the cerebellar tonsils, or impingement of the posterior columns and paraspinal tracts with associated weakness, hyperreflexia, and spasticity. The vertebral arteries may be compressed directly or may be congenitally malformed in association with basilar impression and atlantooccipital fusion. Indications for surgical intervention are based on the patient's neurologic involvement.

Occipitalization of the Atlas

Occipitalization of the atlas (atlantooccipital fusion, assimilation of the atlas) may be detected as an incidental radiographic finding in the neurologically intact individual. When it is associated with congenital fusion of C-2 and C-3 or with anomalies of the odontoid, there is a significant risk of atlantoaxial instability with resultant neurologic compromise (Fig. 2).

In the child younger than 10 years of age, plane radiographic diagnosis may be difficult because of the incomplete ossification of the posterior ring of the atlas. Lateral flexion-extension radiographs, lateral tomography, CT, and MRI are helpful in making the diagnosis and determining the existence of spinal-cord compression.

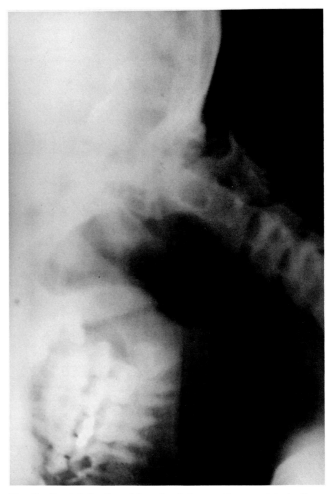

Fig. 2 Occipitalization of the atlas is frequently associated with instability when combined with congenital fusion of C-2 and C-3.

Half the patients with occipitalization of the atlas have relative basilar impression because of diminished vertical height of the ring of the atlas. If the odontoid projects into the foramen magnum, spinal-cord compromise may develop and require treatment. If the odontoid remains at a level below the foramen magnum, neurologic compromise is unusual. In the presence of occiput-atlas-axis instability, the space available for the spinal cord will be significantly decreased by the odontoid, and myelopathy can occur.

If instability is documented, arthrodesis of the occiput-atlas complex to the axis is necessary. If fixed subluxation exists, surgical reduction is frequently associated with significant complications and should be avoided. Suboccipital craniectomy with excision of the posterior arch of the atlas and removal of any coexisting dural bands, followed by posterior arthrodesis, is preferred for patients in whom posterior spinal cord compression is demonstrated. If symptoms originate from anterior spinal cord compression, anterior decompression may be considered. This is a formidable procedure and is rarely indicated.

Congenital Anomalies of the Odontoid

Anomalies of the odontoid include complete aplasia, hypoplasia, and os odontoideum. Aplasia of the odontoid is a rare condition. Hypoplasia of the odontoid may be seen in conjunction with dysmorphic conditions such as achondroplasia or spondyloepiphyseal dysplasia. Os odontoideum, the most common anomaly, occurs on both a congenital and traumatic basis. All three conditions can produce symptoms and serious neurologic sequelae as a result of atlantoaxial instability.

Many congenital anomalies of the odontoid are discovered incidentally on routine radiographic studies of asymptomatic patients. Instability of the atlantoaxial joint may be manifested by local pain, headache, torticollis, and neurologic symptoms that include spasticity, hyperreflexia, clonus, and sphincteric dysfunction. Vertebral artery compression may occur and be made evident by seizures, mental deterioration, syncope, vertigo, and vestibular disturbances.

Lateral flexion-extension radiographs of the cervical spine may show hypermobility and can document the degree of displacement of the atlas on the axis. A CT scan or polytomography occasionally is needed in the presence of os odontoideum to more clearly demonstrate the degree of displacement. In patients with a stable atlantoaxial articulation and minor mechanical symptomatology, nonsurgical treatment often is sufficient. Surgical stabilization is required in patients who have significant instability at the atlantoaxial junction accompanied by compromise of the space available for the spinal cord, particularly when there is history of progressive neurologic deterioration.

The atlantoaxial articulation may be reduced by simple positioning or traction before surgery. Close attention must be given to the tightening of wires in atlantoaxial posterior arthrodesis using iliac bone graft and wiring. The atlantoaxial junction may be unstable in either flexion or extension, and overzealous tightening of the wire passed beneath the laminae of C-1 and C-2 can translate the anterior ring of the atlas posteriorly, resulting in impingement of the spinal cord. In patients in whom the ring of C-1 is deficient or malformed, arthrodesis is extended to the occiput, and maintenance of proper alignment may require a halo cast.

When an irreducible atlantoaxial dislocation exists, manipulative or open reduction should be avoided. In patients who are neurologically intact, posterior atlantoaxial arthrodesis without internal fixation is effective and safe. Passing a wire under the arch of the atlas involves considerable risk and should be done cautiously. In patients with anterior cord compression, anterior decompression should be considered following posterior stabilization.

Posterior decompression and laminectomy without associated arthrodesis has been associated with increased instability and significant morbidity and mortality. Instability is defined as an abnormal atlantodens interval greater than 5 mm in children.

Asymptomatic instability presents the greatest difficulty in decision making. In individuals who are neurologically intact but have more than a 5 mm atlantodens interval, CT and MRI have been very helpful in determining the physiologic state of the spinal cord and determining the need for operative stabilization.

Posterior arthrodesis of the pediatric cervical spine has been generally successful with the use of autogenous bone graft with or without internal fixation. Use of halo cast or Minerva cast has been successful for temporary extension of stabilization. However, the use of cadaver allografts, which has been associated with an increased incidence of nonunion in children, is not recommended in posterior arthrodesis of the cervical spine.

Klippel-Feil Syndrome

The term Klippel-Feil Syndrome includes all variations of congenital failure of segmentation of cervical vertebrae, from simple fusion of two segments to involvement of the entire cervical spine (Fig. 3). Failure of segmentation occurs during the third to eighth week of gestation. Klippel-Feil syndrome is associated with Sprengel's deformity and with a host of congenital anomalies occurring in the genitourinary, nervous, cardiopulmonary, and auditory systems. Classic signs of Klippel-Feil syndrome include low posterior hairline, short neck, and limited range of motion of the neck, but these classic signs are found in fewer than one half of patients. The most common finding is limitation of neck motion, especially in lateral side bending. Many patients with marked cervical involvement have excellent range of motion when tested in flexion and extension.

In the young child, unossified endplates may give the false impression of normal disk space. Lateral flexion-extension radiographs are most helpful in differentiating true from false disk spaces in the young child. Fusion of lamina posteriorly may occur before fusion of anterior elements in the young child.

Scoliosis is found in 60% of patients with Klippel-Feil syndrome, and more than half of these individuals require treatment. One third of those with Klippel-Feil syndrome have significant urinary tract anomalies, which can be detected by renal ultrasound. Fourteen percent have congenital heart disease, and 30% have varying degrees of hearing loss, on either a conductive or a neural basis. Although symptoms are unusual in these patients, neurologic compromise has been reported in a significant number of individuals with Klippel-Feil syndrome. Neurologic impairment has been associated most frequently with upper cervical anomalies, especially involving fusion of C-2 and C-3.

Most individuals with this syndrome have a normal appearance and lead normal, active lives with minimal or no restrictions or symptoms. If cervical spine symptoms develop, they usually occur later in life in association with

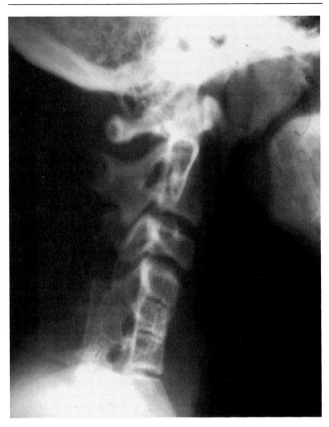

Fig. 3 Klippel-Feil syndrome describes a variety of complex patterns of congenital fusion of the cervical spine. Note that congenital vertebral bodies of C-4, C-5, and C-6 are significantly smaller in height and width compared with normal vertebra above.

degenerative spondylosis. The majority of these older individuals may be successfully treated using nonsurgical methods and will rarely require surgical intervention.

Congenital Muscular Torticollis

Congenital muscular torticollis is a painless condition that usually is discovered in the first two months of life. It involves contracture of the sternocleidomastoid muscle with the head tilted toward the side of contracture and the chin rotated to the contralateral shoulder. Congenital muscular torticollis is not associated with bony abnormalities or neurologic deficit and probably results from ischemia of the sternocleidomastoid muscle.

A nontender enlargement may be palpated in the body of the sternocleidomastoid muscle. The mass resolves within the first year of life and often has disappeared by six months of age. Pathologic studies of surgical specimens suggest fibrosis of the sternal head, which may compromise a branch of the accessory nerve to the clavicular head of the muscle, thereby increasing the deformity.

Differential diagnosis of torticollis in the newborn includes pterygium colli, tumors in the region of the sternocleidomastoid (for example, cystic hygroma, bronchial cleft cysts, and thyroid teratomas), congenital anomalies of the cervical spine (for example, unilateral absence of the lateral mass of the atlas), posterior fossa masses, and superior oblique palsy of the ocular muscle. Evaluation of the newborn with congenital muscular torticollis should include a detailed evaluation of the hips, because 20% of affected individuals have associated congenital hip dysplasia.

With persistent contracture of the sternocleidomastoid, deformities of the face and skull (plagiocephaly) result and are apparent within the first year of life. Flattening of the face is noted on the side of the contracted sternocleidomastoid and is probably caused by the child's sleeping position. Flattening may also be noted at the back of the head as the child tends to sleep supine.

In the first year of life, treatment consists of stretching the sternocleidomastoid muscle by trying to rotate the head to the opposite position. Stretching exercises should include not only lateral rotation, but also side bending to the opposite shoulder. Approximately 90% of patients will respond to this simple regimen if treatment is started before 1 year of age. If nonsurgical measures have not succeeded by 12 to 24 months of age, surgical intervention is needed to prevent further facial deformity. Surgical treatment involves resection of a portion of the distal sternocleidomastoid muscle through a transverse incision in the normal skin fold of the neck. Skin incisions immediately adjacent to the clavicle may result in unsightly hypertrophic scars. Transverse skin incisions in skin folds 1.5 cm proximal to the clavicle result in imperceptible scars. Occasionally, distal resection is insufficient and proximal release of the sternocleidomastoid is needed.

Developmental Problems

Atlantoaxial Instability

Atlantoaxial instability is also associated with many developmental conditions, such as Morquio syndrome, spondyloepiphyseal dysplasia, Larsen's syndrome, and achondroplasia. The most common association is with Down syndrome (trisomy 21) in which 25% of patients have both conditions. Attention has been focused on atlantoaxial instability since the advent of screening for individuals with Down syndrome who participate in the Special Olympics. Individual recommendations have been developed by each state Committee on Special Olympics; all require at least one set of lateral flexion-extension radiographs of the cervical spine to rule out instability. An atlantodens interval greater than 5 mm in the asymptomatic Down syndrome athlete results in a recommendation to avoid activities involving high-impact flexion loading on the cervical spine. Although there is not universal agreement among physicians, individuals with 10 mm or more of atlantodens interval and/or neurologic signs and symptoms require surgical stabilization. Attempts at surgical stabilization of the upper cervical spine in children with Down syndrome are

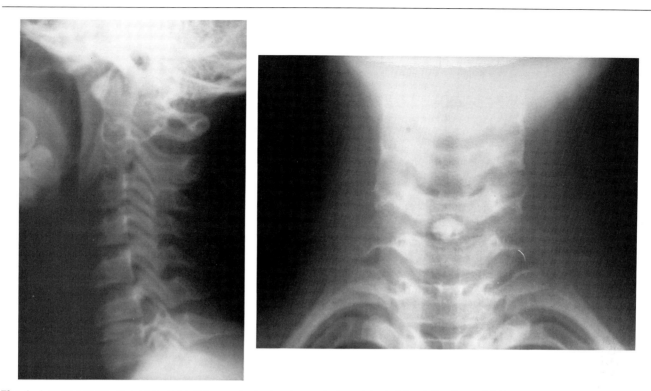

Fig. 4   Lateral and anterior radiographs of the cervical spine demonstrate vertebral disk calcification at C6-C7.

fraught with significant complications. Fixed dislocation at the junction of C-1 and C-2 should not be treated by open reduction because of the high incidence of mortality. In the face of fixed dislocation, laminectomy of C-1 with posterior arthrodesis from occiput to C-2 results in a satisfactory outcome.

Atlantoaxial instability may also be noted in the normal child in association with pharyngeal infection (Grisel's syndrome). Anatomic studies involving injection of the pharyngeal veins have shown retrograde filling, with a lymphovenous anastomosis draining from the posterior pharynx. Hyperemia causes demineralization of the attachment of the transverse ligament to the anterior arch of the atlas, with subsequent rotary subluxation of the atlas on the axis or anterior atlantoaxial subluxation. The vast majority of patients with torticollis from this cause improve spontaneously. In those few cases in which persistent significant instability is present, stabilization by posterior atlantoaxial arthrodesis is required.

Cervical Kyphosis

Extensive laminectomy of the cervical spine in the growing child significantly increases the risk of postlaminectomy cervical kyphosis. Kyphosis may also occur in young patients with intact posterior elements as a result of congenital, traumatic, metabolic, or neoplastic processes. Early recognition and surgical intervention are extremely important in arresting progression and improving neurologic signs and symptoms.

Inflammation

Juvenile Rheumatoid Arthritis

Juvenile rheumatoid arthritis may involve the cervical spine. In contrast to rheumatoid arthritis of the adult cervical spine, involvement at the atlanto-occipital junction or at the atlantoaxial junction is rare in childhood. Children with polyarticular involvement or with systemic onset (Still's disease) frequently complain of stiffness and have radiographic changes in the cervical spine. Spontaneous fusion of posterior elements of the cervical vertebrae is more common than atlantoaxial instability in juvenile rheumatoid arthritis. Even in the presence of extensive radiographic involvement, neck pain is not common. If pain is present, fracture or infection should be considered as potential causes.

Vertebral Disk Calcification

Vertebral disk calcification is an uncommon childhood problem. Cervical involvement typically occurs at the C-6 to C-7 level (Fig. 4). Thirty percent of patients have a history of trauma and 15% have a history of upper respiratory tract infection. The onset of symptoms is abrupt, and symptoms consist of neck pain, limited motion, and torticollis. Fever is present in 25% of patients. The typical course of the illness involves rapid clinical resolution, but radiographic resolution is slower. Two-thirds of children are asymptomatic by three weeks, and 95% are

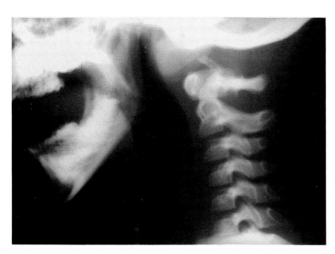

Fig. 5 Minimal traction may result in complete distraction when occipitocervical instability exists.

asymptomatic within six months. Neurologic deficits, if present, improve in 90% of patients. Disk herniation is rare. Posterior herniations cause spinal cord compression and anterior herniations result in dysphagia. The appropriate treatment in the vast majority of cases is rest and cervical immobilization until symptoms resolve.

Neoplasms

Primary neoplasms of the cervical spine are relatively rare in childhood. Benign lesions include osteochondromas, hemangiomas, and osteoblastomas; these may be defined by radiographs, tomography, bone scan, CT scan, and MRI. Spontaneous collapse of the vertebral body with no history of significant trauma should suggest the presence of a neoplasm or infection. Invasion of the vertebral body by an eosinophilic granuloma typically results in complete flattening (vertebral plana). Wedge-shaped bodies are more typical of infection or Ewing's tumor. Neurofibromatosis may be devastating, with considerable loss of bone substance in the cervical spine. Modern imaging techniques allow a high degree of reliability in diagnosis; however, needle or open biopsy of a lesion may still be required for definitive diagnosis. When the decision for biopsy is made, the treating physician, rather than the referring physician, is the most logical individual to perform this procedure.

Fractures

Cervical spine fractures in children are uncommon and represent 3% of all spine trauma. In children under 8 years of age, the upper cervical spine from occiput to C-2 is most frequently involved. In children older than 8 years of age, subaxial fractures and dislocations resemble the adult patterns of injury.

Cervical spine injury should always be suspected in children with head injury, significant facial lacerations, loss of consciousness, neck pain, head cradling, or torticollis following injury. Until the age of 7 years, the size of the skull is large in relation to the child's thorax. Careful management of a child with a suspected cervical injury is mandatory and differs from that of an adult. If the injured child is immobilized in the supine position on a standard spine board, the large skull will force the cervical spine into flexion. Juvenile spine boards with a recessed area for the skull or the use of supports under the shoulders allow the head to extend and thus place the

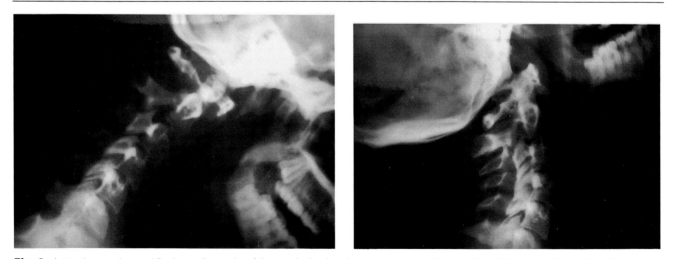

Fig. 6 Lateral extension and flexion radiographs of the cervical spine demonstrate marked translation of the occiput in relationship to the tip of the odontoid.

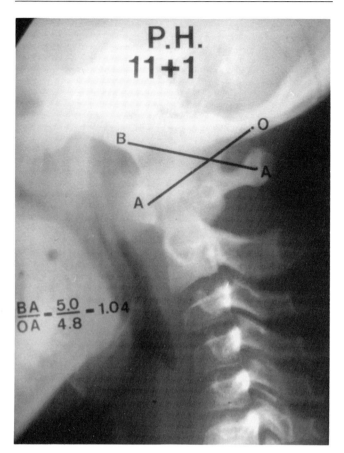

Fig. 7 Power's ratio is the ratio of the distance from the basion (B) to the posterior arch of the atlas over the distance from the opisthion (O) to the anterior arch of C1. A ratio greater than 1 is indicative of instability.

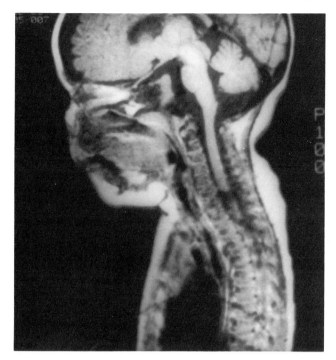

Fig. 8 In the absence of radiographic evidence of injury to the spinal column, MRI demonstrates severe injury to the cervical spinal cord.

cervical spine in a neutral position for safe transport and evaluation.

Traumatic atlanto-occipital injury is the result of severe vehicular injury and is usually fatal. It is extremely important to diagnose this injury in children who have survived such trauma in order to preserve neurologic function and avoid progressive neurologic deterioration and/or death. Lateral radiographs may reveal dissociation at the occipitocervical junction upon application of only minimal amounts of traction or distraction in a halo-device (Fig. 5). More subtle degrees of instability may be documented by computing Power's ratio on lateral flexion-extension radiographs or CT sagittal reconstructions of the occipitocervical junction (Fig. 6). Power's ratio is derived by dividing the distance from the basion to the posterior margin of the anterior march of the atlas by the distance from opisthion to the posterior arch of the axis (Fig. 7). A ratio of one or more is indicative of atlanto-occipital instability.

Spinal cord injury without radiographic abnormality (SCIWORA) may occur in up to 20% of spine injuries in children because of the extreme elasticity of the vertebral column in relation to the less elastic spinal cord. In cases of neurologic injury without radiographic changes, MRI has been helpful in detecting occult injury to the spinal column and spinal cord injury (Fig. 8).

Odontoid fractures in children occur at an average age of 4 years and usually represent epiphyseal fracture through the basilar synchondrosis. The basilar synchondrosis is fused by 6 years of age. Fractures of the odontoid frequently occur in association with head trauma following falls or motor vehicle accidents, in which force is transmitted to the upper cervical spine, and result in anterior displacement of the odontoid. Nonsurgical management is usually successful when the injury is recognized early.

Fracture of the posterior elements of C-2 (hangman's fracture) are reported with increasing frequency and must be differentiated from C-2 to C-3 pseudosubluxation. Early recognition results in successful reduction and healing of the fracture.

Injuries of the subaxial spine occur in children older than 8 years of age and can be treated as adult fractures. Increased awareness and follow-up radiographs are required to monitor for the development of late angulation and instability. Compression fractures are rare and may be confused with the normal anterior wedge-shaped appearance of unossified vertebral bodies. By 10 years of age, the cervical spine has attained the adult radiographic appearance except for fusion of the vertebral endplates. Injuries caused by distraction and/or sheer force tend to involve the cartilaginous vertebral endplates and, most commonly, the pars interarticularis. The intervertebral disks in children are stronger than bone and consequently are rarely disrupted.

Annotated Bibliography

General Considerations

Raynor RB: Congenital malformations, in Sheck HH, Dunn EJ, Eismont GJ, et al (eds): *The Cervical Spine*, ed. 2. Philadelphia, JB Lippincott, 1989, pp 226-285.

This is a detailed reference source for upper cervical anomalies.

Atlantoaxial Instability

Davidson RG: Atlantoaxial instability in individuals with Down syndrome: A fresh look at the evidence. *Pediatrics* 1988;81:857-865.

This review of published cases reveals no evidence that current radiographic criteria are predictive of instability. Those who suffered dislocation had preceding neurologic signs for at least several weeks. No atlantoaxial dislocations were reported in 500,000 individuals with Down syndrome while participating in competitive sports.

Pueschel SM, Findley TW, Furia J, et al: Atlantoaxial instability in Down syndrome: Roentgenographic, neurologic, and somatosensory evoked potential studies. *J Pediatr* 1987;110:515-521.

This combined assessment approach, using roentgenographic, CT scan, neurologic, and neurophysiologic investigations, provides information about the risk status of patients with Down syndrome and atlantoaxial instability.

Torticollis

Phillips WA, Hensinger RN: The management of rotary atlanto-axial subluxation in children. *J Bone Joint Surg* 1989;71A:664-668.

Rotary atlantoaxial subluxation was reviewed in 23 children. If symptoms had persisted less than a month, the subluxation reduced either spontaneously or after a brief period of traction. Three of the seven were seen more than a month after the onset of symptoms and required C1-C2 arthrodesis. Dynamic computed tomographic scans proved the most satisfactory method of documenting this condition.

Trauma

Herzenberg JE, Hensinger RN, Dedrick DK, et al: Emergency transport and positioning of young children who have an injury of the cervical spine: The standard backboard may be hazardous. *J Bone Joint Surg* 1989;71A:15-22.

The relatively large circumference of the head in children younger than seven years forces the cervical spine into flexion when they are transported on a flat spine board. To maintain a neutral position of the cervical spine, the authors recommend a recess for the occiput in the transport board or some other adaption such as shoulder rolls.

Georgopopoulos G, Pizzutillo PD, Lee MS: Occipito-atlantal instability in children: A report of five cases and review of the literature. *J Bone Joint Surg* 1987;69A:429-436.

Five patients with this rare problem are reported. Three have traumatic lesions typified by cardiorespiratory arrest, weakness, neck pain, and torticollis, and two have nontraumatic problems characterized by vertebrobasilar signs such as vertigo, nausea, and vomiting. The authors recommend posterior arthrodesis as the treatment of choice.

Birney TJ, Hanley ENJ Jr: Traumatic cervical spine injuries in childhood and adolescence. *Spine* 1989;14:1277-1282.

Eighty-four children are reported with cervical spine injuries. Forty-four percent incurred neurologic injury. Four groups of injury were identified: atlanto-axial rotary subluxation, upper cervical fracture or dislocation, lower cervical injury, and spinal cord injury without radiographic abnormality. Prognosis is good except in those with initial complete neurologic deficits.

34

Cervical Spine: Trauma

Cervical spine trauma continues to be a significant musculoskeletal problem. Use of seatbelts and airbags in motor vehicles, use of helmets by motorcyclists, and improvements in emergency care between the time of injury and arrival at the hospital have all improved the initial survival of persons with cervical spine injuries, who might otherwise have died from respiratory insufficiency, head injury, or other causes. Careful management of individuals who have a potential cervical spine injury is essential because of the devastating effects of spinal cord injury, the close tolerances and complex structure of the cervical spine, and the frequent association of this injury with altered levels of consciousness. Care of those with spine injuries has benefited from modern imaging methods, computed tomography (CT) and magnetic resonance imaging (MRI); greater understanding of injury biomechanics; and improvements in treatment methods.

Patient Evaluation

General Issues

Patients with cervical spine injuries frequently have other injuries. More urgent or life-threatening problems (airway, breathing, circulation—"the ABCs") clearly take priority; while these are being handled, adequate protection for the potentially-injured cervical spine is essential. Tape and sandbags restrict neck motion better than a hard collar, which in turn is better than a soft cervical collar. Suspicion of a cervical-spine injury should be high in the patient with head injuries (scalp, face, brain) or an altered level of consciousness following trauma. It is essential to keep track of whether or not the spine has been "cleared" in the multitrauma patient with life-threatening injuries.

Distinguishing between hypovolemic and neurogenic shock is important; however, it can be difficult when significant blood loss may have occurred and the patient is comatose. Of all patients with spinal cord injuries, approximately 20% are brought in with hypotension, of which 70% to 80% is neurogenic in origin. Bradycardia suggests that a neurogenic component is present. Diaphragmatic breathing indicates a cervical cord injury. Treatment of hypovolemia may help cord perfusion, although overhydration may increase cord swelling or cause pulmonary edema.

Even transient neurologic signs or symptoms (for example, stingers) may be important indicators of injury severity; therefore, these should be sought in the history.

Documentation of the history and physical examination, including repeated examinations, will make it possible to detect changing neurologic status, especially in patients who have been transferred from one treatment center to another.

Physical Examination

Details and timing of the examination must be placed in the context of overall patient management. Scalp, facial, or head injuries increase the likelihood of cervical spine trauma, although many significant fractures and dislocations occur without head impact. Brain stem, cerebellar, and certain cranial nerve dysfunctions can be indicative of vertebral artery occlusion, although this is rare. Certain cranial nerve deficits can also result from upper cervical dislocations. Neck tenderness may indicate and help localize a spine injury, although false negative findings are not uncommon.

Neurologic examination of the limbs and trunk is essential. The C-4 dermatome spreads down over the chest to the nipple (the "C-4 cape"). Because of variability between individuals and in order to reduce ambiguity, sensory changes should be referenced to specific body parts (for example, thumb instead of C-6 distribution). The possibility of a concomitant thoracic or lumbar spine injury should be considered. It is important to check for sacral sensory sparing because its presence indicates the potential for some recovery.

Spinal shock, in contrast to systemic neurogenic shock from spinal cord injury, is defined by the current absence of reflexes in a patient who subsequently has return of them. The first reflex to return is usually the bulbocavernosus reflex. Diagnosis of spinal shock is important because its presence limits the ability to predict recovery of cord function, at least in terms of spasticity and certain aspects of bladder and bowel function. Although there have been reports of dramatic recovery from severe subtotal deficits, there is no well-documented case of cord recovery in a patient with total deficit persisting for 24 hours after spinal shock has resolved.

Imaging Studies

Imaging studies are particularly important for spine injuries because of the spine's limited access for palpation, because of the potential for further subluxation of an injury missed on examination, and because many patients initially may not cooperate with the examination. Additionally, there is not a strong correlation between neurologic deficit and radiographic appearance. Appropriate radiographic technique and interpretation are essential. Although CT and MRI scanning may help diagnostically, these studies are only adjunctive to a good series of plain radiographs (lateral, anteroposterior, obliques), which is the foundation for imaging of the cervical spine. If no abnormality is seen after initial evaluation, although suspicion of injury remains, repeat evaluation may be indicated.

Lateral View There are few significant injuries that cannot be detected with this view alone (Fig. 1) if it is properly obtained. The entire cervical spine must be visualized, and both the head and thorax should be properly aligned to the x-ray beam. Pulling down of the shoulders will often help visualize C-7. A swimmer's view also is useful, and arm positioning for this need not place the cervical spine at risk. This view frequently will visualize the upper thoracic vertebrae.

The major features to be assessed on the lateral view are soft tissue swelling, particularly above the epiglottis; intervertebral alignment (anterior cortex, posterior cortex, dorsum of lateral masses, parallelness and overlap of articular facets, spinolaminar line); bone fragmentation; and spinal canal size. The latter correlates with risk of injury, although it does not correlate with likelihood of recovery. The normal value for the ratio of canal diameter to body diameter is 0.8 or greater.

Anteroposterior View Certain types of lateral mass fractures and sagittal plane fractures (also called vertical compression fractures) may be visualized on the anteroposterior view. Additionally, this view may show the altered separation between spinous process tips caused by flexion-induced injuries (Fig. 2).

The mandible must be held open (open mouth anteroposterior) to see C-1 and C-2. In a comatose patient, this can be accomplished by placing a gauze roll between the teeth. Shooting one view with the beam slightly angulated cephalad and another with it slightly caudad increased the likelihood of visualizing C-1 and C-2 well, especially in a patient with limited mandibular excursion.

Oblique View A trauma oblique is obtained with the x-ray beam 45 degrees off vertical, the patient supine, and an ungridded cassette horizontal and located towards the opposite side of the patient. This view shows the pedicles and articular process well (Fig. 3), although the appearance of the spine is slightly spread out. A major benefit of the oblique view is that the patient can remain supine; no rotation of the torso or head is required. Furthermore, oblique views often are superior to any other technique, including CT or MRI scans, for visualizing articular process fractures and subluxations. In difficult questions of facet subluxations, flexed oblique views also can be obtained.

CT Scan CT scanning should be considered an adjunct to plain radiographs in cervical spine trauma. Often plain

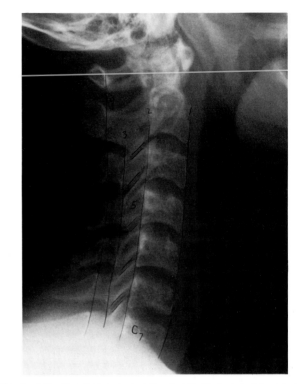

Fig. 1 Lateral radiograph reveals normal alignment of 1, anterior cortices; 2, posterior cortices; 3, dorsum of lateral masses; 4, spinolaminar junctions; and 5, parallel articular process facets. There is a mild compression fracture at C-6.

radiographs are more than sufficient to define the structural damage. CT scans may define certain longitudinally oriented fractures that are not seen well on plain radiographs (for example, nondisplaced laminar fractures), but CT scans are much less sensitive for detecting fractures in the transverse plane (for example, articular process fractures). Oblique plain radiographs probably are more sensitive than reformatted, overlapping, transverse CT cuts for detecting certain articular process injuries, and certainly are more readily available. CT scans may be useful in delineating injuries to the atlantoaxial complex, particularly rotatory subluxation and C-1 ring fractures.

Tomography Excellent visualization of the lateral masses is possible with this technique, using either linear or nonlinear motion patterns. Tomography is helpful in defining the extent of a facet injury (fracture/subluxation). However, most available units have a vertical beam, requiring that the patient be positioned lying on the side to obtain lateral views; this can be awkward or dangerous with an acute spine injury. Tomography is particularly helpful in determining the anatomic level of a dens fracture.

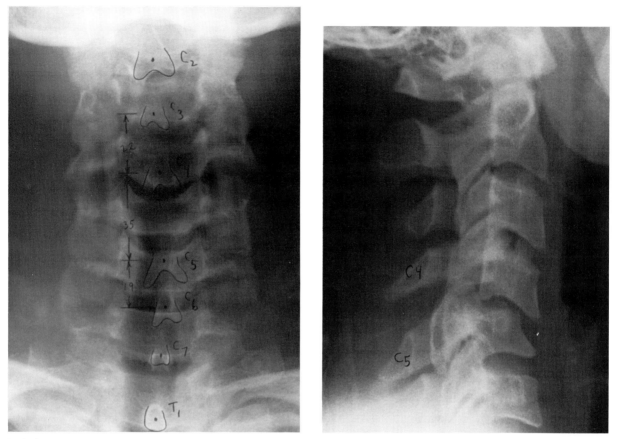

Fig. 2 **Left**, Anteroposterior view. Spinous process separation may be seen even at the cervicothoracic junction. If an interspinous-process distance is more than 50% greater than both the one above and the one below it, there is a high probability of a significant flexion injury. (Reproduced with permission from Naidich JB, Naidich TP, Garfein C, et al: The widened interspinous distance: A useful sign of anterior cervical dislocation in the supine frontal projection. *Radiology* 1977;123:113-116.) **Right**, Lateral view reveals C-4 and C-5 bilateral perched facets.

Myelography Traditional myelography involves prone positioning with the neck in extension and, thus, has limited use in management of acute spine injuries. Computed tomography with intrathecal contrast may be useful in determining the integrity of the intervertebral disk or evaluating for cord compression.

Magnetic Resonance Imaging The exact role for MRI scanning is not yet clear. Advantages include visualization of not only the surface but also the interior of the cord and disk. Cord hematomas, syringomyelia, and subtle disk tears can be detected. Evaluation of disk integrity may be particularly important following a facet injury. Some muscle and ligament injuries may be visualized. Multilevel injuries may be apparent on MRI. An MRI is more effective than a CT scan in assessing cord abnormalities. Disadvantages include less optimal bone detail than CT scanning and the fact that internal cord and disk changes may require hours or days after injury to become apparent. If a patient requires monitoring and respiratory support, special equipment must be used in the magnetic fields.

Dynamic Lateral Radiographs Although these often are referred to as flexion/extension views, it is usually the flexed view that is helpful in detecting a ligamentous injury that is not apparent on the neutral view. When significant trauma is suspected and neutral radiographs are normal, this view may be helpful. Physician supervision is advisable when instability is suspected. An adequate amount of flexion is necessary for the test to be meaningful. One convenient and safe method is to support the head with a lead-gloved hand or small pillow after flexed posture is actively achieved by the patient in the supine position. Interpretation of results is based on comparing the motion at each segment to that at adjacent levels. Muscle splinting may prevent sufficient flexion for detection of structural damage, which may become detectable only on repeat radiographs taken a few days later.

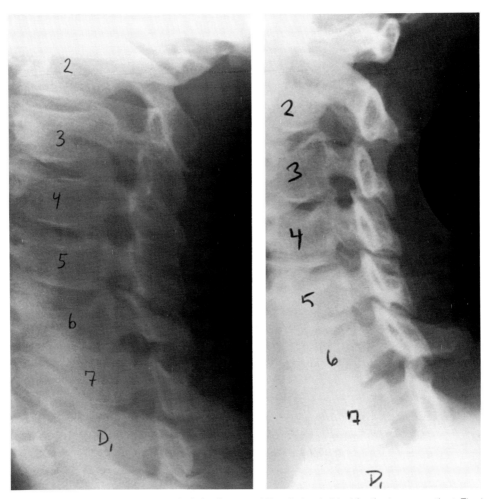

Fig. 3 **Left**, Because no neck or body rotation is needed, the "trauma oblique" view is ideal for the trauma patient. The lateral masses and foramen are well seen, despite the 45-degree angle between beam and cassette. **Right**, Standard oblique view, with cassette perpendicular to x-ray beam.

Other Modalities Technetium bone scanning may be useful under certain limited circumstances, such as when preexisting cervical spine trauma may be present. Ultrasonography is useful for intraoperative imaging of the spinal cord after a laminotomy is performed.

Classification of Injuries

Classification involves description of both of the two major components involved: neural and osteoligamentous.

Neural Spinal cord injuries are divided into complete and incomplete injuries. Incomplete injuries include nerve root injury, anterior cord syndrome, central cord syndrome, and Brown-Sequard syndrome. Functional and quantitative criteria can be used to classify injuries.

The most widely used system for evaluation of functional recovery is the Frankel scale, which consists of five grades (A-E), based on motor and sensory deficits. Fran-

kel A is complete paralysis; Frankel E is normal function. Grades B through D have sensory preservation below the level of injury and vary according to motor deficit: B, no voluntary motor function; C, useless motor function; and D, useful voluntary motor function.

A more quantitative system of motor and sensory evaluation, which assigns points for motor and sensory preservation, has been developed for evaluating the efficacy of therapy, based on standardized muscle testing techniques. This system allows more precise evaluation of function and recovery; however, it is more time consuming. Naming of cord injury level by the distal-most level with fully normal function has become widely accepted.

Osteoligamentous Various classification systems have been proposed, most of which have been based on the presumed injury mechanism. Consensus still has not been reached. There is a growing body of biomechanical literature that characterizes the behavior of cadaveric spines subjected to various injuries. However, the relation of these to the in vivo situation is not clear.

Classification systems for cervical trauma have become more complex as our understanding has improved. The early system of flexion, compression, extension, lateral bend, and rotation injuries has been expanded by the addition of more categories, all of which include subcategories arranged by severity of injury. The concept of anterior, middle, and posterior columns has also been helpful.

The term instability has been used widely to try to characterize the magnitude of mechanical insufficiency. When the bony vertebrae are unable to protect the vital cord, support the remainder of the spine, or allow it to move, instability may exit. However, because consensus has not been reached over the definition of instability and how to quantitate it accurately, the relation between instability and treatment is not clear. The ultimate clinical decision is not whether or not the injured spine is stable, but which treatment is best.

Drug Treatment for Spinal Cord Injury

Corticosteroids have been considered for use in an effort to reduce the severity of spinal cord injury. The first National Acute Spinal Cord Injury Study (NASCIS 1) was performed in the early 1980s. This large, multicenter, prospective, randomized double-blind study compared high dose (1,000 mg bolus, then daily for ten days) and standard dose (100 mg bolus, then daily for ten days) administration of methylprednisolone. The results were that the high-dose group: (1) was no better in neurologic recovery; (2) had a statistically significantly higher wound infection rate; and (3) had a higher (although not statistically significant) acute mortality rate.

Because animal studies suggested that yet higher doses might be effective, the NASCIS 2 was performed. The study design was similar to that of NASCIS 1, except an even higher methylprednisolone dose was used (30 mg/kg body weight), and this was compared to naloxone as well as to a placebo. The major results were (1) methylprednisolone treatment begun within eight hours of injury produced significant improvement in both motor and sensory measures, and treatment begun after eight hours produced significant sensory but not motor improvement; (2) naloxone was no better than placebo; and (3) there was no increase in infection, gastrointestinal bleeding, or mortality rates with methylprednisolone.

More recently, GM-1 ganglioside was compared to placebo in a prospective, double-blind, randomized single-center study. The major findings were: (1) motor recovery was significantly improved; (2) for quadriplegia, the recovery was in the legs rather than the arms; and (3) no drug complications occurred. Because the number of subjects was small, 16 in the active and 18 in the placebo group, further study is needed.

General Treatment Issues

Objectives

For the osteoligamentous component of the injury, the objectives are to minimize residual neck pain, loss of motion, and risk of reinjury. For the neural component of the injury, the objectives are to prevent worsening and to optimize the likelihood of improvement. Recovery of even a single nerve root may have major functional implications.

Methods

Osteoligamentous Recovery Realignment may result in improved comfort. Realignment facilitates solid healing (for example, dens fracture). Improved range of motion may result from joint alignment. The risk of further injury is reduced if solid healing is obtained and spinal cord or foraminal encroachment is minimized (for example, facet subluxation).

One method for accomplishing realignment is postural (for example, hyperextension) during bed rest; however, the prolonged time and attendant risks make widespread use of this method impractical. Traction is widely used in the acute phase. Halter traction is possible, but it obstructs access to the mouth, and adequate traction forces are seldom tolerated. Skeletal (cranial) traction is a safe technique that has many advantages. It may be maintained continuously, even during patient transport. Gardner-Wells tongs are perhaps the quickest to apply. In addition, their strength is high and their placement forgiving. Placement of halo rings and 4-point tongs is more time-consuming; however, they provide more control and may be attached to a vest to provide ongoing treatment.

A number of issues regarding skeletal traction are not resolved: (1) how much force should be used initially; (2) how quickly should the force be increased; (3) what is maximum force; and (4) how much, if any, muscle relaxant and/or anesthesia should be used. In addition, the possibility of creating or worsening a neural deficit by increasing extrusion of a disk during realignment raises the issue of whether to perform an MRI scan or myelography before realignment. Manipulation as a sole or major component of the realignment process is not well accepted, although it may have a role as an adjunct to skeletal traction in selected cases. Surgically-obtained realignment may consist of unlocking facet joints, reapproximating spinous processes (for example, by wiring), or restoring anterior body height (for example, anterior interbody graft after burst fracture).

The intent of immobilization is to prevent loss of alignment and to improve bony and ligamentous healing. The three basic methods are bed rest, orthoses, and reconstruction of load-bearing capacity by means of strut grafting and/or internal fixation. Orthoses may be categorized by the body part they contact: cervical (soft collar), occipitomandibular cervical (Queen Anne collar), occipitomandibular high thoracic (Philadelphia collar), occipitomandibular low thoracic (skull-occipitomandibular immobilization, SOMI), and craniothoracic (halovest). Recent developments have occurred, especially in the area of halovests and in the area of internal fixation. Anterior interbody grafting in the presence of posterior ligamentous disruption often does not fully address the mechanical injury and may lead to failure.

Supplementing normal healing is done by bone grafting. Direct repair of ligament or disk damage is not currently feasible. An autogenous bone graft is generally preferred to autologous bone because it is considered to provide a higher rate of incorporation. Bone grafting is particularly appropriate when significant ligamentous and little or no bone damage is present. Satisfactory healing is less likely to occur in ligamentous injuries treated without grafting. Polymethylmethacrylate does not provide the long-term solution needed for acute trauma management.

Neural Recovery Realignment to obtain decompression and immobilization to prevent neural damage are the most direct methods for optimizing neural function. Rarely is there significant residual encroachment on the cord or roots once bony realignment is accomplished, although encroachment may occur from extruded disk material. Even late removal of compressive tissue may be helpful. Laminectomy is indicated only rarely and may significantly increase the mechanical insufficiency.

How rapidly realignment should be accomplished is not well established. One recent study suggests that speed is important: 70% of quadriparetics improved when realignment was performed within six hours of injury, while only 12% improved when realignment occurred later.

Selection of Treatment

Treatment should be selected based on the specific structural abnormality and should address both osteoligamentous and neural treatment objectives. Before selection, the risks of each treatment should be balanced against the benefits for each individual patient. Good comparative studies of outcome are needed. When short-term costs and length of hospital stay were considered in recent comparisons of surgical and nonsurgical management, surgical treatment showed superior results.

Upper Cervical Injuries

The occipital-atlantoaxial complex (Occiput to C-2) differs substantially from the subaxial (C-3 to C-7) region. The synovial joints at C-1 and C-2 are transversely oriented, and there is no intervertebral disk between the occiput and C-1 or C-1 and C-2. Injuries to this area typically involve impact to the head. Neural deficit in surviving patients is uncommon, partly because the ratio of canal to cord diameter is large, and because of the high mortality rate from paralysis at this location.

Occipital Condyle

Occipital condyle fractures are quite rare and can be caused either by avulsion from the alar ligament insertion or by axial compression of the laterally flexed neck. Typically, treatment for several weeks in a occipito-mandibular high thoracic orthosis is sufficient.

Occipital-Atlantal Joint

These also are rare injuries. Subluxations tend to reduce spontaneously, and dislocations typically are fatal. The Powers' ratio (Fig. 4) is quite helpful in confirming the diagnosis on the lateral x-ray. A ratio of more than 1.0 suggests anterior dislocation, while a value of much less than 1.0 suggests a posterior dislocation.

Because traction can overdistract, early immobilization by halovest may be preferable. Occipitocervical arthrodesis (occiput to C-1) may be necessary to prevent late redisplacement.

Atlas (C-1)

Bilateral Posterior Arch Fracture This injury often is seen readily on the lateral radiograph. There is approxi-

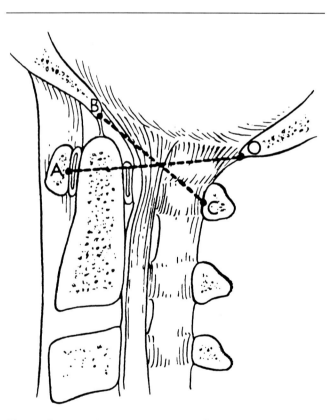

Fig. 4 Powers ratio to detect occipital—C-1 dislocation. The distance between the basion and C-1 posterior arch (BC) is divided by the distance between the opisthion and anterior arch (OA). Normal value is 1.0. (Reproduced with permission from Powers B, Miller MD, Kramer RS, et al: Traumatic anterior atlanto-occipital dislocation. *Neurosurg* 1979;4:12-17.)

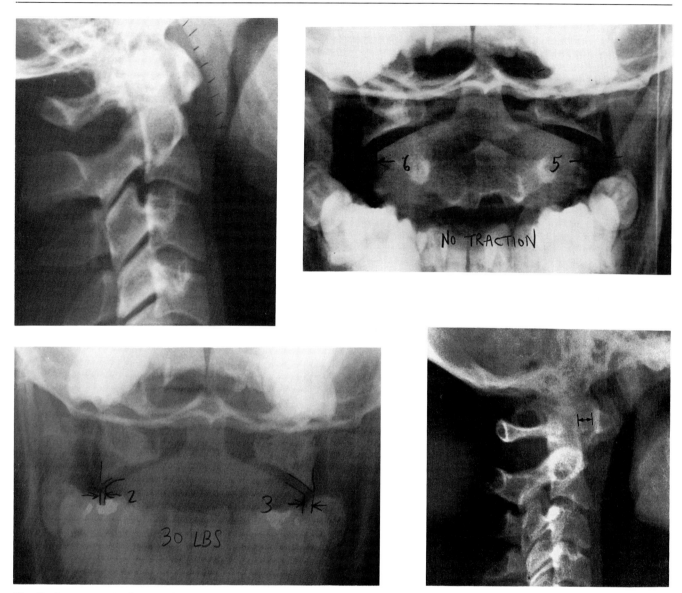

Fig. 5 Anteroposterior C-1 arch (Jefferson) fracture. **Top left**, Lateral view does not visualize anterior arch fractures. Note soft-tissue swelling anteriorly. **Top right**, Combined lateral mass displacement >7 mm suggests transverse ligament is torn. Displacement here is 6 + 5 = 11 mm. **Bottom left**, Cranial traction significantly reduces lateral mass displacement from 11 mm to 2 + 3 = 5 mm. **Bottom right**, Anterior C-1 subluxation with flexion may result from a C-1 ring fracture, but is uncommon. (Reproduced with permission from White AA III, Panjabi MM: *Clinical Biomechanics of the Spine*, ed 2. Philadelphia, JB Lippincott, 1990.)

mately a 50% chance that some other cervical spine injury is present. Thus, further workup may be necessary including CT scan to detect anterior C-1 arch fractures and dynamic lateral radiographs to detect anterior hypermobility. Soft-collar treatment is probably sufficient for isolated posterior arch fractures.

Combined Anteroposterior Arch Fractures (Jefferson Fracture) The original description by Jefferson emphasizes the causative role of axial compression. These injuries can be two-, three-, or four-part fractures (Fig. 5, *top*

left), and the diagnosis is suggested on the anteroposterior open mouth radiograph. Lateral mass displacement of C-1 relative to C-2 is the major finding (Fig. 5, *top right*), and prevertebral soft-tissue swelling is often present. Axial rotation of C-1 on C-2 can cause an apparent displacement. Any displacement of the lateral masses relative to C-2 suggests a fracture of the C-1 ring. Anatomic studies indicate the transverse atlantal ligament is intact if the sum of the lateral mass displacement is less than 7 mm. A displacement greater than 7 mm is strong evidence for ligament disruption, although this does not necessarily result in anterior subluxation (Fig 5, *bottom left*). Additional information may be provided by a CT scan, which may detect a ligament avulsion fracture, even if the displacement is less than 7 mm. Dynamic lateral radiographs (physician-supervised) may also suggest transverse ligament disruption; an atlantodens interval (ADI) greater than 3 mm indicates hypermobility.

The treatment aim of protecting the cord depends on ligamentous healing. The transverse atlantal ligament is the most important. Although late subluxation of C-1 is not common, it should be assessed following bony healing.

The relation between realignment of the C-1 fragments and subsequent neck pain and loss of range of motion is unclear, although at least one recent report shows that realignment by sustained traction improves outcome. Prolonged cranial traction is the only method that will significantly reduce lateral mass displacement (Fig. 5, *bottom right*), because the halovest does not dependably produce sustained traction.

A nondisplaced or minimally displaced injury is often managed with an orthosis; a halovest is recommended by some. For the significantly displaced fracture, the halovest is usually preferred although late atlantoaxial instability may occur.

Other A transverse plane (horizontal) fracture through the anterior arch results from an avulsion injury of the longus colli. This rare injury can be managed with a cervical orthosis. Dynamic lateral radiographs are appropriate to check for hypermobility.

Atlantoaxial (C-1 to C-2) Fixation, Subluxation, and Dislocation

Rotary Fixation (Within the Normal Range of Motion) The structural abnormality of this injury, which also is known as Fielding and Hawkins type I, consists of partial capsular ligament disruption without transverse atlantal ligament disruption. The atlantodens interval is ≤3 mm. The transoral anteroposterior radiograph may show asymmetry between the C-1 lateral masses and the dens, because the C-1 ring has rotated about the dens. This can be seen well on a CT scan.

Unilateral Anterior Subluxation This results from a unilateral capsular tear and a transverse ligament tear. Rotation occurs about the opposite intact lateral joint (Fielding and Hawkins type II). The atlantodens interval is usually increased to 3 to 5 mm.

Bilateral Anterior Subluxation or Dislocation This results from transverse atlantal ligament disruption as well as unilateral or bilateral capsular damage. If the subluxation is symmetric, no rotatory component is present. Asymmetric subluxation is a Fielding and Hawkins type III injury. The atlantodens interval usually is > 5 mm,

and a "wink" sign may be seen on the anteroposterior radiograph if the C-1 lateral mass rides forward and down far enough over the C-2 lateral mass. Diagnosis by radiograph is difficult because C-1 may be rotated about all three axes (flexion, lateral bend, and axial rotation).

These three injury types, Fielding and Hawkins types I through III, usually result from a blow to the head, such as from a fall backward or a car accident. They may be treated initially by traction, but with caution against overdistraction. Supplemental manipulation across the topically anesthetized oropharynx has been described to reduce a dislocated (locked) joint. Reduction may not be maintained in a halovest because of the saddle shape of the joint between C-1 and C-2. If closed reduction cannot be obtained or maintained, open reduction and posterior wiring with a bone graft is usually effected. Reduction may not be possible in late cases.

Posterior Subluxation This Fielding and Hawkins type IV is a rare injury, and includes damage to the dens (for example, a fracture) that allows C-1 to shift posteriorly. Treatment is directed toward both injury components.

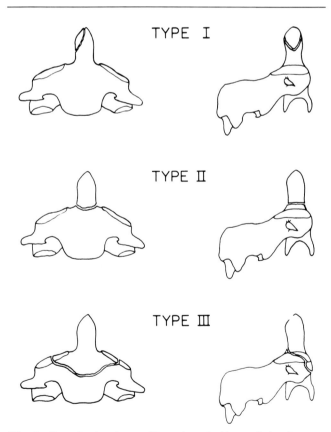

TYPE I

TYPE II

TYPE III

Fig. 6 Dens fracture types. (Reproduced with permission from Anderson LD, D'Alonzo RT: Fractures of the odontoid process of the axis. *J Bone Joint Surg* 1974;56A:1663-1674.)

Axis (C-2) Fractures

Dens Fractures Three types of dens fractures (Fig. 6) have been described based on the anatomic level of injury.

The type I fracture is an avulsion of the alar ligament off one side of the tip of the dens. The alar ligaments connect the dens to the occiput. Evaluation should include dynamic lateral views to rule out anterior subluxation of C-1. A cervical collar for symptomatic management is usually sufficient. This injury, however, may be associated with occipitoatlantal dislocation.

The type II fracture occurs at the base of the dens and, typically, the fracture plane is transverse. When dens displacement occurs, the C-1-dens-transverse ligament complex usually remains intact; the ligamentous disruption may involve the thick atlantoaxial capsular ligaments. The type II fracture is the most common and troublesome, and it has the highest rate of nonunion. Reported risk factors for nonunion include: older age, initial displacement amount, initial displacement direction (posterior worse than anterior), delay in diagnosis, and redislocation in a halovest. Results of one study indicated that 93% of patients healed solidly in a halovest when a number of these risk factors were absent: age under 65; displacement anterior, none, or ≤2mm posterior; and diagnosis within one week. Another study revealed that a significantly greater rate of nonunion occurred in patients who had significant displacement (angulation >10 degrees or translation >5 mm) and were treated with a halo device compared to treatment with surgical arthrodesis.

Generally accepted treatment alternatives include use of a halovest, posterior wiring and arthrodesis of C-1 to C-2, and anterior C-2 screw fixation. Prolonged traction may lead to overdistraction and nonunion. The halovest is widely used, particularly for nondisplaced fractures. There are numerous posterior wiring techniques (Fig. 7) including the Brooks, Griswold, and "Gallie" (apparently first described by Willard). Special caution is needed with posteriorly displaced dens fractures to avoid further displacement.

Management with a halovest for three months is often successful if initial dens displacement is <5 mm, a good reduction can be maintained, and the patient is younger than 50 years old. Posterior atlantoaxial arthrodesis with wire and bone graft has a 95% fusion rate, although an intact C-1 posterior arch is a prerequisite. Anterior screw fixation of the dens has the potential advantage of preserving atlantoaxial motion; however, the procedure has several significant risks.

If the C-1 arch is also fractured, alternatives include: (1) halovest until the C-1 arch is healed, then a posterior C-1 and C-2 arthrodesis if the dens has not healed, (2) anterior screw fixation of the dens (Fig. 8); or (3) Magerl type C-1 and C-2 posterior screw fixation and grafting (Fig. 9). Both the dens screw and C-1 and C-2 screw techniques are technically demanding and should proba-

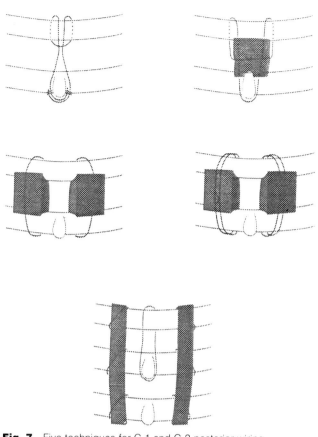

Fig. 7 Five techniques for C-1 and C-2 posterior wiring. Techniques were developed by: Willard and associates in 1941 (often referred to as the Gallie method) (**top left**), McGraw and associates in 1973 (**top right**), Brooks and associates in 1978 (**center left**), D. Griswold and associates in 1978 (**center right**), and E. Forsyth and associates in 1959 (**bottom**). (Reproduced with permission from Krag MH: Biomechanics of the cervical spine, including bracing, surgical constructs, and orthoses, in Frymoyer JW, Ducker TB, Hadler NM, et al (eds): *The Adult Spine: Principles and Practice.* New York, Raven Press, 1991, p 946.)

bly be done by surgeons with significant experience in this area. All three of these options are preferable to initial fusion to the occiput, because of the increased loss of motion with the later.

In type III fractures, the fracture plane passes through the vertebral body. Any combination of angulation and translation can occur. The most typical treatment is 12 weeks of immobilization with a halovest, and the majority of patients heal by bony union. Healing in a fully anatomic position is not likely without prolonged traction. A cervical orthosis may be most appropriate in select patients with stable, impacted fractures, particularly elderly patients. Frequent follow-up is recommended for patients treated in this manner.

Bilateral Pars Interarticularis ("Hangman's" Traumatic Spondylolisthesis of the Axis) Fracture Although this fracture is through the pars interarticularis, it may not

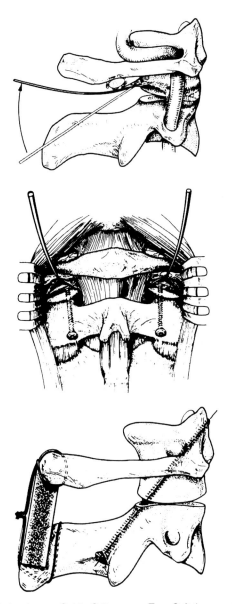

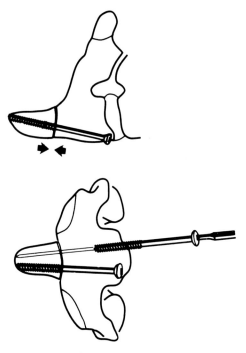

Fig. 9 Anterior screw fixation of dens type II fracture. (Reproduced with permission from Etter C, Coscia M, Jaberg H, et al: Direct anterior fixation of dens fractures with a cannulated screw system. *Spine* 1991;16 (suppl 3):S25-S32.)

Fig. 8 Lateral mass C-1 to C-2 screws. **Top,** Soft tissue retracted by flexible K-wire; **Center,** Posterior view; **Bottom,** Lateral view. (Reproduced with permission from Magerl F, Seemann P: Stable posterior fusion of the atlas and axis by transarticular screw fixation, in Kehr P, Weidner A (eds): *Cervical Spine I.* New York, Springer-Verlag, 1987, p 322.)

This injury is readily seen on a plain lateral radiograph. A common classification includes four subgroups. Type I is minimally displaced and may be treated in an extended or regular Philadelphia-type collar. Type II has significant angulation and translation and typically is treated with a halovest for 12 weeks. Type IIA, in addition to the fractures of type II, has widening of the posterior part of the C2-3 disk with traction, and should be treated in a halovest. Halo traction may cause overdistraction of this injury. Type III has angulation, translation, and also unilateral or bilateral facet dislocation at C2-3.

Type II injuries may be difficult to manage. Following reduction, a halovest trial is reasonable, but this device may not maintain alignment. Open reduction and internal fixation may be necessary to obtain and maintain reduction. Internal fixation techniques include posterior oblique wiring, which resists rotational forces, and screw fixation of C-2 posterior elements to the C-2 body. This latter technique depends on integrity of the C-2 and C-3 capsules and ligaments, which is usually the case.

Lateral Mass Compression Fracture These uncommon injuries result from a compressive load to the laterally flexed neck and may include varying amounts of C-2 lateral mass comminution. Treatment is largely symptomatic, although a halovest may be helpful for large

necessarily involve the C2-3 disk and thus really is not a spondylolisthesis. The term "hangman's fracture" is not accurate for the majority of cases, because the mechanism of injury for clinically encountered fractures often lacks the large traction force present in judicial hangings. Forceful extension of an already extended neck is the most commonly described mechanism of injury, but other causes include flexion of a flexed neck and compression of an extended neck.

amounts of comminution and vertebral height loss. Late C-1 and C-2 arthrodesis may be needed for chronic pain management.

Lower Cervical (C-3 to C-7) Injuries

The C-3 to C-7 vertebrae are fairly uniform and quite different, morphologically and functionally, from C-1 and C-2. The ratio between cord and canal diameters is less in the subaxial spine than that at C-1 and C-2, and there is correspondingly decreased intervertebral mobility. Lower cervical injuries can be divided into three subcategories: (1) Minor compression and avulsion fractures have no facet, spinal canal, or significant ligamentous involvement. These injuries do not involve significant disruption of the posterior tensile or anterior compressive loadbearing capacity. (2) Facet joint injuries include subluxation, dislocation, and fracture. If the displacement is large enough, disk disruption is also present and nerve roots or the spinal cord are at risk for impingement. (3) Complex fractures involve substantial disruption of tensile elements (anterior or posterior), loss of anterior compressive loadbearing capacity, and/or compromise of the spinal canal. Burst and tear drop fractures/dislocations are examples of complex injuries.

Minor Compression and Avulsion Fractures

Spinous Process Fracture These fractures occur most frequently at C-7 and are known as "clayshoveler's fracture." A sudden, single overload is a common cause. The site of occurrence relates to the manner in which the ligamentum nuchae attaches to C-6 and C-7. Dynamic lateral radiographs are useful to check for hypermobility. Treatment is usually symptomatic. It is common for the spinous process not to unite.

Transverse Process Fracture This fracture is an uncommon injury, presumably caused by a muscle pull, and is treated symptomatically.

Teardrop Avulsion Fracture This fracture involves the anterior, inferior corner of the vertebral body (Fig. 10), and is a very different and much less disruptive injury than the teardrop fracture-dislocation described later. The teardrop avulsion fracture probably is caused by hyperextension, and dynamic lateral radiographs rule out hypermobility. A neck collar for comfort and mild activity restriction for a few weeks are probably appropriate. Late degeneration of the subjacent disk may result.

Wedge Compression Fracture This fracture involves loss of vertebral body height anteriorly; the posterior wall remains intact, and the upper vertebra rotates downward about the two facet joints. The posterior ligaments become taut when the anterior height loss is approximately 25%. Compression of more than 50% without compression of the posterior wall may indicate

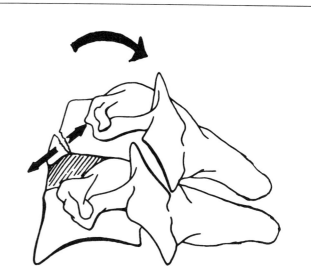

Fig. 10 "Teardrop" avulsion fracture. (Reproduced with permission from Krag MH: Biomechanics of the cervical spine, including bracing, surgical constructs, and orthoses, in Frymoyer JW, Ducker TB, Hadler NM, et al (eds): *The Adult Spine: Principles and Practice.* New York, Raven Press, 1991, p 943.)

posterior ligamentous instability, which may convert this into a complex fracture.

Fractures with up to 25% compression and an intact posterior wall can be treated with an orthosis. If dynamic lateral radiographs reveal instability, posterior interspinous wiring with a bone graft should be considered to stabilize the disrupted posterior ligamentous complex.

Facet Joint Injuries

These are the most frequently missed injuries on radiographic evaluation of acute cervical spine trauma. Trauma oblique radiograph views are important here.

Subluxation (unilateral or bilateral) Structural damage includes partial tearing of the posterior ligaments on the affected side(s), including, to some extent, the posterior portion of the disk. A lateral view radiograph may show mild anterior subluxation of the vertebral body above and soft-tissue swelling anteriorly. Also, there may be a decreased amount of overlap of the articular processes relative to the facet joint above. Dynamic lateral radiographs (physician supervised) may determine if there is hypermobility.

Tomography is useful to determine the presence of a fracture and the extent of displacement. Minimal subluxation is often treated with a Philadelphia-type collar for six weeks. Careful follow-up is appropriate to ensure that progressive subluxation does not occur. Posterior wiring with iliac graft should be performed for progressive subluxation.

Various patterns of posterior wiring have been described. No clear difference between these various meth-

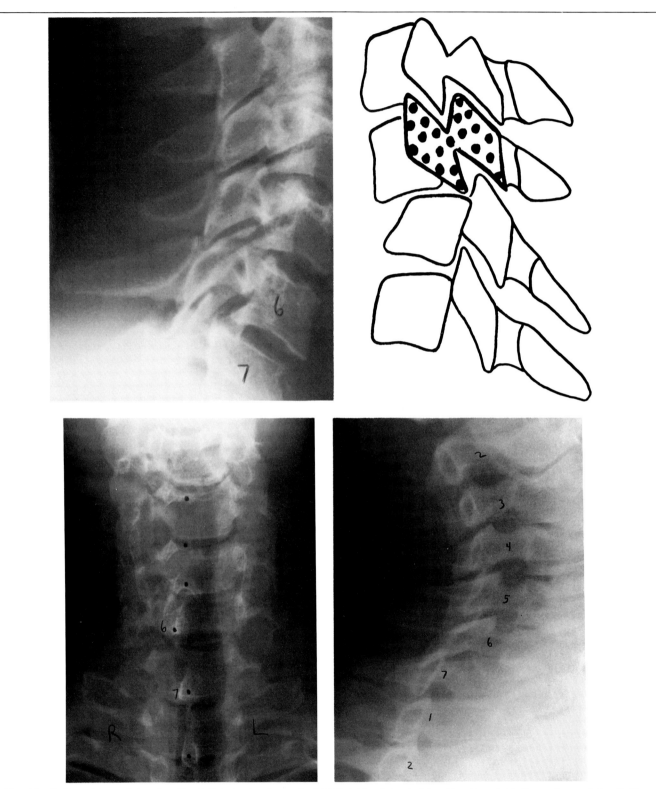

Fig. 11   Unilateral facet dislocation. **Top left**, Lateral radiograph of C6-7 right unilateral dislocation. **Top right**, Same view as left, with "bow-tie" sign shown. Note entire spine above dislocated vertebra is rotated, while below it, right and left lateral masses are superimposed. (Reproduced with permission from Gerlock AJ Jr: *The Cervical Spine in Trauma: Advanced Exercises in Diagnostic Radiology*. Philadelphia, WB Saunders, 1978, vol II.) **Bottom left**, Anteroposterior radiograph shows deviation of C-6 spinous process towards the side of the dislocation (right). **Bottom right**, "Trauma" oblique view shows C-6 dislocated forward on C-7.

ods has been shown in terms of clinical outcome. All are associated with a low failure rate.

Unilateral Facet Dislocation This injury involves forward rotation of one side of the vertebra about the contralateral facet joint. This causes the central portion of the vertebral body to subluxate approximately 25% of the anteroposterior body diameter (Fig. 11, *top left*), and the two lateral masses of the dislocated vertebra to overlap only partially on the lateral view radiograph, giving a "bow-tie" sign (Fig. 11, *top right*). The anteroposterior radiograph shows the spinous process deviated towards the dislocated side (Fig. 11, *bottom left*). The anteriorly dislocated inferior articular process is forced down into the lower half of the neuroforamen, typically causing nerve root compression. This may readily be seen on the trauma oblique radiograph (Fig. 11, *bottom right*). Nonetheless, delays in diagnosis are not rare (40% of patients in one study). Clinically, patients may have torticollis: axial rotation to the contralateral side and lateral bend to the injured side.

Treatment is somewhat controversial. Skeletal traction is recommended by many, followed by open reduction if unsuccessful. The use of closed reduction by manipulation under general anesthesia has been recommended by some and condemned by others. Because of a substantial rate of unsuccessful reduction with traction alone, some recent reports recommend gentle manipulation with radiographic guidance as an adjunct.

Because realignment increases the likelihood of neurologic improvement and may reduce postinjury pain, open reduction is preferred when a closed reduction cannot be obtained. Open reduction is generally performed posteriorly, which allows direct visualization of the articular processes. The anterior approach for this problem provides a limited view and involves additional disruption to the already traumatized disk. However, it does allow complete removal of the disk, which eliminates the risk of inducing paralysis from disk extrusion during reduction. Disk herniation can be identified either by magnetic resonance imaging or by myelography. Anterior diskectomy and interbody fusion may be necessary if significant disk extrusion is present. Failure to recognize a significant disk extrusion, which more commonly occurs with bilateral facet dislocation, can result in a catastrophic neurologic deficit.

Successful closed reduction may be followed either by halovest treatment, typically for three months, or by posterior wiring and bone grafting. Because spontaneous bone fusion may not occur after this injury, many authorities recommend internal fixation and bone grafting, even after successful closed reduction, especially in the presence of neurologic deficit.

Spinous process wiring and grafting is widely used for this injury. Articular process interlocking combines with the tension-band effect of the wire to provide good protection against flexion, anterior subluxation, or axial rotation. If there is an articular process fracture or a "float-ing" lateral mass (ipsilateral lamina and pedicle fractures), the bony block resisting anterior shift on the affected side may be lost, and additional control may be needed (see the section on articular process fractures).

Bilateral Facet Dislocations These dislocations are associated with a high incidence of cord injury. There is approximately 50% anterior displacement of the upper vertebral body with respect to the lower on the lateral radiograph. This injury involves disruption of virtually all ligaments and the disk. Recently, attention has focused on the detection of disk disruption associated with cervical trauma. A case of quadriplegia has been reported, which developed during open reduction, after which a large disk protrusion into the canal was detected. Disk herniation is often associated with bilateral dislocations and may be exacerbated by reduction, leading to neurologic deficit. Magnetic resonance imaging or myelography is useful in this regard. An important unresolved issue is how to predict which patient is at sufficient risk to warrant anterior diskectomy before realignment (Fig. 12).

Initial treatment usually involves skeletal traction in an attempt to obtain reduction, which usually succeeds. The

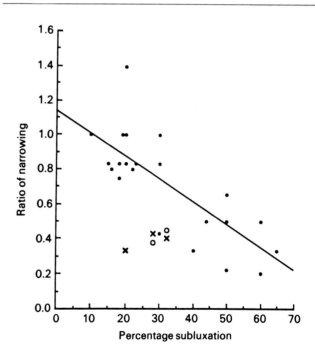

Fig. 12 Disk height ratio versus amount of anterior subluxation (both measured before realignment) for patients with facet dislocations. Three patients who had worsened neurologic deficits after realignment and had a disk herniation are shown by "X." Note these have only a modest amount of subluxation, yet quite a reduction in disk height, apparently because of disk material loss into the spinal canal. (Reproduced with permission from Robertson PA, Ryan MD: Neurological deterioration after reduction of cervical subluxation: Mechanical compression by disc tissue. *J Bone Joint Surg* 1992;74B:224-227.)

amount of force needed is variable; up to one third of body weight is frequently recommended. Safe upper limits have not been well-established, although published reports include forces up to 60 to 75 lbs. Redislocation is occasionally encountered; moderate cervical extension and traction weight reduction will tend to prevent this. Neurologic recovery may improve with realignment. The usual treatment for this injury following reduction is spinous process wiring and arthrodesis with mobilization in the upright posture as rapidly as tolerated postoperatively. Halovest management after closed reduction has also been used; however, potential problems include redislocation, inadequate healing, and scapular or other decubiti in patients with insensate skin.

Articular Process Fractures These are often accompanied by unilateral or bilateral facet joint subluxation or dislocation. The presence of a fracture of the articular process and subluxation or dislocation may significantly alter treatment because the bony resistance to forward subluxation (superior articular process of the lower vertebra) is compromised. With high-grade anterior subluxation ($\geq 50\%$), there remains little, if any, anterior shear resistance by the disk or ligaments. Interspinous wiring alone may not be sufficient treatment.

Articular process fractures can be readily overlooked, especially if intervertebral realignment has already occurred spontaneously. Lateral and oblique radiographs, however, will often demonstrate the injury. Apical fractures of the superior process are usually associated with transient high-grade bilateral facet subluxation and cord injury. The fracture fragment may be small enough that the remaining part of the superior process provides an adequate bony block. Basal fractures of the superior process typically are associated with root or cord deficit because the vertebral subluxation cannot be resisted by the incompetent superior articular process. Flexion of the superior vertebral body usually does not occur, because the subluxing inferior articular process does not have to ride up an intact superior process. Inferior process fractures are typically at the base of the process and tend not to be associated with neurologic deficit, because the neuroforamen is not narrowed. Typically there is no flexion with the anterior subluxation of the superior vertebral body.

A small apical fracture of the superior process without subluxation on dynamic lateral radiographs may be treated with an orthosis. Other articular process fractures are typically managed with posterior wiring and grafting, because an orthosis, including the halovest,

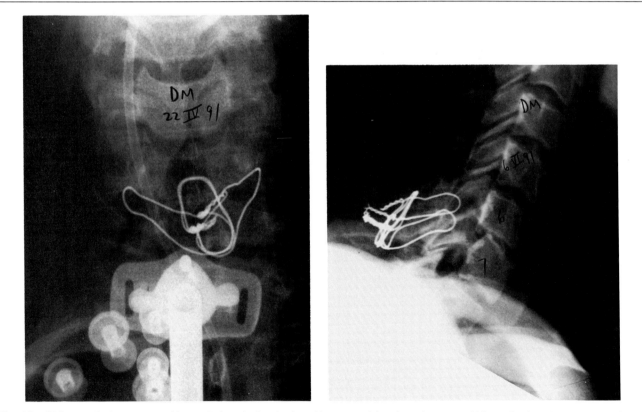

Fig. 13 Oblique articular process wiring technique for interior basal fracture subluxation, shown used bilaterally, for added strength. **Left,** Anteroposterior radiograph taken ten days after surgery. **Right,** Lateral radiograph taken two months after surgery.

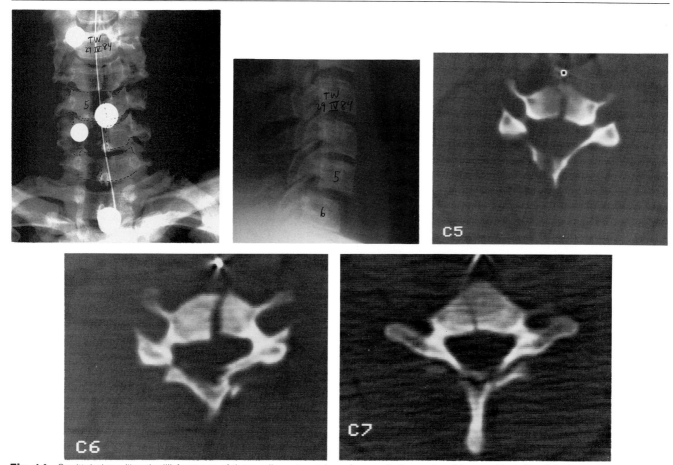

Fig. 14   Sagittal plane ("vertical") fractures of three adjacent vertebrae from a shallow water diving accident. **Top left**, Anteroposterior radiograph. **Top center**, Lateral radiograph. **Top right**, CT scan of C-5. **Bottom left** and **right**, CT scans of C-6 and C-7.

may not maintain the reduction and prolonged traction may not be practical. Spinous process wiring alone may not provide the derotating force needed to maintain realignment. Thus, an oblique facet wiring technique has been developed to manage these injuries. In this technique, the wire passes through the inferior articular process then around the spinous process of subjacent vertebra. It resists both forward and upward motion of the inferior articular process (Fig. 13). Interspinous process wire only resists upward and not forward motion. A more recent, somewhat controversial alternative is posterior cervical plates.

Complex Fractures

These involve the spinal canal, as well as substantial disruption of compressive and anterior or posterior tensile loadbearing elements. Most commonly fractured is the vertebral body, followed by the lamina, and then the pedicle.

Vertebral Body Fractures Without Facet or Laminar Involvement   These may involve a significant axial com-

pressive force applied with the neck in a nearly straight posture. Three subgroups, arranged by increasing injury severity, are sagittal plane fracture, burst fracture, and tear-drop fracture-dislocation.

The sagittal plane fracture has previously been described as a vertical compression fracture, but more specifically it is sagittally and not coronally oriented. This fracture often occurs in combination with other fractures in the same or an adjacent vertebra (for example, laminar fracture, facet dislocation, or teardrop fracture-dislocation), extensive ligamentous damage, and paralysis. The key feature is a midsagittal fracture plane extending from one vertebral end plate to the other, which is best seen on the anteroposterior radiograph (Fig. 14). The lateral radiograph may show no abnormality at all.

The burst fracture (Fig. 15) includes retropulsion of bone fragments into the spinal canal, usually from the superior endplate of the lower vertebra. This may occur with or without involvement of the inferior endplate or the lamina. This injury is considered by some to be a variant of a tear-drop fracture-dislocation.

Treatment alternatives include prolonged traction until sufficient bone union occurs to sustain axial compres-

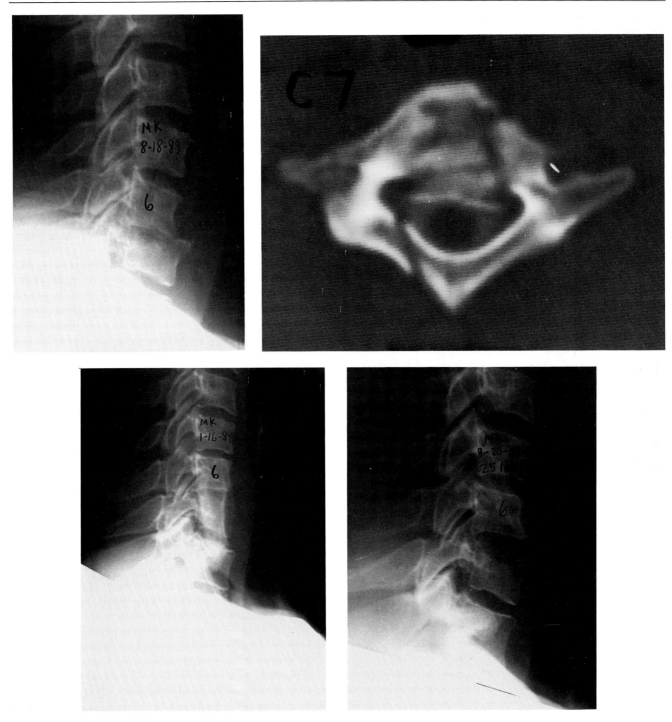

Fig. 15 Burst fracture of C-7. Note retropulsion of body fragment with no apparent disruption of posterior elements. **Top left**, Lateral radiograph. **Top right**, CT transverse cut at C-7. **Bottom left**, Lateral radiograph in traction. The fragment is reduced and there is no posterior ligament disruption. **Bottom right**, Lateral radiograph five months after corpectomy and strut graft.

sive forces, or an anterior strut graft. Orthoses, including the halovest, do not provide significant resistance to axial compressive loads. Traction alone may not produce adequate canal decompression. Removal of bone fragments at the time of strut graft placement may be appropriate. Addition of an anterior cervical plate may be considered, especially if posterior ligamentous disruption is present. This latter treatment is somewhat controversial.

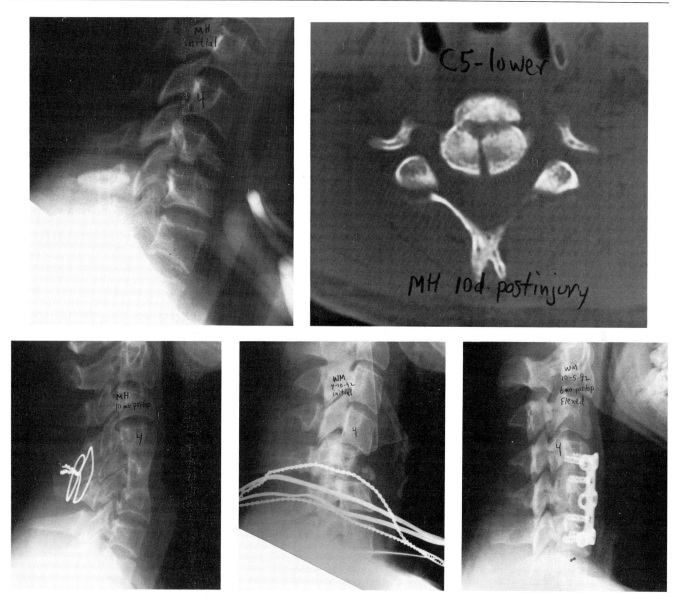

Fig. 16 Complex fracture-dislocations. **Top left**, "Teardrop" fracture-dislocation consisting of comminution of the body (including the anterior-interior fragment) and disruption of posterior ligaments sufficient to produce facet subluxation. **Top right**, CT transverse cut of C-7 shows typical three-part body fracture. **Bottom left**, Surgical repair by anterior corpectomy and strut graft plus posterior spinous process wiring. **Bottom center**, Similar to top left, except worse retropulsion. **Bottom right**, Surgical repair by corpectomy, strut graft and anterior plate attached by screws, which are locked to the plate by recessed, tapered set screws.

The tear-drop fracture-dislocation (Fig. 16, *top left*) was originally described by Schneider and Kahn and is a very different injury from the tear-drop avulsion fracture shown in Figure 10. This fracture-dislocation involves a major compressive force, and much more disruption than is seen in the avulsion fracture. Although the name of this injury has focused attention on the anteroinferior body fragment, the original report emphasized the importance of the posteroinferior fragment. It is this fragment that encroaches into the canal and causes the paralysis that frequently accompanies this injury. Careful examination of the facet joints and articular processes should be made to determine whether or not facet joint disruption is also present (see below).

Treatment for this severe disruption typically involves at least anterior strut grafting. The role of anterior plating is similar to that for treatment of burst fractures. Prolonged traction can also be used, but may not be practical.

Body Fractures with Facet or Laminar Involvement Any of the above body fractures can occur along with facet

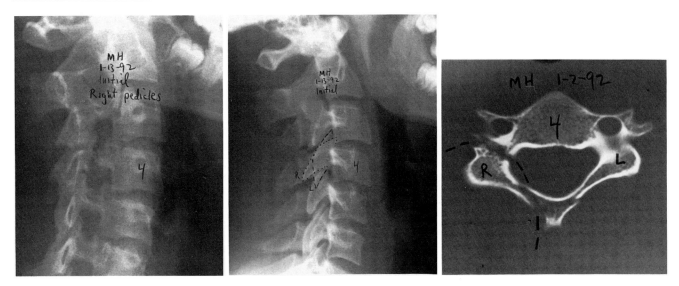

Fig. 17   "Floating" lateral mass. **Left**, Lateral radiograph; note rotated orientation (horizontalization) of right lateral mass. **Center**, Oblique radiographic view. **Right**, CT scan, transverse cut.

disruption or laminar fractures. The mechanism involves severe compression, although the posture of the neck and point of load application may vary.

These injuries involve the most severe mechanical insufficiency in the cervical spine, and the preferred treatment usually includes reconstruction of a compressive loadbearing capacity by means of a strut graft, and of flexion and anterior loadbearing capacity by means of posterior wiring and articular process interlocking (Fig. 16, *top right*). However, anterior plating along with a strut graft (Fig. 16, *bottom*), though somewhat controversial, appears promising according to one recent report.

Other Fractures   Bilateral laminar fractures usually accompany other significant injuries, such as a burst fracture at the same vertebral level, or a bilateral facet subluxation at the subjacent facets. Their presence may significantly alter treatment, such as requiring extension of the posterior wiring up to the next intact level. Bilateral articular process wiring (Fig. 13) or posterior plates may avoid longer instrumentation.

The floating lateral mass fracture (Fig. 17) involves a pedicle fracture and ipsilateral laminar fracture, which completely detach the entire lateral mass from the vertebral body and the remainder of the posterior elements. Often there are other significant associated injuries, such as bilateral facet subluxation or dislocation. This injury involves not only the facet joint above, but also the one below the floating lateral mass. Because disk injury usually is present also, there is a significant tendency for forward subluxation, which cannot be well controlled by an orthosis. Thus, internal fixation is usually the treatment of choice.

Ankylosing spondylitis is relatively rare and fracture of the cervical spine is an uncommon injury if one considers an entire population of spine injuries (eight out of 300 cervical spine injuries in one series). However, there is a very high rate of spinal cord injury associated with fractures in ankylosing spondylitis patients (11 out of 12 patients in a recent series). Fractures in these patients may be difficult to visualize on plain radiographs, because they frequently occur at or near the cervicothoracic junction and there may be no or little displacement. Bone scanning or tomography may be necessary to confirm the diagnosis.

Treatment options include halo traction, cervical orthosis (halovest or sterno-occipitomandibular orthosis), and internal fixation. Halo traction, if used, should initially be applied in the direction of the preexisting deformity. Vigorous attempts to correct a preexisting deformity may lead to neurologic compromise. Alignment must be monitored with periodic radiographs if treatment with an orthosis is selected. Morbidity may be significant with surgical intervention.

Gunshot Wounds

These seldom cause sufficient osteoligamentous damage to warrant surgical treatment. Halovest treatment is sometimes used, although other orthoses often suffice. A recent large multicenter study revealed that bullet removal did not improve neurologic recovery for thoracic spine injuries, as assessed by motor and sensory recovery and by pain reduction. There were too few cases with cervical injuries to allow meaningful conclusions, but there are no clear reasons why the cervical spine should respond differently from T-1 through T-11. Broad spectrum antibiotics alone seem to provide sufficient protection against infection, even when the gastrointestinal canal has been violated. Cerebrospinal fluid leaks have been more of a problem with bullet removal than without, and lead poisoning does not seem to be a problem. However, there may be a role for removal of the compressive mass in cases of incomplete spinal cord injury.

Internal Fixation with Plates and Screws

Anterior Cervical Plates   The role of anterior plating for management of acute trauma is evolving. Initially, plates used for cervical spine problems were designed for other purposes. These allowed only one screw per vertebra, and screw loosening was a problem. Plates designed specifically for the cervical vertebrae include at least two screws per vertebra and the loosening rate is now less than 3% regardless of whether or not the screws were placed through the posterior cortex. Further reduction of the loosening rate may be possible through use of screws that can be expanded within bone or against the plate through which they pass, or that have a rough plasma-sprayed surface. Such screws are intended not to penetrate the posterior cortex and may be safer. Experience with these methods is limited.

Intact posterior elements combined with a well-fitted strut graft provide a dependable surgical construct, and addition of an anterior plate may preclude the need for posterior stabilization when moderate amounts of posterior damage are also present. Biomechanical tests reveal that anterior plating alone is not sufficient when extensive posterior disruption is present. However, a growing clinical experience shows that, even for very unstable three-column injuries, anterior plating and grafting, combined with mobilization in a skull-occiputomandibular immobilization or plastizote collar, produce excellent results.*

Lower Cervical Posterior Plates   Various designs of posterior plates have been developed. These include plates that can be attached both above and below by screws into the lateral masses (Fig. 18), and plates that are attached above by screws into the lateral masses and below by hooks under the lamina (Fig. 19). Multilevel posterior plates may have a role in stabilizing patients with deficient posterior elements (for example, following multilevel laminectomy). Biomechanical comparative testing has been done for various types of posterior as well as anterior plate methods. Screws placed obliquely to the transverse plane (parallel to the facet joint plane) have a longer screw length and, thus, are stronger. The optimal balance among strength of fixation, safety, and ease of implantation remains to be established.

---

*The various devices designed to restore alignment of the spine include some that are in varying stages of approval by the Food and Drug Administration.

Injuries Without Fracture or Subluxation

No Cord or Root Dysfunction

Sprains and Strains   These injuries are caused by overstretching of a muscle or ligament and may result in pain, localized tenderness, and reduced range of motion. Radiographs are frequently normal or may only reveal loss of the cervical lordosis, which is a nonspecific indicator of muscle spasm.

A recent study of all patients treated in an emergency department for neck pain revealed that 82% of injuries were caused by vehicle accidents (54% were rear-end collisions) and 11% resulted from falls. On initial examination, 48% had no posterior midline tenderness, and 60% had no impairment of motion. Pain onset was delayed in 64%. Only 2% had radiographically apparent bony or ligamentous injury. At six-month follow-up, 43% had persistent moderate or severe pain.

Traditionally, the principles of treatment are the same as for sprains and strains elsewhere in the body, including short-term immobilization followed by graded motion, and nonsteroidal anti-inflammatory medication. Few randomized prospective comparative treatment studies have been performed.

Vehicle Acceleration and Deceleration ("Whiplash") Injuries   These injuries overlap the previous category, but are discussed separately because (1) at least one aspect of the mechanism is clearly defined; (2) the injuring forces typically are applied rapidly and unexpectedly, and may be quite large; and (3) medical-legal issues frequently are involved.

This condition may result in symptoms the pathophysiology of which is not well understood, and which may be difficult for the patient to describe: headaches, visual blurring, diplopia, nausea, vertigo, impaired balance, retro-orbital or retro-auricular pain, dysphagia, hoarseness, and jaw pain. Structures that may be involved in addition to skeletal muscles and ligaments include cranial nerves, vestibular apparatus and other intracranial structures, sympathetic nerve fibers, esophagus and trachea, temporomandibular joint, and intervertebral disks.

A significant percentage of patients have long-lasting symptoms: 42% persist beyond 12 months and 36% persist beyond 24 months. However, of those patients with symptom resolution by 12 months, 88% became symptom-free within the first eight weeks.

There are a number of risk factors for a poor outcome. Initial presence of occipital headaches, suprascapular or arm symptoms, abnormal nerve root signs, and interscapular pain indicate a poor likelihood for recovery. Females are twice as likely as males to have persistent symptoms at six months follow-up, although there is no difference at two years. Preexisting cervical spondylosis and a sedentary occupation are risk factors.

Treatment modalities include initial management with

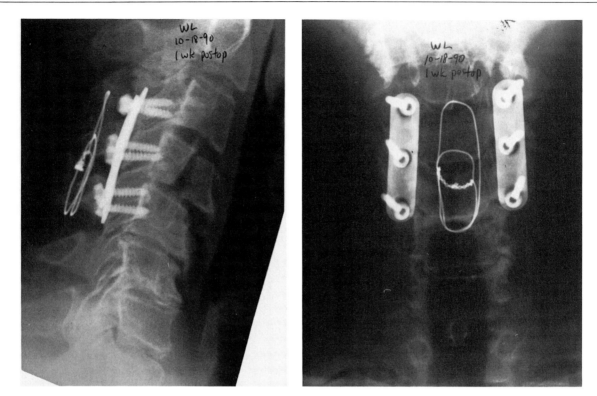

Fig. 18   Posterior plates. **Left**, Lateral radiograph. **Right**, Anteroposterior radiograph.

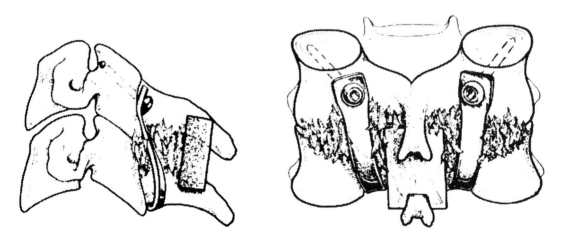

Fig. 19   Posterior hook plates. No screws are needed for the lower end of the plate. There is no disruption to the subjacent facet joint. (Reproduced with permission from Magerl L, Grob D, Seeman P, et al: Stable dorsal fusion of the cervical spine (C2-TH-1) using hook plates in Kehr P, Weidner A (eds): *Cervical Spine I.* New York, Springer-Verlag, 1987, p 217.)

anti-inflammatory medication, careful but progressive muscle activation, return to function starting soon after injury, and appropriate amounts of reassurance and encouragement.

Cord or Root Dysfunction

The most common cause of this injury is a fall that produces hyperextension in an older patient with preexisting cervical spondylosis and increased cervical lordosis. Excessive anterior buckling of the ligamentum flavum into a canal already compromised by posterior vertebral body osteophytes probably is the cause of the often-associated central cord syndrome: greater motor loss in arms than in legs, and variable sensory loss. Typically, patients are managed nonsurgically with an orthosis, and their neurologic status is carefully monitored.

Annotated Bibliography

General

Bohlman HH: Acute fractures and dislocations of the cervical spine: An analysis of 300 hospitalized patients and review of the literature. *J Bone Joint Surg* 1979;61A:1119-1142.

A comprehensive and detailed review of a large series of patients with a wide spectrum of injury types is presented. Well-established treatment principles are presented and discussed.

Sherk HH, Dunn EJ, Eismont FJ, et al (eds): *The Cervical Spine*, ed 2. Philadelphia, JB Lippincott, 1989.

This general resource of up-to-date information on the cervical spine, prepared by the Cervical Spine Research Society, includes extensive groups of chapters on radiology, fractures and dislocations, and injuries to the spinal cord.

White AA III, Panjabi MM (eds): *Clinical Biomechanics of the Spine*, 2 ed. Philadelphia, JB Lippincott, 1990.

The second edition of this well-established work includes material on cervical spine trauma and related topics.

Patient Evaluation

Allen BL Jr, Ferguson RL, Lehmann TR, et al: A mechanistic classification of closed, indirect fractures and dislocation of the lower cervical spine. *Spine* 1982;7:1-27.

This classification scheme defines not only major categories of injuries, but subcategories within which injury types are arranged by hypothesized gradually increasing severity.

Bracken MB, Separd MJ, Collins WF, et al: A randomized, controlled trial of methylprednisolone or naloxone in the treatment of acute spinal-cord injury: Results of the Second National Acute Spinal Cord Injury Study. *N Engl J Med* 1990;322:1405-1411.

This multicenter, double-blind study of methylprednisolone (MP), naloxone, and placebo showed definite effectiveness for MP but not for the other two. If the MP was given less than eight hours after injury, the improvements were in both motor and sensory function. If it was given more than eight hours after injury, then only sensory improvements resulted.

Geisler FH, Dorsey FC, Coleman WP: Recovery of motor function after spinal-cord injury: A randomized, placebo-controlled trial with GM-1 ganglioside. *N Engl J Med* 1991;324:1829-1838.

The number of patients involved is small enough (23 cervical, 11 thoracic) that definitive conclusions cannot be drawn. However, results suggest that GM-1 may produce significantly improved recovery, without drug complications.

Robertson PA, Ryan MD: Neurological deterioration after reduction of cervical subluxation: Mechanical compression by disc tissue. *J Bone Joint Surg* 1992;74B:224-227.

This paper addresses the important topic of increased neurologic deficit by disk herniation brought on as a result of realignment. All three cases had relatively large disk space height reduction without large subluxation. Of 29 consecutive cervical spine trauma cases, only six had a disk height of 50% or less and a subluxation of 33% or less. Of these six, three were the cases presented, and two others had disk extrusion according to an MRI scan but demonstrated no neurologic deterioration.

General Treatment Issues

Aebi M, Mohler J, Zäch GA, et al: Indication, surgical technique, and results of 100 surgically treated fractures and fracture-dislocations of the cervical spine. *Clin Orthop* 1986;203:244-257.

Most patients were treated within six hours of injury, but only one third of patients (33) had their dislocation reduced within that time. Of these 33, 23 (70%) had some neurologic improvement of one or more Frankel grades. Of the 66 reduced over six hours after injury, only eight (12%) had some improvement. These results indicate that rapid reduction is helpful in neural recovery.

Benzel EC, Larson SJ: Recovery of nerve root function after complete quadriplegia from cervical spine fractures. *Neurosurgery* 1986;19:809-812.

Cord function that is totally absent for 24 hours is not improved by subsequent decompression, however, root recovery is possible. Of 25 patients with internal fixation and nerve root decompression, 15 (60%) experienced some improvement. Of ten patients with stabilization and no decompression, none had improvement. Return of even one nerve root has a large impact on function for a quadriplegic, and may be the difference between independence and dependence on a caretaker.

Krag MH, Beynnon BD: A new halo-vest: Rationale, design and biomechanical comparison to standard halo-vest designs. *Spine* 1988;13:228-235.

Describes the unexpectedly large intervertebral motions and forces that actually occur in halovests. Comparative vest-thorax mobility testing shows that an improved fit of the vest on the thorax can better control cervical motion.

Krag MH, Monsey RD, Fenwick JW: Cranial morphometry related to placement of tongs in the temporoparietal area for cervical traction. *J Spinal Disord* 1989;1:301-305.

The transverse diameter and cranial thickness are measured at multiple sites in the temporoparietal region on cadaveric crania. These data show (1) there is no outward-flaring temporal ridge below which to place traction tong points and (2) tong pin placement is fairly forgiving within a zone 4 cm above, in front, and behind the top of the pinna.

Nielsen CF, Annertz M, Persson L, et al: Posterior wiring without bony fusion in traumatic distractive flexion injuries of the mid to lower cervical spine: Long-term follow-up in 30 patients. *Spine* 1991;16:467-472.

Long-term follow-up in these patients revealed residual pain in 24 (80%), which included pain with motion in 19 (63%). All six of the patients with residual motion had pain that increased with neck movement. The authors conclude long-term results regarding late pain might be improved by adding bony fusion to the stabilizing procedure.

Upper Cervical Injuries

Clark CR, White AA III: Fractures of the dens: A multicenter study. *J Bone Joint Surg* 1985;67A:1340-1348.

This paper reports a multicenter retrospective study sponsored by the Cervical Spine Research Society, involving 144 patients (96 type II). Angulation and displacement were significant factors affecting the outcome of treatment of type II fractures. Patients with significant angulation (more than 10 degrees) or displacement (more than 5 mm) had a significantly greater rate of union with surgical stabilization (posterior orthodesis) compared to treatment with a Halo device.

Fowler JL, Sandhu A, Fraser RD: A review of fractures of the atlas vertebra. *J Spinal Disord* 1990;3:19-24.

Forty-eight consecutive patients with C-1 fractures included two groups of Jefferson fractures: Those with initial lateral displacement of the C-1 lateral masses, and those without. The former group was treated with tong traction for six weeks, the latter group with a sterno-occipitomandibular immobilization (SOMI) brace. At follow-up, three of the traction and four of the SOMI patients were nondisplaced, and had significantly more motion and less pain than patients with displacement at follow-up. None of these 48 patients, even those with large amounts of lateral mass displacement, had anterior subluxation of C-1 on C-2 at follow-up.

Levine AM, Edwards CC: Treatment of injuries in the C1-C2 complex. *Orthop Clin North Am* 1986;17:31-44.

Describes the diagnosis and treatment of the more common types of trauma in this region, based on a very extensive clinical experience. For Jefferson fractures the article notes that anterior C-1 subluxation is very uncommon and that halovests do not provide a distractive component to reduce lateral mass displacement. For certain types of hangman fractures, extended Philadelphia collar wear successfully avoids use of a halovest.

Lower Cervical Injuries

Ostl OL, Fraser RD, Griffiths ER: Reduction and stabilization of cervical dislocations: An analysis of 167 cases. *J Bone Joint Surg* 1989;71B:275-282.

A retrospective comparison of 167 consecutive patients treated by two different methods at two spinal treatment centers, respectively. Gentle manual manipulation to supplement cranial tong traction was found to substantially help in obtaining reduction. Of patients treated nonoperatively, 16% had late fusion for persistent pain. The authors caution against operative treatment in quadriplegics because they encountered a high mortality and pressure sore rate. However, postoperative treatment involved three weeks recumbency with the neck in extension.

Ripa DR, Kowall MG, Meyer PR Jr, et al: Series of ninety-two traumatic cervical spine injuries stabilized with anterior ASIF plate fusion technique. *Spine* 1991;16:S46-S55.

All patients were treated with anterior graft and plate, including 48 grossly unstable three column injuries. Upper and lower screws were placed through the posterior cortex; middle screws were used to secure the graft. A skull-occiput-mandibular immobilization brace was used postoperatively. Fusion rate was 90%.

Soft-Tissue Injuries

LaRocca H: Cervical sprain syndrome: Diagnosis, treatment, and long-term outcome, in Frymoyer JW, Ducker TB, Hadler NM, et al (eds): *The Adult Spine: Principles and Practice*. New York, Raven Press, 1991, chap 50, pp 1051-1062.

This review provides a rational approach to dealing with these injuries. Specific points include a frequent delay in symptom onset: 20% of patients will have symptom onset 3 to 48 hours after injury, and 7% will have onset after 48 hours. Preexisting spondylosis decreases the chances of a good recovery. The role of litigation in impending functional recovery is shown to be much less important than is widely believed.

35

Cervical Spine: Reconstruction

Degenerative Conditions

Cervical Spondylosis and Radiculopathy

Neck Pain Neck pain is commonly believed to be caused by muscle strain or overuse, or by age-related changes in the intervertebral disks and other structures that comprise the functional spine unit.

Physical examination reveals local tenderness and diminished motion. In the absence of referred pain or neurologic symptoms, results of the neurologic examination are usually normal. Radiographs may reveal no abnormality, or they may show disk space narrowing and osteophyte formation. Initial treatment includes short-term rest, immobilization with soft collars, local application of heat or cold, home traction, and nonsteroidal anti-inflammatory agents. Manipulative therapy is unproven in its efficacy and has been associated in a few case reports with tragic complications. The benefits of trigger point or facet injection therapy are controversial. In the absence of neurologic symptoms and signs, further testing with myelography, computed tomography (CT), or magnetic resonance imaging (MRI) is of little or no benefit and may be misleading. A recent study of asymptomatic subjects, using MRI, showed that 19% had either a herniated disk, bulging disks, or foraminal stenosis. In individuals younger than 40 years of age, these findings were present in 14% of those studied, but in those older than 40, the prevalence rose to 28%. Disk degeneration was seen in 25% of asymptomatic subjects under 40 and 57% of those over 40 (Table 1). Levels most commonly involved, in order of involvement, were C5-6, C6-7, and C4-5. These findings emphasize that it is important to correlate clinical symptoms and signs with radiographic and imaging findings.

Surgical treatment (anterior disk excision and fusion) for patients with persistent neck pain without instability or neural symptomatology is controversial, as is the use of diagnostic diskography and diskometry. Anterior disk excision and fusion has been reported to be successful in patients with chronic neck pain in whom diskography has shown morphologic changes called internal disk derangement and in whom the injection reliably reproduces the patient's symptoms.

Radiculopathy

Cervical disk herniation occurs frequently and can cause radicular symptoms if there is impingement of a nerve root. These symptoms are usually isolated to one dermatome or sclerotome, but may not follow strict anatomic

Table 1. Major MRI abnormalities in 63 asymptomatic subjects

Major Abnormality	<40 Yrs. Old (N = 167)	>40 Yrs. Old (N = 97)
Herniated disk	5 (3%)	1 (1%)
Bulging disk	0	1 (1%)
Foraminal stenosis	5 (3%)	9 (9%)
Disk space narrowing	3 (2%)	15 (16%)
Degenerated disk	13 (8%)	36 (37%)
Spurs (spondylosis)	5 (3%)	6 (6%)
Abnormal cord	15 (9%)	1 (1%)

(Adapted with permission from Boden SD, McCowin PR, Davis DO, et al: Abnormal magnetic-resonance imaging scans of the cervical spine in asymptomatic subjects: A prospective evaluation. *J Bone Joint Surg* 1990;72A:1178-1184.)

patterns because of intrathecal rootlet overlap. Herniation is most common at the C5-6 level (C-6 nerve root symptoms), followed by C6-7 and C4-5. As demonstrated by MRI, these are the same levels where degenerative changes are most frequent.

The posterolateral disk is the typical site of herniation, although central posterior and anterior herniation may occur. Frank extrusion of a disk fragment is less common than in the lumbar region. Disk herniation with imaging studies demonstrating apparent nerve root compression can occur without any symptoms or signs of neural dysfunction. At the other extreme, large, centrally located herniations can cause spinal cord compression and result in myelopathic symptoms and findings.

When patients present with radicular symptoms, initial treatment is similar to that for patients with spondylotic neck pain and includes rest, traction, nonsteroidal anti-inflammatory medications, and analgesics. The majority of patients respond to these measures, and neurologic deficits related to root compression improve over a few weeks. If the radicular symptoms persist for six to 12 weeks, or if a major neurologic deficit exists, further diagnostic evaluation and even surgery may be appropriate. The essential clinical exercise is to correlate these findings and symptoms with disk herniation demonstrated by myelography/CT, CT alone, or MRI. In these instances, surgery may be beneficial. For soft posterolateral disk herniation, successful results ranging from 75% to 95% have been reported when either anterior or posterior procedures are used.

Orthopaedic surgeons usually favor anterior disk excision combining the decompression with interbody fusion to maintain disk space height and provide stability. Of 94 patients who underwent this procedure for radiculopathy caused by either disk herniation or spondylotic change, satisfactory results were reported for 88% of these patients, when no other levels of degenerative change were noted. When adjacent asymptomatic spondylotic levels were present and only the symptomatic site was decompressed and fused, only 60% of patients who underwent surgery had satisfactory results at follow-up. These symptoms were presumably caused by accentuated stress concentration at the degenerative levels adjacent to the stabilized segment.

Although complete disk excision is not mandatory for a satisfactory result, the trend in recent years has been to excise protruding and free disk fragments and osteophytes to insure root/cord decompression. Posterior laminotomy-foramenotomy can produce acceptable results without fusion-immobilization when the herniation is lateral and/or significant foraminal stenosis is present.

In a prospective study of a group of patients with soft disk herniations where either an anterior or posterior surgical approach was used, root decompression was performed in both groups, but the disk fragment was excised in the posterior group only when it was easily accessible. A satisfactory result was achieved in 94% of patients who underwent anterior disk excision and interbody fusion and in 74% of those treated with posterior decompressive foramenotomy. Thus, depending on training and experience, a surgeon may elect either approach. However, the anterior surgical approach should always be used for treatment of central disk herniation with cord compression.

Cervical Spondylotic Myelopathy

Compression of the cervical spinal cord can occur as a result of degenerative changes in the cervical spinal column that cause narrowing of the spinal canal. The causes are multifactorial and result in progressive degenerative changes at multiple levels, particularly in the midcervical region. Disk narrowing, osteophyte formation, buckling of the ligamentum flavum, facet hypertrophy, and vertebral subluxation are factors that influence the development and severity of this disorder. Ossification of the posterior longitudinal ligaments is a common cause in Oriental patients. Most of these changes are age-related, and it is not surprising that myelopathy is most prevalent in the elderly. Individuals with congenitally small canals may be predisposed to the disorder. Loss of cervical lordosis can exacerbate the problem by permitting the spinal cord to drape over prominent anterior structures. Compromise of blood supply, resulting from compression of the anterior spinal artery, may influence the disease process. Abnormal motion of the vertebrae or of the spinal cord within the spinal canal may also play a role.

Anterior column dysfunction is common and may be accompanied by a mixed pattern of anterior and central cord involvement. Posterior column function is generally preserved. Compression of the cell body and nerve root will produce lower motoneuron problems in the upper extremities. Lower extremity problems, such as weakness, spasticity, and poor limb control, are common. De-

lay in diagnosis can occur because of the insidious onset of early symptoms.

Myelographically enhanced CT and/or MRI delineate the levels of disease and may provide some information on the condition of the spinal cord. Electrophysiologic tests (electromyography and sensory or motor-evoked potentials) may aid in delineating the degree of dysfunction. Somatosensory potentials may also be useful for monitoring spinal cord function during surgery.

The use of motor-evoked potentials in diagnosis has been studied extensively in recent years. They appear to be quite sensitive in detecting, confirming, or localizing the anatomic site of neural dysfunction within the cervical spine. As an intraoperative monitoring method, their efficacy is less clear, but they have been useful during upper cervical spine surgery. Muscle contraction resulting from this technique may interfere with the surgery, and can produce artifact when it is used intraoperatively.

The natural history of myelopathy is not fully understood. Nonsurgical treatment may provide temporary and sometimes lasting benefit in patients with spondylotic myelopathy. Surgery may be indicated for incapacitating symptoms and progressive neurologic deterioration.

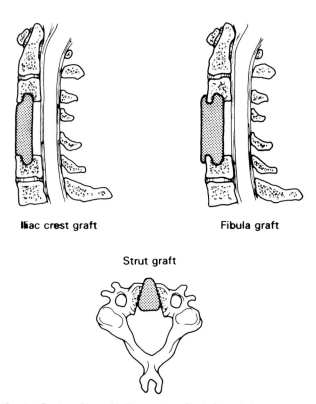

Iliac crest graft   **Fibula graft**

Strut graft

Fig. 1 Strut grafting with iliac crest or fibula for anterior corpectomy and decompression for cervical kyphosis and myelopathy. (Reproduced with permission from Zdeblick TA, Bohlman HH: Cervical kyphosis and myelopathy: Treatment by anterior corpectomy and strut-grafting. *J Bone Joint Surg* 1989;71A;170-182.)

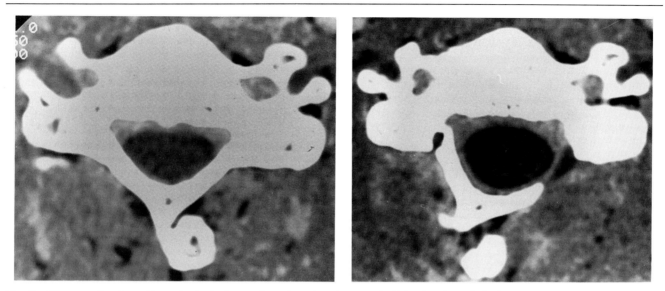

Fig. 2 CT scans of patient with cervical spinal stenosis and myelopathy treated with laminoplasty. **Left**, Preoperative CT at C4-5 level. **Right**, Postoperative CT at same level. Note how canal has been expanded by hinging lamina.

Goals of the procedure are stabilization and, hopefully, improvement of cord function. Anterior decompression usually consists of vertebrectomy and strut grafting with iliac crest or fibula (Fig. 1). This approach is best for patients with straight or kyphotic necks, whose compression is primarily anterior and whose disease is limited to two or three motion segments. Posterior decompression via laminectomy or laminoplasty is probably best reserved for patients with concentric stenosis, preserved lordosis, and multiple level involvement. Laminoplasty has the appeal of canal expansion combined with preservation of stability and some motion (Fig. 2).

A group of 75 patients treated for myelopathic disease with either anterior decompression and fusion, cervical laminectomy, or cervical laminectomy with durotomy and dentate ligament sectioning showed, after a brief follow-up period, that patients with a kyphotic neck deformity did better when an anterior procedure was performed. In the other patients, some benefit from dentate ligament sectioning was seen in selected individuals but no criteria could be found that could help determine those most likely to benefit from this procedure.

The benefits of an anterior procedure in patients with myelopathy and a preexisting kyphosis, even when a prior laminectomy has been performed have also been reported. A study of anterior surgery noted less satisfactory outcomes when preoperative studies showed evidence of spinal cord atrophy, indicating that relief of extrinsic compression will not correct established neural changes.

Laminoplasty has previously been shown to be similar in effectiveness to anterior and other forms of posterior surgery, but the expected benefits of motion retention have not been found. It appears that surgical exposure of the cervical spine for decompressive measures is in itself enough of an insult to limit motion after healing has occurred.

Inflammatory Conditions

Rheumatoid Arthritis

Most patients with rheumatoid arthritis have cervical spine involvement. Progressive, erosive changes of ligaments, bone, and cartilage can cause instability and subluxation of both the upper and lower cervical regions, resulting in neck pain and, later, neural compression and compromise. Hypertrophic pannus may extend into the spinal canal, further influencing neurologic function.

In the upper cervical spine, atlantoaxial instability occurs as a result of transverse ligament erosion by pannus. Subluxation beyond 10 mm implies involvement of the transverse, apical, and alar ligaments. With translation of C-1 on C-2, spinal cord compression and myelopathy can ensue. As the disease progresses, erosion at the occipitocervical and atlantoaxial articulations may produce cranial settling and intrusion of the odontoid process into the foramen magnum, with compression of the upper cord and brain stem. This may be exacerbated by intruding pannus and debris from the inflammatory process. With time, atlantoaxial subluxation, initially dynamic, may become fixed in a pathologic position.

Lower cervical involvement consists primarily of destructive changes at the facet joints, which lead to collapse, incompetence, and subluxation. Intravertebral cysts, end plate collapse, and inflammatory disk destruction can also occur.

Diagnosis and assessment of the severity of the condition are based on clinical history and examination; radiographs reflect neutral as well as flexion-extension postures. Myelography with CT has been the diagnostic method of choice for further evaluation. However, some authorities now believe MRI is best in determining the extent and degree of involvement, particularly in defining the status of the soft tissues and spinal cord. Tomography, MRI, or CT with image reconstruction may be helpful, particularly at the craniocervical junction. Electrophysiologic testing may also be beneficial.

A study of 34 patients with rheumatoid arthritis, using plain radiographs, MRI, and transcranial motor-evoked potentials, showed hypertrophic pannus of more than 3 mm posterior to the odontoid in two thirds of these patients. Abnormalities in neurophysiologic function and evidence of canal compromise were seen when the neck was flexed. Another study, which compared results from MRI with plain radiography in 55 patients, confirmed spinal cord compression when less than 13 mm of space was available for the spinal cord. When erosive disease resulted in intrusion of the odontoid process into the foramen magnum, cord compression was frequently noted.

Nonsurgical treatment focuses on continuous medical management of systemic disease and the use of collars and braces. Clinical decisions should be based on the natural history of the disease, which often is unpredictable. Of 41 patients with rheumatoid arthritis with atlantoaxial subluxation studied over a ten-year period, 61% showed no change in the amount of subluxation, and 12% showed a decrease in the amount of subluxation. Therefore, careful clinical examination is the central means for evaluating disease progression.

Surgical treatment may be indicated for progressive instability, neurologic deficit, or, on occasion, for pain alone. Nonfixed subluxations should be reduced posturally or by traction before surgery. Poor healing of both bone and soft tissues makes pseudoarthrosis and wound problems more common than in healthier individuals. Anesthetic management at the time of surgery can be difficult. Electrophysiologic monitoring may be of assistance during the procedure. Posterior procedures are indicated in the majority of situations, with the rare exception of anterior decompression for fixed subluxation with anterior spinal cord compression. Anterior decompression may further destabilize the spine, and arthrodesis usually is required. In such cases, combined anterior and posterior procedures may be necessary to adequately decompress and stabilize the spine.

In the upper cervical region, posterior C1-2 wiring and arthrodesis are used to stabilize pathologic motion after reduction is accomplished. Supplementary methylmethacrylate fixation may help provide immediate stability in selected circumstances, but bone graft should always be employed to accomplish long-term stabilization. When performed early, this procedure may allay or prevent cranial settling and its potentially catastrophic neurologic sequelae. Occipitocervical arthrodesis is performed when instability is present at the craniocervical level, when the posterior elements of C-1 are deficient, or if needed to control cranial settling.

A recent MRI study demonstrated shrinkage of the periodontoid pannus after posterior atlantoaxial arthrodesis performed for instability. A review of a large long-term follow-up of patients who had undergone atlantoaxial or occipitocervical arthrodesis showed the halovest to be a useful postoperative immobilizing device with minimal associated complications. The rate of arthrodesis was 90% in occipitocervical fusion and 80% in atlantoaxial fusions. Remarkably, cranial settling seemed to be halted by C1-2 fusion. However, occipitocervical fusion more often was followed by lower cervical instability, which required later treatment.

Surgery for lower cervical (subaxial) disease generally consists of selective fusion of involved, subluxated segments. Multiple levels may need to be addressed. That this procedure restricts motion is not a major problem, because these patients usually had marked motion restriction before treatment.

Although associated with a higher complication rate than in nonrheumatoid individuals, the halo device may be used after surgery for supplemental external immobilization; however, close monitoring of the skin and pin site is necessary if it is used.

Ankylosing Spondylitis

Ankylosing spondylitis of the cervical region usually fixes the spine in a flexed position. In severe situations, a chin-on-chest deformity can occur. Functional incapacity is usually caused by an inability to visualize the horizon and is most often seen in patients with a combination of hip flexion contracture and fixed flexion deformities of the cervical, thoracic, and lumbar spine.

When the resultant functional incapacity is major, the hip and lumbar conditions are addressed first, usually with total hip arthroplasty, and/or extension lumbar osteotomy. In certain situations an osteotomy performed under local anesthesia at the cervicothoracic junction can improve sagittal alignment of the head and neck. This operation involves substantial risk but is effective in correcting deformity.

Acute neck pain in a patient with ankylosing spondylitis is usually caused by a fracture through the ankylosed spine. This fracture involves all columns and may be associated with a dramatic change in neck alignment. The site of involvement is most commonly near the cervicothoracic junction. Spinal cord injury can occur as a result of translational deformity, instability, or epidural hematoma. Suspicion of the condition, early recognition, and stabilization with halo immobilization or surgery with stable internal fixation constructs is recommended. Attempts to correct neck deformity through the site of fracture may result in catastrophic neurologic occurrences. It is usually best to immobilize or stabilize the spine in the prefracture position. Unstable segments of the spine associated with hypertrophic inflammatory changes ("spondylodiskitis") are probably sites of previous fracture and nonunion.

In a study of 11 patients with ankylosing spondylitis who sustained cervical fractures, three patients died from pulmonary problems during the period when symptoms were most acute. The other eight were treated with surgical stabilization, and neurologic improvement was seen in six. In another study, 15 patients with such problems were treated nonsurgically (traction from four to six weeks followed by bracing), with results similar to those reported with surgery.

Infection

Hematogenous osteomyelitis of the cervical spine is relatively uncommon. Diagnosis and treatment are similar to those used in other regions of the spine. Clinical indications, appropriate laboratory studies, and radionuclide scanning and MRI help to establish diagnosis and determine extent of the disease. Controlled needle aspiration and culture confirm the diagnosis and may identify the causative organism.

Surgery is indicated for abscess drainage, gross deformity, or epidural abscess with neural compromise. The anterior approach is most often appropriate because, in most instances, the anterior elements are the site of the disease. Primary bone grafting can be employed safely after debridement of involved tissue. Postoperative immobilization in a halo device and appropriate parenteral antibiotic therapy are indicated in such situations.

If surgical indications do not exist, immobilization and appropriate antibiotic treatment usually suffice. Persistent infection after appropriate nonsurgical treatment or the development of any of the indications noted previously are best treated with surgery.

Management of postoperative infections is similar to that used for hematogenous infection. Abscesses should be drained, neural compression relieved, and antibiotics administered that will penetrate into the cerebrospinal fluid. As with other infections, clinical symptoms and signs, the erythrocyte sedimentation rate, and radiographic findings assist in monitoring response to treatment.

Neoplastic Conditions

The majority of neoplasms seen in the cervical spine are metastatic. Replacement of osseous tissue with neoplastic tissue often results in mechanical insufficiency, progressive instability, and kyphotic deformity. Neural compression, usually related to spinal cord compression from deformity caused by pathologic fracture, may also be related to direct extension of tumor into the spinal canal.

Nonsurgical treatment is used in patients with limited involvement (<50%) of the vertebral body and no deformity. Radiation therapy and chemotherapy combined with external support may improve the condition.

As surgical techniques have improved in recent years, a more aggressive approach appears justified in many patients. Patients with involvement of more than 50% of the vertebral body, and pain, deformity, and/or neurologic dysfunction are treated surgically via the anterior approach with vertebral body resection and replacement with bone graft or methylmethacrylate and bone graft constructs. Methylmethacrylate alone should probably be reserved for use in the anterior aspect of the spine and in situations where expectant survival is limited. However, it should be emphasized that limited life expectancy is not a contraindication to surgery, because such intervention can return many patients to a functionally independent status.

In 28 patients with metastatic spinal lesions, surgical treatment involving decompression and reconstruction resulted in improved neurologic function and an extended functional ambulatory period. In another group of patients with neoplastic involvement of the cervical and thoracic spine treated with vertebrectomy and methylmethacrylate stabilization supplemented with anterior plate fixation, results were satisfactory, with no loss of fixation or recurrent deformity. A similar group treated with posterior surgical stabilization with wire and methylmethacrylate stabilization had consistent relief of pain and prevention of neurologic deterioration, but with no change in survival time.

Although neoplastic lesions of the upper cervical spine are uncommon, symptoms and neurologic function can be controlled with appropriate treatment. Sixteen patients with involvement at C-1 or C-2 were treated by posterior surgical stabilization for patients with C-1 lateral mass involvement or C-2 vertebral body destruction, and external immobilization and radiation therapy for other lesions. An aggressive treatment program for pathologic dens fractures has also been reported. These lesions were stabilized with methylmethacrylate and screws from an anterior, high cervical approach.

Primary malignancies of the cervical spine are rare in adulthood. Chordoma has a predilection for the craniocervical region and upper cervical area. Plasmacytoma and myeloma compose the most common group of primary malignancies. Surgery, when employed, should address the area of involvement by an anterior, posterior, or combined approach. Complete resection of the tumor is desirable but often is not possible.

Miscellaneous Considerations

Diagnostic and Monitoring Techniques

Over the past few years, the major advances in diagnosis have been in the application of MRI techniques to the cervical spine and in neurophysiologic testing and monitoring. Of 268 patients with cervical spine disorders studied using transcranial magnetic stimulation of motor-evoked potentials, abnormalities were noted in 72% of 127 patients with degenerative changes of the cervical

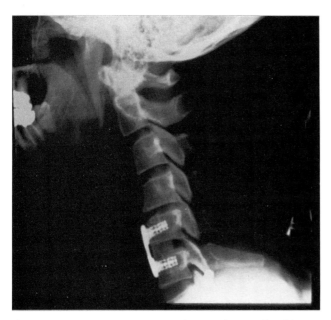

Fig. 3 Lateral cervical radiograph of spine after anterior disk excision, bone grafting, and stabilization with a locking hollow screw plate fixation device. Note that the screws do not penetrate the posterior cortex.

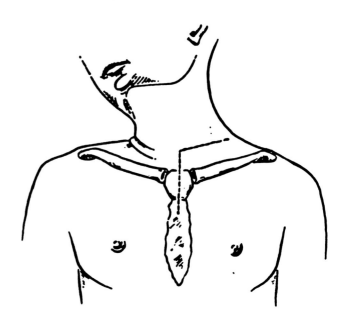

Fig. 4 Modified anterior approach to the cervicothoracic junction. This permits exposure of the spine from C-3 to T-4. The medial portion of the clavicle and part of the manubrium are resected in this approach. (Modified with permission from Kurz LT, Pursel SE, Herkowitz HN: Modified anterior approach to the cervicothoracic junction. *Spine* 1991;16 (suppl 10):S542-S547.)

spine, 67% of 55 patients with rheumatoid arthritis, and 57% of 51 patients with trauma. The magnetic stimulation technique has a high sensitivity for use in confirming diagnoses and symptoms. In a similar study involving 20 patients with cervical spine or cord lesions, multiple muscles in the C-5 to C-8 myotomes were evaluated. There was a strong correlation between clinical muscle weakness and abnormalities in motor-evoked potentials and no correlation with sensory abnormalities. Magnetic stimulation provided an objective assessment of motor function and helped localize the levels of dysfunction.

New Surgical Techniques

Clinical trials, using an anterior cervical plate with hollow titanium screws, allowed what appeared to be satisfactory fixation of the anterior cervical spine region without penetration of the screws through the posterior vertebral body wall. No complications were reported in 13 patients studied and arthrodesis was performed in all patients. This device is recommended for situations where traditional techniques might be unsatisfactory; such as multilevel anterior spine defects, posttraumatic cervical kyphosis, and cervical fractures with posterior disruption requiring anterior fusion (Fig. 3).

The use of allograft bone continues to be debated. Of 87 patients treated with anterior cervical disk excision and fusion, using either freeze-dried tricortical iliac crest bone or autologous iliac crest bone, nonunion for one-level procedures was 5% for both autograft and allograft. For two-level procedures it was 17% for autograft and 63% for allograft. Graft collapse was seen more commonly with the allograft bone. Relief of neck and arm pain was similar in both groups. Results of this study suggest that freeze-dried iliac crest allograft bone should not be used for multilevel fusions. Other researchers have shown less collapse and fewer healing problems with the use of fibular allograft. The issue of infectious disease transmission with allograft materials remains controversial and potentially worrisome.

A new surgical approach that provides access to the anterior spine from C-3 down to T-4 (Fig. 4) involves resection of a portion of the manubrium and medial clavicle, which can then be used as a structural bone graft.*

Biomechanical Considerations

New information concerning bone graft and implant mechanical properties has recently been made available. A study of the compressive strength of various autologous and autogenous bone grafts for use in spinal fusion showed that the fibular strut graft was significantly stronger than anterior and posterior iliac grafts and rib

*The various devices designed to restore alignment of the spine include some that are in varying stages of approval by the Food and Drug Administration.

Table 2. Summary of complications from cervical spine surgery over a five-year period from a total of 5,356 major surgical procedures

Complications of Cervical Spine Surgery (1982-1987)	Total
Major procedures	5,356
Anterior procedures	3,494 (64%)
Posterior procedures	1,862 (36%)
Neurologic complications	1.04%
Anterior procedures	0.64%
Posterior procedures	2.18%
Graft complications	1.64%
Anterior procedures	1.64%
Posterior procedures	0.39%

(Reproduced with permission from Graham JJ: Complications of cervical spine surgery: A five-year report on a survey of the membership of the Cervical Spine Research Society by the Morbidity and Mortality Committee. *Spine* 1989;14:1046-1050.)

grafts. Ethylene oxide sterilization had no effect on immediate compressive strength. All of the cervical graft types studied were thought to be sufficiently strong to support physiologic loads.

A study of various instrument stabilization devices for the lower cervical spine involved nondestructive tests of sublaminar wiring, Rogers wiring, Bohlman's triple wire technique, Roy-Camille posterior plate fixation, AO posterior hook-plate fixation, Caspar anterior plate fixation, and a combination of an AO posterior hook-plate with an anterior Caspar plate. No significant differences in resistance to loading in flexion or torsion were noted between any of the posterior constructs. However, there was a significant increase in posterior strain with the Caspar plate alone. The conclusion was made that there is little biomechanical justification for use of potentially dangerous sublaminar wire fixation and posterior plating methods in patients with distractive-flexion injuries of the lower cervical spine.

A similar study of constructs used in the upper cervical spine showed no significant difference with the fixation techniques in axial translation but did note in shear that the Magerl screw fixation technique was significantly better than the Gallie technique. The Brooks sublaminar and Halifax clamp techniques were not significantly different from one another or from the Magerl or Gallie techniques.*

Complications

In 1989 the Cervical Spine Research Society published a five-year report on a survey of its membership regarding spinal surgery complications as shown in Table 2. The frequency of neurologic complications was notably lower with anterior than with posterior approaches (0.64% versus 2.18%). There were a small number of miscellaneous neurologic complications related to bone graft procurement or to skull penetration, and meningitis related to the use of halo pins. Most complications with halo devices were related to pin loosening and infection. Posterior cervical complications occurred in cases of stenosis with preoperative myelopathy. A few were caused by trauma with a power drill. Bone graft complications averaged 1.64% for anterior procedures, compared with 0.39% for posterior procedures. The Cervical Spine Research Society continues to gather information in an attempt to determine the frequency of complications for various cervical spine surgical procedures.

New information was also reported on halo device complications, cervical spine pseudarthrosis, esophageal perforation after anterior surgery, and airway problems following cervical spine surgery.

---

*The various devices designed to restore alignment of the spine include some that are in varying stages of approval by the Food and Drug Administration.

Annotated Bibliography

Cervical Spondylosis and Radiculopathy

Boden SD, Weisel SW: Conservative treatment for cervical disk disease. *Seminars in Spine Surgery* 1989;1:229-232.

The authors present a concise overview of the rationale and effectiveness of commonly employed nonsurgical measures for neck pain and radiculopathy.

Clements DH, O'Leary PF: Anterior cervical diskectomy and fusion. *Spine* 1990;15:1023-1025.

This study retrospectively reviews 94 patients who underwent anterior cervical diskectomy and fusion for spondylosis, disk herniation, or both. Two patients had dysphagia following surgery. The rate of pseudarthrosis was 4%. Results were

satisfactory in 88% of patients in whom no additional spondylosis was present, and in 60% of patients in whom symptomatic levels alone were addressed, leaving unoperated adjacent levels of spondylosis.

Gore DR, Sepic SB, Gardner GM, et al: Neck pain: A long-term follow-up of 205 patients. *Spine* 1987;12:1-5.

This long-term study revealed that most neck pain improves or resolves with time. Seventy-nine percent of patients experienced decreased pain, 43% were pain free. However, 32% had moderate or severe residual pain.

Herkowitz HN, Kurz LT, Overholt DP: Surgical management of cervical soft disk herniation: A comparison between anterior and posterior approach. *Spine* 1990;15:1026-1030.

This prospective study compares anterior diskectomy and fusion (28 patients) with posterior laminotomy (16 patients) for the management of soft cervical disk herniation with radiculopathy. The disk fragment was not always removed in the posterior surgical group. Satisfactory results were 94% in the anterior surgical group and 74% in the posterior surgical group.

Whitecloud TS, Seago RA: Cervical diskogenic syndrome: Results of operative intervention in patients with positive diskography. *Spine* 1987;12:313-316.

This study reviews 34 patients who underwent cervical arthrodesis for neck pain after concordant diskography. Satisfactory results were 70%.

Cervical Spondylotic Myelopathy

Benzel EC, Lancon JA, Kesterson L, et al: Cervical laminectomy and dentate ligament section for cervical spondylotic myelopathy. *J Spinal Dis* 1991;4:286-295.

Seventy-five patients who underwent treatment for cervical spondylotic myelopathy with laminectomy plus dentate ligament section (40), laminectomy alone (18), and anterior decompression and fusion (17) were compared. Results indicated that myelopathic patients with a cervical kyphosis are best treated with anterior surgery and that patients with a normal cervical lordosis are best treated with posterior decompression surgery. No predictable benefit was seen in treatment with dentate ligament section.

Herkowitz HN: A comparison of anterior cervical fusion, cervical laminectomy, and cervical laminoplasty for the surgical management of multiple level spondylotic radiculopathy. *Spine* 1988;13:774-780.

Forty-five patients treated with anterior fusion (18), cervical laminectomy (12), and cervical laminoplasty (15) for multiple level cervical radiculopathy were compared at least two years after treatment. The success rate was 92% for anterior fusion, 66% for laminectomy, and 86% for laminoplasty. Range of motion was limited most by laminoplasty.

Hirabayashi K, Satomi K: Operative procedure and results of expansive open-door laminoplasty. *Spine* 1988;13:870-876.

This study of 90 patients treated with this technique for myelopathy revealed 75% satisfactory results. Postoperative deformity was not a problem.

Okada K, Shirasaki N, Hayashi H, et al: Treatment of cervical spondylotic myelopathy by enlargement of the spinal canal anteriorly, followed by arthrodesis. *J Bone Joint Surg* 1991;73A:352-364.

Thirty-seven patients treated with this technique were reviewed. A satisfactory neurologic outcome was reported in 29 patients. Atrophy of the spinal cord noted during preoperative studies contributed to an unsatisfactory result.

Zdeblick TA, Bohlman HH: Cervical kyphosis and myelopathy: Treatment by anterior corpectomy and strut-grafting. *J Bone Joint Surg* 1989;71A:170-182.

Fourteen patients with severe cervical kyphosis and myelopathy treated with anterior decompression and arthrodesis with iliac crest or fibula were reviewed. Eight patients had undergone a previous laminectomy. Kyphosis was corrected from an average of 45 degrees to 13 degrees. Arthrodesis

consolidation was achieved in all patients but two of three dislodged grafts required revision in the early postoperative period. Neurologic improvement was seen in all but one patient.

Inflammatory Conditions
Rheumatoid Arthritis

Clark CR, Goetz DD, Menezes AH: Arthrodesis of the cervical spine in rheumatoid arthritis. *J Bone Joint Surg* 1989;71A:381-392.

Forty-one patients with rheumatoid arthritis who underwent surgical arthrodesis were reviewed. The arthrodesis rate was 88%, with 5% of patients having a fibrous union and 7% a nonunion. All problems with union occurred in patients who underwent isolated atlantoaxial arthrodesis. Neurologic status was unchanged or improved in all patients. Four patients later died of unrelated causes.

Dvorak J, Grob D, Baumgartner H, et al: Functional evaluation of the spinal cord by magnetic resonance imaging in patients with rheumatoid arthritis and instability of the upper cervical spine. *Spine* 1989;14:1057-1064.

Thirty-four patients with rheumatoid arthritis with atlantoaxial instability were studied with plain radiographs, MRI, and motor-evoked potentials via transcranial stimulation (25 patients). Inflammatory tissue thicker than 3 mm was noted behind the odontoid in 22 patients. Spinal cord diameter and neurophysiologic function were noted to be significantly affected by the flexed position.

Kawaida H, Sakou T, Morizono Y, et al: Magnetic resonance imaging of upper cervical disorders in rheumatoid arthritis. *Spine* 1989;14:1144-1148.

Fifty-five patients with rheumatoid arthritis were studied with MRI and conventional radiography. In patients with cranial settling, medullary compression was frequently demonstrated. In patients with anterior atlantoaxial subluxation, cord compression was identified when the space available for the spinal cord was 13 mm or less.

Kraus DR, Peppelman WC, Agarwal AK, et al: Incidence of subaxial subluxation in patients with generalized rheumatoid arthritis who have had previous occipital cervical fusions. *Spine* 1991;16:S486-S489.

Seventy-nine patients with rheumatoid arthritis were reviewed at an average of over five years after atlantoaxial fusions for isolated C1-2 subluxation (55 patients) or after occipitocervical fusion for C1-2 subluxation with cranial settling (24 patients). Fusion occurred in 80% of patients with atlantoaxial fusion and in 90% with occipitocervical fusion. Subaxial subluxation later occurred in 36% of the occipitocervical fusion group and 5% of the atlantoaxial fusion group. Early atlantoaxial fusion seemed to prevent the development of cranial settling caused by erosive disease changes.

Milbrink J, Nyman R: Posterior stabilization of the cervical spine in rheumatoid arthritis: Clinical results and magnetic resonance imaging correlation. *J Spinal Dis* 1990;3:308-315.

Thirteen patients with rheumatoid arthritis and atlanto-axial subluxation underwent clinical and magnetic resonance evaluation before and after posterior stabilization. Patients with anterior instability were noted to have large periodontoid pannus formation. This granuloma decreased in size or disappeared after posterior fusion.

Rana NA: Natural history of atlanto-axial subluxation in rheumatoid arthritis. *Spine* 1989;14:1054-1056.

Forty-one patients with rheumatoid arthritis and atlantoaxial subluxation were studied between 1971 and 1981. Radiographically, 61% remained unchanged, 27% exhibited progressive subluxation, and 12% showed a decrease in subluxation. Twelve patients died: two had evidence of neurologic problems, and ten died of unrelated causes. Only three patients underwent surgical stabilization for progressive neurologic problems. Indications for surgical treatment of atlantoaxial subluxation in rheumatoid arthritis are presented.

Ankylosing Spondylitis

Detwiler KN, Loftus CM, Godersky JC, et al: Management of cervical spine injuries in patients with ankylosing spondylitis. *J Neurosurg* 1990;72:210-215.

Eleven patients with ankylosing spondylitis sustained traumatic cervical spine injuries over a 10-year period. Minor trauma was implicated as the mechanism of injury in most instances. Fracture occurred most often between C-5 and T-1. Three patients, with acute symptoms related to pulmonary complications, died. The other eight patients underwent early posterior stabilization and mobilization in a halo or cervical thoracic brace. Neurologic improvement was achieved in six of these cases. The authors advocate initial axial traction and early surgical stabilization for these injuries.

Graham B, Van Peteghem PK: Fractures of the spine in ankylosing spondylitis: Diagnosis, treatment, and complications. *Spine* 1989;14:803-807.

Fifteen patients with ankylosing spondylitis sustained fractures of the spine after minimal trauma. Twelve had fractures involving the cervical spine, with 10 of these between C-5 and C-7. Minor trauma was implicated as the mechanism of injury in most instances. Eleven of the 12 cervical injuries resulted in neurologic deficits. Nonsurgical treatment methods were employed for patients with cervical injuries (halo or skull tong traction for four to six weeks, followed by bracing). Total healing time averaged 17 weeks. Neurologic improvement was seen in four of eight patients with incomplete fractures and one of four patients with complete fractures. Two patients died.

Infection

Emery SE, Chan DP, Woodward HR: Treatment of hematogenous pyogenic vertebral osteomyelitis with anterior debridement and primary bone grafting. *Spine* 1989;14:284-291.

Of 23 adult patients treated for pyogenic vertebral osteomyelitis of the spine, 21 were followed for more than two years after surgical debridement and primary bone grafting with iliac crest or rib strut. Eleven lesions involved the lumbar spine, nine the thoracic spine, and one, the cervical region. All patients with neurologic deficits recovered without functional motor or sensory deficits. Of the 19 patients with bone grafts, 18 showed radiographic evidence of fusion. Average increase in kyphosis at the infection site was three degrees. Supplementary intravenous antibiotics were given for two to six weeks.

Neoplastic Conditions

Hall DJ, Webb JK: Anterior plate fixation in spine tumor surgery; Indications, technique, and results. *Spine* 1991;16:S80-S83.

Fifteen patients with tumor involvement of the cervical or thoracic spine underwent single stage vertebrectomy, canal decompression, filling of the defect with bone graft or methylmethacrylate, and anterior plate stabilization. Neurologic status either remained stable or improved. No loss of fixation or recurrent deformity occurred.

Manabe S, Tateishi A, Abe M, et al: Surgical treatment of metastatic tumors of the spine. *Spine* 1989;14:41-47.

Of 28 patients with metastatic lesions of the spine, 25 with vertebral body involvement underwent direct decompression by removal of the tumor followed by vertebral reconstruction. In six patients, the cervical region was involved. Of nine surviving patients with improved neurologic function at the time the article was written, seven were ambulatory for an average duration of 13 months. For the 19 patients who died, average survival time was eight months and the average postoperative ambulatory period was six months. Of these patients, 26% exhibited recurrent neurologic deficits.

Phillips E, Levine AM: Metastatic lesions of the upper cervical spine. *Spine* 1989;14:1071-1077.

Sixteen patients with metastatic lesions of C-1 and C-2 were studied. Most had severe pain. Neurologic involvement was rare. Diagnosis was delayed in half of the patients. Radiation therapy and external mobilization yielded satisfactory results for minor fractures or diffuse involvement without instability. In patients with C-1 lateral mass involvement or severe destruction of the C-2 body with instability (six patients), posterior surgical stabilization provided excellent relief of pain. Mean survival was nine months.

Sherk HH, Nolan JP Jr, Mooar PA: Treatment of tumors of the cervical spine. *Clin Orthop* 1988;223:163-167.

Thirty-four patients with primary or metastatic lesions of the cervical spine were evaluated. The presenting symptom was neck pain, but 11 patients exhibited neurologic symptoms or deficits. Surgical stabilization successfully relieved pain and prevented further neurologic deterioration in 17 of 18 patients. Complications included tumor progression in two patients and methylmethacrylate dislodgement in one patient. Mean patient survival was not significantly increased by surgical intervention (26 weeks versus 20 weeks). The authors suggest that most lesions of the cervical spine can best be managed nonsurgically but in selected patients, long posterior fusion with wires and methylmethacrylate appears to be successful in relieving pain, halting progress of neurologic deficits, and facilitating early mobilization.

Sjöström L, Olerud S, Karlström G, et al: Anterior stabilization of pathologic dens fractures. *Acta Orthop Scand* 1990;61:391-393.

Six pathologic dens fractures were stabilized with screws and methylmethacrylate via an anterior approach. Patients experienced immediate pain relief and could be mobilized without external support. One patient exhibited subglottic swelling, necessitating ventilator support for one week after surgery. No other complications occurred.

Diagnostic and Monitoring Techniques

Boden SD, McCowin PR, Davis DO, et al: Abnormal magnetic-resonance imaging scans of the cervical spine in asymptomatic subjects: A prospective investigation. *J Bone Joint Surg* 1990;72A:1178-1184.

Asymptomatic volunteers (63) underwent MRI scans of the cervical spine, and the results were compared with scans of 37 patients with symptomatic lesions. An abnormality (herniated nucleus pulposus, bulging disks, or foraminal stenosis) was identified in 19% of asymptomatic patients, 14% of those under

40 years of age, and 28% of those over 40. Disk degeneration or narrowing was noted in 25% under 40 and 56% of those over 40. The C5-6 level was most frequently involved, followed by C6-7 and C4-5.

Dvořák J, Herdmann J, Janssen B, et al: Motor-evoked potentials in patients with cervical spine disorders. *Spine* 1990;15:1013-1016.

Transcranial motor-evoked potential studies were performed in 268 patients with cervical spine disorders. Seventy-two percent of the 127 patients with degenerative changes of the cervical spine, 67% of the 55 patients with rheumatoid arthritis, and 57% of the 51 patients with trauma of the cervical spine showed a pathologic delay of central motor latency. The authors suggest that this method has a high sensitivity in the diagnosis of cervical spine disorders with suspected compression of neural structures.

Kitagawa H, Itoh T, Takano H, et al: Motor evoked potential monitoring during upper cervical spine surgery. *Spine* 1989;14:1078-1083.

Intraoperative motor-evoked potential correlated with clinical outcome and was a useful monitoring technique for upper cervical spine surgery in 20 patients.

Machida M, Yamada T, Krain L, et al: Magnetic stimulation: Examination of motor function in patients with cervical spine or cord lesion. *J Spinal Dis* 1991;4:123-130.

Twenty patients with cervical spine or cord lesions were evaluated using motor-evoked potentials from muscles covering the C-5 to C-8 myotome distribution. Motor-evoked potential abnormalities correlated well with clinical muscle weakness. The authors suggest this technique as a useful adjunct in confirming an objective finding of motor weakness and in localizing the level of dysfunction in cervical spine lesions.

Surgical Techniques

Kurz LT, Pursel SE, Herkowitz HN: Modified anterior approach to the cervicothoracic junction. *Spine* 1991;16:S542-S547.

The authors describe a new approach that provides access to the anterior spine from C-3 to T-4 by resection of the medial portion of the left clavicle and manubrium. Its use in four metastatic lesions for spinal decompression and stabilization is detailed.

Suh PB, Kostuik JP, Esses SI: Anterior cervical plate fixation with the titanium hollow screw plate system: A preliminary report. *Spine* 1990;15:1079-1081.

Thirteen patients were treated with an anterior cervical plate system using a screw design that does not require purchase of the posterior vertebral cortex. This design eliminates potential neurologic complications that can be associated with anterior plate systems while maintaining the mechanical advantages of internal fixation. Indications included acute trauma, subacute trauma, and spondylosis. All patients went on to arthrodesis. No neurologic injuries were noted. The applications of this design are discussed.

Weiland DJ, McAfee PC: Posterior cervical fusion with triple-wire strut graft technique: 100 consecutive patients. *J Spinal Dis* 1991;4:15-21.

One hundred patients were treated with this technique for traumatic conditions, rheumatoid arthritis, congenital arthritis, congenital deformity, and neoplasms. Sixty patients underwent subaxial fusion; 20 atlantoaxial fusion; and 20 stabilization to the occiput. The fusion rate for subaxial arthrodesis was 100%. One pseudarthrosis occurred in an occipitocervical fusion. There were no neurologic complications and no infections. The authors recommend this as a predictable and safe technique for posterior cervical arthrodesis.

Zdeblick TA, Ducker TB: The use of freeze-dried allograft bone for anterior cervical fusions. *Spine* 1991;16:726-729.

Eighty-seven patients underwent Smith-Robinson type anterior cervical fusion with either freeze-dried tricortical iliac crest bone or tricortical autograft bone. After one year, the nonunion rates for autograft and allograft were 8% and 22%, respectively. Nonunion in one-level procedures was 5% for both autograft and allograft. For two-level procedures, the nonunion rate was 17% for autograft, 63% for allograft. Graft collapse was more commonly seen with freeze-dried allograft (30%) than with autograft (5%). Relief of neck and arm pain was similar in both groups. Two percent of the autograft group had donor site complications. Freeze-dried iliac crest allograft bone is not recommended in multilevel fusions.

Biomechanical Considerations

Coe JD, Warden KE, Sutterlin CE III, et al: Biomechanical evaluation of cervical spinal stabilization methods in a human cadaveric model. *Spine* 1989;14:1122-1131.

Human cervical spine specimens were biomechanically tested after destabilization and then after simulated surgical stabilization using cyclic loads. Eight constructs were tested nondestructively, including the intact spinal segment, sublaminar wiring, Rogers wiring, Bohlman's triple wire technique, Roy-Camille posterior plates, AO posterior hook-plate, Caspar anterior plate fixation, and AO posterior hook-plate with Caspar anterior plate fixation. No significant differences were demonstrated between any of the posterior stabilization methods tested but anterior plating was shown to be an inferior method of stabilization.

Crisco JJ III, Panjabi MM, Oda T, et al: Bone graft translation of four upper cervical spine fixation techniques in a cadaveric model. *J Orthop Res* 1991;9:835-846.

Biomechanical testing was performed on cervical spine specimens after the performance of four C1-2 posterior stabilization techniques: Gallie, Brooks, Magerl screw technique, and Hallifax clamps. No significant difference was found with the fixation techniques in axial translation. In shear, the Magerl screw technique was significantly more stable than the Gallie construct. No differences could be shown between the Brooks and Hallifax techniques or the Magerl or Gallie constructs.

Wittenberg RH, Moeller J, Shea M, et al: Compressive strength of autologous and allogenous bone grafts for thoracolumbar and cervical spine fusion. *Spine* 1990;15:1073-1078.

The potential immediate postoperative compressive strengths of various types of bone grafts were tested under axial compression in a materials testing machine. The fibular strut graft was significantly stronger than the anterior and posterior iliac crest and rib grafts. Hydroxyapatite grafts with a smaller pore size were stronger than those with a larger pore size. Ethylene oxide sterilization had no significant effect on the immediate compressive strength. The authors believe that all cervical graft types studied may be sufficiently strong to support sizeable loads.

Complications

Baum JA, Hanley EN Jr, Pullekines J: Comparison of halo complications in adults and children. *Spine* 1989;14:215-252.

Ninety-three of 128 patients who underwent halo vest application for a variety of cervical spine problems were reviewed to determine complications associated with use of this device. Eight percent of adults had major problems consisting of pin track infection and significant pin loosening requiring replacement. Thirty-nine percent (5 of 13) of children had major problems. Recommendations are made concerning halo application and follow-up care.

Emery SE, Smith MD, Bohlman HH: Upper-airway obstruction after multilevel cervical corpectomy for myelopathy. *J Bone Joint Surg* 1991;73A:544-551.

Seven patients are described who experienced upper airway obstruction immediately after an anterior procedure on the cervical spine. All had moderate to severe myelopathy and all had undergone a multilevel anterior cervical corpectomy followed by arthrodesis. Airway compromise was believed to be caused by edema rather than formation of a hematoma. Five patients had no sequelae from this occurrence but two died of complications related to this problem. Six patients had a history of heavy smoking and one of asthma. The authors recommend extra precautions in patients undergoing this procedure with the noted risk factors.

Farey ID, McAfee PC, Davis RF, et al: Pseudarthrosis of the cervical spine after anterior arthrodesis: Treatment by posterior nerve-root decompression, stabilization, and arthrodesis. *J Bone Joint Surg* 1990;72A:1171-1177.

Nineteen patients with a symptomatic pseudarthrosis after failed anterior cervical arthrodesis were treated with posterior nerve decompression and arthrodesis. A solid fusion was achieved in all patients and radiculopathy relieved in all but one. Motor weakness present in four patients resolved.

Graham JJ: Complications of cervical spine surgery: A five-year report on a survey of the membership of the Cervical Spine Research Society by the Morbidity and Mortality Committee. *Spine* 1989;14:1046-1050.

This article presents five years' experience with cervical spine surgery and results from 5,356 major surgical procedures performed by members of the Cervical Spine Research Society. Sixty-four percent of the procedures were anterior operations. The overall incidence of neurologic complications averaged 1.04%. There was a lower incidence of neurologic complications with anterior than with posterior procedures (0.64% versus 2.18%). Bone graft complications were largely in the anterior surgical group, averaging 1.64%, compared with 0.39 percent in the posterior group. Further research is being conducted by this organization concerning surgical rates and complications.

Newhouse KE, Lindsey RW, Clark CR, et al: Esophageal perforation following anterior cervical spine surgery. *Spine* 1989;14:1051-1053.

Twenty-two cases of esophageal perforation following anterior cervical spine surgery are reported. Six occurred at the time of surgery, six during the immediate postoperative period, and ten later. Instrumentation was implicated in 25% of the cases occurring after surgery. Diagnosis was confirmed most often by direct vision at re-exploration or esophagography. Treatment usually consisted of drainage, repair, and parenteral antibiotics. One patient died, and all patients required prolonged hospitalization.

Smith MD, Phillips WA, Hensinger RN: Complications of fusion to the upper cervical spine. *Spine* 1991;16:702-705.

Of 47 patients undergoing upper cervical spine fusions, only 11 had an uncomplicated course. Most complications were minor. There were four nonunions. Seven patients had increased neurologic deficits after surgery but only one was permanent. One death occurred because of a technical error. Patients with significant instability, myelopathy, prior failed fusions, or unreducible dislocations are at high risk for perioperative neurologic complications.

Miscellaneous Conditions

Hadjipavlou A, Lander P: Paget disease of the spine. *J Bone Joint Surg* 1991;73A:1376-1381.

Seventy patients who had the radiographic features of Paget disease of the spine were evaluated clinically and with CT with the objective of correlation of symptoms with lesions. Of 45 symptomatic patients, 21 had pain in the back or neck, and 24 had spinal stenosis with or without pain in the back or neck. Seven patients had a neurologic deficit without pain. Fifteen cervical, 51 thoracic, 104 lumbar, and 16 sacral vertebrae were involved. The fourth and fifth lumbar vertebrae were involved most often. The most common cause of spinal stenosis was expansion of bone that led to compression of the thecal sac and its neural elements because of abnormal hyperactive bone remodeling. In this series one of three patients who had Paget disease of bone had spinal involvement, one of three who had spinal involvement had clinical spinal stenosis, and approximately one of two who had spinal involvement had pain in the back or neck.

36

Thoracolumbar Spine: Pediatric

Congenital Deformity of the Spine

Congenital Scoliosis

The prognosis for progression of congenital scoliosis depends on the type of congenital deformity present, its location in the spine, and the age of the patient at presentation. A progressive spinal deformity is rarely produced by block vertebrae, which are secondary to bilateral failure of segmentation. Single hemivertebrae may produce a progressive spinal deformity; however, their behavior is unpredictable, making radiographic analysis over time necessary before surgery can be considered. Some hemivertebrae are incarcerated (tucked into the spine) and cause no deformity; others are nonincarcerated and cause a curvature. Hemivertebrae with open disks on both sides are referred to as fully segmented; those with one open disk, semisegmented; and those with no open disks, nonsegmented. Because the open disk usually has an active growth plate, prognosis for curve progression can sometimes be predicted; fully segmented hemivertebrae will progress more than those that are semisegmented; these in turn will progress more than the nonsegmented ones, which should not progress. Double hemivertebrae that are ipsilateral and adjacent to one another are more likely to produce a progressive scoliosis and require arthrodesis. Unilateral unsegmented bars are a frequent congenital cause of progressive spinal deformity. The deformity produced by a unilateral unsegmented bar is relentlessly progressive; once a unilateral unsegmented bar is identified, arthrodesis is required to prevent a severe deformity. If a unilateral unsegmented bar is associated with a contralateral hemivertebra, the progression of the deformity is even more rapid.

Magnetic resonance imaging has been recommended as a diagnostic tool for patients with congenital scoliosis being treated by arthrodesis, and for all patients with deformity of the congenital spine and accompanying pain, abnormal neurologic findings, or cutaneous hairy patch. Surgical treatment of a congenital deformity of the spine depends on its severity and the patient's age. In the case of progressive congenital scoliosis, it is generally recommended that posterior arthrodesis be performed as soon as it is diagnosed, and on both the convex and the concave sides of the spinal deformity because posterior arthrodeses performed on the convex side only tend to bend with time.

In the younger child, isolated posterior arthrodesis of a lordotic curve may act as a posterior tethering bar, producing more lordosis or even a rotatory lordosis-scoliosis (the "crankshaft phenomenon") as the unfused anterior vertebral bodies continue to grow. Therefore, anterior as well as posterior arthrodesis is advised for progressive congenital scoliosis associated with lordosis. Other indications for anterior spinal arthrodesis include: (1) deformities with known high risk of progression (such as concave bar with convex hemivertebrae); (2) severe deformity (greater than 50 degrees), which is at risk for the crankshaft phenomenon with posterior arthrodesis alone; and (3) progression of an already posteriorly fused deformity secondary to crankshaft phenomenon.

Two other options exist for patients with hemivertebrae only. During hemiepiphysiodesis, the convex one third to one half of the vertebral end plates are removed and fused anteriorly, and only the convex half of the posterior spine is fused. Some curve correction is achieved with a postoperative cast. Curve stabilization can be accomplished and approximately 50% of the patients achieve modest correction (averaging 10 degrees). Any additional risk in hemiepiphysiodesis, except that associated with a thoracotomy, seems minimal. Currently, the ideal candidate for hemiepiphysiodesis is a patient younger than 5 years of age with a short curvature of less than 70 degrees and no excessive kyphosis or lordosis.

The other option is hemivertebral excision, the procedure of choice for an L-5 deformity. An anterior and posterior lumbar (L-1 to L-4) hemivertebral excision should be considered if significant cosmetic deformity or decompensation of the trunk is present.

In general, correction of congenital scoliosis with instrumentation carries a higher risk of neurologic injury. In older children with congenital scoliosis, instrumentation and correction of the deformity may be done if tethering of the spinal cord has been ruled out by myelography or magnetic resonance imaging. Curve correction occurs through the angulated vertebrae adjacent to the actual congenital bar or hemivertebrae, and not through the actual congenital deformity.

Congenital Kyphosis

Progressive congenital kyphosis is caused by failure of formation or failure of segmentation. Failure of formation of the anterior elements produces the worst deformity and can be associated with paraplegia. Posterior arthrodesis alone may be effective for kyphosis less than 55 degrees in a growing child younger than 5 years of age. If the deformity is greater than 55 degrees, both anterior and posterior arthrodesis will be required. The anterior arthrodesis should be a combination of a strut graft and an interbody arthrodesis. An anterior unsegmented bar will develop in the growing child if an interbody arthrodesis is not added to strut grafting, because the growth of the unfused vertebral bodies has not been arrested. A strut graft should be placed as close to the vertebral bodies as possible because pseudarthrosis is more likely to develop if the graft is more than 4 cm from the apical vertebra. Correction of a congenital kyphosis carries with it the highest risk of paraplegia. A congenital kyphosis may be corrected intraoperatively if great caution is used, but correction should not be attempted preoperatively with traction because the spinal cord will be stretched over the kyphos, which is fixed, thereby producing paraplegia. Decompression of the spinal cord anteriorly is necessary if myelopathic signs are present preoperatively or if correction of the kyphotic deformity is necessary.

Adolescent Idiopathic Scoliosis

Prevalence

Curves of greater than 10 degrees occur in 1.9% to 3% of the population in North America, decreasing to 0.2% to 0.3% for curves greater than 20 degrees. Curves less than 10 degrees should be considered normal and insignificant. There is an increasing prevalence in females for larger, progressive curves. The ratio of female to male for curves 11 to 20 degrees is 1.4:1, for curves greater than 21 degrees 5.4:1, and for curves requiring treatment 7.2:1. Scoliosis occurs in 15% to 20% of children with a parent who had adolescent idiopathic scoliosis, suggesting a dominant or multiple gene inheritance.

Etiology

The cause of adolescent idiopathic scoliosis remains unknown. It continues to be debated whether or not these children have abnormal balance and whether the imbalance is caused by the labyrinthine or ocular systems. When results of these studies are positive, this does not appear to be secondary, because patients with scoliosis caused by other factors (such as congenital) do not have the abnormality. Normal siblings of patients with scoliosis also show abnormal sway tests. The etiologic importance of this postural dysfunction has been debated in the literature. A decrease in perception of vibratory stimuli, as well as a decrease in proprioception, in both the upper and lower extremities has been noted in patients with scoliosis.

The sagittal plane deformity has received much attention in recent years. The apex of a thoracic scoliosis shows that the spine is truly lordotic. The visible posterior deformity is actually the rotational deformity of the ribs on the convex side of the scoliosis. The lordosis of the apex of a scoliosis has been shown to be the first change seen in a child who has a straight spine that progresses to scoliosis. Some have speculated that this small area of lordosis produces a rotation of the spine, which evolves into scoliosis. Why the thoracic spine rotates to the right in the majority of cases is unclear. The lack of association of left thoracic curves with left-handedness rules out handedness as the reason. Left thoracic curves are not idiopathic in a high percentage of cases, and patients should have a thorough neurologic examination, a bone scan, and magnetic resonance imaging to rule out other causes. A recent magnetic resonance imaging study of adolescent patients believed to have idiopathic scoliosis, including both right and left thoracic curves, showed a higher prevalence of Arnold-Chiari abnormalities and syringes than expected, but the true significance of these results can be determined with a prospective study of a large number of patients.

Screening

Screening for scoliosis at school has been advocated and even mandated in some states. A variety of instruments have been developed to measure trunk asymmetry at the apex of the curvature in forward flexion. The sensitivity, specificity, reproducibility, and predictive values remain variable and unproven. Most patients with scoliosis severe enough to require treatment will exhibit a visible trunk asymmetry by age 10; consequently, screening should concentrate on children at this age.

Natural History

Progression is related to the size of the curve, the area of the spine involved, and the physiologic age of the child. Larger curves progress to a greater degree than smaller curves, and thoracic and double primary curves progress to a greater degree than single lumbar or thoracolumbar curves. The curves of children with skeletal maturity levels of Risser grade 0 (in which the iliac apophyses are not visible) or grade 1 progress much more than those in children with Risser grades 2, 3, or 4, as determined by the lateral to medial ossification of the iliac apophyses. The absence of menarche at presentation is an important risk factor for progression. Progression of curves between 20 and 29 degrees has been well studied, with a patient at Risser grade 0 to 1 having a 68% risk of progression and a patient at Risser grade 2 to 4 having a 23% chance of progression. Follow-up examinations are suggested every four to six months. The prevalence of scoliosis is reportedly decreasing; however, a recent cross-sectional and longitudinal survey showed no tendency toward a change in natural history.

Because skeletal maturity of the male spine occurs later, males seem to show more curve progression later in adolescence (between ages 16 and 19), compared with females, and require closer observation. A recent study determined that curves in males progressed significantly until skeletal maturity (Risser grade 5) and concluded that males with curves grater than 20 degrees should be followed radiographically until Risser grade 5 is reached.

Cardiopulmonary function in patients with idiopathic scoliosis has been of much concern. Studies on the work capacity of adolescents with scoliosis of greater than 25 degrees showed some vital capacity measurements one or more standard deviations below normal. Although reductions are present, a classic study shows that curves must be severe (greater than 80 degrees) to produce clinically significant reductions in pulmonary function. Pulmonary symptoms and vital capacity correlate well with the degree of thoracic curvature. With thoracic curves greater than 78 degrees, 93% of patients will have a vital capacity of less than 75%. With curves between 100 and 140 degrees, the average vital capacity is 60%.

Radiology

The range of error in the measurement of Cobb angles is at least 5 degrees, but it can vary to as much as 10 degrees. The most important variable for accurate measurement is selection of end vertebrae. The use of standardized, precision goniometers has also been shown to increase accuracy of measurement, especially with smaller curves.

The most radiosensitive tissues appear to be those of the breast, thyroid, and bone marrow. A recent study from Minneapolis with long-term follow-up reviewed 1,000 women, and evaluated the radiation hazard to the breasts according to the number of radiographs taken. The risk of cancer was significant only if the patient had 60 or more radiographs with a total dose of 20 rads or more. In this study, the dose of radiation per radiograph was 333 mrad. The simplest step to reduce breast and thyroid exposure to radiation has been to change the patient from the anteroposterior to posteroanterior position, which greatly reduces radiation to the breast. Using lead bras as shields during anteroposterior radiographic analysis will also reduce radiation exposure. High-speed rare earth screens, tube head filters, fast x-ray film, and x-ray beam columnization can also be used to reduce the total radiation dosage. Using these new techniques, the aforementioned Minneapolis study reduced the average radiation dosage of a posteroanterior radiograph to 2.2 mrad, meaning that thousands of radiographs could be taken before reaching the risk levels for breast cancer found in their study.

Treatment

Bracing Natural history studies have led to recommendations that nonsurgical treatment be used for curves between 20 and 40 degrees when spinal growth remains (Risser grade 0, 1, or 2). Although some flexible curves between 40 and 45 degrees can be treated successfully, brace treatment is not used for most curves in excess of 45 degrees. Documented progression of 5 degrees over 12 months or less in patients with curves less than 30 degrees is recommended before beginning brace treatment. In skeletally immature patients (Risser grade 2 or less), bracing is used for curves 30 degrees or greater even if there has been no evidence of progression. By using these criteria, physicians can eliminate much unnecessary bracing; bracing during adolescence reportedly has adverse physiologic and psychological effects. In

a study on the psychological, functional, and family impact of brace treatment, 84% of parents described the initial bracing period as stressful. No evidence of overt psychopathology was noted in the child, but the initial bracing period was associated with lower levels of self-esteem. In one study, application of a brace resulted in a significant reduction in vital capacity (14%), functional residual capacity (22%), and total lung capacity (12%).

The Milwaukee brace has largely been replaced by underarm braces, either custom-made (such as the Wilmington brace) or prefabricated (such as the Boston brace), which seem to be as effective in treating curves with apices of T-8 or lower. Bracing is used to prevent progression of the curve until skeletal maturity is achieved (Risser grade 4 or 5). Continued follow-up after brace treatment is necessary. In one study of patients who completed treatment with a Wilmington brace, 16 of 67 patients (21%) experienced 5 to 16 degrees of curve progression following discontinuance of brace treatment, and several eventually required surgery. Low compliance with brace wear has been reported, and, on average, patients wore their braces only 65% of the time they were instructed to do so. These reports have prompted studies of part-time bracing (16 to 18 hours per day), which have revealed results at short-term follow-up equal to those in a similar group of patients who wore their braces full-time (23 hours). These results should be interpreted with caution because they are preliminary. Early results of wearing the Charleston nighttime bending brace in the position of maximum side bend were positive, with 115 of 138 patients (83%) showing improvement or less than 5 degrees change in curvature. Although this treatment is considered to be justified, patients should be observed for an increase in their compensatory curve. Again, part-time bracing programs should be employed with caution until long-term results are available.

Exercise Exercise treatment alone is of no proven value in preventing progression of curves.

Electrical Stimulation Enthusiasm for treatment of progressive curves with transcutaneous electrical stimulation was generated by successful preliminary reports and the desire to rid adolescents of the psychologic and social burdens of wearing a brace. Published reports of good results with electrical stimulation often included patients still being treated or those with small, nonprogressive curves, making it difficult to ascertain the effect of electrical stimulation on larger curves. A well-controlled study found no statistical difference in outcome between patients who had completed electrical stimulation treatment and patients who had no treatment at all, and the failure rate exceeded that found in studies of orthotic treatment.

Surgery For 25 years, use of the Harrington distraction rod combined with a thorough posterior arthrodesis, including the facet joints, followed by immobilization of the patient in a cast or brace for four to nine months has been the standard surgical treatment for adolescent idiopathic scoliosis. The incidence of neurologic injury is less than 1%, and the pseudarthrosis rate is less than 10%. For a new procedure to become standard, it must provide a significant improvement on these results. Multisegmental hook systems, such as the Cotrel-Dubousset (C-D), and Texas Scottish Rite Hospital (TSRH), provide multiple points of fixation to the spine and allow both compression and distraction on the same rod. The theoretical advantages of these systems include improved correction of thoracic hypokyphosis, preservation of lumbar lordosis when instrumentation extends into the lower lumbar spine, and cosmetic improvement in the rib prominence deformity via their derotation effect. The major advantage of multisegmental hook systems is that no postoperative immobilization is required.

Analysis of preoperative and postoperative computed tomographic scans suggests that a preoperative hypokyphosis can be improved an average of 10 degrees using a multisegmental hook system in patients whose preoperative sagittal-thoracic Cobb angle is less than 25 degrees.

For lumbar or thoracolumbar curve patterns and for the lumbar curve of a double-major, anterior spinal arthrodesis with an anterior flexible rod and screw system (Zielke system) or anterior rigid rods and screws (TSRH) have been advocated for theoretical improvement in trunk and pelvic symmetry, better derotation, and preservation of mobile lumbar segments. The disadvantages of the Zielke system include kyphosis across the fused segment, a higher rate of pseudarthrosis, and the need for postoperative immobilization. The anterior rigid rod system should theoretically prevent these problems, but the follow-up data are not yet available (Fig. 1). For flexible curves, posterior multisegmental hook instrumentation systems appear to be as effective as anterior systems when the lumbar segments cannot be saved by Zielke's criteria of determining the lower instrumented vertebrae. Zielke's criteria require that the lower instrumented vertebrae have less than 15 degrees of tilt and less than 20% rotation on the preoperative bending films. For stiff larger thoracolumbar or lumbar idiopathic curves, anterior diskectomy and arthrodesis without instrumentation, followed by posterior instrumentation, is effective.

When using the Harrington rod system, arthrodesis of only the thoracic curve is necessary (King type II), in which the compensatory lumbar curve is smaller and more flexible on bending. The bottom of the arthrodesis should extend to the stable vertebra (the vertebra that is bisected by a line drawn through the middle of the spinous process of S-1 perpendicular to the iliac crestline). The lower level of arthrodesis in lumbar curves should not extend to the lower lumbar region unless it is absolutely necessary. In follow-up studies of patients who have undergone spinal arthrodesis for scoliosis, the lower

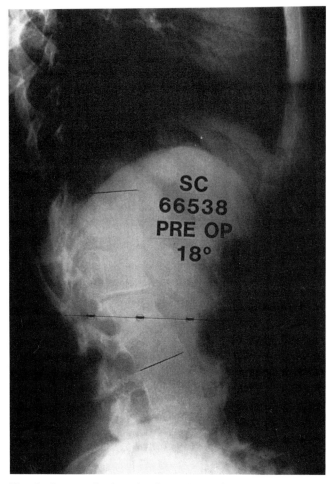

Fig. 1 Preoperative lateral radiograph showing an 18-degree thoracolumbar kyphosis secondary to rotation.

the level of arthrodesis, the higher the incidence of back pain; however, there are some conflicting results. A recent study of Dr. Harrington's patients showed that compared to a control group, there was no difference in low back pain, and the patients were functioning well 21 years after arthrodesis. However, other studies have shown a connection between low back pain and how distal an arthrodesis extends into the lower lumbar (L3-5) region. Avoiding arthrodesis to L-5 and L-4, if possible, seems appropriate.

Principles of instrumentation levels using multisegmental hook systems are different and have yet to be defined. Selective arthrodesis of the thoracic curve in King type II curves can result in larger residual lumbar curves postoperatively and loss of balance. Overcorrection of the main thoracic curve may be one of the problems, because in the lumbar curve, spontaneous correction is not sufficient to restore balance. A recent study also cautions that overcorrection of the main thoracic curve beyond the spontaneous correctability of the upper compensatory thoracic curve can lead to an undesirable asymmetric neck and shoulder contour. Advanced training is necessary to learn about and use these multisegmental hook systems. Anterior instrumentation for thoracic curves (King types II, III, and IV) is being investigated in a few centers, with the theoretical advantages of a shorter fusion length, restoration of a normal kyphosis because of removing the disks, and fewer problems with balance.

The crankshaft phenomenon reportedly occurs following the use of posterior instrumentation alone in the skeletally immature patient. This progression is a consequence of continued anterior growth following posterior spinal arthrodesis even in cases where there is no instrument failure or pseudarthrosis. To achieve a stable correction, an anterior and posterior arthrodesis should be considered in young patients (girls younger than 11 years old, boys younger than 13 years old) with progressive scoliosis over 50 degrees and a significant amount of growth remaining (Risser grade 0 or 1).

Neurologic injury is a feared complication. Monitoring somatosensory-evoked potentials (SEPs) during surgery has been helpful in preventing neurologic injury, but the accuracy of this technique has not yet been firmly established. Temperature and blood pressure have been shown to affect evoked potentials. SEP monitoring continues to improve; epidural electrode leads are less affected by anesthesia. Motor-evoked potentials, now being used along with SEPs in several centers, appear to improve the accuracy of predicting neurologic injury. The wake-up test, as described by Stagnara, is frequently used to determine if neurologic injury is present.

The rib prominence deformity produced by spinal rotation in scoliosis is usually not corrected at all by the Harrington rod procedure but is corrected modestly with multisegmental hook systems in patients with flexible curves. Radiographic analysis suggests improvement in rotation of 40% of thoracic and 22% of lumbar curves. Computed tomography indicates rotational correction of less than 24% in the apical vertebra. Partial rib resection on the convex side as an adjunctive procedure has been recommended as a means of improving the cosmesis of the rib prominence deformity in some patients. Concave rib osteotomies in patients with severe deformities can help with curve correction and improve the trunk wall asymmetry with elevation of the cut rib.

Infantile and Juvenile Idiopathic Scoliosis

The onset of infantile scoliosis occurs between birth and 3 years of age; juvenile scoliosis between 4 and 10 years of age. The incidence of infantile idiopathic scoliosis is consistently higher in Great Britain than in the United States. It has been postulated recently that this scoliosis is related to positioning of the infant. European children are routinely placed in the supine position whereas American infants are usually placed in the prone posi-

tion. When infants are supine or, more correctly, turned slightly from supine, excessive force appears to be placed on the immature spine, producing scoliosis. British children are increasingly being placed prone, and the incidence of infantile idiopathic scoliosis is decreasing in Great Britain.

Rib vertebral angles at the apex of the curve and their difference (RVAD) of greater than 20 degrees is strongly associated with the prognosis of infantile scoliosis. In juvenile idiopathic scoliosis, an RVAD greater than 10 degrees is associated with an increased risk of progression. The presence of thoracic hypokyphosis may be a risk factor for progression in patients with juvenile idiopathic scoliosis.

Bracing is the primary treatment for patients with infantile and juvenile idiopathic scoliosis. Part-time bracing in patients with juvenile scoliosis is reportedly as effective as full-time bracing, and permanent correction can sometimes be achieved. (Again, these preliminary reports should be interpreted with caution.) Infantile and juvenile scoliotic curves that are relentlessly progressive beyond 50 degrees despite bracing are very difficult to treat. The use of a subcutaneous Harrington rod, which involves exposure of the spine at the ends of the rod for hook insertion, has been successful when the vertebrae adjacent to the hooks are fused. The rod must be distracted periodically (every six months) and the spine must be braced until an arthrodesis of the remainder of the curve is performed when the child is older (10 years of age or older). Another effective method in halting progression of infantile scoliosis is to apply posterior segmental spinal instrumentation (SSI) without arthrodesis and anterior apical growth arrest as a separate procedure. Surgical treatment without arthrodesis cannot be regarded lightly, because the complications are many.

Neuromuscular Scoliosis

Cerebral Palsy

Scoliosis is rare in ambulatory patients with mild cerebral palsy but very common in children with severe spastic quadriplegia. Many patients can achieve functional sitting with body jackets or molded wheelchair inserts. The decision to surgically stabilize the spine should be made jointly by the patient's physician, family or caretakers, and therapists. When fusing with segmental instrumentation including multiple hooks or sublaminar wires, the spine is instrumented from the upper thoracic area to the sacrum. Rods may be secured to the pelvis using the Galveston technique to help obtain an arthrodesis across the sacrum. Curves that have progressed beyond 80 degrees and those that cause severe pelvic obliquity require combined anterior and posterior arthrodesis for adequate results. Treatment is directed toward functional goals, such as sitting balance and pain relief, rather than cosmesis.

Myelodysplasia

Scoliosis may be either congenital or paralytic in patients with spina bifida. Progressive paralytic scoliosis may be caused by disturbed ventricular shunt mechanics, a progressive hydromyelia, syringomyelia or tethered cord, or compression from the Arnold-Chiari syndrome, all of which can usually be detected with magnetic resonance imaging. It may be possible to relieve this problem by revision of the ventricular shunt or releasing a tethered cord, thus halting or occasionally reversing progressive scoliosis, particularly if detected before the curve reaches 50 degrees. Treatment for congenital curves in patients with spina bifida is similar to the treatment of congenital scoliosis without a paralytic component. Kyphectomy for severe congenital kyphosis in patients with thoracic-level myelomeningocele is indicated for sitting balance or when skin problems occur over the apex. A patent shunt is essential to prevent acute hydrocephalus, which can result from the spinal sac excision usually necessary with the kyphectomy. For established paralytic scoliosis, best results are obtained by anterior arthrodesis combined with posterior arthrodesis and secure internal fixation, plus bone grafting. Aggressive evaluation of the urinary tract, treatment of urinary tract infection, and perioperative antibiotics are important in reducing wound infections.

Spinal Muscular Atrophy

There are three forms of spinal muscular atrophy. Type I, or Werdnig-Hoffmann, appears between birth and 6 months of age, and the prognosis for survival is guarded. Type II, or chronic Werdnig-Hoffmann, appears between 6 months and 5 years of age. The onset of the mildest form, type III or Kugelberg-Welander, is between 2 and 17 years. Spinal muscular atrophy is an autosomal recessive disease typified by loss of anterior horn cells of the spinal cord. Scoliosis develops in a large number of these patents, and surgery is necessary to prevent progression of the curve and to improve sitting comfort. Bracing is poorly tolerated in these patients. As soon as the curve reaches 40 degrees, it should be treated surgically with instrumentation and arthrodesis. The bone may be too weak for sublaminar wires, and mersilene tapes passed sublaminarly can be helpful. Even though instrumentation without arthrodesis (for example, subcutaneous Harrington rod) to allow continued spinal growth is effective in animal studies and in children who are neurologically intact, this treatment has been ineffective and has a high complication rate in children with paralytic disorders.

Duchenne Muscular Dystrophy

Duchene muscular dystrophy is a sex-linked recessive, relentlessly progressive muscle disease. Children with this disease usually lose their ability to walk by age 12 to 14 years. Once confined to a wheelchair, approximately 50% to 80% of these children develop a collapsing scolio-sis that eventually becomes extremely severe. This scoliosis limits the child's ability to sit, which further complicates an already deteriorating pulmonary status. Bracing is poorly tolerated by these children. When a patient's curve exceeds 35 degrees, the vital capacity is usually less than 40% of predicted normal. A posterior spinal arthrodesis with instrumentation should be considered as soon as the child stops walking, even in children with curves less than 35 degrees. If the curve is allowed to progress, the pulmonary function will deteriorate rapidly, precluding the opportunity to stabilize the curve. In patients with pulmonary function less than 50%, respiratory exercise programs begun before surgery may improve the pulmonary function and decrease the incidence of postoperative pulmonary problems. In patients with smaller curves, the distal level of arthrodesis may stop at L-4 or L-5, because minimal pelvic obliquity seems to be well tolerated by these patients.

Miscellaneous Spine Problems

Neurofibromatosis

Two types of spine deformity, dystrophic and nondystrophic, are associated with neurofibromatosis. Dystrophic neurofibromatosis is characterized by rib penciling, vertebral body scalloping, dural ectasia, and adjacent soft-tissue masses. The indications for treatment of nondystrophic curves are the same as for idiopathic scoliosis. In contrast, dystrophic curves do not respond to any form of bracing and require surgical stabilization. For scoliosis alone, posterior arthrodesis (preferably with internal fixation) is satisfactory. For kyphoscoliosis, anterior disk excision and bone graft, followed by posterior arthrodesis with instrumentation, are indicated if the kyphotic angle is greater than 50 degrees or if the scoliosis is greater than 80 degrees. For failed arthrodeses or severe kyphotic curves, a vascularized rib strut can be effective. Neurologic deficits may occur because of intraspinal neoplasms, kyphosis, or both. Preoperative MRI scans or myelograms are recommended before surgical treatment of dystrophic curves.

Marfan Syndrome

Scoliotic curves of less than 25 degrees should be closely monitored in the growing child. Scoliosis in Marfan syndrome generally does not respond well to orthotic treatment; however, if curve progression is less than 45 degrees without thoracic lordosis or lumbar kyphosis, orthosis is used. Arthrodesis is recommended for adolescents with curves greater than 45 degrees, painful curves, or rapidly progressing curves, or for adults with curves greater than 50 degrees. In these patients, thoracic lordosis may be more of a problem than the scoliosis because of reduced pulmonary function. Posterior spinal arthrodesis with sublaminar wires to correct thoracic lordosis has been effective. A preliminary anterior approach with diskectomy is used for rigid curves. With thoracic lordosis or lumbar kyphosis, maximum flexion and extension radiographs obtained before surgery with the patient lying supine are advised to assess sagittal flexibility. Flexible curves respond to posterior spinal arthrodesis, whereas rigid curves may be corrected with anterior diskectomy and arthrodesis followed by posterior spinal arthrodesis.

Spinal Cord Injury

Children with spinal cord injury have a very high (greater than 95%) prevalence of scoliosis if they are injured before their adolescent growth spurt, regardless of the level of injury. If injury occurs more than one year before the growth spurt, two thirds of these children will require arthrodesis to prevent severe curve progression. Anterior and posterior arthrodesis usually are recommended, along with antibiotic prophylaxis, to prevent urinary tract infection before and after surgery. Subcutaneous rodding or Luque rodding with sublaminar wires without arthrodesis to allow for growth is not recommended because of the high complication rate.

Dwarfism

Thoracolumbar kyphosis in achondroplasia usually improves spontaneously in 70% to 90% of cases when the child is walking independently, but must be monitored and brace treatment used if the curve progresses. Progressive kyphosis that occurs despite bracing requires early surgery. Surgery must be performed both anteriorly with soft-tissue release and strut grafting and posteriorly with spinal arthrodesis. Posterior instrumentation that invades the spinal canal is associated with significant risk of neurologic compromise, and postoperative casting is necessary. The hip flexion contractures seen in these patients may cause increased lumbar lordosis and aggravate the thoracolumbar kyphosis.

Stenosis of the foramen magnum may contribute to a ventilatory insufficiency such as sleep apnea, or even cause sudden death in infants with achondroplasia. Stenotic deformity in the lumbar spine of patients with achondroplasia occurs with increasing age. Compared to normal patients, there is a 30% decrease in cross-sectional area secondary to both abnormal endochondral ossification of the posterior vertebral growth centers and degenerative changes. If myelography is necessary for evaluation of a neurologic deficit, it should be performed via a cisternal puncture above the suspected lesion to avoid the technical difficulty of inserting a needle into a small canal. Also, removal of cerebrospinal fluid may exacerbate neurologic symptoms in an already compromised small spinal canal. Nonsurgical brace treatment of spinal stenosis should be aimed at decreasing the lumbar lordosis with flexion, thereby "opening up" the spinal canal.

Osteogenesis Imperfecta

The incidence of scoliosis in patients with severe osteogenesis imperfecta is very high, perhaps 50% or more. Bracing has been ineffective in preventing progression. Early spinal arthrodesis has been advocated for curves that progress beyond 50 degrees. Instrumentation with sublaminar wires or mersilene tapes has been effective.

Bone Tumors

Osteoblastomas and aneurysmal bone cysts usually occur in the posterior elements of the spine. Magnetic resonance imaging has been helpful in defining lesions by showing enhancement of the septations of aneurysmal bone cysts.

Giant cell tumor, an uncommon tumor of the spine, usually involves the vertebral body. Complete surgical excision and grafting is the recommended treatment, depending on the location of the tumor. Irradiation is not usually recommended because of the risk of inducing a sarcoma.

Eosinophilic granuloma of the spine usually produces a characteristic picture, known as vertebra plana, on a lateral radiograph. Because the lesion is self-limiting, it should be kept under observation unless it causes a neurologic deficit, in which case surgical decompression and arthrodesis are recommended. In cases of vertebra plana where decompression is not feasible for neurologic deficits, low-dose irradiation of the lesion (500 to 900 rads) is justified to prevent paraplegia.

Problems With Treatment

Laminectomy Patients with neurologic deficits can be treated with decompressive laminectomy from L-2 to S-2. Adequate decompression of the lateral recess and neural foramina is imperative. Laminectomy should not extend cephalad of L-2 for fear of worsening an existing kyphosis. The facet joints must be maintained for spinal integrity.

In children who have had extensive laminectomies, especially when facet excision is included, long-term follow-up care is necessary because these children may develop severe kyphotic deformities. Prophylactic arthrodesis of the thoracic spine should be considered at the time of extensive laminectomy. Although not common, spine deformity after lumbar laminectomy for selective posterior rhizotomy in cerebral palsy patients has been reported.

Irradiation A scoliosis can develop long after a child is exposed to radiation for treatment of a tumor (such as Wilms' tumor), with marked increases in the deformity occurring at the adolescent growth spurt. The convexity usually develops toward the side of the radiation. Careful monitoring of such patients until growth ends is necessary.

Infection

Disk Space Infection Disk space infection is usually caused by *Staphylococcus*. Infection probably begins in one of the contiguous vertebral end plates, and the disk is infected as a result. The characteristic finding is the child's refusal to flex the spine. Children with diskitis usually are not systemically ill. They are rarely febrile and their peripheral leukocyte count is frequently normal; however, the erythrocyte sedimentation rate is usually increased. Lateral radiographs of the spine will occasionally reveal disk space narrowing with erosion of the vertebral end plates of the contiguous vertebrae. Lateral tomography may be necessary for better definition of the lesion. Technetium bone scanning can be helpful; however, false-negative bone scans do occur, and the diagnosis of disk space infection should not be excluded simply because a bone scan reveals no abnormality. Magnetic resonance imaging is very helpful in identifying a disk space infection.

Some authors recommend plaster cast immobilization alone; others believe that antibiotics should also be administered because diskitis is probably caused by *S. aureus* infection, but the use of antibiotics is still controversial. Aspiration biopsy is usually not necessary, because in at least one third of cases an organism is never identified, and in the others, *S. aureus* is usually present. In adolescents, a biopsy may be necessary for diagnosis, especially if drug abuse is suspected, because of the possible presence of organisms other than *S. aureus*.

Vertebral Osteomyelitis Vertebral osteomyelitis differs markedly from disk space infection, and it is much less common. Children with vertebral osteomyelitis are systemically ill; symptoms include fever and increased leukocyte count. These symptoms are usually caused by *S. aureus* infection. Long-term antibiotic therapy is necessary and, if there has been significant bone destruction, anterior debridement and arthrodesis probably will be required to prevent kyphosis. Iliac crest or vascularized rib should be used for the anterior arthrodesis, because nonvascularized rib or fibula may induce formation of a sequestrum.

Tuberculosis of the Spine

Although still rare, tuberculosis of the spine is becoming more common in the United States. Unlike disk space infection in children, tuberculosis affects the vertebral bodies and does not destroy the disk until very late in the disease. Neurologic deficit is uncommon in children. If detected early (before collapse of more than one vertebral body), treatment with antituberculous therapy and plaster cast immobilization may suffice. More advanced disease, characterized by an abscess and a kyphosis, usually requires anterior abscess removal, anterior spinal arthrodesis, posterior spinal arthrodesis, and antituberculous therapy. A recent long-term study found that, after 20-year follow-up, both surgical and conservative treat-

ment had resulted in arthrodesis, but all patients treated conservatively ended up with a kyphosis associated with trunk shortening and a higher incidence of back pain.

Disk Herniation

Only 2% of all herniated disks occur in children and adolescents, but the risk of developing a herniation is approximately five times greater in those with a positive family history. There are fewer objective neurologic deficits in children than in adults, but nerve root tension signs are usually more strongly positive. Children often experience little or no back pain, but sciatica is common. Early surgical results are good, but these results seem to deteriorate with time. Surgeons need to be aware of posterior vertebral body apophyseal avulsion fractures causing sciatica. These are the so-called "hard disks" seen at surgery and should be removed via osteotomies. Sciatica is more common in avulsion fracture of the cephalic posterior vertebral body than in the caudal portion. Computed tomography is the most reliable way to diagnose an avulsion fracture, but slices of both end plates (in addition to soft tissue) must be viewed, or this entity will be missed.

In a study of young, competitive gymnasts, magnetic resonance imaging was used to detect the presence of disk degeneration and other disorders of the lumbar spine. Despite excessive range of motion and strong axial loading of the lumbar spine, which are characteristic of gymnastics maneuvers, incurable primary damage to the disks during growth was not common in young gymnasts.

Spondylolysis

Spondylolysis is classified as one of five types: degenerative, dysplastic, traumatic, isthmic, or pathologic. Some isthmic spondylolytic defects usually appear by 5 to 7 years of age and are strongly influenced by genetic factors. Others are seen more commonly in teenagers and are thought to be the result of repetitive microtrauma, which produces fatigue fractures. This problem is more common in gymnasts and other athletes whose activity requires repetitive flexion-extension. A study of adolescent athletes showed progression from a stress reaction of the pars interarticularis without radiographic findings to an isthmic spondylolytic defect noted on radiographs. In patients older than 25 years of age, spondylolysis is associated with a higher prevalence of disk degeneration than is seen in a normal aging population.

The treatment of acute isthmic or traumatic spondylolysis is controversial; nonsurgical management is appropriate for most patients. Most authors recommend treatment with a brace or cast if the lesion has been recently acquired. The probability of healing can be determined with bone scintigraphy. If increased uptake can be seen on bone scan, healing of the stress fracture is possible. Bone scanning with single photon emission computed tomography should be performed in order to diagnose a stress fracture accurately. Immobilization or avoidance of the inducing stress may be all the treatment needed to allow healing.

Nonsurgical treatment of pain secondary to chronic isthmic spondylolysis is usually continued for at least six months. Surgical treatment is then considered for persistent back pain or hamstring tightness. Excision of the posterior elements alone is not recommended in children, because further slip has been documented. The technique of direct repair using cerclage wire or screws is potentially advantageous for midlumbar spondylolysis in which maximum preservation of mobility is desired, but simple posterolateral arthrodesis is still probably the conventional treatment.

Spondylolisthesis

Treatment of spondylolisthesis depends on symptoms and the degree of the slip. In most instances, nonsurgical treatment is effective. In one study of 149 children and adolescents who were treated with surgery or conservatively, there were no statistical differences between the two groups regarding total progression of the slip. Several studies have concluded that nonsurgical treatment of spondylolisthesis of grade I or less can relieve pain in a majority of patients. Once the patient is asymptomatic, normal activities, including contact sports, may be allowed, although bracing may be necessary.

Intractable pain and neurologic compromise in spite of an adequate trial of nonoperative treatment are the principal indications for surgery. A relative indication may be a severe, progressive slip. The traditional indications, grades III and IV spondylolisthesis in an immature adolescent, is currently being questioned. Conventional surgical treatment for L-5 to S-1 spondylolisthesis consists of posterolateral arthrodesis from L-5 to S-1 for grades I and II and L-4 to S-1 for grades III and higher.

Reduction of forward translation and of the lumbosacral kyphosis that accompanies severe slips has been accomplished by various means, including serial casting, traction, external fixators, and a variety of implanted posterior devices such as pedicle screws, plates, and rods. These treatments are now controversial. Further progression of severe slips after apparently solid in situ arthrodesis is one rationale for reduction and instrumentation. A risk factor to predict postoperative progression is a preoperative slip angle greater than 35 degrees. The slip angle is measured by drawing a line perpendicular to a line drawn along the posterior aspect of the first sacral vertebral body and measuring the angle between that and a line parallel to the inferior end plate of L-5 (Figs. 2 and 3). Another rationale for reduction of the slip is improvement in the cosmetic appearance of the trunk.

The major cause of failure of spondylolisthesis surgery is thought to be the lack of high-quality alar-transverse process arthrodesis and inadequate postoperative immobilization of the patient. Most studies of spondylolisthesis reductions report new L-5 root deficits, some of which are permanent. The major problem with these reduction techniques is that nerve root injuries are not only at the

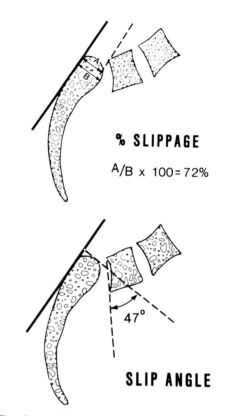

Fig. 2 The slip angle is measured by drawing a line perpendicular to a line drawn along the posterior aspect of the first sacral vertebral body, and measuring the angle between that and a line parallel to the inferior end plate of L-5. (Reproduced with permission from Bradford DS, Hensinger RN (eds): *The Pediatric Spine*. New York, Thieme, Inc, 1985, p 406.)

level of spondylolisthesis but also throughout the lumbosacral plexus because of the trunk lengthening that occurs. Nerve root injury is rare when in situ arthrodesis alone is performed. The issue of reduction versus in situ arthrodesis has not been resolved.

The occurrence of acute cauda equina syndrome after in situ arthrodesis for spondylolisthesis has been reported. Preoperative evaluation for clinically unapparent neurogenic bladder in patients with grades III and IV spondylolisthesis is recommended. If the cauda equina syndrome occurs after arthrodesis in situ, the posterior aspect of the S-1 vertebral body should be removed. Partial reduction of the spondylolisthesis should also be considered.

In a large number of patients, sciatic lumbar scoliosis associated with spondylolisthesis appears to correct itself spontaneously following arthrodesis.

Scheuermann's Disease

Normal kyphosis ranges from 20 to 45 degrees in the thoracic vertebrae, if end vertebrae of the Cobb measurement are not specified. Because the upper thoracic

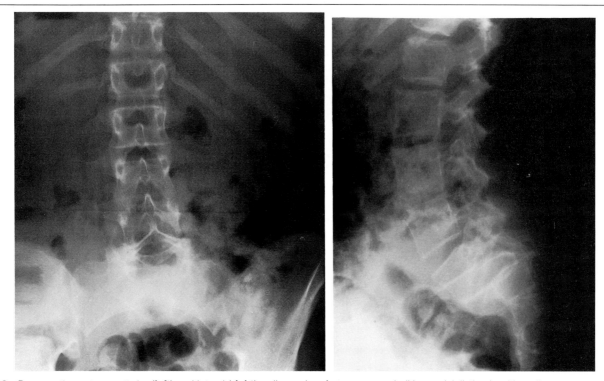

Fig. 3 Preoperative anteroposterior (**left**) and lateral (**right**) radiographs of a severe grade IV spondylolisthesis with a slip angle of 55 degrees.

spine (T-1 to T-5) cannot always be seen on a routine lateral radiograph, a curve measuring more than 33 degrees from T-5 to T-12 should be considered suspicious for abnormal kyphosis and warrants additional, better-quality lateral thoracic spine radiographs. Scheuermann's disease of the thoracic spine is defined as an excessive thoracic kyphosis (Cobb angle greater than 45 degrees) with wedging of 5 degrees or more of at least three adjacent apical vertebrae and vertebral end-plate irregularities. The prevalence of abnormal kyphosis is approximately 1% of the general population, with a slight female-to-male dominance of 1.4:1. Although its etiology is not known, histologic and histochemical studies of Scheuermann's disease indicate a marked alteration in the cartilage growth plate of the vertebral bodies. Bone growth is stunted in these areas, and disk material penetrates into the vertebral bodies (Schmorl's nodes). There have been no inflammatory findings and no evidence of necrotic bone. Density of trabecular bone of the lumbar vertebrae in patients with Scheuermann's disease was not significantly different from that of a group of controls.

Kyphosis in this area is rarely painful, but treatment is indicated if the deformity is cosmetically unacceptable. In skeletally immature patients with curves greater than 50 degrees, treatment with a Milwaukee brace is recommended until skeletal maturity is reached. An underarm

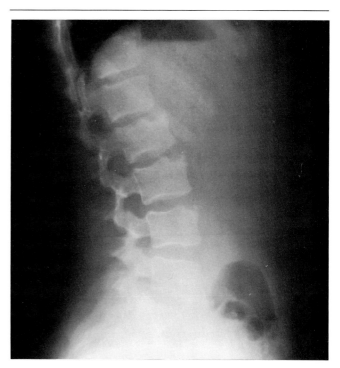

Fig. 4 Lateral radiograph of a 15-year-old male with low back pain. The patient is an active weightlifter. Radiograph reveals lumbar Scheuermann's epiphysitis with defects in the secondary ossification centers.

orthosis also may be used for flexible curves. Progressive curves greater than 75 degrees, or those with an unacceptable cosmesis, require anterior release and spinal arthrodesis and posterior spinal arthrodesis with instrumentation to achieve permanent correction.

The thoracolumbar spine is normally straight; therefore a kyphosis deformity of only 30 degrees can be distinctly abnormal. Scheuermann's disease of the thoracolumbar spine is frequently painful and cosmetically unacceptable. Radiographs reveal anterior deficits in the affected vertebral bodies. Pain associated with this disease is treated conservatively, and most patients are asymptomatic within several months. Occasionally, short-term cast or brace immobilization is necessary for complete pain relief. Cosmetic disfigurement may be severe in spite of a small angle of kyphosis because of its location in the thoracolumbar region, and surgery may be necessary.

Lumbar Scheuermann's epiphysitis is a separate entity, producing pain but not deformity. Defects are seen in the secondary ossification centers of the lumbar vertebrae on lateral radiographs (Fig. 4). Although the pain usually abates with reduced activity (especially reduced weight-lifting), occasionally bracing may be necessary.

Annotated Bibliography

Congenital Deformity of the Spine

Bradford DS, Boachie-Adjei O: One-stage anterior and posterior hemivertebral resection and arthrodesis for congenital scoliosis. *J Bone Joint Surg* 1990;72A:536-540.

Seven children with a fully segmented lumbar hemivertebrae were treated successfully with a single-stage anterior and posterior vertebral resection and arthrodesis.

Bradford DS, Heithoff KB, Cohen M: Intraspinal abnormalities and congenital spine deformities: A radiographic and MRI study. *J Pediatr Orthop* 1991;11:36-41.

Patients with congenital spinal deformity were studied with magnetic resonance imaging, revealing intraspinal abnormalities in 16 of 42 patients (38%), including a tethered cord, diastematomyelia, diplomyelia, syringomyelia, low-lying clonus, and teratoma of the sacrum.

Winter RB, Lonstein JE, Denis F, et al: Convex growth arrest for progressive congenital scoliosis due to hemivertebrae. *J Pediatr Orthop* 1988;8:633-638.

A detailed description of the surgical technique is included in this article. Five patients showed correction as a result of the epiphysiodesis (average 10 degrees) and only one curve progressed further. The absence of excessive kyphosis or lordosis, a short curve, and an age of less than 5 years were associated with postoperative correction.

Natural History

Betz RR, Bunnell WP, Lambrecht-Mulier E, et al: Scoliosis and pregnancy. *J Bone Joint Surg* 1987;69A:90-96.

In adult females with idiopathic scoliosis, just as many curvatures progressed in patients who were pregnant as in those who had never been pregnant.

Radiology

Morrissy RT, Goldsmith GS, Hall EC, et al: Measurement of the Cobb angle on radiographs of patients who have scoliosis: Evaluation of intrinsic error. *J Bone Joint Surg* 1990;72A:320-327.

When the examiners used the same end vertebrae, the range of error was 6.3 degrees, but when each examiner was permitted to select end vertebrae, the error increased to 7.2 degrees. When a single observer measured the same radiograph with consistent end vertebrae and a precision goniometer with extrinsic error eliminated, there was a 95% chance of the error in measurement being less than 3 degrees. The three main causes of extrinsic error are patient positioning, position of the radiographic tube, and the time of day the radiograph was obtained. Error can also be increased when measuring thoracolumbar and lumbar curves because of the poor vertebral landmarks caused by rotation.

Treatment: Bracing

O'Donnell CS, Bunnell WP, Betz RR, et al: Electrical stimulation in the treatment of idiopathic scoliosis. *Clin Orthop* 1988;229:107-113.

In patients treated with electrical stimulation, results were no better than those of control patients who were not treated.

Treatment: Surgery

Dickson JH, Erwin WD, Rossi D: Harrington instrumentation and arthrodesis for idiopathic scoliosis: A twenty-one-year follow-up. *J Bone Joint Surg* 1990;72A:678-683.

A questionnaire was sent to 206 patients with idiopathic scoliosis who were treated surgically by Dr. Paul R. Harrington between 1961 and 1963. Eighty-three percent of patients responded, and 111 patients also sent recent radiographs. A control group of 100 individuals matched for age and sex who did not have scoliosis were sent the same questionnaire. There was no difference with respect to pain in the lumbosacral area or the low back. Twenty-one years after the operation, the patients were functioning quite well compared with the control subjects.

Lagrone MO, Bradford DS, Moe JH, et al: Treatment of symptomatic flatback after spinal fusion. *J Bone Joint Surg* 1988;70A:569-580.

Although this article concentrates on the reconstruction of symptomatic flatback after arthrodesis, it also addresses its causes, noting a relationship with Harrington distraction instrumentation placed in the lower lumbar spine or sacrum. Avoidance of distraction instrumentation in the lower lumbar spine is advised.

Patterson JF, Webb JK, Burwell RG: The operative treatment of progressive early onset scoliosis: A preliminary report. *Spine* 1990;15:809-815.

Thirteen patients were studied who had undergone posterior segmental spinal instrumentation (SSI) without arthrodesis or SSI and anterior apical growth arrest as a separate procedure. The authors concluded that surgical treatment is successful in the short term in all but the most malignant forms of infantile scoliosis.

Mannherz RE, Betz RR, Clancy M, et al: Juvenile idiopathic scoliosis followed to skeletal maturity. *Spine* 1988;13:1087-1090.

Forty-three patients with onset of idiopathic scoliosis between 4 and 9 years of age were studied until skeletal maturity was achieved to document the natural history, effects of bracing, and factors associated with progression (including rib vertebral angle differences and thoracic hypokyphosis).

Neuromuscular Spine Deformity

Padman R, McNamara R: Postoperative pulmonary complications in children with neuromuscular scoliosis who underwent posterior spinal fusion. *Del Med J* 1990;62:999-1003.

Low preoperative vital capacity was shown to correlate with the need for longer postoperative ventilatory assistance. Patients with a preoperative vital capacity of 44% spent an average of 60 hours on a ventilator after surgery. A vital capacity of 59.2% was associated with atelectasis, and these patients spent 44 hours on a ventilator after surgery. Patients with a vital capacity of 64.6% had no complications and spent 26.8 hours on the ventilator after surgery. The preoperative vital capacity is an important prognostic parameter in evaluating postoperative pulmonary recovery.

Phillips DP, Roye DP Jr, Farcy JP, et al: Surgical treatment of scoliosis in a spinal muscular atrophy population. *Spine* 1990;15:942-945.

Scoliosis developed in 34 of 78 patients with spinal muscular atrophy. The prolonged survival rate in these patients justifies aggressive orthopaedic treatment of scoliosis, both to prevent progression and deformity and to improve sitting comfort.

Smith AD, Koreska J, Moseley CF: Progression of scoliosis in Duchenne muscular dystrophy. *J Bone Joint Surg* 1989;71A:1066-1074.

When the curve of a patient with Duchenne muscular dystrophy exceeded 35 degrees, the vital capacity was usually less than 40% of normal. Therefore, when walking becomes impossible, spinal arthrodesis should be considered.

Bell DF, Moseley CF, Koreska J: Unit rod segmental spinal instrumentation in the management of patients with progressive neuromuscular spinal deformity. *Spine* 1989;14:1301-1307.

Stability and curve correction were obtained using unit rod segmental spinal instrumentation in patients with neuromuscular spine deformity.

Dwarfism

Mador MJ, Tobin MJ: Apneustic breathing: A characteristic feature of brainstem compression in achondroplasia? *Chest* 1990;97:877-883.

The authors suggest that cervicomedullary compression may be capable of producing apneustic breathing in patients with achondroplasia.

Lonstein JE: Anatomy of the lumbar spinal canal. *Basic Life Sci* 1988;4:219-226.

This study found decreased cross-sectional area in the lumbar spinal canal of patients with achondroplasia, in addition to associated thoracolumbar kyphosis and a lumbosacral hyperlordosis. On aging, there is disk degeneration with disk space narrowing and osteophyte information. In acknowledging the normal spinal anatomy in the patient with achondroplasia, surgeons can plan treatment accordingly.

Neurofibromatosis

Crawford AH: Pitfalls of spinal deformities associated with neurofibromatosis in children. *Clin Orthop* 1989;245:29-42.

If the kyphotic angle is greater than 50 degrees or if scoliosis is greater than 80 degrees, anterior disk excision and bone graft followed by posterior arthrodesis with instrumentation are indicated. Even these combined operations did not guarantee successful permanent spine stability in young patients with neurofibromatosis.

Spondylolysis and Spondylolisthesis

Bell DF, Ehrlich MG, Zaleske DJ: Brace treatment for symptomatic spondylolisthesis. *Clin Orthop* 1988;236:192-198.

At the conclusion of brace treatment, all 28 patients with grades I and II spondylolisthesis were pain-free, and none had demonstrated a significant increase in slip percentage.

Cohen BA, Huizenga BA: Dermatomal monitoring for surgical correction of spondylolisthesis: A case report. *Spine* 1988;13:1125-1128.

Routine somatosensory-evoked potential (SEP) studies are probably not accurate enough to detect damage to nerve roots during surgical correction of spondylolisthesis. This study reports dermatomal monitoring as an alternative to SEPs.

Harris IE, Weinstein SL: Long-term follow-up of patients with grade III and IV spondylolisthesis: Treatment with and without posterior fusion. *J Bone Joint Surg* 1987;69A:960-969.

Patients with and without arthrodesis were both symptom-free, although those with arthrodesis showed some advantage.

Schoenecker PL, Cole HO, Herring JA, et al: Cauda equina syndrome after in situ arthrodesis for severe spondylolisthesis at the lumbosacral junction. *J Bone Joint Surg* 1990;72A:369-377.

This report identified 12 patients who developed acute cauda equina syndrome after surgery. The authors recommend immediate decompression that includes resection of the posterior-superior rim of the dome of the sacrum and possible internal fixation.

Seitsalo S: Operative and conservative treatment of moderate spondylolisthesis in young patients. *J Bone Joint Surg* 1990;72B:908-913.

This is a retrospective study of 149 children and adolescents with a slip less than or equal to 30%. Patients who were treated surgically compared to those treated nonsurgically had better clinical results and less pain at current review, but the total progression of the slip over the entire follow-up period showed no statistical differences between the two groups. Spontaneous segmental stabilization seemed to occur as a result of degeneration of the disk at the slip level.

Seitsalo S, Osterman K, Poussa M: Scoliosis associated with lumbar spondylolisthesis: A clinical survey of 190 young patients. *Spine* 1988;13:899-904.

Sciatic lumbar scoliosis associated with spondylolisthesis disappeared in 25 of 39 patients following lumbosacral arthrodesis, suggesting the "sciatic muscle spasm" as a causative factor. The torsional type of curve resulting from asymmetrical slipping of the vertebra was also corrected after arthrodesis in 19 of 28 cases.

Szypryt EP, Twining P, Mulholland RC, et al: The prevalence of disc degeneration associated with neural arch defects of the lumbar spine assessed by magnetic resonance imaging. *Spine* 1989;14:977-981.

The intervertebral disks of 40 patients with mild spondylolysis and spondylolisthesis were studied with magnetic resonance imaging. The results suggest that after 25 years of age, a neural arch defect is associated with an increased prevalence of disk degeneration, greater than that seen in a normal aging population.

van den Oever M, Merrick MV, Scott JH: Bone scintigraphy in symptomatic spondylolysis. *J Bone Joint Surg* 1987;69B:453-456.

In a series of patients with back pain and suspected spondylolysis, bone scintigraphy proved useful in detecting stress fractures and fresh spondylolysis and helped distinguish these from established spondylolysis.

Bodner RJ, Heyman S, Drummond DS, et al: The use of single photon emission computed tomography (SPECT) in the diagnosis of low-back pain in young patients. *Spine* 1988;13:1155-1160.

Single photon emission computed tomography (SPECT) is a method of scintigraphy that provides sectional and multiplanar imaging that improved the diagnosis of stress fractures or stress reactions of the spine.

Scheuermann's Disease

Blumenthal SL, Roach J, Herring JA: Lumbar Scheuermann's: A clinical series and classification. *Spine* 1987;1;929-932.

The diagnosis of "lumbar Scheuermann's" is reviewed and a classification proposed.

Lowe TG: Scheuermann disease. *J Bone Joint Surg* 1990;72A:940-945.

This is a comprehensive review of Scheuermann's disease.

Ogilvie JW, Sherman J: Spondylolysis in Scheuermann's disease. *Spine* 1987;12:251-253.

Increased lumbar lordosis and a 50% incidence of asymptomatic spondylolysis were found in 18 patients with Scheuermann's kyphosis.

Gilsanz V, Gibbens DT, Carlson M, et al: Vertebral bone density in Scheuermann disease. *J Bone Joint Surg* 1989;71A:894-897.

The density of trabecular bone in the lumbar vertebra in patients with Scheuermann's disease was not significantly different (p = 0.28) from that in controls.

Disk Disease

Tertti M, Paajanen H, Kujala UM, et al: Disc degeneration in young gymnasts: A magnetic resonance imaging study. *Am J Sports Med* 1990;18:206-208.

Magnetic resonance imaging was performed on 35 young competitive gymnasts and ten control subjects. Despite the excessive range of motion and strong axial loading of the lumbar spine that are associated with gymnastic maneuvers, incurable primary damage to the intervertebral disks is uncommon during growth in young gymnasts.

Hashimoto K, Fugita K, Kojimoto H, et al: Lumbar disc herniation in children. *J Pediatr Orthop* 1990;10:394-396.

This article discusses an important area of differential diagnosis in the treatment of sciatica in adolescents. This series of 12 patients showed no statistically significant difference in age, history of trauma, or symptoms between patients with an apophyseal fracture and patients with herniated nucleus pulposus.

Takata K, Inoue S, Takahashi K, et al: Fracture of the posterior margin of a lumbar vertebral body. *J Bone Joint Surg* 1988;70A:589-594.

This study showed that end-plate fractures at the caudal rim of the lumbar vertebrae were different symptomatically than those at the cephalad end. The authors found sciatica in all patients who had an apophyseal fracture of the cephalad end but in only two of eight patients with fractures of the caudal rim. They recommend further investigation of the cause of sciatica when an avulsion fracture of the caudal rim of the lumbar vertebrae is present, because the causes of sciatica differ in these two groups.

Varlotta GP, Brown MD, Kelsey JL, et al: Familial predisposition for herniation of a lumbar disc in patients who are less than twenty-one years old. *J Bone Joint Surg* 1991;73A:124-128.

The relative risk for development of herniation of a lumbar disk before the age of 21 is approximately five times greater in patients with a positive family history.

Heller RM, Szalay EA, Green NE, et al: Disc space infection in children: Magnetic resonance imaging. *Radiol Clin North Am* 1988;26:207-209.

Magnetic resonance imaging is a noninvasive technique that is very sensitive to disk space infection in children and is helpful in establishing the correct diagnosis.

37

Thoracolumbar Spine: Trauma

Introduction

Approximately 162,000 Americans annually sustain a fracture of the vertebral column, and the thoracolumbar spine is the predominant site for injury. The primary goals in managing these injuries are preservation of life, protection of neurologic function, minimization of the risk of further spinal column or neurologic injury, and maintenance or restoration of spinal stability and alignment.

The management of spine fractures is both similar to and markedly different from the management of long-bone fractures. While the principles of reduction, stabilization, promotion of fracture healing, preservation of joint motion, and early patient mobilization are shared, most spine fractures differ from long-bone fractures in that they involve multiple structures, including articular facets, which may be subluxated or dislocated; intervertebral disks, which may be disrupted; and ligaments, which may be injured. Consequently, union of the vertebral fracture may not be sufficient for full functional restoration of the patient. Recovery from incomplete neurologic injury has not been consistent despite early and adequate decompression, the use of increasingly efficient devices for internal immobilization, and the attainment of arthrodesis.

Approach to the Patient With Thoracolumbar Spine Injury

Prehospital Care

The management of a patient with an injured spine, with or without neurologic deficit, starts at the scene of the accident. Emergency personnel must maintain a high index of a suspicion for spinal cord injury. Improved training of paramedical personnel and great attention to immobilization have resulted in a significant reduction of complete spinal cord injuries over the last two decades. Accident scene investigation and injury mechanism reconstruction can often aid in determining whether the victim is at risk for spinal column injury. The lap seat belt may be associated with a characteristic thoracolumbar flexion-distraction type of injury. The addition of a shoulder harness has decreased the injuries to the thoracolumbar junction; however, these restraints increase the forces about the upper thoracic and cervical levels. When a person is thrown from a motor vehicle, thoracolumbar fracture dislocation frequently occurs. Any unconscious victim of a traumatic event should be approached as though a spinal injury is present until proven otherwise.

Acute Hospital Evaluation

Upon arrival at the Emergency Room, the patient is kept rigidly immobilized on a spine board until the vertebral column can be definitively assessed. If neurologic deficit is present or if significant spine instability exists, a rotating bed will help protect the spine and decrease pulmonary and skin complications prior to surgical stabilization. Even if the injury appears to be limited to the spine, it is important to remember that thoracolumbar fractures are commonly associated with abdominal trauma, and the risks for such injuries are greater when there is an associated neurologic deficit. It is also important to evaluate carefully the entire spine; it has been shown that there is a 10% to 20% likelihood of contiguous or remote associated spinal fracture.

Spine injuries are frequently overlooked initially. The most common predisposing factors associated with a missed or delayed diagnosis include patient intoxication, multilevel spinal fractures, multiple trauma, and head injury.

History and Physical Examination

A complete and documented history and physical examination must be conducted at the time of the initial hospital evaluation and repetitively over time. Essentials of the physical examination include inspection and palpation of the back, because injuries to the skin can dictate the time course of management.

The neurologic assessment includes deep tendon reflexes, elicitation of plantar, bulbocavernosus, and abdominal reflexes, and motor and sensory evaluation. Sensory sparing, which suggests an improved prognosis for the patient, is important to document. The bulbocavernosus reflex involves the S-1, S-2, and S-3 nerve roots and is a spinal cord-mediated reflex arc. The presence or absence of this reflex carries great prognostic significance. Its absence documents the continuation of spinal shock or spinal injury at the level of the reflex arc itself. Rarely does spinal shock last beyond 48 hours. The return of the bulbocavernosus reflex signals the termination of spinal shock. A complete absence of distal motor or sensory function or perirectal sensation, together with recovery of the bulbocavernosus reflex, indicates a complete cord injury, and in such cases it is highly unlikely that significant neurologic function will ever return. Incomplete cord lesions are present when there is any distal sparing of motor or sensory function along with sparing of perirectal sensation. The return of the bulbo-cavernosus reflex has less prognostic significance in an incomplete cord lesion.

Of patients sustaining spine fractures, 10% to 15% have associated major visceral disruption. In patients with head and spinal cord injuries, the reported incidence of undetected fractures is 11%; the incidence of peripheral nerve injuries is also 11%. Truncal and extremity injuries must be suspected and excluded, particularly below the insensate level in a patient with a cord injury or head injury.

Radiographic Examination

The initial assessment consists of anteroposterior and lateral radiographs of the spine. At the present time computed tomography (CT) is superior to other techniques for demonstrating bone impingement on the neural canal and for assessing stability. It is highly recommended that any young adult involved in a high-energy injury who appears on plain films to have just a compression fracture have CT scanning. The major advantage of axial CT is its ability to visualize the spinal canal, the degree of neural compromise, and to delineate clearly posterior element involvement, particularly in a burst fracture. The disadvantage of axial CT is its inability to detect subtle horizontally oriented fractures of the vertebral bodies, pedicles, or lamina. Minimal vertebral body compression fractures may be missed. However, many of these problems can be overcome by accurate frontal and sagittal reformation.

A dural laceration with impaled nerve roots can be anticipated at the time of surgery if a patient with neurologic injury has a burst fracture of the vertebral body combined with a laminar fracture at the same level. This is often best seen on a CT study. However, plain films often suggest the laminar fracture.

Conventional tomography is particularly advantageous in the evaluation of transverse or axially oriented injuries, horizontal laminar fractures, and some facet injuries. However, CT reconstruction formats using thin-slice sagittal and/or coronal modes may negate the need for conventional tomography.

Magnetic resonance imaging (MRI) is often complementary to rather than a replacement study for CT scanning. CT scanning clearly defines osseous anatomy; MRI better demonstrates the status of the intervertebral disk, potential sites of ligamentous injury, and epidural hematoma, and more precisely defines the extent of spinal cord injury.

Patterns of MRI signal abnormality in spinal cord injury can have prognostic significance by differentiating cord edema from hemorrhage or vascular infarction. Indications for MRI include spinal cord injury without obvious explanation (fractures of insufficient magnitude to produce neural injury) or clinical progression of a neural deficit. MRI is particularly useful when traumatic disk herniation may accompany an injury. Despite the many

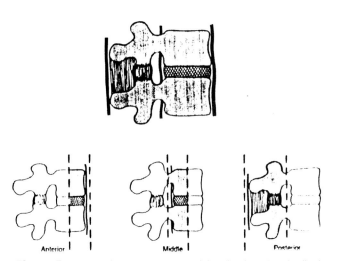

Fig. 1 The anatomic structures comprising the three longitudinal columns of stability in the thoracolumbar spine (Denis three-column model). **Bottom left**, Anterior column comprising the anterior longitudinal ligament, anterior aspect of the vertebral body, and anterior aspect of the annulus fibrosis. **Bottom center**, Middle column comprising the posterior longitudinal ligament, posterior aspect of the vertebral body, and the posterior annulus fibrosis. **Bottom right**, Posterior column comprising the pedicles, facet joint and facet capsules, ligamentus flavum, osseous neural arch, and interspinous and supraspinous ligaments. (Reproduced with permission of Eismont F, Garfin S, Abitbol J-J: Thoracic and upper lumbar spine injuries, in Browner BD, Jupiter JB, Levine AM, et al (eds): *Skeletal Trauma.* Philadelphia, WB Saunders, 1992, vol 1, p 744.)

advantages of MRI, it cannot be used for patients who have cardiac pacemakers, ferromagnetic implants, or claustrophobia. In addition, it is difficult to image a patient who requires mechanical ventilation and other life support systems in an emergency situation.

Myelography alone is rarely indicated for the acute evaluation of spine trauma since the advent of MRI, but it may be helpful in evaluating nerve root avulsions or suspected dural tears. CT enhanced with intrathecal contrast is superior to myelography alone in localizing soft tissue compromise of the spinal cord.

Classification of Fractures

Several classifications of thoracolumbar spine fractures have been proposed. Holdsworth's description was based on a two-column model, in which the posterior longitudinal ligament and all structures anterior to it made up the anterior weightbearing column, and a posterior column consisting of the neural arches and ligaments resisted tension. Although this model helped to explain the chronic instability often seen after many spinal injuries, especially those resulting in a kyphotic deformity, it was not able to fully explain all cases of acute instability. Experiments had shown that complete section of the posterior elements alone did not result in acute instability in flexion, extension, rotation, and shear. To better reconcile

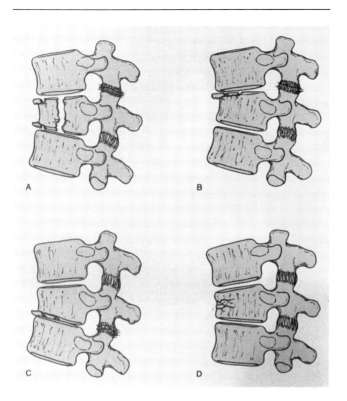

Fig. 2 Four types of compression fractures according to the Denis classification. Type A, involvement of both endplates. Type B, involvement of superior endplate only. Type C, inferior endplate only. Type D, buckling of the anterior cortex with both endplates intact. (Reproduced with permission of Eismont F, Garfin S, Abitbol J-J: Thoracic and upper lumbar spine injuries, in Browner BD, Jupiter JB, Levine AM, et al (eds): *Skeletal Trauma.* Philadelphia, WB Saunders, 1992, vol 1, p 746.)

these clinical and biomechanical observations, Denis proposed a three-column model of the spine, which has achieved wide acceptance (Fig. 1). This classification system is simple to understand and is useful in its application. The middle column, with osteoligamentous and neural elements, consists of the posterior longitudinal ligament, the posterior portions of the vertebral body, and the posterior annulus, along with the spinal cord or cauda equina. Columns can fail individually or in combination by four basic mechanisms of injury—compression, distraction, rotation, and shear. These mechanisms can displace the spinal column beyond its physiologic range in translation, in angulation, or in some combination of these. The resulting thoracolumbar spine injuries are of four major types—compression, burst, flexion distraction (seat belt type), and fracture dislocations. Each of these has a specific mechanism of injury.

Compression Fractures

Compression fractures injure the anterior portion of the vertebral body as a result of anterior or lateral flexion that causes failure of the anterior column (Figs. 2 and 3).

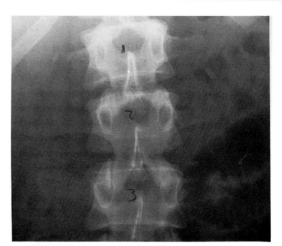

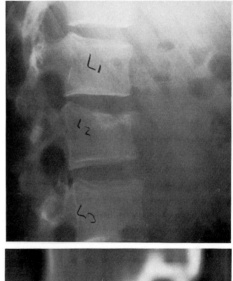

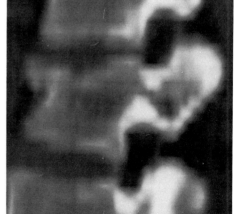

Fig. 3 **Top,** Anteroposterior and (**center**) lateral radiographs of a compression fracture of L2. Note the intact posterior vertebral body cortex, less than 40 degrees anterior vertebral body height, no pedicular widening, no lateral shift, and no anteroposterior translation. **Bottom,** Computed tomographic scan reveals involvement of anterosuperior endplate only—a Denis type B compression fracture.

The middle column remains intact. In some cases, there may be disruption of the posterior column in tension, as the upper segments hinge forward on the intact middle column. Radiographically, the anterior height of the vertebral body is diminished, while the posterior height remains normal. There is no anterior or posterior translation of vertebral bodies. The amount of anterior compression is less than 40 degrees of the posterior body height. These fractures are normally stable and rarely involve a neurologic deficit.

Burst Fractures

The essential feature of a burst injury (Fig. 4) is disruption of the middle column with varying degrees of retropulsion into the neural canal, best identified on a CT scan. There may be spreading of the posterior elements, seen on the plain anteroposterior radiograph of the spine as a widening of the interpedicular distance. When the posterior elements are involved, neurologic injury is present in 50% of cases. In these instances, it is important to recognize that neural injury may be caused by neural element entrapment in laminar fractures. Dural laceration should be suspected. Five subgroups have been identified by Denis, based on which end plate is involved, whether both end plates are involved, and on the rotational or lateral flexion component.

Dislocations

These injuries are considered to be unstable, because all three columns have failed. Multiple forces are involved, including rotation, distraction, compression, and shear. Complete dislocation or subluxation may occur, but some may reduce spontaneously. The magnitude of the injury may not be apparent on the initial evaluation. Fracture dislocations are highly unstable and are often associated with neurologic deficit, dural tears, and intra-abdominal injury (Fig. 5).

Flexion-Distraction Injuries

Chance first described this injury in 1948 as a fracture that involves the upper half of the spinous process and extends anteriorly through the pedicles to emerge on the superior aspect of the vertebral body. Stability depends on the magnitude of the forces, the integrity of the anterior longitudinal ligament, and the pattern of structural involvement, which may be purely ligamentous, purely osseous, or mixed. Osseous injuries have the potential for bony union. Pure ligamentous and mixed lesions lack this potential and involve an increased risk of long-term instability. Radiographic findings include an increased interspinous process distance on the anteroposterior and lateral views, as well as some increased posterior height of the vertebral body relative to the anterior portion of the vertebral body on the lateral film. Flexion-distraction injuries of the Chance type are seldom associated with neurologic compromise, unless a significant amount

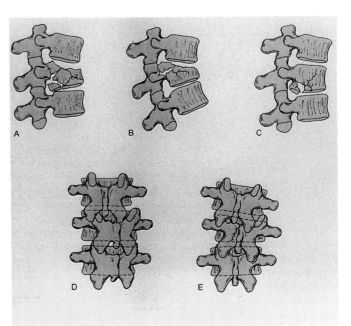

Fig. 4 Burst fractures as classified by Denis. **A**, retropulsion of bone into the canal with fractures of both endplates. **B**, superior endplate. **C**, inferior endplate. **D**, a combination of type A with rotation and best appreciated on the anteroposterior view. **E**, a laterally directed fracture with retropulsion and involvement of endplates. (Reproduced with permission of Eismont F, Garfin S, Abitbol J-J: Thoracic and upper lumbar spine injuries, in Browner BD, Jupiter JB, Levine AM, et al (eds): *Skeletal Trauma.* Philadelphia, WB Saunders, 1992, vol 1, p 753.)

of translation is noted on the lateral radiograph. If this is the case, the injury is probably a true fracture dislocation rather than a simple flexion-distraction injury.

Extension Injuries

In extension injuries, the trunk or head is forced backward, which applies tensile forces to the anterior longitudinal ligament and anterior disk, and compression forces to the posterior elements. An extension injury may result in radiographic evidence of an anterior vertebral body avulsion fracture, as well as fractures of the spinous processes, lamina, and, occasionally, the pedicles. These fractures are usually stable.

Transverse Process Fractures

These injuries are the result of blunt trauma or violent contraction of the paraspinal musculature. When multiple fractures are present as the result of blunt trauma, particularly when the L-5 transverse process is fractured, there is frequent association with intra-abdominal (particularly renal) injuries and pelvic disruption. Occasion-

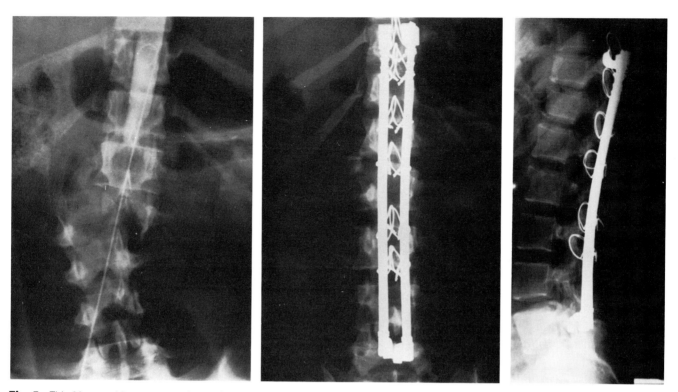

Fig. 5 This 30-year-old woman was thrown from her vehicle and suffered intra-abdominal trauma in addition to near complete paraplegia. This injury requires rotational as well as flexion and translation forces. She was treated with rodding and sublaminar segmental fixation very early in her hospital course.

ally neuropraxias result, typically involving the L-3 and L-4 nerve roots.

Spinous Process Avulsions

Spinous process avulsions are fairly rare in the lumbar spine and are usually the result of direct trauma. These are generally considered stable unless they are associated with a more complex pattern of involvement, such as flexion distraction.

Isolated Facet Fracture

These fractures are uncommon, but may occur in patients with prior laminectomies, most commonly as a result of a fatigue mechanism rather than an acute injury.

Pharmacologic Treatment

Deleterious metabolic and histologic changes occur within seconds of injury to the spinal cord. Whether neurologic injury occurs or not depends on numerous factors. These include: (1) the level of injury— T-1 to T-10 (cord level), T-11 to L-2 (mixed conus medullaris and spinal roots), L-2 to sacrum (cauda equina); (2) the amount of initial displacement of the vertebral components relative to one another that occurs at the time of injury; (3) the amount of spinal canal reserve; and (4) the degree of canal encroachment by vertebral fragments. In general, lesions in the upper thoracic spine associated with significant translation and fragments in the canal tend to be associated with a greater degree of neurologic involvement than is seen in less displaced fractures of the lower lumbar area.

The vascular compromise associated with spinal trauma in conjunction with the inflammatory and reparative reactions affect the extent of neurologic injury. The microvasculature of the neurologic structures can be disrupted by mechanical deformation, motion stresses, edema, thrombosis, or vasoconstriction induced by local and systemic biochemical compounds. Hemodynamic changes resulting from loss of vasomotor activity, lack of response to carbon dioxide, decreased blood flow, and decreased oxygen can produce devastating effects. Maintenance of perfusion at the cellular level of the spinal cord is important to protect remaining viable tissue and allow for recovery. Agents such as norepinephrine produce vasoconstriction and diminished perfusion; whereas lysosomes, hydrolases, and lactic acid can significantly disrupt cell metabolism. Many therapies attempted to arrest or reverse ischemic insults, and despite encouraging experimental results, clinical efficacy has not been unequivocally demonstrated.

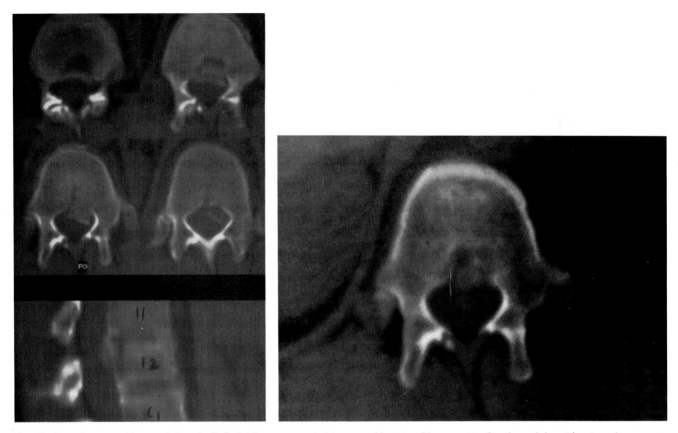

Fig. 6   Burst fracture with remodeling. **Left**, Serial 3-mm computed tomographic cuts with reconstruction through burst fracture shows one-third canal compromise by retropulsed fragments, intact pedicles, no laminar fracture, and facet joints intact. There was less than 20 degrees of kyphosis and on the lateral view. The patient was treated with 3 weeks of bed rest, followed by 2 months of immobilization in TLSO in an outpatient ambulatory setting. **Right**, Computed tomographic scan 9 months post injury with near complete restoration of canal dimensions secondary to resorption of retropulsed bone.

Medications of potential benefits to the patient with an injured spinal cord include glucocorticoids or corticosteroids, opiate antagonists (thyrotropin-releasing hormone), and opiate receptor antagonists, such as naloxone. Used in animal studies, all of these have been much superior to controls in promoting recovery from neurologic injury. Clinical studies are currently underway that seek to correlate the efficacy of naloxone, thyrotropin-releasing hormone, and oxygenated fluorocarbons. The clinical use of corticosteroids is based initially on the observation that their use significantly reduced cerebral edema around brain tumors.

A recent published multicenter randomized, double-blind, placebo-controlled trial in patients with acute spinal cord injury used a bolus (30 mg/kg body weight) of methylprednisolone, followed by an infusion (5.4 mg/kg per hour) for 23 hours. In patients with acute spinal cord injury, treatment with methylprednisolone in these high doses improved neurologic recovery when the medication was given in the first eight hours following injury. A large multicenter study is currently underway to further evaluate the use of high-dose methylprednisolone.

Management of Specific Fractures

Compression Fractures

Compression fractures are generally stable and rarely involve neurologic compromise. For the most part they can be treated symptomatically with a short period of bed rest for pain control only. Depending on the degree of compression, the patient may be treated effectively by hyperextension exercises and the avoidance of compression overloads for a period of approximately 12 weeks. Early ambulation is encouraged in a hyperextension orthosis. However, if there is loss of greater than 50% of vertebral body height, angulation greater than 20 degrees, or multiple adjacent compression fractures, the injury is considered to be potentially unstable. These injuries usually require treatment in a hyperextension cast, or possibly an open reduction and internal fixation using posterior instrumentation and arthrodesis, depending on the severity of the injury. Therefore, compression fractures with greater than 50% compression and 20 degrees of angulation treated in a hyperextension cast require close follow-up; if follow-up evaluation four to six weeks

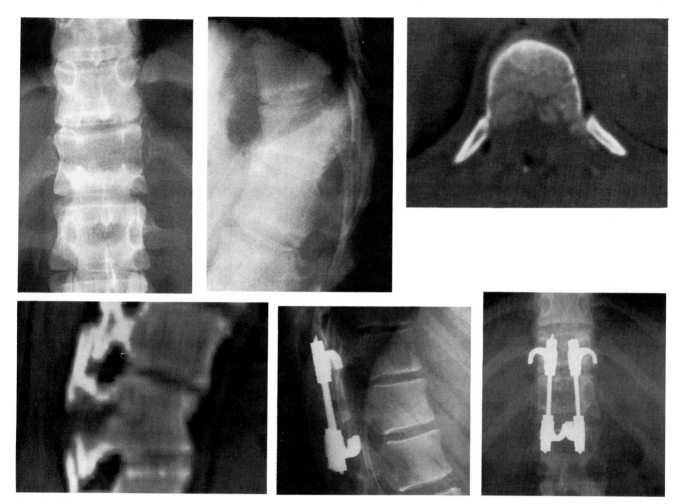

Fig. 7 This 18-year-old neurologically intact female was not seatbelted in the back seat of a vehicle that became airborne. Her abdomen struck the top of the front seat. **Top left**, Anteroposterior view demonstrating fractures through both pedicles of T-12, spinous process widening between T-11 and T-12. **Top center**, Lateral view with apparent increased posterior height as a result of the distraction component of this injury. **Top right**, Computed tomographic scan through T-12 shows comminution of the vertebral body and no osseous structures present posterior to the dural sac. At time of surgery, in fact, dura was easily visualized after incision through skin, subcutaneous fat, and thoracolumbar fascia. The supraspinous and interspinous ligaments were torn and widened as was the ligamentum flavum, so as to easily expose the dorsal aspect of the dura. **Bottom left**, Computed tomogram with reconstruction (plain tomography would likely reveal the same image) shows the marked transpedicular fracture widening through the vertebral body and into the intervertebral disk. **Bottom center** and **bottom right**, Surgical management involved insertion of Harrington rods from T-11 transverse processes to the inferior lamina of T-12 with reduction of fracture. This was combined with a posterolateral fusion. She went on to uneventful healing and return to full activity.

following the injury shows increasing kyphotic deformity or if the patient's pain has not resolved, elective stabilization and arthrodesis should be considered.

Burst Fractures

Management of burst fractures is based on the assessment of stability and the presence of a complete or incomplete neurologic injury. The nonsurgical approach originated by Guttman is still followed in many centers for patients who are neurologically intact (Fig. 6). Such treatment can be effective for these fractures in the long term. Long-term surveillance (20 years) of patients with burst fractures and no neurologic involvement has demonstrated that most patients are working, and most residual backache was mild. No long-term neurologic deterioration was identified. Residual kyphosis averaged 26.5 degrees with no correlation between kyphotic deformity and pain. Retropulsed fragments can gradually reabsorb with time; however, reabsorption varies depending on size, position, and amount of comminution. The development of posterior stabilization devices, beginning with Harrington rods, allowed many to conclude that these fractures could be predictably stabilized with some reduction of the retropulsed fragments being observed.

A traditional posterior approach, still favored by many surgeons, allows a variety of strategies for stabilization. The Harrington distraction implant, or one of its modifications such as the Wisconsin, Jacobs, or Edwards sleeves, is commonly used. The underlying principle is three-point fixation, which is enhanced by placing the rods at least three levels above and two levels below the level of injury. Enhanced stabilization may be obtained by the addition of sublaminar or spinous process wires. Although sublaminar wires give more rigid fixation, their passage in a neurologically compromised patient increases the risk of further injury, particularly if spinal cord edema is present. When using distraction instrumentation, intraoperative radiographs should be obtained to confirm that sagittal plane alignment has been restored and to avoid overdistraction, which is a particular risk when there is evidence of three-column failure.

When neurologic injury is present, and there is loss of vertebral body height greater than 50%, angulation greater than 20%, or canal compromise greater than 40%, early posterior stabilization is advocated to restore sagittal plane alignment. In 75% of the cases, adequate canal decompression can be achieved by posterior instrumentation alone. Repeat CT scan is then performed following surgery and the adequacy of canal decompression is determined. Intraoperative ultrasound may also play a role in this regard. In the event that residual canal compromise is greater than 25% with an incomplete neurologic injury, strong consideration should be given to a secondary anterior decompression.

Pedicle screw implants* have the advantage of controlling the anterior column via the posterior approach. They also provide four-point fixation and significantly reduce the number of levels that must be incorporated in the construct, although there is considerable variation in the rigidity of the fixation provided. The screws provide lever arms, which facilitate reduction maneuvers and allow lordosis to be maintained. The large variety of implants available vary in linkage systems, screw design, and flexibility of application. Disadvantages include commercial unavailability of many devices and the possibility of screw penetration of the pedicle, which provides the potential risk of further neurologic damage.

Laminectomy alone, without stabilization, is rarely warranted, but laminectomy is important when the preoperative status and imaging studies indicate significant posterior neural arch comminution. In these instances, removal of entrapped neural elements from within the arch may improve neurologic status. The accompanying dural leak should be repaired and stabilization with instrumentation then carried out.

Flexion-Distraction Injuries

Flexion-distraction injuries can occur through bone or soft tissue and can involve one or several levels. When these injuries occur entirely through bone, treatment is in a hyperextension cast. When the posterior and middle

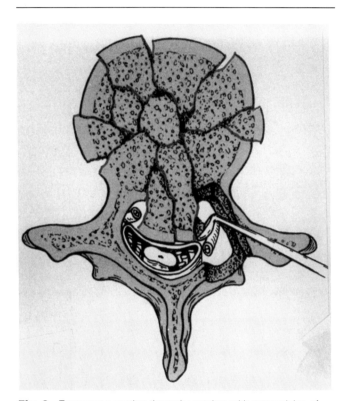

Fig. 8 Transverse section through vertebra with retropulsion of bone into the canal. After partial laminectomy, the medial portion of the pedicle is burred and resected down into the vertebral body, placing the surgeon lateral to the compromised thecal sac and retropulsed bone. A reverse-angle curette can then be used to tap bone out of the canal into the drilled vertebral body. Loose smaller fragments may be extracted and removed through the lateral pedicular trough. Care must be taken not to inadvertently hood the anterior aspect of the dura. (Reproduced with permission of Eismont F, Garfin S, Abitbol J-J: Thoracic and upper lumbar spine injuries, in Browner BD, Jupiter JB, Levine AM, et al (eds): *Skeletal Trauma*. Philadelphia, WB Saunders, 1992, vol 1, p 777.)

columns fail by ligamentous disruption, posterior spinal arthrodesis using a compression system is advocated (Fig. 7). However, it is important to determine that the middle column, specifically the posterior vertebral body, is capable of loadbearing. If it is not, use of a compression system could cause further retropulsion of bone or disk fragments into the canal.

Fracture Dislocations

Fracture dislocations are usually associated with severe neurologic impairment. The goal of treatment is to realign the spinal column and to provide adequate posterior stabilization, so as to allow early mobilization. Early mobilization has been shown to decrease morbidity and mortality while enhancing the ability of the patient to return to a productive lifestyle. The posterior approach with instrumentation is usually advantageous in dealing with facet injuries and correcting rotational deformity.

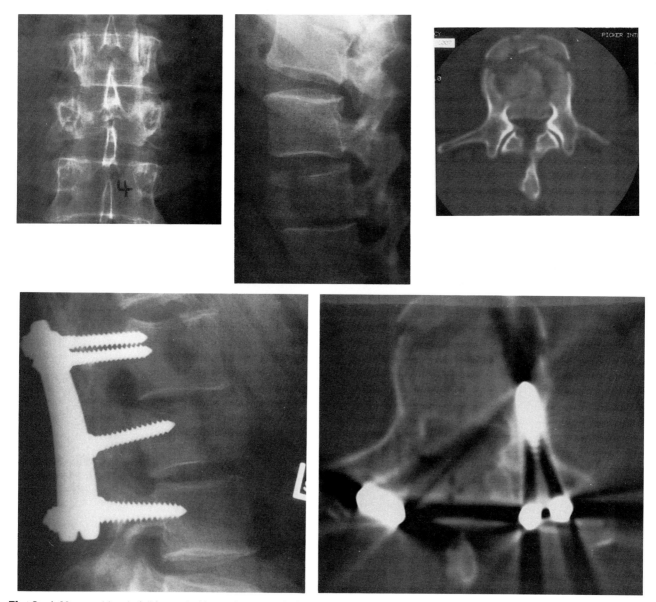

Fig. 9 A 28-year-old male fell from a ladder and presented with bilateral incomplete weakness of L-4, L-5, and S-1. **Top left** and **top center**, Plain films show minimal body fracture of L-3, and very difficult to assess retropulsion between pedicles, no kyphotic deformity, but widening of pedicles. **Top right**, Computed tomographic scan showed more than 50% canal compromise in this partially neurologically compromised patient. **Bottom left**, The patient underwent posterolateral decompression of L-3, pedicle fixation from L-2 to L-4, and posterolateral bone grafting. **Bottom right**, Postoperative CT of L-3 shows partial resection of pedicle unilaterally, insertion of pedicular screw into intact pedicle of L-3 for added stability, and adequate canal clearing.

However, it must include segmental fixation and axial distraction forces to increase rotational and translational control.

Extension Injuries

These injuries are usually stable and can be managed with a flexion cast or orthosis for a period of up to 12 weeks, depending on the patient's comfort.

Timing of Surgery

Emergency decompression is indicated in the presence of a cauda equina syndrome or progressive neurologic deficit. In patients with complete spinal cord injuries or static incomplete spinal cord injuries, some authorities advocate delaying surgery for several days to allow reduction of cord edema, whereas others favor early surgical stabilization. There is no clear evidence that the results of

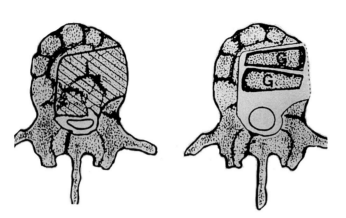

Fig. 10 Through an anterior approach, a partial corpectomy and resection of retropulsed bone can be performed to decompress the spinal canal. The bone resection at the end of the decompression should extend from pedicle to pedicle. Reconstruction of the partial corpectomy utilizes tricortical iliac strut graft and/or rib graft.

decompression of neural structures are enhanced by early reduction, or that they are significantly compromised by a one-week delay. Some studies have documented some return of neurologic function after anterior decompression done more than a year after the initial injury. For neurologically normal patients with unstable spinal injuries and those with nonprogressive, static neurologic injuries, it is preferable to carry out open reduction and internal fixation as soon as the medical and surgical conditions are optimal.

Decompression

Compression of the neural elements by retropulsed bone fragments can be relieved indirectly by the insertion of posterior instrumentation or directly by exploration of the spinal canal through a posterolateral or anterior approach. There is no universal agreement as to indications for these alternatives. The indirect method from the posterior approach usually involves distraction instrumentation and three- or four-point fixation to realign the spine (Fig. 8). These reductions usually are performed with hooks and contoured rods or hook-rod-sleeves to create distraction and provide an anterior vector force across the fracture. The reduction of retropulsed bone from the canal requires that the posterior longitudinal ligament be intact to provide tension. When stretched, the ligament pulls bone out of the canal anteriorly towards the body. Problems with this technique occur if surgery is delayed for several weeks or in severely comminuted fractures. Multiple pieces of bone retropulsed into the canal may not be completely reduced by distraction instrumentation. Further, intraoperative assessment of the adequacy of reduction by this technique is difficult. Intraoperative myelography lacks resolution, and enlargement of the

laminectomy to afford direct visualization increases the instability. Intraoperative ultrasonography, which has been advocated, also requires creation of a laminotomy defect to allow insertion of the transducer head, and the results can be difficult to interpret.

The posterolateral technique for decompression of the spinal canal is effective at the thoracolumbar junction and in the lumbar spine as a more direct means of reducing the bony fragments (Fig. 9). This procedure involves hemilaminectomy and removal of portions of one pedicle with a high speed burr to allow posterolateral decompression of the dura along its anterior aspect. With angled instruments, the bone can be curetted out of the canal or tapped back into the vertebral body. In the thoracic spine, where less room is available for the cord, this technique may involve increased risk to the neural elements.

The anterior approach allows the most direct visualization for decompression of the thecal sac (Fig. 10); however, many surgeons are unfamiliar with this approach. Visceral and vascular structures may be injured, and this approach carries the greatest potential morbidity. If there is significant kyphotic deformity, the degree of correction of the alignment of the vertebral column may be less than with posterior techniques. Anterior strut grafting with iliac crest is required but often provides only minimal immediate stability. In most cases, after an anterior procedure, posterior compression instrumentation and arthrodesis will help increase the stability of the anterior graft, increase the probability of successful fusion, and help minimize residual deformities. Numerous anterior internal fixation devices have been developed, and many studies are currently underway to evaluate the stability of anterior instrumentation without additional posterior stabilization.* If complications occur, additional surgery to remove implants from the anterior aspect of the spine is more difficult than for posterior implants. Adequate correction of kyphosis may be impossible with anterior instrumentation alone if the posterior supporting structures are incompetent.

Multisegmented Hook Instrumentation

The multisegmented hook systems (MSHS) were developed for use in treatment of spinal deformities, and have more recently been applied to the treatment of spine trauma with increasing frequency. The primary advantage of these systems is that multiple hooks can be used in both distraction and compression modes, allowing complex curve correction and providing stability with segmental fixation. The increased stability is obtained without the apparent risk of neurologic damages reported with sublaminar segmented systems. Those systems are further strengthened with the use of several transverse traction devices, which convert the system to a rigid rectangle.

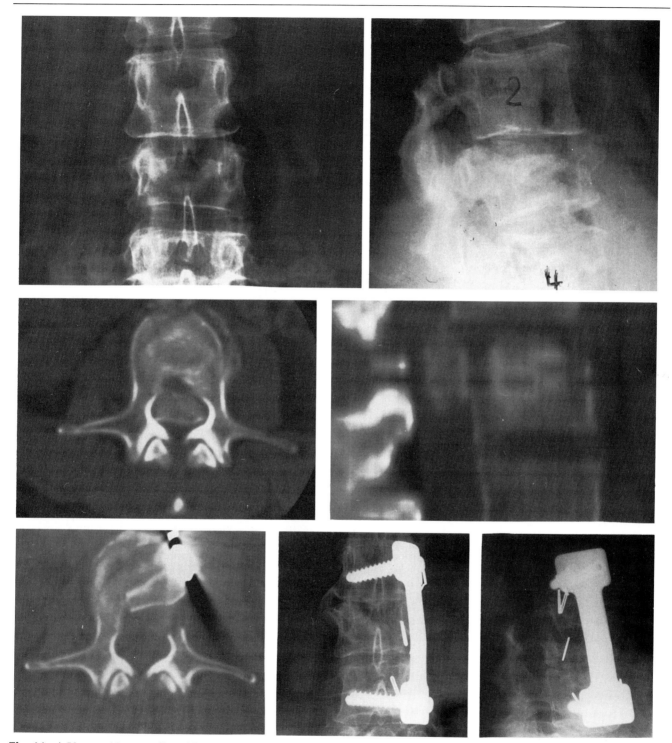

Fig. 11 A 53-year-old woman flipped her riding lawnmower into a ditch, with the machine landing on her. She suffered closed chest injury, left femur fracture, and presented with incomplete, though significant, neurological compromise. **Top left** and **top right**, Plain radiographs show pedicular widening, burst fracture of L-3 with probable retropulsion of bone posteriorly between pedicles and minimal kyphotic deformity. **Center (left** and **right)**, Computed tomographic scanning with reconstruction shows near-complete obliteration of spinal canal, pedicles intact, and facet joints not disrupted. **Bottom left,** The patient underwent anterior decompression through a retroperitoneal approach and tricortical iliac strut grafting. **Bottom center** and **bottom right,** Since the elements of the posterior column appeared to be intact, neutralization plate fixation to the vertebral body above and below were employed. She began weightbearing six days postoperatively and lateral radiograph shows satisfactory incorporation of strut grafting.

One disadvantage of the multisegmental hook systems is that they require more time to insert than do the other posterior systems. A second disadvantage is that a moderate amount of manipulation is required to connect multiple hooks to rods while simultaneously reducing the unstable spine injury. However, one advantage is that postoperative bracing may be minimized without jeopardizing the reduction and eventual fusion. In addition, the systems may allow the use of shorter instrumentation, thus immobilizing fewer segments. It is generally recommended that the length of the lever arms be equal above and below the fracture and that double lamina claws be applied at both the cephalic and caudal extremes of instrumentation.

Pedicle Screw Instrumentation

Many plate-screw, rod-screw and internal fixation systems employing pedicle screws are being evaluated for use in the spine. These systems improve sagittal-plane translational correction, in addition to securing segmental bony fixation. Their most desirable asset is that they limit the number of spinal levels required to manage a spinal fracture. This is a particular advantage in the lower lumbar spine. Because limitations are imposed by pedicle diameter, these systems are best used for L-2 to L-5 levels (Fig. 11). Risks of pedicle screw fixation include the possibility of neurologic and vascular injury caused by the screws. The ability of the pedicle screw systems to distract and significantly improve the amount of canal compromise varies. The improvement is not marked in the patients who initially have moderate spinal canal encroachment (34% to 64% canal compromise) and is even less in those patents with mild or severe spinal canal compromise. Rates of screw breakage and dislodgement have been reported to be as high as 15%, which suggests a possible need for supplemental anterior bone grafting for thoracolumbar fractures treated by pedicle fixation alone. The appropriate rigidity and its affect on the underlying fusion mass and the levels above and below the instrumented levels are yet unresolved questions.*

---

*The various devices designed to restore alignment of the spine include some that are in varying stages of approval by the Food and Drug Administration.

Annotated Bibliography

Aebi M, Etter C, Kehl T, et al: The internal skeletal fixation system: A new treatment of thoracolumbar fractures and other spinal disorders. *Clin Orthop* 1988;227:30-43.

A new internal skeletal fixation system (ISFS) for stabilizing thoracolumbar fractures and other spinal disorders was developed by Dick in Switzerland. The ISFS is a modification of the Magerl external skeletal fixation system of the spine. The indications, techniques, and surgical results are described.

An HS, Vaccaro A, Cotler JM, et al: Low lumbar burst fractures: Comparison among body cast, Harrington rod, Luque rod, and Steffee plate. *Spine* 1991;16:S440-S444.

A review of 31 low lumbar burst fractures stressing the importance of maintenance of vertebral height and restoration of lumbar lordosis in the prevention of disability from back pain.

Anderson PA, Henley MB, Rivara FP, et al: Flexion distraction and chance injuries to the thoracolumbar spine. *J Orthop Trauma* 1991;5:153-160.

Twenty cases of Chance-type thoracolumbar flexion-distraction fractures were reviewed retrospectively.

Bleasel A, Clouston P, Dorsch N: Post-traumatic syringomyelia following uncomplicated spinal fracture. *J Neurol Neurosurg Psychiatry* 1991;54:551-553.

Reports two cases of posttraumatic syringomyelia presenting ten and 41 years after spinal injuries that had caused lumbar vertebral fractures but no lasting neurological deficits.

Bracken MB, Shepard MJ, Collins WF, et al: A randomized controlled trial of methylprednsolone or naloxone in the treatment of acute spinal-cord injuries: Results of the Second National Acute Spinal Cord Injury Study. *N Engl J Med* 1990;322:1405-1411.

A multicenter randomized, double-blind, placebo-controlled trial concluded that in patients with acute spinal cord injury, treatment with high-dose methylprednisolone given in the first eight hours improves neurologic recovery.

Bradford DS, McBride GG: Surgical management of thoracolumbar spine fractures with incomplete neurologic deficits. *Clin Orthop* 1987;218:201-216.

The results of surgical decompression (SD) in 59 patients with neurologic deficits secondary to thoracic or lumbar fractures were evaluated at a mean of 3.7 years after injury. The purpose was to determine whether SD could be correlated with subsequent neurologic outcome. The inferior results in the posteriorly treated SD group appeared to correlate with a high incidence of bony stenosis as measured on postoperative commuted axial tomography.

Cammissa FP Jr, Eismont FJ, Green BA: Dural laceration

occurring with burst fractures and associated laminar fractures. *J Bone Joint Surg* 1989;71A:1044-1052.

This article emphasizes the importance of the association of preoperative neurologic deficit, burst fracture, and laminar fracture being a predictor of dural tear and entrapped neural elements.

Crawford AH: Operative treatment of spine fractures in children. *Orthop Clin North Am* 1990;21:325-339.

This article presents concise methods of evaluation and management of these injuries with regard to their alignment, stability, and possible spinal canal compromise. The role of radiographic imaging is defined and illustrated by example.

Denis F, Burkus JK: Lateral distraction injuries to the thoracic and lumbar spine: A report of three cases. *J Bone Joint Surg* 1991;73A:1049-1053.

Three patients sustained a unique lateral distraction injury to the thoracic or lumbar spine. These injuries were associated with multiple fractures of the ribs and extremities as well as with thoracic and abdominal visceral injuries. Fusion was achieved with the spine in anatomic alignment, without any complications, in all three patents.

Esses SI, Botsford DJ, Kostuik JP: Evaluation of surgical treatment for burst fractures. *Spine* 1990;15:667-673.

The authors instituted a prospective, randomized study of patients presenting with acute burst fractures of the thoracolumbar and lumbar spine. Patients were alternately treated by posterior distraction using pedicle instrumentation or anterior decompression and instrumentation.

Farcy JP, Weidenbaum M, Glassman SD: Sagittal index in management of thoracolumbar burst fractures. *Spine* 1990;15:958-965.

In an effort to quantify the risk for late progression in burst fractures, the sagittal index (SI) was defined to help to assess the segmental deformity at the level of the fracture.

Gardner VO, Armstrong GW: Long-term lumbar facet joint changes in spinal fracture patients treated with Harrington rods. *Spine* 1990;15:479-484.

This is the report on a retrospective analysis of 20 of these patients with an average follow-up period of 8.0 years, radiographically evaluating the status of unfused facet joints with the rod-long, fuse-short technique.

Gertzbein S: Scoliosis Research Society: Multicenter Spine Fracture Study. *Spine* 1992;17:528-540.

A prospective multicenter study of over 1,000 spine fractures assessing surgical versus nonsurgical outcome, neurologic injury and fracture pattern, kyphotic deformity, and persistent pain.

Haas N, Blauth M, Tscherne H: Anterior plating in thoracolumbar spine injuries: Indication, technique, and results. *Spine* 1991;16:S100-S111.

The authors describe their experience from treating 39 patients with anterior decompression and stabilization. One of 19 patients with Frankel grades A and B, and 50% of the remaining 20 patients had improved one Frankel grade.

Johnsson R, Herrlin K, Hägglund G, et al: Spinal canal remodeling after thoracolumbar fractures with intraspinal bone fragments: 17 cases followed 1-4 years. *Acta Orthop Scand* 1991;62:125-127.

The long-term fate of nonreduced intraspinal bone fragments in 17 thoracolumbar fractures was studied with CT. The reduction of the spinal canal area was measured in conjunction with the trauma in the nonoperated cases and immediately after surgery in the operated cases.

Keenen TL, Antony J, Benson DR: Dural tears associated with lumbar burst fractures. *J Orthop Trauma* 1990;4:243-245.

A retrospective review of 817 spinal fracture patients revealed a 7.7% (20 of 258) incidence of dural tears in surgically treated patients. An initial posterior approach with inspection of the dura and stabilization of the fracture is recommended when treating lumbar burst fractures with a neural deficit.

Keenen TL, Antony J, Benson DR: Non-contiguous spinal fractures. *J Trauma* 1990;30:489-491.

A retrospective review of 817 spinal fracture patients revealed a 6.4% (52/817) incidence of noncontiguous spine fractures.

Kostuik JP: Anterior fixation for burst fractures of the thoracic and lumbar spine with or without neurological involvement. *Spine* 1988;13:286-293.

This report details the use of the anterior approach for burst fractures of the thoracic and lumbar spine.

Krag MH, Weaver DL, Beynnon BD, et al: Morphometry of the thoracic and lumbar spine related to transarticular screw placement for surgical spinal fixation. *Spine* 1988;13:27-32.

CAT scan combined with cadaveric measurements were made to delineate pedicular morphology from T-9 to L-5.

Krag MH: Biomechanics of thoracolumbar spinal fixation: A Review. *Spine* 1991;16 (suppl 3):S84-S99.

Reviewed are various devices and the major biomechanical issues relevant to them, categorized by site of attachment. Emphasis is placed on current knowledge and unresolved issues.

Patwardhan AG, Li SP, Gavin T, et al: Orthotic stabilization of thoracolumbar injuries: A biomechanical analysis of the Jewett hyperextension orthosis. *Spine* 1990;15:654-661.

Spinal orthoses have been traditionally used in the management of thoracolumbar injuries treated with or without surgical stabilization. However, the orthotic treatment modality in the management of spinal fractures remains subjective, because few objective data are available on the effectiveness of orthoses in stabilizing injured segments. This study used a finite element model of the spine to evaluate the effectiveness of a hyperextension orthosis in controlling the progression of deformities at the injury site under gravitational and flexion loads.

Tencer AF, Allen BL Jr, Ferguson RL: A biomechanical study of thoracolumbar spinal fractures with bone in the canal: Part I. The effect of laminectomy. *Spine* 1985;10:580-585.

A simulation of thoracolumbar spinal fractures with bone in the canal was performed using fresh cadaver spines. The results indicated that laminectomy had no decompressive effect with up to 35% occlusion of the canal.

Tencer AF, Ferguson RL, Allen BL Jr: A biomechanical

study of thoracolumbar spinal fractures with bone in the canal: Part II. The effect of flexion angulation, distraction, and shortening of the motion segment. *Spine* 1985;10:586-589.

Contact force on the spinal cord-meningeal complex was measured with relation to varying fractures, wedge depth, flexion angulations, and distraction and shortening of the fracture model motion segment.

Transfeldt EE, White D, Bradford DS, et al: Delayed anterior decompression in patients with spinal cord and cauda equina injuries of the thoracolumbar spine. *Spine* 1990;15:953-957.

Describes 49 patients with complete and incomplete injuries of the spinal cord or cauda equina who had undergone anterior decompression at a minimum of three months after injury.

38

Thoracolumbar Spine: Reconstruction

The primary goals in reconstructive surgery of the thoracolumbar spine are (1) preservation or improvement of neurologic function, (2) maintenance or restoration of spinal stability, (3) preservation of the maximum number of vertebral levels of motion (particularly the lower lumbar and lumbosacral joints), and (4) when possible, relief of pain.

Diagnosis and Anatomy

Initial radiographic analysis of the thoracolumbar spine includes standing posteroanterior and lateral films. Focal, coned down views may be useful to evaluate the facets, congenital anomalies, and disk narrowing in patients with significant pain. Oblique radiographs, using Stagnara views, are useful to assess the rotational deformity, particularly when kyphosis is present.

Lateral bending radiographs may indicate the flexibility of a spinal deformity, but do not predict the degree of surgical correction that might be obtained. Traction films occasionally may be of value in determining whether distraction may overcome decompensation.

Once routine radiographs are obtained, a variety of ancillary imaging studies may be considered. Bone scans are rarely indicated, except in the younger adult with pain and a minor curve that may be caused by an osteoid osteoma.

Technologic advances in imaging of the thoracolumbar spine have made possible a more thorough understanding of the interrelationship of the spinal column, the neural axis, and other adjacent soft-tissue structures. Magnetic resonance imaging (MRI) has been heralded as one of the greatest advances in recent years in the diagnosis of thoracolumbar pathology, because of its ability to visualize soft-tissue structures in greater detail than had been possible with any previous radiographic modality (Table 1).

Magnetic resonance imaging is often the first diagnostic study considered when contemplating thoracolumbar spine reconstruction procedures. It is the imaging study of choice when herniated disk, spinal stenosis, and tumors are suspected. However, the images produced using this technique become more difficult to interpret in the presence of major spinal deformity or multiplanar anatomic aberrations. Because of these problems, myelography is often considered as a useful imaging technique, particularly when there are neurologic findings or surgical correction is contemplated. A major objective is to determine any areas of actual or potential compres-

Table 1. Tissue and body fluid signal intensity on T1- and T2-weighted images

Tissue or body fluid	T1-weighted	T2-weighted
Cortical bone	Low	Low
Tendons and ligaments	Low	Low
Fibrocartilage	Low	Low
Hyaline cartilage	Intermediate	Intermediate
Muscle	Intermediate	Intermediate
Non-neoplastic tumor	Low-intermediate	Low-intermediate (Occasionally high)
Neoplastic tumor	Low-intermediate	Intermediate-high (Occasionally low)
Free water (CSF)	Low	High
Proteinaceous fluid (abscess)	Intermediate	High
Adipose tissue	High	Intermediate-high
Hemorrhage	Variable	Variable

sion, which might increase when corrective forces are applied. Although computerized tomographic (CT) scans are very useful for studying the bony structures of the spine, the myelographically enhanced CT scan is particularly helpful in determining the level and extent of required decompression.

Deformity

Adult Scoliosis

The four etiologies of adult scoliosis that are generally considered are: idiopathic, congenital, paralytic, and degenerative. Another subset of patients are those who underwent fusion as adolescents and who develop new problems later in life.

Idiopathic Scoliosis Idiopathic scoliosis is by far the most common form of adult scoliosis, with a reported prevalence of 4% to 6%. The major problem in adult scoliosis is pain, and the diagnostic goal is to determine the exact origin of the pain. The presumption that back pain is derived from degenerative facet joint disease remains plausible, but other conditions, such as spinal stenosis, lumbar disk herniation, and lateral recess stenosis are more definitive causes of pain. The disk is also considered as a source of pain, but surgical intervention for diskogenic pain remains controversial and has unpredictable results. Cosmesis is of concern to some patients and may be an indication for surgical intervention; yet, in long-term follow-up studies, the deformity per se is not commonly a major complaint.

The role of idiopathic scoliosis in the production of adult mechanical low back pain is controversial. The prevalence of low back pain is not increased compared with age-matched controls in some studies. In other studies, low back pain is seen as a potential problem.

Idiopathic scoliosis has been demonstrated to progress after skeletal maturity. The greatest progression is found in thoracic curves greater than 50 degrees and lumbar curves greater than 30 degrees, particularly when associated with a high-riding L-5 (at or above the intercrestal line), greater than 30% rotation, and a right convex deformity. A general rule of thumb is that the curve progresses 1 degree per year. More disabling than curve progression is lateral translation or rotational olisthesis, which often occurs at the inferior end of the lumbar curve. Superimposition of degenerative changes and facet hypertrophy may predispose the adult scoliosis patient to spinal stenosis. In these patients, surgical decompression of the lumbosacral nerve roots may lead to rapid sagittal (acquired spondylolisthesis) and coronal (lateral olisthesis) spinal subluxation. Concomitant fusion with instrumentation should be considered in patients with disabling symptoms.

Additional mechanisms of neurologic compression are: (1) lateral recess stenosis, (2) herniated intervertebral disk at the inferior end of the deformity, and (3) progressive myelopathy caused by spinal cord compression if there is a significant associated kyphosis.

Paralytic Curves Pelvic obliquity is a serious problem for the wheelchair-bound patient with paralytic curves. This deformity, combined with hyperlordosis or kyphosis, requires considerable careful planning, if surgery is contemplated. In adults with paralytic curves, one must always assess pulmonary function, particularly when considering surgical intervention. Indications for surgical treatment of the adult who has scoliosis include: pain, progression of deformity, neurologic compromise, and compromise of respiratory function.

Degenerative Adult Scoliosis Scoliosis also is a problem for older adults. The age of onset varies but is generally reported to be in the fifth and sixth decades of life. These cases are discovered incidentally. Sometimes the patient experiences an acute backache, which may or may not be accompanied by a traumatic event. In the latter instance, a compression fracture may be observed, particularly in postmenopausal females. Later degenerative scoliosis is often associated with radicular symptoms, suggestive of spinal stenosis. Radiographically, the curves measure in the range of 15 to 50 degrees. Lateral translation is a common finding, often with L-3 on L-4 or L-4 on L-5. There is also an association with degenerative spondylolisthesis. The indications for surgical treatment of the adult who has scoliosis include pain, progression of deformity, neurologic compromise, and compromise of respiratory function.

The development of Harrington instrumentation was a major advance in scoliosis surgery, improving fusion rates and significantly increasing the amount of correction. However, the good results achieved using this system of instrumentation in adolescents were not obtained in adults with scoliosis. Adult scoliosis surgery is associated with at least three persistent problems: (1) instrumentation failure, reported by the Scoliosis Research Society to occur in 32% of patients; (2) pseudarthrosis; and (3) degenerative changes in the remaining mobile segments above and below the fusion, in the case of thoracolumbar curves. Attempts to prevent the degenerative changes by fusion to the sacrum have been accompanied by even higher rates of instrumentation failure and pseudarthrosis, in addition to significant flattening of the lumbar lordosis. These problems are even greater in patients older than 50 years of age, whose curves are almost always rigid. Patients with severe rigidity often require multilevel osteotomies posteriorly with associated rib releases and/or resections on the concavity and convexity, respectively. Additionally, some patients require anterior releases followed by posterior instrumentation and fusion. In a prospective study of 37 patients undergoing staged anterior and posterior spinal reconstructive procedures, with stringent criteria for nutritional and immunologic incompetency (serum albumin <3.5 g/dl and total lymphocyte count <2,000/μl), 87% of the patients became malnourished at some time during hospitalization. For this reason, it is better to combine the reconstructive procedures in one operation and obtain enough stability to allow early postoperative ambulation.

Osteopenia, which can cause instrumentation problems, is of great concern because of the combination of weak bone and rigid instrumentation. Complications in these patients are higher (20% to 40%), and curve correction is difficult despite the surgeon's choice of instrumentation. Clearly, the newer devices allow for greater correction, but long-term outcomes remain unknown. Complications include a 20% pseudarthrosis rate, a more than 20% pulmonary complications rate, and an increased risk of late instrumentation failures. Pain relief is unpredictable and has been reported in as few as 30% to 40% of patients.

Recent advances in surgical correction of scoliosis have centered on segmental instrumentation in order to provide more rigid internal stabilization, better rotational correction of the deformity, and limitation of the levels of fusion and instrumentation to as few lumbar vertebrae as possible.

Numerous devices now available allow reconstruction heretofore not achievable. Knowledge of the placement, design, and biomechanics of pedicle screws and of their relationship to their connecting longitudinal devices is critical to proper use of these devices. There is a definite learning curve in placement of pedicle screws, and misdirection of screws can cause significant risks to neurologic structures. Therefore, these devices require significant

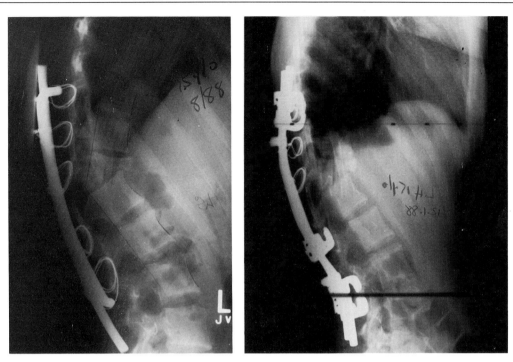

Fig. 1 This is a 15-year-old female who had a burst fracture dislocation at L-1. **Left**, The patient underwent a multilevel laminectomy and posterolateral bone grafting, both anteriorly and posteriorly, with Luque instrumentation and sublaminar wiring. Unfortunately, this patient had collapse of her deformity with progression of her deficit and increasing pain that necessitated reoperation. **Right**, This radiograph was taken following a secondary procedure in which an anterior decompression and strut graft followed by posterior stabilization with CD instrumentation was performed.

training and experience, and roentgenographic assistance during placement is recommended.

Conservative Treatment There are few well-established treatment methods for symptomatic adult scoliosis. Currently acceptable treatments include nonsteroidal anti-inflammatory medications and exercise programs designed to maintain aerobic capacity, maintain or increase flexibility, and strengthen muscles of the spine, extremities, and abdomen. In the female, particular attention is paid to the prevention of osteoporosis. Braces may provide symptomatic relief in some patients. Short-term bed rest may also be useful when there is an acute exacerbation of symptoms. The efficacy of these treatments is largely unstudied, and the natural history of symptomatic patients is not well established.

The Effects of Prior Fusion Long-term studies of young patients who have undergone posterior instrumentation and fusion for scoliosis have shown no increase in disability, provided the fusion extends only to the upper lumbar spine. However, if the fusion extends below L-3, there is a definite tendency toward chronic low back disability and pain. When the fusion extends down to L-4, 62% report pain, and for fusions extending down to L-5, 82% have significant complaints. Problems that can develop in patients that have undergone fusion for scoliosis include:

(1) loss of correction, (2) pseudarthrosis, (3) loss of lumbar lordosis caused by failure of the rod to contour to the normal lumbar lordotic curvature, (4) failure of fusion, and (5) technical complications in patients with lumbosacral fusion.

Degenerative Scoliosis Operative indications for these cases are usually for their stenotic symptoms and not for their deformity. Various approaches have been tried, including posterior decompression, as for any patient with spinal stenosis, and decompression and fusion, with or without instrumentation. It appears that fusion with instrumentation allows for better rates of fusion. The results of surgery are less predictable for degenerative scoliosis than for spinal stenosis without deformity.

Postlaminectomy Deformity

Total laminectomy is rarely indicated in thoracolumbar reconstructive procedures. The biomechanical consequences of a wide laminectomy, which includes facet joint excision, often lead to progressive deformity. Most often the primary deformity is kyphosis.

Prevention is the key. Realization of the biomechanical consequences of decompression and an adequate attempt at reconstruction during laminectomy may prevent future problems (Fig. 1). Preservation of at least one half

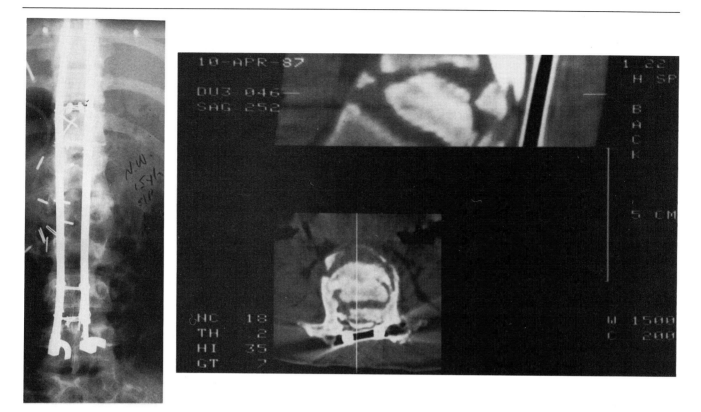

Fig. 2   This 15-year-old male had a thoracolumbar burst fracture of L-2 treated by Harrington instrumentation from T-10 to L-5. **Left**, An anteroposterior radiograph following that surgical procedure shows the right lower hook dislodged. The patient went on postoperatively to have further progression of his neurologic deficit. The retropulsed fragments continuing to impinge on the thecal sac can be seen on both anteroposterior (**top right**) and lateral (**bottom right**) images. With this patient's worsening neurologic deficit and bony impingement a difficult reconstruction was necessitated.

of each facet joint is recommended when possible. If it is not possible to preserve one whole facet or one-half of each facet, arthrodesis is indicated.

Post-Traumatic Kyphosis and Incomplete Paraplegia

Usually these are fixed deformities, which often will not need to be corrected. The indications for surgery for late posttraumatic thoracolumbar kyphosis include increasing kyphotic deformity, pain, or increasing neurologic deficit (Figs. 2 and 3). Despite casting or bracing, ligamentous injuries of the middle and posterior spinal columns in translational or flexion-distraction injuries may result in pain and/or progressive kyphosis. When there is anterior thecal impingement, a two-stage treatment often is recommended: initial anterior decompression followed by posterior stabilization. A single-stage posterior closing wedge osteotomy is a technically demanding option. This usually is achieved at the L2-3 or L3-4 level or below the level of the spinal cord, similar to "spontaneously fused" thoracolumbar kyphosis in ankylosing spondylosis (Fig. 4).

Anterior spinal exposure can be important in thoracolumbar reconstructive surgery for kyphosis. Once the periosteum is reflected, the fractured vertebrae are visu-

alized. Hemorrhage is minimized by performing complete diskectomies and anterior releases before excising the vertebral body and inserting the prosthesis or bone graft. All displaced bone and soft tissue anterior to the posterior longitudinal ligament at the kyphosis is debrided. Tricortical iliac crest bone and fibula are commonly used as grafts to reconstruct anterior defects.

Kyphosis

Symptomatic kyphosis is relatively rare in adults. However, ankylosing spondylitis leads to kyphotic deformities that require a special approach. Because of the high neurologic risk of thoracic osteotomy, lumbar osteotomy, sometimes followed by cervical osteotomy, is the preferred surgical strategy for the majority of patients. Most commonly, the osteotomy is carried out at L2-3, which avoids potential neurologic compromise of the conus medullaris. This procedure has undergone very little modification since it was initially described in 1945. The facet joints are resected at L2-3 or L3-4 in a diagonal fashion, at an angle of approximately 45 degrees to the longitudinal axis of the spine. The amount of bone resected is directly proportional to the amount of correc-

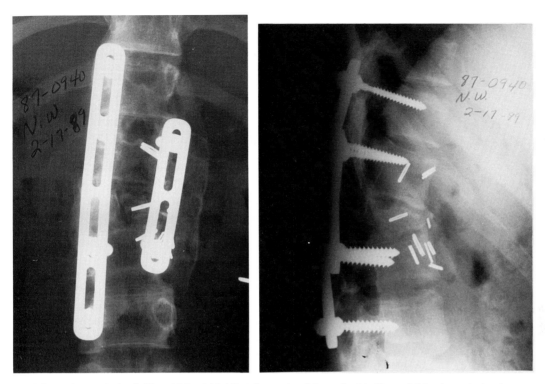

Fig. 3 Representative anteroposterior (**left**) and lateral (**right**) radiographs of the patient in Figure 2 following anterior decompression and posterior stabilization with pedicle fixation. The patient regained complete neurologic function and has retained it for four years postoperatively.

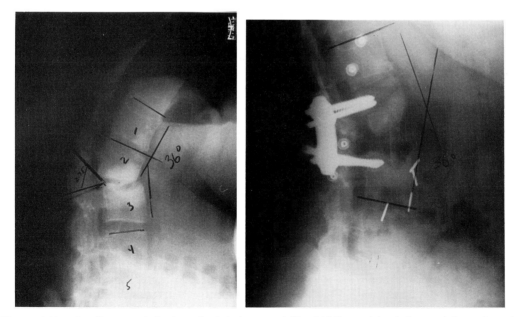

Fig. 4 This 43-year-old female with a pseudo fracture of ankylosing spondylitis at L2-3 complained of excruciating pain and of having to sit in a chair in order to sleep. Her pain had progressed over the past five years to the point of intolerability. She was currently taking narcotic analgesics and able to look at the floor only during ambulation. **Left**, This shows an acute kyphosis at L2-3 of 36 degrees with a pseudo fracture. **Right**, Postoperative lateral radiographs following posterior wedge osteotomy and anterior strut grafting. Four years later, the patient has healed nicely.

tion anticipated, based on preoperative radiographs. A correction of more than 45 to 50 degrees at any one level is probably unrealistic and increases the neurologic risk. The advent of pedicle fixation devices, however, has added the advantage of segmental fixation with greater assurance of sagittal-plane stability and the possibility of increasing lumbar lordosis. Because patients with ankylosing spondylitis are relatively osteoporotic, instrumentation failures are common. Pedicle fixation provides an opportunity for potentially greater mechanical fixation in such cases, but caution must be exercised. Normal anatomic landmarks are absent or obscure, and the quality of bone is poor. Improvement in functional status can be anticipated after a successful osteotomy. Risk versus benefits, however, must be reviewed with the patient in each case.

Tumors

Metastatic Tumors

Although primary tumors of the spine are rare, the increased longevity secondary to advances in medical oncology has made metastatic tumors of the thoracolumbar spine an increasingly common problem. Despite improved chemotherapeutic and radiation therapy techniques, the incidence of and morbidity from metastatic tumors to the spine have been increasing. In a detailed study of 322 patients with metastatic bone disease, the seven most common sites of tumor origin with spinal metastasis were breast (31.2%), lung (21.8%), prostate (20.1%), kidney (6.7%), colon (5.6%), bladder (3.4%), and head and neck (2.2%). More than half of patients who have metastatic bone disease have involvement of the spine, and neurologic deficits occur in 20% of these patients.

Radiotherapy Despite the favorable results obtained by surgical decompression, radiotherapy historically has been the treatment of choice for spinal osseous metastases, and still remains the most reasonable treatment option for many patients. Patients with spinal pain alone and, occasionally, patients with neurologic compromise without vertebral collapse will receive significant benefit from radiotherapy alone. The preoperative neurologic status of the patient dictates the likely outcome. Although 70% of patients who are ambulatory will retain that functional ability following radiotherapy, rarely will patients who have lost this ability regain it following radiation alone. The nature of the metastasis is also important to the outcome following radiotherapy because of the significant difference in radiosensitivity among tumor types and among different clones of the same tumor type. Prostatic and lymphoreticular tumors are usually quite radiosensitive, and excellent clinical results can be obtained by radiation alone in most patients. Metastases

from breast carcinoma often are responsive to irradiation, but as many as 30% of patients treated may be unresponsive to radiation alone. Gastrointestinal and renal tumors usually are quite resistant to radiotherapy.

Surgical Indications Improved therapies for systemic disease, more sophisticated preoperative evaluation and staging, new surgical techniques and materials, and the trend toward a more aggressive surgical approach have improved surgical outcomes for patients with spine tumors. However, the lack of uniform treatment and uniformity in reporting outcome make comparison of treatment protocols difficult. Despite questions regarding definitive management, surgical treatment, in appropriately selected patients, now offers a reasonable likelihood of functional improvement, pain relief, and, in some cases, cure of disease.

The indications for vertebral body resection for epidural compression include: (1) the need for tissue diagnosis, which may require concomitant reconstruction; (2) treatment of radioresistant tumor; (3) pathologic fracture-dislocation; and (4) neurologic deterioration following radiation therapy or while the patient is receiving this treatment.

A series of 40 patients was analyzed who had a neurologic deficit. Following anterior decompressions, 80% had enough motor recovery to regain the ability to walk and 93% regained bowel and bladder sphincter control. In the past it had been customary not to consider operation if paraplegia had been present for 48 to 72 hours. Two patients who had been paraplegic for an extended period (up to 14 days) regained both the ability to walk and sphincter control after anterior decompressions. Therefore, recovery from incomplete neurologic deficit is possible following anterior decompression. The indications for laminectomy are rare in the surgical treatment of tumor patients. The results following laminectomy are significantly worse than those following anterior surgery. Table 2 represents the clinical outcomes reported for anterior compared to posterior surgery, and Figure 5 is an algorithm formulated as an approach to the patient with metastatic spine tumors. Figures 6 through 9 represent one of the more difficult metastatic spine tumors, metastatic renal cell carcinoma. Consideration should be given to whether surgical management will affect outcome and prognosis in these difficult cases.

Table 2. Maintenance and recovery of neurologic function in patients treated surgically (anterior versus posterior decompression) for cord compression due to metastatic or primary spinal tumor

Decompression Route	Number of patients	% Improvement	% Satisfactory Outcome
Anterior	427	78	80
Posterior	746	33	37

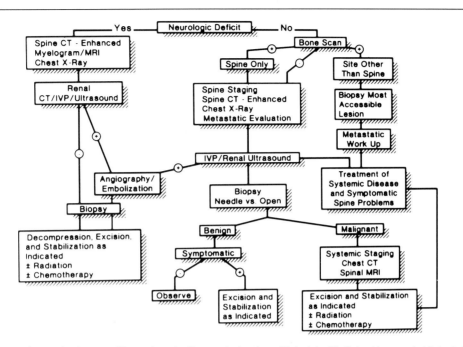

Fig. 5 Algorithm; approach to spine tumors. (Reproduced with permission from Weinstein JN: Spinal tumors, in Weinstein JN, Wiesel S (eds): *The Lumbar Spine*. Philadelphia, WB Saunders, 1990, pp 741-759.)

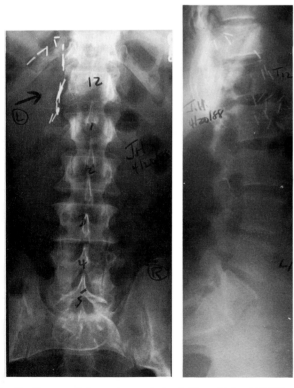

Fig. 6 Representative anteroposterior (**left**) and lateral (**right**) roentgenograms of a 54-year-old male with a history of metastatic renal cell carcinoma to T-12 and L-4. Patient had progression of pain with quadriceps weakness on the right.

Anatomic Extent of Spinal Tumors

If spinal tumors are to be surgically treated, it is evident that a logical and consistent approach is needed. To this end, an anatomically based scheme has been developed to help the surgeon approach these most difficult lesions (Table 3). Surgical outcome is ultimately affected by the anatomic zones involved (Fig. 10); by whether the lesion is intraosseous (A), extraosseous (B), or metastatic (C); and by the type of tumor and its grade.

Primary Tumors

Primary tumors of the spine are rare. Certain tumors (chordoma, osteoblastoma) show a predilection for the spinal column, but these still make up a very small proportion of all spinal tumors. In a review of 82 primary neoplasms of the spine seen over a 50-year period, 31 benign and 51 malignant lesions were identified, which represent eight benign and nine malignant tumor types. In the vertebral body, 75% of the tumors were malignant, compared to only 35% of those in the posterior elements. For patients older than 18 years of age, 80% of primary tumors proved to be malignant, while in children and adolescents, only 32% of lesions were malignant. The five-year survival in these series was 86% of patients with benign tumors and 24% of patients with malignant tumors.

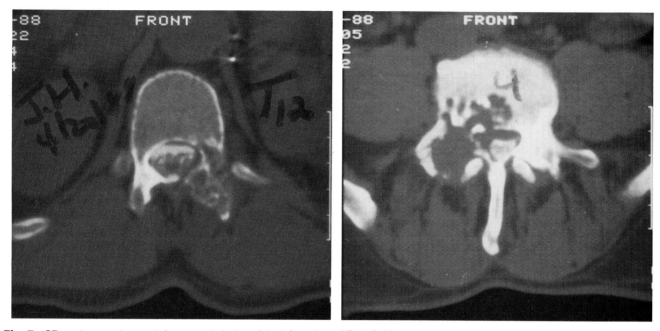

Fig. 7   CT myelogram shows a left metastatic lesion of the left pedicle of T-12 (**left**) and a metastatic lesion of the right pedicle and body of L-4 (**right**).

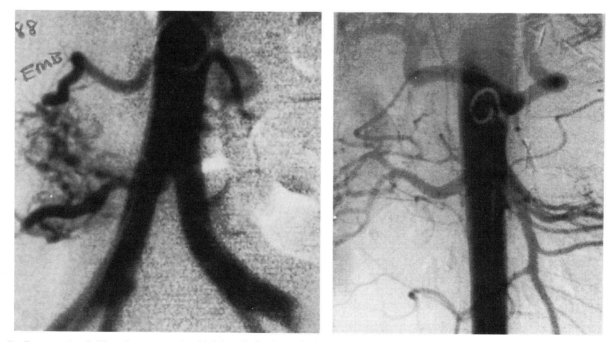

Fig. 8   Preoperative (**left**) and postoperative (**right**) embolization at L-4.

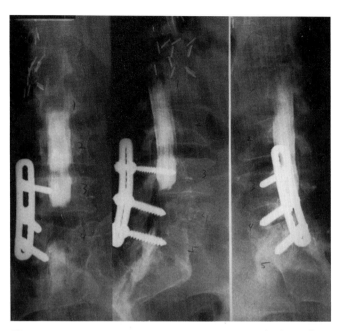

Fig. 9 Following decompressive surgery, the patient had excellent relief of his symptoms; however, within 12 months he had recurrence of his disease as demonstrated on myelogram at L-4. Renal cell carcinoma is one of the more difficult metastatic lesions of the spine to treat, and surgical extirpation should be done only with the realization that a high recurrence rate is probable.

Table 3. Anatomic extent by zone

Zones I to IV	Site A—intraosseous; site B—extraosseous; site C—regional or distant metastasis.
Zones IA to IVA	Intraosseous lesions confined within the cortical boundaries.
Zones IA	Includes spinous processes to the pars interarticularis and inferior articular processes.
Zones IIA	Includes the transverse processes, superior articular processes, and the pedicles to their junction with the vertebral body.
Zones IIIA	Anterior three fourths of the vertebral body.
Zones IVA	Posterior and medial one fourth of the vertebral body.
Zones IB to IVB	Extraosseous extension beyond the cortical boundaries. Lesions having extraosseous extension extend beyond the bony margins of their respective zones.
Zones IC to IVC	Intraosseous or extraosseous lesions associated with regional or distant metastases.

Surgical treatment can have a dramatic impact on function and outcome in selected patients with primary tumors of the spinal column and should never be dismissed as an option without serious consideration. Advances in fixation systems, in local and systemic therapy, and in our understanding of cancer, in general, promise even greater improvements for the future. Figures 11 through 13 represent a 52-year-old male with a space-occupying lesion of L-3, which proved to be primary chordoma.

Infections

Infections of the spine are not uncommon. The incidence of tuberculosis relative to pyogenic infection varies among countries. Patients from poorer countries with poorer environmental hygiene and dense populations tend to develop tuberculosis. Pyogenic infections are less influenced by these factors. The incidence of tuberculosis in the United States has risen recently because of immigration from third-world countries, as well as chronically debilitating conditions such as alcoholism and the immune compromise seen in patients with acquired immune deficiency syndrome (AIDS). Although pyogenic infections can occur in otherwise healthy individuals, patients at risk include those with an aseptic focus elsewhere in the body, drug addicts, and the immunocom-

promised. The diagnosis of vertebral infection with brucellae, candidae, or coccidiomycosis should not be overlooked in individuals with a suggestive occupational history, impaired immunity, or exposure to an endemic area.

One of the largest reported series of nontuberculous spinal infections included 61 patients with pyogenic and fungal vertebral osteomyelitis with paralysis. Factors that predisposed to paralysis were diabetes, rheumatoid arthritis, increased age, and cephalad level of infection. The cause of paralysis was almost always anterior to the neural elements, that is, the abscess generally is formed anterior to the thecal sac. In such cases, the anterior approach provides better exposure for draining associated psoas and paraspinal abscesses. Provided the spine was debrided adequately and patients were given appropriate intravenous antibiotic therapy, spine arthrodesis was performed safely with an autogenous iliac bone graft placed in the site of infection.

Pyogenic infections are often diagnosed late. Eight- to 13-week delays in diagnosis have been reported, and 25% of patients in one series waited more than two years for a correct diagnosis. Many factors are responsible for this delay. Often, patients with vertebral osteomyelitis have few systemic symptoms such as fever or sepsis and cannot localize their pain accurately. Many have normal complete blood cell counts. Additionally, symptoms may be attributed to concurrent infection or a disease process such as carcinoma. In one report, three of seven patients with thoracic osteomyelitis underwent cholecystectomy for chronic pain before their disease was diagnosed correctly. Technetium bone scans reportedly have a sensitivity of more than 90% in patients whose symptoms have lasted more than two days. In animal experiments, magnetic resonance imaging (MRI) has been found to be much more sensitive than bone scanning in the diagnosis

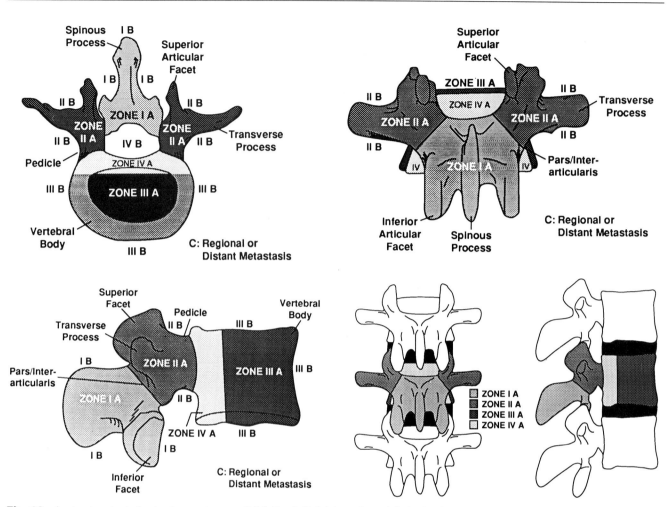

Fig. 10 Anatomic extent of spine tumors by zone (I-IV). **Top left**, Axial cut through L-1, showing zones IA through IVA: Intraosseous lesions are confined within the boundaries of the cortical spine. **Top right**, Posterior view of L-1, showing zones I through IVB: Extraosseous extension is beyond the boundaries of the cortical spine. **Bottom left**, Lateral view of L-1. **Bottom right**, Posterolateral view of L-1 through L-3.

of disk-space infection, making possible diagnosis several days earlier. However, MRI is at least as sensitive as, and more specific than radionucleotide uptake scanning for diagnosis of disk space infection. Specifically, MRI has a reported sensitivity of 96%, a specificity of 93%, and an accuracy of 94%, equaling the results of a combined bone scan and gallium study. MRI more accurately locates the disease process in the disk space, when compared with a bone scan, and MRI has the added advantage of being completely noninvasive.

The diagnosis of vertebral osteomyelitis based on MRI includes: (1) confluent decreased signal intensity in the vertebral bodies and intervertebral disk with inability to discern a margin between the disk and adjacent vertebral bodies on T1-weighted images, (2) increased signal intensity in the vertebral bodies adjacent to the intervertebral disk on T2-weighted images (TR 2,000 to 3,000 milliseconds, TE 120 milliseconds), and (3) abnormal configura-

tion and an increased signal intensity of the intervertebral disk along with the absence of intranuclear cleft on a T2-weighted image (TR 2,000 to 3,000 milliseconds, TE 120 milliseconds).

The initial approach is to identify the organism by needle or open biopsy, or to infer the diagnosis from a positive blood or urine culture. Appropriate intravenous antibiotics should be instituted along with spinal immobilization, including bed rest, bracing, or a combination of both. Surgical debridement is indicated when systemic signs continue despite antibiotic treatment, vertebral-body collapse continues, or evolving neural deficits occur. If surgical debridement is indicated, autogenous bone grafting is generally appropriate as long as intravenous antibiotics are administered. Anterior decompression is often the most appropriate approach because abscesses most often form anterior to the thecal sac. Decompression via laminectomy has been shown re-

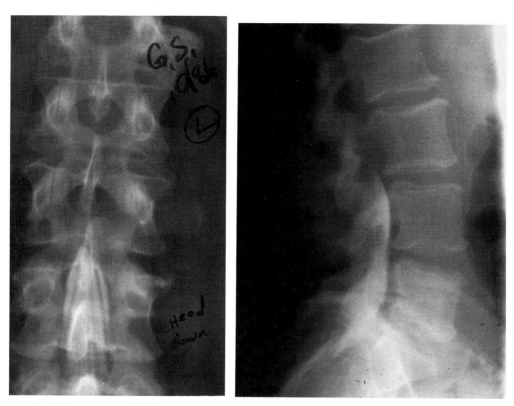

Fig. 11 Anteroposterior (**left**) and lateral (**right**) myelographic views of a 52-year-old man who had a space-occupying lesion of L-3. The myelograms show an incomplete block of the myelographic dye.

peatedly to be ineffective and should be avoided except for patients with diffuse epidural empyema. Costotransversectomy is preferred by some, particularly for patients with thoracic infections, when limited decompression and grafting can be considered. If extensive resection of the necrotic bone with strut graft is needed, then transthoracic or extraperitoneal approaches are preferable. The role of spinal instrumentation in such cases is controversial; however, when there is a large deformity, posterior instrumentation may be indicated.

The development of neurologic complications in vertebral osteomyelitis is often directly related to how soon treatment is initiated. The reported incidence varies from 3% to 40%. Several predisposing factors include: increased age, more cephalad location (cervical, thoracic) of lesions, systemic disease (especially diabetes and chronic steroid therapy), and virulence of the organism, with *Staphylococcus aureus* being implicated most often. Treatment consists of early decompression with appropriate intravenous antibiotic coverage, autogenous bone grafting, and appropriate spinal stabilization and/or bracing. Nonoperative treatment of such cases offers little hope for neurologic recovery.

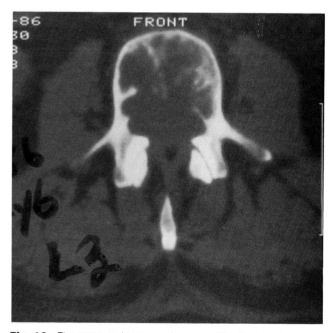

Fig. 12 The computed tomography scan without contrast demonstrates a space-occupying lesion through the posterior cortex of the body of L-3. Biopsy revealed a primary chordoma.

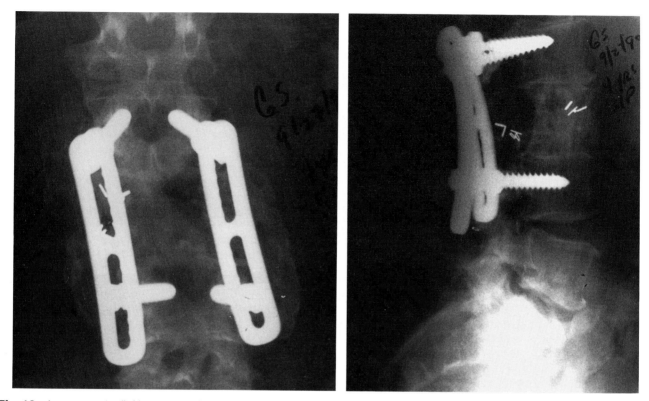

Fig. 13 Anteroposterior (**left**) and lateral (**right**) film taken four years after surgical extirpation or vertebrectomy of L-3.

Tuberculosis of the spine can mimic other infections or tumorous conditions. Tuberculosis causes erosion of the vertebral bodies and can strip the anterior longitudinal ligament and periosteum of adjacent vertebrae. An extensive anterior debridement of abscesses, sequestrated bone, and intervertebral disks is recommended by many, particularly when paraplegia is present. However, some authors report satisfactory results with antituberculosis therapy alone in patients without significant deformity and no neurologic compromise. If surgery is indicated, extensive anterior (usually transthoracic) debridement is performed and anterior strut grafts are inserted in order to obtain tissue for diagnosis, decompress the spinal cord anteriorly, drain abscesses, and prevent postinfection kyphosis. The surgery is performed under cover of antituberculous therapy.

Thoracic Disk Herniation

The prevalence of clinically significant thoracic disk herniation is about one in one million people and between 0.2% and 1.8% of all disk operations. However, a number of studies have suggested that asymptomatic herniations are not uncommon.

Thoracic disk herniations are usually diagnosed late, because the diagnosis is not considered. The radiologic method of choice is either magnetic resonance imaging or high-resolution computed tomographic myelography (Fig. 14).

Neurologic findings may include nonspecific lower extremity weakness, spasticity, ataxia, numbness, and bowel and bladder disturbance with associated sphincter dysfunction. One or more of these symptoms and signs may be present in any combination. Depending on the combination of symptoms, the differential diagnosis can be quite large and includes various causes of thoracic pain, such as infection and neoplasia, as well as such neurologic problems as demyelinating diseases and spinal cord infarction.

The surgical treatment preferred by many for a herniated thoracic disk is an anterior diskectomy with generous removal of bone (hemicorpectomies) superiorly and inferiorly to provide adequate visualization. Neurologic recovery often follows even when there is significant preoperative paralysis.

Anterolateral approaches using variations in the costotransversectomy also have been employed and include pedicle excision and division of the erector spinal muscle mass to improve visualization.

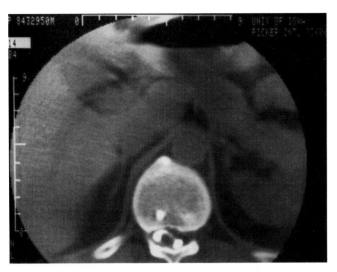

Fig. 14 A T-11 left, lateral thoracic disk herniation. Patient had paraparesis and problems with bladder control. Patient underwent an anterior diskectomy and interbody fusion at T10-11.

In a review of thoracic disk herniations in which anterior approaches by either a costotransversectomy or a thoracotomy were compared, the thoracotomy seemed better. Interestingly, a fusion was not performed routinely following the diskectomy.

Spinal Cord Monitoring

During complex spinal surgery, limiting the risks of neurologic injury is paramount. Spinal cord monitoring has evolved with this in mind. However, to be clinically useful, spinal cord monitoring must be accurate and sensitive, must indicate a preinjury state or at least an injury to the cord that is reversible, and must not increase surgical time and risks.

The ideal form of spinal cord monitoring is not yet available. Limitations in the two currently used major categories, the wake-up test and electrophysiologic monitoring, have prompted the search for more sophisticated monitoring techniques. The use of somatosensory evoked potentials has had the widest application. This technique tests the dorsal columns of the spinal cord (sensory paths). The status of the motor tracks is inferred. The mechanisms responsible for changes in evoked potentials, however, have not been fully elucidated.

Although not yet widely available clinically, motor evoked potential monitoring appears to be a promising alternative. This technique allows the stimulation of the motor cortex and the measurement of potentials from a distal site. These data may more accurately depict the integrity of the motor tracks and, thus, provide a more reliable measure of motor function.

Annotated Bibliography

Diagnosis and Anatomy

Forristall RM, Marsh HO, Pay NT: Magnetic resonance imaging and contrast CT of the lumbar spine: Comparison of diagnostic methods and correlation with surgical findings. *Spine* 1988;13:1049-1054.

Thirty-two patients with suspected lumbar disk herniation underwent magnetic resonance imaging and computed tomographic evaluation of 100 disk levels, and the results were compared with the surgical findings. Surgical findings supported the magnetic resonance imaging diagnosis in 90.3% of cases and the computed tomographic diagnosis in 77.4% of cases. The authors conclude that surface coil magnetic resonance imaging is superior to contrast-enhanced computed tomography in the diagnosis of disk herniation.

Deformity

Byrd JA III, Scoles PV, Winter RB, et al: Adult idiopathic scoliosis treated by anterior and posterior spinal fusion. *J Bone Joint Surg* 1987;69A(6):843-850.

Twenty-six adults were treated for idiopathic scoliosis by two-stage anterior and posterior spinal fusion. It was concluded that a two-stage anterior and posterior fusion is of value for the treatment of adults who have rigid curves that require maximum correction to allow the head, shoulders, and torso to be centered over the pelvis. The authors of this article do not recommend anterior instrumentation for anterior fusion because it did not increase curve correction in their patients.

Ginsberg H, Scoles P: Scoliosis Research Society, Morbidity and Mortality Committee, 1990, Complication Report.

Complications reports were submitted for approximately 147 individuals or centers for the reporting period between January 1, 1990, through December 31, 1990. Complications were analyzed in two categories—procedures and complications. Approximately 512 posterior procedures and 146 anterior procedures were done for adult idiopathic scoliosis, with 95 having combined anterior and posterior procedures during the same anesthetic. From these data, various complications are reported in the following categories of neurologic deficits; spinal fluid leak, infection, instrument failure, death, pseudarthrosis, and other. For example, there were 21 spinal fluid leaks out of 5,269 laminectomy cases, for a prevalence of .003%, or one in 250 cases.

and other. For example, there were 21 spinal fluid leaks out of 5,269 laminectomy cases, for a prevalence of .003%, or one in 250 cases.

Sponseller PD, Cohen MS, Nachemson AL, et al: Results of surgical treatment of adults with idiopathic scoliosis. *J Bone Joint Surg* 1987;69A:667-675.

Forty-five patients with adult scoliosis were interviewed at least three years after surgery to determine the long-term results. There was a reduction in the severity of peak and constant pain, but no change in the frequency of peak pain. Similarly, functional impairment caused by scoliosis was lessened and the ability to perform common activities of daily living was improved, but no important changes in occupation or recreational activity were recorded. A high complication rate and limited gains suggested that patient information and selection are important factors to be considered.

van Dam BE, Bradford DS, Lonstein JE, et al: Adult idiopathic scoliosis treated by posterior spinal fusion and Harrington instrumentation. *Spine* 1987;12:32-36.

Ninety-one adult patients with idiopathic scoliosis underwent posterior spinal fusion and Harrington rod instrumentation. Indications for surgery included pain, progressive deformity, and pulmonary symptoms. The average correction was 38% at the time of surgery and 32% at the time of follow-up (average, 3.5 years). Seventy-nine percent of the patients reported complete relief of the symptoms for which they underwent surgery. The complication rate was 33%, including a 15% pseudarthrosis rate and a 5% instrumentation failure rate.

Posttraumatic Kyphosis

Bradford DS, McBride GG: Surgical management of thoracolumbar spine fractures with incomplete neurologic deficits. *Clin Orthop* 1987;218:201-216.

The results of surgical decompression in 59 patients with neurologic deficit secondary to thoracic or lumbar fractures were evaluated at a mean of 3.7 years after injury. More neurologic recovery occurred in patients who underwent anterior decompression (88%) than in those who underwent posterolateral or posterior decompression (64%).

Transpedicular Approaches and Fixation

Weinstein JN, Spratt KF, Spengler D, et al: Spinal pedicle fixation: Reliability and validity of roentgenogram-based assessment and surgical factors on successful screw placement. *Spine* 1988;13(9):1012-1018.

Roentgenograms were determined to be unreliable for determining angle screw entry and for evaluating placement success. However, success rates without the use of roentgenograms to assist in placement of angle screws may have proved even worse. Spinal pedicle fixation represents a difficult surgical procedure even in the ideal conditions provided by cadaveric specimens. Traditional training methods and surgical experience may not provide the quality feedback necessary to develop mastery skill levels. Experienced surgeons might expect to have significant learning curves if trained according to procedures used in this study. Small pedicle sizes may preclude successful fixation even when using very small screws, especially at T-11 to L-2, where pedicle widths of less than 0.5 mm have been reported.

Metastatic Tumors

Kostuik JP, Weinstein JN: Differential diagnosis and surgical treatment of metastatic spine tumors, in Frymoyer JW, Ducker TB, Hadler NM, et al (eds): *The Adult Spine, Principles and Practice.* New York, Raven Press, 1991, pp 861-888.

The authors review the pathophysiology and tumor biology of metastatic spine tumors as well as the prognosis and surgical and nonsurgical options. The authors have expanded the surgical recommendations for intervention to include (1) an isolated primary and some isolated metastatic lesions or solitary site of relapse, (2) pathologic fracture or deformity producing neurologic symptoms and/or pain, (3) radio-resistant tumors, metastatic or primary, and (4) segmental instability following radiotherapy.

Primary Tumors

Weinstein JN, McLain RF: Primary tumors of the spine. *Spine* 1987;12(9):843-851.

Of 82 cases of primary spine neoplasms reviewed, 31 were benign and 51 malignant. Plain roentgenograms demonstrated the spinal lesion in 99% of all cases. Malignancy proved to be associated with an older age at diagnosis, a higher incidence of neurologic deficit, and a higher incidence of occurrence in the vertebral body. Five-year survival for patients with benign tumors was 86%, five-year survival for malignant lesions correlated with the extent of initial surgery and with tumor type. Patients having complete excision had the best surgical outcome. In this series, the prolonged survival seen with complete excision where possible justified the aggressive surgical approach to the treatment of such tumors. Spine tumors should only be biopsied and treated by surgeons experienced in the approach and management of these most difficult problems.

Weinstein JN: Differential diagnosis and surgical treatment of primary benign and malignant neoplasms, in Frymoyer JW, Ducker TB, Hadler NM, et al (eds): *The Adult Spine—Principles and Practice.* New York, Raven Press, 1991, pp 829-860.

The goals of treatment should be to: (1) obtain a definitive diagnosis through biopsy or primary excision, (2) the institution of appropriate surgical or medical treatment according to tumor type and the patient's condition, (3) preservation of neurologic function, and (4) the maintenance of spinal column stability. Although the treatment of patients with spinal tumors must be individualized, specific principles should be observed in managing tumors in general and for specific tumor types, in order to meet these goals.

Infection

Szypryt EP, Hardy JG, Hinton CE, et al: A comparison between magnetic resonance imaging and scintigraphic bone imaging in the diagnosis of disc space infection in an animal model. *Spine* 1988;13:1042-1048.

A series of 33 rabbits was used to compare the efficacy of magnetic resonance imaging with that of scintigraphy in the diagnosis of pyogenic infection of the intervertebral disk. Magnetic resonance imaging was found to be more sensitive, particularly in the early stages of the disease. The overall results showed that magnetic resonance imaging had a sensitivity of 93%, a specificity of 97%, and an accuracy of 95%.

Thoracic Disk Herniation

Bohlman HH, Zdeblick TA: Anterior excision of herniated thoracic discs. *J Bone Joint Surg* 1988;70A:1038-1047.

The incidence of clinically significant thoracic disk herniations is about one in one million or about 0.25% to 1.8% of all disk operations. They concluded that in thoracic disk herniations treated anteriorly via either a costotransversectomy or a thoracotomy, a thoracotomy approach seemed best. Interestingly, they did not routinely perform a fusion following the diskectomy.

Spinal Cord Monitoring

Lieponis JV, Jacobs K, Bunch WH, et al: The effect of spinal cord blood flow on evoked potentials, in Ducker TB, Brown RH (eds): *Neurophysiology and Standards of Spinal Cord Monitoring*. New York, Springer-Verlag, 1988.

An overview of intraoperative spinal cord monitoring is presented. Altered primate spinal-cord blood-flow states demonstrated significant changes in evoked potentials. Study conditions mimicked actual operating room settings.

Brown RH, Nash, CL Jr: Intra-operative spinal cord monitoring, in Frymoyer JW, Ducker TB, Hadler NM, et al (eds): *The Adult Spine, Principles and Practice*. New York, Raven Press, 1991, pp 549-564.

The authors review the indications for intraoperative spinal cord monitoring as well as the nomenclature. They discuss in depth somatosensory cortical evoked potentials as well as the somatosensory spinal evoked potentials, the applications thereof, and the need for further work.

39
Lumbar Spine

Low back pain is a common symptom, affecting 60% to 80% of individuals at some time in their lives. Disorders of the back and spine are the most frequent and most costly musculoskeletal impairments and rank third behind arthritis/rheumatism and heart disease as a cause of disability in people in their working years. The natural history of low back pain is that 50% of patients recover by two weeks and 90% by three months. Nevertheless, the total medical cost attributable to this condition has been estimated at between $16 billion and $50 billion annually. Individuals having persistent and disabling back pain account for 85% to 90% of this cost. The rate of disability attributable to low back pain has exceeded the growth of the general population 14 fold, contributing to the escalation of treatment costs.

Epidemiology

Low Back Pain

The lifetime incidence of low back pain has been reported at 60% to 80%. In a study of 10,404 adults (25 years and older) the second National Health and Nutrition Examination Survey (NHANES II) discovered a point prevalence of adult back pain of 6.8%. The cumulative lifetime prevalence of low back pain lasting at least two weeks was 13.8%, and 5% of the respondents reported chronic symptoms. Extrapolated to the total United States population, these figures yield an estimated 10 million persons with chronic back pain symptoms. Other data suggest a prevalence of low back pain of any duration of 12% to 52%. The annual incidence has been reported to be anywhere from 1% to 20%, the actual incidence being a function of the type of industrial population surveyed.

Sciatica

The lifetime incidence of sciatica has been reported to be as high as 40% in the adult population. In the NHANES II study, only 1.6% of the population reported sciatica, which represented approximately 12% of the individuals with low back pain. The natural history of sciatica, like that of low back pain, favors recovery, with approximately 50% of patients relieved of their symptoms within 1 month and 96% functioning fully by six months.

The incidence of surgical treatment of lumbar disk herniations varies among countries: 0.8% of Swedish adults versus 2.0% of United States adults report they have had surgical diskectomy. In the United States, 188,000 procedures were performed for lumbar disk herniation in 1983, and the annual rate is increasing.

Diagnosis

In the evaluation of the patient with low back pain, it is imperative that all diagnostic imaging studies be placed in the proper perspective. In a group of 300 patients who had no symptoms of spinal pathology and underwent posterior fossa myelography to establish a diagnosis of acoustic neurilemmoma, there was some degree of disk abnormality in 37%. In the lumbar spine alone, 24% of the individuals had a disk abnormality. Similar data were reported for computed tomography (CT), with 35% of asymptomatic individuals having abnormal lumbar scans. Not surprisingly, the results varied with age. In subjects aged 20 to 39 years, the rate of abnormal findings averaged 19.5%; in subjects over 40, abnormalities were found in 50% of the group. In a recent study in which magnetic resonance imaging (MRI) was performed on 67 asymptomatic individuals, one third of the subjects were seen to have a substantial abnormality, and 20% of these under 60 years of age had a disk herniation. In subjects older than 60 years, 57% of the scans were interpreted as abnormal, with 36% of the subjects having a disk herniation and 21% spinal stenosis.

Thus, abnormal morphology is not always productive of symptoms, particularly in degenerative spinal conditions. The problem that the clinician faces is in trying to ascribe symptoms to a morphologic abnormality. In the absence of correlative data such as a positive straight leg-raising sign or a neurologic deficit, the clinician cannot be sure that the abnormalities seen radiographically cause or explain the patient's symptoms. The diagnostic imaging study although important, is but a single facet of the overall evaluation of patients with suspected disk herniation or spinal stenosis, which must include thorough history taking and physical examination.

History

A good presumptive diagnosis of many disorders of the back may be obtained from a careful medical history. The presumptive diagnosis is then refined by the physical examination and imaging studies.

Pain is the usual complaint in most back disorders. It is helpful to determine first whether the primary complaint is low back pain or leg pain. Leg pain may be referred from the back or it may be radicular pin or claudication. Referred pain extending into the buttocks, down the posterior thigh, and, occasionally, into the calf can be elicited by injecting hypertonic saline into the interspinous ligaments and facet joints. Such pain reflects the mesodermal nature of the anatomic structures involved, which are related embryologically to the sclerotome. True radicular pain, on the other hand, generally radiates below the knee in a dermatomal pattern.

It is useful to determine whether back pain or radicular leg pain is the predominant complaint and to note the relative intensities of each. For example, patients with low back problems often complain of pain in the coccyx. Although coccygectomy usually is viewed as having a high failure rate in producing relief of coccygeal pain, one researcher reported satisfactory results in 89% of patients undergoing this procedure. That report examined the anatomic configuration of the coccyx in asymptomatic subjects and compared the results of coccygectomy with the type of configuration.

Patients with radiculopathy have well-described pain, the distribution of which depends on the particular nerve root involved. Lateral calf pain radiation to the dorsum of the foot and the big toe is typical of an L-5 radiculopathy, whereas posterior calf pain extending to the sole and the lateral aspect of the foot suggests an S-1 radiculopathy. Pain in the anteromedial thigh often suggests an L-3 or L-4 pattern. Anterior thigh pain can reflect conditions such as hip disease or a retroperitoneal neoplasm or other mass compressing the lumbar plexus.

Night pain is an unusual complaint with common spinal disorders. It may portend a more sinister condition such as malignancy or infection.

Perianal numbness and urinary symptoms such as retention, overflow incontinence, or loss of desire to void suggest a cauda equina syndrome, which is one of the rare emergencies in spinal surgery, demanding rapid diagnosis with surgical decompression if a compressive cause can be demonstrated. However, the mere presence of muscle weakness is not a surgical emergency, as several studies have shown that the ultimate return of muscle strength is independent of the treatment rendered. That is, statistically, strength is just as likely to return with conservative treatment as it is with surgery. Documented progressive weakness of functionally significant muscles, on the other hand, usually is considered an indication for surgical decompression if a compressive cause for the weakness can be demonstrated.

The *mode of onset* of the pain is relevant. Mechanical low back pain usually is characterized by a vague long history of intermittent attacks, sometimes interspersed with diminishing intervals of relief. Often, low back pain is succeeded by leg pain, with the original pain diminishing or disappearing. This picture suggests that the original pain was caused by compression of the innervated outer layers of the annulus fibrosus, with subsequent rupture of the disk through the annulus, resulting in compression of the nerve root and predominance of leg over low back pain.

Although sudden strenuous events occasionally produce low back or leg pain, many episodes of disk hernia-tion occur as the result of relatively innocuous actions such as bending over or picking up a light-weight object. When there is a history of an apparently well-defined work-related injury, caution should be exercised, as all forms of treatment, including surgery, have a poorer success rate in worker's compensation cases.

The next step in history taking is to elicit any *provocative or palliative factors*. Patients with disk herniations frequently give a history of leg pain that is aggravated by sitting or car riding and relieved by lying down or standing. This pattern of complaints reflects the biomechanics of the disk. The pressure in the L-3/L-4 disk varies with position, ranging from 20 kg in the supine position to 270 kg while sitting forward 20 degrees with a 10-kg load in each hand. The pressure during upright sitting is 43% greater than that during upright standing. These data help explain the preference of the patient with a disk herniation for standing rather than sitting.

Patients with mechanical low back pain often report a long history of pain that is related to activity. That is, the more they do, the more they hurt. Activities such as lifting, bending, or changing position often produce back pain that abates with rest.

Patients with stenosis of the lumbar canal (neurogenic claudication) typically give a history of back, buttock, or leg pain with standing or walking that is relieved by sitting down or bending forward. Often, a positive "grocery cart" sign can be elicited: the patient leans over a cart while shopping to obtain immediate pain relief. Neurogenic claudication may be explained in part on a mechanical basis. The increased lumbar lordosis that is normal with standing and walking can produce symptoms in a spine whose neural foramen is already narrowed by age-related changes in the adjacent disk and facets. The claudication may also be explained on vascular basis, in that obstruction to venous outflow from the nerve roots, which increases with lordosis, produces pressure changes or ischemia within the nerve-root blood vessels.

It is important to distinguish neurogenic claudication from the vascular type. In either condition, leg pain is provoked by walking. However, standing produces leg pain only in neurogenic claudication. Indeed, the leg pain associated with vascular claudication frequently is relieved by standing, whereas with neurogenic claudication, relief is obtained only by a positional change that reduces lumbar lordosis, such as sitting, bending forward, or leaning against an object. A useful provocative study is the Van Gelderan bicycle test. With vascular claudication, pain is provoked, because bicycle riding increases the demands on the vascularly impaired leg muscles. With neurogenic claudication, however, pain is not provoked because sitting reduces lordosis, thereby opening the neural foramen and relieving neural compression. Walking may also distinguish the two types of claudication. Because the lesion in vascular claudication is fixed, the distance a patient can walk without pain is relatively constant. With neurogenic claudication, on the other hand, the distance the patient can walk before experiencing leg pain typically is variable.

Complaints of morning stiffness should be sought, particularly in young men. This symptom raises the possibility of seronegative spondylarthropathy such as ankylosing spondylitis.

An increasingly recognized complaint is Vesper's curse, characterized by night cramps. There is some evidence that these symptoms worsen when patients have incipient congestive heart failure.

The medical history also must encompass psychosocial factors. Because the most common presenting symptom of back disorders is pain, and because the most common indication for surgery is relief of pain, it is important to keep in mind the factors that can alter a patient's perception of pain and impair the clinician's ability to render an unbiased judgment about its origin. Psychosocial factors such as depression, drug addiction, litigation, or worker's compensation must always be sought when taking the history. The effect of worker's compensation was studied in 103 industrial compensation patients in whom one operation had failed to produce relief of pain and who underwent a second procedure. Follow-up for one to two years revealed improvement on only 40% to 50% of patients and deterioration in 20%. Similarly poor results have been shown for primary disk excision and fusion in spondylolisthesis in the presence of pending litigation.

Because in some studies as many as 50% of depressed patients reported pain as a prominent symptom, depression should be looked for in patients with long-standing pain. Five simple questions can give the clinician a clear indication of possible depression and should be asked whenever that emotional state is suspected: questions about anergia (lack of energy), anhedonia (inability to enjoy oneself), sleep disturbances, spontaneous weeping, or a general feeling of depression. Indeed, when the latter two questions are posed, a depressed patient will frequently become tearful. Other useful clinical indicators of emotional distress are the Waddell signs: skin tenderness, simulation, distraction, regional disturbances, and overreaction to stimuli.

Finally, the physician must inquire about previous lumbar surgery. In the patient who has been operated on previously, the examiner should first try to determine whether there were clear indications for the initial operation. If the initial procedure was not clearly indicated, additional surgery is unlikely to be palliative. On the other hand, if the initial surgery was indicated, it should be determined whether or not there was a pain-free interval following the surgery. If there was no pain-free interval, then it is likely that the lesion was missed at surgery, and additional surgery may be helpful. On the other hand, if the patient had a relatively short pain-free interval, (six to 12 months), scar tissue must be seriously considered at the cause of the pain. If scar is confirmed by gadolinium-enhanced MRI, it is unlikely that additional surgery will help the patient's pain. If the patient had a long pain-free interval, typically longer that a year, then it is possible that the disk has reherniated at the level operated on or that there is a compressive lesion elsewhere in the spine. Under these circumstances, the neurologic examination results may differ from those prior to the initial surgery, and diagnostic imaging should confirm the presences of such a lesion. Again, gadolinium-enhanced MRI is the imaging technique of choice. If a lesion can be demonstrated, surgery is likely to be palliative.

Physical Examination

The physical examination refines the presumptive diagnosis made from the medical history. The patient should be examined for fixed or postural disturbances such as a sciatic list (Fig. 1). Palpation and percussion should also be performed to elicit sites of tenderness. The presence of skin tenderness is one of Waddell's nonorganic physical signs.

Range of motion should be examined next. Patients with a disk herniation frequently complain of leg pain on forward flexion, whereas patients with spinal stenosis often have leg pain on back extension. The latter movement is believed to cause further mechanical narrowing of the neural foramen and spinal canal, thus compressing the involved spinal nerve and producing leg pain (Fig. 2). Indeed, this single finding may be the only abnormality easily elicited on the physical examination of the patient with spinal stenosis.

A precise neurologic examination is necessary. Usually, the patterns of individual nerve root compression syndromes are easily recognized.

The presence or absence of a tension sign is the most important finding in patients suspected of having a disk herniation, as has been emphasized repeatedly. For example, in a series of 2,157 patients with surgically verified disk herniation, Lasegue's sign was positive in 97%, being positive in 98% of patients with verified disk herniations at L-5/S-1 and 97% of those with herniations at L-4/L-5. The frequency of a positive sign decreased with increasing age. Therefore, the absence of a positive tension sign in a young patient with suspected disk herniation at L-4/L-5 or L-5/S-1 should raise the possibility that a condition other than herniation is the cause of the patient's symptoms. The contralateral straight leg-raising (cross Lasegue) sign, in which radiating pain is produced in the symptomatic leg when the painless leg is elevated, is uncommon, being present in approximately 20% of patients with surgically verified lumbar disk herniation.

For levels above L-4/L-5, particularly for lesions involving the L-3 or L-4 nerve root, the femoral nerve stretch test is the equivalent of the straight leg-raising sign for lower lumbar herniations.

In patients with claudication, it is important to check the peripheral pulses, as it occasionally is difficult to differentiate neurogenic and vascular etiologies. In the clinical setting of an equivocal history, diminished or absent pulses in the affected leg indicate a need for further vascular evaluations.

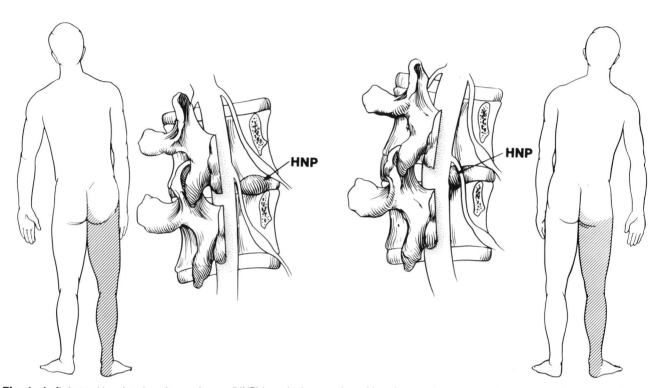

Fig. 1 **Left,** Lateral herniated nucleus pulposus (HNP) in typical posterolateral location causing compression and medial deviation of the affected spinal nerve. The patient lists to the left in an involuntary maneuver to relieve compression on the nerve. **Right,** HNP in more unusual axillary location causing lateral deviation and compression of the affected spinal nerve. The patient lists to the right in this situation. Shaded area indicates pain. (Reproduced with permission from Bell GR: *Semin Spine Surg* 1989;1:8-17.)

Finally, it is important to recall that there are non-spinal causes of back pain, such as abdominal aortic aneurysm, ulcer disease, a retroperitoneal mass or neoplasm, or hip disease. Indeed, the differential diagnosis of anterior thigh or groin pain includes, in addition to an L-3 or L-4 radiculopathy, hip disease and a retroperitoneal lesion.

Imaging Techniques

Only one of 2,500 plain radiographic examinations of the lumbar spine yields clinically unsuspected findings in patients 20 to 50 years old. Most studies have found no association between low back pain and disk space narrowing, transitional vertebrae, Schmorl's nodes, lumbar lordosis, disk vacuum sign, claw spurs, scoliosis, the level of the pelvic intercrestal line, disk space wedging, the relative lengths of the L-3 and L-5 transverse processes, or spina bifida occulta.

The reported accuracy of myelography with water-soluble contrast medium for the diagnosis of lumbar disk herniation ranges from 67% to 100%. This study is no longer the imaging technique of choice in most patients, although some experts believe that myelographically enhanced CT is valuable in the preoperative evaluation of spinal stenosis.

The advantages of CT over myelography include better visualization of lateral lesions, such as foraminal stenosis and lateral disk herniations, a lower radiation dose, the absence of known adverse reactions, and the ability to perform the procedure on an outpatient basis. In addition, CT allows discrimination between neural compression caused by soft tissue (eg, a disk) and that caused by bony pathology (eg, facet hypertrophy or osteophytes of posterior vertebral bodies). Like myelography, CT can provide orthogonal views. When necessary, CT data can be reformatted for three-dimensional surface reconstruction.

Computed tomography is useful in the diagnosis of extreme lateral or foraminal herniation of lumbar disk. One study found only a 58% accuracy rate for metrizamide myelography in the diagnosis of such lesions, compared with 71% for CT. Contrast CT is more sensitive (78% versus 71%), as specific as (76% versus 76%), and slightly more accurate than (77% versus 74%) noncontrast scanning in the diagnosis of lumbar disk herniation.

An inherent drawback of CT is that axial imaging is typically performed only at the lower three lumbar levels (from L-3 to S-1) because many cuts would be required to image the entire spine. There is, therefore, the possibility

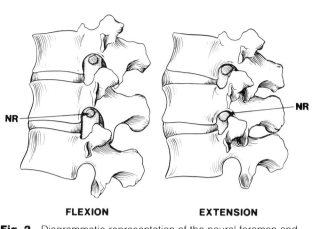

FLEXION   **EXTENSION**

Fig. 2 Diagrammatic representation of the neural foramen and nerve root (NR) in flexion and extension. Note that in flexion the neural foramen is more patent and the spinal nerve root (NR) is free of compression. In extension, the neural foramen narrows and the nerve root (NR) becomes compressed, typically by the superior articular facet. (Reproduced with permission from Bell GR: *Semin Spine Surg* 1989;1:8-17.)

of missing unsuspected pathology at higher levels. Both myelography and MRI are superior to CT in this regard, providing sagittal imaging of the entire lumbar spine and thoracolumbar junction.

Computed tomography following diskography (disko-CT) may have a place in the diagnosis of lumbar spine disorders. The injection of contrast agents into the disk allows better distinction between the disk and other structures on subsequent CT examination. In one study, disko-CT proved to be more accurate than either myelography (87% versus 70%), CT (87% versus 74%), or contrast-enhanced CT (87% versus 77%) in the diagnosis of lumbar disk herniation.

Magnetic resonance imaging is similar to CT in that it provides cross-sectional images based on a matrix of numbers, each assigned to a shade of gray and each representing a physical property of the tissue it depicts. As with CT, MRI provides orthogonal imaging with both sagittal and axial images. More than other imaging modalities, MRI shows normal and abnormal structures of the spine and provides the ability to delineate anatomically intimate structures such as the annulus fibrosus and the nucleus pulposus. It can reveal pathological states of the lumbar spine such as degeneration, which causes a signal change in the vertebral body marrow adjacent to the end plate of degenerative disks. The images also can reveal changes within the disk itself, which usually are depicted as decreased signal intensity on the T2-weighted spin-echo sequence.

The use of paramagnetic contrast agents such as gadolinium diethylenetriamine pentaacetic acid (Gd-DTPA) provides information not obtainable with other imaging modalities. Gadolinium has been particularly useful in evaluation of the postoperative lumbar spine. Recent data suggest that Gd-DTPA examination has a 96% agreement with surgery in distinguishing epidural fibrosis from recurrent disk herniation. Epidural scar tissue, which has a vascular supply, enhances after injection of Gd-DTPA, whereas disk herniations do not enhance.

Diskography has been the subject of considerable interest and debate since the original reports on the technique were published in 1948. Proponents of diskography emphasize two important aspects: the morphology of the disk as seen on contrast-enhanced radiography and the use of diskography in an attempt to reproduce the patient's usual type of pain. In a series of asymptomatic volunteers, 37% had abnormal diskograms. In another study, seven patients with low back pain and ten volunteers without back pain had injections at three levels while their responses were videotaped. In the asymptomatic population, the diskogram was interpreted as abnormal in 17% of the 30 disks injected, although none of the asymptomatic individuals exhibited a pain response to the injection. In the seven patients with low back pain, the diskogram was abnormal in 13 of the 20 disks (65%) with a positive pain response involving at least one level in all seven patients. Thus, if an individual had no back pain, the diskogram was negative and in this respect exhibited a 0% false-positive rate. The question not answered by this study was the precise source of the pain in those individuals exhibiting an abnormal pain response. Until this question is answered, and until an outcome study is completed showing the effect of surgery performed on the basis of an abnormal diskogram, the ultimate role of diskography as an aid in surgical decision-making will remain unanswered.

The role of electrodiagnostic studies in spinal stenosis and disk herniation is limited, particularly after surgery entailing denervation of the paravertebral muscles. Electromyography (EMG) enables the surgeon to assess the physiologic integrity of the nerve root and thus can reveal evidence of root dysfunction caused by conditions other than compression. This is particularly true in patients with diabetes, in whom nerve fiber infarction can cause lumbosacral root syndromes. Situations in which the EMG can provide useful information include distinguishing a peroneal neuropathy from an isolated L-5 radiculopathy, identifying upper motor neuron lesions, and determining the presence or absence of generalized myopathy. The EMG also is useful in identifying a peripheral polyneuropathy and plexus or peripheral nerve lesions such as might be present in patients having a retroperitoneal neoplasm causing compression of the lumbosacral plexus.

Somatosensory evoked potential (SEPs) are used to evaluate the function of both central and peripheral somatosensory pathways. Electrical stimulation of the peripheral nerve excites the large, fast-conducting group Ia and group II afferent fibers. Responses are recorded with either surface or needle electrodes from a more proximal portion of the nerve and over the spine and scalp. The SEPs provide a noninvasive method for evaluating the function of the sensory fibers of nerve roots. There are a number of theoretical limitations in the use of SEPs, however, and their utility in compressive lumbosacral radiculopathies is limited.

Isolated cutaneous nerve stimulation, as opposed to stimulation of a multisegmental nerve trunk, has been reported to be sensitive to compressive radiculopathies, although this view is not universally accepted. Similarly, dermatomally elicited SEPs, whereby recording is performed over the scalp during stimulation in the cutaneous distribution of an individual nerve root, are only marginally sensitive to compressive root lesions of L-5 and S-1.

Other Diagnostic Tests

Other methods used to localize a source of pain have included injections, rhizotomy, and arthrography of the facets. Most studies indicate that these tests are unreliable. Facet injection, although once popular, now appears to have little benefit. In a prospective study of 97 patients randomly assigned to facet injection with either methylprednisolone or isotonic saline with a six-month follow-up, only 22% of the former group and 10% of the latter obtained relief. There likewise is little evidence that thermography is sufficiently specific to make it useful.

Treatment

Acute Low Back Pain

Irrespective of treatment, the vast majority of patients with low back pain will get better within two months. Such a favorable natural history makes evaluation of treatment methods difficult. In an analysis of 59 therapeutic trials for their adherence to 11 methodological criteria, it proved impossible to substantiate the efficacy of corsets, bedrest, transcutaneous nerve stimulation, or conventional traction for the treatment of back pain. There was some evidence that flexion exercises provide benefit, but the difference in the results was not statistically significant. "Autotraction" showed some superiority over a corset at one week but not at three months' follow-up. Some studies have shown short-term but no long-term benefits from manipulation. No drug has proved superior to aspirin alone, although some medications have fewer side effects. Two days of bedrest is as effective as seven days in patients with acute low back pain. In addition, patients receiving two days of bedrest miss 45% fewer days of work than those receiving seven days of bedrest, yet without any increase in symptoms, dysfunction, or health-care use.

Chronic Low Back Pain

Chronic low back pain is defined as pain that is persistent after three months. Fewer than 5% of patients with low back pain develop a chronic pain syndrome, yet it is this group of patients that accounts for at least 85% of the total cost of back pain in terms of compensation and loss of work. As with acute low back pain, there are many potential causes for chronic pain, such as the disk, annulus fibrosus, facet joint, muscles, ligaments, and tendons, but a structural diagnosis is usually absent. Unlike acute low back pain, chronic pain frequently has a significant psychosocial component. Psychosocial factors include depression, narcotic and alcohol addiction, and litigation and compensation issues.

The chemical mediators of pain are a current focus of study in patients with chronic pain, and there is some suggestion that endogenous opiates have a significant role in pain inhibition. Substance P, a neuropeptide stored in the dorsal root ganglion, is present in lower concentration in the cerebrospinal fluid of patients with chronic pain.

The treatment of chronic back pain must be directed to the underlying physical and psychosocial factors. Surgery is rarely palliative. Nonsurgical treatment might include detoxification and the use of antidepressants, not only for those individuals who are depressed, but occasionally for those who are not. Other treatments that have shown some benefit include biofeedback training to produce muscle relaxation and functional restoration programs that emphasize reconditioning and work hardening. Transcutaneous nerve stimulation has shown no efficacy in randomized studies.

Surgery for Low Back Pain

Surgical treatment of low back pain is a controversial issue that often fails to address the primary problem: inability to determine the exact source of the pain in most instances. In most patients, precise anatomic localization of the pain source is not important, as the intermediate-term outcome is generally favorable. However, when considering surgical treatment, it becomes important to define the anatomic site of the pathology accurately. A common method is diskography. However, this study has a significant number of false-positive and false-negative results, regardless of whether the findings are judged by the radiographic image or the pain response. The definitive study correlating abnormal diskography findings with surgical outcome has yet to be done.

The theory behind lumbar fusion for back pain is that immobilization of the offending spinal segment will alleviate the pain. Unfortunately, as the literature attests, there are many patients with continued pain after solid fusion as well as those with pseudarthrosis after spinal fusion who have symptomatic improvement.

Despite the lack of definitive efficacy information, lumbar spinal fusion continues to gain popularity. For unexplained reasons, the popularity of the procedure varies significantly in different geographic regions of the United States. There also is increasing popularity for pedicle fixation and combined anteroposterior fusion. Although surgeons report a high level of success, there are no carefully controlled analyses. However, laboratory experiments do confirm more predictable and earlier fusion.

Radicular Pain

Lumbar disk herniation is thought to represent the final step along a continuum of degeneration that is a normal part of aging. Degeneration or bulging of at least one lumbar disk was found in 35% of 35 asymptomatic individuals between 20 and 39 years of age but in 13 of 14 asymptomatic individuals between 60 and 80 years of age. More impressively, a herniated nucleus pulposus (HNP) was found in 20% of asymptomatic individuals less than 60 years old and in 36% of asymptomatic subjects more than 60 years of age. A similar incidence of disk herniation in asymptomatic individuals has been found by CT (35%) and oil-based myelography (24%). Thus, it is clear that the mere presence of a disk herniation does not necessarily result in symptoms and that factors other than compression can be a source of pain. The current focus is on inflammatory causes and non-neurogenic mediators such as substance P, vasoactive intestinal peptide (VIP), and calcitonin gene-related peptides (CGRP). These peptides have been identified in the outer layers of the annulus fibrosus, as well as in the supraspinous and intraspinous ligaments. The dorsal root ganglion seems to serve as a warehouse for these peptides and may play an important, yet incompletely understood, role in modulating pain at each segmental level. Such factors may help explain the generally favorable prognosis of symptomatic disk herniation.

In a controlled prospective ten-year study of 280 patients with lumbar disk herniation treated either conservatively or surgically, the surgically treated group was doing better at one year. However, comparison of the results at four years and ten years revealed no statistically significant difference in outcome, although there was a slight tendency to a more favorable outcome with surgery. It appears that although surgery may provide a more rapid end point (relief of pain), the ultimate end point is approximately the same, regardless of treatment.

As in the case of acute low back pain, the generally favorable natural history of symptomatic disk herniation makes it difficult to determine the efficacy of the various treatment modalities. Nonsurgical treatments include bedrest, oral medication, epidural steroids, physical therapy, bracing, traction, manipulation, and techniques such as transcutaneous nerve stimulation, most of which have not been proved effective. Most studies indicate that a brief period of rest should be the mainstay of initial treatment, with non-narcotic analgesics and nonsteroidal anti-inflammatory drugs used to control pain. Although epidural steroids may play a role, they have not been shown conclusively to produce a long-term benefit. Manipulative therapy has been advocated, but although short-term success has been reported in some studies, no long-term benefit has been documented consistently.

The generally good prognosis for conservatively treated symptomatic disk herniations (92%) indicates that no more than 10% of patients with symptoms and signs should ultimately require surgery. This finding contrasts sharply with the reported number of surgical procedures performed in the United States, which numbered 188,000 in 1983.

Results of surgical diskectomy have generally been quite favorable, with reported success rates being in the range of 90% to 95%. In a one-year follow-up of 274 patients with lumbar disk herniation meeting the criteria of leg pain in excess of back pain, an abnormal neurologic examination including a positive tension sign, and a positive imaging study, the success rate in the relief of leg pain was 93% and that for relief of low back pain was 80%. Although some surgeons advocate radical extirpation of the disk, most prefer to perform a limited diskectomy in which only the extruded fragment is removed. The results of this more limited surgery are similar to those of the more radical removal of the disk, but the limited approach entails less risk of vascular injury.

Microdiskectomy offers the benefit of a magnified illuminated field and the theoretical advantages of minimal dissection, preservation of normal anatomy, and gentle manipulation of the neural elements. Williams advocated removal of the ligamentum flavum only and reported a 91% success rate. Modifications of his technique have produced success rates of 96% and 88%. A collation of published reports of 1,257 patients undergoing microdiskectomy reveals excellent or good results in 97%, with a 4.5% recurrence rate and a 0.9% complication rate. The problems with such studies include the generally short follow-up and the evaluation of the results by the surgeons themselves.

Chemonucleolysis is an alternative to surgery with a reported success rate of approximately 75%. The principal concern is complications associated with the use of chymopapain. When this product first received approval for use within the United States, there were 19 deaths in the first 95,000 injections as a result of anaphylaxis, infection, cerebral hemorrhage, cardiovascular or pulmonary problems, and hepatic coma. In addition, there were 49 neurologic complications consisting of cerebral hemorrhage, cerebrovascular accident, coma, hemiplegia, quadriplegia, seizures, and paraparesis. The overall rate of anaphylactic reaction was 0.3%. It should be noted that not all the deaths, or even all the complications, were necessarily attributable to the chymopapain itself; and the overall rate of anaphylactic reaction has been diminished significantly by performing the procedure under local rather than general anesthesia. Furthermore, most of the complications of the procedure itself appeared to be technique related and therefore potentially avoidable. Nevertheless, the initial concern about such complications, particularly in the face of an alternative procedure (surgical diskectomy) that gave an overall higher success rate, led most physicians and patients in the United States to abandon chymopapain as an alternative to surgical diskectomy. However, this drug continues to be popular in Europe. New enzyme products are being developed but are still experimental.

Like chemonucleolysis, percutaneous lumbar diskectomy is an alternative to surgical diskectomy for symptomatic disk herniation failing to respond to conservative treatment. The purported advantages of the percutaneous procedure include its theoretically less invasive nature. The exact mechanism by which the procedure works is not entirely known, although it likely involves altered biomechanics of the disk itself. Like chymopapain, percutaneous diskectomy should be reserved for a contained disk herniation and should not be used in the presence of an extruded or sequestered disk. Most uncontrolled studies report a success rate for percutaneous lumbar diskectomy similar to that of chymopapain (75%). However, in one series of 38 patients, postoperative leg pain was present in 56% and postoperative back pain in 64%, with only 55% ultimately returning to work. Of the 17 patients with failed procedures, 13 ultimately underwent surgery, all of whom eventually returned to work and 85% of whom had relief of leg pain. Those investigators concluded that percutaneous diskectomy is not as predictable or successful as surgical diskectomy in the treatment of HNP. Moreover, a randomized prospective study has shown chymopapain to be significantly more effective than percutaneous diskectomy.

Spinal Stenosis

The most common cause for neurologic leg pain in the older population is spinal stenosis. The pathology of this disorder involves the three-joint complex (disk and facet joints) with the intervertebral disk usually undergoing significant degenerative changes before the facet joint does. With subsequent degeneration of the three-joint complex, there is collapse of the disk and subsequent facet arthritis, both of which tend to narrow the neural foramen progressively. The pathology thus involves not only posterior bony impingement but also soft tissue compression by either the disk anteriorly or the ligamentum flavum posteriorly. On a purely mechanical basis, the neural foramen is more narrowed with lumbar lordosis than it is with lumbar flexion. More recent work suggests that factors other than pure mechanical occlusion of the neural canal or foramen may play a role in symptom production. Impedance of the venous outflow of the intrinsic circulation of the nerve root can produce neuroischemia and impair cerebrospinal fluid circulation.

The site of neural compression may be either centrally within the canal, more laterally within the lateral recess, within the neural foramen, or some combination of these. It is important to know the exact site of neural compression when surgical decompression is considered.

Although most cases of spinal stenosis reflect primarily a degenerative involvement of the three-joint complex, other factors may contribute to this syndrome. Canal narrowing may be on a congenital basis, including genetic conditions such as achondroplasia. It also can occur on the basis of degenerative scoliosis or degenerative spondylolisthesis, in which spinal deformity compresses neural structures.

The natural history of spinal stenosis is unknown, and there is little information about the efficacy of conservative treatment. Initial treatment is symptomatic and includes nonsteroidal anti-inflammatory medication and restriction of those activities that aggravate the symptoms. However, aerobic conditioning such as bicycling is promoted. Epidural steroids can provide short-term relief, but there are no data to suggest that they provide any significant long-term benefit.

Surgical treatment depends first on documenting the nature and extent of the lesion. Imaging by MRI, myelography, or CT is effective in depicting the morphology of the stenosis. Surgical decompression involves removal of all compressing elements, whether they be bone or soft tissue. Where possible, care should be taken to preserve the integrity of the facet joint on at least one side. Removal of more than one whole facet, either by complete ablation unilaterally or by 50% removal bilaterally, risks late instability. If some extensive removal is necessary, consideration should be given to a prophylactic intertransverse process fusion. Attempts should be made to preserve the disk, because violation of the disk increases the risk of subsequent late instability. Reported short-term success rates from simple decompression range from 71% to 85%. However, the results deteriorate during long-term surveillance. Predictors of higher failure rates are increasing length of follow-up, the presence of comorbid conditions such as cardiac disease and diabetes, and use of more extensive decompression. The best results have been reported in patients with one- or two-level disease in whom there is no concomitant spondylolisthesis.

The issue of whether to perform a concomitant fusion for patients with both spinal stenosis and degenerative spondylolisthesis has been evaluated, with the conclusion that concomitant fusion increases the success rate. In a series of 50 patients with both spinal stenosis and degenerative spondylolisthesis randomized to either intertransverse process arthrodesis with decompression or decompression alone, 96% of the arthrodesis group had excellent or good results, whereas only 44% achieved such results in the other group. These results strongly suggest that spinal stenosis with associated degenerative spondylolisthesis should be treated by surgical decompression and intertransverse process fusion. Whether the results can be improved by the additional use of hardware fixation or by reduction of the slip remains to be answered.

Annotated Bibliography

General Information

Frymoyer JW: Back pain and sciatica. *N Engl J Med* 1988;318:291-300.

This well-referenced review article deals with the epidemiology, natural history, and treatment of low back conditions.

Frymoyer JW, Gordon SL (eds): *New Perspectives in Low Back Pain.* Park Ridge, IL, American Academy of Orthopaedic Surgeons, 1989.

This book presents clinical syndromes and manifestations of low back disorders as a backdrop for basic science information, and it outlines future directions for research.

Epidemiology

Deyo RA, Tsui-Wu YJ: Descriptive epidemiology of low back pain and its related medical care in the United States. *Spine* 1987;12:264-268.

The authors examined data from NHANES II to obtain information on the epidemiology of low back pain. The cumulative lifetime prevalence of pain lasting at least two weeks was 13.8%.

Diagnosis

History

Bell GR: Diagnosis of lumbar disc disease. *Semin Spine Surg* 1989;1:8-17.

This article summarizes the interrelations between history, physical examination, and diagnostic imaging, emphasizing the important part each of them plays in overall surgical decision making in lumbar disk disease.

Waddell G, Kummel EG, Lotto WN, et al: Failed lumbar disc surgery and repeat surgery following industrial injuries. *J Bone Joint Surg* 1979;61A:201-207.

Of 179 patients who failed to achieve relief from their initial back surgery, 103 had a second operation and were followed for one to two years. Beyond the second operation, patients were more likely to be made worse than to be helped by subsequent surgery. Good results of repeat surgery generally were associated with six to 12 months of pain relief after the initial operation, a predominance of leg pain over back pain, and unequivocal evidence of recurrent disk herniation. These results, like those of 11 other studies analyzed by the authors, suggest that in the presence of worker's compensation issues, any form of treatment for low back pain has one third poorer results than in patients who are not candidates for compensation.

Wiesel SW, Boden SD: The multiply operated low back patient, in Herkowitz HN, Garfin SR, Balderston RA, et al (eds): *The Spine,* ed 3. Philadelphia, WB Saunders, 1992, pp 1899-1906.

The authors outline an algorithm for evaluating the patient who has already had multiple back operations and who either continues to have back or leg pain or presents with new onset of such pain. They offer a precise description of the thinking involved in working through the differential diagnoses.

Physical Examination

Offierski CM, MacNab I: Hip-spine syndrome. *Spine* 1983;8:316-321.

The authors examined 35 patients with concurrent disease of the hip and spine and developed a three-part classification to aid in the management of such cases. This article emphasizes the importance of considering hip disease and the differential diagnosis in patients suspected of having an L-4 radiculopathy.

Spangfort EV: The lumbar disc herniation: A computer-aided analysis of 2,504 operations. *Acta Orthop Scand* 1972;142(suppl):1-95.

This benchmark study reviewed the medical records of 2,504 consecutive operations for lumbar disk herniation performed at two hospitals in Sweden. The analysis showed clearly that the amount of relief of sciatica was directly proportional to the magnitude of the pathology found intraoperatively. The Lasegue sign was positive in 97% of the patients with surgically verified disk herniation, and the incidence of positivity decreased with increasing patient age. The author emphasized the value of diagnostic myelography with water-soluble contrast medium, with 82% of the myelograms predictive of the surgical findings.

Imaging Techniques

Jackson RP, Cain JE Jr, Jacobs RR, et al: The neuroradiographic diagnosis of lumbar herniated nucleus pulposus: I. A comparison of computed tomography (CT), myelography, CT-myelography, discography, and CT-discography. *Spine* 1989;14:1356-1361.

In a correlation of surgical findings and preoperative imaging studies in 124 patients, CT-diskography was the most accurate, with lower false-positive and false-negative rates than the other studies.

Jackson RP, Cain JE Jr, Jacobs RR, et al: The neuroradiographic diagnosis of lumbar herniated nucleus pulposus: II. A comparison of computed tomography (CT), myelography, CT-myelography, and magnetic resonance imaging. *Spine* 1989;14:1362-1367.

In 59 patients with surgically confirmed disease and preoperative imaging studies, MRI was the most accurate, with the lowest false-positive rate. However, CT-myelography had the lowest false-negative rate. Overall, the authors believe MRI is the imaging study of choice for diagnosing most lumbar disk herniations.

Wiesel SW, Tsourmas N, Feffer HL, et al: A study of computer-assisted tomography: I. The incidence of positive CAT scans in an asymptomatic group of patients. *Spine* 1984;9:549-551.

Fifty-two patients without symptoms of back disorders underwent CT of the lumbar spine. Regardless of age, 35% were found to have abnormalities. Spinal disease was identified in an average of 19.5% of individuals less than 40 years of age and in 50% of the older patients. This study, like others, emphasizes the potential fallacy in basing a diagnosis purely on an imaging study such as CT.

Boden SD, Davis DO, Dina TS, et al: Abnormal magnetic resonance scans of the lumbar spine in asymptomatic patients: A prospective investigation. *J Bone Joint Surg* 1990;72A:403-408.

Sixty-seven asymptomatic subjects underwent lumbar MRI, with approximately one third having a substantial abnormality noted. Of subjects younger than 60 years, 20% had a disk herniation, and one had spinal stenosis. Abnormal scans were seen in 50% of the older subjects, with 36% having a disk herniation or bulging and 21% having spinal stenosis.

Boden SD, Davis DO, Dina TS, et al: Contrast-enhanced MR imaging performed after successful lumbar disk surgery: Prospective study. *Radiology* 1992;182:59-64.

Areas of intermittent signal intensity with peripheral enhancement and a mass effect suggesting disk herniation were present in 38% of the patients three weeks after surgery had rendered them pain free; by three months, similar findings were present in only 12%. This article emphasizes the importance of waiting before obtaining a gadolinium-enhanced MRI scan postoperatively.

Nachemson A: Lumbar discography—Where are we today? *Spine* 1989;14:555-557.

The author summarizes much of what is known about diskography and reviews the studies that support or dispute its value. The basic problem with diskography is that at present it is impossible to state whether the pain that follows disk injection originates in the injected disk.

Walsh TR, Weinstein JN, Spratt KF, et al: Lumbar discography in normal subjects: A controlled prospective study. *J Bone Joint Surg* 1990;72A:1081-1088.

In a carefully controlled investigation, seven patients with low back pain and ten asymptomatic volunteers had diskography with injection at three lumbar levels, with the sessions being videotaped to examine the subject's facial response. If a positive diskogram is defined as significant pain associated with the injection, there were no positive studies in the asymptomatic subjects (specificity 100%). Abnormal radiographic images were obtained in 13 of 20 disks in symptomatic individuals and at one or more levels in all seven patients. Although it was carefully performed, this study, like prior ones, did not address the issue of what actually was responsible for the pain.

Other Tests

Saal JA, Dillingham MF, Gamburd RS, et al: The pseudoradicular syndrome: Lower extremity peripheral nerve entrapment masquerading as lumbar radiculopathy. *Spine* 1988;13:926-930.

In 36 patients with lower extremity pain who were found to have peripheral nerve entrapment as the sole cause of that pain, the diagnosis was established by electrophysiologic studies and nerve blocks. Lesions distal to the neural foramen must be considered as a potential cause of radiculopathy.

Treatment

Acute Low Back Pain

Deyo RA: Fads in the treatment of low back pain. *N Engl J Med* 1991;325:1039-1940. Editorial.

The author summarizes current thinking on the treatment of back pain, emphasizing the scientific pitfalls in the assessment of newer modalities.

Deyo RA, Diehl AK, Rosenthal M: How many days of bed rest for acute low back pain? A randomized clinical trial. *N Engl J Med* 1986;315:1064-1070.

The authors report on 203 patients with mechanical low back pain, 78% of whom had acute pain of less than 30 days' duration, who were randomized to either two days (group I) or seven days (group II) of bedrest. The patients assigned to group I missed 45% fewer days of work than patients in group II, with no other differences noted between the groups in terms of functional, physiologic, or perceived outcomes. The authors question the traditional recommendation of long-term bedrest for the treatment of acute low back pain.

Chronic Low Back Pain

Carette S, Marcoux S, Truchon R, et al: A controlled trial of corticosteroid injections into facet joints for chronic low back pain. *N Engl J Med* 1991;325:1002-1007.

This randomized study compared injections of methylprednisolone acetate or isotonic saline (placebo) into the facet joints of 95 patients. After six months, 22% of the methylprednisolone group and 10% of the placebo group had less pain and limitation of function and greater back mobility. The authors conclude that the injection of methylprednisolone acetate into the facet joints is of little value in the treatment of patients with chronic low back pain.

Radicular Pain

Garfin SR, Rydevik BL, Brown RA: Compressive neuropathy of spinal nerve roots: A mechanical or biological problem? *Spine* 1991;16:162-166.

In four patients, nerve root-related pain gradually resolved with no change in the mechanical deformation of the involved nerve root being seen by CT and MRI. Mechanical compression may not be the only cause of pain and dysfunction with disk herniation.

Saal JA, Saal JS, Herzog RJ: The natural history of lumbar intervertebral disk extrusions treated nonoperatively. *Spine* 1990;15:683-686.

Eleven patients with disk extrusions noted on CT, MRI, or both were treated nonoperatively for their radiating leg pain and neurologic loss. Lumbar intervertebral disk extrusions changed morphologically in a manner that was consistent with resorption. These data, like those of Garfin and associates, suggest that nonmechanical factors may be important in the pain response.

Weinstein J, Claverie W, Gibson S: The pain of discography. *Spine* 1988;13:1344-1348.

Changes in substance P (SP) and VIP after diskography in normal and abnormal lumbar intervertebral disks were studied in dogs. Dorsal root ganglion SP and VIP were indirectly affected by manipulation of the disk during diskography, suggesting that the pain sometimes associated with an abnormal diskographic image may be related in part to the chemical environment within the intervertebral disk and the sensitized state of its annular nociceptors.

Wiesel SW, Feffer HL, Borenstein DG: Evaluation and outcome of low-back pain of unknown etiology. *Spine* 1988;13:679-680.

This study prospectively evaluated 5,362 patients with low back pain, 2% of whom failed to improve or could not be given a specific diagnosis. This subset of patients, defined as having chronic low back pain of unknown etiology, was referred to a rheumatologist for evaluation, and a specific diagnosis was obtained in 13%.

Wiskneski RJ, Rothman RH: Microdiscectomy techniques. *Semin Spine Surg* 1989;1:54-59.

This article reviews the history and the current techniques of microdiskectomy and presents data on the outcome of various techniques.

Brown MD, Cammisa FP: Role of chemonucleolysis for lumbar disc disease. *Semin Spine Surg* 1989;1:43-46.

This review article outlines the status of chemonucleolysis in the treatment of disk herniation.

Kahanovitz N, Viola K, Goldstein T, et al: A multicenter analysis of percutaneous discectomy. *Spine* 1990;15:713-715.

In this study, 38 patients underwent percutaneous diskectomy at L-4/L-5 or L-5/S-1 for a documented disk herniation. Only 21 patients (55%) returned to work, and 13 (34%) ultimately underwent successful surgical diskectomy for continued symptoms. The 25 patients who did not undergo subsequent surgical diskectomy had more pain, weakness, and numbness than the 13 patients having surgery. Percutaneous diskectomy did not appear to be as predictable or successful a treatment for disk herniation as was traditional surgical diskectomy.

Garfin SR, Glover M, Booth RE, et al: Laminectomy: A review of the Pennsylvania Hospital experience. *J Spine Dis* 1988;1:116-173.

The authors present a one- to five-year follow-up of laminectomy for spinal stenosis or disk herniation. Overall, 90% to 95% of patients noted good or excellent relief of their leg pain, with 80% reporting relief of their low back pain. The results of surgery are gratifying when the operation is performed for the appropriate indications.

Songer MN, Ghosh L, Spencer DL: Effects of sodium hyaluronate on peridural fibrosis after lumbar laminectomy and discectomy. *Spine* 1990;15:550-554.

The authors demonstrate the effectiveness of sodium hyaluronate in preventing peridural fibrosis in an experimental model. Unlike previous investigators, Songer and associates combined laminectomy with diskectomy, and they postulate that the scar arises from the disk rather than the muscle adjacent to the laminectomy.

West JL III, Bradford DS, Ogilvie JW: Results of spinal arthrodesis with pedicle screw-plate fixation. *J Bone Joint Surg* 1991;73A:1179-1184.

This clinical report covers the problems and benefits of pedicle fixation. Most of the patients had degenerative spondylolisthesis or pseudoarthosis. There was a 47% failure rate in patients who underwent pseudoarthrosis repair, although 65% achieved solid fusion. The overall rate of solid arthrodesis was 90%. Complications occurred in 25% of patients, and 7% suffered neurologic compromise.

Spinal Stenosis

Herkowitz HN, Kurz LT: Degenerative lumbar spondylolisthesis with spinal stenosis: A prospective study comparing decompression with decompression and intertransverse process arthrodesis. *J Bone Joint Surg* 1991;73A:802-808.

In this randomized study of 50 patients with spinal stenosis and degenerative spondylolisthesis, patients having intertransverse process arthrodesis and decompression obtained significantly better results than those undergoing decompression alone (96% versus 44% good outcome).

Katz JN, Lipson SJ, Larson MG, et al: The outcome of decompressive laminectomy for degenerative lumbar stenosis. *J Bone Joint Surg* 1991;73A:809-816.

This clinical study suggests a somewhat bleak outlook for decompressive laminectomy when follow-up is extended for four years. Older patients and those with comorbid conditions or longer follow-up had less favorable results. Reoperation was necessary in 17% of patients, usually because of recurrent stenosis or instability.

Ryan J, Zwerling C: Risk for occupational low-back injury after lumbar laminectomy for degenerative disc disease. *Spine* 1990;15:500-503.

The authors analyzed patients who had undergone successful laminectomy and returned to work comparing them with a control group. The postlaminectomy patients sustained a 25% reinjury rate, versus 6% in the controls. The risk of reinjury increased as a function of the job requirements for heavy lifting.

V
Lower Extremity

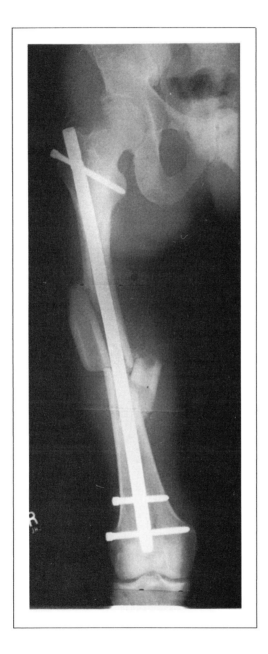

40

Hip: Pediatric Aspects

The child's hip may be affected by a range of disorders from the perinatal period through adolescence. The most common of these are developmental dysplasia (formerly called congenital dislocation of the hip, or CDH), femoral anteversion, Legg-Calvé-Perthes disease, slipped capital femoral epiphysis, transient synovitis, the late sequelae of septic arthritis, and neuromuscular conditions such as cerebral palsy and spina bifida. Of particular note is the recent international acceptance of the substitution of the term "developmental dysplasia" for "congenital dislocation" of the hip. This change recognizes that the disorder is of variable degree and pathology, does not always result in dislocation, and even when it does, may not be congenital.

Developmental Dysplasia of the Hip (DDH)

Developmental dysplasia of the hip encompasses a wide spectrum, from the rare fixed prenatal "teratologic" dislocation to postnatal instability of the hip to dysplasia (inadequate development) to subluxation (where the initial cartilage-to-cartilage contact is nonconcentric and can become incongruous later in childhood) to complete dislocation (where no cartilage contact exists between the femoral head and the acetabulum). The etiology is multifactorial, with genetic, mechanical (prenatal and postnatal position), and hormonal (affecting the ligamentous complex of the hip) factors involved to various degrees in a given individual. A positive family history, breech position in utero, torticollis, plagiocephaly, hyperextension, and congenital dislocation deformities of the knee and foot at birth are significant risk factors, some of which are associated with developmental displacement of the hip in as many as 50% of patients. A positive family history carries the highest risk.

Diagnosis

Early diagnosis by postnatal screening with the Ortolani or Barlow tests is essential to detect hip instability or dislocation. The Ortolani maneuver and the second part of the Barlow test involve detection of a sensation of reduction of a dislocated hip when the hip is placed in 90 degrees of flexion and then abducted. The first part of the Barlow test provokes dislocation of an unstable hip by gently adducting the flexed hip while pushing posteriorly in the line of the shaft of the femur. The implications of positive Ortolani and Barlow tests are quite different. The Barlow test identifies an unstable hip that requires splintage and close observation over time to make sure

that it does not dislocate. The Ortolani maneuver identifies a dislocated hip that can still be reduced in the early weeks of life and requires active treatment with proof of reduction, whether the treatment is by a Pavlik harness or by closed reduction and spica casting.

Dynamic real-time ultrasonography (Fig. 1) is valuable in detecting dislocation, subluxation, and acetabular dysplasia but is time consuming and costly and requires that an experienced examiner be available. Ultrasonography probably results in the treatment of a significant number of hips that would spontaneously develop normally, and therefore, its cost effectiveness remains unclear.

Radiographs are of little value for screening until 4 to 6 months of age, which is beyond the ideal period for treatment. However, radiographs may be useful in confirming the position of hips undergoing treatment and when teratologic dislocation is suspected.

To date, no hip screening program has been 100% successful in eliminating late presentation of displaced hips. Whether these hips are "missed" at birth or were normal at that time and later developed displacement remains unresolved.

Treatment

Early treatment of the displaced or unstable hip is based on the principle of concentric reduction in the position of abduction and flexion of the hip. Although a number of devices capable of achieving this position are available, the Pavlik harness is the most widely used for children younger than 6 months of age because of its ease of adjustment and the control it provides of the range of motion of the hip. Regardless of the type of device used, proof that the hip is concentrically reduced during treatment is necessary. This may be achieved by plain radiograph, by ultrasound, or, in difficult cases, by computed tomography. Extremes of position, particularly wide abduction, must be avoided. Among patients with frank dislocation, the Pavlik harness fails to reduce the hip in 25%. The chest straps of the harness must not be applied distal to the nipple line, or reduction will not be achieved. Excessive flexion can result in femoral nerve palsy or fixed posterior dislocation that may be difficult to recognize and treat. Excessive abduction causes avascular necrosis. Children with a greater degree of displacement and those in whom treatment is commenced after 7 weeks of age are at particular risk of developing these complications.

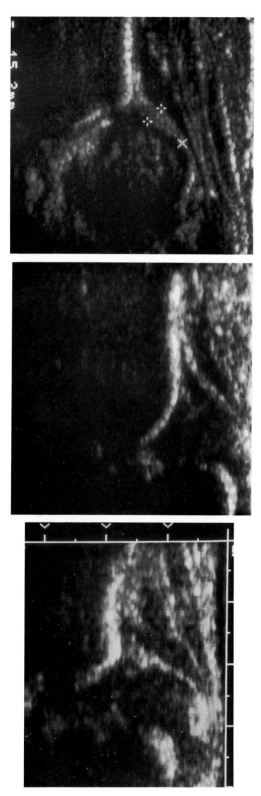

Fig. 1 Ultrasound of the hip. **Top,** Normal hip; + is acetabular labrum and x is superior capsule. **Center,** Nonconcentric reduction of hip with marked acetabular dysplasia. **Bottom,** Dislocated hip.

The Pavlik harness is seldom effective after 6 months of age. Closed reduction with general anesthesia following a period of skin traction and adductor tenotomy to reduce the frequency of avascular necrosis is the usual initial management in the child between 6 months and 2 years of age. This method will result in concentric reduction in 60% to 80% of patients, depending on where the child is in this age spectrum. Once again, it is essential that the concentricity of the reduction be confirmed by arthrography or computed tomography, because plain radiographs taken through a spica cast may be misleading. The need for preliminary traction is currently questioned by some authors.

If reduction cannot be achieved easily and the hip is not stable in 90 to 100 degrees of flexion and 45 to 55 degrees of abduction (ie, the use of force and immobilization in wide abduction are to be avoided), then open reduction is necessary. After 2 years of age, the risk of avascular necrosis and failure to maintain reduction by closed means increases, so that open reduction through an anterolateral approach is generally preferred. Some authors advocate the medial adductor approach through which the impediments to obstruction can be released. This procedure is of more value in the child younger than 18 months old in whom concentric reduction cannot be achieved by closed means. In the child older than 2 years, correction of secondary skeletal deformity about the hips by redirectional innominate osteotomy or varus derotational osteotomy of the femur is usually required, either at the time of or subsequent to open reduction. The choice between femoral and innominate osteotomy depends more on the training and experience of the surgeon than on any evidence of superiority of one or the other in the literature. However, innominate osteotomy can more readily be done simultaneously with an anterolateral open reduction. There is considerable debate about whether open reduction and osteotomy should be concurrent or staged, as there are arguments favoring both approaches: the risk of redislocation and stiffness with simultaneous surgery versus the morbidity and repeat hospitalization of staged procedures.

In children older than 3 years, open reduction, femoral shortening, and acetabular redirection are required simultaneously to maintain concentric reduction, to reduce the frequency of avascular necrosis, and to achieve a functional range of motion. The upper age limit after which reduction of the hips is less favorable than the natural history of untreated dislocation is controversial. A general rule is 8 to 9 years for unilateral dislocation and 5 to 6 years for bilateral dislocation.

The type of reconstruction for hips with subluxation recognized late, residual dysplasia after treatment, or the sequelae of avascular necrosis depends on the type of abnormality of the acetabulum and proximal femur, which is best determined by computed tomography with three-dimensional reconstructions. Deformity should be corrected by femoral or pelvic osteotomy, either alone or in combination, maintaining cartilage-to-cartilage contact rather than resorting to salvage procedures such as the Chiari medial-displacement interpositional osteotomy, which relies on fibrocartilaginous metaplasia for coverage rather than redirected acetabular hyaline articular cartilage.

It is imperative that all hips requiring treatment be followed until skeletal maturity. There is a risk of deterioration in adolescence secondary to late arrest of proximal femoral or acetabular growth, particularly failure of development of the lateral acetabular epiphysis and asymmetric closure of the proximal femoral physeal plate.

The adolescent or young adult with symptomatic subluxation requires detailed imaging studies to aid in predicting whether postoperative congruence may be achieved by acetabular redirection, varus derotation osteotomy of the proximal femur, or both. The choice of procedure is determined by an assessment of which side of the joint is more abnormal, but in practice, at least half of the patients require both procedures to achieve congruence. The selection of the single innominate osteotomy of Salter, the double osteotomy of Sutherland, or the triple osteotomy of Steel depends on the amount of redirection of the acetabulum required and the experience of the surgeon in achieving the requisite amount of coverage. However, it is important to realize that the factor limiting success is more often the available area of articular cartilage on the acetabulum than the degree to which the acetabulum may be rotated. Because this patient population often has early signs of degenerative arthritis, it also is preferable to select a procedure that avoids postoperative immobilization by achieving stable internal fixation. If imaging studies predict that congruence cannot be achieved by acetabular redirection or varus derotation osteotomy of the femur, and if the hip is painful with early degenerative arthritis, then a salvage procedure may be indicated. The Chiari osteotomy is the usual choice, but an acetabular shelf procedure may be an acceptable alternative.

If there is a large osteophyte on the medial aspect of the femoral head, improved congruence on a radiograph taken with the leg in adduction, and preservation of at least 50% of the joint cartilage space, a valgus osteotomy of the proximal femur may relieve the symptoms and delay the need for total hip arthroplasty.

Patients with avascular necrosis and arrest of proximal femoral physeal growth often have a pronounced Trendelenburg gait, pain from abductor fatigue after only moderate activity, and a greater trochanter at the level of or proximal to the superior aspect of the femoral head. This situation may be substantially improved by transfer of the greater trochanter laterally and distally to restore the normal articulotrochanteric distance (the superior tip of the greater trochanter should be at the level of the center of the femoral head) and the abductor lever arm (the medial-to-lateral distance from the center of the head to the trochanter). The lateralization of the trochanter is perhaps more important than the distal displacement and may necessitate an interpositional bone graft. Internal fixation should be sufficiently stable to obviate external immobilization.

Anteversion of the Femur

Intoeing secondary to femoral anteversion is probably the most common hip problem. Recent studies have confirmed that there is no relation between femoral anteversion and an increased risk of arthrosis of the hip. Although intoeing is only a cosmetic problem, it can be significant. Bracing is ineffective. Spontaneous improvement may be expected until 8 years of age, with conscious compensation occurring in adolescence. Therefore, any surgery should be deferred until adolescence; ultimately, it is seldom, if ever, necessary. The relation between anteversion of the femur and patellofemoral pain and instability is not clear.

Legg-Calvé-Perthes Disease

Legg-Calvé-Perthes disease is the least understood of pediatric hip disorders. Controversy exists about almost all its aspects, including etiology, pathogenesis, classification, management, natural history, and the results of treatment or no treatment.

Necrosis of the bony nucleus of the proximal femoral epiphysis, impairment of the growth of the physis, and subsequent remodeling of regenerated bone are the essential elements of Perthes disease. Evidence supports loss of blood supply to the epiphysis as a significant factor in the pathogenesis, but whether this loss is extraepiphyseal or intraepiphyseal and primary or secondary has not been proved. There also is evidence that more than one episode of infarction may be necessary before the full clinical picture develops. There appears to be little relation to transient synovitis of the hip, which seldom leads to Perthes disease.

The Catterall and Thompson/Salter classifications of Perthes disease are the most widely used, but both have significant limitations when applied early in the disease. The predictive value of each classification for the individual patient is limited, and neither is clearly superior to the other. These classifications are based on the degree of involvement of the epiphysis (Catterall) or on the extent of the subchondral fracture seen on the plain radiographs (Thompson/Salter). More recently, maintenance of 50% of the normal height of the lateral portion of the epiphysis (the lateral pillar), regardless of the degree of involvement of the remainder of the epiphysis, has been suggested as an important favorable prognostic factor. Bone scans and magnetic resonance imaging are sensitive in establishing the diagnosis, but the images have not yet been shown to be of prognostic value.

The prognosis for Perthes disease depends on the age at onset, the degree of epiphyseal involvement, the ability to maintain hip motion, the shape of the femoral head after healing, and the development of subluxation of the joint. Of the numerous clinical and radiographic at-risk signs only subluxation can be convincingly related to prognosis. Studies of the natural history reveal that at least 50% of involved hips do well with no treatment. The remainder, with various degrees of asphericity and incongruity, do well functionally into the fifth decade. The exception to this statement is that children older than 9 years at onset do poorly, with significant symptoms and restriction of motion at skeletal maturity.

The goal of treatment is a spherical, well-covered femoral head with a range of motion of the hips approaching normal. The principles of treatment are maintenance of range of motion and containment of the femoral head through the evolution of healing of the epiphysis. In the younger child (less than 5 years of age), this goal may be achieved by relief of weightbearing and supervising of range-of-motion exercises. In the child older than 5 years who has more than half of the epiphysis involved, abduction bracing or surgery are the methods of treatment currently employed. There is considerable debate about whether innominate or femoral osteotomy is the better operative procedure or whether either is superior to bracing. The weightbearing abduction orthosis has been the most popular brace for the treatment of Perthes disease, but recent studies have failed to establish any advantage over other methods of management. The current view is that this orthosis should not be used for severely involved hips.

The initiation of bracing or surgical intervention when the hip is irritable and stiff should be avoided. A full range of motion should be regained before proceeding to definitive treatment. A return to these methods may be necessary during abduction bracing or after surgery to maintain range of motion. Definite radiographic signs of reossification signal the point at which weaning from bracing and a return to normal activity after surgery may be considered.

Treatment of the child presenting with significant femoral head deformity (Mose sphericity greater than 4 mm out of round) and evidence that the reparative phase has commenced should be mainly symptomatic, reserving salvage procedures (excision of the extruded portion of the head when there is hinge abduction, Chiari osteotomy to cover the femoral head, valgus osteotomy to increase abduction and bring the more normal medial femoral head into the weightbearing area, and arthrodesis near to or at skeletal maturity in unilateral involvement) for patients with severe functional impairment. The child older than 9 years at presentation may benefit from combined innominate and femoral osteotomies if done in the earliest stages of the disease and if the preceding guidelines are followed.

Slipped Capital Femoral Epiphysis

Mechanical and constitutional factors combine to produce slipped capital femoral epiphysis. Patients with a slipped epiphysis may exhibit physical findings that suggest a subtle endocrinopathy, but testing for an endocrine disorder is seldom productive and therefore not recommended routinely. Patients with an underlying endocrine cause are usually recognizable because of features of renal, pituitary, or thyroid disease or significantly retarded bone age.

Experimental investigations have shown that with removal of the perichondral ring, even normal activity can generate forces close to those necessary to produce a slipped epiphysis. It also has been suggested that patients with slips may have a relative retroversion of the femoral neck that may increase the shear across the physis and that the epiphysis rotates posteriorly rather than inferiorly or medially around the axis of the femoral neck.

Treatment of a slipped epiphysis is designed to stabilize the epiphysis on the femoral neck and prevent further slipping while avoiding the complications of chondrolysis and osteonecrosis. This may be achieved, without attempting to manipulate the epiphysis, by inserting a single strong screw into the center of the epiphysis from the anterior aspect of the greater trochanter or femoral neck (depending on the degree of slip), avoiding penetration into the hip joint by careful radiographic imaging. Although bone graft epiphysiodesis is a more extensive procedure and the subject of considerable debate, the published results make it a reasonable alternative in severe slips. Fixation in situ by whatever method is strongly supported by the literature.

Osteonecrosis results from manipulation or open reduction of the epiphysis and intracapsular osteotomies of the neck. In the acute or acute-on-chronic slip, reduction may be accomplished by preoperative skeletal traction in flexion and internal rotation or by gentle intraoperative manipulation, but all of these maneuvers carry considerable risk of inducing osteonecrosis. Forceful manipulation must be avoided. In the chronic slip, repositioning of the epiphysis should not be attempted. When inserting pins or screws, the superior quadrant of the femoral head, where the retinacular vessels enter, should be avoided. There is a clear, although not perfect, correlation between pins penetrating the joint and chondrolysis. Even if chondrolysis is not induced by a pin penetration, the acetabular articular cartilage may be abraded, leading to early degenerative arthritis. However, penetration of the joint by a single screw with immediate recognition and screw removal probably does not cause chondrolysis.

In the absence of complications, patients with slipped epiphyses do quite well in the long term. However, if either chondrolysis or osteonecrosis develops, early osteoarthritis is more likely. Those patients developing chondrolysis may function reasonably well in the short term with partial reappearance of the joint cartilage space on plain radiographs, remarkably little pain, and recovery of a portion of the range of motion. Even when the problem is recognized early, no treatment has been proven effective for either osteonecrosis or chondrolysis.

Recent investigators have claimed that significant remodeling of the proximal femur will occur for at least two years after treatment of slipped epiphysis. Range of motion and gait improve, which leads to acceptable function in most patients. However, there is controversy about whether true remodeling occurs or whether bone on the anterolateral aspect of the neck of the femur, impinging on the margin of the acetabulum, is simply resorbed over time, thereby permitting an increased range of motion. The resolution of muscle spasm, synovitis, and fluid in the joint in the early months after fixation is undoubtedly responsible for some increase in the range of motion and improvement of gait. Osteotomies should therefore be reserved for hips with unacceptable function after the remodeling period and certainly should not be performed earlier than one year after the slip.

Transient Synovitis

Transient synovitis is a benign, self-limited condition of unknown etiology that is manifested by hip or knee pain, restricted range of motion, and a limp. The challenge to the surgeon is to differentiate this condition from septic arthritis and Perthes disease. The child's temperature, leukocyte count, and erythrocyte sedimentation rate are helpful, but if there is any doubt, aspiration of the hip joint is essential to rule out septic arthritis.

If the initial radiographs are normal and there is strong suspicion of Perthes disease, bone scanning and magnetic resonance imaging may be helpful. The likelihood of transient synovitis leading to Perthes disease is small, certainly less than 3%. Routine follow-up radiographs probably are not necessary in children younger than 5 years old if they remain asymptomatic after recovery from synovitis. Treatment of transient synovitis is symptomatic, with a response expected within a week. The recurrence rate is approximately 5% with no change in the benign prognosis.

Septic Arthritis

Septic arthritis of the hip is a surgical emergency. The infant or child presenting with painful restriction of movement requires careful assessment, which should include recording of body temperature, white blood cell count, erythrocyte sedimentation rate, blood culture, ultrasound examination, and isotope bone scan. However, none of these investigations is a substitute for clinical judgment, because the results of all of them may be normal in the early stages before there is damage to the articular cartilage or the blood supply to the epiphysis. This is particularly true in the neonatal infant.

Septic arthritis may be difficult to distinguish from transient synovitis. Needle aspiration of the hip is helpful if either pus or normal synovial fluid is obtained. If any pus is obtained, then immediate arthrotomy is indicated, regardless of the Gram stain or culture results. The re-

sults of early arthrotomy and antibiotic therapy are good; complications are inevitably the result of late diagnosis or delay in arthrotomy.

The preferred surgical approach is by an oblique anterior incision separating the tensor fasciae femoris and sartorius, reflecting the rectus femoris, and incising the anterior capsule. It is best to avoid drilling a hole in the neck of the femur: either decompression into the joint has already occurred, or a primary osteomyelitis of the metaphysis of the proximal femur may be treated by antibiotic therapy, which should be commenced immediately after fluid and synovium are obtained for culture. An opening through the incision should be maintained by placement of a drain to the level of the capsule. The drain should be removed in 24 to 48 hours. Suction drainage and irrigation with antibiotics are not necessary. Cefuroxime is the initial systemic antibiotic of choice; it may be changed according to the results of the cultures and sensitivity studies.

Septic arthritis of the hip may lead to dislocation, subluxation, acetabular dysplasia, coxa vara, coxa breva, absence of the head and neck of the femur, and degenerative (postinfectious) arthritis. Numerous reconstructive procedures, such as open reduction, pelvic osteotomy, femoral osteotomy, and greater trochanteric arthroplasty, have been advocated to treat the residual deformity. However, two recent long-term studies suggest that the results of these procedures performed at any stage are less favorable than the natural history of the deformity. In particular, those patients with great degrees of deformity did poorly after reconstruction.

Cerebral Palsy

The pattern of hip deformity in cerebral palsy depends on the type and extent of neurologic impairment. Flexion-adduction contracture, rotational malalignment, subluxation, coxa valga, acetabular dysplasia, and femoral anteversion occur alone or in combinations in the ambulatory child with spastic diplegia. More severe contractures with unilateral or bilateral hip dislocation occur in the nonambulatory child with spastic quadriplegia. Hip deformity is more likely to be asymmetric in spastic quadriplegia and in association with pelvic obliquity and scoliosis. The hip on the high side of the pelvis is usually dislocated, adducted, and internally rotated, whereas the hip on the opposite side is located, abducted, and externally rotated, producing perplexing problems with seating. There is little doubt that there is an interaction among the spinal, pelvic, and hip deformity, but the temporal relation is variable.

For the child with spastic diplegia, adductor tenotomy or posterior transfer, with iliopsoas lengthening when the adduction deformity is accompanied by flexion contracture, typically is done between 4 and 9 years of age. Overzealous lengthening and obturator neurectomy, particularly in the presence of spastic hip extension, many result in a severe deformity that is more disabling and difficult to treat than the original problem. In the older child, rotational deformity may interfere with gait and contribute to tripping. Derotational osteotomy may produce a more normal gait but does not necessarily increase the stride length or cadence and should be deferred until 8 to 10 years of age. This operation can be done at the supracondylar level, but if there is significant valgus or subluxation of the hip, it should be done in the intertrochanteric region.

In the severely affected child, pain in a dislocated hip may be a significant problem and can limit the child's ability to sit. Careful monitoring and judicious soft-tissue releases followed by nighttime abduction bracing may prevent dislocation if done before the femoral head is 50% uncovered. Typically, the hip dislocates when the child is between 5 and 7 years of age, taking approximately two years in evolution from the first evidence of subluxation. Unilateral soft-tissue surgery has a definite untoward effect on the opposite hip, so preoperative planning should address the issue of symmetry. Careful monitoring of the opposite hip is essential if the decision has been made for unilateral surgery.

In the older child with greater than 50% subluxation, concentric reduction, soft-tissue release, and capsular repair with correction of both the acetabular and the femoral deformity, preferably done in one stage, are all essential to achieve long-term stability of the hip. In the postoperative period, abduction splinting while in bed and early wheelchair positioning are preferable to spica cast immobilization, which typically is poorly tolerated in these children and may lead to the disabling complication of a stiff hip.

Despite surgical intervention, a significant number of patients have pain in the hip in their adolescent and young adult years that limits their function. Alternatives for salvage include resection arthroplasty, total hip arthroplasty, and arthrodesis. The magnitude of the surgery, the difficulties with postoperative immobilization, and the issue of ongoing spasticity, muscle imbalance, and recurrent deformity make these procedures unattractive. Proximal femoral resection distal to the lesser trochanter with careful soft-tissue interposition is the option most frequently chosen but only after extensive discussion with the patient (if cognitive ability permits) and consultation with those who provide the patient's other daily care.

Spina Bifida (Myelomeningocele)

The importance of dislocated hip to the long-term well-being of children with spina bifida is the subject of debate. Dislocated hips do not appear to have any relation to the ability to walk and rarely cause pain. However, there is a definite relation between inability to walk and the level of paralysis, the presence of syringohydromyelia and the Arnold-Chiari malformation, scoliosis, and the function of the upper extremities.

Dislocated hips in the child unable to walk require no treatment. Dislocation of the hip, particularly unilateral, in a child with the potential for ambulation is the focus of considerable debate. Children with strong quadriceps muscles and, especially, those with functional hamstrings may well benefit from surgical correction of subluxating or dislocated hips.

Fixed flexion deformity of the hip interferes with fitting of a standing frame, parapodium, or reciprocating gait orthosis, and there is general agreement that this problem requires correction. The question is whether this correction is best achieved by soft-tissue release alone or in combination with relocation of the hip, and which is more likely to result in long-term correction. It would seem that the individual circumstances of the child and, especially, factors other than the hip should prevail in making the difficult decision about whether to relocate the hip in the patient with spina bifida.

Annotated Bibliography

Developmental Dysplasia of the Hip

Galpin RD, Roach JW, Wenger DR, et al: One stage treatment of congenital dislocation of the hip in older children, including femoral shortening. *J Bone Joint Surg* 1989;71A:734-741.

Children who are 2 years of age or older can safely be treated with an extensive one-stage operation consisting of open reduction combined with femoral shortening and, often, pelvic osteotomy without increasing the risk of avascular necrosis.

Grill F, Bensahel H, Canadell J, et al: The Pavlik harness in the treatment of congenital dislocating hip: Report on a multicenter study of the European Paediatric Orthopaedic Society. *J Pediatr Orthop* 1988;8:1-8.

A total of 3,611 children with dysplastic and dislocated hips were treated at an average age of 4.1 months. Those with higher grades of dislocation (Tonnis 3 and 4) had a failure rate of 14% or more and an osteonecrosis rate of 10% to 16%.

Kahle WK, Anderson MB, Alpert J, et al: The value of preliminary traction in the treatment of congenital dislocation of the hip. *J Bone Joint Surg* 1990;72A:1043-1047.

In 41 children, 47 dislocated hips were treated by attempted closed reduction with general anesthesia but without preliminary traction.Twenty hips (43%) could not be reduced, and open reduction was necessary. Osteonecrosis of the femoral head had developed in only two hips (4%) at a minimum follow-up of two years. The authors concluded that dislocated hips could be treated safely by either open or closed reduction without preliminary traction in patients younger than 2 years.

Klisic PJ: Congenital dislocation of the hip: A misleading term. *J Bone Joint Surg* 1989;71B:136.

Dissatisfaction is expressed with the term CDH because the disorder is of variable pathology, does not always culminate in dislocation, and often happens postnatally (ie, it is not truly congenital). The author recommends the terms "developmental displacement" or "dysplasia" of the hip (DDH) rather than CDH.

Lang P, Genant HK, Steiger P, et al: Three dimensional digital displays in congenital dislocation of the hip: Preliminary experience. *J Pediatr Orthop* 1989;9:532-537.

Three-dimensional computed tomography and three-dimensional magnetic resonance imaging were used to study children with CDH. Both appear promising in confirming the pathological anatomy and facilitating the choice of treatment.

O'Hara JN: Congenital dislocation of the hip: Acetabular deficiency in adolescence (absence of the lateral acetabular epiphysis) after limbectomy in infancy. *J Pediatr Orthop* 1989;9:640-658.

Excision of the limbus in infancy was associated with failure of appearance and development of the lateral acetabular epiphysis in adolescence. This failure was associated with loss of cover of the femoral head and late deterioration of the hip. This paper reinforced the importance of following dislocated hips to skeletal maturity after treatment, showing that the results of a particular form of treatment cannot be fully assessed until that time.

Viere RG, Birch JG, Herring JA, et al: Use of the Pavlik harness in congenital dislocation of the hip: An analysis of failure of treatment. *J Bone Joint Surg* 1990;72A:238-244.

The criteria for the use of the harness in patients with dislocatable and dislocated hips were age less than 7 months, the femoral head pointed to the triradiate cartilage on anteroposterior radiographs with the child wearing the harness, and no evidence of neuromuscular disease or teratologic dislocation. The harness failed in 26% of the patients.

Williamson DM, Benson MK: Late femoral osteotomy in congenital dislocation of the hip. *J Bone Joint Surg* 1988;70B:614-618.

After the age of 5 years, femoral osteotomy alone was inadequate for true subluxation of the hip unless there was already good acetabular development (acetabular angle less than 25 degrees).

Yngve D, Gross R: Late diagnosis of hip dislocation in infants. *J Pediatr Orthop* 1990;10:777-779.

In a study of 26,455 newborns, the incidence of dislocated or dislocatable hips was 3.8 per 1,000. The incidence of known late cases was 0.2 per 1,000, leading the authors to conclude that screening programs with direct pediatric orthopaedic supervision can be successful but that late diagnoses will still occur.

Anteversion of the Femur

Hubbard DD, Staheli LT, Chew DE, et al: Medial femoral torsion and osteoarthritis. *J Pediatr Orthop* 1988;8:540-542.

Anteversion was measured by biplanar radiography both in patients with idiopathic osteoarthritis and in controls. No significant difference was found.

Kitaoka HB, Weiner DS, Cook AJ, et al: Relationship between femoral anteversion and osteoarthritis of the hip. *J Pediatr Orthop* 1989;9:396-404.

Anteversion was measured by computed tomography in patients with idiopathic osteoarthritis and in controls. No significant difference was found.

Wedge JH, Munkacsi I, Loback D: Anteversion of the femur and idiopathic osteoarthritis of the hip. *J Bone Joint Surg* 1989;71A:1040-1043.

The authors studied the radiographs of 220 consecutive cadavers that were used for anatomic dissection over an 11-year period. Anteversion was measured directly after dissection, and the authors were unable to find a significant difference between the degree of anteversion in the osteoarthritic and control groups.

Legg-Calvé-Perthes Disease

Coates CJ, Paterson JM, Woods KR, et al: Femoral osteotomy in Perthes disease: Results at maturity. *J Bone Joint Surg* 1990;72B:581-585.

Of 48 hips with Catterall II, III, or IV disease, 58% were Stulberg class I or II at maturity; 29% of the patients had significant shortening, and 25% had a positive Trendelenburg sign.

Crutcher JP, Staheli LT: Combined osteotomy as a salvage procedure for severe Legg-Calvé-Perthes disease. *J Pediatr Orthop* 1992;12:151-156.

Combined innominate and varus femoral osteotomies were done for 14 children with a mean age of 8 years and 4 months and severe Perthes disease. The combined osteotomies were safe and effective salvage procedures in this group with a poor prognosis.

Evans IK, Deluca PA, Gage JR: A comparative study of ambulation— abduction bracing and varus derotation osteotomy in the treatment of severe Legg-Calvé-Perthes disease in children over 6 years of age. *J Pediatr Orthop* 1988;8:676-682.

In 36 patients, bracing and femoral osteotomy gave similar results.

Henderson RC, Renner JB, Sturdivant, MD, et al: Evaluation of magnetic resonance imaging in Legg-Perthes disease: A prospective, blinded study. *J Pediatr Orthop* 1990;10:289-297.

Magnetic resonance scanning and serial radiographs to assess the extent and course of the disease were compared. Although magnetic resonance often delineated the extent and location of the area of involvement more clearly, plain radiographs were as good or better for following the course of the disease and were considerably less costly.

Herring JA, Neustadt JB, Williams JJ, et al: The lateral pillar classification of Legg-Calvé-Perthes' disease. *J Pediatr Orthop* 1992;12:143-150.

The authors applied a three-group classification system based on the height of the lateral 15% to 30% of the epiphysis, as seen on the anteroposterior radiograph, in 93 involved hips in the active phase of the disease. When this classification was combined with the age at onset, it could be used to predict the natural history of the disease.

Martinez AG, Weinsten SL, Dietz FR: The weight-bearing abduction brace for the treatment of Legg-Perthes disease. *J Bone Joint Surg* 1992;74A:12-21.

Neither of these studies was able to demonstrate any improvement in the outcome with brace treatment compared with the published natural history of Perthes disease. Both are retrospective studies without controls.

Meehan PL, Angel D, Nelson JM: The Scottish Rite abduction orthosis for the treatment of Legg-Perthes disease: A radiographic analysis. *J Bone Joint Surg* 1992;74A:2-11.

After evaluating a series of 34 patients, the authors concluded that the Scottish Rite weightbearing abduction orthosis did not appear to offer an advantage compared with other methods of management.

Sponseller PD, Desai SS, Millis MB: Comparison of femoral and innominate osteotomies for the treatment of Legg-Calvé-Perthes disease. *J Bone Joint Surg* 1988;70A:1131-1139.

Objective ratings showed no difference between the two operations. Patients more than 10 years old had poor results with both procedures.

Weiner SD, Weiner DS, Riley PM: Pitfalls in treatment of Legg-Calvé-Perthes disease using proximal femoral varus osteotomy. *J Pediatr Orthop* 1991;11:20-24.

Problems, which occurred in 19% of patients, included excessive varus (neck-shaft angles less than 105 degrees), Trendelenburg gait, shortening (greater than 2.5 cm), premature growth-plate closure, and subluxation. The authors recommend epiphysiodesis of the greater trochanter at the time of the osteotomy.

Wenger DR, Ward WT, Herring JA: Legg-Calvé-Perthes disease. *J Bone Joint Surg* 1991;73A:778-788.

This well-referenced review concludes by stating that there is skepticism concerning the efficacy of treatment in all age groups but that the current literature appears to support treatment of children who exhibit at-risk signs.

Slipped Capital Femoral Epiphysis

Carney BT, Weinstein SL, Nobel J: Long-term follow-up of slipped capital femoral epiphysis. *J Bone Joint Surg* 1991;73A:667-674.

In this latest report on patients treated 35 to 72 years previously, the authors conclude that the natural history of the malunited slip is mild deterioration related to the severity of slip, attempts at realignment, and complications (osteonecrosis 12%; chondrolysis 16%). Regardless of the severity of the slip, pinning in situ provided the best long-term function and the greatest delay in the appearance of degenerative arthritis.

Jones JR, Paterson DC, Hillier TM, et al: Remodeling after pinning for slipped capital femoral epiphysis. *J Bone Joint Surg* 1990;72B:568-573.

Remodeling occurred in 50% of hips with a head-shaft angle of 30 degrees or more; the probability of remodeling was significantly less with greater degrees of slip but was increased if the triradiate cartilage was open at the time of presentation.

Nguyen D, Morrissy RT: Slipped capital femoral epiphysis: Rationale for the technique of percutaneous in situ fixation. *J Pediatr Orthop* 1990;10:341-346.

Through the use of radiographs of models and of patients in various positions, the authors concluded that the femoral head in most cases of chronic slipped capital epiphysis rotates around its axis and does not slip inferiorly. Therefore, the starting point for an in situ fixation device is the anterior femoral neck.

Riley PM, Weiner DS, Gillespie R, et al: Hazards of internal fixation in the treatment of slipped capital femoral epiphysis. *J Bone Joint Surg* 1990;72A:1500-1509.

Complications developed in 80 of 308 hips fixed with pins or screws, and 18% of patients required an additional procedure to correct a pin- or screw-related complication.

Siegel DB, Kasser JR, Sponseller P, et al: Slipped capital femoral epiphysis: A quantitative analysis of motion, gait and femoral remodeling after in situ fixation. *J Bone Joint Surg* 1991;73A:659-666.

The majority of motion returned within six months of treatment, which was attributed to relief of pain, spasm, and synovitis rather than to changes in the relation of the femoral head to the shaft or in the neck-shaft angle. The authors speculate that soft-tissue stretching and resorption of bone in the anterolateral part of the femoral neck may account for a further increase in internal rotation and the foot-progressive angle.

Wong-Chung J, Strong ML: Physeal remodeling after internal fixation of slipped capital femoral epiphyses. *J Pediatr Orthop* 1991;11:2-5.

Remodeling of the physeal shaft angle averaged 11.7 degrees in 55 hips. The authors recommend a wait of at least two years after initial fixation before considering realignment osteotomies.

Zionts LE, Simonian PT, Harvey JP Jr: Transient penetration of the hip joint during in situ cannulated-screw fixation of slipped capital femoral epiphysis. *J Bone Joint Surg* 1991;73A:1054-1060.

None of 11 patients followed for a minimum of two years after transient intraoperative penetration of the hip joint developed clinical or radiographic evidence of chondrolysis. This result suggests that a single episode of penetration with immediate removal from the joint is not associated with chondrolysis.

Septic Arthritis of the Hip

Betz RR, Cooperman DR, Wopperer JM, et al: Late sequelae of septic arthritis of the hip in infancy and childhood. *J Pediatr Orthop* 1990;10:365-372.

This multicenter review found poor radiographic appearance and hip rating scores at long-term follow-up but with minimal pain and activity restriction. Patients who were not treated operatively tended to function better than patients who underwent operative reconstruction.

Choi IH, Pizzutillo PD, Bowen JR, et al: Sequelae and reconstruction after septic arthritis of the hip in infants. *J Bone Joint Surg* 1990;72A:1150-1165.

The authors propose a complex classification system based on the severity of residual deformity. The functional result of surgery was satisfactory in less severe deformity but poor in those with more severe deformity.

Cerebral Palsy

Cooke PH, Cole WG, Carey RP: Dislocation of the hip in cerebral palsy: Natural history and predictability. *J Bone Joint Surg* 1989;71B:441-446.

The acetabular index was the most powerful single predictor of dislocation among a number of radiographic features studied. Measurement of this index at 2 and 4 years of age could identify patients who would suffer dislocation unless effective treatment was undertaken, those at risk only if scoliosis developed, and those who would not have dislocations.

Gamble JG, Rinsky LA, Bleck EE: Established hip dislocations in children with cerebral palsy. *Clin Orthop* 1990;253:90-99.

In 31 occurrences of established hip dislocation in 24 patients, the most successful operations were a combination of soft-tissue release, open reduction, femoral varus derotation and shortening osteotomy, and pelvic osteotomy.

Pritchett JW: Treated and untreated unstable hips in severe cerebral palsy. *Dev Med Child Neurol* 1990;32:3-6.

The author compared 50 patients with severe cerebral palsy and dislocated hips who had soft-tissue releases about the hip and anterior branch obturator neurectomy with 50 patients who had received no treatment. No significant differences were found in the frequency of pain or other complications. The findings suggest that soft-tissue releases alone are not helpful in patients with already dislocated hips and severe cerebral palsy.

Spina Bifida (Myelomeningocele)

Beaty JH, Canale ST: Orthopaedic aspects of myelomeningocele. *J Bone Joint Surg* 1990;72A:626-630.

The best candidate for operative correction is a child who has a unilateral dislocation, is between 1 and 3 years old, and has an established neurosegmental level and stable neurologic status. However, dislocation of the hip does not affect the child's ability to walk, as the neurologic level of involvement is the primary influence.

Fraser RK, Hoffman EB, Sparks LT, et al: The unstable hip and mid-lumbar myelomeningocele. *J Bone Joint Surg* 1992;74B:143-146.

In this study of 55 patients followed for an average of ten years, the neurologic level was the most significant determinant of walking ability. All patients with L-4 neurologic levels could walk (45% of the hips were subluxated or dislocated), but only one third of those with L-3 lesions could do so (86% of the hips were dislocated and subluxated). Hip stability, intelligence quotient, and fixed deformity did not influence walking ability.

Samuelsson L, Eklof O: Hip instability in myelomeningocele: 158 patients followed for 15 years. *Acta Orthop Scand* 1990;61:3-6.

Children were assessed at 2 and 15 years of age to assess the prevalence of hip dislocation. In infants examined during the first 10 weeks after birth, 10% of the hips were dislocated. In children with L-3 and L-4 levels of involvement, 25% of the hips were dislocated and 50% subluxated. Spasticity promoted dislocation with involvement above L-3, and there was little risk of developing dislocation below L-4.

Sherk HH, Uppal GS, Lane G, et al: Treatment versus nontreatment of hip dislocations in ambulatory patients with myelomeningocele. *Dev Med Child Neurol* 1991;33:491-494.

The authors compared 30 children with untreated hip dislocations with 11 patients who underwent open reduction of a dislocated hip with a 2-year follow-up and concluded that surgical reduction of paralytic hip dislocations in ambulatory myelomeningocele patients is costly and offers little obvious benefit.

41

Pelvis and Acetabulum: Trauma

Disruption of the pelvic ring traditionally has been associated with a significant risk of nonunion, malunion, and leg-length discrepancy. The evolution of surgical techniques continues to improve the orthopaedist's ability to manage bony injuries and any accompanying visceral and neurologic complications.

Pelvic Fractures

High-energy trauma severe enough to cause a pelvic fracture carries a significant risk of associated injury to neurologic, urologic, gynecologic, gastrointestinal, and vascular structures. Any associated injury to skin and subcutaneous tissues further complicates treatment.

The initial treatment, therefore, often involves an emergency resuscitation protocol. Intrapelvic bleeding, a major cause of shock, can result in death. Typically, the bleeding occurs from veins lacerated by bony spicules; arterial hemorrhage is less common. The greatest risk for such bleeding is to the patient with displaced and unstable disruption of the posterior pelvic ring. In addition to the usual volume replacement by intravenous crystalloid solutions and whole blood, specific strategies in these patients may include the temporary use of military anti-shock trousers (MAST suit), angiography and transarterial embolization, vascular repair, and external or internal stabilization of the pelvic ring.

External Fixation

Unstable pelvic ring injuries, particularly those that increase the diameter and volume of the pelvis, may benefit from external fixation placed during the first few hours after injury. In most cases, such devices are considered one component of the resuscitation effort, rather than a method for definitive fixation. Their use has been shown to decrease initial blood loss in unstable fractures. Fractures that are amenable to external fixation include some sacral fractures, sacroiliac dislocations and fracture dislocations, ilium fractures, and dislocations of the pubic symphysis. External fixation is not indicated as a strategy for resuscitation in patients with stable pelvic ring injuries or acetabular fracture.

When indicated, the usual approach is to apply the frame to the anterior portions of both iliac crests through stab wounds. A variety of configurations can be used to provide adequate initial stability. The timing of placement varies according to the situation. In some patients attempts are made to control shock with fluid and blood replacement, followed by external fixation if these ef-

forts are not successful. A second course is to apply the frame for prophylaxis before the patient shows signs of progressive hemodynamic instability. Proponents of the first course argue that many patients with unstable pelvic ring injuries respond to fluid replacement alone, and do not require immediate stabilization. Furthermore, the pins can provide an avenue for bacteria to invade subcutaneous hematoma, and they increase the risk of infection at the time of definitive internal fixation. The argument for the second course is that application of the fixator in a patient who is currently hemodynamically stable may prevent subsequent severe blood loss, which is more difficult to control if the patient does become hemodynamically unstable.

Angiography

Angiography of the pelvic arteries should be performed in patients who do not respond to fluid resuscitation and external fixation, or in those patients for whom external fixation is not applicable. If the bleeding is only venous, then angiographic embolization will be of no benefit. However, in many patients with continued and uncontrolled hemorrhage, arterial injuries may be identified and controlled. The superior gluteal artery is the most common culprit. The embolization should be localized in order to minimize subsequent tissue ischemia, which can be an important factor affecting tissue healing following later surgical repair. If major arteries are involved, embolization is unlikely to give permanent control, and surgical repair is indicated.

Military Anti-Shock Trousers (MAST)

Temporary use of the MAST, applied by paramedical personnel, can be an important factor in controlling hemorrhage. However, it does not allow full examination of the patient, and it can obscure such injuries in the lower extremities as open fracture, vascular injury, or compartment syndrome.

Associated Injuries

Skin and Subcutaneous Tissues

Injury can occur in two ways: as a laceration producing an open fracture, or, more commonly, as a closed degloving injury with fat necrosis and hematoma, which can occupy a large cavity. When present, these cavities usually require surgical debridement and drainage because they serve as a nidus for infection, which can develop hematogenously or can be introduced through a fixation pin or traction pin tract. The extent of these cavities must also be considered in planning for internal fixation.

Visceral Injuries

Urologic   Disruptions of the bladder and urethra are commonly associated with pelvic fractures. The mechanism of injury can be direct laceration by fracture fragments or pressure and tension stresses that occur during deformation of the pelvic ring.

Intravenous pyelograms, or transurethral cystograms and retrograde urethrograms, usually are required to make a definitive diagnosis. If possible, the orthopaedist and urologist should collaborate in a plan to manage the urologic injury and, at the same time, protect the surgical approach for future internal fixation of the pelvic fracture. For example, if suprapubic drainage is the best treatment from the urologist's perspective, the drain should be placed so that it will not interfere with the later approach to internal fixation.

Gynecologic Injury   Gynecologic injury may involve lacerations of the vagina, which most commonly occur in dislocations of the symphysis pubis or fractures of the pubic rami. Larger peritoneal lacerations can involve the perineum and rectum. Although the more extensive injuries are usually obvious, isolated vaginal lacerations may be overlooked because vaginal bleeding is attributed to menstruation.

Gastrointestinal Injury   Gastrointestinal injury may include lacerations of the rectum, or less commonly, perforations of the small and/or large bowel. The latter may be overlooked initially, because the mechanism of injury is indirect. When a rectal laceration is present, a diverting colostomy is indicated, accompanied by thorough irrigation and debridement of the fracture(s) communicating with the laceration. There is some controversy regarding the best method for stabilizing associated unstable fractures or fracture/dislocations in this situation. Because internal fixation is the most definitive, many orthopaedists advocate its use even in the presence of bacterial contamination, but this requires extensive irrigation, and debridement. However, others feel that external fixation, which carries less risk of infection, is preferable.

Neurologic Injury   Neurologic injuries occur more often than was appreciated in the past. The mechanism of injury can be direct, commonly with fractures of the sacrum, or indirect, resulting from nerve root and/or peripheral nerve traction accompanying pelvic displacement. The distribution of injury can involve any of the nerves represented by the femoral and lumbosacral plexus (L-2 to S-4) but L-5 and S-1 are at greatest risk. Although the initial examination may be difficult because of pain and associated injuries, every effort should be made to assess the sciatic, femoral, and obturator

nerve functions. A rectal examination should be included to assess the lower sacral nerve roots. This baseline information is important because the neurologic function may improve or deteriorate as a result or complication of treatment.

Relatively few nerve injuries should be treated surgically, because most of them are caused by traction rather than laceration. Exceptions to this general rule include some sacral fractures with bony compromise of the spinal canal or neural foramina, and displaced acetabular fractures, posterior hip dislocations, or other posterior column injuries compressing the sciatic nerve.

Evaluation of the Patient With Suspected Pelvic Fracture

In addition to the complete clinical evaluation, which has been described, radiologic examination should include anteroposterior, 40-degree cephalad (outlet), and 40-degree caudad (inlet) projections, often complemented by 45-degree oblique views. The cephalad view best demonstrates the sacral foramina, as well as displacements of the ischial tuberosities. The caudad view best visualizes deformities of the pelvic inlet and the true magnitude of sacroiliac dislocations or sacral fractures. The 45-degree oblique views may demonstrate acetabular fractures not visible on other views, and they can further define involvement of the sacroiliac joint, iliac wing, and obturator foramen.

If there is any doubt about the displacement or instability, a computed tomographic scan should be obtained (Fig. 1). This scan further delineates fracture dislocations of the sacroiliac joint. It also defines sacral fractures that are unstable, despite a plain radiographic appearance suggestive of stability. In selected patients, three-dimensional reconstructions are useful, particularly in planning surgical interventions in patients with malunions or nonunions of pelvic fractures.

Treatment Principles

The basic principles are similar for all fractures—fracture union in a satisfactory position and rapid rehabilitation. Most pelvic ring injuries are stable and are treated by closed methods, which include bedrest, for initial comfort, and protected ambulation until full weightbearing is tolerated. If there is any question about stability, serial radiographs should be obtained to ensure that displacements are not occurring.

For unstable fractures, the critical factors are careful definition of instability and displacement. Failure to recognize significant instability or displacement can cause later nonunion or instability, which can lead to problems such as sacroiliac pain, leg-length discrepancy, difficulties in sitting, and functional impairment. Women may have additional problems relating to parturition and dys-

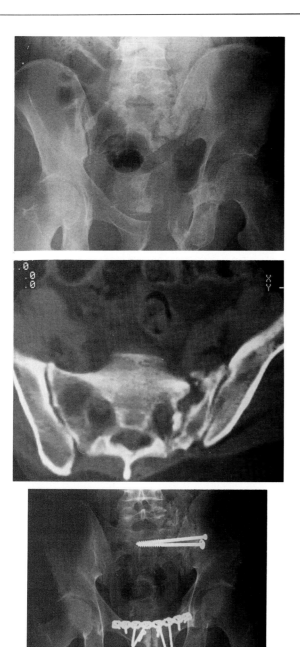

Table 1. Tile classification of pelvic ring disruptions

Classification	Description
Type A	Stable
A1	Fracture of the pelvis not involving the ring
A2	Stable, minimally displaced fracture of the ring
Type B	Rotationally unstable but vertically stable
B1	Open book
B2	Lateral compression (ipsilateral)
B3	Lateral compression (contralateral)
Type C	Rotationally and vertically unstable
C1	Unilateral
C2	Bilateral
C3	Associated with an acetabular fracture

pareunia. The Tile classification, given in Table 1, is very useful in planning treatment.

Treatment of Unstable Injuries

When instability is identified, the preferred treatment is surgical stabilization, particularly if the posterior pelvic ring is involved or if the patient has an associated fracture of the acetabulum or extremities. Although alternative treatments such as closed reduction and skeletal traction have been used, malunion, nonunion, or later instability are more common than with surgical stabilization. Furthermore, skeletal traction must be maintained for eight to 12 weeks, which increases debilitation and loss of joint motion in the ipsilateral joints. Such closed methods have little chance of success when the sacroiliac joint is involved, because the major injury is to ligamentous structures. Although a pelvic sling has been used in rotationally unstable but vertically stable injuries with 3 cm or more of diastasis of the symphysis, the efficacy of open treatment usually makes conservative methods less attractive.

Surgical Approaches to Open Reduction and Internal Fixation

Posterior Injuries

The choice of incision depends on associated injuries, soft-tissue contusion, abrasion, laceration, or hematoma cavities, as well as placement of other devices, such as a suprapubic catheter.

Virtually all posterior injuries can be accessed through a posterior surgical incision which begins 2 cm lateral and proximal to the posterior iliac crest, and extends vertically across the buttock to a point distal to the greater sciatic notch. After the gluteal muscles are mobilized from their origins on the iliac wing and sacrum (gluteus maximus) the pyriformis is mobilized from the greater sciatic notch so that palpation can be performed anteriorly along the sacrum and sacroiliac joint. An alternative anterior approach starts along the iliac crest and continues slightly distal to the anterior iliac crest. The iliacus is mobilized to expose the sacroiliac joint.

Fig. 1 **Top,** Anteroposterior pelvis radiograph of a 58-year-old man six months after a motor vehicle accident. The symphysis remains dislocated and a fracture through the left sacrum is ununited and displaced. Shortening of the extremity secondary to pelvis displacement was measured at 36 mm. The patient complained of pain in the sacral area, a short leg, and sitting difficulties. Initial treatment was by 12 weeks of skeletal traction. **Center,** Computed tomography of the sacrum demonstrating the left sacral nonunion. **Bottom,** 1.5 years following operative reduction and fixation of the pelvic nonunion. Shortening is now 10 mm. The patient has no symptoms referable to his pelvis. Late reconstruction of the nonunion was successful; however, early internal fixation is the preferred treatment.

Fractures of the Sacrum The patient is positioned prone on a radiolucent table. A posterior incision is made; if fixation is planned, an additional vertical incision is made on the opposite side, extending between the two iliac wings. An alternative approach is a transverse incision, crossing the sacrum and both posterior iliac crests. The sacral nerve roots and fracture site are visualized by placing a laminal spreader at the fracture site or between the two posterior superior iliac crests. Reduction is performed using forceps spanning from the spinous processes of the sacrum to the iliac crest. The sacral nerve roots are palpated after the reduction to be certain they have not become entrapped.

One strategy is direct fracture fixation from the iliac crest into the sacrum. Under radiographic control, long, 6.5-mm cannulated lag screws transfix the fracture from the iliac wing to the body of S-1. Because of risk to neural structures, a Kirschner guide wire usually is inserted, and its position is confirmed before the screw is placed. An alternative approach with less potential for neurologic injury is to place the fixation device between the two posterior iliac crests. Large diameter threaded sacral bars or double cobra plates are commonly employed.

Sacroiliac Dislocations These injuries are managed in a fashion similar to that used for a sacral fracture. An alternative is anterior reduction and stabilization using two three-hole plates spanning from the anterior surface of the sacral ala to the internal iliac fossa. Care must be taken to avoid stretching the L-5 nerve root which passes across the anterior aspect of the sacral ala. A second approach is to perform anterior reduction followed by screw fixation placed percutaneously from the iliac wing across the joint.

Fracture Dislocations of the Sacroiliac Joint These injuries are approached, and the sacroiliac dislocation managed, in a fashion similar to that used for a sacral fracture. Before sacroiliac reduction, the iliac fracture is reduced and fixed, typically with long lag screws between the two tables of the ilium.

Fractures of the Ilium and Iliac Wing An incision is made parallel to the crest, allowing access to the external and internal surfaces of the iliac wing. Depending on the type of fracture, long lag screws can be placed between the two tables of the ilium, spanning the fracture site, or screws can be supplemented by plates.

Anterior Injuries (Approach)

Transverse or vertical incisions are made, according to the individual patient's problem. A transverse incision is more cosmetic, and is best for managing an associated bladder rupture. A vertical, midline incision can be extended for management of associated intra-abdominal injuries. In either incision, the two heads of the rectus abdominis are split along the linea alba.

Dislocation of the Symphysis Pubis Reduction is usually made using forceps, or two-screw technique. A four- or six-hole plate stabilizes the fracture and allows the best control of vertical translations. When the symphysis displacement is minimal, it is sometimes possible to use a two-hole plate.

Fractures of the Pubic Ramus These fractures rarely require fixation, except when there is very wide displacement.

Combined Injuries

Combined pelvic injuries can involve the pelvic ring and acetabulum, or anterior and posterior pelvic ring. In patients with acetabular injuries, posterior pelvic fixation is performed first, followed by management of the acetabulum. If the lesion is a combined anterior-posterior injury, the anterior injury can be stabilized without compromising the posterior reduction and stabilization.

In patients with a symphysis dislocation and sacroiliac joint dislocation or a fractured ilium, an anterior approach can be used to manage the combined injury. However, if the posterior injury is a fracture dislocation or sacral fracture, the patient must be repositioned.

Postoperative Management

The benefit of stable internal fixation is that it allows rapid mobilization of the patient. Depending on the patient's associated injuries, gait training usually can begin two to five days postoperatively, protecting unilateral injuries with partial weightbearing. In bilateral injuries, gait training is not started for six weeks. In unilateral and bilateral injuries, full weightbearing typically can begin six to eight weeks postoperatively.

Management of Nonunions and Malunions

Nonunions and malunions pose a major surgical challenge. The usual indications for surgical repair relate to pelvic instability, pain, leg-length discrepancy, or, for women, anticipated difficulties in pregnancy and delivery. The risks attendant to surgical reduction and stabilization are greater than in the acute injury. Nerve roots may be bound down by scar, and must be mobilized with care to avoid stretch injury. The bladder, internal iliac vessels, or femoral arteries and veins likewise may be adherent and easily transgressed during exposure and mobilization. The preoperative evaluation, therefore, should include careful assessment of these structures using cystograms, and arteriograms. Intraoperatively, cortical evoked potential monitoring may be required to monitor the effects of neurologic manipulation. Three-dimensional reconstructions of computed tomographic scans and plastic models created by CAD-CAM are extremely useful for determining the full extent of deformity and the position of fracture fragments.

Acetabular Fractures

Acetabular fractures are usually best seen on anteroposterior views of the pelvis and hip and 45-degree oblique views of the pelvis. Computed tomographs are indicated in most patients, because they reveal hidden fractures of the posterior pelvic rings, such as a minimally displaced sacral fracture. In addition, the computed tomographic scan gives full information regarding minimally displaced fractures of the ilium, fractures involving the quadrilateral space, rotational displacements of the anterior and posterior columns, and fragments incarcerated between the femoral head and the walls of the acetabulum.

Classification

The Letournel classification includes ten fracture types subdivided by five simple fracture types—fractures of the posterior wall, the posterior column, the anterior wall, the anterior column, transverse fractures, and five combined fracture types. This classification best guides the indications for surgery and the surgical approach. Posterior wall fractures always involve the posterior articular surfaces, often accompanied by a portion of the retroacetabular surface and sometimes the entire surface. However, the ilioischial line remains intact. Posterior column fractures involve not only the posterior articular surfaces, but also the ilioischial line. Anterior wall fractures involve the central portion of the anterior column, whereas anterior column fractures involve varying amounts of the anterior column based on a high or low fracture line. In both cases, the iliopectineal line is involved. Transverse fractures involve both the anterior and posterior acetabulum and divide the innominate bone into a superior segment containing the acetabular roof and intact ilium, and an inferior segment consisting of a single ischiopubic fragment. Combined fracture types include combined posterior wall and posterior column fractures, or posterior wall and transverse fractures as well as several more complex patterns. A T-shaped fracture combines a transverse component and a vertical component that separates the lower ischiopubic segment into the anterior and posterior columns. A second type combines anterior and posterior hemitransverse fractures, with the anterior column or anterior wall predominating in displacement. A low and usually minimally displaced posterior hemitransverse component is present. In both column fractures, all segments of the articular surface are detached from the ilium.

Treatment Principles

As with any articular injury, the goal is to restore function and to prevent late osteoarthritis. Most osteoarthritis is caused by imperfect reduction. Residual displacements as small as 1 to 2 mm, particularly in weightbearing surfaces, can lead to degenerative changes. Other, less

common causes are incarcerated osteochondral fragments, or articular surface damage that is not evident radiographically.

Determining which fractures can be treated without surgery requires plain radiographs and computed tomography. Of particular importance is the measurement of the amount of acetabular dome that is intact. Three radiographic measurements guide this determination. The medial roof arc is determined from the anteroposterior radiograph. A vertical line is drawn from the roof of the acetabulum to the geometric center of the femoral head. A second line is drawn from the fracture to the geometric center. The angle subtended by these lines forms the medial roof arc. Similar measurements are made to determine the anterior and posterior roof arcs. The former is made on the obturator oblique view, and the latter on the iliac oblique views. Despite the utility of these measurements, they have a limited role in assessing two-column and posterior wall fractures.

A candidate for nonsurgical treatment should fulfill the following criteria: (1) the anterior roof, medial roof, and posterior roof arcs should all be greater than 45 degrees; (2) the posterior acetabular wall should be adequate; and (3) the femoral head should remain congruent with the acetabular roof when traction is removed.

Fracture patterns amenable to nonsurgical treatment include very low transverse fractures not involving the weightbearing dome, and two-column fractures without wide displacement, as determined by the three arc measurements. If nonsurgical treatment is selected, Neufeld type roller traction has the advantage of permitting active lower extremity exercises. Traction must be maintained from four to eight weeks to achieve bony union.

Surgical Treatment

Urgent surgical treatment is warranted when a patient has anterior or posterior dislocations that cannot be reduced by closed means. A delay of two to three days, with the patient maintained in distal femoral traction, is appropriate for all other fractures. However, a delay longer than ten days makes reduction more difficult, and by three weeks callus formation significantly complicates reduction. If such delays are unavoidable, open reduction and internal fixation should be undertaken in younger patients, particularly those with simple fracture configurations. Osteotomy of the fracture fragments may be required to effect reduction. In older patients, particularly those with complex fractures, surgery can be deferred with the anticipation that later total joint replacement may be required.

The incision chosen is based on the location of the fracture(s) and surgical strategy. Alternatives include the Kocher-Langenbeck, the ilioinguinal, extended iliofemoral, or triradiate incisions. The expectation should be that the entire operation can be accomplished through the chosen incision. Usually intraoperative traction is employed either through the distal femoral pin and fracture table, or an ASIF femoral distractor. It is important to flex the knee to at least 60 degrees to relax the sciatic nerve. The lateral position allows a simultaneous anterior and posterior approach.

Treatment

Specific Fractures

Posterior Wall Fractures After exposure through the Kocher-Langenback incision, the joint is debrided and irrigated to remove all loose osteocartilaginous fragments. The articular surfaces are inspected and impactions of the articular surface elevated and supported by bone graft, depending on the magnitude of depression. The fracture is then fixed with lag screws and a posterior buttress plate along the posterior rim of the acetabulum.

Posterior Column Fractures The Kocher-Langenback incision is used with the patient in the prone position. After reduction and visual assessment of the retroacetabular surfaces, fixation is obtained with a dynamic compression or small reconstruction plate applied from the ischial tuberosity to the lateral ilium along the retroacetabular surfaces.

Transverse Fractures The approach is similar to that used for posterior wall and column fractures, and the posterior column is reduced and fixed. A long, 6.5-mm cancellous screw transverses the anterior portion of the fracture into the superior pubic ramus. However, a high transverse fracture is best exposed through the ilioinguinal approach.

Associated Transverse and Posterior Wall Fractures For most patients, the approach is similar to that used for the posterior wall fracture and requires distraction of the femoral head, removal of all osteocartilaginous fragments, and correction of femoral head depressions. After transverse fracture has been reduced and provisionally fixed, the posterior wall fracture is reduced, the buttress plate is applied, and a long cancellous screw is transfixed into the superior pubic ramus. In patients with remote or difficult fractures, an extended iliofemoral or triradiate approach may be necessary.

T-Shaped Fractures The fracture may be approached and reduced as a posterior column injury. The anterior column is manipulated through the sciatic notch, or through the joint. If these maneuvers do not produce adequate reduction, a subsequent ilioinguinal approach is required. An alternative and sometimes preferable approach uses the extended iliofemoral or triradiate incision at the outset.

Anterior Column and Anterior Wall Fractures The ilioinguinal approach is preferred, followed by reduction and fixation with lag screws and application of a plate along the pelvic brim.

Associated Anterior Column and Posterior Hemitransverse Fractures The approach and anterior column fixation is the same as for the isolated injury. Following anterior stabilization the posterior column is reduced by manipulation of the quadrilateral surface and is fixed by long lag screws placed from the pelvic brim to the posterior column near the ischial spine.

Two-Column Fractures These difficult fractures can be treated by the ilioinguinal approach, or an extended iliofemoral approach. The latter is preferable when there is a complex posterior column fracture or when fracture lines cross the sacroiliac joint. The anterior column is reduced and fixed to the ilium. The posterior column is then reduced and fixed, using interfragmentary lag screws and reconstruction or buttress plates. Because the acetabular reconstitution can only be inferred by the external appearance of the fracture fragments, radiographic evaluation must be performed before closure to insure adequate reduction.

Postoperative Management

Closed suction drainage and antibiotic therapy is used for 48 hours. Passive motion is initiated after drain removal, and crutch walking with 15 kg weightbearing starts as soon as pain is diminished, usually two to five days postoperatively. Eight weeks after internal fixation, weightbearing is increased progressively, assuming the fracture shows evidence of healing.

Complications

Infection The risk of infection is similar to that for all hip surgery, providing there are no associated injuries. The risk of infection is significantly increased by associated urologic and gastrointestinal injuries, as well as skin lacerations and closed degloving lesions. Like all pelvic injuries, degloving injuries require debridement, and they may influence the placement of incisions or delay definitive surgical stabilization. If infection is suspected, the treatment should include debridement, irrigation, and antibiotic treatment.

Thromboembolism As in all hip surgery, the risks of thromboembolism are significant. The best prophylaxis is debatable, the choices being pneumatic compression boots or anticoagulation. Anticoagulation is particularly warranted for those at risk, such as the elderly.

Nerve Palsy The most common cause is retraction of the sciatic nerve in a posterior approach. Flexion of the knee to at least 60 degrees reduces the risk of this complication.

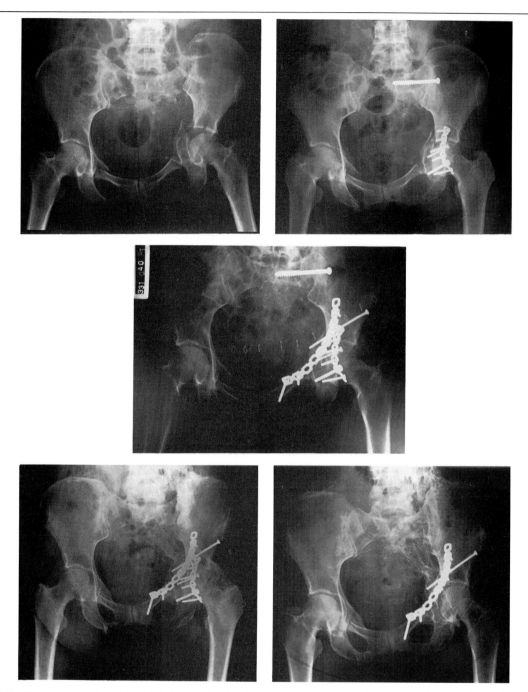

Fig. 2 **Top left**, Anteroposterior pelvis radiograph of a 60-year-old woman after a motor vehicle accident. The radiograph demonstrates a displaced left sacrum fracture adjacent to the sacroiliac joint, a displaced T-shaped fracture of the left acetabulum, and bilateral pubic ramus fractures. The patient also had a closed degloving injury over the entire buttocks bilaterally. **Top right**, Five days after the injury and transfer to another hospital, the patient underwent drainage and debridement of the closed degloving injury, fixation of the sacrum with an iliosacral screw, and fixation of the posterior column of the acetabulum. **Center**, One week after the initial surgery the anterior column of the acetabulum was reduced and fixed through the ilioinguinal approach. **Bottom left**, Anteroposterior pelvis radiograph nine months after the injury. The patient's postoperative course was complicated by a deep infection involving the left sacrum and sacroiliac joint. Intermittent drainage was present until a final debridement and screw removal were performed at six months after the injury. The hip joint was not infected; however, it fused spontaneously secondary to heterotopic ossification. **Bottom right**, Anteroposterior pelvis radiograph at seven years following the injury. The patient underwent ectopic bone excision and posterior plate removal at 18 months after the injury. At seven years she has no pelvis or hip pain and has normal hip motion. The patient had two significant complications (infection and heterotopic ossification). The risk of complication was greatly increased by the patient's associated soft-tissue trauma. The final result was good, however, following successful treatment of the complications.

Ectopic Bone   This complication most commonly occurs following lateral exposure of the innominate bone, and is most likely with an extended iliofemoral approach, less likely with the Kocher-Langenbeck approach, and negligible with the ilioinguinal approach (Fig. 2). Prophylaxis includes indomethacin (25 mg three times daily for several months) or postoperative irradiation. If ectopic bone does occur, its excision should be delayed for at least 15 to 18 months.

Osteoarthritis   Posttraumatic degenerative changes are the most common long-term complication. Although osteoarthritis can occur despite accurate bony reduction, the best strategy is to achieve maximal reduction and stable fixation.

Combined Acetabular and Pelvic Injury

Combined acetabular and pelvic injuries should be treated first by reduction and stabilization of the pelvic ring, followed by acetabular reduction and internal fixation. The choice of incision depends on the particular combination of injuries.

Annotated Bibliography

Pelvic Ring Injuries

Burgess AR, Eastridge BJ, Young JW, et al: Pelvic ring disruptions: Effective classification system and treatment protocols. *J Trauma* 1990;30:848-856.

A treatment protocol was followed in 210 patients (1985 to 1988) with high-energy pelvis fractures. The expanded mechanism of injury classification (Dalal, et al) was used. A variety of treatment methods including bed rest, traction, external fixation and internal fixation were used. The authors concluded that the classification system effectively directed treatment that decreased morbidity and mortality.

Dalal SA, Burgess AR, Siegel JH, et al: Pelvic fracture in multiple trauma: Classification by mechanism is key to pattern of organ injury, resuscitative requirements, and outcome. *J Trauma* 1989;29:981-1002.

A retrospective analysis was performed of 343 patients (1983-1985) with pelvis fractures. A modification of the mechanism of injury classification system of Pennal and Tile was used. Severe anteroposterior compression injuries were found to have the highest requirement for transfusion and resuscitation and a high incidence of adult respiratory distress syndrome and other organ injury.

Denis F, Davis S, Comfort T: Sacral fractures: An important problem: Retrospective analysis of 236 cases. *Clin Orthop* 1988;227:67-81.

Sacral fractures, often undiagnosed and untreated, frequently result in neurologic symptoms and deficits in the lower extremities and urinary, rectal, and sexual dysfunction. This retrospective study included 236 patients with sacral fractures in a series of 776 patients with pelvic injuries. The sacral fractures were classified on the basis of their direction, location, and level. Injuries in zone I, the region of the ala, were occasionally associated with partial damage to the L-5 nerve root. Injuries in zone II, the region of the sacral foramina, were frequently associated with sciatica but rarely with bladder dysfunction. Injuries in zone III, the region of the central sacral canal, were frequently associated with saddle anesthesia and loss of sphincter function.

Ganz R, Krushell RJ, Jakob RP, et al: The antishock pelvic clamp. *Clin Orthop* 1991;267:71-78.

A new antishock pelvis clamp, which provides external fixation of the posterior pelvic ring, is described. Early clinical trials indicate probable effectiveness in achieving provisional stability and controlling hemorrhage in patients with sacroiliac dislocation and sacrum fractures.

Isler B: Lumbosacral lesions associated with pelvic ring injuries. *J Orthop Trauma* 1990;4:1-6.

Displaced vertical sacral fractures can produce a dislocation of the L-5/S-1 facet joint. This dislocation can make retraction of the sacral fracture more difficult and may lead to late pain.

Matta JM, Saucedo T: Internal fixation of pelvic ring fractures. *Clin Orthop* 1989;242:83-97.

Fifty-four patients with unstable pelvic injuries were treated by one of three methods—skeletal traction, external fixation, or open reduction and internal fixation. A comparison of results demonstrated that internal fixation was superior for anatomic results, union rate, and functional results. Of 32 injuries treated by internal fixation, 22 were fixed initially and ten were fixed after failure of traction or external fixation. One deep wound infection was the only surgical complication. The authors describe current treatment protocols and fixation techniques.

Shaw JA, Mino DE, Werner FW, et al: Posterior stabilization of pelvic fractures by use of threaded compression rods: Case reports and mechanical testing. *Clin Orthop* 1985;192:240-254.

Threaded compression rods were placed between the posterosuperior spines as a means of posterior stabilization of pelvic fractures. Malgaigne fractures with sacroiliac disruptions were created in four cadaveric pelvises. Anterior frames alone provided little stabilization of the disrupted sacroiliac joints with either longitudinal or torsional loading. Markedly improved stabilization in both loading modes was achieved with posterior augmentation. Two typical cases are presented to demonstrate that posterior stabilization is as effective in clinical practice as in the biomechanics laboratory.

Simpson LA, Waddell JP, Leighton RK, et al: Anterior approach and stabilization of the disrupted sacroiliac joint. *J Trauma* 1987;27:1332-1339.

The authors describe their technique for and excellent results with anterior sacroiliac fixation.

Tile M: *Fractures of the Pelvis and Acetabulum.* Baltimore, MD, Williams & Wilkins, 1984.

This text details the radiologic study, classification, and surgical and nonsurgical treatments of fractures of the acetabulum and pelvis.

Tile M: Pelvic ring fractures: Should they be fixed? *J Bone Joint Surg* 1988;70B:1-12.

Of 494 fractures treated over five years, only 19% needed stabilization (5% by internal means). External fixation should be used initially, followed by internal fixation posteriorly for unstable or unreduced fractures.

Acetabular Fractures

Bosse MJ, Poka A, Reinert CM, et al: Heterotopic ossification as a complication of acetabular fracture: Prophylaxis with low dose irradiation. *J Bone Joint Surg* 1988;70A:1231-1237.

In a retrospective review of 37 patients who underwent surgery for 38 complex acetabular fractures, postoperative low dose irradiation was administered to 17 patients (18 fractures) done through either an extended iliofemoral incision or a modified extended iliofemoral incision. Most received 10 GY in 2-GY increments, starting on the third postoperative day. The incidence of heterotopic ossification in the 18 irradiated limbs was much lower than that in the 20 patients in the control group (50% versus 90%). The difference in the incidence of severe (class III or class IV) heterotopic ossification between the two groups of patients was significant.

Bosse MJ, Poka A, Reinert CM, et al: Preoperative angiographic assessment of the superior gluteal artery in acetabular fractures requiring extensile surgical exposures. *J Orthop Trauma* 1988;2:303-307.

The authors review eight cases in which a preoperative arteriogram was performed prior to performing their "Modified Extensile Exposure" for acetabulum fractures to assess the superior gluteal artery. They conclude that this approach may cause ischemic necrosis of the abductor musculature if the superior gluteal artery blood flow is not intact.

Burk DL Jr, Mears DC, Kennedy WH, et al: Three-dimensional computed tomography of acetabular fractures. *Radiology* 1985;155:183-186.

Computer programs that produce three-dimensional surface reformations from sets of contiguous axial computed tomographic scans were used in evaluating various acetabular fractures in 20 patients. The three-dimensional images were easily correlated with plain radiographs, and new views were produced that provided a unique perspective not obtained by conventional radiography. The three-dimensional images were useful in complex displaced fractures. Plain radiographs and conventional computed tomographic scans were more sensitive than the three-dimensional images in detecting undisplaced fractures.

Epstein HC: *Traumatic Dislocation of the Hip.* Baltimore, MD, Williams & Wilkins, 1980.

Posterior dislocation of the hip combined with acetabular fracture leads to a high incidence of posttraumatic arthritis. The long-term results were best in those patients who underwent primary open reduction of the dislocation with removal of the intra-articular bone fragments and internal fixation of the fracture.

Heeg M, Oostvogel HJ, Klasen HJ: Conservative treatment of acetabular fractures: The role of the weight-bearing dome and anatomic reduction in the ultimate results. *J Trauma* 1987;27:555-559.

A retrospective study of 57 conservatively treated acetabular fractures with an average follow-up of 7.9 years found that the overall functional results were satisfactory in 75%. The least satisfactory results were seen in fractures crossing the weightbearing dome of the acetabulum in which congruency could not be achieved. Fractures crossing the weightbearing dome that could be reduced by traction to less than 2 mm had good or excellent results in seven patients. The authors concluded that conservative treatment of acetabular fractures can be very successful, even in fractures crossing the weightbearing dome, provided that congruence is preserved during the period of traction.

Hesp WL, Goris RJ: Conservative treatment of fractures of the acetabulum: Results after long time follow up. *Acta Chir Belg* 1988;88:27-32.

Of 79 patients with 81 fractures of the acetabulum, 83% had multiple injuries. The mean injury severity score was 34 (range, nine to 75). Involvement of the dorsal column or roof of the acetabulum produced moderate or bad results in 79%. In such cases, surgical repositioning and fixation should be considered.

Judet R, Judet J, Letournel E: Fractures of the acetabulum: Classification and surgical approaches for open reduction: Preliminary report. *J Bone Joint Surg* 1964:46A:1615-1646.

This classic article presents the initial findings in the techniques for open reduction and internal fixation of acetabular fractures. The anatomic classification provided continues to be the most useful acetabular fracture classification available.

Keith JE Jr, Brashear HR Jr, Guilford WB: Stability of posterior fracture-dislocations of the hip: Quantitative assessment using computed tomography. *J Bone Joint Surg* 1988;70A:711-714.

This paper investigates the stability of cadaver hips after osteotomy of progressively larger segments of the posterior wall of the acetabulum. This model simulated fractures of the posterior wall that may allow posterior hip instability. The width of the fragment was measured on CT scan as a percentage of the depth of the acetabulum. Defects up to 20% were stable. Defects over 40% were unstable.

Letournel E, in Judet R (ed): *Fractures of the Acetabulum.* Berlin, Springer-Verlag, 1981.

Thorough anatomic and radiographic descriptions of the ten major types of acetabular fractures are given. After analysis of an acetabular fracture and assignment of the classification, decision making proceeds to selection of a surgical approach for open reduction and internal fixation. The long-term functional results are highly correlated with the accuracy of surgical reduction.

Matta JM, Merritt PO: Displaced acetabular fractures. *Clin Orthop* 1988;230:83-97.

The rate of satisfactory surgical reductions improved gradually over the first 50 operations in a prospective study of 121 displaced acetabular fractures. Overall, clinical results were satisfactory in 80% of this series. Complications included a 3% infection rate and a 5% incidence of nerve palsy. Open reduction and internal fixation is indicated for most displaced fractures. However, closed treatment can produce satisfactory results in selected patients.

Mayo KA: Fractures of the acetabulum. *Orthop Clin North Am* 1987;18:43-57.

Open reduction and internal fixation is now the preferred treatment for most displaced fractures of the acetabulum. Long-term follow-up of a large number of cases operated on within the first three weeks of injury showed excellent clinical and radiographic results in about 74% of cases. The outcome after anatomic reduction is significantly better than in cases in which there is residual deformity. Reported complications included a 2% to 4% infection rate and nerve palsy in 3% to 6% of patients. Heterotopic bone formation occurred in almost one half of surgically treated cases, but required secondary resection in only 1% to 2%.

McLaren AC: Prophylaxis with indomethacin for heterotopic bone after open reduction of fractures of the acetabulum. *J Bone Joint Surg* 1990;72A:245-247.

Fifty percent of 26 patients operated for acetabulum fractures developed Brooker grade 2 or greater ectopic bone. 5.5% of 18 patients treated postoperatively with indomethacin (25 mg 3 times daily for 6 weeks) developed grade 2 or greater ectopic bone.

Reinert CM, Bosse MJ, Poka A, et al: A modified extensile exposure for the treatment of complex or malunited acetabular fractures. *J Bone Joint Surg* 1988;70A:329-337.

A modification of the extended iliofemoral incision facilitates the surgical exposure of T-shaped, complex transverse, and two-column fractures and malunions. The modification includes the use of a T-shaped skin incision with large flaps and osteotomies of the iliac crest, greater trochanter, and anterosuperior iliac spine.

Webb LX, Bosse MJ, Mayo KA, et al: Results in patients with craniocerebral trauma and an operatively managed acetabular fracture. *J Orthop Trauma* 1990;4:376-382.

Hip function was found to be significantly compromised in 23 patients with significant craniocerebral trauma who were treated operatively for acetabulum fractures. Symptomatic ectopic bone occurred in 61%. Three patients suffered a loss of reduction and fixation.

42

Hip: Trauma

Trauma of the hip, particularly that occurring in the elderly, remains a major challenge to our health care system, one that continues to accelerate as a greater number of hip fractures occur each year and as the age and frailty of those patients sustaining fractures also increase. In the 1980s, improved medical and surgical management of hip trauma significantly decreased mortality. Technical advances in fracture fixation and in prosthetic design and replacement have decreased complications and improved functional outcomes. Hip dislocations and femoral neck, intertrochanteric, and subtrochanteric fractures will be discussed in this chapter.

Hip Dislocations

Hip dislocations are typically caused by high-energy trauma, usually from motor-vehicle accidents. They occur most frequently in young patients. In 35% to 95% of cases, severe associated injuries occur, including craniofacial, chest, abdominal, and other musculoskeletal injuries. Radiographs of the pelvis and entire femur are taken to identify the most commonly associated musculoskeletal injuries that occur with hip dislocations.

Hip dislocations are classified as either anterior or posterior; each is discussed separately. Principles of treatment include (1) careful evaluation of the patient for associated injuries; (2) immediate gentle closed or, if necessary, open reduction, with assessment of stability following reduction; (3) careful radiographic evaluation (including a postreduction computed tomographic scan); and (4) evaluation for congruency of reduction and any associated fractures of the femoral head or acetabulum.

In general, if a concentric, stable reduction is obtained, treatment should include a brief period of bed rest until symptoms subside, followed by protected weightbearing for four to six weeks. If the reduction is concentric but unstable and there are no associated fractures, traction should be maintained for four to six weeks until soft-tissue healing occurs. In a nonconcentric reduction, intra-articular osteochondral fragments, interposed soft tissue, or malreduction of associated femoral head fractures can be responsible, necessitating open reduction, joint exploration, and removal of osteochondral fragments. The location and size of the fragments and the stability of the reduction determine the treatment approach for associated fractures of the femoral head and acetabulum.

Complications of hip dislocation may be immediate or late. Femoral artery and nerve injuries, while uncommon, can be associated with anterior dislocations. Sciatic nerve injuries are associated with approximately 10% of posterior dislocations. Osteonecrosis, which may occur up to five years after injury, increases in incidence with delay of reduction. Posttraumatic degenerative arthritis following hip dislocation is more common with associated femoral head or acetabular fractures.

Anterior Dislocations

Approximately 10% to 18% of all hip dislocations are anterior and can be classified as either superior or inferior. Both types of anterior dislocation result from abduction and external rotation. In addition, superior dislocations occur in extension and inferior dislocations, which are far more common, in flexion. The femoral head is displaced anteriorly and may compress the femoral neurovascular bundle. Closed reduction is achieved by traction, followed by extension and internal rotation.

Femoral head fractures occur in 22% to 77% of cases and are either transchondral or indentation fractures; they may be difficult to diagnose without tomograms or computed tomographic scans. Transchondral fractures that result in a nonconcentric reduction require open reduction and either excision or internal fixation of the fragment, depending on size and location. Indentation fractures, more common and also typically superior on the femoral head, require no specific treatment, but their location has significant prognostic implications.

Osteonecrosis occurs in approximately 10% of anterior dislocations; risk factors include a delay in reduction or repeated reduction attempts. Posttraumatic degenerative arthritis occurs in most cases; transchondral fractures, indentation fractures deeper than 4 mm, and osteonecrosis are primary risk factors.

Posterior Dislocations

Posterior dislocations, classified by Epstein on the basis of associated femoral head and/or acetabular fractures, account for up to 90% of all hip dislocations. Posterior dislocations are the result of a force applied to the flexed knee along the axis of the femur. If the hip is in a neutral position or in adduction, a simple dislocation results; if the hip is in abduction, an associated posterior acetabular rim fracture occurs. Closed reduction may be achieved by traction on the adducted and flexed hip; postreduction radiographs should be evaluated carefully for concentricity of reduction. A computed tomographic scan should be performed in all cases to identify intra-articular fragments or associated fractures. If closed re-

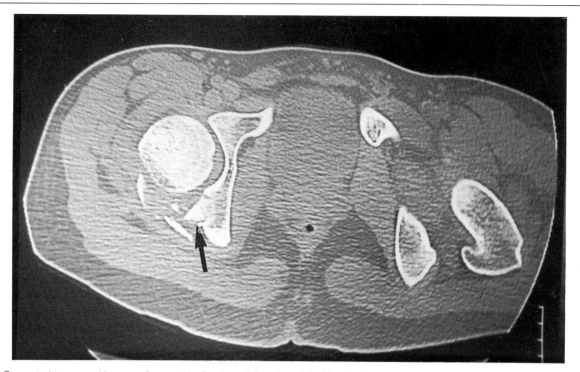

Fig. 1 Computed tomographic scan of a posterior fracture-dislocation of the hip showing an acetabular depression fracture involving a large portion of the posterior wall (black arrow).

duction with the patient under general anesthesia is unsuccessful or nonconcentric, open reduction is indicated. At that time, the joint should be explored and any osteochondral fragments internally fixed or removed.

Assessment of stability following either closed or open reduction is essential. Computed tomography (CT) can assist in the assessment of stability after reduction of posterior fracture-dislocations of hip. Stability is inversely related to the size of the posterior acetabular fragment. CT studies in cadaveric models have demonstrated that fragments involving less than 20% to 25% of the acetabular wall do not affect hip stability, while those involving more than 40% to 50% result in instability. Fragments of transitional size may or may not result in instability, depending on the status of the posterior capsule. To restore stability, hips in which the posterior acetabular fragments are large should undergo posterior joint irrigation and debridement, followed by open reduction and internal fixation of the acetabular fragment. The surgeon should avoid dissection around the quadratus femoris to prevent injury to the medial femoral circumflex artery.

An acetabular depression fracture representing a rotated, impacted, osteocartilaginous fracture of the posteromedial articular surface has been described (Fig. 1). It occurs as a result of a posterior fracture-dislocation. This fracture is not uncommon (an incidence of 23% has been reported when CT evaluation is used) and may be a factor in posterior instability after reduction. Operative

management consisting of elevation with bone graft added to maintain the reduction is indicated.

Osteonecrosis of the femoral head, reported in 10% to more than 50% of posterior dislocations and fracture-dislocations, usually occurs within two to three years of injury, but may develop up to five years after the injury. The risk of osteonecrosis depends on the severity of the injury, delay of reduction (that is, for longer than six to 12 hours), and repeated attempts at closed reduction. Simple dislocations without acetabular fractures have the lowest incidence of osteonecrosis. The risk factors for posttraumatic degenerative arthritis include the severity of the initial injury, nonconcentric reduction, the time interval between injury and reduction, and the development of osteonecrosis.

Delayed diagnosis of posterior dislocations decreases the chance of a successful outcome. If the injury is three or more weeks old, closed reduction is usually not possible because of periarticular soft-tissue contracture. Open reduction is required but increases the risk of osteonecrosis. In young patients, open reduction and internal fixation of associated fractures is indicated. In elderly patients, primary prosthetic joint replacement is preferred.

Posterior Dislocations with Femoral Head Fractures

Associated fractures of the femoral head occur in approximately 10% of all posterior dislocations. Epstein type V injury has been further categorized by Pipkin. Femoral head fractures occur when a force is applied to the flexed knee with the hip adducted and flexed less than 50 degrees. The femoral head is driven into the posterosuperior portion of the acetabular rim, shearing off a fragment.

Identification and sizing of the femoral head fragment may be difficult with standard radiographs; CT scanning usually will provide this critical information. Radiographs should be evaluated carefully prior to closed reduction so that a nondisplaced femoral neck fracture is not overlooked. Nondisplaced femoral neck fractures that become displaced as a result of attempted closed reduction significantly worsen the prognosis for this injury. Gentle closed reduction should be attempted for Pipkin types I, II, and IV injuries; type III injuries require open reduction. Postreduction radiographs, including computed tomographic scanning, should be evaluated for concentricity and reduction of the femoral head fragment.

If a closed reduction is unsuccessful (including under general anesthesia) or nonconcentric, then open reduction is indicated. Once again, treatment depends on both the type and size of the fracture. Types I and II fractures generally require an open reduction and internal fixation from an anterior approach. Type III fractures should be treated by primary open reduction and internal fixation of the femoral neck fracture, followed by excision or internal fixation of the femoral head fracture, depending on size and location. Primary prosthetic replacement is preferred for type III fractures in the elderly. Treatment of type IV fractures depends on the stability and concentricity of the reduction. If the reduction is unstable or nonconcentric, open reduction, joint exploration, excision or fixation of the femoral head fracture, and internal fixation of the posterior acetabular fracture are indicated.

Posterior dislocations with femoral head fractures present particular risk for osteonecrosis and posttraumatic degenerative arthritis. The prevention of concomitant osteonecrosis may depend on prompt reduction, within six to 12 hours of injury. The prognosis for these fractures varies. Types I and II injuries have the same prognosis as simple dislocations. Type IV injuries have the same prognosis as posterior dislocations with acetabular fractures, but without femoral head fractures. Type III injuries have a poor prognosis.

Bilateral hip dislocations result from high-energy trauma and account for 1% to 2% of all hip dislocations. Fifty percent are bilateral posterior dislocations, 40% are anterior and posterior dislocations, and 10% are bilateral anterior dislocations. Treatment for these injuries follows what was described previously.

Hip Fractures

Risk Factors

The incidence of hip fractures increases with increasing age, doubling for each decade beyond 50 years of age.

Among patients 90 years of age and older, one third of women and one sixth of men will have sustained a hip fracture. Women are more commonly affected, by a ratio of 2 or 3 to 1. The incidence among white women is two to three times higher than that reported for black and Hispanic women. Urban dwelling, excessive prolonged alcohol intake, physical inactivity, previous hip fracture, use of psychotropic medication (hypnotics or anxiolytics, tricyclic antidepressants, and antipsychotic), and senile dementia are all additional risk factors. The relationship between hip fracture and osteoporosis or osteomalacia has been studied extensively. The relationship between osteoporosis and hip fracture remains unclear; in two large series, bone density between patients with hip fracture and age-matched controls displayed no significant difference. Osteomalacia has not been shown to be a risk factor for hip fracture.

Nutritional copper deficiency or excessive caffeine intake may increase the risk of hip fracture. A recent study reported that patients with hip fracture had significantly lower mean serum copper levels than did controls (20.5 vs 26.9 mol/L). Copper is a coenzyme for collagen cross-linking, and deficiencies compromise bone strength, predisposing to fracture and interfering with fracture healing. Caffeine intake greater than two units per day (two cups of coffee or four cups of tea) has been reported to increase the risk for hip fracture by 53% during a two-year period. The highest relative risk identified was in caffeine users younger than 65 years of age.

Several age-related changes in neuromuscular function may increase the likelihood of a fall resulting in a hip fracture. These changes include slowing of the gait, which increases the probability that the point of impact from a fall will be near the hip, and slowing of reaction time, which limits the potential for a protective response.

The morphology of the proximal femur may influence whether a patient sustains a femoral neck or intertrochanteric hip fracture. One study reported that patients with intertrochanteric fractures had a significantly shorter femoral neck than did patients with femoral neck fractures.

Supplemental estrogen has been found to protect against hip fracture in women with diminished estrogen level. Replacement therapy decreases the risk of hip fracture in all age groups but most significantly in women younger than 60 years of age.

Mortality

Hip fractures occur primarily in elderly patients who often have comorbidities, increasing the risk of mortality. In the 1980s, the mortality for elderly patients with hip fractures was approximately 20% for the first year after fracture and 13% for the second year after fracture. There is general agreement that increased mortality is seen primarily in the first year after injury. After one year, the mortality rate returns to that for age- and sex-matched controls. Advanced age, significant medical comorbidities, male sex, institutionalized living, and dementia are factors associated with increased mortality. Disagreement exists as to whether fracture type, delay in surgical treatment, or type of surgical procedure present consistent risk factors for increased mortality.

The influence of nutrition on the morbidity and mortality following hip fracture is well documented. Serum albumin levels have been found to correlate closely with mortality. One study reported 70% mortality for patients with albumin levels less than 3.0 g/dl compared with 18.2% for patents with albumin levels greater than 3.0 g/dl. A recent study reported the value of total lymphocyte counts as a prognostic indicator of survival following femoral neck fracture. A low lymphocyte count was found in 82% of patients with femoral neck fractures who died before discharge but in only 36% of patients who survived at least six months after fracture.

Principles of Treatment

Surgical management, followed by early patient mobilization, is generally accepted treatment for adult hip fractures. Historically, nonsurgical management resulted in an excessive rate of medical morbidity and mortality, as well as malunion and nonunion. Nonsurgical management may, however, be appropriate in selected elderly demented patients who were nonambulators prior to the fracture and who experience minimal discomfort from the injury. Such patients should be mobilized as soon as possible to avoid the complications of prolonged recumbency. Nonsurgical management should be approached cautiously and in carefully selected patients.

Before surgery, elderly patients with hip fractures should be medically stabilized. The vast majority of patients can undergo surgery within 24 hours of injury; longer delays necessary for stabilization of medical problems have not been shown to increase morbidity or mortality. Conversely, the surgical treatment of medically unstable patients significantly increases the risk of mortality. The choice of anesthesia (spinal versus general) has not been shown to affect postoperative confusion or mortality in elderly patients with hip fractures.

While broad-spectrum antibiotics have been shown to decrease significantly the incidence of postoperative infection, their prolonged use, that is, longer than 24 hours, has not been demonstrated to be advantageous. Postoperative management is directed at early mobilization and the avoidance of the complications of recumbency. The ability to ambulate within two weeks of surgery has been correlated with living at home one year after surgery. Prevention of decubitus ulcers, which occur in up to one third of patients, usually within the first week after admission, is extremely important. Patients with decubiti have a significantly longer length of stay and a higher mortality rate. Meticulous nursing care remains the best approach for the prevention of decubiti.

Thromboembolic Disease

Compression ultrasonography has been shown to be a very effective technique for diagnosing venous thrombo-sis in patients with hip fractures. It has a reported accuracy of 97%, a sensitivity of 100%, and a specificity of 97% compared with standard venography. It is a safe, quick, and easily repeated diagnostic test with minimal risks.

The significant incidence of thromboembolic disease (deep venous thrombosis, pulmonary emboli) in patients with hip fractures has generated several different prophylactic regimens. The efficacy of some regimens in these patients has been extrapolated from their use in patients undergoing total hip replacement. Aspirin is generally effective and has the advantages of low cost and easy administration; its efficacy has been demonstrated primarily in men. Warfarin has been shown to be effective, but results in an increased incidence of bleeding problems (hematoma), particularly if the prothrombin time exceeds 1.5 times control. Dextran alone, or in combination with dihydroergotamine, also has been shown to be effective, but its use requires a large fluid administration, which increases the risk of fluid overload. Low-dose intravenous heparin or heparin in combination with dihydroergotamine have been effective, specifically in patients with hip fractures; low-dose subcutaneous heparin has not been shown to be effective. Intermittent external pneumatic compression also may be of value, but the cost of specialized equipment and the physical restraint it places on a patient must be considered.

Imaging Studies

Among elderly patients with normal radiographs and persistent hip pain following a fall, bone scanning is useful in identifying occult fractures. It has been generally accepted that two to three days may be required for bone scanning to become positive in an elderly patient with a hip fracture. However, a recent study reported that the overall sensitivity of bone scanning was 93.3% with a specificity of 95.0% for the diagnosis of hip fracture regardless of the age of the patient or time interval after injury.

The vitality of the femoral head after surgery, as determined by radionuclide scanning within three weeks of surgery, may be predictive of healing complications. Femoral neck fractures with femoral head uptake greater than or equal to the nonfractured side can be expected to heal uneventfully. Those with a lower uptake than the nonfractured side carry a high risk of segmental collapse or nonunion. The usefulness of preoperative radionuclide scanning in predicting the development of these complications is, however, controversial. Thus far, it has not been used to determine choice of treatment (internal fixation versus prosthetic replacement).

Magnetic resonance imaging (MRI) within 48 hours of injury does not appear to be useful for assessing femoral head viability and vascularity. In a prospective study of 15 patients with femoral neck fractures (12 of 15 displaced), all MRI scans were normal and without evidence of osteonecrosis. However, based on its incidence in other large series, the probability that osteonecrosis would not develop in any of the displaced fractures is 4%. Two explanations suggested for the normal scans were the relative paucity of hematopoietic elements in the femoral head and the lack of adequate time for the repair response to develop.

Functional Recovery

The success of treating an elderly patient with hip fracture is frequently measured using the prefracture level of function as a standard. The goal of management, to restore a patient's prefracture level of function, is difficult to achieve. Of patients who were functionally independent and living at home prior to hip fracture, 15% to 40% will require institutionalized care for more than a year after fracture. Only 50% to 60% will regain their prefracture ambulatory status within a year after fracture. Approximately 50% to 83% of patients will regain independent ambulation with assistive devices. The vast majority of patients will require assistance in performing activities of daily living (ADLs). Among those who were independent in ADLs prior to fracture, only 20% to 35% will regain their prefracture ADL independence.

Functional recovery following hip fracture is not complete until at least six months after surgery. A follow-up study of 92 patients with surgically treated intertrochanteric hip fractures assessed walking ability using walkway tests and found that less than half of the patients had achieved their preoperative levels within three months of surgery. This was particularly true for those with unstable fractures. Walking capacity improved in more than one third of patients between the third and sixth months. The significant factors associated with improvement in walking capacity during this period were unstable fracture type, continued improvement in hip strength, and continued reduction of pain.

Stress Fractures

Stress fractures of the femoral neck are relatively uncommon injuries, with most reports involving military recruits and athletes. Initial radiographs are often normal and a bone scan or MRI is necessary to identify the fracture. Stress fractures are classified as either tension or compression fractures. Tension fractures occur on the superior aspect of the femoral neck; they are potentially unstable and should undergo internal fixation. Compression fractures occur on the inferior aspect of the femoral neck; they are more stable than tension fractures and generally can be treated without surgery (initially with bed rest followed by protected weightbearing). Radiographic evidence of disruption of both cortices or fracture widening is an indication for prompt internal fixation to prevent displacement. Nonsurgical treatment must include frequent serial radiographs to detect any changes in fracture pattern or displacement.

Pathologic Fractures

Metastatic lesions that result in pathologic fractures or impending fractures are commonly found in the proximal femur. The indications for stabilization of impending fractures include a lesion larger than 2.5 cm in diameter or with destruction of 50% or more of the cortex of a long bone. Patients treated prophylactically for impending fractures have reduced operative mortality, fewer complications, less stabilization failures, and more successful rehabilitation outcomes than those with pathologic fractures who underwent surgery. Stabilization of an impending fracture spares the patient the pain and disability associated with fracture. Life expectancy is sometimes regarded as an indication for surgical treatment, with some recommending a life expectancy of at least 90 days, and others of 30 days. The surgical treatment of impending and pathologic fractures is indicated in patients whose quality of life will be enhanced, regardless of the anticipated life expectancy. Surgical management provides for pain relief and patient mobilization.

Preoperative evaluation and preparation must be meticulous because patients with pathological fractures are often extremely debilitated. Serum calcium levels require particular attention, because hypercalcemia is common in such patients. Radiosensitive metastatic lesions should undergo radiotherapy preoperatively or immediately following stabilization of the fracture. Although radiotherapy has not been demonstrated to decrease soft tissue healing, it does interfere with the incorporation of bone graft. Methylmethacrylate is used to fill defects resulting from tumor resection and for fixation of prostheses; it is an important adjunct for stabilizing pathologic fractures. Surgical management usually consists of internal fixation using adjunctive methylmethacrylate or prosthetic replacement, depending on the location and size of the lesion and its sensitivity to radiotherapy. The treatment of pathologic femoral neck, intertrochanteric, and subtrochanteric fractures is discussed elsewhere.

Femoral Neck Fractures

The Garden classification of femoral neck fractures is the system most commonly cited in the literature, but difficulties persist in differentiating the four fracture types. It may be more accurate to classify femoral neck fractures as nondisplaced/impacted (Garden types I and II) or displaced (Garden types III and IV).

Treatment

Treatment of nondisplaced/impacted femoral neck fractures (Garden types I and II) should consist of internal fixation with multiple parallel lag screws or pins. There is no consensus as to the optimal number of pins, although most authors report successful treatment using three or four pins or screws for both nondisplaced and displaced fractures. Sliding screw devices were used previously, but reported results have been inferior.

A relatively new device, the telescoping, variable-length compression screw (VLCS), applies the principles of sliding and compression used in intertrochanteric fractures to femoral neck fractures. A recent biomechanical study compared three telescoping screws to three cannulated cancellous screws in both normal and osteoporotic bone. There was no significant biomechanical difference in normal bone; in osteoporotic bone, the telescoping screws had a significantly greater load-to-failure. However, thus far the clinical efficacy of this new device has not been sufficiently evaluated. Following nondisplaced fractures, nonunion and osteonecrosis are uncommon complications, with nonunion occurring in fewer than 5% of cases and osteonecrosis in fewer than 8%.

The treatment of displaced femoral neck fractures remains controversial. Most authors advocate closed reduction or open reduction and internal fixation in younger, active patients and primary joint replacement in older, less active patients. When internal fixation is used, successful anatomic reduction is probably the most important factor in avoiding complications during healing. An acceptable reduction may have up to 15 degrees of valgus angulation and less than 10 degrees of anterior or posterior angulation. Prompt reduction of displaced fractures has been advocated, but has not been consistently demonstrated to decrease the rate of nonunion or osteonecrosis. Following closed reduction, anteroposterior and lateral radiographs are necessary to determine the adequacy of reduction. If a closed reduction is not acceptable, open reduction may be required.

Nonunion and osteonecrosis continue to be problematic following displaced femoral neck fractures. The incidence of nonunion has ranged from 10% to 30% and the incidence of osteonecrosis, from 15% to 33%. Adequate reduction has consistently been reported to be the single most important prognostic factor influencing the development of these complications. The need for reoperation following internal fixation of displaced fractures is variable. Approximately one third of patients with osteonecrosis will require additional surgery; approximately 75% of patients with nonunion or early fixation failure will require reoperation.

Increased intracapsular pressure and capsular distention may decrease perfusion through the capsular vessels and contribute to the development of osteonecrosis. Preoperative intra-articular pressure measurements in a series of 19 patients with femoral neck fractures averaged 66.4 mm Hg for Garden types I and II fractures and 28 mm Hg for Garden types III and IV fractures. The lower readings in displaced hip fractures were thought to be secondary to capsular rupture. Blood flow to the femoral head after fracture was recorded indirectly in 50 femoral neck fractures by intraosseous pressure measurement using a transducer. Significant increases in intracapsular and intraosseous pressures, as well as a decrease in intraosseous pulse pressure (a measure of bone blood flow), occurred after fracture. All of these findings were reversed following needle aspiration of the hip. These results support the clinical usefulness of immediate joint aspiration following femoral neck fracture.

An important predictor of internal fixation complications is fracture stability. The influence of femoral neck fracture stability and intraoperative impaction on healing was studied in 41 patients. A metal probe fitted with strain gauges was used intraoperatively to measure the effect of the impaction maneuver. Patients with healing complications (early loss of fixation or nonunion) had fractures that were less stable than did those patients with fractures that progressed to uneventful union. Intraoperative impaction using a mallet improved stability in only 23 of 41 fractures; in the others, stability either remained unchanged or worsened.

A stepwise logistic regression analysis has been reported that is designed to assess the influence of various factors on the incidence of healing complications following internal fixation of femoral neck fractures using three pins or screws. Healing complications (displacement, nonunion, or late segmental collapse) occurred in 34% overall: 12.5% for Garden type I fractures, 7.8% for Garden type II fractures, 37.5% for Garden type II fractures, and 52.5% for Garden type IV fractures. The most important factor influencing healing was the quality of reduction. The amount of initial displacement and implant position were less important.

Primary prosthetic replacement for displaced femoral neck fractures has been advocated to avoid the problems of nonunion and osteonecrosis in older, less active patients, but specific indications have not been defined. It should be considered in elderly patients when an adequate closed reduction cannot be obtained or when severe posterior comminution of the neck precludes stable internal fixation. Different types of prostheses have been used successfully, including uncemented and cemented unipolar and bipolar endoprostheses.

Earlier studies on prosthetic replacement reported increased morbidity and mortality compared with patients undergoing internal fixation. This probably reflected the seriously debilitated condition of these patients and the lack of antimicrobial and antithrombotic prophylaxis. More recent studies comparing prosthetic replacement with internal fixation have reported significant benefits with the former. Following prosthetic replacement, pain relief was improved, need for reoperation was decreased, and function was improved both one and two years after the fracture was repaired.

Progressive acetabular erosion has been reported to be a problem following cemented unipolar hemiarthroplasties. A retrospective study of 72 cemented Thompson hemiarthroplasties followed for an average of 7.7 years reported that the severity of acetabular erosion most consistently correlated with patient activity level and duration of follow-up. Erosion progressed at an average rate of 3% per year in active patients. However, the Thompson hemiarthroplasty had consistently good results in patients with low activity levels.

The exact role of the bipolar prosthesis, designed to decrease the incidence of acetabular erosion, remains unclear. A retrospective study of 49 cemented Bateman bipolar prostheses followed for an average of 7.5 years reported that 52% had acetabular erosion of 2 mm or less; there were no cases of protrusio. The failure rate at 7.5 years was 10.4%. A ten-year prospective study of 561 displaced fractures treated with a cemented bipolar prosthesis identified significant acetabular erosion (greater than 3 mm) in 5.6% of 243 hips followed for at least one year; however, there was no significant association between pain and acetabular erosion. Of the 91 patients followed for three to nine years, 95% had only slight or no hip pain.

Controversy continues regarding the amount of motion that occurs at the inner and outer surfaces of the bipolar prosthesis. In a series of 65 Hastings bipolar prostheses examined radiographically, 70% functioned as a unipolar prosthesis with motion occurring only between the acetabulum and prosthetic shell. However, a study of 26 bipolar prostheses reported that motion occurred at both the inner and outer bearing surfaces.

The need for cement in prosthetic replacement after hip fracture was evaluated in a prospective randomized study of cemented versus noncemented bipolar hemiarthroplasties in previously ambulatory individuals. The incidence of postoperative complications and early mortality, the duration of surgery, and the amount of blood loss were not significantly different between individuals. However, there was a significant difference in the incidence of pain at 18 months: 32% of patients in the cemented group and 80% of patients in the noncemented group experienced pain.

The results of primary cemented total hip replacement following acute femoral neck fracture have been disappointing. At an average follow-up of 56 months, 18 (49%) of 37 patients younger than 70 years of age had undergone or were awaiting revision surgery; in addition, four (11%) had definitive radiologic signs of loosening. Activity level correlated with early failure. A prospective study comparing the range of hip motion following total hip replacement for arthritis and fracture reported significantly greater range of motion in the fracture group, a possible predisposing factor for dislocation and early loosening.

The results of secondary total hip replacement performed after failed internal fixation of femoral neck fractures have been reported to be similar to the results of primary total hip replacement for femoral neck fracture. However, the failure rate is greater than twice that reported for elective total hip replacement performed for osteoarthritis.

Young Adults

In most cases, femoral neck fractures in young adults occur as a result of high-energy trauma (motor vehicle accidents, falls from heights). In those that occur from a simple fall, a predisposing factor (intoxication, medication use) is often present. When these fractures result from high-energy trauma, careful evaluation for other injuries should be performed. Specific consideration should be given to the possibility of ipsilateral femoral neck and shaft fractures.

Nondisplaced fractures should be treated by multiple lag screw or pin fixation. Care should be taken to avoid any loss of reduction during the surgical procedure. Nonunion and osteonecrosis are very uncommon following nondisplaced fractures, except in cases where the fracture was not initially identified. The successful treatment of displaced fractures is related to achieving anatomic reduction and stable internal fixation as soon as possible after the injury. A gentle closed reduction should be attempted. If the reduction is unacceptable, an open reduction followed by multiple lag screw or pin fixation should be performed. When prompt anatomic reduction and internal fixation are achieved, the incidence of nonunion should be less than 10%, and that of osteonecrosis, 20% to 33%.

The treatment of acute displaced femoral neck fractures using a muscle pedicle graft with or without bone graft to reduce the incidence of nonunion and osteonecrosis remains controversial. Initial successful results have not been reproduced in a large series. This procedure may be useful as treatment for ununited femoral neck fractures.

Intertrochanteric valgus osteotomy is indicated in young and active patients with a nonunion of the femoral neck. A recent series followed 50 patients younger than 70 years of age for an average of 7.1 years after osteotomy and found that 86% of fractures united an average of 3.6 months after surgery; seven (14%) patients required prosthetic replacement. The presence of osteonecrosis was not found to be a contraindication to osteotomy, providing there was no collapse.

Special Problems

Neurologically impaired patients include those with Parkinson's disease who sustain a femoral neck fracture, both internal fixation and prosthetic replacement have been recommended. A retrospective review of 94 patients compared the results of internal fixation with hemiarthroplasty. Nondisplaced fractures generally underwent internal fixation; displaced fractures were treated by prosthetic replacement. The complication rate was much greater in the hemiarthroplasty group; the use of anti-Parkinson's medication did not affect the complication rate. The treatment chosen in these patients should be based on patient age, fracture type, and disease severity. All of these patients require meticulous medical and nursing care to avoid complications.

If prosthetic replacement is chosen, correction of a hip adduction contracture by tenotomy and an anterior surgical approach should be considered. Both measures may decrease the risk of dislocation. Patients with previous strokes are at increased risk for hip fractures, primarily because of residual balance and gait problems and osteoporosis of the paretic limb. The treatment approach depends on fracture type and functional status. When the fracture occurs within one week of the stroke, poor functional recovery can be anticipated. If prosthetic replacement is chosen, hip contractures may require tenotomy and an anterior approach may be preferred. Institutionalized patients with severe dementia present a particular challenge. In-hospital mortality as high as 50% has been reported. Nondisplaced fractures should be treated by internal fixation. An anterior approach should be used for displaced fractures requiring prosthetic replacement to decrease the risk of dislocation and infection from wound contamination. In nonambulatory patients with severe dementia who do not experience significant discomfort from the injury, nonsurgical management with early bed-to-chair mobilization should be considered.

Femoral neck fractures in patients with rheumatoid arthritis are associated with a high complication rate. In general, nondisplaced fractures can be treated successfully by internal fixation. Total hip replacement is recommended for displaced fractures. Femoral neck fractures are very uncommon in patients with underlying osteoarthritis of the hip. When they do occur, total hip arthroplasty is preferred.

Displaced and nondisplaced femoral neck fractures in patients with chronic renal disease or hyperparathyroidism are at increased risk for complications of internal fixation because of associated metabolic bone disease. In these patients, cemented primary prosthetic replacement is recommended.

Femoral neck fractures in patients with Paget's disease should be evaluated carefully because of the potential for preexisting acetabular degeneration and deformity of the proximal femur. Nondisplaced fractures can be treated by internal fixation. For displaced fractures, prosthetic replacement is preferred. If there were prefracture symptoms of hip pain in the presence of acetabular degeneration, total hip arthroplasty is recommended; if no acetabular degeneration is present, cemented hemiarthroplasty should be performed. Deformity of the proximal femur and the tendency for excessive bleeding are technical difficulties that are often encountered.

Femoral neck fractures that occur as a result of metastatic disease require prosthetic replacement. Involvement of the entire proximal femur may require a calcar or proximal femoral replacement. For patients with acetabular involvement, a cemented acetabular component should be used. If acetabular involvement is extensive, portions of the ilium may have to be reconstructed using methylmethacrylate, wire mesh, and specialized acetabular components. Before prosthetic replacement for pathologic fractures of the proximal femur is performed, it is important to identify any metastatic lesions that may be present in the femoral shaft. This will decrease the risk of intraoperative fracture or shaft perforation.

Intertrochanteric Fractures

Intertrochanteric fractures occur with approximately the same frequency as femoral neck fractures in patients with similar demographic characteristics. The most important aspect of fracture classification is determination of stability. In 1949, Evans introduced a classification system based on fracture pattern and on stability of the fracture after reduction. This system recognized that stability is provided by the presence of an intact posteromedial cortical buttress. Comminution of this area or inability to restore a medial buttress permits the fracture to collapse into varus. Unstable fracture patterns also include intertrochanteric fractures with subtrochanteric extension and reverse obliquity fractures.

Surgical treatment of intertrochanteric fractures has undergone an important evolution over the past 40 years. Operative management using rigid nail-plate devices, which did not allow impaction at the fracture site, resulted in complication rates of up to 40% for unstable fractures. Mechanical complications, including nail penetration, nail breakage, and superior cut out, resulted as unstable fractures impacted into a more stable position. In the 1960s, in an effort to overcome these mechanical problems, displacement osteotomies were developed to convert unstable fractures to more stable patterns. The Dimon and Hughston medial displacement osteotomy and the Sarmiento valgus osteotomy successfully decreased the rate of mechanical complications when rigid nail-plate devices were used. However, because additional impaction occurred after osteotomy and fixation, mechanical problems persisted when these devices were used.

Sliding nail and screw devices, which developed in the 1970s, provided secure fixation of the proximal (head and neck) fragment to the distal (shaft) fragment, but more importantly, they allowed controlled impaction at the fracture site. Sliding screw devices were preferred over sliding nail devices, because the screw provided better fixation in the proximal fragment. These sliding devices are load-sharing devices, compared to rigid nail plates, which were load-bearing devices. They permit early mobilization and weightbearing without the high risk of fixation failure associated with rigid nail-plate devices. Intramedullary fixation of intertrochanteric fractures also became popular in the 1970s. These condylocephalic nails were inserted in a retrograde manner through an insertion point in the distal aspect of the femur. It was hoped that a less-extensive surgical procedure, which avoided exposing the fracture site, would decrease postoperative morbidity. In the 1980s, calcar replacement endoprostheses were used to treat selected, comminuted, intertrochanteric fractures.

Sliding Hip Screws

The sliding hip screw remains the implant of choice for the treatment of both stable and unstable intertrochanteric hip fractures (Fig. 2). Available in 5-degree

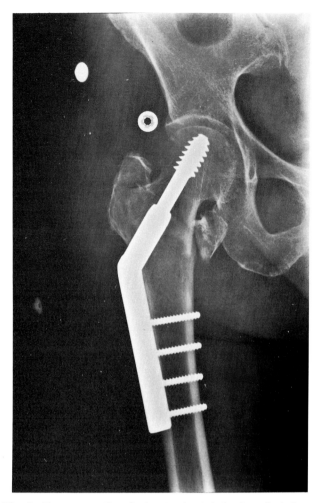

Fig. 2 Treatment options for intertrochanteric fractures include internal fixation, which is most commonly performed using a sliding hip screw.

increments from 130 degrees to 150 degrees, the 135-degree and 150-degree plate angles are the most commonly used sizes. The 150-degree angle plate has certain theoretical advantages: it more closely approximates the resultant forces acting across the hip, thereby facilitating sliding and fracture impaction. In addition, a smaller varus moment arm acts on this device, reducing the risk of implant failure. It is, however, difficult to insert a 150-degree device consistently into the center of the femoral head and neck; newer implant designs have almost eliminated the problem of implant breakage. The 135-degree plate is easier to insert in the desired central portion of the femoral head and neck. In addition, it has an insertion point in metaphyseal bone, which produces less of a stress-riser effect than the diaphyseal insertion point required for 150-degree devices. Clinical studies have not shown a significant difference in the amount of sliding and impaction for these two plate-angles.

Based on available information, the most important aspect of device insertion is secure placement of the screw within the proximal fragment. This requires insertion of the screw to within 1 cm of the subchondral bone. A central position within the femoral head and neck is most commonly recommended. If a central position is not possible, a posteroinferior position is preferred. Anterosuperior positions should be avoided, because the bone is weakest in this area, which increases the risk of superior cutout of the screw.

The necessity of a medial displacement osteotomy with use of the sliding hip screw remains controversial. Because the sliding hip screw allows controlled collapse at the fracture site, unstable fractures that are anatomically reduced can be expected to impact spontaneously to a stable and often medially displaced position. This usually results in less shortening of the extremity than a formal medial displacement osteotomy.

Sliding hip screw fixation of intertrochanteric fractures is associated with an incidence of loss of fixation of between 4% and 12%, occurring most commonly in unstable fractures. Most fixation failures can be attributed to the technical problems of fracture reduction and screw placement. Although the sliding hip screw allows postoperative impaction at the fracture site, it is essential to obtain an impacted reduction at the time of surgery. This impacted position avoids excessive postoperative collapse that may exceed the sliding capacity of the device. If screw sliding brings the threads in contact with the plate barrel, additional impaction will not be possible and the device becomes the biomechanical equivalent of a rigid nail-plate (Fig. 3). A recent study advocated the use of a short-barrel dynamic hip screw sideplate when a screw 80 mm or shorter was inserted to maximize the available sliding capacity.

Axial loading studies of unstable fractures have confirmed that the posteromedial fragment (PMF) is the keystone to mechanical stability. When anatomic reduction is possible, fixation of the PMF becomes progressively more important as its size increases. According to a recent study, anatomic reduction of a large PMF increased load resistance by 57% over identical fractures with the fragment excluded. Fixation of a small PMF increases load resistance by only 17%.

Methylmethacrylate has been advocated as an adjunctive fixation agent in extremely osteoporotic, unstable fractures treated by a sliding hip screw. Currently, its routine use with sliding hip screw fixation for nonpathologic fractures is not recommended.

Intramedullary Devices

Intramedullary devices have been used extensively for the treatment of intertrochanteric fractures. The largest experience has been with the Ender nail. The results have been variable and generally disappointing. Among the stated advantages of these devices are decreased operative time, minimal blood loss due to the distal insertion, and unexposed fracture site. This technically de-

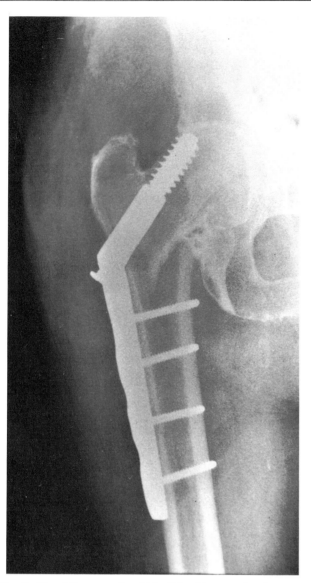

Fig. 3 The sliding capacity of this sliding hip screw has been exceeded, resulting in superior screw cut out.

manding procedure requires use of the image intensifier. Complication rates have ranged from 16% to 71%, with varus deformity being the most common, along with external rotation deformity and knee pain caused by distal migration of the nails. Early reoperation has been required in up to 19% of cases. The highest complication rates were reported when these devices were used for unstable fractures.

At present, the indications for Ender nailing of intertrochanteric fractures remain undefined. It may be most useful in elderly, debilitated patients with stable fractures who can tolerate only minimal operative intervention. An adequate number of nails must be used and they should be driven deeply into the femoral head with ante-

version prebending to prevent postoperative external rotation deformity. They should not be used for unstable intertrochanteric fractures.

The Gamma nail, a new device that has been used for the treatment of intertrochanteric hip fractures, has, in theory, technical (limited exposure, closed insertion, reduced time in the operating room, decreased blood loss) and mechanical (shorter lever arm and bending moment on the device due to its intramedullary placement) advantages over the sliding hip screw. However, a recent prospective, randomized study comparing the Gamma nail and the sliding hip screw for the treatment of 100 intertrochanteric hip fractures found no difference with respect to operating time, blood loss, duration of hospital stay, infection rate, wound complications, implant failure, screw cut out, or screw sliding. The major difference was that four Gamma nail patients sustained femoral shaft fractures at the nail tip or at the distal locking bolts. The Gamma nail may be best used in the treatment of comminuted intertrochanteric fractures with subtrochanteric extension, reverse obliquity fractures, or high subtrochanteric fractures. However, additional clinical studies are necessary to show the efficacy of the device over those already available.

Prosthetic Replacement

Prosthetic replacement for intertrochanteric fractures has been used successfully to treat postoperative loss of fixation when repeat open reduction and internal fixation is not possible or desirable. A calcar replacement prosthesis is necessary because of the fracture level. The role of primary prosthetic replacement for the treatment of unstable intertrochanteric hip fractures remains unclear. Primary replacement of comminuted unstable intertrochanteric fracture has the theoretical advantage of allowing early full weightbearing and rapid rehabilitation (Fig. 4). Its disadvantages include a more extensive surgical procedure and the potential for dislocation. Two series reported good results using a bipolar hemiarthroplasty for the treatment of unstable intertrochanteric fractures. However, neither was a prospective, randomized study comparing hemiarthroplasty with the use of the sliding hip screw.

Subtrochanteric Fractures

Subtrochanteric fractures account for approximately 15% of all proximal femur fractures. These fractures start at or below the lesser trochanter and involve the proximal femoral shaft. They are generally seen in three groups: young patients with normal bones involved in high-energy trauma; older patients with weakened bone whose fracture is the result of a minor fall; and older patients with pathologic or impending pathologic fractures from metastatic lesions. The subtrochanteric area experiences some of the highest biomechanical stresses in the body. The medial and posteromedial cortex is a

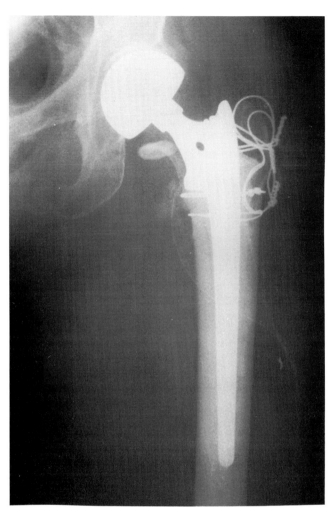

Fig. 4 Calcar replacement hemiarthroplasty can be considered for primary treatment of intertrochanteric fractures in selected cases. However, it is usually reserved as a salvage procedure following failed internal fixation.

site of high compressive forces, while the lateral cortex experiences high tensile stresses. This stress distribution has important implications in fracture fixation and healing.

Fracture stability is based on the presence or absence of a posteromedial buttress. In stable fractures, medial and posteromedial cortical support is intact or can be reestablished. In unstable fractures, comminution results in loss of medial cortical continuity. These fractures present the highest risk for healing complications and implant failure.

Among the various implants available for surgical management of subtrochanteric fractures are intramedullary devices, sliding hip screws, and plate or screw assemblies. Intramedullary devices were a significant improvement over rigid nail-plates. Available devices include the Zickel nail, Ender nails, and interlocking

rods, although the Zickel nail has been used most extensively. Insertion was initially described as an open procedure with exposure of the fracture site. For unstable fractures, supplemental fixation (cerclage wires) is necessary to restore stability and prevent shortening. When significant medial comminution is present, bone grafting should be performed. This procedure also can be performed using a closed technique, which avoids exposure of the fracture site and also might shorten operating time and decrease blood loss and postoperative morbidity.

Removal of the Zickel nail has also caused problems. At the time of nail removal, a small but significant number of patients developed a subtrochanteric fracture at a level different from that of the original fracture. This complication may require reevaluation of the use of the Zickel nail in younger patients, in whom the nail can be expected to be removed eventually.

The results of Ender nailing of subtrochanteric fractures continued to be varied. Early reoperation rate has ranged from 10% to 32%. Interlocking nails have been used for subtrochanteric fractures when the lesser trochanter remains attached to the proximal fragment. Since the development of second generation nails, comminution around the trochanters is no longer a strict contraindication to the use of intramedullary devices.

Sliding hip screws also have been used for the treatment of subtrochanteric fractures. One series reported a rate of union at 95%. For this device to function optimally, the sliding component must cross the fracture site. Therefore, subtrochanteric or intertrochanteric fractures are most suitable for this device. More distal fractures can be treated using a 95-degree fixed angle plate. This device improves the fixation of the proximal fragment and acts as a lateral tension band if the medial cortex is intact. Indirect reduction of bony fragments with minimal soft-tissue striping may optimize the treatment of these difficult fractures by maintaining the vascular supply to comminuted fragments. If medial cortical comminution is present, bone grafting should be performed.

Postoperative management depends on fracture pattern and method of fixation. For subtrochanteric or intertrochanteric fractures treated with a sliding hip screw that allows impaction at the fracture site, weightbearing may be started early. Stable fractures treated with intramedullary devices also can be treated with early weightbearing. Fractures with medial or segmental comminution must be protected, regardless of the device used, for at least six to eight weeks until early healing is radiographically evident.

Pathologic fractures and impending pathologic fractures in the subtrochanteric region have been treated successfully with Zickel nailing, both with and without adjunctive methylmethacrylate. Insertion via a closed technique has been particularly beneficial for the treatment of impending fractures in this patient population. The Zickel nail provides the benefits of proximal fixation with an intramedullary rod that can bridge more distal lesions.

Annotated Bibliography

Hip Dislocation

Brumback RJ, Holt ES, McBride MS, et al: Acetabular depression fracture accompanying posterior fracture dislocation of the hip. *J Orthop Trauma* 1990;4:42-48.

Seventy-five posterior fracture-dislocations of the hip were retrospectively reviewed. An acetabular depression fracture was identified in 17 cases (23%), primarily by computed tomographic scanning. Preoperatively, each of these injuries demonstrated posterior instability with hip flexion less than 90 degrees. Treatment consisted of fragment disimpaction and reduction, bone grafting, and stabilization.

Vailas JC, Hurwitz S, Wiesel SW: Posterior acetabular fracture-dislocations: Fragment size, joint capsule, and stability. *J Trauma* 1989;29:1494-1496.

In a study involving 22 cadaveric specimens, the authors removed increasing amounts of the posterior wall, leaving the joint capsule intact. The amount of posterior wall remaining was measured by computed tomography. Fragments involving less than 25% of the posterior wall did not affect joint stability; those involving more than 50% resulted in instability. The significance of transitional fragments (25% to 50% of the posterior wall) was determined by the stability provided by posterior capsule.

Hip Fractures

Risk Factors

Cummings SR, Nevitt MC: A hypothesis: The causes of hip fractures. *J Gerontol* 1989;44:M107-111.

The authors propose that the exponential increase in the incidence of hip fracture with aging has causes other than just osteoporosis and increasing falls. They identified four preconditions for a hip fracture: (1) a fall oriented to impact near the hip; (2) failure of protective responses; (3) inadequate energy absorption by soft tissues to prevent fracture; and (4) residual energy of the fall exceeding the strength of the bone. The authors suggest modes of study and preventive measures aimed at each step in the sequence of events from fall to hip fracture.

Ferris BD, Kennedy C, Bhamra M, et al: Morphology of the femur in proximal femoral fractures. *J Bone Joint Surg* 1989;71B:475-477.

This study compared the morphology of proximal femur in patients with femoral neck fractures, intertrochanteric fractures, and unilateral osteoarthritis. Patients with intertrochanteric fractures had a significantly shorter femoral neck than did those with femoral neck fractures or osteoarthritis.

Thromboembolic Disease

Froehlich JA, Dorfman GS, Cronan JJ, et al: Compression ultrasonography for the detection of deep venous thrombosis in patients who have a fracture of the hip: A prospective study. *J Bone Joint Surg* 1989;71A:249-256.

The effectiveness of compression ultrasonography in the detection of femoral and popliteal venous thrombosis was prospectively evaluated and compared with standard venography. The incidence of venous thrombosis in 112 hip fractures (detected by venography) was 12.5%. The compression ultrasonic technique had an accuracy of 97%, a sensitivity of 100%, and a specificity of 97%.

Femoral Neck Fractures

Chen SC, Badrinath K, Pell LH, et al: The movements of the components of the Hastings bipolar prosthesis: A radiographic study in 65 patients. *J Bone Joint Surg* 1989;71B:186-188.

In 65 patients, nonweightbearing movement of the Hastings bipolar prosthesis was assessed radiographically; in 70% of patients, the only movement was between the acetabulum and the prosthetic shell, representing the equivalent of a unipolar prosthesis.

Emery RJ, Broughton NS, Desai K, et al: Bipolar hemiarthroplasty for subcapital fracture of the femoral neck: A prospective randomised trial of cemented Thompson and uncemented Moore stems. *J Bone Joint Surg* 1991;73B:322-324.

This prospective randomized study compared cemented Thompson with noncemented Moore hemiarthroplasties. Differences in operating time and blood loss were not significant. Results at follow-up favored the use of a cemented prosthesis; 68% of the cemented prostheses were painless 1.5 years after surgery compared with only 20% of the noncemented group. Deterioration of ambulatory status was greater in the noncemented group: 80% vs 42%.

Franzén H, Nilsson LT, Strömqvist B, et al: Secondary total hip replacement after fractures of the femoral neck. *J Bone Joint Surg* 1990;72B:784-787.

The rate of revision in 84 consecutive total hip replacements performed for failed osteosynthesis of femoral neck fractures was compared with that of primary arthroplasty for osteoarthritis. The age- and sex-adjusted risk of prosthetic failure was 2.5 times higher after failure of fixation.

Greenough CG, Jones JR: Primary total hip replacement for displaced subcapital fracture of the femur. *J Bone Joint Surg* 1988;70B:639-643.

In this series, 37 patients younger than 70 years of age who had displaced femoral fractures and no preexisting degenerative changes of the acetabulum underwent primary total hip replacement. At average follow-up of 56 months, 49% had undergone or were awaiting revision. An additional 11% had radiographic signs of loosening.

Harper WM, Barnes MR, Gregg PJ: Femoral head blood flow in femoral neck fractures: An analysis using intra-osseous pressure measurement. *J Bone Joint Surg* 1991;73B:73-75.

The authors studied 50 patients with femoral neck fractures (33 intracapsular and 17 extracapsular) and analyzed the intraosseous and intracapsular pressures using transducers. The mean intracapsular pressure was lower in the extracapsular fractures. In these, the mean intraosseous pressure in the femoral head was unchanged by joint aspiration. In intracapsular fractures, however, joint aspiration produced a significant decrease in intraosseous pressure and an increase in pulse pressure (a measure of bone blood flow) within the femoral head. This study confirms the usefulness of hip joint aspiration following fracture, possibly reducing the incidence of osteonecrosis.

Holder LE, Schwarz C, Wernicke PG, et al: Radionuclide bone imaging in the early detection of fractures of the proximal femur (hip): Multifactorial analysis. *Radiology* 1990;174:509-515.

The authors report the results of 179 radionucleotide bone scans, 105 of which were collected retrospectively from the records of 97 patients referred for assessment of suspected hip fracture and 74 performed prospectively on 63 patients with a diagnosis of either definite or suspected hip fracture. Thirty-one examinations were performed within 24 hours of injury. For the diagnosis of hip fracture in any individual patient, sensitivity was 93.3%; specificity, 95.0%; positive predictive value, 91.8%; and negative predictive value, 96.0%. For the subgroup of patients with normal or equivocal radiographs, the sensitivity was 97.8% with a specificity of 95.0%. The authors conclude that bone scans are an effective method of identifying suspected hip fractures regardless of patient age or time after injury.

LaBelle LW, Colwill JC, Swanson AB: Bateman bipolar hip arthroplasty for femoral neck fractures: A five- to ten-year follow-up study. *Clin Orthop* 1990;251:20-25.

A retrospective study of 49 cemented Bateman bipolar hemiarthroplasties followed for an average of 7.5 years reported that 52% had acetabular erosion of 1 to 2 mm, and 18% had femoral subsidence of at least 2 mm. Survivorship analysis revealed a failure rate of 10.4% at 7.5 years. Femoral stem loosening was attributed to inadequate cement technique (only five cement restrictors were used in this series).

Neustadt JB, Tronzo R, Hozack WJ, et al: Femoral neck fractures: A biomechanical study of a new form of internal fixation using multiple telescoping variable length compression screws. *Clin Orthop* 1989;248:181-188.

The authors introduce a new form of fixation for femoral neck fractures, which utilizes the principles of the sliding hip screw. In a biomechanical study, the variable length compression screws provided a significantly higher load-to-failure than Asnis screws in osteoporotic bone. However, no significant difference was found in normal bone.

Phillips TW: Thompson hemiarthroplasty and acetabular erosion. *J Bone Joint Surg* 1989;71A:913-917.

Acetabular erosion was measured in 72 hips treated with cemented Thompson hemiarthroplasties. Follow-up averaged 7.7 years. Acetabular erosion was correlated with level of activity and duration of follow-up, occurring in 34 of 38 active patients and in none of the 34 inactive patients. Severity of erosion increased with time, but only in active patients. The Thompson hemiarthroplasty had consistently good results in inactive patients.

Rehnberg L, Olerud C: The stability of femoral neck fractures and its influence on healing. *J Bone Joint Surg* 1989;71B:173-177.

This study measured the stability of screw fixation in 41 patients with femoral neck fractures, investigated the influence of fracture impaction on stability, and correlated perioperative stability with clinical results. Stability was measured intraoperatively using a metal strain gauge probe anchored in the subchondral bone of the femoral head. Fractures with early loss of fixation or nonunion had significantly poorer stability than the fractures that had healed. Impaction at surgery improved stability in 23 of 41 fractures; in the others, impaction decreased stability or was unchanged.

Speer KP, Spritzer CE, Harrelson JM, et al: Magnetic resonance imaging of the femoral head after acute intracapsular fracture of the femoral neck. *J Bone Joint Surg* 1990;72A:98-103.

Magnetic resonance imaging of the femoral head was performed within 48 hours of injury in 15 patients who had a subcapital fracture of the femoral neck (12 displaced and 3 nondisplaced) but it did not identify osteonecrosis of the femoral head in any patient. Based on the anticipated incidence of osteonecrosis in a large series, the probability that osteonecrosis would not develop in any of the displaced fractures is 4%. The authors conclude that magnetic resonance imaging is inadequate to determine the inability of the femoral head within 48 hours of injury. They postulate that the factors resulting in the normal scans are the relative paucity of hematopoietic elements in the femoral head and the lack of adequate time for a repair response to develop.

Wetherell RG, Hinves BL: The Hastings bipolar hemiarthroplasty for subcapital fractures of the femoral neck: A 10-year prospective study. *J Bone Joint Surg* 1990;72B:788-793.

In a ten-year prospective study, 561 patients were treated with a Hastings bipolar hemiarthroplasty for a displaced femoral neck. In 243 hips followed for at least one year, 14 (5.6%) showed acetabular erosion. In 91 patients followed for three years or longer (mean, 4.8 years), 95% had slight or no hip pain.

Intertrochanteric Fractures

Apel DM, Patwardhan A, Pinzur MS, et al: Axial loading studies of unstable intertrochanteric fractures of the femur. *Clin Orthop* 1989;246:156-164.

An experimental four-part, unstable intertrochanteric hip fracture was created with either a large or small posteromedial fragment (PMF). Load studies were performed in 68 embalmed femora after fixation. In the presence of a large posteromedial fragment, anatomic reduction and fixation allowed the femur to resist an average maximum load that was 57% greater than identical fractures with the fragment excluded. Fixation of the small posteromedial fragment increased construct strength by an average of 17% over no fixation. The authors concluded that when anatomic reduction is possible, fixation of the posteromedial fragment becomes progressively more critical as its size increases.

Bridle SH, Patel AD, Bircher M, et al: Fixation of intertrochanteric fractures of the femur: A randomised prospective comparison of the gamma nail and the dynamic hip screw. *J Bone Joint Surg* 1991;73B:330-334.

The study compared the results of fixation of 100 intertrochanteric hip fractures using the dynamic hip screw and Gamma nail but could not confirm the proposed advantages of the Gamma nail (decreased operative time, blood loss, infection rate, and implant failure rate). The major finding was a significant incidence of femur fractures at the nail tip or distal locking bolts when the Gamma nail was used.

Hopkins CT, Nugent JT, Dimon JH III: Medial displacement osteotomy for unstable intertrochanteric fractures: Twenty years later. *Clin Orthop* 1989;245:169-172.

Fifty-five unstable intertrochanteric fractures fixed with a sliding hip screw were reviewed; 37 cases were treated by anatomic reduction and 18 by primary medial displacement osteotomy. Eighty-nine percent of anatomically reduced fractures collapsed into a medially displaced position, 97% healing without complications. The authors conclude that medial displacement osteotomy has no advantage over anatomic reduction.

Meislin RJ, Zuckerman JD, Kummer FJ, et al: A biomechanical analysis of the sliding hip screw: The question of plate angle. *J Orthop Trauma* 1990;4:130-136.

   This cadaver-based biomechanical cadaver study analyzed the effects of plate angle on proximal femoral strain distribution in stable and unstable intertrochanteric fractures. There was no statistical difference in strain disruption among plate angles ranging from 130 degrees to 150 degrees although there were mechanical complications with the 130-degree and 150-degree plates. The 130-degree plate had a tendency to jam during testing of unstable fractures while the 150-degree plate had a propensity for cut out. The authors conclude that the 135-degree or 140-degree plates are preferable for the fixation of intertrochanteric fractures.

43

Hip: Adult Joint Reconstruction

Orthopaedic Knowledge Update 1 summarized information published until mid-1982. The early good results of cemented total hip replacement and the significant complications occurring with hip replacement were discussed, and the initial results obtained with revision total hip replacement were reported. *Orthopaedic Knowledge Update 2* covered information published up to mid-1986. It focused primarily on complications and long-term results with cemented total hip replacement, and contained an initial discussion of the first phases of uncemented arthroplasty of the hip. In reviewing information published until 1989, *Orthopaedic Knowledge Update 3* again focused on cemented and uncemented total hip replacements, contained more extensive material on revision total hip replacements, and included a section on hip reconstruction without implants. That chapter concluded with controversies, including the causes of loosening in cemented total hip replacement, indications for cemented versus uncemented total hip replacement, autografts versus allografts, and the treatment of osteonecrosis.

This chapter covers information published from 1989 through 1991 and is again focused on the long-term results of total hip replacement, the controversy of primary cemented versus uncemented total hip replacement, and the complexities of revision total hip replacement surgery.

Cemented Total Hip Replacement

Long-term Follow-up

Clinical studies show dramatic results in the first two years after total hip replacement, with a very low incidence of death (0.1% to 0.5%), infection (0.5% to 4%), and mechanical problems necessitating revision surgery (less than 5%). Studies of five years showed an increased incidence of mechanical loosening. At ten to 15 years, loosening emerges as the most common complication. Two categories of loosening have been identified in long-term studies: radiologic and clinical. Clinical loosening describes those hips that are significantly painful and frequently require revision surgery. Partly because different authors have defined it differently, the reported incidence of radiologic loosening has ranged from 10% to 40%. All authors agree that a change in the position of the prosthesis represents definite radiologic loosening. Most also agree that a circumferential radiolucency of 2 mm or more surrounding the acetabular cup or circumferential lucency around the femoral component represent probable radiologic loosening. Possible radiologic loosening usually has been defined as incomplete radio-

lucent lines around either the femoral or acetabular component that encompass up to 50% of the bone-cement interface. Clearly, the most definitive radiologic sign of loosening of the prosthetic component, other than actual change of position of the component itself, is a progressively enlarging radiolucent line on serial radiographs.

Table 1 (from OKU 3) summarizes data published before 1989 from several long-term follow-up studies of cemented total hip replacements. Since then, a study of the first 333 consecutive Charnley total hip arthroplasties performed at a major institution and followed a minimum of 15 years revealed that 80% of the living patients had no pain. On the basis of radiographic evaluation, the probability of loosening was 3% one year after surgery, 13% five years after surgery, 19% at ten years, and 32% at 15 years. The probability of failure based on a need for revision or symptomatic loosening was 0.9% at one year, 4.1% at five years, 8.9% at ten years, and 12.7% at 15 years.

Long-term studies reflect the outcome of surgical techniques and experience, and the prosthesis and patient-selection decisions of the early 1970s. The early choice of available prostheses had significant bearing on long-term outcome. For example, in contrast to 12.7% revision and 32% radiologic loosening for Charnley prostheses at 15 years, a shorter ten-year follow-up of first generation curved stem Mueller prostheses revealed a revision rate of 20% and signs suggestive of radiologic loosening in 40% (Figs. 1 and 2).

Improved Surgical Techniques and Prosthesis Designs

Improvements in the Femoral Prosthesis Numerous laboratory and clinical studies have addressed improvement in design and materials composition of the femoral prosthesis. Super alloys of forged cobalt chromium and titanium have fatigue strengths several times greater than those of earlier stainless steel or cast alloys of cobalt chromium. Published clinical case reports of stem breakage with these new metals are rare, indicating that the use of these stronger metals markedly decreases the incidence of stem breakage. Results of geometric design laboratory studies, including three-dimensional finite stress analyses, support eliminating sharp corners of the prosthesis and broadening the femoral component in the anteroposterior dimension to distribute stresses to the cement more broadly. Autopsy material from 16 cemented total hip replacements that were functioning well clinically up to 17 years after insertion had microfractures in the cement and the junction of sharp corners of the prostheses.

Table 1. Long-term follow-up studies of cemented total hip replacements

Site of Study	No. of Hips	Follow-up (yrs)	Revision Rate (%)	Radiographic Failure Rate (%)
New York	100	15	9	13
Exeter	426	11 to 16	11	65
California	700	14	17	54
California	479	11	8	21F; 45 A*
New York	122	11	12	25
Eugene	156	12	15	20
San Francisco	100	15 to 17	16	20
Sweden	325	10 to 14	14	50
Wrightington	116	15 to 21	"Very low"	52
Wrightington†	49	10 to 15	18	26
South Africa	98	12	15	12

*F, femoral; A, acetabular.
†Patients less than 30 years old.

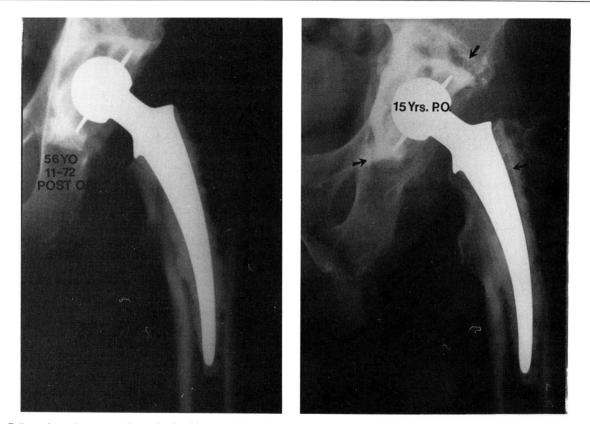

Fig. 1 Failure of poorly cemented prosthesis with poor design characteristics. **Left**, A 56-year-old male six weeks after receiving a Mueller prosthesis. Minimal cement was used, especially distally, and the prosthesis is positioned in varus. **Right**, Fifteen years later, both components are loose with large radiologic lucencies around cup and stem and change of position. Patient has pain that requires revision surgery.

Data are inconclusive regarding the appropriate modulus of elasticity of the femoral component. A high modulus (stiffer material such as cobalt chrome) will increase stresses in the stem and decrease stresses in the cement. Transfer of the stress into the distal stem might stress shield the proximal femur and lead to disuse bone resorption. A lower modulus (more flexible material such as titanium) can increase stress on the proximal bone but might also increase the stress on, and thus fatigue, the proximal cement increasing the incidence of loosening. Laboratory studies establish that a more flexible stem stresses the cement more. However, the use of femoral components large enough to fill the femoral canal may result in stems of such large cross-sectional area and, thus, of such rigidity that elastic modulus differences may be inconsequential in the clinical setting.

Improvements in the Acetabular Component In the early 1980s, laboratory studies indicated that metal backing of cemented polyethylene acetabular components would re-

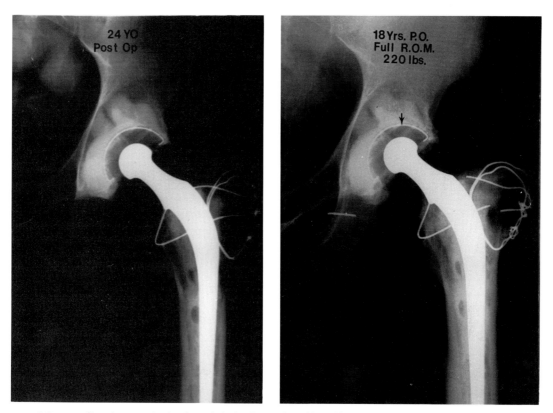

Fig. 2 Long-term follow-up. Charnley prosthesis of good design in good position with reasonable cement technique. **Left,** Immediate postoperative revision of a painful hemiarthroplasty. **Right,** Eighteen years later in a heavy active male, the only findings are 2 mm of acetabular polyethylene wear.

duce peak stresses in the cement and trabecular bone. Results of subsequent clinical studies have failed to meet expectations. In one clinical study, the radiologic failure rate increased when the surgeon changed from a non-metal-backed to a metal-backed acetabular component; the surgeon concluded that cemented metal-backed components should not be used.

Bearing Surfaces

The material for the bearing surface of the acetabular component is of major concern. To date, polyethylene has been the most frequently used material. Recently, a polyethylene material with straighter molecular chains has been introduced with the idea that it will have better wear characteristics, but clinical experience has been limited. To date, attempts to use ceramics have resulted in significantly higher acetabular loosening rates. Because many of these cups have been nonhemispherical or fixed to bone with large external threads, this increased loosening has resulted from the geometric design of the cup and its fixation to bone rather than from the bearing surface. Certainly, ceramic materials are harder and will have less wear than polyethylene. One study from France

indicates that coupling alumina/alumina acetabular and femoral surfaces resulted in a 94% probability of keeping the prosthesis for eight years in a group of 76 patients less than 50 years of age. In several studies, titanium has been shown to be an inappropriate bearing surface against polyethylene. Two recent reports of favorable long-term use of metal-on-metal bearing surfaces in Europe suggest that early bad results with these surfaces may have resulted from the prosthetic design and not the bearing surface.

Prosthesis Selection and Placement The femoral stem should be placed in neutral or slight valgus. The acetabular component must be positioned in the anatomic position at the level of the true notch to reduce stresses and increase longevity. Orientation of the cemented cup so that it is contained by surrounding bone has significant implications for long-term results. In one study of nearly 1,100 hips, cups completely contained by bone had a significantly lower incidence of complete cement-bone radiolucencies and of wear (p = 0.02 and 0.09, respectively). The authors concluded that vertical cup orientation (>55 degrees) with full bony coverage was better than more horizontal orientation with only partial bone containment. Dislocation in these vertically oriented cups was not a problem, but there is a possibility of increased polyethylene wear.

In another study of 385 hips followed at least 9.5 years, the least wear on the polyethylene occurred when a femoral head diameter of 28 mm was used. The greatest amount of linear wear occurred in the 22-mm components. The greatest volumetric wear and mean rate of wear were seen in 32-mm components. There also seemed to be a greater resorption at the proximal femur in hips in which volumetric wear was calculated to be the greatest; this was postulated to be a reaction to polyethylene debris. Uncemented acetabular components, used routinely by many surgeons, are discussed later in this chapter.

Optimal Cementing Technique   Reports suggest slower mixing of the cement over a shorter time decreases the air voids within cement and thus improves the strength characteristics. The physical characteristics of polymethylmethacrylate are markedly improved by centrifugation. In one study, there was a 24% increase in ultimate tensile strength, a 54% improvement in mean ultimate tensile strain, and a 136% increase in mean fatigue life. Mixing the cement under vacuum with reduced pressure also decreased retained air and increased cement strength. Results of one laboratory study established that different brands of polymethylmethacrylate respond differently to vacuum mixing and that chilling of the monomer significantly alters the working time and intrusion qualities.

To prepare the bone bed for the cement, loose cancellous bone debris, blood, and tissue are removed. The femoral cortex should not be perforated, and the acetabular subchondral bone should be preserved. Cleansing the bone bed with a water pick is helpful, and routine mechanical drying of both acetabular and femoral surfaces is important. Applying a dilute solution of adrenaline with a moist sponge helps prevent blood interposition. Some authors also use hypotensive anesthesia to reduce blood at the bone cement interface during cementing. Mechanical compression of the cement to facilitate its intrusion into the bony bed is important. This compression can be facilitated on the femoral side by distally plugging the canal with Silastic, polyethylene, bone, or cement, and delivering the cement with a syringe to allow retrograde filling and better pressurization. In one study of 105 hip replacements done using cement in the doughy stage, plugging of the femoral canal, retrograde cement injection, and a femoral component of improved design, after follow-up of ten to 12.7 years, authors found only three definitely loose femoral components. Despite anatomic positioning and good cementing techniques, the radiologic failure rate of the acetabular component was 42%.

Uncemented Total Hip Replacement

The findings of a significant need for revision and serious loss of bone stock on long-term follow-up of cemented total hip arthroplasty have led to heavy use of uncemented total hip replacements in the 1980s. Because none of these uncemented systems has been subjected to the long-term follow-up of the cemented systems, the results are not directly comparable (Table 2). Although the most popular femoral components have a porous ingrowth surface, a few surgeons have used a smooth surface press-fitted stem. After four- to five-year follow-up (average of 4.8 years) of 39 such hips, only one hip was revised for femoral loosening. These implants require aggressive femoral canal filling, which increases the risk of fracture of the femur during insertion. Results of previous studies in dental science establish that bone grows directly on the metal nonporous surfaces. Smooth implants potentially decrease the problems of particle debris formation as compared with the microstructured surfaces.

Most uncemented devices used in the United States have a microporous surface with ideal pore size reported as 200 to 500 microns (Fig. 3). Design appears to be an especially critical factor in these prosthetic components. For example, a number of centers report significant failure rates with attempts to use peripherally threaded screw-in type cups, even if they have porous surfaces. In one European study, a 33% loosening rate was reported for 100 hips in which large-threaded type screw-in cups were inserted between 1980 and 1985. Similar dismal results were reported from the United States. Eleven of 27 hip replacement patients with a self-locking, nonhemispherical threaded ceramic cup, who were followed up for an average of 51 months, complained of enough pain to limit activities, although only three hips had been revised.

Early clinical success has been reported for numerous designs of hemispheric porous-ingrowth noncemented cups. Surface materials used include cobalt beads, titanium mesh, and plasma spray material. Many short-term successful results have been reported for such cups that were fixed to the pelvis with rigid hemispheric press fitting, often supplemented with screw, fin, or lug fixation.

The newer uncemented systems have had the most questionable results, predominantly on the femoral side. Most developers of uncemented porous-surfaced femoral components have reported early (three- to seven-year) good results; however, other investigators using the same prosthesis have not always confirmed these good results. Nearly all porous-surfaced systems have had an incidence of thigh pain ranging from 5% to 25%. This thigh pain has been characterized as start-up pain and ranges from a very mild pain that does not limit activity to a disabling discomfort. In the majority of hips, it diminishes in intensity after a year or two. Many investigators have found it difficult to correlate radiologic findings with this thigh pain.

Table 2. Results of cementless total hip replacement

| Site of study | Prosthesis | | Follow-up (yrs) | Comments |
	Type	No.		
Washington, D.C.	PCA	50	>2	Pain, 16%; limp, 28%
Multicenter	PCA	118	>2	Pain, 4%; limp, 5%; failed, 6%
Arlington	AML	100	1	Pain, 14%; limp, 21%
Boston	HGP	—	1	Pain, 5%; limp, 9%
	Isoelastic	34	3.5	Revised, 32%

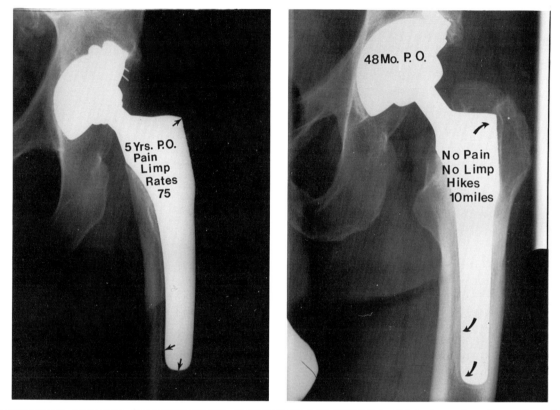

Fig. 3 Similar radiographic findings: One patient with pain, another without. **Left**, Patient five years postoperative with prosthesis tipped in varus and reactive sclerotic radiodense line and distal density with significant pain and limp. **Right**, Another patient four years postoperatively has similar radiographic findings but has no pain or limp.

If a reactive sclerotic line is seen parallel to the porous metal surface, the fixation is probably fibrous rather than bony ingrowth. A sclerotic pedicle of bone distal to the tip of the stem also suggests lack of bone ingrowth. Densification and bridging of the bone between the cortex and porous ingrowth surfaces suggests bone ingrowth fixation. The bone proximal to these areas may atrophy, presumably because it is stress shielded. Radiographic confirmation of lack of bone ingrowth exists when the prosthesis either has subsided measurably or is noted to have divergent sclerotic lines surrounding the stem. These findings usually correlate with clinical symptoms (Fig. 4).

Two different geometric designs of uncemented porous ingrowth stems have been used—curved and straight stems. The curved-stem prostheses are considered anatomic, because they fit to the anatomic bow of the proximal femur. When using the straight stems, the surgeon machines the curved bony anatomy to fit the prosthesis. Primary fixation to bone of either curved or straight stems is obtained in two ways: proximal fixation with wedge fitting in the metaphyseal region and diaphyseal fixation, which requires a significantly longer prosthesis. Results were reported for 64 diaphyseal-fixed prostheses and 20 metaphyseal (anatomic) prostheses. The diaphyseal-fixed prostheses had been in place 36 months, and the curved prostheses 40 months; recipients were of similar age groups. Both the diaphyseal and metaphyseal fixed prostheses had a 30% incidence of thigh pain. Radiographically, however, no component was thought to

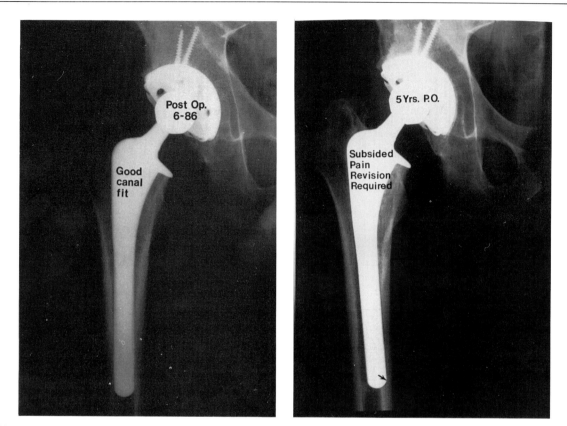

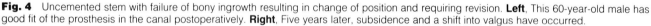

Fig. 4 Uncemented stem with failure of bony ingrowth resulting in change of position and requiring revision. **Left**, This 60-year-old male has good fit of the prosthesis in the canal postoperatively. **Right**, Five years later, subsidence and a shift into valgus have occurred.

demonstrate complete radiolucency and all were thought to have radiographic evidence of bone ingrowth. The authors concluded that these results were inferior to those for cemented total hip placement. Later, the same authors reported only an 8% incidence of significant pain using their own noncemented prosthetic design.

The uncemented prosthesis in longest clinical use is a diaphyseal-fitted, long, straight-stemmed prosthesis. At ten years, 959 primary arthroplasties show a 96% survivorship of the femoral component. When radiographic loosening is added to revision, the survivorship is 90.8%. There were no radiographic failures in prostheses that filled the entire canal and were bony ingrowth. These large stems do, however, increase the potential of proximal stress shielding, and 75% revealed this radiographic finding. Fortunately, less than 5% had a severe degree of stress shielding. In 110 stems thought not to be fixed by bone ingrowth, survivorship rate when revision and radiologic loosening were added was 51.3%.

Hybrid Total Hip Replacement

Improvements in implant design and cementing technique have not improved the results of cemented acetabular components. This knowledge, coupled with the infrequent failures seen in the early (three- to eight-year)

results with porous surfaced hemispheric cups fixed by accurate, secure, press-fitting into the acetabular bone stock, has led many surgeons to use this type of cup component in most total hip replacement. These cups have been successful with both titanium and cobalt chrome porous surfaces. Auxiliary fixation with pegs, screws, and fins is frequently used.

Improved implant design and cementing technique have clearly improved the results of cemented femoral components. This improvement, coupled with the inability of many surgeons to obtain excellent early results in their patients with uncemented components as compared with cemented stems, has led many researchers to recommend use of a cemented system on the femoral side in older patients. The definition of older has varied from over 50 years of age to over 70, but the most usual has been 60 years of age. In one study, cemented, uncemented, and hybrid prostheses were followed prospectively for two to four years. Fifty-two cemented prostheses had hip ratings of 91 points and 42 hybrid prostheses had ratings of 90. Sixty-five hips that were uncemented on both acetabular and femoral sides had ratings of 95. However, two uncemented stems had aseptic loosening and one of these required revision; 24% had slight but nondisabling thigh pain. In another study, 126 hybrid total hips were followed up a minimum of two years and a mean of 42 months in patients who underwent surgery at an average age of 63 years. Pain was rated as none or slight in 94% of the cases. No components were revised and radiographic examination found no femoral component definitely or probably loose. The authors concluded that the selective use of cement provided excellent results at 5.5 years.

Comparison of the early results of these new methods of hip replacement is nearly impossible. One author indicated that in order to have large enough groups to show statistical differences, assuming that uncemented hips had a lack of early biologic fixation rate in 1% of the patients and a revision rate of 0.5% per year, a five-year study would have to include at least 1,400 hips if the cemented group had a 1% failure rate per year. A ten-year evaluation would require 350 hips in each group. Another author stated that with two different prostheses and failure rates of 3% and 5%, it would take 2,960 hips to obtain a significance level of 0.05.

Total Hip Replacement in Young People

Clearly, the heavier use to which young people subject their hips and the increased years of use place greater demands on a hip joint replacement in a young person. In an initial study of cemented total hip replacements in patients younger than 30 years, there was a 57% failure rate as early as five years following surgery. Subsequent authors have clearly indicated that patients younger than 30 are at extreme risk of failure, but found more favorable results in patients in their 30s and 40s. In a series from a large institution, the success rate for cemented total hip replacements in patients under 45 years of age was 77% at 4.5 years follow-up. However, when this same group of patients was followed to an average of 9.2 years, the revision rate had tripled from 11% to 33%, and 56% of the remaining hips were on the verge of failure. The initial study of these hips suggests results depended on the original operative technique, but this was not confirmed with the latest study. In a series of 51 cemented total hip replacements followed for 12 to 18 years, there was a 69% survivorship of the prosthesis at 14.9 years.

Currently, most surgeons suggest that uncemented femoral components be used for patients younger than 60 years of age. The longest published follow-up of uncemented total hip replacements in younger people is of 150 hips in patients younger than 40 years of age who had extensively coated large diaphyseal-fitted femoral components. Only three stems required revision. Survivorship analysis, with revision as the end point, found a 94.9% survivorship at seven years.

In the 1970s and early 1980s, surface arthroplasty was thought by many to be the most appropriate replacement for young patients, but failure rates as high as 70% are now reported. Before any replacement prosthesis is used in young people, alternatives of osteotomy, fusion, or nonsurgical care must be considered carefully.

Custom Implants

The difficulty of fitting the component in the femoral canal has led some investigators to develop custom implants. These have not been in use long enough for appropriate follow-up. However, this procedure would seem to be appropriate in certain unusual anatomic circumstances. Cost factors will probably prevent routine use of these prostheses.

Hydroxyapatite

Coating the surface of the metal with materials such as hydroxyapatite is still in its early investigation phases. Two-year follow-up data from Europe suggest rapid bony ingrowth and good early clinical results. Study in the United States has shown excellent early clinical results. The hydroxyapatite must be the appropriate thickness, and commercial technique for bonding to the substrate metal is critical. The possibility certainly exists for fracture or for delamination of the hydroxyapatite from the surface. Adsorption of this material with replacement by fibrous tissue may be found on long-term follow-up. These problems have not been seen in short-term follow-up.

Modularity

Recent designs of both ingrowth and cemented total hip components have led to nearly universal acceptance of modular systems. For successful use of an uncemented polyethylene acetabular component, the metal backing must be in place. Disassociation of the polyethylene material from its metal backing, which has been reported, results in the need for surgical revision. On the femoral side, disassociation of the modular head from the trunnion of the stem has been reported. This construction also poses the problem of fretting and corrosion at the interface of the two parts. In addition, the increased size of the neck portion of the head-neck component, which must fit over the trunnion, may increase the likelihood of impingement, which may cause dislocation.

Total Hip Replacement—Special Problems

Studies have indicated excellent long-term results in patients with rheumatoid arthritis who have undergone total hip replacement. In a recent study of 75 total hip replacements in patients with rheumatoid and juvenile rheumatoid arthritis, who were followed an average of 7.4 years, there were four acetabular revisions and one femoral revision for loosening and four revisions for infection. A survivorship analysis showed 93% survival at seven years, falling to 77% at 12 years. In juvenile rheumatoid arthritis patients, 62 total hip replacements were followed six years with only one revision. In another study of 75 hips, there were two revisions at 5.4 years. Total hip replacement in patients with tuberculosis resulted in reactivation of the disease in 25% according to one report and 14%, another. There was less reactivation if the disease had been inactive for ten years. Eight patients with Paget's disease followed for ten years showed an incidence of 15% aseptic loosening requiring revision and 30% with radiographic evidence of loosening. These numbers were not significantly different from the overall experience with total hip replacement at the same institution. Patients with lupus erythematosus had excellent clinical results, but a higher incidence of delayed wound healing (15%) and wound infection (10%). In Jehovah's Witnesses, patients having total hip replacement did well under hypotensive anesthesia. Of 15 patients with cerebral palsy who had total hip replacements, only two required revision for recurrent dislocation. One other patient had progressive femoral loosening. An early study of total hip replacement following surgical fusion had shown a 33% failure rate at 10.4 years. A recent study of 39 ankylosed hips converted to total hip replacement showed an excellent range of motion. There was a significantly better survivorship of the implant in total hip replacement following spontaneous fusion, with 96% survival at 13 years compared with 62% survival of the implant after only four years in those that had been surgically fused.

Total Hip Replacement for Osteonecrosis

A 37% failure rate was reported for 28 total hip replacements followed an average of 7.6 years. Patients with idiopathic osteonecrosis who avoided alcohol or corticosteroids fared much better than the overall group, with only an 11% failure rate.

In a recent comparative study of 29 patients with osteonecrosis and 63 with osteoarthritis, all of whom had total hip replacements, there were 14 (48%) unsatisfactory clinical results and, radiographically, all showed aseptic component loosening. In another European study following 73 total hip replacements, there was a 10% revision rate at an average of 4.9 years.

Conversion of Osteotomy to Total Hip Replacement

In a recent European study 112 consecutive cemented total hip replacements performed after medial displacement intertrochanteric osteotomy were compared with 262 primary total hip replacements that served as a control. Pain was relieved in 89% of the osteotomy group and 91% of the control group. The femoral component was more frequently in varus position in the control group. Radiographic evidence of migration and radiolucency was similar in the two groups. There was a higher rate of interoperative fracture in the conversion group. The need for revision, 1.5 in the osteotomy group and 0.9% in the control group, was similar in both groups.

In a recent study of 27 patients who had sickle cell anemia with avascular necrosis of the femoral head and who were treated with total hip replacement, there were significant technical difficulties with sclerotic bone and tight medullary canals. These difficulties resulted in four femoral fractures and in a high rate of loosening of both cemented and uncemented prostheses, with a 59% revision rate at 5.5 years.

The most recent data indicate that patients with renal transplants actually fare better following total hip replacement than do those who are undergoing renal dialysis. This is not an unexpected finding, given the significant chance of infection with ongoing dialysis and the markedly variable systemic blood chemistries.

Complications

Infection

Prevention Antimicrobial agents should be given prophylactically when the patient has dental or urologic procedures or any other potential source of bacteremia. However, recent articles and editorials question the scientific evidence for and, therefore, the cost benefit of prophylaxis for dental work. To date, one case has been published in which infection was probably secondary to dental work.

In many total hip replacement series in which prophylactic antimicrobial therapy was used, infection rates were less than 1%. In a large multicenter retrospective study of 8,000 joint replacements in England, use of ultraclean air and body exhaust systems decreased the infection rate to 0.14%. Use of ultraviolet light decreased the incidence of postoperative infection to 0.15% after 1,322 total hip replacements. One recent report indicates that using special nonwoven polyglycal gowns decreased bacteria in the air, but the gowns caused increased heat for the wearer. In another study, a history of previous surgery on the hip, failure to use prophylactic antimicrobial therapy, failure of the surgical wound to heal within three to four weeks, and the presence of postoperative infections elsewhere in the body all were related to an increased incidence of deep wound infection after total hip replacement. Current evidence suggests that the use of antimicrobial agents in the cement in uncomplicated primary total hip replacement decreases the infection in the first year after surgery, but not thereafter. One article reports the development of organisms resistant to gentamicin when it was used prophylactically in cement.

Diagnosis Numerous authors have indicated that unexplained pain after total hip replacement must arouse suspicion of infection. Indium-111 has been reported by some as reliable for making a definitive diagnosis of infection, but its use is being questioned at this time. Aspiration of the joint itself, often under image intensification, remains the most definitive diagnostic test. However, even culture of material taken at operation, which microscopically shows the presence of infected material, fails to grow microorganisms in up to 10% of cases.

Treatment In most patients with chronic infection, surgeons continue to advocate complete removal of the prosthesis and the cement. It is becoming accepted treatment to use antibiotic-impregnated methylmethacrylate beads as an interim procedure before implantation of new prosthetic components. If gross purulence is present, delayed primary or secondary wound closure is appropriate. Primary closure over one or two closed suction drains has proved to be effective in the treatment of an increased total hip arthroplasty in which only granulation (without gross pus) is present. Parenteral antimicrobial therapy is recommended for several weeks, followed by oral therapy for one to several weeks. In one study, such excisional arthroplasty was found to be effective in eradicating infections in 27 of 33 hips. In a study with six-year follow-up after resection arthroplasties, sepsis was controlled in 97% of the patients. Although the patients were left with shortened extremities and the need for external support in walking, the results seemed to improve over time.

Recommendations for timing of the reimplantation vary from several weeks to several months, depending on the extent of the infection, the causal organism, and the surgeon's preference. Most surgeons use gentamicin, tobramycin, or other heat-stable antimicrobial agents with acrylic cement at the time of reimplantation. In all series, gram-negative infections had a poorer prognosis for successful reimplantation. In fact, successful reconstruction can be done earlier (three months) with the less virulent microorganisms. When the causal organism is a gram-negative bacillus, reconstruction should be delayed for 12 months.

Primary exchange arthroplasty, although popular in Europe, has had little advocacy in the United States.

Adequate soft-tissue coverage after resection arthroplasty can be achieved by the use of a vastus lateralis flap. The vastus lateralis is dissected in a distal-to-proximal direction and is vascularized by the descending branch of the lateral femoral circumflex artery, which emerges proximally from beneath the rectus femoris. The distal portion of the vastus lateralis is secured to the acetabular area and the bulk of the muscle can then be rolled into the wound. Primary closure with or without skin grafting over drains completes the procedure.

Heterotopic Ossification

Heterotopic ossification frequently occurs following total hip replacement. Up to 60% of patients show some degree of this complication. Fortunately, the amount of bone formation that occurs usually is not clinically relevant; only 1% to 5% of patients have pain or decreased range of motion secondary to heterotopic bone. Surgical excision is rarely necessary. Patients in high-risk categories, such as men with hypertrophic osteoarthritis, patients with ankylosing spondylitis, or patients in whom previous hip surgery has resulted in heterotopic bone formation may be candidates for prophylaxis against this complication.

Indomethacin (25 mg 3 times daily for six weeks) has been shown in a randomized double-blind study to be significantly effective (p = 0.0005) in preventing heterotopic ossification.

Other anti-inflammatory agents and, possibly, aspirin may also be effective. Because data from animal studies show that these agents also decrease bony ingrowth into porous surface metals, these agents must be used cautiously when this type of prosthetic device is used.

Some studies have shown that low-dose radiation can prevent heterotopic bone in patients who have undergone total hip replacement. Some recent data suggest that very low doses, as low as 600 rads, given in a single dose within three days of surgery can be effective. If bony ingrowth type prostheses have been used, these areas of the prosthesis must be shielded.

Trochanteric Nonunion

An ever-increasing number of surgeons report using the trochanteric osteotomy approach only in the most complicated cases because of problems in obtaining union of the greater trochanter. Approaches have been developed to avoid the complications of nonunion of the trochanter and proximal displacement and subsequent weakness in abduction. Trochanteric slides in which a continuous sleeve of abductor muscle, trochanteric bone, and vastus lateralis muscle origin is displaced have been found to have a very low incidence of abductor dysfunction. Various trochanteric reattachment methods have been described. A special circumferential cable system threaded through a special clamp over the trochanter recently has been reported to be effective in reducing nonunions. However, according to one early report, the use of this method in complex cases resulted in 33% trochanteric nonunion. In this series, use of vertical stainless steel cables rather than circumferential chrome cobalt cable may have led to the high failure rate.

Dislocation

Postoperative dislocation has been reported in 1% to 5% of total hip replacements. In nearly all studies, there was a higher dislocation rate with the posterior approach than with the anterior lateral or transtrochanteric approaches. In recent studies describing improved soft-tissue repair, dislocation rate following the posterior approach was comparable to that for the anterolateral approach. Other causes of postoperative dislocations include malposition of components, failure of the greater trochanter to unite after a trochanteric approach, and failure to obtain adequate leg length. Most dislocations occur in the weeks immediately after surgery and can be treated by simple reduction, with the expectation of lasting stability. Casting or bracing has been reported to be effective, and these methods may allow the patient to regenerate a stabilizing hip capsule. If dislocations recur, surgical treatment may be necessary. When obvious correctable prosthetic positioning or anatomic deficiencies are not present, revision surgery results in dislocation in up to one third of the patients. Late dislocations that occur five to ten years after the operation may represent aging soft-tissue deficiencies and may be very difficult to treat.

Neurovascular

The incidence of sciatic and/or femoral palsies after total hip replacements ranges from 1% to 3% in various series. In a recent study of 3,126 total hip replacements at one institution, incidence of nerve palsy was 1.3% of primary total hip replacement, 3.2% after revision, and 5.2% in total hip replacement for congenitally dislocated hips. Fortunately, the majority of these nerve deficits were partial, and recovery was significant, if not complete. All patients initially retained some motor function or recovered some function while still in the hospital. One electromyographic study showed a 77% incidence of subclinical injury to the superior and inferior gluteal innervated muscles with use of the posterior and lateral approaches.

Intraoperative somatic sensory-evoked potential may be used to monitor the sciatic nerve during total hip arthroplasty. The incidence of sciatic nerve injury is so low that the effectiveness of this method is difficult to demonstrate, and its use should probably be limited to high-risk reconstructive surgery. Arterial injuries, even rarer than neurologic deficits, have been reported in 0.1% to 0.2% of all total hip replacements. Recent studies have established that the use of screws to fix an uncemented cup to the acetabulum represents a special threat to the intrapelvic neurovascular structures. Anatomic dissections have indicated that the anterior and anterosuperior quadrants of the acetabular wall should not be perforated because of their close proximity to the neurovascular structures. One major institution reported 11 neurovascular injuries in orthopaedic procedures over a ten-year period. Only three of the 11 occurred during total hip replacement. These authors concluded that injuries manifested themselves primarily as hemorrhage or ischemia, that excellent results could be obtained with prompt recognition and treatment, and that angiography was useful mainly in those with mild ischemia and those in whom the diagnosis was delayed.

Femur Fractures

Fractures of the femur during total hip replacement can almost always be avoided by careful surgical technique, notably with good exposure, careful hip dislocation, careful use of power tools, and appropriate bone preparation to allow easy insertion of the prosthetic devices. Fractures that occur during surgery are usually treated by using a longer or larger prosthesis, some other form of internal fixation, or both. Most postoperative femoral fractures can be prevented by avoiding injury to the bone during the original hip replacement procedure. Bone lysis from secondary aseptic loosening may significantly compromise the strength of the femur and can lead to eventual fracture (Fig. 5). Fractures distal to the prosthe-

sis may be treated with traction or cast-brace if good alignment can be maintained. If, indeed, the femoral prosthesis is loose, it should be replaced at the time of the fracture. Using a large uncemented prosthesis and obtaining stability in the diaphyseal region is often successful treatment of these fractures. Occasionally bone destruction is such that a large allograft is necessary. A cemented femoral component may be required, particularly in the elderly patient. The use of circumferential large cortical allografts secured with cerclage wiring to support the deficient proximal bone stock has been reported.

Loosening and Failures of Materials and Bone Loss

The most significant and common complication following total hip replacement is loosening of the component and the potential for resultant bone loss. Because of both the long-term use of cemented systems and the inferiority of the early cementing techniques, the most frequently observed form of loosening is that seen with methacrylate failure. Once loose, either at the bone-cement or the prosthesis-cement interface, polymethylmethacrylate is structurally weak and tends to fracture into even smaller pieces. These small pieces produce a histologic response of macrophages and histiocytes, which results in a characteristic synovial-like membrane with few inflammatory cells. Studies of the tissue reveal that it has the capacity to generate interleukin I, prostaglandin E_2, and collagenase and that these may cause the progressive lysis of bone that occurs. Particles of titanium and cobalt chromium were found to produce this histiocytic response, but seemingly to a lesser extent than polymethylmethacrylate. Polyethylene debris may stimulate an even greater response (Fig. 6).

In one study the immunopathologic response of six aggressive granulomatous lesions that caused marked bone osteolysis was compared with that of tissues found with revisions done for common loosening of the prosthetic stem. A relative lack of activated fibroblasts was found in the aggressive lesions, and the authors suggested that these granulomas involved an uncoupling of the normal sequence of monocyte-and macrophage-mediated clearance of tissue debris that is normally followed by a fibroblastic mediated synthesis and remodeling. Particles of titanium and cobalt chromium have also been found in these granulomatous lesions. Large quantities of particulate titanium were found in five patients who underwent revision. Two of 16 hips revised for aggressive granulomatous lesions following cemented total hip replacement had recurrence of the aggressive granulomatous lesions at the original sites 4.5 and 6.5 years after revision. In a further study of six patients with aggressive granulomas around cementless total hip replacement prostheses, the granuloma showed a uniform pathology that included histiocytosis presumably caused by polyethylene debris from acetabular sockets. Fracture of a ceramic head on a femoral component in one study resulted in increased polyethylene wear of the acetabular component. Sixteen

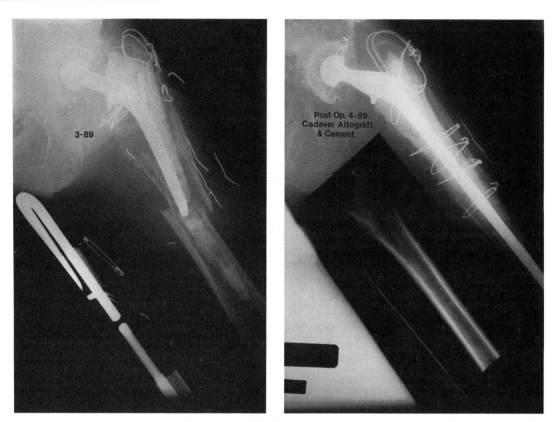

Fig. 5 Recementing a stem using large cadaver allograft. **Left**, This 79-year-old male has marked proximal bone lysis and a fractured femur distally. **Right**, Revision was done with a large cadaver allograft and cement.

cases of femoral osteolysis were found, in a retrospective review of 475 consecutive total hip replacements without cement. Fourteen of the 16 patients had excellent clinical results; two required revision. No osteolysis was identified before two years postoperatively, but in most cases it had appeared by three years.

In a study of 16 postmortem specimens from symptomless patients, it was postulated that the failure of the cemented components was primarily mechanical, starting with debonding at the interface between the cement and the prosthesis and slowly continuing as fractures developed in the cement mantle. A study of 13 femoral titanium alloy components requiring revision for loosening revealed a fibroblastic reaction, with abundant titanium lying free within the histiocytes and scanty foreign body cell reaction.

The body's reaction to foreign materials seems to be basically a granulomatous reaction, and a similar response is seen to cobalt chromium, nickel, methacrylate, and polyethylene. There has been more concern with the long-term debris products of the polyethylene worn from acetabular components, because there appears to be a greater volume of these particles. A definite relationship has been noted between particle size and foreign body reaction; particles smaller than 10 microns seem to incite

the greatest tissue reaction. Smaller particles stimulate a macrophage response; larger particles have a giant cell reaction. Greater reaction may occur where the products of several different materials are present at the same biologic site.

Revision Total Hip Replacement

Indications

The most common indication for revision total hip replacement is loosening of the prosthesis with subsequent pain and varying degrees of bone loss. These are major procedures, and pain is usually so great that hip function is significantly limited. However, radiologic signs of loosening in hips with little pain should be watched carefully, and serial films taken. If major bone destruction progresses, even when pain is not too disabling, revision should be done before bone destruction proceeds to the extent that successful revision is less likely. The expected clinical results of revision surgery must be considered before undertaking these procedures, because they are often inferior to those of primary surgery. One series that compared 184 primary and 227 revision total hip replacement revealed no difference in relief of pain if the

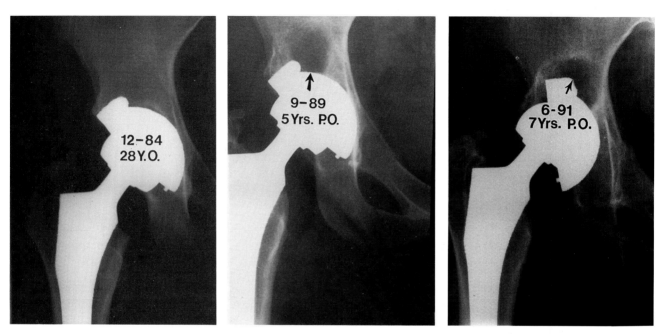

Fig. 6 Osteolysis of bone resulting in implant failure. Microscopic polyethylene debris was found in the bony defect. **Left**, Postoperative uncemented total hip replacement was done for rheumatic arthritis (RA). **Center**, Five years after surgery, bone destruction is seen. **Right**, After seven years, prosthetic displacement is seen.

surgery was successful. The failure rates of primary and revision total hip replacement were significantly different, with 7% revisions (11/156) in the primary series versus 27% (54/195) in the revision series. Complications were also significantly higher in the revision series, with a 16% incidence of interoperative fracture of the femoral shaft and a 6% incidence of postoperative dislocation. .

Surgical Techniques (Removal)

These lengthy, complex procedures should be undertaken by an experienced surgical team in a hospital that has numerous specialized pieces of equipment for prosthetic and cement removal and a large inventory of revision prosthetic components. Some authors recommend routine trochanteric osteotomy; all recommend wide exposure of the hip with removal of the pseudocapsule, exposing the entire proximal end of the femur and the entire circumference of the acetabulum to permit careful implant removal. The acetabular cup can often be removed intact with large curved gouges passed between the cup and the bone, but occasionally it must be split into segments and removed in pieces. All acetabular cement must be removed, including cement plugs, which often remain firmly fixed to bone. Care must be taken to avoid removal of the remaining bone stock. If the acetabular component is not loose and is fixed to bone by cement or bony ingrowth, its removal may be a significant challenge. Smooth gouges must be passed between the outer shell of the prosthesis and bone, avoiding the cortex of the inner pelvis.

Removal of a loose femoral component usually is accomplished readily. If the prosthesis was cemented, some of the remaining cement mantle may be tightly attached to the bone and must be removed with great care to avoid penetration of the femoral shaft. High-speed drills are available for cement removal; however, these drills remove bone more easily than they do the harder methacrylate. Specially designed hand chisels and osteotomies are available for cement removal. Image intensification is extremely useful in avoiding bone damage, but it introduces increased risks of radiation and potential contamination of the surgical site. Special lights are available for exposing the inner endosteum of the femur.

Animal studies are being done on use of lithotriptor to loosen the bone-cement interface preoperatively. The efficacy of the CO_2 laser to facilitate removal of the cement from the cement-bone interface during surgery is being investigated. Ultrasound equipment appears promising for making cement removal easier, but clinical trials are just beginning. Another recently described method involves bonding freshly mixed methacrylate to the old cement and using a special extraction rod tapped into the new cement.

Removal of broken femoral stems poses a special problem because the remaining distal portion of the stem may be held rigidly in its cement bed. Windows can be made in the anterior aspect of the femur to remove these distal methacrylate pieces. The distal stem can be successfully removed by drilling with high-speed drills into the fractured surface of the metal and attaching an extraction device to it. This method requires special equipment and is very technique dependent. Distal stem pieces can also be removed using a large trephine saw drilled over the length of the distal stem. This method may be especially helpful in removing uncemented ingrowth stems. These long stems may even require sectioning of the prosthesis and windowing or sectioning of the femur to remove the stem in pieces. Special thin-bladed osteotomies and high-speed drills may be used to separate the bone or fibrous tissue from the metal.

Reimplantation—Femoral Component (Results)

The basic choice of implants for revision surgery is between an uncemented and a cemented stem. Results of cemented revisions done with techniques of the early 1970s were not good. In one study of 166 hips followed 4.5 years, only 52% had good or excellent results, and 15 of the hips required re-revision. Of 99 revisions followed 8.1 years, results were good or excellent for 63%, and 29% were failures (revisions). Among 139 revisions done at the same institution with the improved surgical techniques of 1970 to 1982 and followed 3.6 years, 59% had excellent results, 29% had progressive radiolucency, and 8.6% required a second revision. Of 43 hips revised using cement techniques and femoral components developed after 1976, only one femoral component required revision and only four hips had definite radiologic loosening after 74 months average follow-up. One recent report of cemented revisions in a European center revealed a survivorship in 80 hips of 85% at 14 years. This group consisted of predominantly older patients. A report of 138 revisions done by a single surgeon and followed 7.4 years revealed good results with good to excellent Mayo hip scores in 62% and little or no pain in 86%. These authors recommend replacing both components, even when careful assessment before and during surgery shows that one component seems to be securely fixed, because subsequent loosening frequently occurs.

Revisions because of loosening were required in 4% of 57 uncemented stems followed an average of 2.8 years. An additional 12% were radiologically loose (subsided), but functioned well. Of these patients, 17% had some pain, 30% had moderate or severe limps, 27% used canes regularly, and only 60% could walk six blocks. The longest published follow-up of uncemented revision arthroplasty is that of 204 long straight-stemmed femoral components. The majority of these stems were porous coated over an extensive area, although 19 only had the porous coating on the proximal aspect. The eight-year survivorship in this group of patients was 91.7% with revision as the end point and 81.4% if loosening was added.

Femoral Component Revision (Technique)

The use of cement for reimplantation on the femoral side frequently requires a stem of greater length and should always bypass femoral cortical defects by two to three diameters of the femur. The modern techniques described in the section on "Cemented Total Hip Replace-

ment" should be used. In patients over 60, if good bone stock exists, recementing a stem can result in good long-term hip function. Some of the best results are seen in revisions done for femoral stem fractures where significant osteolysis of the bone has not taken place. In very elderly patients, even moderately poor bone stock can support the use of a cemented stem. For patients in whom severe osteolysis has occurred or there has been femoral shaft fracture, significant allografting may be necessary, possibly including use of a proximal femur replacement. When using these large allografts in older patients, cement around the proximal portion is appropriate, because there is no chance of bone ingrowth into a porous-surfaced device.

In younger patients, structural allografting may be used in the hope that eventually some of this dead bone may be revascularized, providing a potential source of bone stock for subsequent re-revisions. Large fragment proximal femoral allografts and cortical strut allografts were successful in 85% of 78 proximal femoral allografts followed an average of 36 months. Calcar grafts of less than 3 cm were clinically successful in 81%, but 50% underwent significant radiographic resorption. Several authors report success with external cortical allografts stabilized to the deficient femur by cerclage wiring techniques. The long-term fate of these structural allografts currently is unknown. One case has been reported in which a failed cemented total hip replacement was treated with a matched pair allograft hip. Seven years later, this hip required re-revision, and a new prosthetic hip was placed into the old allograft bone.

Acetabular Component Revision (Technique)

Several reports indicate high failure rates when large peripherally threaded screw-in type cups are used in acetabular revision surgery. Most authors report only fair results when using a bipolar type component in revision total hip surgery even when supplemental bone graft is used (Fig. 7). Most have reported a high incidence of bone resorption with morselized as well as structural bone graft. One study of 106 bipolar revisions revealed a need for re-revision in 29 hips. Success was obtained in 14 of these by using a fixed cup on the second revision.

Numerous studies indicate successful use of femoral head autografting for acetabular deficiency. In one study, good results were obtained using an L-shaped proximal head-neck fragment for acetabular augmentation in congenital hip dysplasia. Among 42 hips studied over a 12-year period, all grafts were united and, at an average follow-up period of 5.7 years only two acetabular components were found to be loose. One study of 38 dysplastic hips in which femoral head autografts were used with cemented acetabular components revealed that at 5.9 years, 12 components (32%) had become loose. In a series of 39 hips followed an average of 12.8 years after acetabular autografting for dysplasia, radiologic loosening rates were 20% definite, 10% probable, and 60% possible. The authors concluded that the bone grafting

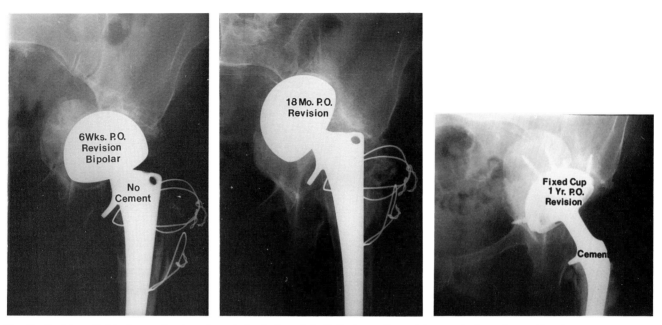

Fig. 7 Revision with bipolar prosthesis and poorly fixed allograft. **Left,** Postoperative revision used a large femoral head allograft and a bipolar uncemented hemiprosthesis. **Center,** The allograft is not rigidly fixed and quickly fails. **Right,** Re-revision is done with more allograft and a fixed acetabular component with screw fixation.

was effective in arresting the progression of the acetabular protrusion in 90%.

Most surgeons no longer use peripherally threaded cups and bipolar components in acetabular revision. Although some surgeons still recommend a cemented cup for acetabular revision, most use a fixed uncemented cup. Efforts should be made to fix the cup to primary bone. Structural stability is obtained by using a hemispherical cup, frequently with additional screws or lugs. When bone deficiency is extensive, use of an autograft is recommended, and when autograft bone is not available, allograft may be necessary. Morselized bone is incorporated most readily. If structural pieces of autograft or allograft are necessary, they should be rigidly fixed to the primary bone stock with screws or plates.

The surgeon also may obtain structural stability by placing a smaller acetabular component in a higher position. Currently, there are no definitive data that indicate a preference for either of these uncemented methods or fixation with cement.

Bipolar Arthroplasty

Except for rare cases of massive acetabular bone loss, use of bipolar arthroplasty in hip surgery seems limited to treatment of fresh femoral neck fracture. Reports indicate results of bipolar arthroplasty for aseptic necrosis are not as good as results for a standard total hip replacement. Replacement of the acetabulum with a fixed cup acetabular replacement prosthesis appears to be appropriate.

Hip Reconstruction Without Implants

Biomechanics of the Hip

A telemeterized femoral head replacement articulating with the acetabular cartilage has been used to measure contact forces in vivo. The data reveal very high (up to 18 MPa) local and nonuniform pressures with abrupt spatial and temporal gradients. These figures correlate well with in vitro data and computerized simulations of joint mechanics. However, peak pressures are much higher than those measured in vitro. Because of these high peak pressures, rehabilitation protocols and design criteria for hemiarthroplasties and total hip replacements may need reevaluation.

Intraosseous pressure in the femoral head in response to compressive loading of the joint was measured in vitro. The juxta-articular cancellous bone of the femoral head becomes pressurized with compressive loading in vitro. In vivo, cyclic changes in intraosseous pressure may play a major role in the remodeling, perfusion, and load transmission of bone. In addition, load-induced pressure pulses may play a role in the development of atraumatic osteonecrosis.

Arthrodesis

Energy expenditure after arthrodesis of the hip has been measured. The average walking speed was 84% of normal gait velocity and the mean oxygen consumption was 14.9 ml/kg of body weight per meter, which is 32%

greater than normal. The oxygen cost, 0.223 ml/kg per meter, represented a gait efficiency of 53%. The physiologic energy expenditure after hip arthrodesis is greater than that reported after unilateral total hip arthroplasty for osteoarthritis.

A 35-year follow-up study of hip arthrodesis revealed generally satisfactory results. Ipsilateral knee and back pain were present in 60% of patients, with onset at about 25 years postoperatively. Pain in the contralateral hip was present in 25%, with onset about 20 years after the arthrodesis. Only one patient had severe pain. Seventy percent of patients were able to walk a mile and to sit for two hours. Six patents underwent total hip replacement because of back pain; all cases were successful.

A Japanese study of 40 patients in whom arthrodesis was done more than 15 years earlier revealed no case in which position of the fusion was unsatisfactory. However, 26 patients had back pain, nine had knee pain on the same side and two on the other side, and three had pain in both knees. All patients could walk for more than 30 minutes, but 35 had difficulty with sitting. All but two were satisfied with the operation, and none wanted a total hip replacement.

The technique of hip fusion varies. Many authors recommend a cobra-shaped plate applied along the lateral shaft underneath the trochanter and fixed to the side of the ilium after removal of residual cartilage from the joint. Others recommend fixation with a long nail and plates or screws. Most recommend that a spica cast be worn for several months postoperatively.

Osteotomy

A computer-generated 3-D model has been developed to improve the results of osteotomy for hip dysplasia. The technique clearly delineates both deficiencies of osseous and cartilaginous coverage and congruence of pathologic hips. It thus can be used to create a more precise definition and treatment of multiple congenital abnormalities.

A new periacetabular osteotomy has been described in which cuts are made through a Smith-Peterson approach. The advantages include maintenance of the pelvic outlet, enhanced stability and vascularity of the acetabular fragment, and elimination of the significant pubic and ischial displacement seen with the Steele osteotomy. Complications in 75 patients included two intra-articular osteotomies, one femoral nerve palsy, one nonunion, and four cases of heterotopic ossification. The screws used for fixation of the acetabular fragment required removal in 13 patients.

A follow-up of 50 patients (average age, 42 years) three years and three months after rotational osteotomies of the acetabulum revealed 82% satisfactory results. Few recent reports are available of follow-up of femoral osteotomies. One large European study of 1,200 osteotomies revealed good results, but the authors did not recommend osteotomy in elderly patients.

Osteonecrosis

Diagnosis

Bone scanning with technetium detects osteonecrosis of the femoral head before changes appear on conventional radiographs. The intensity of the increased isotope uptake does not correlate with the stage of the disease.

Magnetic resonance imaging (MRI) has been shown to be very sensitive to early changes that occur within the marrow elements in osteonecrosis of the femoral head and is the standard for early diagnosis of osteonecrosis. The marrow cavity in normal femoral heads emits a strong magnetic resonance signal because it contains large amounts of hydrogen-rich fat. In the early stages of osteonecrosis, MRI detects changes arising from necrosis of marrow and ingrowth of vascularized mesenchymal tissue. These changes occur sometime before any alteration in trabecular architecture. Later, as the disease progresses, localized increases in bone density resulting from biologic and mechanical compaction further reduce the magnetic resonance signal. If one hip has been diagnosed as having osteonecrosis, there is a 50% incidence of the other hip developing the condition within a few months.

Although MRI is the most sensitive diagnostic technique and provides the earliest diagnosis, it is not useful for staging the disease. Seven stages have been proposed: 0, negative radiograph and negative MRI (diagnosis made by positive biopsy); I, negative radiograph and positive MRI; II, positive radiograph and positive MRI; III, crescent sign on radiograph; IV, femoral head flattening; V, degeneration changes in the acetabulum; and VI, advanced degenerative arthritis of the hip.

Treatment

A retrospective review of 50 femoral heads revealed that only 6% stabilized with conservative management consisting of crutches and nonweightbearing. However, many of these heads had already reached stage III at the time treatment was begun. A prospective study of stage I and, perhaps, stage II lesions is necessary to define the natural history of osteonecrosis and to determine whether or not conservative management is effective.

Reviews of the results of core decompression have not supported previous work suggesting success rates of 80% to 90%. A 69% failure rate at 18 months with a 10% femoral fracture rate was noted in one group of 40 hips. A 60% failure rate was noted in a review of 21 core decompressions performed in Cincinnati.

A five-year study of core decompression in 39 hips supported its use in Ficat stages 0, I, and IIA disease. Of hips with stage I disease, only 17% showed progression of the disease; of those with stage IIA disease, 58% showed disease progression. In contrast, 100% with stage IIB and 82% with stage III showed disease progression.

Review of a series of patients who underwent core decompression and bone grafting with or without electrical stimulation via an implantable electrode showed no benefit from the electrode treatment.

Transtrochanteric rotational osteotomy was performed in 17 patients with stage III disease. Within three years, 56% of the patients required total hip arthroplasty. Failures were highest in patients with large necrotic fragments, degenerative joint disease, and steroid- or alcohol-related disease.

Coring and grafting of avascular necrosis often fails because it has been implemented too late, that is, after the hip has reached stage III and fracturing of the femoral head has occurred. Some authors have been using vascularized bone grafting for the femoral head for osteonecrosis. To date, long-term follow-up is not yet available for this extensive surgical procedure. Simple drilling of the femoral head seems to be successful in the early stages of osteonecrosis.

Cemented total hip replacement for osteonecrosis in 28 hips followed up for five to ten years (average 7.6 years) had a failure rate of 37%. There is some hope that use of uncemented devices will improve these results.

Miscellaneous Considerations

Resection of the proximal end of the femur and interpositional arthroplasty were used in patients with cerebral palsy to enable them to sit. Of these patients, 97% had successful and durable results after two years.

Sepsis of the hip in nine paraplegic patients was treated successfully by resection of the head and neck of the femur, transposition of the vastus lateralis into the void, and external fixation across the resection for three to six weeks.

Annotated Bibliography

Cemented Total Hip Replacement

Ahnfelt L, Herberts P, Malchau H, et al: Prognosis of total hip replacement: A Swedish multicenter study of 4,664 revisions. *Acta Orthop Scand Suppl* 1990;238:1-26.

The large numbers in this extensive data base from combined hospitals in Sweden allowed study of two different types of prosthesis. With a probability of failure rates of 5% and 3% in two different prostheses followed over a five-year period; 2,960 patients are needed to obtain a significance level of 0.05.

Dorr LD, Luckett M, Conaty JP: Total hip arthroplasties in patients younger than 45 years: A nine- to ten-year follow-up study. *Clin Orthop* 1990;260:215-219.

Eighty-one cemented total hip replacements in patients under 45 were compared at 9.2 years follow-up with the same group at 4.5 years follow-up. Satisfactory results dropped from 78% to 58%, and the revision rate tripled to 33%. The impending failure rate was 56%. Best results were obtained in patients from age 30 to 45 with inflammatory collagen disease.

Hozack WJ, Rothman RH, Booth RE Jr, et al: Survivorship analysis of 1,041 Charnley total hip arthroplasties. *J Arthroplasty* 1990;5:41-47.

Survivorship analysis of 1,041 Charnley total hip replacements found a 92% probability of survival at ten years. Radiographic evidence of femoral component loosening occurred in 9.6%, with a revision rate of 1.8%. Given these results, the authors concluded that it was difficult to justify the widespread use of noncemented total hip systems, except in identifiable high-risk patients whom they found to be young, heavy, active males.

Kavanagh BF, Dewitz MA, Ilstrup DM, et al: Charnley total hip arthroplasty with cement: Fifteen-year results. *J Bone Joint Surg* 1989;71A:1496-1503.

Follow-up of 333 Charnley total hips indicated 80% of the living patients had no pain. Radiographic evaluation revealed the probability of loosening was 3% at one year, 13% at five years, 19% at ten years, and 32% at 15 years. Probability of revision and symptomatic loosening was 0.9% at one year, 4.1% at five years, 8.9% at ten years, and 12.7% at 15 years.

Mulroy RD Jr, Harris WH: The effect of improved cementing techniques on component loosening in total hip replacement: An 11-year radiographic review. *J Bone Joint Surg* 1990;72B:757-760.

One hundred and five hips were followed-up for an average of 11.2 years (range, 10 to 12.7). These total hip replacements were performed with improved cementing techniques, including use of medullary plug, cement gun, doughy Simplex, and an improved stem design. Follow-up revealed three definitely loose stems, no probably loose stems, and 24 possibly loose stems. In contrast, there was an acetabular radiologic loosening rate of 42%.

Mulroy RD Jr, Harris WH: Failure of acetabular autogenous grafts in total hip arthroplasty: Increasing incidence: A follow-up note. *J Bone Joint Surg* 1990;72A:1536-1540.

Although autogenous femoral head acetabular allografts seemed successful at seven years, at 11.8 years, nine of the 46 hips (20%) had required a second operation because of acetabular fixation failure. In 12 of the remaining 36, there was definite radiographic evidence of acetabular loosening. Thus, 46% showed signs of failure.

Newington DP, Bannister GC, Fordyce M: Primary total hip replacement in patients over 80 years of age. *J Bone Joint Surg* 1990;72B:450-452.

In 107 patients over the age of 80, the authors identified increased risks in primary total hip replacement. The dislocation rate was 15%, of which nine became chronic. Femoral shaft fractures occurred in 4.6%, although 75% had satisfactory outcomes.

Russotti GM, Harris WH: Proximal placement of the acetabular component in total hip arthroplasty: A long-term follow-up study. *J Bone Joint Surg* 1991;73A:587-592.

This is a retrospective review of 37 hips, which required the center of the hip to be placed proximally, followed-up seven to 17 years (11 years average). Thirty-three of the 37 components had been replaced superiorly with no lateral displacement. Only 6 of 37 (16%) were loose and only one needed revision, indicating this position can give acceptable results in cemented total hip replacement.

Semlitsch M, Streicher RM, Weber H: The wear behavior of capsules and heads of CoCrMo casts in longer-term implanted all-metal hip prostheses. *Orthopade* 1989;18:370-381.

Follow-up of metal-on-metal total hip replacements done ten to 20 years ago showed very low wear. A comparative polyethylene metal articulation showed a wear rate 40 times greater.

Wixson RL, Stulberg SD, Mehlhoff M: Total hip replacement with cemented, uncemented, and hybrid prostheses: A comparison of clinical and radiographic results at two to four years. *J Bone Joint Surg* 1991;73A:257-270.

Cemented, uncemented, and hybrid total hips with comparable clinical Harris hip ratings in all were followed-up for two to four years. In 65 uncemented stems, two had aseptic loosening. Twenty-four percent had thigh pain, which usually was slight and not disabling, and the prevalence had declined after one year. Radiolucent lines and incidences of migration were greater in acetabular components fixed with cement than in those allowing bone ingrowths.

Uncemented Total Hip Replacement

Bargar WL: Shape the implant to the patient: A rationale for the use of custom-fit cementless total hip implants. *Clin Orthop* 1989;249:73-78.

One hundred fifty-six cases of custom femoral components were followed six weeks to three years, with only 48 hips followed more than two years. Use of custom components decreased the need for structural bone grafts. Revision for aseptic loosening was required in one of 81 primary and one of 75 revisions. Subsidence of more than 3 mm was seen in the collarless design in 8%.

Engh CA, Glassman AH, Suthers KE: The case for porous-coated hip implants: The femoral side. *Clin Orthop* 1990;261:63-81.

Follow-up of 1,163 uncemented THAs (AML type). Nine hundred fifty-nine primary total hip replacements followed two to 12 years had a survivorship rate of 96%. In 204 revision total hip replacements, the survivorship rate was 91.7% at eight years and 81.4% if loosening was added to revisions. Stress shielding was noted in more than 75%, but was graded severe in less than 5%.

Engh CA, Massin P: Cementless total hip arthroplasty using the anatomic medullary locking stem: Results using a survivorship analysis. *Clin Orthop* 1989;249:141-158.

A study of 343 hips followed for five years revealed a cumulative survival rate for stable fixation of 94% at five years and 88% at eight years. Of 143 stems that did not fill the canal, 17 showed late migration and a survivorship of 77% at eight

years; 200 complete canal filling stems showed no radiographic failures. Proximal stress shielding, seen when bony ingrowth occurred, was slightly progressive.

Geesink RG: Hydroxyapatite-coated total hip prostheses: Two-year clinical and roentgenographic results of 100 cases. *Clin Orthop* 1990;261:39-58.

This is a follow-up report of 100 consecutive cases of hydroxyapatite coated uncemented total hip arthroplasties. Average follow-up was two years, incidence of pain was 4% at one year, radiographic exams showed rapid bony integration within six months, and no radiolucent lines were detected on the hydroxyapatite-coated areas. Positive roentgenographic evidence of femoral ingrowth was seen in 97% of patients.

Haddad RJ, Cook SD, Brinker MR: A comparison of three varieties of noncemented porous-coated hip replacement. *J Bone Joint Surg* 1990;72B:2-8.

This is a review of 134 noncemented total hip replacements: 64 AML, 20 PCA, and 50 LSF followed 36, 40, and 24 months, respectively. Harris scores were 80.7%, 83.8%, and 91.5%; there was groin pain in 30%, 30%, and 8%, respectively.

Haddad RJ Jr, Skalley TC, Cook SD, et al: Clinical and roentgenographic evaluation of noncemented porous-coated anatomic medullary locking (AML) and porous-coated anatomic (PCA) total hip arthroplasties. *Clin Orthop* 1990;258:176-182.

Eighty-four noncemented total hip replacements (64 AMLs and 20 PCAs) were reviewed at an average follow-up of 37 months in patients at an average age of 51.9 years. Most of the AMLs were 5/8 coated. Postoperative hip scores were comparable and 30% had pain related to the implant in both devices. All components demonstrated radiographic evidence of bone ingrowth.

Maloney WJ, Jasty M, Harris WH, et al: Endosteal erosion in association with stable uncemented femoral components. *J Bone Joint Surg* 1990;72A:1025-1034.

Sixteen hips showed focal femoral osteolysis after uncemented total hip replacement. Fourteen had excellent clinical results; two required revision. Osteolysis was not identified before two years, but usually was identified within two and three years. Histologic evaluation showed macrophages and particulate polyethylene and metallic debris.

Sedel L, Kerboull L, Christel P, et al: Alumina-on-alumina hip replacement: Results and survivorship in young patients. *J Bone Joint Surg* 1990;72B:658-663.

Review of 86 ceramic hips implanted between 1977 and 1986 in patients under 50 years of age showed 98% survivorship of prosthesis retention at ten years. Fifteen acetabular components and one femoral component had radiographic instability.

Revision Total Hip Replacement

Allan DG, Lavoie GJ, McDonald S, et al: Proximal femoral allografts in revision hip arthroplasty. *J Bone Joint Surg* 1991;73B:235-240.

Follow-up of 78 proximal femoral autograft revision total hip replacements for 36 months revealed large fragment proximal femoral allografts and cortical strut allografts were successful in 85%. Small calcar grafts were successful in 81%, but 50% had significant radiographic resorption.

Marti RK, Schüller HM, Besselaar PP, et al: Results of revision of hip arthroplasty with cement: A five to fourteen-year follow-up study. *J Bone Joint Surg* 1990;72A:346-354.

Follow-up of 60 revision cemented total hip replacements for five to 14 years revealed two infections and four revisions for aseptic failure. Three cups migrated, and seven were radiologically loose. Five femoral components subsided, and 11 were radiologically loose. Survivorship analysis showed 85% cumulative survival at 14 years in this relatively old group of patients.

Kershaw CJ, Adkins RM, Dodd CAF, et al: Revision total hip arthroplasty for aseptic failure: A review of 276 cases. *J Bone Joint Surg* 1991;73B:564-568.

Results of 276 cemented revisions done between 1977 and 1986 were reviewed an average of 75 months after surgery. Eighteen required further revision: 12 for loosening, two for sepsis, two for pain, one for fracture, and one for dislocation. Pain was mild or absent in 83%. Survival at five years was 95% and at ten years 77%. The authors conclude the failure rate of revision operations is not as great as originally feared.

Murray WR: Acetabular salvage in revision total hip arthroplasty using the bipolar prosthesis. *Clin Orthop* 1990;251:92-99.

Average follow-up was 2 years 11 months for 106 revision total hip replacements using a bipolar device for acetabular salvage. Of 29 that failed and required reoperation, 14 were successfully revised using a fixed cementless cup. Although somewhat disappointing, the results were superior to those of excision arthroplasty.

Nonimplant Hips

Garvin KL, Pellicci PM, Windsor RE, et al: Contralateral total hip arthroplasty or ipsilateral total knee arthroplasty in patients who have a long-standing fusion of the hip. *J Bone Joint Surg* 1989;71A:1355-1362.

In this study of 13 total hip replacements in patients who had had a hip fusion in acceptable position on the opposite hip, average time from arthrodesis to arthroplasty was 32 years. Hip ratings for the total hip replacements were excellent, five; good, five; fair, one; and poor, three. The poor results have each been revised twice for mechanical loosening.

Lack W, Windhager R, Kutschera HP, et al: Chiari pelvic osteotomy for osteoarthritis secondary to hip dysplasia: Indications and long-term results. *J Bone Joint Surg* 1991;73B:229-234.

The outcome was good in 75% of 142 Chiari pelvic osteotomies, most performed by the originator, followed an average of 15.5 years. Twenty hips had undergone secondary total hip replacement.

Sofue M, Kono S, Kawaji W, et al: Long term results of arthrodesis for severe osteoarthritis of the hip in young adults. *Int Orthop* 1989;13:129-133.

Forty hips were followed 15 years or more after hip arthrodesis. There was no case in which the fusion was unsatisfactory. Twenty-six patients had backache, nine had ipsilateral knee pain, two contralateral knee pain, and three pain in both knees. All patients returned to their previous occupation and could walk more than 30 minutes.

Steinberg ME: Management of avascular necrosis of the femoral head: An overview, in Bassett FH III (ed): *Instructional Course Lectures XXXVII*. Park Ridge, IL,

American Academy of Orthopaedic Surgeons, 1988, pp 41-50.

This is a good review of avascular necrosis of the femoral head. The results of established surgical procedures have been inconsistent and frequently disappointing, often because they are instituted too late. Early diagnosis is essential.

Watillon M, Maquet P: Indications des ostéotomies fémorales intertrochantériennes pour séquelles arthrosiques de la dysplasie de hanche. (Indications for femoral intertrochanteric osteotomy for arthritis sequelae of hip dysplasia.) *Acta Orthop Belgica* 1990;56:371-377.

The authors recommend varus osteotomy for subluxation coxa valga when the joint is congruent in abduction and valgus osteotomy when the acetabulum and femoral head are considerably deformed when the joint surfaces are congruent in adduction. If congruency is not obtained radiographically or in older patients, they suggest total hip replacement.

Complications

Brien WW, Salvati EA, Wright TM, et al: Dissociation of acetabular components after total hip arthroplasty: Report of four cases. *J Bone Joint Surg* 1999;72A:1548-1550.

This is a report of four cases having dissociation of the acetabular plastic liner in modular uncemented total hip arthroplasty requiring major revision surgery.

Livermore J, Ilstrup D, Morrey B: Effect of femoral head size on wear of the polyethylene acetabular component. *J Bone Joint Surg* 1990;72A:518-528.

The least amount of linear wear was found in 385 hips followed-up for 9.5 years when 28-mm diameter heads were used and the greatest amount when 22-mm heads were used. The greatest volumetric wear was with 32-mm components. The resorption of the proximal part of the femoral neck and proximal femur correlated positively with the extent of linear and volumetric wear, suggesting that polyethylene debris was the cause of this bone resorption.

Basic Science of Total Hip Replacement

Galante JO, Lemons J, Spector M, et al: The biologic effects of implant materials. *J Orthop Res* 1991;9:760-775.

This has an excellent reference list and discussions of common implant materials, corrosion, biodegradation, tissue response to implant materials, carcinogenicity, and bone loss and remodeling in uncemented total hips, as well as causes of osteolysis and metal ion migration.

Huiskes R: The various stress patterns of press-fit, ingrown, and cemented femoral stems. *Clin Orthop* 1990;261:27-38.

This is a finite element analysis studying load-transfer mechanisms and stress patterns in cemented, uncemented, and press-fitted stems. Titanium would be expected to produce better results in noncemented stems and cobalt-chrome in cemented stems. Stress shielding effects are most severe in fully ingrown stems and milder in cemented proximally ingrown stems.

Jasty M, Maloney WJ, Bragdon CR, et al: Histomorphological studies of the long-term skeletal responses to well fixed cemented femoral components. *J Bone Joint Surg* 1990;72B:1220-1229.

Thirteen autopsy specimens from patients who had well-functioning total hip replacements showed a dense shell of substantial new bone around the cement mantle with substantial osteoporosis in the adjacent femoral cortex. The dense shell of new bone and internal remodeling helped maintain the femoral components.

Johnston RC, Fitzgerald RH Jr, Harris WH, et al: Clinical and radiological evaluation of total hip replacements: A standard system of terminology for reporting results. *J Bone Joint Surg* 1990;72A:161-168.

This article is a combined effort of several societies, including the Hip Society and the American Academy of Orthopaedic Surgeons, to provide a standard system of data collection and reporting for clinical results in total hip replacement.

Wickland I, Romanus B: A comparison of quality of life before and after arthroplasty in patients who had arthrosis of the hip joint. *J Bone Joint Surg* 1991;73A:765-769.

Quality before and after total hip arthroplasty in 56 patients was studied and was found significantly improved at the 0.0001 level in energy, sleep, and social isolation. There also was a reduction in frequency of health-related problems pertaining to housework, holidays, hobbies, social life, sexual function, and family life in patients who were 65 years old or less.

Loosening

Santavirta S, Hoikka V, Eskola A, et al: Aggressive granulomatous lesions in cementless total hip arthroplasty. *J Bone Joint Surg* 1990;72B:980-984.

This is a description of six hips with aggressive granulomatous lesions forming around cementless chrome-cobalt stems. Pain developed in an average of 3.2 years and revision was done at 4.8 years. The granuloma was thought to be caused by plastic debris from the acetabular socket.

44

Femur: Trauma

Introduction

Fracture of the femoral shaft in an adult is an orthopaedic emergency. These fractures are generally the result of high-energy trauma, can be both life- and limb-threatening injuries, and almost always require surgical treatment and stabilization. Major improvements in surgical technique, implants, and instrumentation have led to dramatic improvement in the outcome of management.

Femoral Shaft Fractures

Patients With Multiple Injuries

Early stabilization of femoral shaft fractures (within the initial 24 hours) is desirable in patients with multiple injuries. This aggressive approach decreases the incidence of pulmonary complications such as adult respiratory distress syndrome, fat emboli, pneumonia, and pulmonary failure. This advantage of early surgical intervention is especially evident in patients with multiple injuries (Injury Severity Score >18) involving the head, chest, spinal column, or abdomen, or in those with multiple fractures.

Classification of Injuries

Femoral shaft fractures are categorized by their location, fracture pattern, degree of comminution, associated soft-tissue injury, and mechanism of injury. The usual locations are the subtrochanteric, the mid-diaphyseal, or the distal third (infraisthmal) areas. Spiral and oblique fracture patterns characteristically occur in elderly patients as a result of low-energy injuries. High-energy shaft fractures are classified by Winquist by the degree of comminution (Fig. 1). Type I comminution is defined by a small butterfly fracture involving less than 25% of the width of the bone. A larger butterfly fracture involving 50% or less of the circumference of the bone defines a type II fracture. Type I and II fractures have axial and rotational stability after intramedullary nailing if there is good apposition between the major proximal and distal fragments and if the fracture is located near the femoral isthmus. Type III comminuted fractures have a large bony fragment of more than 50% of the circumference of the bone with only a small spike of remaining proximal and distal fragments in contact. Type IV comminuted fractures have segmental comminution with no contact between the major proximal and distal fragments. Type III and IV fractures are always unstable in length and rotation. Open fractures with segmental bone loss are classified as type V.

The AO group has proposed a new classification system for femoral shaft fractures. The system defines 27 distinct patterns of fractures which are based on fracture location (proximal, midshaft, or distal), anatomy (transverse or oblique), and degree of comminution. This classification is complicated and does not have therapeutic or prognostic implications.

Common Related Injuries or Complications

Vascular Injuries Vascular injuries are clinically evident in approximately 2% of femoral shaft fractures. Many minor injuries to the femoral vessels may go undetected, because intimal tears do not always result in lessening of palpable distal pulses. Arteriography is indicated in any fracture secondary to penetrating trauma. Blunt trauma causing a fracture of the distal fourth of the shaft of the femur can also result in arterial injury by tearing the femoral artery at the level of the adductor canal. The intimal tears may go undetected and produce later occlusion, as long as 48 hours after injury. Arteriography is, therefore, indicated in such fractures if there is any suspicion of an arterial injury, and careful monitoring is necessary.

Treatment of arterial injuries depends on the severity of vascular compromise and the amount of time that has elapsed since the injury. If arterial compromise is severe, eg, a complete laceration, arterial flow must be reestablished within six hours. The artery is temporarily shunted, the femoral fracture stabilized by internal fixation, and then arterial repair is performed. Four-compartment fasciotomy routinely should be performed.

Open Fractures All open fractures in the femur require irrigation and debridement. Surgical extensions of the traumatic wound can be closed, but the original wound must be left open.

The traditional treatment of initial debridement with delayed wound closure after five to seven days and surgical stabilization of the fracture after ten to fourteen days is acceptable in patients with isolated open femoral shaft fractures. Current recommendations for treatment of open fractures are based on the presence or absence of multiple injuries and the severity of soft-tissue injury to the thigh. Grade I, II, and IIIA open fractures preferably are treated by thorough irrigation and debridement of the wound followed by immediate intramedullary nailing, whether the patient is multiply injured or has an isolated injury. There appears to be no significant increased risk of wound infection compared to the traditional treatment. Intramedullary nailing or alternative

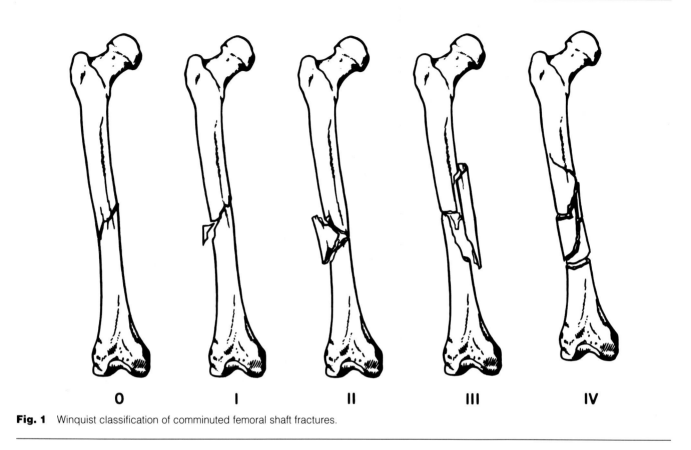

Fig. 1   Winquist classification of comminuted femoral shaft fractures.

forms of fracture fixation should be delayed in grade IIIB and IIIC fractures in patients with an isolated injury. The fracture care of multiply injured patients with grade IIIB and IIIC fractures must be individualized. External fixation is reserved for grade IIIB and IIIC open fractures and severely contaminated wounds (such as those secondary to close-range shotgun blasts or farm injuries). Patients with multiple injuries that include an open femoral fracture benefit from immediate fracture stabilization.

Compartment Syndrome   Compartment syndrome of the thigh is a relatively rare phenomenon. In a series of 21 compartment syndromes, ten were associated with an ipsilateral femoral shaft fracture. Five of the ten were open. The remaining 11 compartment syndromes followed blunt trauma to the thigh with prolonged compression by body weight (a comatose or pinned patient) or vascular injury. Thigh compartment syndrome is a serious medical problem that carries a high risk of death or infection and is predisposed to by multiple injuries, systemic hypotension, external compression, coagulopathy, vascular injury, and thigh trauma with or without fracture. Thigh compartment pressures should be measured in any patients suspected to be at risk.

Gunshot Fractures   Gunshot fractures are generally treated in the same manner as a closed femoral shaft fracture, with similar results. When the bullet is low velocity, the track is debrided locally at the skin level, but a formal, extensive debridement of the wound usually is not required.

The minority of gunshot fractures to the femoral shaft are secondary to high-velocity bullets, such as close-range shotgun blasts and high-velocity rifles. Their management is similar to that of a type III open fracture as previously described. Delayed internal fixation or, perhaps, external fixation, along with radical wound debridement, are preferred treatment methods.

Ipsilateral Fractures

Hip and Shaft   Ipsilateral hip fracture occurs in as many as 5% of all femoral shaft fractures, and is initially overlooked in 20% to 30% of cases. The common fracture site is the femoral neck. Less frequently the intertrochanteric area is involved. All severely traumatized patients, with or without a femoral shaft fracture, should have an anteroposterior radiograph of the pelvis performed as part of the initial diagnostic evaluation.

In these fractures, management of one fracture significantly affects the management of the other. Simultaneous stabilization of both hip and shaft fractures yields the best clinical results. Management of the femoral shaft fracture, however, should not compromise the optimal management (anatomic reduction and rigid internal fixation) of the femoral neck fracture.

The surgical treatment of this combined injury is based on the fracture patterns and the experience of the treating surgeon. Preliminary stabilization of the femoral neck with pins or screws, followed by intramedullary nailing of the femoral shaft and then placement of parallel interfragmental screws into the femoral head has been recommended.

The use of a single implant to fix both of these fractures simultaneously is extremely difficult because both fractures must be anatomically reduced at the same time. Ender nails and second-generation locked nails have been tried, but abandoned by most investigators because of inadequate stabilization of the femoral neck. Such surgical implants are recommended only when anatomic reduction of both femoral neck and shaft fractures can be achieved and maintained during insertion of the device.

Femoral Shaft and Tibial Shaft A floating knee injury, with ipsilateral fracture of the femoral shaft and tibia, occurs in about 10% of all femoral shaft fractures. The mortality rate of these high-energy injuries is 5% to 15%, and fat emboli syndrome is reported in 9% to 13% of patients. Prompt resuscitation, diagnosis, and treatment of life-threatening injuries is thus imperative for these severe combined injuries. Because most life-threatening complications are worsened by prolonged recumbency, fracture stabilization should be performed in the first 24 hours. The best functional results have been reported with early stabilization of both the femur and tibia and early restoration of knee motion.

Open fractures are common in this combined injury (20% femur, 50% tibia). Ideally, the femur is stabilized with closed locked intramedullary nailing whenever possible and the tibia is stabilized by internal or external fixation depending on the severity of the soft-tissue injury. Grade I and II open and unstable closed tibial fractures are best treated by intramedullary nailing with reamed or unreamed nails. Grade III open or severely contaminated fractures of the tibia should be treated by external fixation. Satisfactory results have been reported for external fixation of both the femur and tibia when open, contaminated fractures are present at both sites. Intra-articular fractures (distal femur, proximal or distal tibia) should be managed by primary anatomic reduction and stable internal fixation that allows active knee range of motion as soon as possible.

Femoral Shaft and Knee Ligaments Ipsilateral knee ligament injury should be suspected in all patients with femoral shaft fractures, even though it is present in only 5% of fractures. After femoral fracture fixation, the knee should be reexamined to assess ligamentous stability. If the shaft fracture has been rigidly fixed and the patient's condition is stable, repair of all ligamentous injuries can proceed.

Adolescent Femoral Shaft Fractures

Although treatment of shaft fractures by traction and casting is satisfactory in younger children, it is less useful in obtaining and maintaining satisfactory alignment in adolescent patients. Surgical treatments carry the risks of growth-plate damage and infection. These risks, however, are low. Patients over the age of 12 are preferably treated by intramedullary nailing with care taken to avoid damaging the distal femoral physis. Small diameter cloverleaf nails or Ender pins can be used. Patients younger than 12 years of age with severe head trauma and signs of posturing or with fractures that are irreducible should also be considered candidates for surgery. Most patients younger than 12 years of age should be treated with 90/90 femoral pin traction, followed by spica cast or cast brace. The treatment for femoral shaft fractures should allow for early mobilization of the patient, restoration of the length and alignment of the femur, and early knee motion.

Alternatives to Intramedullary Nailing

Traction and some form of cast or brace have traditionally been used for fractures of the femoral shaft. Although this treatment has a high rate of union with a low risk of infection, the results are often unacceptable because of excessive knee stiffness and fracture malalignment. Most surgeons now limit traction and cast bracing treatment to those rare patients who have infected fractures or some other condition that contraindicates intramedullary fixation.

External fixation of femoral shaft fractures has limited applications. External fixators are easily and quickly applied with low risk, and they allow early mobilization of the patient, but late problems include knee stiffness, pin-tract infection, delayed union, and malalignment. The ideal indication for an external fixator is the severely contaminated grade III open fracture. The fixator may be used as the definitive form of fixation or as a temporary fixation until soft-tissue healing is achieved. However, once an external fixation has been used, the risks involved in delayed internal fixation are increased, especially if colonized pin sites are present. External fixation can also be useful in a multiply injured patient who cannot tolerate prolonged anesthesia. The external fixator can be applied in 15 to 20 minutes using a limited open operative technique.

Compression plates provide stable fixation of femoral shaft fractures and permit early mobilization of patients. The disadvantages of compression plates include infection, screw and plate fatigue, refracture at the end of the plate, and slow fracture healing. For these reasons, compression plates should be used only in intra-articular fractures that extend into the knee joint, fractures associated with ipsilateral proximal femoral fractures, or in patients undergoing vascular repair associated with a distal-third femoral fracture. When these indications are present, a single broad compression plate is applied to the lateral aspect of the femur and a cancellous bone graft routinely applied along the medial aspect of the femur. Two plates cause excessive stress-shielding, require extensive dissection, and should be avoided. Devices that apply intraoperative distraction can be helpful when a plate is applied. A broad plate is used to bridge comminuted fractures. Stable fixation is provided by screws that engage eight cortices both proximally and distally. Soft-tissue dissection should be minimized.

Intramedullary Nails

Intramedullary nailing is the treatment of choice for most femoral shaft fractures. Closed nailing is preferred over open nailing, but similar results can be achieved with an open technique if the incision is used primarily to obtain reduction and minimal soft-tissue dissection is performed. Fracture fixation is enhanced by reaming of the femoral canal, which permits the placement of a stiffer nail of larger diameter, and by the use of interlocking nails, which allow for locking of the major fracture fragments to the nail.

The use of small diameter intramedullary nails in the unreamed femur is advocated by some authors, especially for use in open fractures. The technique uses either a single nail of small diameter or multiple round nails of even smaller diameter. The use of these types of nails in the unreamed femur should be reserved for simple fracture patterns (transverse or short oblique) that occur in the midshaft area. When these nails are used for proximal, distal, or more comminuted fractures, fracture shortening and malalignment can occur.

Reamed, Locked Intramedullary Nails   The use of reamed, locked intramedullary nails has proliferated in the past ten years (Fig. 2). These nails require reaming to allow placement of a nail with a relatively large diameter (12-16 mm) and holes for locking of the proximal and distal fracture fragments to the nail. They adequately stabilize most fractures of the shaft of the femur and allow early mobilization of the patient and limb. Closed nailing requires the use of special equipment, including an image intensifier, a radiolucent fracture table, and a large inventory of nails and locking screws. The use of locked nails requires an experienced surgeon's assistant and expert radiologic technical support.

Recently, changes have been introduced in the design of intramedullary nails. Closed section nails, which lack the longitudinal slot of the Küntscher nail, possess increased torsional stiffness and, to a lesser degree, increased bending strength. The increased strength lessens the risk of nail fatigue, but the increased stiffness can increase the risk of fracture comminution during nail insertion. It is recommended that the canal be overreamed 2 mm greater than the diameter of the selected nail. Closing the cross section of the nail also allows variations in the wall thickness and make thick-walled, smaller diameter, unreamed, locked nails a reasonable alternative for certain fractures.

Other design changes have affected the biomechanics of these nails. The radius of curvature of intramedullary nails varies from manufacturer to manufacturer. The anterior bow of the nail allows a more anatomic fit within the femur, but increases the force required for nail insertion. A relatively stiff nail with a large radius of curvature can create large hoop stresses and comminution at the fracture site during insertion if the starting point is not carefully selected, especially when an anterior starting point is used. The stiffer the nail and the larger the radius of curvature, the more attention must be paid to selection of the appropriate starting hole. Fatigue fractures of partially slotted nails can occur at the junction of the slotted and unslotted portions of the nail. Such partially slotted nails are now manufactured with a gun-drill method using solid bar stock metal to enhance their strength. Fatigue fracture of interlocking nails can also occur at the most proximal of the distal screw holes if the fracture site is within 5 cm of this hole. The risk of failure is decreased by avoiding full weightbearing until early fracture union is evident.

Results   The results of closed intramedullary nailing are far superior to those of other forms of treatment. Fracture union within 16 to 24 weeks with a return of near full knee motion can be anticipated in over 90% of patients. Three fourths of patients return to work within six months, and 96% return to work within 12 months.

Complications   The reported infection rates after closed intramedullary nailing vary from 0.5% to 1.5%. The infection rate after intramedullary nailing of open femoral shaft fractures is 2% to 4%, whether the intramedullary nailing is performed immediately after irrigation and debridement or seven to ten days later.

Acutely infected intramedullary nails should be irrigated and debrided at the fracture site as well as in the intramedullary canal. The nail should then be removed and the canal overreamed to remove infected granulation tissue from the canal. A drainage hole in the distal medial aspect of the femur may be created to allow thorough irrigation and drainage of the canal. If the wound appears adequately debrided, a slightly larger nail may then be inserted to stabilize the fracture. After fracture union, which predictably occurs despite the infection, the intramedullary nail is removed and any residual infection is addressed. This treatment is adequate for most infected intramedullary nails and generally results in a healed femoral shaft fracture without chronic osteomyelitis. More extensive or fulminant infection may require alternative types of treatment, which can include nail removal and external fixation.

Delayed union or nonunion after intramedullary nailing is rare, occurring in less than 2% of cases. Nonunion is preferably treated by removal of the intramedullary nail, reaming of the intramedullary canal, and replace-

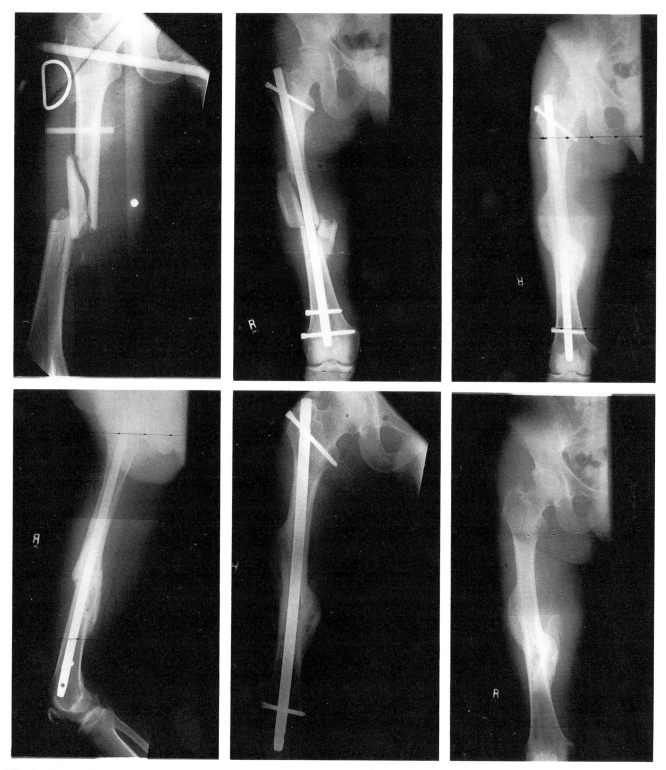

Fig. 2 **Top left**, Comminuted femoral shaft fracture (Winquist IV); **Top center**, One month following closed static locked nailing; **Top right**, Eight months post injury with healed fracture. Note heterotopic ossification. **Bottom left** and **Bottom center**, Lateral and anteroposterior radiographs at one year. Circumferential cortical healing is evident; **Bottom right**, Following nail removal at one year with debridement of heterotopic ossification.

ment with a larger diameter nail. Selected cases of statically locked intramedullary nails with slow fracture healing can be treated simply by removal of the proximal or distal locking screws (dynamization).

Malunion from fracture shortening or malrotation about a nail has been virtually eliminated with the introduction of locked nails. When any type of shortening or malrotation is possible, a static locked nail should be used. If shortening or malrotation is evident about a dynamically locked nail during the immediate postoperative period (one to two weeks), realignment with skeletal traction, followed by placement of static locking screws, is indicated. Recent studies have demonstrated that, in most femoral shaft fractures, the use of static locking eliminates most problems of shortening and malalignment without adversely affecting the union rate.

Heterotopic ossification about the proximal tip of intramedullary nails is quite common (Fig. 2). Mild or minimal heterotopic ossification occurs in approximately 35% of patients, moderate heterotopic ossification is evident in 15% of patients, and severe heterotopic ossification in 10% of patients. There appears to be no correlation between the degree of heterotopic ossification, the age or sex of the patient, the severity of the injury, the presence or absence of head injury, the timing of the nailing, or the type of intramedullary fixation. Irrigation with pulsatile lavage does not lessen the incidence or severity of this complication. Rarely does the ectopic bone limit motion at the hip.

Nerve palsy from excessive traction during the nailing maneuver may involve either the sciatic nerve, or, more commonly, the pudendal nerve. Forced adduction of the hip around the perineal post on the fracture table increases the traction forces on the nerves and should be avoided. Most nerve palsies secondary to compression resolve spontaneously.

Supracondylar Fractures of the Femur

Supracondylar fractures are usually either the result of high-energy vehicular trauma in the younger patient, or the result of low-energy injuries in the elderly, most commonly from a fall. Because of the frequent intra-articular extension of the fracture and the proximity of the fracture to the joint, stiffness and posttraumatic osteoarthritis of the knee are common sequelae. Fractures of the distal femur can be classified as intra-articular or extra-articular and as involving either one or two condyles. The ASIF classification system divides fractures according to whether they are strictly extra-articular (type A), unicondylar (type B), or extra-articular and intra-articular (type C) (Fig. 3). A variety of different nonsurgical and surgical treatments may be considered, depending on the fracture pattern, the patient's age and medical condition, and associated injuries.

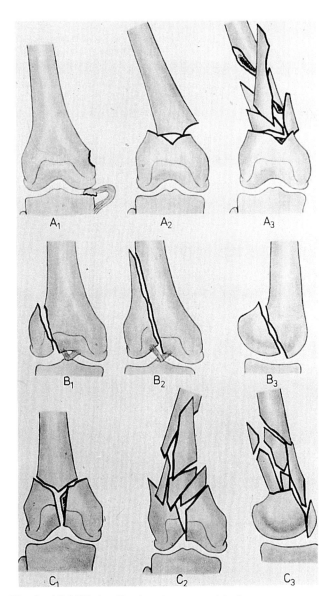

Fig. 3 AO/ASIF classification of supracondylar fractures.

Cast Bracing

Hinged casts or functional bracing are useful in nondisplaced extra-articular supracondylar fractures, especially in elderly osteoporotic patients in whom internal fixation with plates or screws is contraindicated. This treatment can also be applicable to young patients with comminuted extra-articular fractures. Following an initial period of three to four weeks of skeletal traction through a distal femoral pin, either a hinged cast brace or a functional brace is applied. This treatment method is not appropriate for most comminuted and intra-articular supracondylar fractures, because better results have been reported with internal fixation techniques.

Interlocking Intramedullary Nailing

Standard locked intramedullary nailing may be used for type A extra-articular fractures as well as selected C1 and C2 intra-articular fractures. The results of locked intramedullary nails supplemented with intrafragmental screw fixation of intra-articular fragments parallel those following open reduction and internal fixation with plates. Certain modifications of the standard nailing procedure are necessary. These include the use of a distal femoral traction pin, substantial adduction of the distal fragment, the use of a thigh support under the proximal fragment to prevent fracture sagging, absolute central placement of the nail within the distal fragment, and intraoperative verification of anatomic reduction of all intra-articular fractures. The precise measurement of the nail is imperative, and this often necessitates cutting off the distal-most 15 mm of the nail. The use of fully threaded screws is also recommended. This treatment is not recommended for type B or type C3 fractures.

Flexible Intramedullary Rods

Flexible intramedullary rods are indicated primarily for elderly patients with noncomminuted extra-articular distal femoral fractures. Satisfactory axial alignment of the fracture and early mobilization of the patient is possible, but anatomic fracture reduction and rigid stabilization should not be expected. If the fracture is comminuted, shortening usually occurs around the rods. Available implants include Rush rods, Ender nails, and the Zickel supracondylar device.

These devices can be inserted under image intensifier control without opening the fracture site. A functional fracture cast brace often is used for additional stability, because these implants serve only as intramedullary splints. Weightbearing should be avoided until early fracture union has occurred. Deep infections occur infrequently and nonunion is rare.

Condylar Blade Plate and Compression Screw

The condylar blade plate provides rigid stabilization of comminuted, extra-articular and intra-articular fractures and is particularly applicable in young adults. If used in intra-articular fractures, additional lag screws for fixation of the major articular fragments are needed. Its insertion requires an extensive surgical incision. The goblet or "Mercedes" incision has been associated with high incidence of wound breakdown and infection, and is not advocated. A universal longitudinal midline incision over the knee is currently recommended. Separate lateral and medial incisions may alternatively be used.

When the blade plate is accurately inserted, good to excellent results can be expected in 75% of patients. Complications are usually caused by technical errors, and result from inadequate reduction of the articular surfaces, from inaccurate positioning of the blade plate, or from failure to apply a cancellous bone graft. Long-term complications include nonunion, which may result in failure of the implant, knee joint stiffness, and degenerative osteoarthritis.

The condylar compression screw has indications similar to those for the condylar blade plate, but is easier to insert. The lag screw of this implant provides compression across the intercondylar fracture, but supplemental interfragmentary lag screws separate from the plate are recommended. The disadvantage of the condylar compression screw is that stabilization of the distal fragment is less rigid than with the condylar blade plate, and insertion of the lag screw requires removal of a large amount of metaphyseal bone. If the device fails and the fracture does not unite, the loss of metaphyseal bone makes reconstruction difficult. Satisfactory results have been reported in 70% of cases in which the device has been applied correctly.

Condylar Buttress Plate

The condylar buttress plate is designed to fix intra-articular fractures of the femur that have extensive comminution (type C3). It is easy to apply and permits the insertion of multiple lag screws across the intra-articular fracture. Anteroposterior lag screws may be needed to fix fractures of the medial or lateral condyle in the frontal plane. The plate must be applied accurately to avoid fixation of the fracture in varus or valgus alignment. This implant has several mechanical problems. The plate is weaker than either the condylar blade plate or the condylar compression screw. The screw head/plate junction of the condylar buttress plate is not rigidly locked, and thus can slip with early loading of the fracture. Early weightbearing on an unhealed fracture can therefore result in varus deformity. The patient should avoid weightbearing ambulation until the fracture has healed, but early motion of the knee is allowed. All type A2, A3, C1, C2, and C3 fractures stabilized by a plate require a bone graft medially. Occasionally, when comminution is severe, a medial buttress plate is also required to prevent varus settling of the fracture.

Annotated Bibliography

Patients with Multiple Injuries

Bone LB, Johnson KD, Weigelt J, et al: Early versus delayed stabilization of femoral fractures: A prospective randomized study. *J Bone Joint Surg* 1989;71A:336-340.

A total of 178 acute femoral fractures in adults were randomly assigned to early or delayed fracture stabilization. When patients with multiple injuries had delayed fracture stabilization, the evidence of pulmonary complications (adult respiratory distress syndrome, fat embolism, and pneumonia) was higher, the hospital stay was longer, and the number of days in the intensive care unit was increased. The cost of hospital care showed a statistically significant increase for all patients with delayed fracture treatment compared with those with early fracture stabilization.

General Considerations

Bohn WW, Durbin RA: Ipsilateral fractures of the femur and tibia in children and adolescents. *J Bone Joint Surg* 1991;73A:429-439.

Long-term follow-up (7.5 years) was obtained for 32 limbs with ipsilateral fracture of the femur and tibia and open growth plates (average age, 10.5 years). Multiple methods of treatment for fractures were used. Recommendations included 90-90 femoral pin traction and a tibial cast for patients under the age of 10 years. Indications for surgical stabilization of the femoral fracture were severe head trauma, adolescence (age undefined), severe soft-tissue injury, and inability to achieve acceptable closed reduction. Inability to achieve acceptable closed reduction and open fractures were indications for surgical stabilization of the tibial fracture regardless of age.

Brumback RJ, Wells JD, Lakatos R, et al: Heterotopic ossification about the hip after intramedullary nailing for fractures of the femur. *J Bone Joint Surg* 1990;72A:1067-1073.

One hundred consecutive unilateral fractures of the femur were studied prospectively to determine the incidence of heterotopic ossification (HO) about the hip after intramedullary nailing. No HO developed in 40% of patients, minimal or mild in 34%, moderate in 15%, and severe in 11%. Only severe ossification substantially limited hip motion. No correlation was evident between the degree of HO and the age or sex of the patient, the severity of injury, the presence or absence of head injury, the degree of comminution, the timing of nailing, or the type of intramedullary fixation. Irrigation with pulsatile lavage did not affect the incidence or severity of this complication.

Fein LH, Pankovich AM, Spero CM, et al: Closed flexible intramedullary nailing of adolescent femoral shaft fractures. *J Orthop Trauma* 1989;2:133-141.

Twenty-five stable femoral shaft fractures were nailed in patients 10 to 16 years of age using flexible intramedullary nails in each. Nails were inserted using a closed technique from the knee in a retrograde manner through medial and lateral portals 2 to 3 cm proximal to the distal physis. All fractures healed without leg length inequality. Unprotected weightbearing ambulation without assistive devices was possible at an average of 7.7 weeks. All patients had a normal gait at follow-up. Complications were minimal but included intraoperative comminution in three patients, mild angulation in two, and loss of knee motion in one.

Kruger DM, Kayner DC, Hankin FM, et al: Traction force profiles associated with the use of a fracture table: A preliminary report. *J Orthop Trauma* 1990;4:282-286.

A load cell was designed and constructed to use with a fracture table that allowed the determination of forces applied at the peroneal post during intramedullary nailing. Measurements were made on eight patients during actual surgery. Transient pudendal nerve palsy developed in three of eight patients. In both of these cases, relatively high loads were measured (428 to 643 N). Adduction of the hip around a fixed peroneal post during intramedullary nailing caused great increases in traction forces.

Schwartz JT Jr, Brumback RJ, Lakatos R, et al: Acute compartment syndrome of the thigh: A spectrum of injury. *J Bone Joint Surg* 1989;71A:392-400.

This is by far the largest series of thigh compartment syndrome ever reported (21 cases in 17 patients). Ten were associated with an ipsilateral femoral fracture. Predisposing factors for development of the syndrome included: hypotension, external thigh compression (MAST trousers), coagulopathy, vascular injury, and trauma to thigh with or without fracture. One-half of these patients developed a crush syndrome (myoglobinuria, renal failure, and organ collapse), and eight patients died of multiple injuries. Infection developed in six of nine patients who survived. Prompt diagnosis and immediate fasciotomy are imperative.

Wiss DA, Brien WW, Becker V Jr: Interlocking nailing for the treatment of femoral fractures due to gunshot wounds. *J Bone Joint Surg* 1991;73A:598-606.

Fifty-six patients with a low-velocity gunshot fracture of the femur were treated by closed or modified open reduction and interlocking nailing of the fracture. Five patients with a femoral artery injury were nailed acutely (within 48 hours), but the remainder were treated with delayed nailing (10 to 14 days). Intravenous antibiotics were administered for 72 hours, but no formal debridement was performed. All fractures healed (average, 23 weeks). There was no deep wound infection or osteomyelitis. Complications included malalignment (7 patients), broken screws (2), broken nails (3), and heterotopic ossification (2). The incidences of delayed union, nonunion, infection, and blood loss were comparable to reports of closed fractures treated with locked nailing.

Open Fractures

Brumback RJ, Ellison PS Jr, Poka A, et al: Intramedullary nailing of open fractures of the femoral shaft. *J Bone Joint Surg* 1989;71A:1324-1331.

Eighty-nine open femoral shaft fractures were treated with intramedullary nailing (27 grade I, 16 grade II, and 46 grade III open wounds). Treatment was immediate (24 hours) in 33 fractures. The criterion for immediate nailing was that irrigation and debridement (I & D) be done within eight hours of injury. All wounds had immediate I & D. All fractures healed (average, 5.2 months). No infections occurred in 62 grade I, grade II, or grade IIIA open fractures. In 27 grade IIIB open fractures there were three infections (one after immediate and two after delayed nailing).

Lhowe DW, Hansen ST: Immediate nailing of open fractures of the femoral shaft. *J Bone Joint Surg* 1988;70A:812-820.

Debridement of the wound and immediate reamed nailing were performed in 67 patients with open fractures of the femoral diaphysis from 1980 to 1985. There were 15 grade I, 19 grade II, and eight grade III soft-tissue injuries. Perioperative complications included loss of fixation in four patients, infection in two patients, and wound seroma in two patients. Other complications were routine for intramedullary nailing during that period. The authors concluded that immediate reamed nailing of open fractures of the femur was not associated with an increased rate of infection in their series.

Intramedullary Nails

Brumback RJ, Reilly IP, Poka A, et al: Intramedullary nailing of femoral shaft fractures: Part I. Decision-making errors with interlocking fixation. *J Bone Joint Surg* 1988;70A:1441-1452.

The criteria for dynamic intramedullary femoral stabilization should be precise and exact. Dynamic intramedullary femoral stabilization should be performed only for transverse or short oblique fractures of the femoral isthmus, with type I or type II comminution. Any increase in comminution at the site of the fracture noted during the procedure is an indication for static interlocking. The threshold for the use of static interlocking fixation of an apparently stable femoral fracture should be extremely low.

Brumback RJ, Uwagie-Ero S, Lakatos RP, et al: Intramedullary nailing of femoral shaft fractures: Part II. Fracture-healing with static interlocking fixation. *J Bone Joint Surg* 1988;70A:1453-1462.

Of 87 comminuted femoral fractures treated with static interlocking fixation, 98% were followed up. In two cases, conversion from static to dynamic interlocking fixation was required because of inadequate fracture healing; both progressed to uneventful union. Static interlocking of intramedullary nails in femoral shaft fractures does not appreciably inhibit the process of healing of the fracture, and routine conversion to dynamic intramedullary fixation is not needed.

Brumback RJ, Ellison TS, Poka A, et al: Intramedullary nailing of femoral shaft fractures: Part III. Long-term effects of static interlocking fixation. *J Bone Joint Surg* 1992;74A:106-111.

The final installment of this three-part series reviews 214 cases of femoral nailing with static locking. At 30 months of follow-up, two separate groups were reviewed, 111 cases with retained static locking and 103 cases which underwent dynamization at an average of 14 months after injury. Neither stress-shielding nor stress concentration was clinically evident in either group. Conversion to dynamic fixation before nail removal is unnecessary. Nail removal should follow circumferential healing of the femoral cortex.

Bucholz RW, Ross SE, Lawrence KL: Fatigue fracture of the interlocking nail in the treatment of fractures of the distal part of the femoral shaft. *J Bone Joint Surg* 1987;69A:1391-1399.

Fatigue fracture of an interlocking nail at the more proximal of the two distal screw holes was studied in seven patients. In all patients the fracture of the femur was 5 cm or less from the level of the fatigue fracture. Finite-element analysis revealed that the stress on the nail exceeded its fatigue-endurance limit with weightbearing, and that the femur had to regain 50% of its original stiffness through healing to accommodate weightbearing. The risk of fatigue failure may be minimized by using nails that have a larger diameter and by avoiding early weightbearing.

Christie J, Court-Brown C, Kinninmonth AW, et al: Intramedullary locking nails in the management of femoral shaft fractures. *J Bone Joint Surg* 1988;70B:206-210.

A total of 117 patients with 120 femoral shaft fractures were treated with intramedullary locking nails; there were 20 open fractures, 13 pathologic fractures, and two nonunions. No infections occurred. Rehabilitation and union rates were satisfactory. Comminution of the proximal femoral fracture occurred in six patients, and there were three femoral neck fractures. All healed without further complications.

Franklin JL, Winquist RA, Benirschke SK, et al: Broken intramedullary nails. *J Bone Joint Surg* 1988;70A:1463-1471.

Sixty broken intramedullary nails in 56 patients were evaluated. There was a major correlation between the types and diameter of the nails and the incidence of breakage. Locking nails with distal interlocking holes and an anteriorly placed slot may leave too little metal in the anterior aspect of the nail, predisposing them to fatigue fracture. Proximal welds in the nail predispose nails to breakage. The design of the nail is an important factor. Nail design, technical errors in insertion, improper choice of starting point, underreaming the canal, and defects in fabrication can contribute to nail breakage. Recommendations for removal of broken nails are provided.

Supracondylar Fractures of the Femur

Leung KS, Shen WY, So WS, et al: Interlocking intramedullary nailing for supracondylar and intercondylar fractures of the distal part of the femur. *J Bone Joint Surg* 1991;73A:332-340.

Thirty extra-articular (type A) fractures and seven intra-articular (type C1 and C2) fractures were treated with closed locked intramedullary nailing with the addition of percutaneous screw fixation for the intra-articular fractures. Results were 94% good to excellent using the The Hospital for Special Surgery knee-rating system. Complications included one delayed union which healed 2 cm short and local pain around screws in ten patients. No nail breakage occurred. Nails were modified by cutting off the distal 15 mm of the nail. Patients were nailed in the supine position.

Siliski JM, Mahring M, Hofer HP: Supracondylar-intercondylar fractures of the femur: Treatment by internal fixation. *J Bone Joint Surg* 1989;71A:95-104.

Fifty-two fractures treated by a standard technique (angle blade plate and bone graft) were evaluated. Age did not influence results. Results were good to excellent in 75%. Infection accounted for three of four poor results; all were in patients with open fractures.

45

Knee and Leg: Pediatric Aspects

Congenital Abnormalities

Congenital anomalies of the lower extremity are best approached through a classification system that divides such malformations on the basis of the embryologic failure thought to be responsible. The principal categories are failure of formation, failure of differentiation, duplication, hyperplasia, congenital constriction band syndrome, and generalized skeletal abnormalities. Significant longitudinal deficiencies involving the knee and leg represent failures of formation and are named according to the bone(s) that are completely or partially absent.

Paraxial Fibular Hemimelia

Fibular deficiency is the most common congenital long-bone deficiency of the lower extremity. It affects boys almost twice as often as girls, is usually unilateral, and is most commonly a complete terminal deficiency. Fibular hemimelia is often associated with other deformities of the extremity, including femoral shortening, abnormality of the distal tibial physis, and lateral column deficiency of the foot. As a result, the involved extremity is short and bowed, with a skin dimple at the apex of the bow. The foot is in an equinovalgus position, with missing lateral rays.

Clinically, the primary problems related to fibular hemimelia are limb length inequality and foot/ankle instability. The average discrepancy of limb length at maturity is approximately 12 cm. When a normal foot is present, careful consideration should be given to limb lengthening. With extreme limb length inequality, or when gross instability at the foot/ankle is present, Syme amputation may be carried out to allow application of a highly functional below-knee prosthesis.

Paraxial Tibial Hemimelia

The incidence of tibial hemimelia in the United States is estimated at 1 in 1 million. It is the only skeletal deficiency with a documented familial inheritance. Approximately 75% of all patients have associated skeletal anomalies; the incidence of congenital hip dysplasia may be as high as 20%. Tibial hemimelia may be terminal or intercalary, complete or incomplete. Thirty percent of cases are bilateral. Clinically, the affected extremity is shortened, with the foot in a rigid varus and supinated position. The knee joint may be unstable in two planes, and there may be an associated flexion contracture with popliteal webbing.

Clinically, the principal problems are limb length inequality, knee instability/contracture, and foot malrota-

tion. Successful centralization of the fibula has been described, but the procedure is not predictable. Most patients should be treated by amputation.

Congenital Femoral Deficiency

Proximal femoral focal deficiency (PFFD) is the third most common longitudinal deficiency of the lower extremity. The extent of the abnormality ranges from hypoplasia of the entire femur to a complete absence of the proximal end. In approximately two thirds of these patients, there is associated fibular hemimelia. Bilateral involvement is seen in 15% of the patients. The affected extremity has a short thigh, and the hip is held in flexion, abduction, and external rotation. The position and stability of the knee and foot are variable.

The primary clinical problems are limb length inequality, malrotation, instability at the hip (and, to a lesser extent, at the knee), and weakness of the proximal musculature. Treatment options range from limb lengthening or contralateral epiphysiodesis (or both) for mild cases to iliofemoral fusion, knee fusion, Syme amputation, Van Nes rotationplasty, and creative prosthetic application for more severe cases.

Angular Deformities

Angular deformities of the knee and leg may be present at birth. Subsequent angular deformity is developmental and may be either a normal physiologic variation during growth or pathologic as a result of a variety of conditions.

Congenital Angular Deformity

Posteromedial bowing of the tibia may be secondary to either developmental delay of the distal tibial physis or intrauterine malposition. This deformity is associated with calcaneus deformity of the foot, triceps surae weakness, and dorsiflexion contracture of the ankle. Involvement is unilateral, and often there is a posteromedial skin dimple at the apex of the angulation. Spontaneous correction of the angular deformity is often seen with growth. However, a significant number of patients will have limb length discrepancies averaging 4.0 cm at maturity. Determination of the ultimate limb length inequality is based on the observation that the proportional difference in length between the normal and the angulated tibia remains constant throughout growth. Treatment options include contralateral epiphysiodesis or ipsilateral limb lengthening. In the unusual instance of persistent severe, posteromedial bowing, corrective osteotomy should be considered. Bone healing after osteotomy is not a problem in this condition.

Anterolateral bowing of the tibia is a serious condition because of its association with pseudarthrosis. This deformity should be considered part of the spectrum of the bowing-pseudarthrosis disorder seen in neurofibromatosis. Anterolateral bowing of the tibia should be treated as a pre-pseudarthrotic lesion, with early application of a total contact orthosis. In the infant and younger child, the orthosis should include the knee and ankle. In the older child, a high ankle-foot orthosis may be adequate. A corrective osteotomy for the angular deformity is contraindicated because of the high incidence of bone healing problems in this condition.

Pseudarthrosis of the tibia may be present at birth, or it can result from fracture of an anterolaterally bowed tibia. Neurofibromatosis is present in approximately 50% of the patients with a tibial pseudarthrosis, while approximately 10% of patients with neurofibromatosis will have a pseudarthrosis of the tibia. The dysplastic type is characterized by narrowing, sclerosis, and obliteration of the medullary canal (Fig. 1). The cystic type shows no narrowing but instead has cyst-like areas containing tissue that resembles fibrous dysplasia microscopically (Fig. 2). In the latter type, the leg appears normal early in the course, with fracture and pseudarthrosis occurring after 5 years of age.

There are four general options in the treatment of this challenging condition. The first is osteosynthesis, which involves serial procedures to resect the abnormal bone and soft tissues, autogenous bone grafting, application of local muscle flaps, internal fixation, prolonged immobilization, and electrical stimulation to heal the defect. The second is vascularized osteotransfer, in which resection of the abnormal tissues is followed by intercalation of a vascularized fibular graft from the contralateral extremity. Unfortunately, nonunion at the distal anastomosis and fracture of the graft are common complications. The third option is osteotransport, in which a multilevel ring fixator is applied, the abnormal tissue is resected, a proximal corticotomy is performed, and segmental bone transport is used to fill in the defect. Finally, in severe cases or after multiple procedures with persistence of the pseudarthrosis, amputation and prosthesis application are advisable. Syme amputation is preferred to amputation through the lesion because the latter is associated

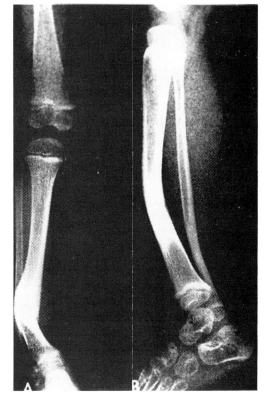

Fig. 1 Anteroposterior and lateral radiographs of dysplastic type of congenital pseudarthrosis of the tibia. Note the anterolateral bowing and the narrowed, sclerotic diaphyseal segment. (Reproduced with permission from Tachdjian MO: Congenital pseudarthrosis of the tibia. *Pediatric Orthopedics*, ed 2. Philadelphia, WB Saunders, 1990, vol 1, p 659.)

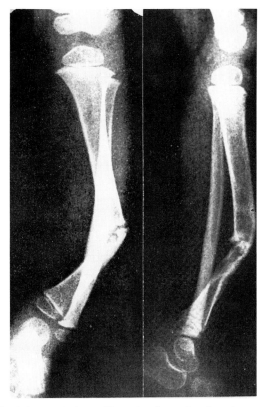

Fig. 2 Anteroposterior and lateral radiographs of cystic congenital pseudarthrosis of tibia. Note the fracture through the diaphyseal cyst. (Reproduced with permission from Tachdjian MO: Congenital pseudarthrosis of the tibia. *Pediatric Orthopedics*, ed 2. Philadelphia, WB Saunders, 1990, vol 1, p 660.)

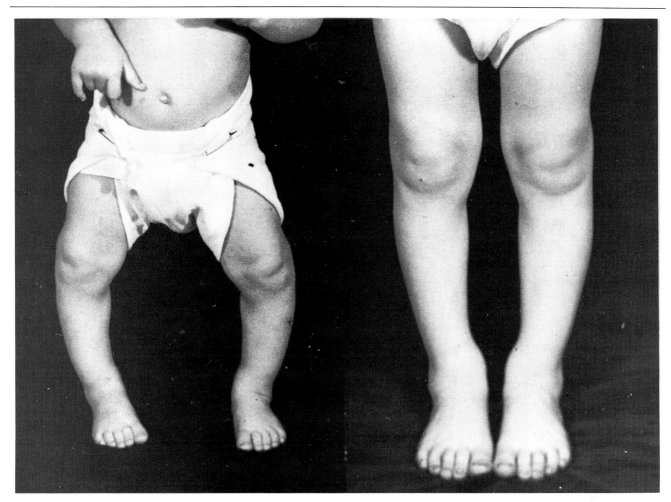

Fig. 3   Spontaneous correction of physiologic genu varum in a child between 1 year of age (**left**), and 3 years of age (**right**).

with bone overgrowth and a need for frequent stump revision of the residual limb in the growing child.

Development Angular Deformity

Physiologic genu varum and genu valgum are common angular deformities seen in infants and children. Early in infancy, lateral bowing of the tibia is common. Subsequent physiologic genu varum, or bowlegs, involves angular deformity of both the tibia and the femur and is maximal at approximately 18 months of age (Fig. 3). Physiologic genu valgum, or knock knees, develops next, with the maximum deformity occurring at 3 years of age (Fig. 4). Gradual correction to the ultimate alignment of slight genu valgum occurs by 9 years of age in the great majority of patients.

Pathologic tibia vara, or Blount's disease, a growth disorder of the medial portion of the proximal tibial physis, is characterized by medial angulation and internal rotation of the proximal tibia. The etiology is related to repetitive trauma to the posteromedial proximal tibia physis from ambulating on a knee with varus alignment.

Children with tibia vara are usually in the upper percentiles of weight for age and began walking early. Their gait is characterized by a painless varus thrust in the stance phase. Early-onset, or infantile, tibia vara is usually seen between 2 and 4 years of age, and early brace treatment is possible. This includes long-leg, locked-knee braces with a pelvic band to control rotation, worn while the child is weightbearing. Nighttime bracing does not address the pathophysiology and is ineffective. In progressive cases, early valgus osteotomy of the tibia is necessary to avoid development of irreversible medial growth-plate arrest. Late-onset tibia vara may be juvenile or adolescent. The pathophysiology remains the same in all types of tibia vara. Juvenile tibia vara has its onset between 4 and 10 years of age, whereas adolescent tibia vara is seen after 11 years of age in association with growth spurts. Prior to development of a physeal arrest, treatment consists of proximal tibial osteotomy. Once a medial physeal arrest occurs, treatment becomes more difficult. Considerations for treatment would be tibial osteotomy with or without completion of fusion of the physeal plate.

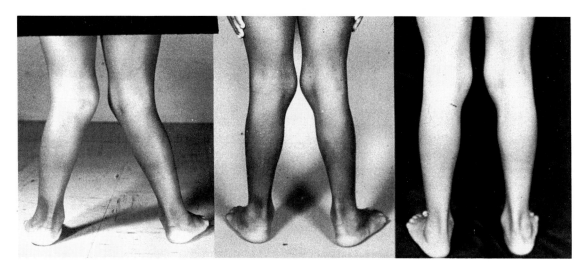

Fig. 4   Natural history of physiologic genu valgum in a child at 3, 5, and 7 years of age (from **left** to **right**).

Physeal bar resection and interposition remains an unproven technique.

Pathologic genu valgum is occasionally seen after unresolved physiologic valgus and can be treated effectively by stapling of the distal, medial femoral physis or hemiepiphysiodesis.

Post-traumatic genu valgum can follow a proximal tibial metaphyseal fracture (Fig. 5). This deformity is thought to be attributable to relative overgrowth of the tibia with respect to the fibula. Progressive valgus alignment may occur as late as two years after injury. Early osteotomy should be avoided, because the deformity usually corrects spontaneously over a three- to four-year period. Any residual deformity can be treated in adolescence by physeal stapling or hemiepiphysiodesis.

Other potential causes of pathologic genu varum or genu valgum are metabolic disorders such as rickets and renal osteodystrophy. Correction of the underlying metabolic condition often leads to spontaneous resolution of the angular deformity and is an absolute prerequisite to surgical correction by osteotomy.

Abnormalities of the Knee

Knee pain is a common complaint in children and adolescents. A systematic evaluation of the pediatric patient with knee pain should begin at the hip, because relatively common disorders of the hip, such as Legg-Calvé-Perthes disease and slipped capital femoral epiphysis, often present as referred pain involving the knee. The knee examination should include the patellofemoral joint, the tibiofemoral joint, the distal femoral and proximal tibial physes, the intra-articular and extra-articular ligaments, and the menisci.

Patellofemoral Disorders

Congenital dislocation of the patella describes a complete, irreducible, lateral dislocation. Clinically, the infant presents with genu valgum, flexion contracture of the knee, and lateral rotation of the tibia. The treatment is surgical, involving quadriceps mobilization, medial advancement, and medial hemitransfer of the patellar tendon. The surgery should be performed as early in infancy as possible.

Recurrent patellar subluxation or dislocation may occur during childhood but is more commonly seen in adolescence. The etiology is multifactorial, involving several predisposing factors in conjunction with a traumatic episode. Significant factors include generalized ligamentous laxity, excessive genu valgum, rotational malalignment (increased femoral anteversion with compensatory external tibial torsion, reflected by an increased Q angle), and patella alta. In the child, patellar subluxation or dislocation is usually associated with several of these pathologic conditions, and surgical treatment usually is necessary. In the adolescent, trauma may be the most significant factor, and after an initial period of immobilization, a vigorous program of quadriceps strengthening is the treatment of choice. Unfortunately, two thirds of patients will have recurrent episodes of patellofemoral instability, and, in this group, surgical correction is indicated. The many surgical techniques described for patellar realignment involve variable combinations of lateral release, medial advancement, distal patellar tendon hemitransfer, and medial semitendinosis tenodesis. Selection of the appropriate procedure requires an appreciation of the significant predisposing factors.

The patella may develop from one or multiple ossification centers. Failure of the separate centers of ossification to fuse may result in the formation of a bipartite, or occasionally tripartite, patella. This condition is usually

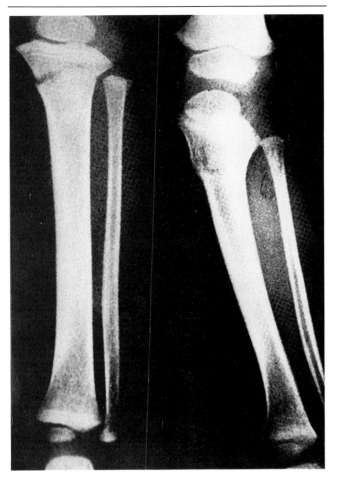

Fig. 5 Radiographs of a left tibial fracture in a 3-year-old girl with a genu valgum deformity at the time of injury (**left**) and 1 year later (**right**). (Reproduced with permission from Staheli LT: The lower limb, in Morrissy RT (ed): *Lovell and Winter's Pediatric Orthopaedics*, ed 3. Philadelphia, Lippincott, 1990, vol 2, p 752.

bilateral and painless. Of the accessory fragments, 75% are superlateral, 20% are lateral, and 5% are found at the inferior pole. Repetitive microtrauma may injure the synchondrosis, resulting in pain. Surgical treatment (excision or internal fixation) is reserved for lesions not responding to a three-week period of immobilization or for those with significant displacement.

Osteochondritis dissecans is characterized by bone necrosis and softening of the overlying cartilage. The fragment may separate and displace to varying degrees. The etiology is multifactorial, and there appears to be a hereditary predisposition. Males are affected three times more commonly than females. Osteochondritis dissecans occurs most frequently on the lateral aspect of the medial femoral condyle, the posterior aspect of the lateral femoral condyle, and the patella. Routine anteroposterior and lateral radiographs of the knee should be supplemented by a tunnel or notch view to best determine the location of the lesion. Bone scanning, magnetic resonance imaging, and arthroscopy are also helpful diagnostic tools. Intact asymptomatic lesions require only observational management. Persistently symptomatic or displaced lesions are best evaluated and treated arthroscopically. Treatment ranges from drilling of in situ lesions to promote revascularization to excision of displaced fragments less than 5 mm in diameter. Open reduction with internal fixation and bone grafting is the treatment of choice for large fragments that are either loose or displaced. Fixation may be obtained with standard Kirschner wires, resorbable Kirschner wires, and AO or Herbert screws.

Physeal Injuries

Physeal fractures about the knee are more common than ligamentous injuries in children. Stress-view radiographs and the presence of circumferential physeal tenderness help to make the diagnosis. Distal femoral physeal fractures account for approximately 5% of all physeal fractures. Displacement in the sagittal plane has been associated with neurovascular injury in the popliteal fossa and instability on closed reduction. Displacement in the coronal plane is not associated with other injuries, and the joint may be stable after closed reduction. Salter-Harris II fractures are the most common fracture pattern of the distal femoral physis. Subsequent growth arrest, partial or complete, with progressive angulation, shortening, or both occurs in between 30% and 80% of patients. Anatomic reduction can usually be obtained by closed means and maintained by percutaneous crossed Kirschner wires and spica cast immobilization.

Proximal tibial physeal fractures are relatively rare, with an estimated incidence of less than 1%. Sagittal plane displacement can injure either the popliteal or the anterior tibial artery. Compartment syndrome has also been described after this injury.

Physes under tension or distraction forces are known as apophyses. Repetitive microtrauma to the tibial tubercle, which may produce a partial avulsion, is known as Osgood-Schlatter's disease. This condition is usually seen in adolescents and is associated with growth spurts and quadriceps tightness. Treatment principles include both reduction of stress on the apophysis by activity modification and quadriceps-stretching exercises. The natural history is usually benign and self-limited, with resolution of symptoms within two years.

A similar mechanism of injury may lead to an apophysitis of the distal pole of the patella, a condition known as Sinding-Larsen-Johansson syndrome. This condition is also seen in patients with cerebral palsy who have a crouched gait and patellar overload. The treatment principles and the natural history are similar to those of Osgood-Schlatter's disease.

Ligamentous Injury

Ligamentous injuries about the knee are less common in children than in adults but may be just as debilitating. The collateral ligaments originate from the distal femoral epiphysis and insert on the proximal tibial epiphysis, with the exception of the superficial portion of the medial collateral ligament, which inserts on the tibial metaphysis distal to the physis. Although the ligaments are stronger than the physis, there have been reports of isolated ligamentous injuries in children, as well as of collateral ligament disruption associated with physeal fracture. Treatment of collateral ligament injuries is controversial and anecdotal and is based on principles established in adults.

Anterior cruciate ligament (ACL) injuries in children are difficult to manage. The prognosis for the ACL-deficient knee in the child is poor, with a significant incidence of subsequent meniscal injury, early degenerative changes, and poor function. Avulsion injuries of the ACL from the tibial epiphysis, and occasionally from the femoral epiphysis, reflect the relative strength of the bone-ligament interface in children. Anatomic reduction, with internal fixation if necessary, is the treatment of choice for this injury. Despite adequate reduction and fixation, a measurable degree of cruciate ligament laxity is seen in 50% of patients. Midsubstance ACL tears in children may be treated by bracing, primary repair, extra-articular tenodesis, or intra-articular reconstructions. A poor functional result, with a high incidence of subsequent reinjury, is seen after bracing and primary repair.

Disruption of the posterior cruciate ligament (PCL) is a rare injury in children. Deficiency of the PCL associated with osteochondral avulsions, primarily from the femoral side, is a consequence of hyperextension and should be repaired primarily. A midsubstance tear of the PCL in an adolescent is treated according to the principles established for adults.

Meniscal Injuries

The menisci, previously considered expendable, actually serve several important functions in the knee. They function as joint stabilizers, transmit and distribute load between the femoral and tibial articular surfaces, and play a role in the nourishment of the articular cartilage by distributing synovial fluid.

A discoid meniscus, instead of being semilunar or C shaped, is thick and wafer shaped (Figs. 6 and 7). This abnormality usually involves the lateral meniscus and is frequently found in both knees. There are two main types of discoid meniscus. The complete type has normal peripheral attachments and normal mobility. It is thought to represent a failure of differentiation in utero and is usually asymptomatic. When symptomatic, a tear is usually present, which should be treated by arthroscopic partial meniscectomy and meniscoplasty. The incomplete, or Wrisberg ligament type, has no posterior attachment to the tibial plateau. Despite the presence of the posterior meniscofemoral (Wrisberg) ligament, there is instability of the meniscus, and on knee extension, the abnormal meniscus is pulled into the intercondylar notch instead of gliding forward. This abnormal motion causes irritation of the initially normal semilunar lateral meniscus, which becomes thickened and irregular in shape.

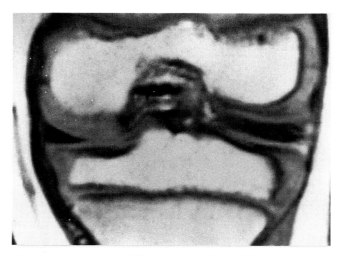

Fig. 6   Anteroposterior MRI scan of a left knee with a discoid lateral meniscus.

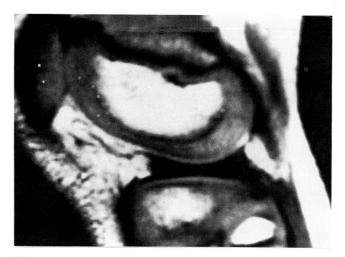

Fig. 7   Lateral MRI scan of a left knee with a discoid lateral meniscus.

The incomplete type of discoid meniscus is usually symptomatic (limited extension, pain, snapping) and should be treated by partial meniscectomy and posterior stabilization via the arthroscope or by a transverse lateral arthrotomy.

The treatment of meniscal tears in children and adolescents, a relatively uncommon injury, is based on an appreciation of the meniscal vascularity. Peripheral detachments and longitudinal tears near the capsular margin can be treated by primary repair. Chronic, complex, central tears should be treated by partial meniscectomy via the arthroscope.

Limb Length Inequality

The many potential etiologies of limb length inequality can be grouped functionally into two types of processes: those that change the length of the leg directly, and those that alter its growth. Examples of the former type include malunited fractures and dislocations. The latter type may reflect growth inhibition by such processes as physeal arrests after trauma; physeal destruction by infection, tumor, or vascular insult; and paralysis. Alternatively, growth may be stimulated by fracture (eg, femoral overgrowth after diaphyseal fracture), tumor (eg, Klippel-Trenaunay-Weber syndrome, neurofibromatosis), and chronic inflammation (eg, juvenile rheumatoid arthritis, hemophilia).

Limb length inequality affects the biomechanics of gait and alters the distribution and transmission of forces across the ankle, knee, hip, and spine. Discrepancies less than 2.5 cm are generally well tolerated and require no treatment. When the discrepancy is less than 5 cm, a shoe lift or a contralateral epiphysiodesis are the simplest, most reliable methods to obtain limb length equality at skeletal maturity. Limb lengthening is reserved for discrepancies greater than 5 and less than 15 cm. Effective lengthening can be accomplished by uniplanar or ring fixators attached to the bone by multiple pins or wires.

Distraction osteosynthesis is obtained by gradual distraction (1 mm/day) across an osteotomy.

To determine the appropriate management of the child with a limb length inequality, it is necessary to estimate the anticipated discrepancy at skeletal maturity. Three methods are used to analyze limb length data: the arithmetic method, the growth-remaining method, and the straight-line graph method. The arithmetic method is the simplest, yet least accurate. It is based on the assumption that the proximal femoral physis grows 4 mm per year, the distal femoral physis 10 mm per year, the proximal tibial physis 6 mm per year, and the distal tibial physis 5 mm per year. The other essential assumptions are that girls stop growing at 14 years and boys at 16 years. In a busy clinic, when surgical intervention is not imminent, this method is the most useful form of analysis. The other two methods, both of which are more complex, are also more accurate. Both include assessment of past growth, prediction of future growth, and prediction of the effect of surgery. The straight-line graph method is the most sophisticated and is widely used. The development of computer software to analyze data by this method has facilitated its application in the clinical setting.

Annotated Bibliography

Congenital Deficiencies

Choi IH, Kumar SJ, Bowen JR: Amputation or limb-lengthening for partial or total absence of the fibula. *J Bone Joint Surg* 1990;72A:1391-1399.

A review of 32 patients with fibular hemimelia compared treatment by Syme or Boyd amputation and early prosthetic fitting with treatment by Wagner-technique limb lengthening. The latter regimen is best suited for patients with a percentage of shortening of less than 15% and stable hips, knees, and ankles. Ablation of the foot and prosthetic fitting yielded excellent results in patients with fibular hemimelia not meeting these criteria.

Epps CH Jr, Tooms RE, Edholm CD, et al: Failure of centralization of the fibula for congenital longitudinal deficiency of the tibia. *J Bone Joint Surg* 1991;73A:858-867.

This study documents the poor outcome after treatment of complete tibial hemimelia by centralization of the fibula. Progressive flexion deformity of the knee occurred after all of the index procedures, necessitating multiple reoperations. Satisfactory results were ultimately reliably obtained after disarticulation at the knee.

Pirani S, Beauchamp RD, Sawatzky B: Soft tissue anatomy of proximal femoral focal deficiency. *J Pediatr Orthop* 1991;11:563-570.

Biplanar MRI evaluation of six patients with PFFD revealed a consistent pattern of soft-tissue anatomy. All muscles are present, most are smaller than normal, and some may have a functional role in the stability of the hip in PFFD, analogous to that of the rotator cuff at the shoulder.

Schoenecker PL, Capelli AM, Millar EA, et al: Congenital longitudinal deficiency of the tibia. *J Bone Joint Surg* 1989;71A:278-287.

A multi-institutional review was conducted of the treatment of all degrees of tibial hemimelia. The authors developed comprehensive treatment guidelines based on the radiographic assessment of the tibial deficiency and the clinical assessment of knee and ankle stability. Knee disarticulation, foot ablation, ankle reconstruction, and limb lengthening are used in various combinations based on the degree of deformity.

Angular Deformities

Crossett LS, Beaty JH, Betz RR, et al: Congenital pseudarthrosis of the tibia: Long-term follow-up study. *Clin Orthop* 1989;245:16-18.

Controversies regarding the treatment of congenital pseudarthrosis of the knee are attributable in part to disagreement about when the result can be considered final. This study reviews 25 patients with congenital pseudarthrosis of the tibia for an average follow-up of 36 years. The authors conclude that the results at skeletal maturity are reliable indicators of long-term results.

Thompson GH, Carter JR: Late onset tibia vara (Blount's disease): Current concepts. *Clin Orthop* 1990;255:24-35.

This paper compares and contrasts the juvenile and adolescent forms of idiopathic tibia vara. With the exception of age at onset, amount of remaining growth, and magnitude of the compressive forces across the medial aspect of the knee, the authors found no significant clinical, radiographic, or physeal-histopathologic differences between the two groups. Recurrence of the deformity after surgical correction was more frequent in the juvenile type, while incomplete surgical correction of the deformity was seen more often in the adolescent type.

Weiland AJ, Weiss AP, Moore JR, et al: Vascularized fibular grafts in the treatment of congenital pseudarthrosis of the tibia. *J Bone Joint Surg* 1990;72A:654-662.

State-of-the-art treatment with a free vascularized fibular graft yielded an ultimate union in 18 of 19 patients. Five nonunions after the index procedure, usually at the proximal end of the graft, required nine bone-grafting procedures. Residual tibial malalignment, anterior bowing or valgus deformity, was a common problem.

Abnormalities of the Knee

Bowen JR, Leahey JL, Zhang ZH, et al: Partial epiphysiodesis at the knee to correct angular deformity. *Clin Orthop* 1985;198:184-190.

The authors review 13 patients treated by partial epiphysiodesis to correct angular deformity before skeletal maturity is reached. The article includes a chart of angular deformity versus growth remaining that can be used to predict the appropriate timing for partial epiphysiodesis.

Gao GX, Lee EH, Bose K: Surgical management of congenital and habitual dislocation of the patella. *J Pediatr Orthop* 1990;10:255-260.

The authors review 12 patients with congenital dislocation of the patella and 23 patients with habitual dislocation of the patella after surgical realignment and stabilization. The underlying disorder was usually contracture of the quadriceps mechanism. Surgical treatment involving various degrees of lateral and proximal release, medial plication, and distal hemitransfer yielded satisfactory results in 88% of the patients.

Grogan DP, Carey TP, Leffers D, et al: Avulsion fractures of the patella. *J Pediatr Orthop* 1990;10:721-730.

This is a comprehensive clinical, radiographic, histopathologic, and biomechanical review of 47 patients with marginal fractures of the patella. Appreciation of the "sleeve" fracture pattern is essential when determining the appropriate treatment of patellar fractures in children.

Hresko MT, Kasser JR: Physeal arrest about the knee associated with non-physeal fractures in the lower extremity. *J Bone Joint Surg* 1989;71A:698-703.

This article describes seven patients with concomitant diaphyseal fracture of the tibia or femur and initially unrecognized physeal injury about the knee. Recognition of the physeal injury was delayed for almost two years, until gross angular deformity occurred. Awareness of this association should lead to careful evaluation of the physes at the time of injury and in the early follow-up period to permit early diagnosis and prevention of angular deformity.

Slough JA, Noto AM, Schmidt TL: Tibial cortical bone peg fixation in osteochondritis dissecans of the knee. *Clin Orthop* 1991;267:122-127.

A review of 10 knees with large, loose, symptomatic osteochondritis dissecans treated by tibial, iliac, or allograft bone pegs. Clinical results at three-year follow-up were excellent; however, magnetic resonance images show poor lesion cartilage and incorporation in almost half of the cases. Magnetic resonance imaging should be the standard on which future analysis of the treatment of osteochondritis dissecans is based.

Sullivan JA: Ligamentous injuries of the knee in children. *Clin Orthop* 1990;255:44-50.

This article is a comprehensive review of the tibial spine avulsions, tears of the anterior and posterior cruciate ligaments, collateral ligament injuries, and associated fractures and ligament injuries about the knee. Extensive references are provided.

Twyman RS, Desai K, Aichroth PM: Osteochondritis dissecans of the knee: A long-term study. *J Bone Joint Surg* 1991;73B:461-464.

A follow-up study to the senior author's classic paper published in 1971. Twenty-two knees with osteochondritis dissecans diagnosed in children were followed for an average of 33.6 years. Fifty percent showed some radiographic signs of osteoarthritis; in 32% this condition was graded as moderate or severe. Larger lesions in a weightbearing position on the condyle had the worst outcome. Classic medial position lesions did the best when any loose fragments were excised.

Wiley JJ, Baxter MP: Tibial spine fractures in children. *Clin Orthop* 1990;255:54-60.

The authors review 45 children with fractures of the tibial spine. Instrumental testing revealed measurable degrees of residual laxity of the anterior cruciate ligament despite the absence of clinical symptoms of instability. Anatomic reduction by arthrotomy did not prevent the cruciate laxity or loss of full knee extension. Concomitant collateral ligament injuries healed well with immobilization, demonstrating no residual laxity.

Yates CK, Grana WA: Patellofemoral pain in children. *Clin Orthop* 1990;255:36-43.

Recognizing that the majority of patellofemoral pain in children is caused by trauma, malalignment, or both, the authors propose a classification system based on etiology rather than symptoms. This systemic approach facilitates the diagnosis and directs treatment, both nonoperative and operative.

Limb Length Inequality

Green SA, ed: Limb lengthening. *Orthop Clin North Am* 1991;22:555-734.

The editor, one of the most experienced North American orthopaedists with respect to the Ilizarov technique, has put together 16 articles that represent the state-of-the-art thinking on limb lengthening. Several articles deal with clinical technical aspects, such as percutaneous osteotomies, avoidance of equinus contracture during tibial lengthening, and management of skin and myofascial complications. Patient selection in general, as well as the role of lengthening in achondroplasia and fibular hemimelia, are also reviewed.

Grill F, Dungl P: Lengthening for congenital short femur: Results of different methods. *J Bone Joint Surg* 1991;73B:439-447.

Thirty-seven patients with unilateral congenital short femur were treated by several different lengthening techniques. Callus distraction with uniplanar or ring fixators utilizing a distal metaphyseal corticotomy proved to be the most effective. The authors suggest that lengthening procedures can be applied successfully to Pappas Class II and IV deformities.

Guidera KJ, Hess WF, Highhouse KP, et al: Extremity lengthening: Results and complications with the orthofix system. *J Pediatr Orthop* 1991;11:90-94.

Early North American experience with limb lengthening by callotasis with a uniplanar fixator showed improvement in length gain and treatment time. Complications were common with this technique. In this series, there were 1.2 major complications per patient, and each patient required an average of 3.4 surgical procedures. Patients with congenital insensitivity to pain or postirradiation syndrome and those whose lower extremities are important for daily activities (eg, bilateral upper extremity amelia) should not undergo lengthening.

Moseley CF: Assessment and prediction in leg-length discrepancy, in Barr JS (ed): American Academy of Orthopaedic Surgeons *Instructional Course Lectures, XXXVIII.* Park Ridge, IL, 1989, pp 325-330.

This is a comprehensive review, with examples, of the three principal methods utilized to predict leg length discrepancy; a clear, precise, "how-to-do-it" article.

Paley D: Problems, obstacles, and complications of limb lengthening by the Ilizarov technique. *Clin Orthop* 1990;250:81-104.

The author provides a somewhat controversial but comprehensive review of clinical difficulties during limb lengthening. This article is one of 19 in a symposium edited by the author on modern techniques in limb lengthening that appear in the same issue of this journal.

Timperlake RW, Bowen JR, Guille JT, et al: Prospective evaluation of 53 consecutive percutaneous epiphysiodeses of the distal femur and proximal tibia and fibula. *J Pediatr Orthop* 1991;11:350-357.

A concise review of this technique, as developed by the senior author, is given. The patients were divided into two groups based on whether the epiphysiodesis was the only procedure or a portion of the overall treatment plan. Both groups had excellent outcomes, with minimal complications. The authors also found a good correlation between the actual discrepancy at follow-up and the discrepancy at maturity as calculated by standard growth charts.

46

Knee and Leg: Bone Trauma

Fractures of the Proximal Tibia and the Tibial Plateaus

In younger patients, most fractures involving the largely cancellous proximal 10 to 12 cm of the tibia are caused by high-energy motor vehicle or industrial accidents. With the exception of the much feared extra-articular bumper injury, fractures of the proximal tibia in the elderly are caused by falls or minor missteps.

Of the intra-articular fractures, 60% involve the lateral plateau. This probably is a result of the valgus alignment of the lower extremity and the fact that most injuring forces are directed laterally to medially. Fractures of the medial plateau make up 15% and bicondylar lesions 25% of all tibial plateau fractures. Split, depression, and split-depression fractures are well recognized unicondylar fracture patterns. Bicondylar fractures combine any of the unicondylar lesions with a fracture of the metaphysis below. Partial or complete ligamentous ruptures occur in about 15% to 45% and meniscal lesions in about 5% to 37% of all tibial plateau fractures. With surgical management, a higher percentage of these lesions is noted. Nerve injuries, vascular disruptions, and compartment syndromes, rarely seen in typical tibial plateau fractures, are the hallmark of fracture dislocations. These lesions, characterized by minor avulsion fractures of the proximal tibia, carry a high incidence of associated injuries to ligaments, vessels, and nerves.

Evaluation

After assessment of the patient's general status and associated injuries, the initial evaluation focuses on location and extent of soft-tissue swelling; tenderness; integrity of muscle compartments, nerves, and vessels; and finally the fracture pattern. Radiographically, anteroposterior and lateral views in line with the tibial plateaus are basic. Traditionally, fracture severity has been further clarified by tomographs in two planes. In many institutions, tomograms have been replaced by computed axial tomography, which gives greater detail (2-D and 3-D reconstructions) and causes less discomfort to the patient. Anteroposterior views of the extended, uninjured knee are obtained as a reference for limb alignment. Preoperative stress films, taken with the patient under anesthesia, will identify associated ligamentous lesions. Stress films also have become an important tool to select between conservative and surgical treatment options, because these films provide an objective measure of the instability caused by the fracture itself. A history or fracture pattern suggestive of a fracture dislocation and di-minished peripheral pulses not restored by longitudinal traction are urgent indications for angiography.

Treatment

Extra-articular fractures of the proximal tibia often are associated with severe soft tissue compromise. In the initial period, they are ideally stabilized with an external fixator, which avoids the additional insult that typically occurs with open reduction and internal fixation. Once the soft tissues have healed, secondary plating or a proximally locked intramedullary nail should be considered if neither the operating field nor the pin tract have been jeopardized by an infection.

Some surgeons advocate open reduction and internal fixation for all tibial plateau fractures that are not anatomically aligned. Yet, most long-term studies indicate that patients who have less than 10 degrees of instability in full extension on initial examination will achieve a good result when treated in a cast or cast brace for 12 weeks. This is particularly true for patients who are older than 50 years of age, have osteopenic bone, a sedentary profession, and mild or moderate recreational needs. Initial immobilization in calcaneal traction and balanced suspension for four to six weeks, followed by transfer to a long leg cast or a cast brace has been, in the hands of some authors, as successful as casting alone or operative management. Major ligamentous disruption, instability of more than 10 degrees with a fully extended knee, age younger than 50 years, firm bone stock, a profession that involves moderate to heavy physical demands, and the enjoyment of vigorous recreational activities are factors that favor open reduction and internal fixation.

For surgical management, the knee joint is approached through a lateral parapatellar or midline incision. Progressively more extensive exposure is facilitated through an osteotomy of Gerdy's tubercle, detachment of the anterior horn of one or both menisci, and elevation of the quadriceps mechanism through an osteotomy of the tibial tubercle. Once anatomic reduction and rigid internal fixation are secured, the knee is clinically and radiographically examined for collateral ligament instability. A completely avulsed ligament should be repaired. Postoperatively, the limb is moved in a continuous passive motion machine. Later, active range-of-motion exercises and, if the fixation was suboptimal or the bone osteoporotic, a cast brace is added. Full weightbearing is rarely possible before eight to ten weeks.

Some simple split and depression fractures can be managed, through use of an image intensifier or an arthroscope, without massive surgical exposure. After reduction and percutaneous fixation of the joint surface with wires and screws, overall limb alignment is often secured with an external fixator. Little has been published on experience with this approach.

For the rare tibial plateau fracture associated with a popliteal artery injury or extensive local soft-tissue destruction, temporary immobilization of the knee joint with an anterior external fixator reaching from the midfemur to the midtibia can be advantageous. Secondary internal fixation with plates and screws can follow healing of the associated soft-tissue lesions.

Comparative Studies

Investigators who have addressed tibial plateau fractures during the past three years were mainly concerned with advantages and limitations of different management options, and the influence of ligamentous injuries, cast braces, bone substitutes, and various combinations of internal and external fixation on final outcomes.

One retrospective review evaluated 128 fractures treated over a 20-year period by either long leg casts and traction or open reduction and internal fixation according to AO principles. There was no algorithm for the choice of treatment modalities. A satisfactory outcome was defined as minimal pain, more than 90 degrees of knee motion, no instability, and no major complications. Satisfactory results were achieved in 85% of undisplaced and in 54% of displaced fractures treated nonsurgically and in 78% of displaced fractures treated with open reduction and internal fixation. The differences in outcome between these treatment groups were not statistically significant for any fracture type. For displaced fractures, results were unsatisfactory for traction alone, but traction followed by cast bracing was as successful as cast immobilization alone. Results were satisfactory for 72% of bicondylar fractures treated surgically and only 25% of those treated with cast immobilization. The choice of implant directly affected outcomes: satisfactory results were seen in 86% of fractures managed with buttress plates, in 80% with the use of cancellous screws, and in only 40% when fixation was secured with bolts, Kirschner wires, or staples. The nonunion rates were between 5% and 6% for either treatment method, but malunions occurred in 12% of surgically and 23% of nonsurgically treated patients. Of 12 nonunions in the nonsurgical group, nine occurred in split-compression or bicondylar fractures. The infection rate was 16% in the surgically treated group, with two patients developing osteomyelitis and one aseptic arthritis. Secondary surgical interventions, needed in 12% of patients after nonsurgical treatment and in 21% after surgery, were mostly open reduction and internal fixation, total knee replacement, fusion, and removal of hardware. Despite the limitations inherent in a retrospective review, the authors were able to document the following conclusions: (1) all patients with nondisplaced fractures treated with casts did well regardless of the period of immobilization; (2) patients with isolated depression or split fractures did equally well with or without surgery; (3) for displaced fractures, traction alone caused uniformly poor results; (4) although superior for split depression and for bicondylar fractures, open reduction and internal fixation had a high infection and reoperation rate; and, (5) if operative care is chosen, buttress plates and cancellous screws give the most secure fixation, bone grafts should be used to fill metaphyseal defects, menisci must be preserved or repaired, and early postoperative motion is paramount for a good outcome.

A fascinating comparison of conservative and surgical management was carried out by two Danish universities. Between the years 1976 and 1982, most patients at one center were treated by calcaneal traction for four to six weeks, followed by a cast brace. At the other center even minimally displaced fractures were treated by open reduction and internal fixation according to AO principles. Demographic and injury parameters were similar for both groups. Sixty-one patients in the traction group and 48 patients in the surgical group were reexamined between five and six years after the initial injury. Traction patients stayed in the hospital for six weeks and surgical patients for four weeks, a significant difference. Overall, functional results were significantly better in the traction group, and radiographic findings were similar in both groups. Seventy-four percent of the patients treated in traction and 54% of those treated by open reduction and internal fixation achieved knee motion from 0 to at least 90 degrees, had less than 5 degrees of valgus or varus, and were able to walk up to three quarters of a mile. However, there were no significant functional differences between patients who were operated on but did not have a meniscectomy and those treated nonsurgically. Osteoarthritic changes were significantly more common after surgery, particularly when the menisci were excised. The authors concluded that traction followed by cast bracing was a valid alternative to surgery but, considering its cost, should probably be reserved for cases where an operation is undesirable.

Ligamentous Injuries To determine the importance of associated ligamentous injuries and the advisability of surgical repair, one group compared charts of 20 patients who did not have surgical repair of the injured ligaments with those of 19 patients who had primary repair. In the first group, 13 patients had open reduction and internal fixation after a plateau fracture; in the second group all plateau fractures were treated surgically. Both groups were immobilized from two to ten weeks. Follow-up was at least one year. Medial collateral injuries accounted for 55%, lateral collateral injuries for 22%, and combined cruciate and collateral injuries for 23% of the lesions. The patients in both groups had comparable overall functional scores and a total range of motion between 113 and 115 degrees. Isolated injuries to the medial collateral ligaments that were repaired had a somewhat better outcome score, less residual instability (2.8 degrees), and no more than 10 degrees of total instability. For unrepaired medial ligaments, the average valgus instability was 6.8 degrees, with 30% of all patients having more than 10 degrees of valgus instability. For isolated lateral collateral injuries, surgical repair resulted in less varus instability (3.8 versus 8.8 degrees) and a better clinical result than no intervention. Isolated injuries to the cruciate ligaments were rare. Nine patients had a combination of injuries to the collateral and cruciate ligaments. Regardless of intervention, they had the lowest score and the highest residual varus/valgus instability (8.1 degrees). Of the 39 patients, 11 had poor results. All but one of these had in excess of 10 degrees of varus or valgus instability resulting from either ligamentous laxity or residual plateau depression. Among the patients who did not have surgical repairs, 50% had a good and 40% a poor result. Of the surgically repaired ligaments, 63% led to good and 15% to poor results.

Nonsurgical Management It appears that cast braces are an ideal adjunct to the management of surgically stabilized tibial plateau fractures, because, according to one study, they provide additional stability and security without restricting the ultimate range of motion. In 42 patients treated with cast braces alone, the brace was applied within a week of the injury, knee motion was initiated at an average of 12 days, and weightbearing was allowed only after fracture consolidation. Cast braces stabilized all fracture patterns successfully, apart from medial plateau lesions where malunions developed in over 20%.

Surgical Management In two smaller series of 20 and 43 patients treated surgically, there was a high incidence of ligamentous and meniscal tears. Open reduction and internal fixation led to satisfactory results in most patients. In one report, four out of five ligamentous injuries that had been repaired led to poor results despite the fact that the knees were clinically stable. The omission of a bone graft in fractures associated with a depressed joint surface also led to lesser outcomes. Implant removal to relieve slight pain or tenderness over plates or screws was demanded by more than a third of the patients.

Because many tibial plateau fractures require bone grafting, several investigators have searched for a substitute off-the-shelf material that would be as effective as bone. Assessment of two groups of comparable tibial plateau fractures, one treated with cancellous bone graft and the other with porous hydroxyapatite, indicated the latter was safe and as effective as autogenous bone. Although it is not osteoinductive, porous hydroxyapatite seems to meet most prerequisites for an effective filling agent: (1) the material is readily available in adequate volume, both in block form and granule size; (2) it can be easily contoured to the defect with a rongeur or a scalpel; (3) it allows adequate bone ingrowth; and (4) it is bioinert. Although biodegradation occurs at a slow pace, porous hydroxyapatite and similar materials are ex-

pected soon to become routine substitutes for the filling of metaphyseal defects. While possibly more costly, this approach will reduce donor site complications and, when compared to allografts, will avoid the transmission of infectious agents.

It has become increasingly evident that the use of indirect reduction techniques reduces morbidity after surgical interventions, increases the healing rate, and possibly improves outcomes. In an attempt to reduce the extent of surgical dissection, a small series of bicondylar plateau fractures were treated with lateral buttress plates in combination with a medial external fixator. This approach was also effective as the method of management for the salvage of secondary varus deformity after lateral plating. External fixation may also have a place in the management of comminuted proximal metaphyseal fractures with extension into the knee joint and minimal displacement at the articular surface. Rather than using buttress plates, one group of investigators is managing these fractures with closed manipulation followed by stabilization with multiple transfixion wires connected to an Ilizarov ring. Distally, this construct then is anchored to a ring or half-pin frame. Although this technique looks promising, long-term outcomes are needed to assess the validity of this approach.

Closed Tibial Shaft Fractures

General Aspects

The tibia is the most commonly fractured long bone. In children, union is quite rapid and complications are rare. Healing delays and unsatisfactory results are seen more often in adults in whom infection, displacement, an open wound, and comminution are the principal variables that lead to these problems. Although open fractures represent only 10% to 20% of all broken tibiae, they have the highest rates of complications and nonunions. The widely held belief that tibial fractures involving the distal third and those associated with an intact fibula heal more slowly remains unsubstantiated. In fact, an intact fibula generally means a shorter healing time but an increased tendency for varus misalignment.

A prospective analysis of 50 consecutive tibia shaft fractures undertaken at two trauma centers indicated that 22% of these fractures were accompanied by one or more ligamentous injuries, resulting at least in a 2 + laxity. More ligamentous tears were seen in closed fractures. The medial collateral ligament was always involved and the posterior cruciate ligament in 6%. The authors recommend that all knees be carefully examined for a ligamentous tear once the fracture is stabilized.

Treatment

The treatment of most closed tibial fractures starts with the application of a long leg cast, which often is replaced, after three to five weeks, by a snugly fitting short leg cast or a cast brace. With this approach, healing times average 16 to 20 weeks. Nonunion occurs in 2% to 5%, malalignment occurs in 3% to 8%, and shortening of more than 1 cm occurs in as many as 10% of patients. Because of associated injuries or unacceptable shortening and displacement in the cast, about 20% to 30% of all closed tibial fractures currently are treated with primary or secondary internal fixation. Plates seem best suited for the proximal and distal tibia; however, when plates are used in tibial shaft fractures, the rate of major complications, such as nonunions, implant failures, and infections, is around 5% to 17%. Intramedullary nails appear to be safer. For transverse fractures with minimal comminution, multiple thin elastic nails or a single stiff nail with and without reaming seem to be equally advantageous. More extensive comminution and/or a proximal or distal metaphyseal lesion, however, are best managed with locking nails. Closed fractures associated with severe skin abrasions or soft-tissue contusion should be treated temporarily with a splint, traction, or an external fixator. After fasciotomies for compartmental syndrome, tibia fractures should be stabilized with internal or external fixation.

Fracture Bracing

For the past three decades immobilization in a short leg walking cast or a functional brace has been the standard of care for most closed and some open tibial shaft fractures. A pioneer of this approach recently reviewed over 700 tibial shaft fractures treated with a long leg cast for three to five weeks followed by a functional brace with a hinged ankle joint until healing. The indications for this approach included most closed fractures, open lesions with minimal soft-tissue damage, and secondary conversion from an external fixator. Bracing was contraindicated for nonambulatory patients and those fractures that initially had a more than 10 mm of shortening or 5 degrees of angulation in any place. Patients with significant neurologic and vascular damage, segmental bone loss, and soft-tissue defects needing flap coverage were also excluded. Three percent of the fractures had to be remanipulated after the initial cast application. Treatment of another 6% was changed because of unacceptable angulation or shortening. The shortest healing times were observed with closed isolated fractures (15 weeks), and the longest with grade III open fractures (25 weeks). Of the fractures, 90% healed with 10 mm of shortening or less. Shortening in addition to that documented on initial radiographs occurred in 3% of the fractures and averaged 4 mm. Angulation in excess of 10 degrees and rotational deformities were rare. Nonunions occurred in 2.5%, mostly after open fractures. The patient's age, fracture location, and the mechanism of injury did not influence fracture healing. The authors concluded that grade III open fractures, displacement greater than one third of the tibial shaft, and comminution at the fracture site significantly prolonged fracture healing and increased the incidence of delayed unions. Fractures with

these characteristics should be considered less suitable for bracing.

Apart from increasing patient comfort, it has been felt that fracture bracing with a freely moving ankle joint will preserve a full range of ankle and subtalar motion. According to a study from Hong Kong that included 97 tibial fractures treated with a fracture brace and followed for about two years, this is not necessarily true. Few of the patients had full ankle and subtalar motion when the brace was removed. After 1.6 years, 60% of the patients had normal inversion and eversion, and about 70% had normal ankle motion. After two years, normal motion in subtalar and ankle joints was noted in 75% and 71% of all patients, respectively. Residual knee stiffness was rare and clinically insignificant. Noting that a hinged joint restricts ankle motion, the authors recommend a modified functional brace that allows full plantarflexion and dorsiflexion in the apparatus.

Intramedullary Nailing

A strong demand for early return to normal activities and the recognition that functional bracing is contraindicated for more complex fracture patterns has rekindled an interest in intramedullary nailing, particularly since locking devices became widely available about five years ago. Traditional nailing was limited to the middle third of the tibia, and locking has extended the functional range of tibial nails from the central one third to the central two thirds of the leg. Nailed tibial shaft fractures with up to grade II soft-tissue injury healed in an average of 15 to 17 weeks for isolated lesions, and 21 weeks for multiply injured patients. With an intact fibula, healing times were reduced by one to two weeks. Immediate weightbearing was possible in about 40% of the patients, 60% were weightbearing at three weeks, and over 90% at six weeks. Complications ranged between 1.6% and 5.3% and included compartment syndromes, deep infections, patellar tendon rupture, and the breakage of screws and nails. Hardware breakage often occurred after the fractures were healed. Shortening in excess of 1 cm was seen in up to 10% and rotational deformities in excess of 10 degrees in 1% to 2%, but angulatory deformities in excess of 10 degrees were rare. Up to 40% of the patients complained about knee pain and a third had the nail removed. Knee pain, in fact, was the most frequent complaint and was not always relieved by nail removal. Ankle motion was normal in about 90% of the patients and loss of knee motion was rare. Authors concluded that intramedullary nailing of closed and grade I open tibial fracture is a safe technique that combines a high rate of union with a low complication rate and early return to function. After a similar, favorable early experience with tibial nailing, a group of orthopaedic surgeons from New Zealand compared cast immobilization with closed intramedullary nailing of tibial shaft fractures in a prospective trial. Only fractures more than 5 cm away from either knee or ankle were entered. All fractures were at least 50% displaced and angulated 10 degrees or more. In addition to closed fractures, grade I open lesions were included. The treatment design was random and the final assessment was by an independent observer. Thirty-three patients were treated initially by a long leg cast, which was, at about four weeks, changed to a below knee walker. After an early review of their results, the authors terminated the trial as they felt it was unethical to continue conservative treatment. With intramedullary nailing, hospital stay was about three days longer, healing times were two weeks shorter (15 versus 18 weeks), the number of outpatient visits was cut almost in half (four versus seven), and return to work was shortened from 23 to 14 weeks. Problems after casting included three superficial peroneal nerve palsies, two pressure sores, and one refracture. Fifteen of the casted patients required surgical intervention to secure acceptable fracture alignment. The outcome of this study is not a complete surprise, because the principal entry criterion of displacement in excess of 50% of the shaft diameter is now a well-accepted contraindication to nonsurgical management.

Less optimistic data are presented in an in-depth review of complications after reamed intramedullary nailing of 60 acute shaft fractures. Although many of these fractures were unusually severe, and 75% were accompanied by one or more associated fractures in the same limb, the rate and nature of complications noted is instructive. Early complications included fractures extending into the tibial plateau, postoperative hematomas requiring surgical drainage, shortening in excess of 1 cm, and paresthesia in the distribution of the superficial or deep peroneal nerve in 20% of the patients. Three had a complete foot drop and two had a combined sensory and motor deficit. Forty-five fractures with more than one year follow-up had the following late complications: persistent neurologic problems (4%), patellar tendinitis (22%), prominent locking screws (4%), nonunion (4%), and two deep infections that ultimately resolved. Overall, 58% of the patients with long-term follow-up developed at least one complication. Although most of them did not affect the final result, they retarded rehabilitation and caused discomfort.

Open Tibial Shaft Fractures

Advanced age, displacement and comminution, the severity of the soft-tissue injury, the extent of bone loss, the disruption of a major artery, and the presence of a superficial or deep infection all adversely affect the outcome of open tibial fractures. Open fractures are classified into three main groups and three subgroups according to the severity of the soft-tissue injury. Grade I fractures have a small skin perforation from inside out. Grade II lesions have a large opening with associated muscle laceration and skin contusions. Grade IIIA lesions are even more extensive, have larger soft-tissue flaps, and a considerable amount of crushed muscle. Grade IIIB indicates initial soft-tissue loss and extensive

areas of denuded bone that make later flap coverage necessary. Grade IIIC fractures are associated with disruption of a major vessel, requiring surgical repair.

As in open fractures elsewhere, antibiotics, extensive and repeated debridements, fasciotomies, early stabilization, the use of local or free muscle flaps, and bone grafts are all crucial to the successful management of a severe open tibial fracture. The initial debridement must be radical, including all dead tissues and foreign material. Because continued soft-tissue swelling can cause additional muscle necrosis after the initial treatment, repeated debridements are needed at intervals of 36 to 48 hours until the wound is clean. Four-compartment fasciotomies are needed in about 5% to 10% of open tibial fractures and are mandatory in grade IIIC lesions. Criteria have been developed for separating those grade IIIB and grade IIIC lesions best managed with extensive soft-tissue reconstruction from those that will do best with early amputation. Most grade IIIC injuries with a warm ischemia time exceeding six hours should be amputated.

Antibiotic coverage starts when the patient arrives in the emergency room and takes into account the characteristics of the patient's injuries and the severity of the wound contamination. For most injuries a broad-spectrum cephalosporin should be supplemented by an aminoglycoside. Penicillin is added for farm-related injures and lesions suspected of major clostridial contamination. Antibiotics are discontinued within three days if the wound appears to be clean, or adjusted according to the results of earlier wound cultures.

Most wounds of grade IIIA severity or less can be closed on a delayed primary basis, or using a split-thickness skin graft. All grade IIIB and many grade IIIC wounds, however, require flap coverage. For the proximal third of the leg, such coverage is best achieved with a gastrocnemius flap; a soleus flap will cover soft-tissue defects extending towards the mid-aspect of the tibia, but a free flap is required for more distal defects. If the soleus or gastrocnemius muscles have been damaged, they are unsuitable for local coverage and a free flap must be substituted.

Although plating of open tibial shaft fractures has led to good results at some institutions, there is increasing evidence that infection rates and such secondary complications as implant failures and nonunions are unacceptably high. Early intramedullary nailing with either unreamed solid nails or thin elastic nails is becoming the method of choice for open tibial shaft fractures up to grade II severity. However, most tibial shaft fractures with grade IIIB and grade IIIC soft-tissue injuries, and less severe lesions unsuitable for internal fixation, are managed best with external fixators (Figs. 1 and 2).

Decision to Amputate

Management of grade IIIB and grade IIIC fractures remains a major dilemma. A high rate of complications and unsatisfactory functional outcomes often leads to secondary amputations. Several groups are working on

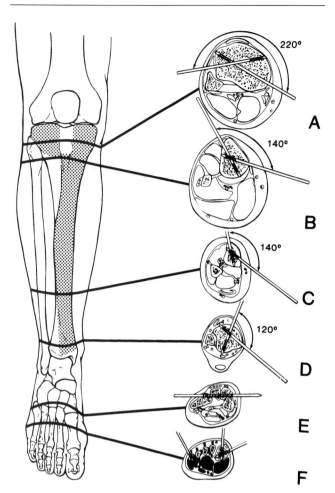

Fig. 1 The "safe corridor" for pin insertion in the lower leg. At level A, proximal to the tibial tubercle, pins can be safely inserted within an arc of 220 degrees. At level B, just below the tibial tubercle, the safe arc decreases to 140 degrees. At C, in the distal third of the leg, the safe arc remains 140 degrees, but the anterior tibial vessels and deep peroneal nerves become vulnerable as they cross the lateral tibial cortex. At levels E and F, pins in the tarsal or metatarsal bones may be used to splint the ankle joint if neurologic or soft-tissue injuries prevent the application of an external support. The dotted area indicates where the tibia lies subcutaneously and pin insertion is safe. (Reproduced with permission from Behrens F, Searls K: External fixation of the tibia: Basic concepts and prospective evaluation. *J Bone Joint Surg* 1986;68B:246-254.)

A			Most mid tibial lesions
B		1	Extensive lesions allowing only short pin–pin spreads Segmental bony defects Large limbs
		2	As above Large segmental or infected bony defects Lesions needing fixator frames for long periods of time

C			Proximal periarticular and undisplaced intra articular fractures
			    Simple lesions
			    Segmental comminution or bone loss
			    Large soft tissue defects

D			Distal metaphyseal fractures
			    Simple lesions
			    Segmental comminution or bone loss
			    Large soft tissue defects

E			Distal intraarticular fractures, often as temporary immobilization preceding internal fixation

Fig. 2 Diagrams showing the recommended configuration of fixator frames for different bone and soft-tissue injuries. The location and extent of the lesion are indicated on the left, by the cross-hatched area. In the middle is the preferred frame with solid bars representing the pins. On the right are the specific indications for the use of the configuration. (Reproduced with permission from Behrens F, Searls K: External fixation of the tibia: Basic concepts and prospective evaluation. *J Bone Joint Surg* 1986;68B:246-254.)

criteria to separate tibial fractures amenable to successful reconstruction from those that do best with immediate amputation. In one recent effort, the severity of the injury, limb ischemia, shock, and age were each rated according to severity. The individual scores were then added to form what the authors' called the Mangled Extremity Severity Score (MESS) (Table 1). When 25 severely injured lower extremities were scored retrospectively, the successfully reconstructed legs had scores from 3 to 6 (mean 4.9) and the amputated limbs had scores ranging from 7 to 11 (mean 9.1). In a second prospective trial, a score of 7 or higher predicted amputations in 26 patients with 100% accuracy. While this and other rating scales may accurately predict the best early treatment for a mangled extremity, they do not address long-term function and the general well-being of the patient.

Wound Management

The dictum to leave open fractures open was recently confirmed by Canadian investigators who evaluated retrospectively the effects of wound closure in 90 consecutive open tibial fractures. The deep wound infection rate was 20% with primary, and 3% with delayed wound closure. Nonunions occurred in 14% after primary and 3% after delayed wound closure. Both findings were statistically significant.

External Fixation

Comparison With Plates   It has long been recognized that casts and braces provide insufficient stabilization for open tibial fractures of grade II and grade III severity. Immediate plate fixation was popular a decade ago, because it facilitated secondary soft-tissue coverage and

Table 1. MESS (mangled extremity severity score) variables

	Points
A. Skeletal/soft-tissue injury	
Low energy (stab; simple fracture; "civilian" gunshot wound)	1
Medium energy (open or multiple fractures, dislocation)	2
High energy (close-range shotgun or "military" gunshot wound, crush injury)	3
Very high energy (above + gross contamination) soft-tissue avulsion	4
B. Limb ischemia	
Pulse reduced or absent but perfusion normal	1*
Pulseless; paresthesias, diminished capillary refill	2
Cool, paralyzed, insensate, numb	3*
C. Shock	
Systolic BP always >90 mm Hg	0
Hypotensive transiently	1
Persistent hypotension	2
D. Age (years)	
<30	0
30-50	1
>50	2

*Score doubled for ischemia >6 hours
(Reproduced with permission from Johansen K, Daines M, Howey T, et al: Objective criteria accurately predict amputation following lower extremity trauma. *J Trauma* 1990;30:568-573.)

provided sufficient rigidity to permit early rehabilitation of adjacent joints. While successful in the hands of some authors, others reported a high rate of infections, soft-tissue complications, and fixation failures. A recent prospective randomized study compared plate fixation and external fixators. The authors felt that both methods yielded acceptable results but found a significantly higher rate of wound infections (35% versus 13%) and chronic osteomyelitis (19% versus 3%) after plating. Nonunions occurred in 4% of plated fractures and in 10% after external fixation. The authors recommended unilateral external fixation as the primary method to stabilize grade II and grade III open tibial fractures.

Micromotion Because a 10% to 30% delayed and nonunion rate typically is seen with traditional external fixators, some authors have long felt that more elastic fixation would lead to faster healing and fewer nonunions. This hypothesis recently has been tested in a prospective randomized trial involving several British centers. Forty-one fractures held with a rigid unilateral fixator until they healed were compared with 39 fractures treated with the same device but receiving, in addition, a controlled program of cyclic axial stimulation. A pneumatic pump was used to provide 1 mm axial displacement at 0.5 Hz in one 20-minute session each day. As soon as each patient was weightbearing, the pneumatic pump was replaced by a spring device that allowed maximum axial deformation of 1 mm with loading in excess of 12 kg. The authors found that unsupported weightbearing and union occurred significantly faster in fractures treated

with micromovement (23 weeks) than in those maintained in a rigid fixator (29 weeks).

Another group evaluated the efficacy of a unilateral fixator that allowed axial motion in 101 grade II and grade III open tibial fractures. Axial sliding was initiated after an average of nine weeks. Of the fractures, 96% proceeded to complete union with the fixator in place, but not before 31% had received a bone graft between four and 14 weeks after the injury. Fractures with grade II and grade IIA soft-tissue injuries healed in an average of 21 weeks, and those with grade IIIB or grade IIIC injuries after an average of 31 weeks. A third of the patients were kept in short leg casts or braces for an additional 11 weeks to provide further protection. The deep infection rate was 6%. Realignment of the fixator was necessary in 20% of the patients who developed angulation in excess of 5 degrees. Thirty-nine percent of the patients had some pin tract problem during the treatment, and in 5% the fixator had to be removed prematurely for this reason. Only 3% of the fractures healed with angulation in excess of 10 degrees but less than 16 degrees. The authors demonstrated that external fixation until union is safe, well-tolerated, and without the secondary deformities so frequently seen after premature transfers to a cast. The clinical effectiveness of the sliding mechanism remains in question, because it did not decrease the need for bone grafting.

Combination With Internal Fixation Rather than rely on elastic fixation, other authors prefer rigid fixation in combination with interfragmental screws as a means to increase the success rates of external fixation. One group of Navy investigators used this approach in 20 patients with comminuted tibial shaft fractures. There were three wound infections, but no major malalignments. All fractures healed after an average of 19 weeks. The authors felt that early cancellous bone grafting and sequential removal of the external fixation were crucial to success. A German group arrived at an opposite conclusion. They compared 44 fractures stabilized with external fixation alone with 55 fractures stabilized with additional lag screw fixation. The two methods were similar with respect to times to full weightbearing, times to union, rates of delayed union, malunion, superficial or deep pin tract infection, and loosening of the pins. However, fractures stabilized with an external fixator and supplemental lag screws had double the infection rate (11% versus 5%) and required bone grafting twice as often to achieve bony union (60% versus 30%) as the fractures treated with external fixation alone.

Secondary Intramedullary Nailing Early fixator removal followed by secondary reamed intramedullary nailing also has been used to increase union rates after external fixation. A report of 24 patients indicated that despite an average interval of 65 days between fixator removal and intramedullary nailing, 20% of the patients developed a deep infection. Further analysis of the data showed that a previous pin site infection was the culprit in most instances. However, a Canadian group found that secondary infections after nailings are rare if the external fixator is removed within three weeks of the injury, and secondary nailing is delayed for one to two weeks. Of 39 patients, only 5% developed a deep infection after secondary nailing. These infections healed with retention of the nail and without chronic osteomyelitis. There were two nonunions. Satisfactory alignment was achieved in 95%. These findings were confirmed by another group of investigators using a similar protocol.

Intramedullary Nailing

With the increasing recognition that external fixators are not without problems, primary stabilization of open tibial shaft fractures with intramedullary nails has gained renewed interest. In one study, open tibial shaft fractures of grade I and grade II severity were prospectively and randomly assigned to stabilization with unilateral external frames or Ender nails. After an average follow-up of 18 months, the authors concluded that Ender nails were a safe alternative to external fixation for lower grade open tibial shaft fractures, but considered the method contraindicated for comminuted lesions. They also found that protruding nails caused pain around the knee in 38% of the patients. Deep infections (14% versus 7%) and malunions (36% versus 12%) were clearly more common after external fixation. Both problems were related to techniques (secondary nailing after external fixation and transfer of the fractured limb to a cast at an average of eight weeks) that now have become problematic.

As a result of this provocative and well-designed study and a confirming retrospective review, many investigators have started to use small diameter unreamed locking nails. Early reports have been encouraging, but larger series and longer follow-ups will be needed to validate this approach.

Large Segmental Defects

During the past decade, the most popular treatment for tibial fractures with soft-tissue loss and segmental defects has been free fibular transfers. Because the method is time-consuming and requires an experienced microvascular team, alternative methods are of interest. In a recent study from the Armed Services, eight patients with grade IIIB open tibial fractures and segmental defects measuring, on the average, 10 cm were managed by: (1) stabilization with stiff half-frame external fixator; (2) serial wound debridement; (3) filling of the osseous defect with antibiotic-impregnated polymethylmethacrylate beads and coverage of the soft-tissue defect by a local myoplasty or a free muscle transfer; (4) elevation of the flap after about four to six weeks and packing of the osseous defect with large amounts of autogenous cancellous bone graft from the iliac crest; and (5) partial weightbearing and gradual disassembly of the external fixator as bony consolidation was noted radiographically. With this approach, all segmental defects healed

after an average of nine months. One deep infection at the bone graft donor site and one at the fracture site were resolved after local drainage. Because it is relatively simple, does not injure the contralateral extremity and, in their hands, had a low complication rate, the authors feel that this method provides a good alternative to free fibular transfer, which has a success rate of about 80% and a secondary amputation rate of 10% to 20%.

Tibial Malunions and Nonunions

Malunions

Symptomatic malunions are rare. The decision to manage a malunion with palliative measures or a corrective procedure must be based on a thorough clinical and radiographic evaluation. This should include an analysis of stance, gait, limb alignment, length, articular change, soft-tissue coverage, and infectious status. After careful preoperative planning, most malunions are corrected with a single or multiplanar osteotomy followed by internal or external fixation and possibly a bone graft. Another option is gradual multiplanar correction with a ring fixator.

Long-Term Studies   There has been a long-standing concern that tibial malunions, particularly those resulting in varus deformities, will eventually lead to degenerative changes in the knee and ankle. To test these hypotheses, two groups of investigators have reexamined patients with tibial deformities exceeding 10 degrees, 10 to 39 years after the original injuries. In one series, between 75% and 80% of the ankles and 90% of the knees had excellent clinical function and no arthritic changes on radiographs. Functional results and radiographic changes suggestive of arthritis occur with equal frequency in patients with minimal angulation and in those with frontal-plane, sagittal-plane, or combined deformities in excess of 10 degrees. In addition, outcomes were not affected by the length of immobilization as long as it did not exceed one year. However, angular deformity alone does not define alignment of the knee and ankle joint in the horizontal plane and, therefore, may be an inappropriate outcome measure.

Another group of investigators used mathematical analysis to show that for any position of the angulation apex along the shaft of the tibia, the horizontal malalignment is always greater for the ankle than for the knee joint. Malalignment in the ankle joint increases as the apex of the angulation moves distally. To gain further information, these authors radiographically and clinically reevaluated 28 angulated tibial fractures, 8.2 years after the initial injury, using a scale that took pain, function, motion, deformity, and radiologic changes into account. Mean joint malalignments were 1.3 degrees (0.2 degrees to 3.8 degrees) for the knee and 6.6 degrees (1.2 degrees to 26.7 degrees) for the ankle joint. Only 19% of the knees and 50% of the ankles were symptomatic.

Knee scores showed no correlation with the degree of knee malalignment, and valgus deformity in the ankle was only weakly correlated with symptoms. However, there was a highly significant relationship between varus ankle deformity and the clinical score. In ankles with a varus malalignment of less than 4 degrees, excellent scores were seen in 83%, but when the varus malalignment increased to 6 degrees or more, the scores decreased to 12%.

Treatment In the past, corrective procedures for complex malunions of the tibia generally have relied on the resection of multiplanar wedges. These were often difficult to calculate and made rigid fixation difficult. A recent analysis suggests an approach that integrates vector trigonometry with proper surgical planning. This method involves only one osteotomy cut without removal of bone or the need for bone grafting. According to the authors, this technique allows simultaneously for the correction of angular misalignment in two planes and torsional deformities. The method was used clinically in four patients and performed according to predictions.

Uninfected Nonunions

Hypertrophic nonunions with an intact fibula initially are best treated with a partial fibulectomy (1 cm) and full weightbearing in a plaster cast. This approach carries little risk, has a success rate of 75% to 80%, and does not preclude later use of more invasive measures. Most other hypertrophic nonunions will consolidate quickly with rigid fixation in the form of a plate, an intramedullary nail, or an external fixator. Hypotrophic nonunions need an osteogenic stimulus in the form of a cancellous bone graft and stabilization with a cast, or internal or external fixation.

Intramedullary Nailing A recent large study documents the advantages and limitations of reamed intramedullary nailing for nonsegmental tibial nonunions. In 66% of the cases, the fracture site had to be opened to remove hardware or to improve the alignment by performing an osteotomy. Iliac crest bone grafts were used in 20% and a fibular osteotomy was done in 66%. Ninety-six percent of the nonunions healed after an average of seven months postoperatively. The rate of major complications was 18% and included deep infections, nail fracture, shortening of more than 1 cm, malrotation of more than 15 degrees, and peroneal nerve palsy. The authors felt that bone grafting was needed only when there was a gap between the main bony fragments and recommend a nail that is at least 2 mm larger than the width of the medullary canal as measured on preoperative radiographs.

Pulsed Electromagnetic Fields The effectiveness of pulsed electromagnetic fields for tibial delayed unions was evaluated in a randomized prospective double-blind, multicentered trial. The study included 45 tibial fractures that had not healed after 16 to 32 weeks. All were immo-bilized in a long leg plaster cast and kept nonweightbearing. The patients were randomly allocated to either an active or a dummy stimulator activated for a total of 12 hours per day, with no individual treatment session being less than one hour. The effectiveness of the intervention was evaluated after 12 weeks. Radiographically, both radiologists and orthopaedic surgeons found that significantly more delayed unions had healed in the treatment than in the control group. On clinical evaluation, however, there were no differences between the two groups as to motion, pain, or tenderness at the fracture site. Thus, the usefulness of pulsed electromagnetic fields for the management of delayed nonunions remains in question. The method is at best marginally effective, is cumbersome, and does not correct concurrent malunions.

Autologous Bone Marrow Numerous animal studies have demonstrated the osteogenic properties of bone marrow stem cells. A recent study evaluated these properties clinically. Autologous marrow injections were used to stimulate healing in 20 ununited tibial fractures, ten immobilized in a cast and ten with intramedullary nails. The bone marrow is aspirated from the posterior iliac wing in an outpatient setting under general anesthesia. The marrow is then injected under fluoroscopic control into the region of the nonunion, preferably into an area surrounded by muscle and good blood supply. Because marrow is not an osteoconductive agent it should not be used for nonunions with larger defects. The average time from injury to marrow injection was 18 months. Median time to union after injection was seven months, similar to the union times required after open bone grafting techniques. The authors felt that bone marrow injection was, in their hands, as effective as autologous bone grafting, but had fewer disadvantages and less morbidity.

Infected Nonunions

For infected nonunions of the tibia, particularly those associated with soft-tissue defects and segmental bone loss, amputation is always an important consideration. Another option is wide local resection, stabilization with an external fixator, coverage with a local or free muscle flap, and application of a local bone graft or a free vascularized fibular graft. Although this approach has a 60% to 80% success rate, the time to union may exceed a year and the result may still be an atrophic limb with stiff joints. A new and exciting technique to treat these difficult problems is local bone transport with the Ilizarov technique.

Classification Based on their experience with over 250 patients with posttraumatic tibial osteomyelitis, a group of authors has proposed a clinical classification that focuses on the reconstruction of the osseous defects, surmising that debridement, bacteriological control of the wound, and soft-tissue coverage are achievable with modern techniques. They suggest five classes of bony defects of increasing severity ranging from unicortical involvement with no structural consequences to tibial defect in excess of 6 cm without a usable fibula.

Intramedullary Nailing   The effectiveness of intramedullary nailing in 19 infected tibial nonunions was assessed. Of the nonunions, 94% had full-thickness involvement of the tibial cortex and moderate size soft tissue defects (about 4 to 6 cm). The authors used the following protocol: (1) complete debridement of necrotic bone and interposed soft tissue; (2) stable fixation with a reamed, locked intramedullary nail; (3) open wound management using occlusive dressings to encourage drainage and growth of granulation tissue until exposed bone and hardware are covered and spontaneous epithelialization has occurred; (4) passive and active range of motion for adjacent joints; and (5) early weightbearing. No rotational free vascularized muscle flaps were used, and bone grafts were applied in only three cases. Ultimately, 18 nonunions healed (95%), four (20%) of which had minimal but persistent drainage.

Ilizarov Technique   Ring fixators such as the Ilizarov device may secure union and proper alignment and length in severe clean or infected tibial nonunions that, in the past, often proceeded to amputations. This method relies on the gradual and progressive correction of deformities through complex hinge systems and the restoration of length by means of distraction osteogenesis. The infected focus is treated by radical resection of the dead bone, which is then replaced by a bony regenerate stemming from the gradually distracted corticotomy site. Twenty-five patients with osteomyelitis and a mean bone loss of 6.2 cm were treated with this approach. The authors felt that 72% of the patients had good results; mean time to union was 14 months. Lesser outcomes were due to persistent infection (12%), deformity (16%), and excessive limb shortening (4%). Although spectacular corrections appear possible, the method is time consuming, requires particular expertise, and carries a high complication rate. The optimal indication for the Ilizarov technique, therefore, will remain unclear until larger patient series with more meticulous follow-up evaluations are available.

Tibial Plafond Fractures

Fractures of the tibial plafond remain among the most challenging intra-articular lesions. Apart from malalignment of the distal tibia and comminution of its talar articular surface, most tibial plafond fractures are accompanied by a crush injury to the local soft tissue that can result in a compartment syndrome. Interruption of major neurovascular structures, however, is rare.

Unless open or complicated by neurovascular compromise or adjacent lesions that may need immediate attention, tibial plafond fractures are managed electively. Initial stabilization can be with a splint, Boehler's traction, an external fixator, or fibular plating. A careful clinical assessment of the lesion and associated injuries is followed by standard radiographs of the leg and ankle joint. Tomograms in two planes or a computed axial tomographic scan with 2-D and/or 3-D reconstruction further clarify the fracture pattern, while standard radiographs of the opposite side provide a template for a difficult reconstruction. Fractures with minimal comminution or displacement do well in a nonweightbearing cast. More severe lesions are managed best with open reduction and internal fixation using, whenever possible, indirect reduction techniques. After fixation of the fibula at the correct length, the tibial articular surface is reconstructed, bony defects are filled with bone graft, and the tibia is finally buttressed with a plate. Weightbearing is not allowed until the fracture is healed.

Open fractures are managed by immediate debridement, reduction, and fixation. The wound is left open and secondary closure or a free flap should follow within three to five days. In the face of massive contamination, it is wise to focus on wound debridement and possibly salvage the extremity with a tibiotalar fusion, generally with the help of an external fixator.

Intra-articular fractures of the distal tibia continue to exert a considerable challenge. One author reviewed outcomes in 42 patients 4.5 years after the initial injury. Some patients were treated nonsurgically, but most were managed according to classic AO techniques. Satisfactory outcomes were achieved in 36% of the fractures with minimal to moderate comminution or intra-articular displacement that were treated nonoperatively and 76% of those treated with open reduction and internal fixation. All fractures with severe intra-articular comminution or displacement that were treated nonsurgically had an unsatisfactory result. Anatomic reduction with stable fixation was achieved in 13% of those treated with AO technique, and 43% had a satisfactory outcome. The reasons for the unsatisfactory results in this group included deep infections (13%), nonunions (25%), malunions (25%), and secondary degenerative arthritis (53%). After an average of 4.5 years, 32% of these patients had undergone ankle arthrodesis to salvage an unsatisfactory clinical result.

Five comminuted plafond fractures, complicated by significant soft-tissue injury and osteopenic bone stock, were managed by one group of investigators using a small pin circular fixator because open reduction seemed contraindicated. In cases with minimal plafond displacement, three sets of wires and rings are used: one just above the plafond, the other in the proximal tibia, and the third through the os calcis. Some distraction is possible between the two distal rings, and reduction of the metaphyseal fragments is facilitated by the application of tension to wires with stop nuts. The calcaneal wires are removed at six weeks, and range of motion exercises are started. In cases with severe articular comminution, the authors proceeded with a second stage at about 15 days when the soft tissues were healed. The distal tibia and fibula were exposed through a posterolateral incision. The fibula was plated, and the tibial fragments were reduced and held with screws. No tibial plates were applied, because the external fixator preserves overall alignment. The calcaneal pins, again, were removed at around six weeks. With this approach, the authors achieved good early results in three out of five cases.

Annotated Bibliography

Tibial Plateau Fractures

Anglen JO, Healy WL: Tibial plateau fractures. *Orthopaedics* 1988;11:1527-1534.

This retrospective review is based on charts and radiographs of 128 patents with tibial plateau fractures treated over a 20-year period. There were no clear criteria for choice of treatment options and no follow-up evaluation. Open reduction and internal fixation was superior to cast treatment for split-depression and bicondylar fractures, but was accompanied by a higher infection and reoperation rate. The use of buttress plates, the preservation of menisci, and early postoperative mobilization were paramount for good outcomes after surgical intervention.

Bucholz RW, Carlton A, Holmes R: Interporous hydroxyapatite as a bone graft substitute in tibial plateau fractures. *Clin Orthop* 1989;240:53-62.

In a comparison of two groups of comparable tibial plateau fractures, one treated with cancellous bone graft and the other with porous hydroxyapatite, the latter appears to be safe and as effective as autogenous bone. Use of this material will reduce donor site complications and, unlike allografts, involves no risk of transmission of infectious agents.

Delamarter RB, Hohl M, Hopp E Jr: Ligament injuries associated with tibial plateau fractures. *Clin Orthop* 1990;250:226-233.

This is an evaluation of 39 patients with tibial plateau fractures and concomitant ligamentous lesions one year after injury. Ligamentous injuries are most common with split-compression and local compression fractures. Poor results in 28% of patients were related to residual varus or valgus instability in excess of 10 degrees caused either by ligamentous laxity or persistent plateau depression. Results were acceptable in 63% after surgical repair and in 50% with nonsurgical management.

Delamarter R, Hohl M: The cast brace and tibial plateau fractures. *Clin Orthop* 1989;242:26-31.

This is a review of 141 patients with tibial plateau fractures treated with cast braces as primary treatment mode or as an adjunct to open reduction and internal fixation. Cast braces stabilized all fracture patterns successfully with the exception of medial plateau lesions, where malunions were noted in over 20%.

Jensen DB, Rude C, Duus B, et al: Tibial plateau fractures: A comparison of conservative and surgical treatment. *J Bone Joint Surg* 1990;72B:49-52.

Traction and operative management from two Danish university hospitals were compared. Traction required a longer hospital stay (seven versus four weeks). Satisfactory results were achieved in 74% of the patients treated in traction and 54% of those treated according to AO principles. Clinical outcomes deteriorated and arthritic changes increased after meniscectomy.

Lachiewicz PF, Funcik T: Factors influencing the results of open reduction and internal fixation of tibial plateau fractures. *Clin Orthop* 1990;259:210-215.

This is a review of 44 tibial plateau fractures treated by open reduction and internal fixation between 1980 and 1987. After an average follow-up of 2.7 years, 91% of the results were rated as good or excellent. Mild to severe degenerative changes occurred in 23%, and implant removal was needed in more than one third of patients because of slight pain and tenderness over implants. Omission of bone grafting was associated with lesser results.

Muller ME, Allgower M, Schneider R, et al: *Manual of Internal Fixation*, 3 ed. New York, Springer-Verlag, 1991, pp 568-574.

A concise description is presented of the principles and techniques of open reduction and internal fixation for most fractures and other orthopaedic lesions.

Murphy CP, D'Ambrosia R, Dabezies EJ: The small pin circular fixator for proximal tibial fractures with soft tissue compromise. *Orthopedics* 1991;14:273-280.

This report of five severely comminuted tibial plateau fractures, mostly bicondylar, managed with closed manipulation and application of a ring fixator is promising, but long-term outcomes are lacking.

Ries MD, Meinhard EP: Medial external fixation with lateral plate internal fixation in metaphyseal tibia fractures: A report of eight cases associated with severe soft-tissue injury. *Clin Orthop* 1990;256:215-223.

Early good results are reported for eight patients with unstable metaphyseal and associated intra-articular tibial plateau fractures treated with a combination of lateral buttress plates and medial external fixation.

Stokel EA, Sadasivan KK: Tibial plateau fractures: Standardized evaluation of operative results. *Orthopedics* 1991;14:263-270.

Surgical management of 20 tibial plateau fractures treated by one surgeon is analyzed, standardized criteria recommended, and a 100-point knee-rating score presented to assess follow-up results.

Closed Tibial Shaft Fractures

Alho A, Ekeland A, Strømsøe K, et al: Locked intramedullary nailing for displaced tibial shaft fractures. *J Bone Joint Surg* 1990;72B:805-809.

This analysis of 93 tibial shaft fractures treated with locked nails includes open grade I and grade II, comminuted, and junctional fractures. There were only two poor results. The deep infection rate was 3.2%.

Collins DN, Pearce CE, McAndrew MP: Successful use of reaming and intramedullary nailing of the tibia. *J Orthop Trauma* 1990;4:315-322.

Review of charts and radiographs of 87 patients with tibial shaft fractures treated with reamed intramedullary nails indicated three major complications: two deep infections and one patellar tendon rupture. Nine patients required reoperations. Overall results were good, but attention to technical details is important to minimize complications.

Court-Brown CM, Christie J, McQueen MM: Closed intramedullary tibial nailing: Its use in closed and type I open fractures. *J Bone Joint Surg* 1990;72B:605-611.

This is a review of 125 closed and open tibial shaft fractures treated with interlocking nails. There were few complications, including a 6% incidence of infection and knee pain in 41% of the patients. Nail removal was requested by 26%.

Hooper GJ, Keddell RG, Penny ID: Conservative management or closed nailing for tibial shaft fractures: A randomised prospective trial. *J Bone Joint Surg* 1991;73B:83-85.

Displaced (closed and grade I open) tibial shaft fractures were prospectively randomized to short leg walking casts or reamed intramedullary nails. Intramedullary nailing carried fewer complications, required fewer outpatient visits, and shortened return to work from 23 to 14 weeks. Of patients treated in casts, 15% needed secondary surgical intervention to secure acceptable fracture alignment.

Koval KJ, Clapper MF, Brumback RJ, et al: Complications of reamed intramedullary nailing of the tibia. *J Orthop Trauma* 1991;5:184-189.

This is an in-depth review of complications that occurred after reamed intramedullary nailing of 60 severe tibial shaft fractures. Early complications included fractures extending into tibial plateau, hematomas, shortening in excess of 1 cm, and peroneal nerve lesion. Of the patients with two-year follow-up, 58% developed some complication related to the nail procedure.

Pun WK, Chow SP, Fang D, et al: A study of function and residual joint stiffness after functional bracing of tibial shaft fractures. *Clin Orthop* 1991;267:157-163.

Review of 97 tibial shaft fractures treated with a fracture brace and followed for two years; indicated that normal motion in subtalar and ankle joint was noted in only 71% to 75% of patients. Knee stiffness, however, was rare. The authors recommend a modified functional brace that permits full plantarflexion and dorsiflexion.

Sarmiento A, Gersten LM, Sobol PA, et al: Tibial shaft fractures treated with functional braces: Experience with 780 fractures. *J Bone Joint Surg* 1989;71B:602-609.

In this review of over 700 tibial shaft fractures treated with a long-leg cast for three to five weeks followed by a functional brace with a hinged ankle joint, average time to union was 18 weeks. The nonunion rate was 2.5%. Ninety percent of the fractures healed with 10 mm of shortening or less. The method is not recommended for grade III open fractures, displacement greater than one third of the tibial shaft, comminution at the fracture site, and nonambulatory patients.

Templeman DC, Marder RA: Injuries of the knee associated with fractures of the tibial shaft: Detection by examination under anesthesia: A prospective study. *J Bone Joint Surg* 1989;71A:1392-1395.

Examination of 50 patients with tibial shaft fractures showed that 22% had sustained an injury to at least one ligament of the knee resulting in laxity of 2+ or more. Routine knee examination is recommended after stabilization of a tibial shaft fracture.

Open Tibial Shaft Fractures

Bach AW, Hansen ST Jr: Plates versus external fixation in severe open tibial shaft fractures: A randomized trial. *Clin Orthop* 1989;241:89-94.

In this prospective study, 59 patients with grade I and grade II open tibial fractures were assigned randomly to stabilization with plates according to AO principles or unilateral external fixation. Both methods rendered good results, but the rate of wound infections (35% versus 13%) and chronic osteomyelitis (19% versus 3%) was significantly higher after plating. Malunions occurred in 4% of plated fractures and in 10% after external fixation.

Blachut PA, Meek RN, O'Brien PJ: External fixation and delayed intramedullary nailing of open fractures of the tibial shaft: A sequential protocol. *J Bone Joint Surg* 1990;72A:729-735.

This is a study of 39 patients, describing a safe method for secondary reamed intramedullary nailing after external fixation. The fixator was removed within three weeks, followed by nailing under ten days of antibiotic coverage. No nailings were done after previous deep or pin tract infections. The deep infection rate was 5% and satisfactory alignment was achieved in 95%.

Bosse MJ, Staeheli JW, Reinert CM: Treatment of unstable tibial diaphyseal fractures with minimal internal and external fixation. *J Orthop Trauma* 1989;3:223-231.

Unstable fractures of the tibial diaphysis were treated with minimal internal fixation and external fixation. All fractures healed. To be successful, this approach requires dynamization of the external fixator and early bone grafting.

Christian EP, Bosse MJ, Robb G: Reconstruction of large diaphyseal defects, without free fibular transfer, in Grade-IIIB tibial fractures. *J Bone Joint Surg* 1989;71A;994-1004.

Eight grade IIIB tibial fractures with large segmental diaphyseal defects (average 10 cm in length) were successfully managed with the use of methylmethacrylate beads as spacers, free tissue flaps, and secondary replacement of the beads with cancellous bone graft. All fractures healed in an average of nine months. One deep infection resolved.

Holbrook JL, Swiontkowski MF, Sanders R: Treatment of open fractures of the tibial shaft: Ender nailing versus external fixation: A randomized, prospective comparison. J Bone Joint Surg 1989;71A;1231-1238.

In this prospective evaluation of grade I and grade II open tibial fractures randomly assigned to unilateral external fixators and Ender nails, healing times were comparable, but deep infections (14% versus 7%), and malunions (36% versus 21%) were seen more often after external fixation. Ender nails are contraindicated for comminuted fractures.

Johansen K, Daines M, Howey T, et al: Objective criteria accurately predict amputation following lower extremity trauma. *J Trauma* 1990;30:568-572.

A mangled extremity severity score (MESS) was developed based on tissue injury, limb ischemia, systemic hypotension, and patient age. A cumulative score of seven and above predicts need for early amputation with 100% accuracy.

Johnson EE, Simpson LA, Helfet DL: Delayed intramedullary nailing after failed external fixation of the tibia. *Clin Orthop* 1990;253:251-257.

Sixteen tibial shaft fractures that had delayed intramedullary nailing after initial placement of an external fixator are reported. Six fractures were closed. All fractures healed without major complications. For this approach to be successful, the authors recommend: nailing within 30 days of initial injury, no evidence of soft-tissue and pin tract infection, and the use of perioperative antibiotics.

Kenwright J, Richardson JB, Cunningham JL, et al: Axial movement and tibial fractures: A controlled randomized trial of treatment. *J Bone Joint Surg* 1991;73B:654-659.

This prospective evaluation of 80 open fractures randomly assigned to a stiff unilateral external fixator or a fixator that permits cyclic axial displacement of 1 m for 20 minutes a day indicated healing times were significantly shorter for fractures treated with micromovement (23 versus 29 weeks).

Khouri RK, Shaw WW: Reconstruction of the lower extremity with microvascular free flaps: A 10-year experience with 304 consecutive cases. *J Trauma* 1989;29:1086-1094.

In this retrospective review of 304 consecutive microvascular flaps to the lower extremity, mostly for grade IIIB and grade IIIC soft-tissue loss, latissimus dorsi and rectus abdominus were most frequently used. Flap failure rate was 8%. Anastomotic failure related directly to the severity of trauma. Amputation rate within the first three months was 6%.

Krettek C, Haas N, Tscherne H: The role of supplemental lag-screw fixation for open fractures of the tibial shaft treated with external fixation. *J Bone Joint Surg* 1991;73A:893-897.

Fifty-five open tibial fractures treated with external fixation and supplemental lag screws were compared with a control group stabilized only with external fixation. Complications and outcome parameters were similar in both groups, with the exception that the refracture rate and the need for bone grafting the achieve union was increased by a factor of two for the group treated with external and lag screw fixation.

Marsh JL, Nepola JV, Wurest TK, et al: Unilateral external fixation until healing with the dynamic axial fixator for severe open tibial fractures. *J Orthop Trauma* 1991;5:341-348.

In this evaluation of 101 grade II and grade III open tibial fractures, stabilized with unilateral fixator allowing axial motion late in the treatment course, 96% of the fractures healed in the fixator after an average of 21 weeks for grade II and grade IIIA lesions, and after an average of 31 weeks for grade IIB and grade IIIC injuries. Bone grafts were applied in 31%. Deep infection rate was 6%. Fixator realignment was needed in 20%. Ninety-seven percent healed with angulation of less than 10 degrees.

Maurer DJ, Merkow RL, Gustilo RB: Infection after intramedullary nailing of severe open tibial fractures

initially treated with external fixation. *J Bone Joint Surg* 1989;71A:835-838.

Twenty-four patients were treated with external fixation and secondary reamed intramedullary nailing. The infection rate after nailing was 71% with a previous history of a pin tract infection, and 14% without.

Russell GG, Henderson R, Arnett G: Primary or delayed closure for open tibial fractures. *J Bone Joint Surg* 1990;72B:125-128.

A retrospective analysis of 110 open tibial fractures treated with primary or delayed wound closure indicated that primary closures increased the infection rate from 3% to 20% and the rate of nonunions from 3% to 14%. Both findings were statistically significant.

Whitelaw GP, Wetzler M, Nelson A, et al: Ender rods versus external fixation in the treatment of open tibial fractures. *Clin Orthop* 1990;253:258-269.

In this retrospective comparison of tibial shaft fractures treated with external fixation or Ender nails, patients treated with external fixation had a higher rate of complications and required more procedures until healed.

Tibial Malunions and Nonunions

Connolly JF, Guse R, Tiedeman J, et al: Autologous marrow injection as a substitute for operative grafting of tibial nonunions. *Clin Orthop* 1991;266:259-270.

Twenty united tibial fractures were treated with local autologous marrow injection and cast or nail immobilization. Eighteen of the 20 fractures healed.

Kristensen KD, Kiaer T, Blicher J: No arthrosis of the ankle 20 years after malaligned tibial-shaft fracture. *Acta Orthop Scand* 1989;60:208-209.

In this reevaluation of 22 patients whose tibial shaft fractures had healed with an angulatory deformity exceeding 10 degrees, 20 to 39 years after injury, none of the patients had degenerative arthritis in the ankle joint. The authors conclude that angular deformity within 15 degrees will not lead to restricted motion, pain, or arthrosis of the ankle.

May JW Jr, Jupiter JB, Weiland AJ, et al: Clinical classification of post-traumatic tibial osteomyelitis. *J Bone Joint Surg* 1989;71A:1422-1428.

This practical classification emphasizes the reconstruction of the osseous tibial defect occurring with tibial osteomyelitis. Five types of bony defects are identified, and the most successful option for reconstruction is analyzed.

Merchant TC, Dietz FR: Long-term follow-up after fractures of the tibial and fibular shafts. *J Bone Joint Surg* 1989;71A:599-606.

This is a review of 37 patients with tibial fractures healed in angulation 29 years after the injury. Varus, valgus, anterior, and posterior angulations up to 15 degrees did not affect clinical and radiographic outcomes, nor did length of immobilization not exceeding one year.

Miller ME, Ada JR, Webb LX: Treatment of infected nonunion and delayed union of tibia fractures with locking intramedullary nails. *Clin Orthop* 1989;245:233-238.

This reports an analysis of 19 infected tibial nonunions treated with complete debridement, reamed locked nail, open wound management to generate granulation tissue, and early weightbearing. Without the use of muscle flaps, 95% of the nonunions healed, 80% being free of drainage.

Paley D, Catagni MA, Argnani F, et al: Ilizarov treatment of tibial nonunions with bone loss. *Clin Orthop* 1989;241:146-165.

In this analysis of 25 patients treated for tibial nonunions (88% atrophic) and a mean bone loss of 6.2 cm with the Ilizarov technique, 52% were infected. Union was achieved in all patients after an average of 14 months. Results were acceptable in 72% despite a high complication rate.

Puno RM, Vaughan JJ, Stetten ML, et al: Long-term effects of tibial angular malunion on the knee and ankle joints. *J Orthop Trauma* 1991;5:247-254.

Analysis of 28 tibial fractures that had healed in malalignment, at a follow-up of 8.2 years emphasizes tibial plateau and tibial plafond malalignment relative to the mechanical axis rather than amount of angulation. Malalignments of the knee and valgus deformity in the ankle only weakly correlated with clinical results, but severity of ankle varus directly affected clinical outcomes. Good results were seen in 83% with ankle varus of less than 4 degrees and in only 12% with ankle varus in excess of 6 degrees.

Sangeorzan BJ, Sangeorzan BP, Hansen ST Jr, et al: Mathematically directed single-cut osteotomy for correction of tibial malunion. *J Orthop Trauma* 1989;3:267-275.

Authors suggest that vector trigonometry and proper surgical planning allow correction of tibial malunion with only one osteotomy cut and without the need to remove bone or the need to bone graft. The method was successfully used in four cases.

Sharrard WJW: A double-blind trial of pulsed electromagnetic fields for delayed union of tibial fractures. *J Bone Joint Surg* 1990;72B:347-355.

This is a report of 45 tibial fractures with delayed union, which were treated with an active or dummy stimulator. Radiographically, it appeared that more fractures had healed in the treatment than in the dummy group, but clinically the two groups were equivalent as to motion, pain, or tenderness at the fracture site.

Tibial Plafond Fractures

Bourne RB: Pylon fractures of the distal tibia. *Clin Orthop* 1989;240:42-46.

Forty-two patients with intra-articular fractures of the distal tibia were reevaluated after a mean followup of 4.4 years. After open reduction and internal fixation, over 80% of patients with minimally and moderately comminuted fractures achieved satisfactory result. In fractures with severe comminution, unsatisfactory internal fixation was common. Only 32% of patients with these fractures retained satisfactory joint function.

Murphy CP, D'Ambrosia R, Dabezies EJ: The small pin circular fixator for distal tibial pylon fractures with soft tissue compromise. *Orthopedics* 1991;14:283-290.

In five patients with closed or open comminuted intra-articular fractures of the distal tibia, early results after stabilization with a circular external fixator appear acceptable.

47

Knee and Leg: Soft-Tissue Trauma

Knee Ligament Injuries

The capsuloligamentous structures about the knee are responsible for knee joint stabilization. After disruption of one or more of these ligamentous structures, abnormal joint motion may be noted. In assessing the knee for ligamentous instability, the following points should be considered: (1) Ligaments may act as primary or secondary stabilizers of knee joints. The four primary stabilizers of the knee are the anterior cruciate ligament (ACL), the posterior cruciate ligament (PCL), the medial collateral ligament (MCL), and the fibular collateral ligament (FCL), which restrain anterior, posterior, medial, and lateral translation, respectively. (2) There are six degrees of freedom in the knee, three in rotation and three in translation; therefore, anterior, posterior, varus, and valgus laxity testing should be performed in various positions of flexion and rotation. (3) During assessment of ligamentous instability, displacement or abnormal motion is defined in terms of the tibia sliding, distracting, or rotating about a stable femur. (4) When a knee is examined for ligamentous instability, the injured knee must always be compared to the contralateral knee. Approximately 90% of ligamentous injuries can be diagnosed by a thorough history and physical examination. In addition to clinical physical examination, instrumented measurements, stress radiographs, and magnetic resonance imaging (MRI) can help diagnose ligamentous disruption.

Measurement of Knee Laxity

The presence of ligamentous instability usually can be determined and may be grossly quantified during standard clinical examination. Instrumented measurement may provide a more accurate quantification of ligamentous instability. All of the instrumented devices that presently are available compare the amount of tibial translation between the involved and uninvolved knees. Reproducibility of measurements among devices has improved. However, clinical examination remains the most successful tool for diagnosis of ligamentous instability. Machine testing is used mainly to further document ligamentous disruption and to help quantify the amount of instability before and after surgery and following rehabilitation.

Magnetic resonance imaging (MRI) is a very sensitive and accurate test for determining ligamentous disruption in both the ACL and PCL. This modality is rarely necessary in isolated ligamentous injury; however, it may be useful to help determine associated meniscal injuries.

Injury Classification and Laxity Grading Ligamentous injury may be partial or complete. Classification of these injuries is based on the amount of translation. Normal laxity is graded 0; translation less than 0.5 cm is graded 1+; translation of 0.5 to 1.0 cm is graded 2+; and translation of 1 to 1.5 cm is 3+. Some authors use grading systems that include an additional group, 4+, which is >1.5 cm translation.

Knee instability can be classified into two major groups: single plane instability (medial, lateral, anterior, and posterior) and rotatory instability (posteromedial, posterolateral, anteromedial, anterolateral, or a combination thereof). Ligamentous instability implies ligament disruption. However, the patient is not always aware of this instability during activities of daily living. If the patient experiences episodes of giving way, ligamentous instability becomes functional instability.

Treatment of Knee Ligament Injuries

Medial Collateral Ligament To test for MCL injury, valgus stress should be applied with the knee in 30 degrees of flexion and in full extension. As the knee moves into extension, the role of secondary restraints greatly increases. Therefore, isolated MCL injury is revealed by instability only at 30 degrees of flexion. Instability in full extension indicates that secondary restraints are also disrupted in addition to the MCL.

Nonsurgical treatment of isolated MCL injury currently is recommended. Depending on the severity of the injury, bracing may be necessary; however, early motion is encouraged in all cases.

If an MCL injury is associated with another major ligamentous injury, for example, ACL or PCL injury, surgical intervention usually is indicated. However, repair of the ACL or PCL may be all that is necessary.

Fibular (Lateral) Collateral Ligament The FCL also should be tested with the knee in 30 degrees of flexion and in full extension while applying a varus stress. In isolated FCL rupture, instability is revealed only at 30 degrees of knee flexion. Isolated FCL ruptures are rare. FCL injury usually is associated with posterolateral corner injury (popliteus tendon and arcuate complex), cruciate ligament injury, or both.

Isolated FCL injuries rarely produce functional instability and, as a general rule, may be treated nonsurgically. However, if associated secondary restraints also are disrupted, surgical repair is recommended.

Posterior Cruciate Ligament Injury to the PCL is about one tenth as common as injury to the ACL. There must be a high index of suspicion for PCL injury.

PCL injury usually occurs secondary to one of three different mechanisms. The most common mechanism involves a posteriorly directed force on a flexed knee, such as when the knee strikes the dashboard. A second mechanism is forced hyperextension of the knee, and, third, a posterior rotatory force may lead to PCL disruption. PCL instability can be assessed using the posterior drawer sign with the knee in 90 degrees of flexion. The Godfrey test, which reveals posterior subluxation of the tibia on the femur at 90 degrees of knee flexion and 90 degrees of hip flexion, also can be used to determine isolated PCL instability. PCL disruption can be assessed by the 90-degrees quadriceps active test.

Whether or not to use surgery for treatment of isolated PCL injuries remains questionable. Isolated PCL injuries rarely are associated with meniscal pathology and result in little functional instability. However, chronic instability may lead to degenerative arthritis of the medial compartment, the patellofemoral joint, and, less often, the lateral compartment. In general, in patients with isolated PCL disruption, a nonsurgical approach, in which quadriceps strengthening is stressed, should be implemented. Surgical intervention should be reserved for patients who fail conservative therapy, patients with combined ligamentous injury, and those with multidirectional instability. In patients with chronic PCL instability, the extent of degenerative changes should be noted because ligament reconstruction probably will not affect the arthritic changes that already are present.

Maintenance of quadriceps strength is crucial in rehabilitation after PCL reconstruction. Hamstring strengthening should be delayed in patients with PCL reconstruction because the pull of the hamstrings, in knee flexion, is posterior. Therefore, most surgeons place the knee in extension for six weeks, allowing quadriceps-strengthening exercises while inhibiting hamstring exercises. Range of motion and progressive rehabilitation are instituted six weeks after surgery.

Anterior Cruciate Ligament The majority of ACL tears occur during noncontact sports that involve jumping or cutting. Deceleration/valgus/rotational injuries and hyperextension injuries are the two most common injury patterns described in ACL disruption. On physical examination, acute traumatic effusion will be seen in approximately 70% to 80% of patients with ACL disruption, assuming there is no intra-articular fracture or patellar injury. Approximately 50% of all acute ACL ruptures are associated with meniscal tears. Acute ACL disruption is best assessed by the Lachman test, which is performed with the knee flexed approximately 30 degrees and an anterior force applied to the tibia. The anterior drawer and pivot shift tests may also help to determine ACL instability in patients with chronic ACL insufficiency.

The true natural history of ACL injuries is unknown. To determine its natural history, a disease process must be allowed to progress without intervention or treatment, and conservative treatment, including rehabilitation, may be considered by some as intervention and treatment of the disease process. What is more important is whether ACL injuries should be treated with or without surgery.

Numerous studies have shown that meniscal injury, degenerative osteoarthritis, and functional loss can result from untreated ACL injuries. On the other hand, many studies have revealed favorable results with conservative management of ACL injuries. Patient selection, surgical indications, and treatment, both conservative and surgical, vary from study to study. In addition, most studies are retrospective in nature.

Treatment of ACL injuries must be individualized. The patient's level of activity before the injury and, more importantly, the patient's expectation for the future must be determined. In general, if patients are willing to modify their activities, nonsurgical treatment and a vigorous rehabilitation program can return them to satisfactory function. Initial treatment is directed at controlling pain and inflammation. Weightbearing as tolerated is permitted and range-of-motion exercises are initiated to help the patient regain full extension and flexion. Once a painless range of motion is achieved, muscle strengthening of the quadriceps and hamstrings is begun. As muscle strengthening progresses, patients are permitted to begin activities that do not stress the ACL, such as swimming, bicycling, and jogging. Activities that involve cutting, jumping, twisting, or turning may exacerbate symptoms of instability.

If patients plan to return to sports requiring jumping, cutting, twisting, or turning, chronic instability can occur, leading to osteoarthritic changes. It is this group of patients who are most apt to benefit from ACL reconstruction. Currently, there is no supportive evidence for repair of midsubstance ACL tears. However, ligament avulsions with attached bone blocks may well be amenable to repair. Otherwise, ACL surgery should be limited to ACL reconstruction.

The goal of ACL reconstruction is to provide a stable knee with normal limits of motion. Many factors are crucial in achieving these goals, including graft selection, graft placement, graft fixation, repair of secondary restraints as well as meniscal tears, and postoperative rehabilitation.

ACL replacement materials presently include autograft, allograft, and synthetic materials. Most experience is with autograft tissue; most often, the central one third of the patellar ligament, the semitendinosus, or the iliotibial band is used. Autogenous tissues are the standard, with allograft and synthetic ligaments considered experimental.

Allograft tissue is a promising alternative to autogenous tissue. Its advantages include: (1) the absence of donor site morbidity; (2) availability in various shapes and sizes; (3) potentially unlimited supply; (4) incorporation and healing similar to autograft tissue; and (5) decreased time in surgery. However, allograft tissues are not without disadvantages.

The main disadvantage of allograft tissues is the possible transmission of infectious organisms, including the AIDS virus. Recent studies have shown that the infectivity of AIDS virus may be decreased by secondary sterilization techniques including gamma radiation and ethylene oxide. However, the virus still could be isolated after treatment with various sterilization techniques. Moreover, sterilization techniques are not without potential problems. Because adverse clinical results recently have been reported for ethylene oxide-treated allografts, they are not recommended for use in ACL reconstruction.

Autograft and allograft tissues are initially strong replacement tissues. However, the grafts undergo necrosis, followed by vascular invasion and cellular proliferation. During these histologic changes, the strength to failure of the graft tissue decreases and then increases, but the ligament may never return to original preimplant strength.

Synthetic replacement materials offer the advantage of immediate strength, allowing quicker return to activity. In addition, there is no risk of infectious disease transmission. Although early results for use of synthetic materials in ACL reconstruction were encouraging, longer term follow-up has been disappointing. In addition, concern has been voiced over wear debris and its possible deleterious effects on the surrounding knee joint.

ACL Graft Placement

Isometric placement of ACL replacement materials is crucial in achieving full range of knee motion without causing long-term ligament deformation. However, isometry as such does not exist because, during the range of motion, there is no one point on the femur that maintains a fixed distance from a single point on the tibia. Elongation always will occur. Therefore, the surgeon should concentrate on the amount of elongation, and try to determine how much elongation is acceptable. Zero to 3 mm of elongation seems acceptable. The graft should appear to tighten as the knee goes into increased flexion. Many researchers have tried to determine which bundle regions of the ACL are most isometric. Previous work suggested that central placement was the closest to being isometric. However, recent work shows that under surgical testing conditions, the anteromedial fibers are closest to being isometric, and it is these fibers that surgeons should be trying to reproduce.

Graft Fixation

There is inherent graft weakness during the period after implantation when allograft and autograft tissues undergo necrosis, revascularization, and cellular proliferation. However, the weakest link initially is the graft fixation sites. Therefore, it is important to achieve strong fixation initially. Bone plugs with interference screws

seem to provide the greatest fixation strength. As healing occurs, strength at the fixation sites exceeds graft strength.

ACL replacement may be performed arthroscopically, by open surgery, or by a combined procedure. The main advantage of arthroscopic, or arthroscopically assisted, ACL reconstruction is potential reduction in surgical morbidity.

A wide spectrum of rehabilitation procedures are available for use after reconstruction. In general, after surgery the knee is placed in a brace in full extension, and weightbearing as tolerated is encouraged. The brace is removed daily and full extension and flexion to 90 degrees is performed. At six weeks after surgery, the brace is removed and muscle-strengthening exercises are begun. Activities are progressively increased, and full activity may be started approximately nine to 12 months after surgery, including sports involving cutting, twisting, and jumping. Trends toward accelerated rehabilitation recently have been introduced. Early protected motion and weightbearing, as well as early strengthening, have proven to reduce limitations of motion and loss of strength without compromising stability. Some patients have been reported to be back to full sports activities by six months; however, it should be emphasized that such a program requires close patient follow-up.

Braces

Braces may be classified into three main groups: rehabilitative, prophylactic, and functional. Rehabilitative braces are those used to protect and limit knee motion. Braces used after ACL reconstruction, in the early postoperative period, are considered rehabilitative braces. Braces of this type usually do not provide any rotational control.

In theory, prophylactic braces were designed to decrease the number and severity of knee ligament injuries. Many studies have been performed both at the college and high school levels to examine the efficacy of prophylactic knee braces. Almost all of these studies reveal methodologic difficulties. The results are mixed, with some showing a decrease in MCL injury and others an increase in MCL injury. In general, results indicate that the use of prophylactic braces has reduced neither the number nor the severity of knee injuries. In addition, there is no evidence to support recommendation of prophylactic knee bracing in tackle football.

Functional braces are used to provide stability in the patient with functional knee instability. There are two types of functional braces with similar design and features. Both use hinges and posts; however, they differ in methods of suspension, which are thigh and calf enclosures or straps. Functional braces are inadequate in and of themselves to control instability at higher loads. However, anterior tibial displacement was reduced at low loads. It is felt that during athletic competition, with activities of high loading, functional braces may provide minimal stability at best.

ACL Injuries in the Skeletally Immature

Tibial spine fractures in children should not be confused with ACL rupture. Tibial spine fractures are always associated with intact ACLs, and, depending on whether the fracture is type I, II, or III, closed or open treatment may be indicated. Despite the treatment, symptomatic cruciate instability does not result.

Midsubstance ACL tears are less common in the skeletally immature. Many of these tears are associated with meniscal lesions. Conservative versus surgical treatment remains open to debate, depending on the child's age, symptoms, and desire to return to sports. In children with a strong desire to return to competitive sports, there is a trend toward surgical reconstruction (extra-articular/intra-articular or both). Despite skeletal immaturity in these patients, there have been few reports of growth arrest or growth disturbance.

Knee Dislocation

Complete knee dislocation results in multiple ligamentous injuries as well as possible neurovascular injuries. Closed reduction and neurovascular evaluation should be performed immediately.

Anterior dislocation can cause a traction injury to the popliteal artery, resulting in an acute intimal tear and, possibly, an intraluminal thrombus. Posterior dislocation can cause complete laceration of the popliteal artery. Popliteal artery injuries occur in 10% to 50% of knee dislocations; therefore, arteriography is recommended as part of the early management. If the leg is clinically ischemic, the arteriogram may be bypassed, and exploration and repair of the popliteal artery as well as fasciotomies should be performed immediately. Vascular injury must be corrected within six to eight hours to decrease the possibility of amputation. Amputation rates following knee dislocation are approximately 10%. Limb salvage is, therefore, a major issue in knee dislocation. Peroneal nerve injury is reported in 20% to 40% of knee dislocations and approximately half of all palsies are permanent. Multiple structures may be injured in all cases of knee dislocation. In all instances both cruciate ligaments and at least one if not both collateral ligaments are disrupted. Surgical repair and/or reconstruction is recommended, and early postoperative motion is encouraged to avoid the complication of knee stiffness.

The Menisci

The menisci are fibrocartilaginous structures that function in loadbearing, shock absorption, joint stability, and lubrication between the femoral and tibial articulating surfaces. An understanding of the vascular supply to the menisci is important when considering meniscal repair. The vascular supply to the meniscus is age dependent; in the adult, the peripheral 3 mm of the menisci as well as the anterior and posterior horns are well vascularized.

The vascular supply to the menisci originates from the geniculate arteries.

Meniscal tears may be isolated or may be associated with ligamentous injuries. In addition they may be degenerative tears, more commonly seen in older patients, or they may be secondary to trauma. Diagnosis of meniscal tears is based on a careful history and physical examination. Mechanical symptoms of pain, catching, popping, or locking are seen in displaceable tears. The findings are more subtle in degenerative tears. Multiple clinical tests can help to increase the accuracy of diagnosis. It probably is best to use three to five currently available tests in every knee examination for meniscal injury.

Diagnosis of meniscal tear can be confirmed by a variety of invasive and noninvasive tests including computed tomographic (CT) scanning, MRI, and arthrogram. Recent studies examined the sensitivity and specificity of MRI in diagnosing meniscal tears. Sensitivity ranges from 69% to 88%; specificity from 57% to 84%. Overall accuracy is between 72% and 89%. Accuracy increased for units with stronger magnetic fields. Because MRI is very expensive, its use as a diagnostic aid must take cost into consideration.

Grading meniscal lesions has decreased the false-positive findings with MRI. Grade I and II lesions are intrameniscal and usually are treated nonsurgically. However, approximately 20% of grade II lesions have been shown arthroscopically to be detectable tears. Therefore, arthroscopy may be indicated if a patient's symptoms persist after appropriate nonsurgical treatment of a grade II lesion.

Treatment options for meniscal tears include leaving the tear alone, meniscal repair, partial meniscectomy, and total meniscectomy. Meniscal transplantation is experimental at this point, but offers hope for the future. Partial thickness tears and full thickness, stable, vertical or oblique tears measuring ≤5 mm may be left alone. Stable radial tears ≤5 mm have a low potential for healing but may be considered for nonsurgical management. However, in each of the above instances, if the tear is the only abnormality that is found and is felt to be causing the patient's symptoms, the decision to leave the tear alone or treat it surgically becomes more difficult and is left to clinical judgment.

If after history, physical examination, and further diagnostic testing it is determined that a meniscal lesion cannot be left alone, it is necessary to decide what surgical intervention is necessary. Meniscal repair should be reserved for traumatic tears in the vascular region of the meniscus. If the tear is within 3 mm of the periphery, it is considered vascular. The area 3 to 5 mm from the periphery is a grey zone, and greater than 5 mm from the periphery is considered avascular. Tears that are unstable or tears within the vascular zone that are larger than 7 mm should be considered repairable. Tears may be repaired arthroscopically (inside-out or outside-in techniques) or open depending on location and the surgeon's preference. If the tear is repaired arthroscopically, care must be taken not to injure the saphenous nerve medially nor the peroneal laterally. Tears that are determined to be irreparable should be treated by partial meniscectomy and, in rare instances, total meniscectomy. To avoid degenerative arthritis after meniscectomy, every effort should be made to preserve as much meniscal tissue as possible when repair is not an option. Degenerative meniscal tears are best treated by partial meniscectomy.

Meniscal Injury in Conjunction with ACL-Deficient Knees

In patients with meniscal injury as well as ACL injury, treatment should be directed toward meniscal repair and stabilization of the knee by ACL reconstruction. A 30% to 40% failure rate has been noted in patients who have undergone meniscal repair without ACL reconstruction. The overall success rate approaches 90% in patients undergoing both meniscal repair and ACL reconstruction. Partial meniscectomy alone may be indicated for those patients in whom meniscal repair is not an option. However, if the patient's symptoms are secondary to instability, partial meniscectomy is not likely to relieve the symptoms and, in addition to meniscal surgery, ACL reconstruction should be performed in these cases. In older, less active patients, partial meniscectomy and ACL rehabilitation may be all that is necessary.

Plica Syndrome

Three different synovial folds or plicae have been identified in the knee: the suprapatellar, medial patellar, and lateral patellar folds. Of the three, the medial patellar fold most often becomes symptomatic; however, it must be remembered that plica syndrome is rare. Plicae may become symptomatic as a result of repetitive trauma. Trauma, whether direct or indirect, causes the fold to become inflamed. Inflammation leads to decreased elasticity, causing the plica to impinge on either the patella or the femoral condyle. Repetitive impingement leads to further inflammation and fibrosis, causing patellofemoral pain. Approximately 60% to 90% of patients respond to conservative therapy. When symptomatic plica fail to respond to long-term conservative therapy, including nonsteroidal anti-inflammatory drugs (NSAIDs) and quadriceps exercise, excision may be indicated. Of patients with medial plica resection, 70% to 80% had good to excellent results.

The Patellofemoral Joint

Patellofemoral disorders can, at times, be difficult to evaluate. Complaints of anterior knee pain almost always are present. Careful history and physical examination as well as radiographic analysis can usually lead the orthopaedic surgeon to a diagnosis. Patellofemoral disorders include trauma, patellofemoral malalignment, and idiopathic chondromalacia patellae.

Trauma

Acute trauma to the patellofemoral joint can result in patellar fracture, extensor mechanism disruption, and, rarely, patellar dislocation. Extensor mechanism rupture may involve either the quadriceps tendon or the patellar ligament and may be either partial or complete. Complete rupture is rare in the young athlete unless associated with steroid use. In general, patellar ligament ruptures usually occur in patients younger than 40 years of age and quadriceps tendon ruptures in patients older than 40 years of age. Extensor mechanism ruptures have been seen in association with rheumatoid arthritis, long-term diabetes mellitus, and long-term steroid use.

Quadriceps Tendon Rupture

Clinical examination findings for a complete acute quadriceps tendon rupture include a large hemarthrosis and, on palpation, a freely mobile patella and an impressive loss of extensor function. Radiographs may reveal a low-riding patella. In partial tears the findings may be less impressive, and extensor function may be near normal although an extensor lag usually is present. In these patients, MRI may delineate the extent of injury. Partial tears of the quadriceps tendon may be treated nonsurgically with immobilization and early range of motion. Surgical intervention is indicated for complete tears. Early intervention allows end-to-end repair of the tendon. The fibers of the rectus femoris tendon should be sutured to the superior pole of the patella through drill holes, because the tendon is pliable and it provides most of the strength of the repair.

In patients undergoing late repair, retraction of the proximal flap becomes a problem. End-to-end repair may be successful if the tissues can be reapproximated. However, if there is tension at the repair site, supplemental fixation or special techniques, including a Scuderi flap or transfer of the biceps and semitendinosus tendons, may be necessary. Postoperative management includes immobilization followed by early passive motion and quadriceps strengthening.

Patellar Ligament Rupture   Patellar ligament ruptures occur mainly at the level of the inferior patellar pole, less often at the level of the tibial tubercle, and, rarely, mid-substance. Tears at the inferior patellar pole usually are associated with previous patellar tendinitis and local steroid injections.

On examination, a defect in the patellar ligament may be palpated, the patella is high riding, and, most importantly, the patient will be unable to extend the knee despite evidence of intact quadriceps mechanism. Radiographs may reveal a small avulsion from the inferior patellar pole, and patella alta may be seen. Partial tears of the patellar ligament may be differentiated from complete tears by the fact that the patella will not be high riding and the patient will be able to extend his/her knee fully. In cases of partial patellar ligament disruption a nonsurgical course of treatment may be followed.

Complete tears of the patellar ligament require surgical repair. Immediate repair may be performed using end-to-end suture technique. Some authors advocate supplemental fixation with pins and wires; however, most feel that this is not necessary if repair is early enough. End-to-end suturing may not be attainable for delayed or late repair. In these cases, a variety of techniques may be helpful, including the Scuderi turn-down flap or reconstruction using the semitendinosus tendon. Postoperative management is the same as that described for quadriceps tendon rupture.

Patellar Tendinitis

Clinically repetitive trauma may result in patellar tendinitis, otherwise referred to as "jumper's knee." This entity is commonly seen in athletes involved in running, jumping, and kicking sports. Pain is insidious and usually is localized to the inferior pole of the patella, although in some cases it is located at the superior pole of the patella. On physical examination, tenderness can be localized to the inferior patellar pole. Usually, there is no effusion, no joint line tenderness, and no loss of motion. Radiographs may reveal traction spurs or calcification in the patellar ligament but most often are normal. Patellar tendinitis has been classified into four groups or phases: phase I, pain only after activity; phase II, some pain/discomfort during activity, but does not interfere with participation; phase III, pain both during and after participation, which interferes with competition; and phase IV, complete tendon disruption. Treatment depends on the phase. Phases I and II can successfully be treated conservatively. Activity modification, preparticipation warm-up, stretching, ice, and anti-inflammatories are the mainstays of therapy. Sometimes, months of therapy are required for resolution. Phase III jumper's knee initially should be treated similarly to phases I and II. However, the patient should be advised to curtail all athletic activity. Cortisone injections should not be administered because they can weaken the patellar ligament, increasing the possibility of disruption. Surgical intervention may be indicated in chronic cases when all conservative measures have failed. Many procedures have been suggested, including incision and resection of the degenerative portion of the tendon, and resection or drilling of the inferior pole of the patella. In phase IV jumper's knee, acute repair of the patellar ligament is indicated.

Patellofemoral Malalignment

Classification and Education Fulkerson recently classified patellofemoral disorders into four types: type I, subluxation alone; type II, subluxation and tilt; type III, tilt alone; and type IV, no malalignment. He further divided each type depending on the absence of an articular lesion (type A), presence of minimum chondromalacia (type B), or presence of osteoarthrosis (type C) found at arthroscopy.

Evaluation of patellofemoral disorders should begin with a thorough history and physical examination. The history should focus on pain and instability. Physical examination includes testing for retinacular tenderness and for pain on patellar compression, as well as to assess for malalignment and instability. The passive patellar tilt test and the patellar glide test assess the tightness/laxity of the lateral and medal retinacula, respectively. The quadriceps angle (Q angle) also should be assessed. An increased Q angle simply indicates an increased lateral quadriceps vector. Deficiency of the vastus medialis oblique is best assessed while the leg is suspended in 15 to 20 degrees of flexion. A large convexity at the superomedial corner of the patella indicates vastus medialis deficiency. Patellar tracking should be assessed during knee flexion and extension, and the presence/absence of a J sign should be noted.

Radiographic evaluation of the patellofemoral joint should include anteroposterior lateral and axial views. The lateral view most effectively assesses patellar height, and the axial view is the most informative. Increased flexion usually results in reduction of a subluxated patella, obscuring findings; therefore, it is crucial that axial radiographs be obtained between 20 and 45 degrees of flexion. On the axial view, the angle of congruence, as described by Merchant, can be used to help determine subluxation. The lateral patellofemoral angle, as described by Laurin, can be used to radiographically assess patellar tilt.

Computed tomography has been shown to precisely reproduce patellofemoral relationships including normal alignment, lateral patellar tilt, and patellar subluxation. CT scanning should be reserved for those difficult cases in which plain radiographs are indeterminate.

Arthroscopy may be used to assess the articular cartilage of the patellofemoral joint, especially in those patients who are in need of surgery. Some authors have shown that surgical success may be correlated with the absence or presence of articular cartilage damage, while others have shown no correlation at all.

Treatment Use of rest, ice, and NSAIDs is the first line of nonsurgical treatment. Next, a rehabilitation program may be started. To avoid unnecessary patellofemoral joint reactive forces and contact stresses, the rehabilitation program should begin with exercises done in complete knee extension with no range of motion (quadriceps setting and straight leg raising without and then with weights). Approximately 90% of patients will respond to conservative treatment.

Surgical intervention may be necessary for patients who do not respond to a detailed, carefully monitored rehabilitation program. Surgical treatment depends on the type of malalignment present; options include any one or a combination of the following procedures: lateral release, proximal realignment, and distal realignment.

Lateral release is most successful in patients with isolated lateral retinacular tightness as evidenced by a negative or neutral patellar tilt. Other predictors of good outcome include preoperative positive Merchant views, arthroscopic evidence of lateral patellar overhang, and toughened lateral retinacular structures. Reduction of the released patella after rehabilitation, as seen on the quadriceps films, also is a predictor of good outcome. In properly selected patients, 85% to 90% good to excellent results can be expected.

If malalignment, as evidenced by an abnormal Q angle, increased medial and lateral patellar glide, and/or positive patellar tilt are present, the prognosis for success of isolated lateral release is lowered significantly. A lateral release clearly is not indicated in patients with lateral retinacular laxity. Lateral release may be performed by open or arthroscopic surgery. Regardless of the technique used, hemostasis is crucial.

The complication rate associated with arthroscopic lateral release is 7%. The most common complication was postoperative hemarthrosis. The incidence of complications was significantly increased with the use of a tourniquet and the use of a postoperative suction drain for more than 24 hours. There also was a higher incidence of complications with the subcutaneous technique of release, but it was not significant.

Depending on the degree of subluxation, lateral release alone may reduce a subluxating patella. However, if inadequate patellar alignment is noted after release, advancement of the vastus medialis or distal realignment procedures must be considered.

Medial advancement of the vastus medialis is necessary for vastus medialis obliquus deficiency. When both lateral tightness and medial laxity are present, both a lateral release and medial advancement are necessary.

Determining the correct surgical procedure for patients with combined patellar tilt and subluxation can be very difficult. Many patients can be treated with proximal realignment procedures. However, in patients who also have an increased Q angle, proximal and distal realignment procedures may be indicated. Distal bony realignment procedures are contraindicated in the skeletally immature.

Idiopathic Chondromalacia Patellae

Chondromalacia patellae is a pathologic diagnosis and should not be used as a diagnosis of anterior knee pain, based solely on clinical criteria. Chondromalacia is normally secondary to instability and/or malalignment, as seen in patellofemoral dysplasia. The patellar compression test and the crepitation test are useful clinically to determine the presence and extent of chondrosis.

Treatment If chondromalacia patellae is secondary to patellofemoral malalignment, correction of the underlying abnormalities should reduce the destructive forces. However, the severity and extent of chondromalacia may lead to a poor result despite successful realignment. If chondromalacia is truly idiopathic, its long-term prognosis is questionable. It is usually a self-limited disease that is best treated nonsurgically. Arthroscopic debridement as treatment is controversial.

Overuse Injuries

Running injuries are common among the overuse injuries, because running is becoming more and more popular. There currently are at least 30 million runners in North America. About 70% will suffer injuries significant enough to prevent running for at least one week, but very few will seek medical attention. Almost all injuries are secondary to training errors. Excessive mileage, a rapid increase in mileage, inadequate warm-up, and improper stretching are a few of the more common training errors.

Running injuries can be correlated with the four levels into which runners can be classified. Level I includes the recreational runner or jogger who runs less than 20 miles a week, at 9 to 18 minutes per mile. These runners usually suffer from patellofemoral stress syndrome, "shin splints," and a variety of ankle and foot disorders. Level II runners are considered sports runners and run approximately 20 to 40 miles a week at 8 to 10 minutes per mile. These runners commonly incur Achilles tendinitis, plantar fasciitis, and stress fractures. Level III includes the long-distance runner who covers 40 to 70 miles a week at an average rate of 7 to 8.3 minutes per mile. Injuries common to these runners include adductor muscle strains, stress fractures, and iliotibial tract friction syndrome. Level IV or elite marathon runners run approximately 70 to 80 miles a week at 5.5 to 6.5 minutes per mile and suffer few injuries, among which are stress fractures and acute muscle strains. Almost all running injuries respond to conservative treatment including rest, ice, NSAIDs, stretching, rehabilitative strengthening exercises, and orthotic devices, followed by a gradual return to running.

Knee Injuries

Injuries to the knee and its surrounding structures are the most common of all overuse injuries. Knee injuries include: (1) Patellofemoral pain syndrome; (2) iliotibial band friction syndrome; (3) popliteal tendinitis; and (4) pes anserine bursitis.

Patellofemoral Pain Syndrome In runners with patellofemoral pain syndrome, the chief complaint is peripatellar or retropatellar pain that usually is absent at the beginning of a run, but becomes evident during the middle and end of a run. Malalignment problems frequently are associated. Conservative management is best for this syndrome. The goal of treatment is to unload the patellofemoral joint.

The management of patellofemoral pain syndrome includes: (1) complete rest or alteration in training routine; (2) ice/heat; (3) NSAIDs; (4) patellar knee orthotic devices; and (5) quadriceps muscle strengthening.

When symptoms improve, short arc quadriceps exercises may begin, progressing to long arc exercises and nonimpact loading activities. When asymptomatic, the patient may slowly begin to return to running. Surgery rarely is indicated, except in cases that fail conservative treatment and where biomechanical correction can correct an underlying malalignment abnormality.

Iliotibial Tract Friction Syndrome   Patients usually have pain over the lateral femoral epicondyle, which is caused by inflammation resulting from friction as the iliotibial tract slides over the condyle. This syndrome can be seen in association with genu varum and hyperpronated feet. Conservative treatment, including stretching exercises, rest, ice/heat, and NSAIDs, is successful in most cases. At times, corticosteroid injections may be necessary. If associated with hyperpronated feet, orthotic devices may provide relief. Surgery rarely is indicated. However, in chronic cases in which conservative therapy has failed, bursectomy and lateral tendon resection may relieve symptoms effectively.

Popliteal Tendinitis   Inflammation in and around the knee is secondary to overuse. Common sites of inflammation are the multiple bursae and tendon insertions present around the knee. Two common inflammatory abnormalities around the knee are popliteal tendinitis and pes anserine bursitis.

Popliteal tendinitis occurs mainly as a result of either hyperpronation or excessive downhill running. Pain is localized over the popliteus tendon just anterior to the fibular collateral ligament. Popliteal tendinitis usually responds to conservative treatment, including rest, ice, NSAIDs, and ultrasound modalities. Refractory cases may benefit from a local injection of steroids with or without local anesthetic. Once symptoms have resolved, patients may return to activities. However, a structured stretching and strengthening program may help prevent further recurrence of the problem.

Pes Anserine Bursitis   Pain, swelling, and tenderness approximately 6 cm distal to the medial joint line at the region of the pes insertion is characteristic of pes anserine bursitis. Pes anserine bursitis responds to conservative treatment as outlined above. If conservative treatment, including steroid injections, fails, surgical excision of the inflamed bursa occasionally may be indicated.

Lower Leg Injuries

The majority of lower leg injuries are secondary to overuse. Injuries can be classified into four major categories: (1) medial tibial stress syndrome; (2) compartment syndrome; (3) Achilles tendinitis; and (4) posterior tibial tendinitis.

Medial Tibial Stress Syndrome   Medial tibial stress syndrome encompasses a wide spectrum of disorders including periostitis near the origin of the soleus and posterior tibial muscle origins and stress fractures.

On physical examination, tenderness is localized to the posteromedial border of the tibia in the mid to distal third regions. Tenderness is usually more localized with stress fractures. Radiographs are usually normal in periostitis, and bone scintigraphy is necessary to make the definitive diagnosis. On bone scan, periostitis appears as linear streaking over the posteromedial aspect of the tibia. Stress fractures differ in that uptake is localized. Rest is the key to treatment of stress fractures and periostitis. Stress fractures may take up to 12 weeks to heal completely. Casting may be indicated.

Compartment Syndrome   Exercise-induced pain that resolves with rest may be a clue to chronic compartment syndrome. In addition, evidence of muscle herniation on physical examination may be seen in patients with chronic compartment syndrome. If there is a high index of suspicion, pressure measurements should be taken of the involved compartments. Pressures should be measured before and after exercise. During the test, exercise should be continued until symptoms are reproduced. Compartment pressures may be measured using a variety of techniques including needle manometer, wick catheter, slit catheter, and microcapillary infusion. Criteria for diagnosis of chronic compartment syndrome vary. For example, according to a recent review, the presence of one or more of the following pressure criteria, measured using a slit catheter, is considered diagnostic of chronic compartment syndrome: (1) pre-exercise pressure ≥ 15 mm Hg; (2) one-minute postexercise pressure ≥ 30 mm Hg; (3) five-minute postexercise pressure ≥ 20 mm Hg.

In general, the anterior compartment is most often involved followed by the deep posterior compartment. Nonsurgical treatment of chronic compartment syndrome is controversial. Surgical treatment involves release of the involved compartment. Good to excellent results following fasciotomy have been reported in 80% to 100% of patients.

Annotated Bibliography

Knee Laxity Measurement

Steiner ME, Brown C, Zarins B, et al: Measurement of anterior-posterior displacement of the knee: A comparison of the results with instrumented devices and with clinical examination. *J Bone Joint Surg* 1990;72A:1307-1315.

Four commercial instrumented devices were tested in patients with chronic anterior cruciate ligament ruptures and in normal controls. Significant differences in reproducibility were found among the devices. Three devices had more reproducible measurements and were as successful as clinical examination for determining ACL rupture. Approximately 80% to 90% of normal and ACL-deficient knees were identified using those devices.

Knee Ligament Injuries

Indelicato PA, Hermansdorfer J, Huegel M: Nonoperative management of complete tears of the medial collateral ligament of the knee in intercollegiate football players. *Clin Orthop* 1990;256:174-177.

Twenty-eight varsity football players who suffered isolated complete MCL tears were managed nonsurgically with early protected motion and physical therapy. Diagnosis was made by physical examination; meniscal and ACL pathology were ruled out by arthroscopy. Patients were evaluated subjectively, objectively, and functionally. The average time from injury to return to full contact sports was 9.2 weeks. The authors concluded that complete isolated tears of the MCL can be successfully managed nonsurgically provided there is no associated ACL or meniscal damage.

Roberts TS, Drez D Jr, McCarthy W, et al: Anterior cruciate ligament reconstruction using freeze-dried, ethylene oxide-sterilized, bone-patellar tendon-bone allografts: Two year results in thirty-six patients. *Am J Sports Med* 1991;19:35-41.

Of 44 patients who underwent ACL reconstruction with freeze-dried, ethylene oxide-treated bone-patellar tendon-bone grafts, 36 were evaluated at two-year follow-up. Nine patients had episodes of recurrent synovitis, and eight had graft rupture and dissolution requiring reoperation. The authors concluded that the most probable cause of the poor results was secondary to ethylene oxide and its by-products and that freeze-dried, ethylene oxide-treated bone-patellar tendon-bone allografts should not be used for ACL reconstruction.

Sapega AA, Moyer RA, Schneck C, et al: Testing for isometry during reconstruction of the anterior cruciate ligament: Anatomical and biomechanical considerations. *J Bone Joint Surg* 1990;72A:259-267.

Instrumented excursion wires were placed in the central portions of the anteromedial, central, and posterior fiber regions of the ACL. Under intraoperative testing conditions, the knee was cycled through a 120-degree range of motion. In no instance did the insertion site centers exhibit isometric behavior. The authors concluded that a residual deviation of up to 3 mm should not be considered nonphysiologic unless its separation does not correlate with the normal pattern of deviation, initial slackening then retightening as the knee progressively flexes.

Shelbourne KD, Nitz P: Accelerated rehabilitation after anterior cruciate ligament reconstruction. *Am J Sports Med* 1990;18:292-299.

In patients undergoing autogenous bone-patellar tendon-bone ACL reconstruction, an accelerated rehabilitation program was instituted and compared to a conventional rehabilitation program. The authors showed that loss of strength, loss of extension, and anterior knee pain were less with the accelerated program when compared with the conventional program, and stated that the accelerated program neither compromises stability nor puts the graft at risk.

Torg JS, Barton TM, Pavlov H, et al: Natural history of the posterior cruciate ligament-deficient knee. *Clin Orthop* 1989;246:208-216.

Forty-three patients with an average of 6.3 years between PCL injury and evaluation were studied. Evaluation included physical and roentgenographic examination, functional assessment, instrumented laxity measurement, and isokinetic and dynametric testing of quadriceps function. The authors concluded that patients with unidirectional instability should be treated nonsurgically. The authors further concluded that because patients with multidirectional instability had a poorer functional result, a higher incidence of degenerative changes on radiographs, and increased incidence of patellofemoral disease, this group of patients should be considered for surgical reconstruction.

Braces

Sitler M, Ryan J, Hopkinson W, et al: The efficacy of a prophylactic knee brace to reduce knee injuries in football: A prospective, randomized study at West Point. *Am J Sports Med* 1990;18:310-315.

Cadets (1,396) were randomized to either brace or no-brace groups. The brace used was a double-hinged, single upright brace. The cadets experienced a total of 21,570 athletic exposures over a two-year period of intramural football. Variables such as athletic shoe, athlete exposure, brace assignment, playing surface, and knee injury histology were all controlled. The authors concluded: (1) a unilateral-biaxial prophylactic knee brace was effective in statistically reducing the total and MCL knee injuries; (2) the reduction in total and MCL knee injuries was dependent on player position; (3) the severity of MCL and ACL knee injuries was not significantly reduced; (4) the mechanism of knee injuries most frequently observed was direct lateral contact; and (5) prophylactic knee braces reduced the number of MCL knee injuries due to direct lateral contact. However, this was not statistically significant.

McCarroll JR, Rettig AC, Shelbourne KD: Anterior cruciate ligament injuries in the young athlete with open physes. *Am J Sports Med* 1988;16:44-47.

Forty patients 14 years of age or younger with ACL tears and open physes were studied. Sixteen were treated conservatively and 24 surgically. Surgical reconstruction was either intra-articular or extra-articular based on the patient's growth potential. In no cases were any growth abnormalities noted. The authors recommend full evaluation of the injury under anesthesia as well as arthroscopy. If the patient has the proper indications and has a desire to continue in competitive athletics, reconstruction is recommended.

The Menisci

DeHaven KE: Decision-making factors in the treatment of meniscus lesions. *Clin Orthop* 1990;252:49-54.

This article presents an overview of meniscal lesions describing criteria for nonsurgical treatment, meniscal repair, partial meniscectomy, and total meniscectomy. The main factors to be considered in the decision-making process are: location of tear, extent of tear, type of tear, associated lesions, and clinical evaluation.

Fischer SP, Fox JM, Del Pizzo W, et al: Accuracy of diagnoses from magnetic resonance imaging of the knee: A multi-center analysis of one thousand and fourteen patients. *J Bone Joint Surg* 1991;73A:2-10.

In this study, 1,014 patents had both a presurgical MRI of the knee and an arthroscopic examination to confirm the diagnosis. The authors showed that the accuracy of diagnosis varied somewhat depending on the location of injury. The authors also revealed that 17% of meniscal lesions reported as grade II lesions were found by arthroscopy to be full thickness tears.

Raunest J, Oberle K, Loehnert J, et al: The clinical value of magnetic resonance imaging in the evaluation of meniscal disorders. *J Bone Joint Surg* 1991;73A:11-16.

In a prospective, double-blind study, 50 patients with symptoms of knee pain first underwent MRI of the involved knee (1.5 tesla magnetic) and then underwent arthroscopic evaluation. This study suggests that MRI is an effective screening measure, but the capability to rule out a meniscal tear is not satisfactory as evidenced by a high false-negative rate.

Warren RF: Meniscectomy and repair in the anterior cruciate ligament-deficient patient. *Clin Orthop* 1990;252:55-63.

The author outlines treatment plans for patients with meniscal tears and associated ACL tears, both chronic and acute. When possible, the author recommends meniscus repair with ACL reconstruction, especially in the young, athletic patient. Overall clinical success approaches 90% with this treatment plan. In patients who undergo meniscal repair without ACL reconstruction, failure rates approach 40%.

Plica Syndrome

Amatuzzi MM, Fazzi A, Varella MH: Pathologic synovial plica of the knee: Results of conservative treatment. *Am J Sports Med* 1990;18:466-469.

Patients (136) with pathologic synovial plicae were reviewed. Patients underwent a detailed rehabilitation program directed at decreasing the compressive forces in the anterior compartment of the knee as well as increasing the structural flexibility of the joint. Of knees, 34% had no associated abnormalities; 66% had either patellofemoral instability, epiphysitis, ligamentous instability, or meniscal pathology. Most associated abnormalities improved with rehabilitation and were not a factor in outcome.

The Patellofemoral Joint

Dzioba RB: Diagnostic arthroscopy and longitudinal open lateral release: A four year follow-up study to determine predictors of surgical outcome. *Am J Sports Med* 1990;18:343-348.

Sixty patients who underwent lateral release were evaluated at mean follow-up of four years. Predictions of good outcome were preoperative reproduction of pain, positive Merchant view, arthroscopic findings of positive lateral patellar overhang, and positive toughened lateral retinacular structures. The author also stated that the best correlation of good outcome was the reduction of the released patella after rehabilitation, as seen on the quadriceps film. Neither abnormal Q angle nor patellar articular changes were predictors of surgical outcome.

Fulkerson JP, Shea KP: Disorders of patellofemoral alignment. *J Bone Joint Surg* 1990;72A:1424-1429.

This is an excellent review of the clinical evaluation, radiographic evaluation, arthroscopic evaluation, and treatment options of the various patellofemoral malalignment disorders.

Kolowich PA, Paulos LE, Rosenberg TD, et al: Lateral release of the patella: Indications and contraindications. *Am J Sports Med* 1990;18:359-365.

The authors retrospectively reviewed the charts of 202 patients who underwent lateral release. The authors concluded that the most predictable criterion for success was a negative patellar tilt. Secondary criteria included medial and lateral patellar glide of two quadrants or less and a normal Q angle. Patients with a positive patellar tilt, three quadrants or greater medial and lateral patellar glide, or an abnormal Q angle at 90 degrees had higher failure rates.

Merchant AC: Patellofemoral malalignment and instabilities, in Ewing JW (ed): *Articular Cartilage and Knee Joint Function: Basic Science and Arthroscopy*. New York, Raven Press, 1990.

Classification, radiographic techniques, diagnosis, and treatment of patellofemoral dysplasias are discussed.

Small NC: An analysis of complications in lateral retinacular release procedures. *Arthroscopy* 1989;5:282-286.

A multicenter study (21 surgeons) reviewing complications associated with arthroscopic lateral release was presented. The two factors associated with a statistically significant higher incidence of complications were the use of a tourniquet and the use of a postoperative suction drain for greater than 24 hours. A trend toward increased complications with subcutaneous release was noted. The use of electrocautery and outpatient versus inpatient procedures had no effect on the incidence of complications.

Overuse Injuries

Martens M, Libbrecht P, Burssens A: Surgical treatment of the iliotibial band friction syndrome. *Am J Sports Med* 1989;17:651-654.

Twenty-three of 24 patients did not respond to conservative treatment for iliotibial band friction syndrome, including rest, anti-inflammatory drugs, physiotherapy, muscle stretching and strengthening, and steroid injection. These patients underwent surgical resection of a portion of the iliotibial tract (the technique is described in detail). All patients were satisfied and all returned to their previous level of sports activity.

Pedowitz RA, Hargens AR, Mubarak SJ, et al: Modified criteria for the objective diagnosis of chronic compartment syndrome of the leg. *Am J Sports Med* 1990;18:35-40.

Of 150 patients referred for evaluation of chronic leg pain, 131 records were available for review. The authors established criteria for the diagnosis of chronic compartment syndrome based on slit catheter measurement of intramuscular pressures.

48

Knee and Leg: Reconstruction

Synovectomy

Synovectomy continues to be a useful option for the management of selected patients with rheumatoid arthritis, pigmented villonodular synovitis, synovial chondromatosis, and hemophilic synovitis.

Synovectomy decreases, at least temporarily, the pain and synovitis of a knee affected with rheumatoid arthritis. It is not clear, however, whether synovectomy prevents or significantly delays the deterioration of the knee joint. Long-term surveillance demonstrates that at least half of patients who undergo synovectomy later require osteotomy or total knee replacement within four years, suggesting that synovectomy is a palliative rather than a curative procedure. Patients selected for the procedure should have a minimum of six months of persistent effusion and synovitis despite comprehensive medical management and meet the American Rheumatological Association's criteria for rheumatoid arthritis with a functional class I or class II.

The advantages of arthroscopic synovectomy are low morbidity, decreased risk of infection, and minimal loss of motion postoperatively. The procedure may be performed on an outpatient basis, unlike open synovectomy, which often requires a hospital stay of seven to ten days. In a study of 96 rheumatoid patients, 56% had moderate to severe pain and 100% had synovitis. Four years postoperatively, 21% of the patients had pain and 24% had synovitis, again indicating that synovectomy is at least a valuable palliative procedure.

An arthroscopic synovectomy is performed systematically using the 5.5-mm full-radius shaver. The superficial layers of the synovium are removed down to the plane between the synovium and subsynovial tissues. Anterolateral and anteromedial portals are used in addition to the posterior portal, which allows the synovium to be removed from the posterior aspect of the joint.

Alternatives to the open and arthroscopic techniques include chemical synovectomy and radiation synovectomy. Chemical synovectomy with alkylating agents or osmic acid now is rarely used because of the potential for articular cartilage damage. Radiation synovectomy with gold or yttrium provides satisfactory results at three years in more than 50% of properly selected patients. As in all synovectomies, the best results are obtained in patients with minimal radiographic abnormalities and low systemic disease activity. The disadvantages of these agents are their long half-lives (two to three days) and some diffusion of the agents to the regional lymph nodes and liver. Dysprosium 165 attached to ferric hydroxide

macroaggregates can be used as an alternative. Its two-hour half-life and larger carrier size minimize diffusion of the agent from the knee. The results seem comparable to those reported with the other chemical agents.

Arthroscopy

Arthroscopic lavage alone appears to provide greater symptomatic relief of the osteoarthritic knee joint in some patients than does physical therapy alone. While the mechanism of pain relief is not known, the removal of cartilage debris, crystals, and inflammatory factors may play a part. Arthroscopy is indicated in patients for whom other procedures are contraindicated.

Arthroscopic debridement with lavage of the osteoarthritic knee is often performed to postpone total knee arthroplasty. However, its efficacy remains unclear. Proponents of arthroscopic debridement stress its low risk and low morbidity and the fact that the knee joint is preserved. However, the procedure fails in half of the patients. The best postoperative results are obtained when preoperatively the pain has not been present for a long time, mechanical symptoms are present, radiographic changes are minimal, and crystal deposits are present. Debridement has little value for the long-standing or severely arthritic knee.

Osteotomy

Despite advances in total knee arthroplasty, the implants still have a limited life span and impose significant restrictions on younger, active patients. An osteotomy may provide pain relief and freedom of activity in the young person or a laborer and may delay total knee arthroplasty for as long as 15 years.

Biomechanics

In the normal knee, loads that are two to four times body weight are imposed on the tibiofemoral joint, with 60% of the load passing through the medial compartment. In the knee with unicompartmental degenerative changes, the altered limb alignment redistributes more load to the affected compartment, which may accelerate the degenerative process and cause severe pain. An osteotomy redistributes the loads to the uninvolved compartment.

The mechanical axis of the limb passes from the center of the femoral head to the middle of the tibial plafond as measured in a full length, weightbearing radiograph.

The axis normally passes through the center of the knee joint but is shifted with varus or valgus malalignment. The mechanical axis of the femur passes from the center of the femoral head to the midpoint of the intercondylar notch. The anatomic axis of the femur passes through the radiographic center of the intramedullary canal of the femur. The average angle between the mechanical and anatomic axes of the femur is 5 degrees in men and 7 degrees in women. The mechanical axis of the tibia passes from the center of the knee to the middle of the tibial plafond. The tibiofemoral angle is the angle between the femoral anatomic axis and the tibial mechanical axis.

Total varus or valgus angulation of the arthritic knee usually results from three components: the geometric alignment of the femur and tibia, narrowing or loss of bone and cartilage in one compartment, and widening of the other compartment's joint space because of slack ligamentous and soft-tissue structures. Widening is detected by measuring the difference between the involved knee and the opposite, uninvolved knee. Each millimeter of excessive joint space separation causes an apparent 1 degree of angular deformity on the weightbearing radiograph. If the contribution of excessive tibiofemoral joint separation is not considered preoperatively when choosing the amount of bone to be resected, the malalignment may be overcorrected.

Valgus-Producing Osteotomy

The high tibial valgus osteotomy is an efficacious procedure for the relief of pain and improvement of function in selected patients with medial compartment osteoarthritis. The ideal candidate is younger than 60 years of age, has symptoms localized to the medial compartment, and a flexion arc of a minimum of 90 degrees. Flexion contracture of more than 15 degrees and a varus deformity of more than 15 degrees are contraindications. Degenerative changes confined to the medial compartment should be apparent in radiographs, although minor arthritic changes in the lateral compartment or patellofemoral joint are not viewed as absolute contraindications by some authorities.

Absolute contraindications to a high tibial osteotomy include inflammatory arthritides, multicompartment symptomatic disease, and subluxation of the tibia greater than 1 cm in relation to the femur. There should not be significant ligamentous instability resulting from more than 1 cm of bone loss from the medial plateau. Relative contraindications include age older than 70 years and severe patellofemoral arthritis.

Preoperative Planning   Full-length, weightbearing radiographs are used to determine the desired amount of correction. To unload the arthritic medial compartment, the angle between the mechanical axis of the tibia and the anatomic axis of the femur should be in 8 to 10 degrees of valgus. Slight overcorrection provides the most reliable long-term results.

Gait analysis is also used to plan this procedure, as it permits a dynamic analysis of the forces created by muscles, the adduction moment at the knee, the upper body positioning, and the walking speed. The success of a high tibial osteotomy may be related to decreasing the postoperative adduction moment at the knee. In one study, there was no correlation between angular deformity measured on plain radiographs and the true distribution of forces across the knee joint.

Technique   The high tibial osteotomy should be performed with fluoroscopic guidance to determine accurate resection levels and angles as defined in the preoperative plan. A wedge osteotomy or a dome-shaped osteotomy can be performed with the aid of various alignment guides. The osteotomy is performed 2 cm distal to the joint line. A more proximal resection causes the proximal fragment to be too thin and at risk for intraoperative fracture or avascular necrosis. An osteotomy site that is too distal disrupts the extensor mechanism at the tibial tubercle. The medial cortex should be drilled and then fractured by closing the angle once the bone fragment is removed, thereby preventing malrotation (Fig. 1).

The method of fixation is controversial. Many authors advocate staple fixation and casting at surgery or shortly thereafter. Others recommend plate fixation, which offers early mobilization of the knee joint and has shortened rehabilitation time and decreased the incidence of patella infera.

Results   High tibial osteotomy for varus deformity has had satisfactory results as high as 60% at a ten-year follow-up. Survivorship analysis demonstrates that 80% of patients did not require further surgery by six years, but by seven years this number drops to 60%. In another series of 128 high tibial osteotomies in 107 patients with osteoarthritis, results were good or excellent in 80% at nine years. Adequate angular correction has the greatest correlation with a good long-term result.

Complications   Inadequate correction at the time of osteotomy, the most frequent complication, occurs in approximately 20% of all patients. Varus deformity, which recurs over time in 5% to 30% of all patients, is probably related to progression of the underlying osteoarthritic disease.

Osteonecrosis of the proximal fragment or nonunion can occur if the proximal fragment is too thin. Delayed union or nonunion occurs in 1% to 3% of patients and is treated by bone grafting or by repeat osteotomy when correction is lost.

Neurologic injuries have been reported in 1% to 10% of patients. The frequency of injury to the peroneal nerve is increased when external fixation is used, osteotomy of the fibular head has been performed, or corrections greater than 15 degrees have been attempted.

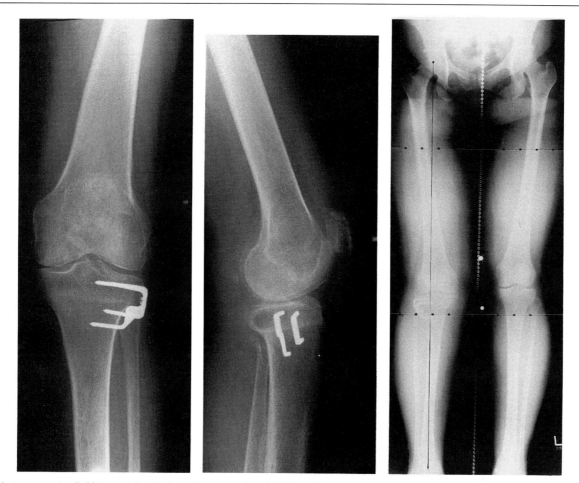

Fig. 1   Anteroposterior (**left**), lateral (**center**), and long standing (**right**) radiographs demonstrating a healed proximal tibial valgus-producing osteotomy.

Infection, a rare complication usually associated with pin sites if external fixation is used, has been noted in 1% to 8%. Compartment syndrome is also a recognized complication of high tibial osteotomy. Anterior compartment pressures are found to be significantly lower in patients for whom wounds are drained postoperatively.

Varus-Producing Osteotomy

Osteoarthritic valgus deformity of the knee is much less common than varus deformity. Genu valgum is more common in patients with a history of trauma, rheumatoid arthritis, renal osteodystrophy, rickets, or infantile poliomyelitis. While high tibial osteotomy has been successful in the treatment of genu varum, its efficacy is limited with genu valgum.

Because of the inherent valgus angulation of the normal distal femur, a medial-based proximal tibial osteotomy results in an oblique joint line tilted superolaterally. Such tilting leads to a shear force across the knee and gradual tibial subluxation laterally, while the distal femur appears to fall off the medial tibial plateau. For these

reasons, a distal femoral osteotomy should be done if the angle between the anatomic femoral axis and the tibial mechanical axis is greater than 12 to 15 degrees of valgus or if the plane of the joint deviates from the horizontal by more than 10 degrees.

The indications for a varus osteotomy are similar to those for valgus osteotomy. The patient should have adequate bone stock, normal circulation, a stable joint with no evidence of subluxation, a range of motion of at least 90 degrees of flexion, and a flexion contracture of no more than 15 degrees. The procedure is contraindicated in patients with inflammatory arthritides or inadequate motion of the knee.

The goal of the procedure is to correct the angle between the anatomic axis of the femur and the mechanical axis of the tibia to 0 to 2 degrees of valgus. Such overcorrection will unload the lateral tibiofemoral joint compartment and help prevent recurrence of the deformity.

Proximal Tibial Varus-Producing Osteotomy   This osteotomy differs from the high tibial osteotomy for varus deformity only in the medial approach and lack of need for fibular osteotomy or resection. The results of high tibial varus osteotomy for degenerative genu valgus deformity in properly selected patients are comparable with those for high tibial valgus osteotomy. Among 49 knees with an average follow-up of 31 months, pain was relieved completely in 53%, partially in 14%, and not at all in 33%. In another series of 31 patients with a mean follow-up of 10.2 years, 35% had no pain, 43% had mild pain not requiring restricted activity, 19% had moderate pain, and 3% had severe pain. Complications are similar to those for the high tibial valgus osteotomy.

Distal Femoral Varus-Producing Osteotomy There is controversy regarding the best surgical approach to the distal femoral varus-producing osteotomy. Although the medial approach is often used, the lateral and the midline approaches are advocated by some authors. Rigid fixation with a device such as the blade plate is recommended at the osteotomy site. Staples are inadequate. If rigid fixation of the osteotomy site is confirmed, it is possible to start early continuous passive motion in conjunction with a hinged fracture brace. However, if the rigidity of the fixation is questionable, it is preferable to keep the knee locked in extension using a knee immobilizer or a fracture brace with the hinge locked.

In a series of 23 distal femoral osteotomies, the tibiofemoral angle was corrected from a preoperative average of 18 degrees of valgus to a postoperative average of 2 degrees of valgus. At a mean follow-up of four years, the outcome was good or excellent for 19 knees (83%), and fair to poor for the remaining four. Three of the four poor outcomes occurred in patients with rheumatoid arthritis. Complications included two nonunions at the osteotomy site and one traumatic nondisplaced fracture through healing callus. In another group of 24 patients, 92% were successful at an average follow-up of four years.

Total Knee Arthroplasty Following Proximal Tibial Osteotomy

High tibial osteotomy provides the properly selected patient with significant pain relief and a durable knee joint. Nevertheless, many patients experience a gradual return of knee pain five to seven years postoperatively. In one series of 95 knees (83 patients), 22 knees (23%) had undergone total knee arthroplasty because of increasing pain an average of 8.9 years after an initially successful high tibial osteotomy.

A successful arthroplasty after high tibial osteotomy is technically more difficult to perform than a primary total knee arthroplasty. In one study of 45 knees, only half of the patients had an excellent result and 29% a good result, which was comparable with the results obtained for revision knee surgery at the same institution. In 21 of the 45 knees, the patellofemoral mechanics (patella infera) had been altered, necessitating a lateral retinacular release. A quadriceps turn down was required in two knees

to avoid avulsion of the patellar tendon at the patellar tubercle. A higher incidence of infection (4.4%) also was noted. In another review of 35 patients, the clinical results of total knee arthroplasty were comparable, but the investigators encountered no technical difficulties.

Unicompartmental Arthroplasty

Unicompartmental knee arthroplasty is a treatment alternative for osteoarthritis limited to the medial or lateral compartment of the knee. Proponents of unicompartmental arthroplasty cite the following benefits: preservation of a greater range of postoperative motion and nearly complete preservation of normal knee kinematics; longer enduring clinical results; fewer postoperative complications; and no required immobilization.

Patient Selection

The ideal patient is older than 60 years and is relatively inactive. Patients who weigh more than 80 kg (180 lbs) are at increased risk for component failure. Pain should be restricted primarily to one compartment and should be relieved by rest. The preoperative range of motion should be at least from 5 to 90 degrees. The maximum angle between the anatomic axis of the femur and the mechanical axis of the tibia should be no more than 15 degrees of valgus or 10 degrees of varus, either of which is passively correctable to neutral. Contraindications for unicompartmental arthroplasty include inflammatory arthritis, ligamentous instability, multicompartmental degenerative changes, and a flexion arc of less than 90 degrees. The procedure is also contraindicated in the patient who is highly active or performs heavy labor.

Intraoperative inspection of the entire knee joint is essential before a final decision is made to proceed with unicompartmental arthroplasty. Minor arthritic changes in the patellofemoral joint and opposite compartment are acceptable as long as they spare the weightbearing regions.

Results

Survivorship analysis of 100 unicompartmental knee arthroplasties has shown that the probability that a prosthesis will not loosen (defined as failure requiring revision) is 90% at nine years, 85% at ten years, and 82% at 11 years. A pattern of failure that accelerated after nine years was recognized in the first 60 knees. In another series of 50 unicompartmental knee arthroplasties that included a metal-backed tibial component, good to excellent results were obtained in 92%. The addition of a metal-backed polyethylene tibial component was credited with the relatively low incidence of failure and tibial component loosening.

Complications

Infection, implant loosening, and subsidence are potential complications of all arthroplasties. Failure mechanisms unique to unicompartmental arthroplasty include progression of degenerative changes to the opposite compartment and impingement of the patella on the edge of the femoral component.

Surgical Technique

The best results are observed following unicompartmental arthroplasties in which the final mechanical axis of the limb passes through the center of the knee or slightly medial to the center. The overcorrection of the deformity required by osteotomies is unnecessary.

The standard method of fixation uses methylmethacrylate bone cement for the femoral and tibial components. Long-term results of cementless unicompartmental arthroplasty have yet to be published, but shorter term surveillance suggests that results are comparable with those seen with cemented procedures. Some investigators believe cementless fixation may be advantageous in the young, heavy, or active patient, in whom biologic fixation may produce a longer-lasting result. Others are concerned that the relatively small surface area of the unicompartmental prostheses may limit the amount of bony ingrowth and make the implants more susceptible to loosening.

Total Knee Arthroplasty

An estimated 129,000 total knee arthroplasties are performed in the United States each year. Successful outcomes depend on patient selection, technique, component design, rehabilitation, and prevention of complications. The etiology, prevention, and treatment of complications related to the extensor mechanism is receiving increased attention because failure due to these complications is common.

Patient Selection

The indications for total knee arthroplasty have remained fairly constant: disabling knee pain, functional impairment, and radiographic evidence of significant arthritis. The most common causes are rheumatoid arthritis and osteoarthritis, but knee arthroplasty has been used successfully to treat a variety of arthritides. The ideal candidate is a thin, relatively inactive, elderly person with low functional demands and no medical illnesses that could impair rehabilitation or preclude safe anesthesia. The patient should not be an appropriate candidate for more conservative procedures, such as realignment osteotomies or synovial debridement, and should have exhausted nonoperative treatment options.

Total knee arthroplasty is contraindicated in a patient who has a nonfunctioning extensor mechanism, active sepsis, a painless, well-functioning arthrodesis, or a neuropathic arthropathy. The procedure is relatively contraindicated in patients with a history of prior osteomyelitis, significant peripheral vascular disease, or an overall medical condition that precludes anesthesia or rehabilita-

tion. Additionally, patients should be aware of the functional limitations imposed by the arthroplasty.

Technical Principals

Despite changes in technology, certain principles continue to apply when performing total knee arthroplasty.

Exposure The surgical incision should incorporate previous incisions where possible. If a new incision must intersect a prior incision, the angle of intersection should be as close as possible to 90 degrees. For the knee without previous incisions, either anterior midline or medial parapatellar incisions are acceptable. Traditionally, the knee joint is entered through an anteromedial capsular incision that proceeds through a longitudinal split in the quadriceps tendon and medial retinaculum. In contrast, with the subvastus, or Southern, approach, the vastus medialis is reflected laterally without interrupting its insertion into the patella and the supreme geniculate arterial supply to the patella is preserved. The lateral approach, which has been advocated in knees with severe valgus deformity, calls for the insertion of the iliotibial band and portions of the patellar tendon to be elevated.

Limb Alignment Varus or valgus malalignment of the limb following total knee arthroplasty is associated with an increased incidence of component loosening. The mechanical axis should pass through the midline of the proximal tibia after arthroplasty is performed. Two techniques to achieve a correct mechanical axis are commonly used. In one technique, the proximal tibia is cut at 3 degrees of varus in relation to its longitudinal axis. This means that the distal femoral cut must be approximately 9 degrees of valgus in relation to the anatomic axis of the femur in order to achieve an overall mechanical axis of 0 degrees. In the second technique, the proximal tibia is cut at 0 degrees to its longitudinal axis and the distal femur at approximately 7 degrees to its anatomic axis. The advantage of the second technique is that it reduces the probability of an inadvertent excessively varus cut and thus the likelihood of varus alignment of the limb.

Extramedullary and intramedullary guides for cutting the femur are available. If properly applied, the intramedullary femoral alignment systems are accurate to within 1 to 2 degrees of varus or valgus, and are more accurate than extramedullary systems. The use of an extramedullary alignment system is necessary in certain circumstances, such as in ipsilateral hip arthroplasty with a long femoral component or malalignment following a femoral fracture. Intramedullary and extramedullary systems are available for aligning the proximal tibial cut. However, the intramedullary system is less accurate, particularly when the tibia has a varus bow.

Ligament Balance The desired stability of the knee during normal activities requires collateral ligaments that have equal tension throughout the entire range of motion. To provide equal collateral ligament tension after the components are in place, the flexion and extension gaps should be inspected intraoperatively to ensure that they are equal in flexion and extension. If ligamentous rebalancing is necessary, it is best achieved by release on the concave side of the deformity rather than ligament advancement on the convex side of the deformity.

Component Orientation   Component orientation in the coronal, sagittal, and axial planes is critical to knee function. The correct coronal alignment of the components is necessary to establish proper overall leg alignment.

The sagittal alignment of the tibial component is determined by the amount of posterior slope of the proximal tibial cut. Most current systems strive for 3 to 7 degrees of posterior slope, because the bone in the anterior portion of the cut surface of the tibia is weaker. If the proximal tibia is cut perpendicular to the long axis of the tibia in the sagittal plane, tibial component subsidence is more likely. Inaccurate sagittal orientation that places the femoral component in too much extension may notch the anterior femur and can lead to later supracondylar fracture of the femur. A femoral component placed in too much flexion alters the kinematics of the knee and may decrease extension.

The proper axial alignment of the tibial and femoral component is still debated. The rotation of the femoral or tibial components cannot be determined from routine radiographs, and is best estimated by intraoperative observation. Although complete data are lacking, some believe errors in rotation of as little as 2 to 3 degrees may be significant. Internal rotation of the tibial component, a common error, causes lateral displacement of the tibial tubercle, which increases the Q angle and makes the risk of patellar instability greater. As a general rule, the tibial component should be aligned such that it points to the medial third of the tibial tubercle. The femoral component is also commonly placed in excessive internal rotation, which significantly affects patella tracking. The axial alignment of the femoral component either is determined by the posterior femoral condyles, or is adjusted to provide equal collateral ligament tension with the knee in flexion. Use of the femoral epicondyles also has been described. Several systems currently call for externally rotating the femoral component 3 to 4 degrees relative to the posterior femoral condyles to aid patella tracking. If the femoral component is rotated to provide equal collateral ligament tension, external rotation of 3 to 4 degrees usually results.

The level of the joint line should be maintained as close as possible to its preoperative position. Restoration of the joint line is more critical for knees in which the posterior cruciate ligament is retained, because the posterior cruciate ligament must be balanced to ensure full range of motion.

Patellar Tracking   Intraoperatively, the patella should track in the trochlear groove without external force. If

necessary, lateral retinacular release should be performed.

Component Design

Posterior Cruciate Ligament   Current knee arthroplasty designs can be generally grouped into three subsets with respect to the posterior cruciate ligament (PCL): PCL sacrificing, PCL sacrificing with substitution (Fig. 2), and PCL preserving (Fig. 3). The advantages of preserving the PCL include the restoration of normal knee kinematics (particularly axial rotation of the tibia and increased roll back of the femur on the tibia), maintenance of the ligament's proprioceptive abilities, and maintenance of load transfers by the PCL. Preserving the PCL also has disadvantages. In addition to more difficult collateral ligament balancing, the preoperative joint line must be reproduced. When the joint line level is not reproduced and the PCL is preserved, increased joint reactive forces and a change in the kinematics of the knee theoretically can lead to increased polyethylene wear. However, attempts to recreate the joint line at its preoperative level may necessitate excessive proximal tibial

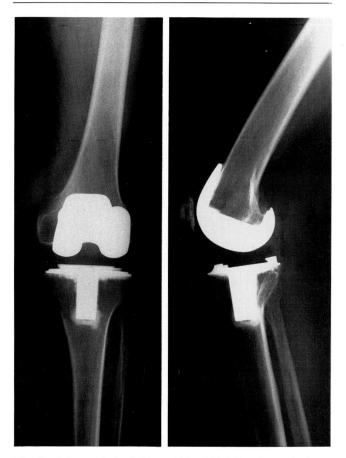

Fig. 2 Anteroposterior (**left**), and lateral (**right**), radiograph of a posterior cruciate ligament substituting total knee arthroplasty. All components are cemented.

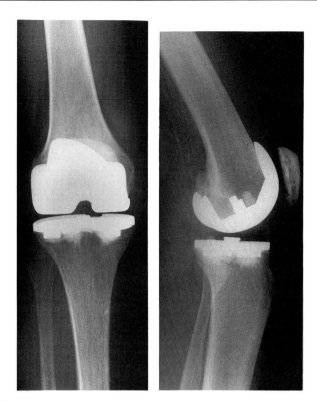

Fig. 3 Anteroposterior (**left**), and lateral (**right**) radiograph of a posterior cruciate ligament retaining total knee arthroplasty. The tibial and patellar components are cemented. The femoral component is porous coated.

bone resection to avoid the use of an excessively thin polyethylene component. Balancing or partial release of the PCL may be necessary for correct ligament balance. Finally, adequate exposure of the proximal tibia may not be possible when the PCL is retained. Substitution of the PCL is accomplished by the addition of a central build-up on the tibial polyethylene, which functions as a cam during movements of the knee. Theoretically, PCL-substituting prostheses allow the exposure and ligament correction of the PCL-sacrificing prosthesis while reproducing the kinematic effects of the PCL.

The difference between patients who have undergone PCL-sacrificing arthroplasty, with or without substitution, and those in whom the PCL is retained is shown using gait analysis. During stair climbing, patients without a PCL shift their weight farther forward with each step. This is thought to be due to the shortened quadriceps mechanism lever arm without the roll back provided by the PCL. Those patients with a retained PCL more closely approximate a normal stair climbing pattern. Little difference between the two groups can be detected during level gait.

It is difficult to otherwise compare the results of PCL-retaining, PCL-sacrificing, and PCL-substituting prostheses. Excellent results have been recorded using all of these techniques. One study of PCL-sacrificing total condylar arthroplasty found an 88% good to excellent clinical result after ten to 12 years. Although radiolucent lines were seen at the tibial bone-cement interface in 54.7%, only five of these knees had required revision arthroplasty. Of the patients in the study, 46% could not climb stairs with a reciprocal pattern. Among series of patients who underwent a PCL-substituting total knee arthroplasty, clinical results at two to eight years were good to excellent in 83%. A study of total knee arthroplasties that preserve the PCL found 88% had good to excellent clinical results and a 3% revision rate after five to nine years. However, 50% of the patients in the study could not climb stairs using reciprocal gait.

Fixation The best technique to achieve durable fixation of the components to bone in knee arthroplasty remains controversial. The longest follow-up data are in knees with cement fixation of the femoral and tibial components. The factors associated with enduring cemented arthroplasties are correct limb alignment, adequate coverage of the cut surface of the tibia, and metal backing of the tibial component. Survivorship analysis of cemented total condylar design knee arthroplasty indicates a 15-year survival rate of 90.6% using an all-polyethylene tibial component. Another survivorship study analyzed a broader spectrum of cemented component designs and found a five-year survival rate of 98% and a ten-year survival rate of 91%. A greater probability of prolonged survival was present in patients who had undergone primary knee arthroplasty, had a diagnosis of rheumatoid arthritis, were older than 60 years of age, or received a metal-backed tibial component. Radiolucent lines at the cement-bone interface, observed in 30% to 78% of cemented knee arthroplasties, did not correlate with clinical results.

Cemented fixation remains the standard against which other modes of fixation should be judged. However, the durability of cemented fixation is suspect because of its time-dependent fatigue properties. Cement also causes heat-induced osteonecrosis, and may contribute particulate debris once failure has begun. Cementless components were developed in an attempt to avoid these and other problems.

The initial clinical results of cementless components are comparable to cemented knee arthroplasties. For example, a prospective study compared cemented and cementless fixation. Patients selected for cementless fixation were relatively young, had no evidence of osteoporosis, were physically capable of more strenuous rehabilitation, and had the prostheses conformed to the bone surface intraoperatively. After three to six years, the average knee score was 89 in the cemented group and 93 in the cementless group. The incidence of radiolucencies under the tibial component was 42% in the cementless group compared to 20% in the cemented group. None of the cemented prostheses and two of the cementless tibial components were revised because of loosening.

Another prospective study randomized patients to receive cemented or cementless fixation without regard to age, rehabilitation potential, or bone quality. Clinical results were nearly identical after two to five years, although the cementless group had a higher frequency of subsidence (50%) and radiolucent lines (44%) compared to the cemented group (8% subsidence and 12% radiolucent lines). Longer term surveillance, however, has shown an increased frequency of metal fatigue, patellar failure, persistent pain, surface debonding, and evidence of inadequate bone ingrowth, particularly at the tibia. These findings continue to promote design changes.

Micromotion greater than 100 to 150 microns between the metal and bone induces fibrous rather than bone ingrowth into the component. In order to obtain the stability necessary to prevent such motion, a component must be secured solidly to a bone foundation that can withstand forces imposed by a patient's activities. A keel, 6.5-mm cancellous screws, and a stem improve the fixation of the tibial component in laboratory studies. A stem appears to contribute more significantly to fixation in osteoporotic bone and less so in strong bone. The use of a central stem and screws in osteoporotic bone can achieve initial fixation equal to cement. Micromotion also occurs when the component sinks on one side and lifts off the bone surface on the other side. Imprecise bone cuts, weak bone, or unbalanced forces contribute to this teeter-totter effect, and any of these factors can magnify the effect of another. Bone of less compressive strength is found with excessive bone resection and in osteoporotic conditions, such as rheumatoid arthritis.

Because loosening of cementless knee implants occurs most frequently in the tibial component, many surgeons perform hybrid total knee arthroplasty, that is, cemented fixation of the tibial component and cementless fixation of the femoral component. In one such group of patients, 93% had a good or excellent clinical result an average of two to eight years postoperatively. Nonprogressive radiolucent lines were found under 30% of the tibial components and 30% of the femoral components. No revisions had been performed because of either femoral or tibial component loosening.

Polyethylene Catastrophic wear of polyethylene inserts, an increasingly prevalent mode of failure in total knee arthroplasty, is influenced by many factors, including limb alignment, articular geometry of the tibial and femoral component, the presence or absence of metal backing, polyethylene thickness, femoral component material, the modular design of the tibial insert, and the material properties of polyethylene itself.

Asymmetric loading of the articular surfaces increases the contact forces transmitted to the polyethylene-bearing surface of the tibial component and leads to high localized stresses at the margin of the polyethylene component. Less-than-conforming articular surfaces reduce the areas where forces are transmitted between the components and increase the contact stresses in the polyethyl-ene. Contact can be increased by using components that provide closer conformity between the femoral and tibial components in both the sagittal and coronal planes. Components with relatively more conforming surfaces maintain larger regions of contact and reduce stress on the polyethylene.

Metal backing of the tibial component has a number of advantages, including enhanced fixation and longer survival of cemented total knee arthroplasty. It also allows porous surface application for uncemented designs, supplemental screw fixation, and trial reduction with components of different thicknesses to assess soft-tissue tension and ligament balance.

A distinct disadvantage of metal backing is the necessity of using thinner polyethylene. The stress generated in thin polyethylene inserts may exceed the yield strength of ultra-high-molecular-weight polyethylene. Finite element analysis has demonstrated that the stress intensity in polyethylene decreases dramatically with increasing thickness of the component. A minimum polyethylene thickness of 6 to 8 mm is suggested in contemporary designs.

An additional problem with metal backing is that motion can occur between the insert and the metallic tray, producing particulate debris. The presence of polyethylene debris at the bone-implant interface is associated with osteolysis and loosening. Inserts that are bonded to the metal backing may decrease peripheral stresses in the polyethylene, as well as motion between the components of the tibial prosthesis.

The material properties of polyethylene continue to undergo extensive scrutiny to determine if altering the fabrication technique can improve wear properties. Heat pressing of the surface has been found to accelerate the initiation and propagation of subsurface cracks that cause delamination and accelerated wear. Carbon fiber reinforcement has not proven advantageous.

Rehabilitation

The factors that affect the range of motion after knee arthroplasty are still being discovered. The final range of motion after knee arthroplasty is fairly similar among the various prosthetic designs, and usually approximates 100 to 115 degrees. Patients with greater than 100 to 115 degrees of motion preoperatively tend to decrease their motion postoperatively, whereas patients with less than 100 to 115 degrees of motion preoperatively tend to increase their motion postoperatively. A flexion contracture of 20 degrees or less immediately postoperatively often corrects with physical therapy. Therefore, inability to obtain full extension intraoperatively should not necessarily be corrected with increased bone resection, although attention should be paid to posterior capsular release and posterior femoral osteophyte excision.

There are conflicting data on the long-term effects of continuous passive motion (CPM) on range of motion, deep vein thrombosis, pulmonary embolus, and pain relief. Several studies have indicated a shorter hospital stay with the use of CPM, but an increased incidence of wound complications also has been reported. The transcutaneous oxygen tension of the skin near the incision for a total knee arthroplasty has been shown to decrease significantly after the knee is flexed past 40 degrees. Therefore, a CPM rate of one cycle per minute and a maximum flexion limited to 40 degrees for the first three days has been recommended.

The indications for and benefits of manipulation following knee arthroplasty have not been clearly established. In general, if a patient has not reached 90 degrees of flexion by three to six weeks postoperatively, manipulation is considered. All other causes of limited range of motion, including infection, reflex sympathetic dystrophy, and component malposition, should be excluded.

Complications

Infection Approximately 250,000 hip and knee replacements are performed annually in the United States. Given an infection rate of 1% to 2%, between 3,500 and 4,000 joint replacements are infected each year. Assuming an average hospital cost of $50,000 to treat an infected joint replacement, the impact of this complication approaches $200 million annually. This statistic emphasizes the need to identify those patients at increased risk for infection and to manage aggressively, before undertaking surgery, any problems that could increase that risk. Patients at increased risk for infection include those who have rheumatoid arthritis (especially males), concurrent skin ulcers, or prior knee surgery. Obesity, concurrent urinary tract infections, and the use of oral steroids are associated with infection, but these associations are not statistically significant.

Perioperative prophylactic measures, including preoperative antibiotics and laminar air flow systems, have been shown to decrease the rate of infection significantly. For maximum effectiveness, intravenous antibiotics should be administered five minutes before tourniquet inflation. In some high-risk patients, antibiotic-impregnated cement has been used to lessen the infection rate following primary and revision knee arthroplasty. However, recent research has suggested that the release of gentamicin from antibiotic cement can depress bone turnover, which may have a later effect on the rate of loosening.

Early diagnosis of an infected prosthesis requires a high index of suspicion. Infection may cause only knee pain, persistent effusion, or early painless loosening, or there may be more obvious signs, including inflammation, drainage, and sepsis. Abnormal laboratory values, such as an elevated serum white blood cell count, C-reactive protein, or sedimentation rate, may help with the diagnosis, but each of these has a high false-negative rate. Although the accuracy of indium scanning in identifying infection of orthopaedic implants has been reported to be as high as 84%, aspiration and culture remains the most accurate method of diagnosis. However,

a 25% false-negative aspiration rate means that positive cultures often will be isolated only after the components are removed and the tissue is cultured.

Options for treatment of an infected prosthesis include antibiotic suppression, debridement with retention of the prosthesis, debridement and removal of the components, or amputation. Antibiotic suppression alone is indicated only in those patients who cannot medically tolerate further surgical procedures. Effective suppression depends on the presence of a well-fixed prosthesis and an infecting organism of low virulence that is sensitive to oral antibiotics. Antibiotics will likely be administered for the rest of the patient's life, and eventual cure should not be expected.

Successful treatment of an infected knee arthroplasty by debridement and retention of the components is associated with an infection of less than two to four weeks duration, a susceptible gram-positive organism, absence of prolonged drainage or sinus tract formation, well-fixed components, and good overall patient health. Debridements should be aggressive and include an open, complete synovectomy. Multiple debridements may be necessary, but if cultures remains positive, the components should be removed.

Debridement and removal of the prosthesis, followed by a course of intravenous antibiotics, remains the most reliable method of eradicating the infection. Debridements should be repeated until cultures are negative. After debridement, the wound is closed over suction drains. Following the last debridement, a six-week course of intravenous antibiotics should be administered, maintaining a bactericidal titer of 1:8. The use of an antibiotic-impregnated methylmethacrylate spacer block inserted between the femur and tibia is an effective way to deliver high concentrations of antibiotic to the tissues and to maintain the ligament tension in preparation for future reimplantation.

Once the infection has been adequately treated, three alternatives remain—resection arthroplasty, reimplantation, or fusion. Resection arthroplasty is appropriate for patients with limited potential function who are generally debilitated or have limited rehabilitation potential. Resection arthroplasty requires prolonged cast and brace immobilization, and functional results are unpredictable.

A candidate for staged reimplantation must be in relatively good health and able to tolerate multiple surgical procedures. The infecting organism may be gram-positive or gram-negative, but it must be sensitive to relatively nontoxic antibiotics. The skin and soft tissues must be healed and supple and the extensor mechanism intact. Preoperative aspiration is mandatory, and a positive culture precludes reimplantation. Reimplantation is a difficult procedure often accompanied by complexities in exposure, bone defects, and ligament instability. Following reimplantation, antibiotic regimens described in the literature vary from 48 hours to a lifetime course of oral antibiotics. Using a two-stage technique, eradication of infection has been reported in up to 95% of patients, with good to excellent clinical results in 65% of cases at an average follow-up of four years (range two to ten years). Longer term analysis is necessary.

Arthrodesis remains a treatment option for patients who have recurrent infection, or who are poor candidates for reimplantation. Results depend on the type of prosthesis used for the knee arthroplasty. Resurfacing implants in general require less initial bone resection than hinged prostheses, and therefore are associated with a higher rate of fusion after their removal. Arthrodesis using external fixation has a published success rate of 70% to 80%, but also an increased frequency of complications, including peroneal nerve palsy and pin tract infections. Internal fixation requires a clean wound that has been adequately treated for infection. Intramedullary nail fixation has become increasingly popular. Fusion rates of 80% to 85% are reported. Although the procedure is lengthy, technically demanding, and associated with significant blood loss, patients are frequently ambulatory on the treated extremity within a short period of time. Successful fusion usually occurs within four to six months. Tension-band plating and dual plating also have been used successfully in the arthrodesis of a previously infected knee arthroplasty.

Amputation is reserved for those patients who have uncontrolled sepsis, multiple failed attempts at less ablative procedures, and for the elderly, nonambulatory patient who cannot withstand reconstruction or who has undergone unsuccessful systematic antibiotic treatment.

Thrombophlebitis Following total knee arthroplasty venous thrombosis reportedly occurs in 50% to 84% of patients; asymptomatic pulmonary embolism, in 8.2% to 17%; symptomatic pulmonary embolism, in 0.5% to 3%; and death, in 0.3%. Thrombophlebitis occurs in the contralateral leg in only 3.2% of patients who have undergone knee arthroplasty, in contrast to hip arthroplasty, in which thrombophlebitis is more common in the nonoperated leg. Fortunately, most thromboses following knee arthroplasty occur in the calf.

Prophylactic measures are either mechanical or pharmacologic. Prophylactic medications include warfarin, low-dose heparin, aspirin, dextran, and antithrombin III; each regimen has proponents. The commonly used mechanical prophylaxes are compressive hose, continuous passive motion, and sequential pneumatic compression devices. Studies can be found that either support or refute the benefit of continuous passive motion, cement fixation, and one-stage bilateral knee arthroplasty on the frequency of vein thrombosis, but the use of a tourniquet seems unrelated. Warfarin, heparin, and sequential compression devices are generally considered to be the most effective of the various modalities.

Three reports specifically compare different techniques for the prevention of venous thrombosis. In each, venography was used to establish the diagnosis. The first study compared dextran to antithrombin III and subcutaneous heparin. Antithrombin III in conjunction with subcutaneous heparin was more effective than dextran in reducing the overall frequency of thrombosis, but not in preventing proximal vein thrombosis. In the second study, sequential compression devices were as effective as, and less expensive than, low-dose warfarin in preventing both calf and proximal vein thromboses. In the third study, the use of sequential compressive devices alone was more effective than aspirin in preventing both calf and proximal vein thrombosis, particularly following bilateral one-stage arthroplasty.

Neurovascular Damage Arterial injury following total knee arthroplasty is a rare event (less than 0.05%), but it can lead to limb ischemia and subsequent amputation. Arterial injuries include femoral or popliteal arterial thrombosis, traumatic aneurysm, arteriovenous fistula, and arterial transection of the vessels. Thrombosis also can be caused by the application of a tourniquet to a vessel affected with atherosclerotic disease. Although usually recognized intraoperatively, arterial laceration or transection may manifest postoperatively as a false aneurysm or an arteriovenous fistula. The absence of pedal pulses, the presence of atherosclerotic vascular disease, or radiographic arterial calcification warrants cautious use of the tourniquet and careful postoperative monitoring of the pulses. These patients should be examined preoperatively and cleared for the operation by a vascular surgeon. In selected patients, arterial reconstruction may be considered prior to the arthroplasty.

Peroneal nerve damage has a reported frequency of less than 3% following total knee arthroplasty and usually occurs when the procedure is done to correct a flexion and valgus deformity. Other possible causes include intraoperative traction, intraoperative or postoperative external compression, and compression secondary to a hematoma. A nerve palsy should be treated by knee flexion and release of compressive dressings or wraps. Among a group of 26 patients with peroneal nerve palsies, all had at least partial recovery, and 54% recovered completely. Of those patients who initially had a partial nerve palsy, 84% recovered completely, whereas only 35% of patients with an initially complete nerve palsy had complete recovery.

Blood Loss Blood loss following total knee arthroplasty averages 1,500 ml. It is unclear whether the magnitude of loss is affected by cement fixation or continuous passive motion. In one study, no significant decrease in blood loss was noted to result from releasing the tourniquet and obtaining hemostasis intraoperatively. However, intraoperative tourniquet release, in conjunction with continuous passive motion begun immediately postoperatively, correlated positively with increased blood loss.

Periprosthetic Fractures A periprosthetic fracture of the femur is defined as a fracture within 15 cm of the joint line or within 5 cm of the proximal extent of an intramedullary component. Such fractures occur in 0.6%

to 1.6% of patients undergoing total knee arthroplasty. Predisposing factors include osteoporosis, anterior femoral notching, and revision arthroplasty in patients with distal femoral bone loss. The trauma causing the fracture is usually minimal. Treatment is aimed at healing the fracture and maintaining knee motion. Revision of the components at the time of fracture treatment is reserved for patients with gross component loosening or those whose fracture cannot be treated by any other method. One proposed algorithm for treatment emphasizes assessment of the amount of displacement, the degree of comminution, and the ability to maintain a satisfactory reduction of the fracture.

Fat Embolism   Fat embolism following total knee arthroplasty is associated with stemmed intramedullary components or intramedullary guides used for tibial and femoral osteotomy. Fat embolism is more common when either of these methods is used during one-stage bilateral total knee arthroplasty. Fat embolism may occur more often than in the reported 3%, because its pulmonary and neurologic symptoms are probably often attributed to atelectasis, pulmonary embolism, sundown syndrome, medication overdose, or senile hospitalization confusion. The treatment is respiratory support as needed.

Wound Healing   Wound complications associated with the patient's nutritional status correlate specifically with the white blood cell count and the albumin level. A preoperative white blood cell count of less than 1,500 cells per mm^3 has correlated with a five-fold increase in major wound complications. An albumin level less than 3.5 g/dl is associated with a seven-fold increase. Clinical factors associated with wound-healing problems include rheumatoid arthritis, diabetes mellitus, and hematoma. Any wound drainage should be treated initially with immobilization. Persistent drainage for more than one or two days is treated by wound debridement.

The routine use of drains to prevent hematoma formation has been questioned. No significant differences were found in rehabilitation or in the frequency of delayed wound-healing when knees that were drained and those that were not were compared after one-stage bilateral total knee arthroplasty. Further, drains may increase the risk of infection. An increased frequency of positive cultures was seen for drains removed after 48 hours, compared with those removed after 24 hours. Draining hematomas should be debrided immediately.

Large areas of skin necrosis require immediate irrigation and debridement followed by a local soft-tissue flap. The medial or lateral head of the gastrocnemius is usually effectively used as a pedicle flap in such circumstances.

Patellofemoral Resurfacing

Despite more than ten years of experience with patellofemoral resurfacing, the procedure is associated with a 5% to 10% rate of related complications and accounts for almost 50% of all long-term complications of total knee arthroplasty. Complications attributed to the patellofemoral joint include the failure of metal-backed components, patellofemoral instability, component loosening, patellar fracture and osteonecrosis, and failure of the extensor mechanism.

Early prosthetic designs did not include patellofemoral resurfacing. Symptoms attributable to the patellofemoral joint occurred in 25% of patients. While most reports suggest that patellar resurfacing can offer the patient improved pain relief and knee strength, selective patellar resurfacing has been advocated as a way of avoiding patellofemoral complications. A reasonable approach to patellofemoral replacement is to perform patellar resurfacing for all patients with rheumatoid arthritis or advanced degenerative changes in the patella. Reasonable indicators for patellofemoral replacement in osteoarthritic patients appear to be preoperative patellofemoral pain, patient height greater than 160 cm, and weight greater than 60 kg.

Failure of Metal-Backed Components

As with the tibial component, metal backing of the patellar polyethylene component is thought to decrease polyethylene deformation and wear, reduce the stress at both the implant-cement and implant-bone interfaces, and enable the application of porous coatings for biologic fixation. Despite the theoretic advantages of this design concept, reports continue to document unacceptable failure rates of the metal-backed patellar components. The mode of failure for metal-backed patellar implants include polyethylene wear through, dissociation of the polyethylene from the metal backing, failure of the patella peg-plate junction, and failure of bony ingrowth into the porous surface. To date, 11 different metal-backed patella designs have been associated with component failure.

Symptoms that indicate possible failure of the metal-backed patellar implant include anterior knee pain, swelling, effusion, and subpatellar crepitus. Anteroposterior lateral radiographs may demonstrate failure, but an axial radiograph of the patella is the most informative. Factors that indicate failure of the implant include contact between the metal endoskeleton of the patellar implant and the anterior phalange of the femoral component, metallic debris within the soft tissues or the patellar bone, or dissociated polyethylene within the suprapatellar pouch. In addition, aspirated synovial fluid from the knee joint may reveal dark stained fluid containing metallic debris. When symptoms persist and the diagnosis remains uncertain, an arthroscopic examination of the knee can be helpful. The diagnosis is confirmed by the presence of fragmented or delaminated polyethylene.

The high incidence of polyethylene failure in metal-backed patellar components has rekindled interest in cemented all-polyethylene designs. Two design features that affect patellar performance are polyethylene thickness and congruity of the patellofemoral joint. Patella maltracking and excessive knee flexion increase forces at the patellofemoral joint. In a laboratory model, a dome-shaped polyethylene patella in an incongruent trochlear groove is associated with stresses that exceeded the yield strength of polyethylene, causing the polyethylene to deform and the underlying bone to fail. Patellar components of congruent patellofemoral design are associated with significantly lower stress levels and less polyethylene deformation and wear than are those of incongruent designs. However, patellofemoral conformity may restrict patellar rotation, which can increase forces on the polyethylene or lead to component loosening. Congruent patellar components have not yet been studied adequately in a long-term clinical setting to determine which type of component is superior.

Under experimental conditions, congruent metal-backed patellar replacements perform better than all-polyethylene models in both contact stress analysis and wear testing. However, eventual wear through of the polyethylene is noted under high-level cyclic testing. Setting the metal-backed patellar component into the patella has enhanced component fixation. An inset patella, however, may be difficult to remove in revision surgery, and requires further follow-up to evaluate its effect on fixation. A metal-backed rotating bearing patellar prosthesis has been reported to yield early good clinical results. In contact stress analysis, this design demonstrated the lowest stress levels of the various patellar prosthetic designs. Further clinical testing of this metal-backed design is necessary to support its further use.

Treatment of a failed metal-backed patellar implant involves revision to a polyethylene component and synovectomy. Malpositioned tibial or femoral components should be revised if they contribute to patellar component failure. Femoral component revision also should be performed if metal abrasion is significant.

Patellofemoral Instability

The function of the patellofemoral joint is largely determined by surgical technique. Function of the extensor mechanism is influenced by each bony cut and by the accuracy of ligament and soft-tissue balancing. A preoperative valgus deformity is common in patients with later patellofemoral instability and represents a failure to adequately release contracted lateral retinacular structures. Residual postoperative valgus limb alignment also can result in an unstable extensor mechanism. Likewise, internal rotation of the tibial component can cause patellar instability. Internal rotation and medial translation of the femoral component increases medial displacement, tilting, and subluxation of the patella, whereas external rotation of the femoral component has produced radiographic patterns of patellar tracking most closely reproducing those of the intact knee. The combined thickness of the patellar bone and the component should not exceed patella thickness preoperatively. On the other hand, to avoid increased patellar strains, the bony patella should not be cut to a thickness of less than 12 to 15 mm.

At the completion of a total knee arthroplasty, patellar tracking should be critically evaluated to insure stability. Patellar tracking may be improved by removal of patellar osteophytes and lateral retinacular release. Although identification and preservation of the lateral geniculate vessels during lateral retinacular release appears prudent, clinical studies have not supported the hypothesis that interruption of the superior geniculate artery causes osteonecrosis of the patella.

When patellar instability occurs, its successful treatment depends on an accurate determination of its etiology. The axial alignment, component position, level of the joint line, and overall thickness of the patella should be evaluated. If possible, the radiographic dimensions of the knee before the index procedure should be measured. Component malposition and malalignment should be corrected. A lateral retinacular release with medial reefing may be the only procedure necessary if component position is correct. Distal realignment may be necessary and is performed by an extended osteotomy of the tibial tubercle with medial translation. Combined proximal and distal procedures should be avoided because of the risk of extensor mechanism failure.

Patellar Component Loosening

Treatment options for a loose patellar component include reimplantation, leaving the unresurfaced patella in place without resurfacing, and patellectomy. If adequate host bone is available with potential interdigitation of the cement, then reimplantation should be performed. If insufficient bone exists, then leaving the patella unresurfaced has been suggested, but sufficient clinical evaluation of this technique is not available. Patellectomy should be reserved as a final option. The quadriceps mechanism should track in the trochlear groove after the patella is removed. Some extensor weakness is expected.

Periprosthetic Patellar Fracture

Undisplaced or minimally displaced fractures not involving the patellar component and presenting with a minimal extensor lag are treated with six weeks of immobilization followed by progressive range of motion. Displaced patellar fractures with a significant extensor lag and no involvement of the patellar component are treated with open reduction and internal fixation of the patella and repair of the torn retinaculum. Often the only internal fixation that can be used is a cerclage wire. Immobilization for six weeks is recommended. Patella fractures with displacement of the patellar button require excision of the loose component and the associated cement. Inadequate bone stock frequently prevents prosthetic replacement. If extensive comminution is present, partial or total patellectomy is performed with repair of the extensor apparatus. Elaborate internal fixation devices are best avoided. In patients with patellar fractures following condylar total knee arthroplasty there is a significant correlation between component alignment and the severity of the fracture. Patients with major component malalignment have more severe fractures with less satisfactory results. The best results were in patients who underwent repair of the fracture with tibial and femoral component revision to achieve neutral alignment.

Patellar Tendon Avulsion

Avulsion of the patellar tendon is a serious complication that is very difficult to treat. When the knee is flexed intraoperatively, the tendon insertion may be stressed to the point of partial or complete avulsion. This is particularly true in patients who have had high tibial osteotomy or who are undergoing revision arthroplasty, because scar tissue makes patella eversion more difficult and the patellar tendon may be shortened. Extensive soft-tissue release from the proximal tibia, a V-Y quadricepsplasty, or elevation of the patellar tendon with a bony block can be used to prevent tendon avulsion and improve the exposure of the knee joint.

Patellar tendon rupture is best treated with primary repair, but knee arthrodesis ultimately may be required. A newly described technique involves use of an allograft extensor mechanism. The early results are promising, but the longer term allograft durability is not known. Quadriceps tendon rupture with loss of function is best treated by repair of the proximal patella with viable tissue. After the scarred area of rupture is resected, the quadriceps is advanced, so that healthy tissue is used for the repair.

Revision Total Knee Arthroplasty

Revision total knee arthroplasty is a technically demanding procedure, requiring the ability to manage severe osseous and soft-tissue defects. Contemporary revision systems can provide varus or valgus constraint, replace inadequate bone stock with wedges and blocks, and augment component fixation with intramedullary stems.

Before performing revision knee arthroplasty, it is essential to understand the failure mechanism of the implant to be revised. The physical examination should thoroughly test for the integrity of the ligaments, as well as assess the quality of the skin and location of previous incisions. Full-length, weightbearing radiographs showing anteroposterior, lateral, and sunrise views should be analyzed for evidence of component loosening, limb alignment, and the position of the patella in relation to the joint line. Joint line analysis should be done of either the uninvolved knee or of the operative knee prior to the initial arthroplasty. Computed tomography can assess component rotation and dimensions of bone architecture. The knee joint should be aspirated to determine whether a subclinical infection is present.

Revision Arthroplasty

The technical principles of exposure, limb alignment, ligament balance, component orientation, and patella tracking that apply to a primary arthroplasty also apply to a revision. The goal is to recreate the joint line in relation to the patella in order to restore tibiofemoral and patellofemoral kinematics. Exposure poses a particular challenge because of capsule scarring and contractures. Extensive soft-tissue dissection on the medial and posterior aspect of the tibia may be necessary to expose the proximal tibia. A V-Y incision in the quadriceps tendon or an osteotomy of the tibial tubercle may be necessary to allow adequate lateral tibial plateau exposure.

Although results for revision knee arthroplasty can be acceptable, they do not equal those of primary procedures because of the increased risk of sepsis and the technical problems created by massive bone loss and ligamentous instability. Hinged components to overcome instability provide less favorable results; an infection rate of approximately 5% is higher than the rate of less than 1% for primary knee arthroplasty. There is an increased frequency of wound-healing problems, deep venous thrombosis, maltracking of the patella, and pulmonary embolism.

In a recent study that compared primary and revision knee arthroplasties, results were good or excellent in 92% of the primary series and good or excellent in 81% of the revision series. Good or excellent clinical results are reported in 70% to 75% of patients using the Total Condylar III implant. In a cohort of patients who underwent revision strictly for aseptic loosening, 5.8% required yet another operation for aseptic loosening. However, the incidence of radiolucent lines beneath the tibial component was 61%, and malalignment was present in 78% of the limbs.

Special Problems in Revision Bone Defects

The choice of technique for managing bone defects is influenced by the location and the depth of the defect, as well as by whether or not the defect is contained by a rim of cortical bone. The defect of a varus deformity is usually located peripherally on the posteromedial aspect of the tibia. A valgus deformity more often produces a contained posterolateral tibial defect in conjunction with a lateral femoral condylar deficiency. During revision surgery, contained defects may be found centrally after the components are removed, or an angular, asymmetric defect may be found, the result of component malalignment or subsidence. The dimensions of the defects frequently cannot be defined preoperatively. Attention to fundamental principles of ligament balance and establishment of a correct mechanical axis are critical to success, regardless of the management option chosen.

Two methods do not involve filling the defect. Bone resection can eliminate the defect, however, tibial bone resection greater than 8 to 10 mm places the component on significantly weaker bone and should be avoided. The component can be displaced from the defect in such a way that a minimal amount of the prosthesis overlies the bone defect. The latter technique, however, is helpful only for peripheral defects and necessitates the use of a smaller component, which changes the distribution of load transfer.

The techniques available to fill defects include cement alone, cement with screw support, an autogenous or allogenic bone graft, modular metal wedges, and custom components. Each technique commonly is used in conjunction with extended intramedullary stems. Methylmethacrylate cement is readily available, and its use is less technically demanding than other techniques. However, laboratory experiments show that cement with or without reinforcing screws provides less mechanical support than do other methods. For this reason, cement filling should be limited to defects less than 1 cm. Defects deeper than 10 mm should use screws to act as reinforcement for the cement. Although the early clinical results using this method are promising, a 26% frequency of radiolucencies at the cement-bone interface at a three-year follow-up makes the longer term results questionable.

Locally obtained autogenic bone graft usually is available in sufficient quantity during primary knee arthroplasty. Fixation of these grafts requires the use of screws or pins, or the graft can be fashioned into a wedge to fit the tibia defect. Intrusion of cement into the host-graft interface must be avoided because it impairs bone union. The clinical results using autogenous bone graft for tibial bone defects have been good. However, radiographic union of the graft has been reported to be as low as 67%. The grafts that fill contained defects provide more reliable support for the tibial component than do grafts that fill uncontained defects. In one series, dissolution and collapse was reported in four of 27 uncontained grafts. More promising results are reported by most other authors. Longer follow-up is necessary to determine if late collapse will be a common finding.

Bulk and morselized allogenic bone are more commonly used in revision arthroplasty, and are fixed with the same techniques described for autologous grafts. The long-term outcomes for allogenic graft are not yet available. In one study of contained and uncontained tibial defects filled with allogenic grafts, radiographic union was evident in 92% of revision knee arthroplasties after two to four years.

Modular metal wedges have been demonstrated in cadaveric models to have more stability than bone graft or cement. The short-term clinical results are promising. However, the amount of debris produced by the metal-to-metal interfaces can theoretically affect the long-term results. Care should be taken to avoid resecting more bone to accommodate the wedge than would be lost by selecting a slightly lower cut on the tibia.

Custom-made components are particularly useful following severe bone loss or major resections in the treatment of tumors. The high cost of these custom implants makes routine use prohibitive. Careful preoperative planning is required, because the bone defect predicted preoperatively often differs from that discovered intraoperatively.

Finally, the addition of a stem to the component generally is desirable in all of the techniques used for bone defects. A stem transfers up to 30% of the force from the bone subtending the component to a point more proximal in the femur or more distal in the tibia. Press-fit prostheses, particularly the femoral component, are often used because of the difficulty in removing a long-stem cemented component should infection occur.

Special Cases

Young Patients Total knee arthroplasty performed on relatively young patients increases the risk for early failure. The results of knee arthroplasty on young patients with rheumatoid arthritis have been comparable to those obtained in elderly patients with osteoarthritis. The results of knee arthroplasty in young patients with rheumatoid arthritis cannot be generalized to all young patients, because localized osteoarthritis is less debilitating than is rheumatoid arthritis. However, cemented knee arthroplasty in osteoarthritic patients younger than 55 years years of age is reported to have radiographic and clinical outcomes after six years that were comparable to the results obtained in younger patients with rheumatoid arthritis and elderly patients with osteoarthritis. These promising results should not dissuade the surgeon from pursuing treatment other than prosthetic replacement in the young active patient.

Obesity One study found comparable clinical results of posterior stabilized cemented knee arthroplasty at two to six years in patients weighing more and less than 150% of their desired body weight. Patellar complications, however, were more common in the obese patients, possibly due to the increased reactive forces at the patellofemoral joint. The frequencies of other complications, including deep vein thrombosis, hematoma, and delayed wound-healing, were about the same in all patients. Another study examined both the clinical and the radiographic findings in obese patients two years after cemented knee arthroplasty. The frequency of radiolucent lines under the tibial component correlated with the patient's weight, a finding that is consistent with previous studies. The obese patients did not demonstrate impaired rehabilitation. Obesity alone should not be considered a contraindication to knee arthroplasty, but longer follow-up may show greater loosening and component wear.

Diabetes Diabetes mellitus has been associated with significant problems in wound healing and infection. After cemented total knee arthroplasty, one study identified an infection rate of 7%, a higher revision rate, and more perioperative mortality. However, deep vein thrombosis and wound complications were comparable to those in nondiabetic patients.

Paget Disease Patients with Paget disease of the tibia or femur often have degenerative changes of the knee.

Among a group of patients with Paget disease who received cemented total knee arthroplasties, function was restored, symptoms were relieved, and seven years postoperatively the loosening rate was comparable to patients without this disease. The tibial and femoral bowing associated with Paget disease often necessitates extramedullary cutting guides. Arthritic knee pain must be differentiated from pain caused by Paget disease. An arthritic knee can be confirmed as the source of pain if that pain is relieved after intra-articular local anesthetic injection or ineffectively relieved following diphosphonate or calcitonin therapy.

Hemophilia The risk for complications from total knee arthroplasty in patients with hemophiliac arthropathy is increased and the likelihood for restoration of knee motion is reduced. A group of such patients followed for a minimum of 5.5 years after total knee arthroplasty had a 53% complication rate, including an increased risk of nerve palsies, bleeding, and infection. When the intraoperative factor VIII level was maintained at 100% and then postoperatively tapered there was a significant decrease in complications compared with a regimen that maintained the intraoperative levels of factor VIII at 80%. The failure rate was reduced from 57% to 16%. Complete synovectomy reduces the probability of recurrent bleeding. The last evaluation, 5.5 years after the index total knee arthroplasty, showed restoration of function and relief of pain. However, radiolucent lines were found under the tibial component in 72% of the patients, which casts doubt on the longevity of total knee arthroplasty in hemophiliacs.

Annotated Bibliography

Synovectomy

Doets HC, Bierman BT, Soesbergen RM: Synovectomy of the rheumatoid knee does not prevent deterioration: 7-year follow-up of 83 cases. *Acta Orthop Scand* 1989;60:523-525.

A retrospective study of 83 knees was conducted in 65 patients three to 11 years after synovectomy. The investigators concluded that open synovectomy did not prevent deterioration of the rheumatoid knee.

Ogilvie-Harris DJ, Basinski A: Arthroscopic synovectomy of the knee for rheumatoid arthritis. *Arthroscopy* 1991;7:91-97.

The authors noted statistically significant decreases in pain and synovitis over a four-year surveillance in 96 patients. They concluded that arthroscopic synovectomy was a valuable palliative procedure for rheumatoid synovitis of the knee.

Sledge CB, Zuckerman JD, Shortkroff S, et al: Synovectomy of the rheumatoid knee using intra-articular injection of dysprosium-165-ferric hydroxide macroaggregates. *J Bone Joint Surg* 1987;69A:970-975.

Results were satisfactory in 66% of patients two years after radiation synovectomy using dysprosium 165. The best results occurred in patients whose disease was in an early stage.

Arthroscopy

Baumgaertner MR, Cannon WD Jr, Vittori JM, et al: Arthroscopic debridement of the arthritic knee. *Clin Orthop* 1990;253:197-202.

The authors retrospectively studied 49 knees in 44 patients who had undergone arthroscopic debridement of the knee joint for severe degenerative disease. Preoperative symptoms of long duration, malalignment, and radiographic evidence of severe arthritis correlated with poor results. Arthroscopic debridement provided good or excellent results in 40% of the patients, but 47% of the procedures were considered failures an average of 33 months postoperatively.

Livesley PJ, Doherty M, Needoff M, et al: Arthroscopic lavage of osteoarthritic knees. *J Bone Joint Surg* 1991;73B:922-926.

Arthroscopic lavage for the treatment of the osteoarthritic knee may provide temporary relief of pain. It is a low-morbidity procedure for patients in whom other procedures are not indicated.

Osteotomy

Berman AT, Bosacco SJ, Kirshner S, et al: Factors influencing long-term results in high tibial osteotomy. *Clin Orthop* 1991;272:192-198.

The authors comprehensively reviewed the current literature on high tibial osteotomy. They also retrospectively studied 39 high tibial osteotomies in 35 patients with an average follow-up of 8.5 years. Results were good for 22 (57%), fair for seven (18%), and poor for ten (25%). Nine of the 35 patients required a total knee arthroplasty an average of 4.7 years after osteotomy.

Dugdale TW, Noyes FR, Styer D: Preoperative planning for high tibial osteotomy: The effect of lateral tibiofemoral separation and tibiofemoral length. *Clin Orthop* 1992;274:248-264.

A study was conducted to determine the increase in varus angulation caused by lateral tibiofemoral separation. Trigonometric analysis was used to subtract the increased varus angulation, which was caused by slack lateral ligamentous structures, from the preoperative calculations, and the results were applied to prevent overcorrection.

McDermott AG, Finklestein JA, Farine I, et al: Distal femoral varus osteotomy for valgus deformity of the knee. *J Bone Joint Surg* 1988;70A:110-116.

Twenty-four patients with degenerative arthritis of the lateral compartment of the knee were treated by distal femoral varus osteotomy. At an average length of follow-up of four years, 22 of the 24 patients had successful results.

Prodromos CC, Andriacchi TP, Galante JO: A relationship between gait and clinical changes following high tibial osteotomy. *J Bone Joint Surg* 1985;67A:1188-1194.

Correlation between the clinical results of osteotomy and preoperative gait analysis revealed that the best results were achieved when the preoperative adduction moment was low. The overall geometry of the joint and alignment did not directly correlate with the dynamic loading that occurred during walking.

Ritter MA, Fechtman RA: Proximal tibial osteotomy: A survivorship analysis. *Arthroplasty* 1988;3:309-311.

Survivorship analysis was used to determine the longevity of the proximal tibial osteotomy. Any osteotomy with a Hospital for Special Surgery knee score of 70 or less or any knee requiring revision surgery was considered a failure. At six years, the survival rate was almost 80%, but by seven years it had dropped to nearly 60%.

Rudan JF, Simurda MA: High tibial osteotomy: A prospective clinical and roentgenographic review. *Clin Orthop* 1990;255:251-256.

A prospective analysis of 79 valgus closing wedge osteotomies of the proximal tibia revealed 80% good or excellent clinical results. Correction to a femorotibial angle between 6 and 14 degrees valgus was associated with an optimal clinical result. Undercorrection to less than 5 degrees of femorotibial valgus alignment was associated with a 62.5% failure rate. Moderate to severe patellofemoral arthritis was associated with a poor clinical outcome.

Staeheli JW, Cass JR, Morrey BF: Condylar total knee arthroplasty after failed proximal tibial osteotomy. *J Bone Joint Surg* 1987;69A:28-31.

Results of condylar-type total knee arthroplasty were satisfactory in 89% of patients who had undergone a previous upper tibial osteotomy. The intraoperative and postoperative complication rates were no higher than those of primary condylar total knee arthroplasty.

Windsor RE, Insall JN, Vince KG: Technical considerations of total knee arthroplasty after proximal tibial osteotomy. *J Bone Joint Surg* 1988;70A:547-555.

Forty-five total knee replacements were performed in 41 patients with failed high tibial osteotomies. Intraoperatively, 80% of the knees were found to have patella infera. The authors found that 80% of the results were good to excellent, which was comparable to results obtained in revision total knee surgery.

Unicompartmental Arthroplasty

Kozinn SC, Scott R: Unicondylar knee arthroplasty. *J Bone Joint Surg* 1989;71A:145-150.

The authors review the indications and technique of unicondylar knee arthroplasty. Postoperative care and a review of clinical results is also included.

Magnussen PA, Bartlett RJ: Cementless PCA unicompartmental joint arthroplasty for arthritis of the knee: A prospective study of 51 cases. *J Arthroplasty* 1990;5:151-158.

The results of the first 51 knees treated with cementless unicompartmental arthroplasties were studied prospectively. In the medial joint replacement group, which consisted of 42 knees, the results were good to excellent in 37 (88%), fair in three (7%), and poor in two (5%). All lateral joint replacements had good to excellent results. The authors concluded that satisfactory early results can be obtained with a cementless unicompartmental arthroplasty.

Scott R, Cobb A, McQueary F, et al: Unicompartmental knee arthroplasty: Eight- to 12-year follow-up evaluation with survivorship analysis. *Clin Orthop* 1991;271:96-100.

A total of 64 knees in 51 patients who underwent unicompartmental arthroplasty were evaluated clinically and radiographically. Survivorship analysis revealed 90% survivorship of the prostheses at nine years, 85% at ten years, and 82% at 11 years. No significant pain was present at last follow-up and the average knee flexion was 115 degrees.

Total Knee Arthroplasty

Collins DN, Heim SA, Nelson CL, et al: Porous-coated anatomic total knee arthroplasty: A prospective analysis comparing cemented and cementless fixation. *Clin Orthop* 1991;267:128-136.

A prospective study compared cemented and cementless fixation of the porous-coated anatomic prostheses in patients randomly selected without regard to age, weight, or functional status. The cemented and cementless groups had comparable clinical results, but radiolucent lines, loose beads, and tibial component subsidence were more common in the cementless group.

Lee RW, Volz RG, Sheridan DC: The role of fixation and bone quality on mechanical stability of tibial knee components. *Clin Orthop* 1991;273:177-183.

The mechanical stability of tibial implants using various modes of fixation to a foam model was studied. "Good" and "bad" density bone were simulated. The addition of a central stem significantly enhances stability only in the case of poor-quality bone. The most rigid noncemented implant fixation was achieved using four peripherally placed 6.5-mm cancellous bone screws.

Moran CG, Pinder IM, Lees TA: Survivorship analysis of uncemented porous-coated anatomic knee replacement. *J Bone Joint Surg* 1991;73A:848-857.

Ninety-six patients who underwent a total of 108 knee replacements with an uncemented porous-coated anatomic prosthesis were followed up for an average of 64 months. Twenty-one implants (19%) failed because of problems with the tibial component. The most common cause of failure was collapse of the prosthesis into the anteromedial tibial plateau.

Rand JA, Ilstrup DM: Survivorship analysis of total knee arthroplasty: Cumulative rates of survival of 9200 total knee arthroplasties. *J Bone Joint Surg* 1991;73A:397-409.

Four independent variables were associated with a significantly lower risk of failure: (1) primary (versus revision) total knee arthroplasty; (2) a diagnosis of rheumatoid arthritis; (3) age of 60 years or greater; and (4) the use of a condylar prosthesis with a metal-backed tibial component. When all four of these variables were present, the survivorship was 97% at both five and ten years.

Rosenberg AG, Barden RM, Galante JO: Cemented and ingrowth fixation of the Miller-Galante prosthesis: Clinical and roentgenographic comparison after three- to six-year follow-up studies. *Clin Orthop* 1990;260:71-79.

Clinical and radiographic findings in younger patients with good bone quality who underwent uncemented total knee arthroplasty were compared with those of older patients who received cemented replacements of the same design. Results showed slightly better knee function in the cementless group, but this group also had a higher (42%) incidence of tibial radiolucent lines than did the cemented group (20%).

Scott WN, Rubinstein M, Scuderi G: Results after knee replacement with a posterior cruciate-substituting prosthesis. *J Bone Joint Surg* 1988;70A:1163-1173.

Of 119 knees treated with a cemented posterior stabilized prosthesis, 83% had good or excellent results after two to eight years. Radiolucent lines were seen in 76% of the knees. Radiolucent lines did not correlate with clinical results.

Scuderi GR, Insall JN, Windsor RE, et al: Survivorship of cemented knee replacements. *J Bone Joint Surg* 1989;71B:798-803.

Survivorship analysis was used to compare the results of 1,430 cemented primary total knee arthroplasties. The total condylar series showed an average annual failure rate of 0.65% and a 15-year success rate of 90.56%. The posterior stabilized prosthesis with an all-polyethylene tibia showed an annual failure rate of 0.27% and a 10-year success rate of 97.34%. The posterior stabilized metal-backed tibial prosthesis had an annual failure rate of 0.19% and a seven-year success rate of 98.75%. Infection was the major cause of failure.

Vince KG, Insall JN, Kelly MA: The total condylar prosthesis: 10- to 12-year results of a cemented knee replacement. *J Bone Joint Surg* 1989;71B:793-797.

Results 10 to 12 years after cemented total condylar arthroplasty for 58 patients are reported. Of the six patients with poor results, five had undergone revisions; 88% of the patients had a good or excellent clinical result. The authors continued to be optimistic about the use of methylmethacrylate fixation.

Wright J, Ewald FC, Walker PS: Total knee arthroplasty with the kinematic prosthesis: Results after five to nine years: A follow-up note. *J Bone Joint Surg* 1990;72A:1003-1009.

A five- to nine-year follow-up of 192 cemented posterior cruciate ligament-preserving total knee replacements showed a 90% rate of good or excellent clinical results. Thin radiolucent lines were seen around 40% of the tibial components, 30% of the femoral components, and 60% of the patellar components. These lines did not correlate with the clinical results.

Wright RJ, Lima J, Scott RD, et al: Two-to-four-year results of a posterior cruciate-sparing condylar total knee arthroplasty with an uncemented femoral component. *Clin Orthop* 1990;260:80-86.

The results of 114 hybrid total knee arthroplasties were reviewed an average of 2.8 years postoperatively. Good or excellent results were found in 93%, and radiographic analysis revealed no signs of component loosening. The authors concluded that hybrid total knee arthroplasty provides a good and predictable outcome, comparable to that with cemented total knee arthroplasty.

Polyethylene

Bloebaum RD, Nelson K, Dorr LD, et al: Investigation of early surface delamination observed in retrieved heat-pressed tibial inserts. *Clin Orthop* 1991;269:120-127.

More than half of the retrieved heat-pressed tibial inserts of porous-coated anatomic knee replacements have shown severe delamination with visible failure of polyethylene. Surface-layer separation from the heat-pressed insert was noted in a majority of retrieval specimens.

Collier JP, Mayor MB, McNamara JL, et al: Analysis of the failure of 122 polyethylene inserts from uncemented tibial knee components. *Clin Orthop* 1991;273:232-242.

A series of 122 tibial inserts were graded for wear based on contact stress films. Significant wear was seen in more than half of the inserts examined. Contact stresses in noncongruent designs exceeded the yield strength of polyethylene in many of the knee-implants tested. Also, in noncongruent designs, thin polyethylene components showed greater wear than did thicker components of the same design.

Landy MM, Waler PS: Wear of ultra-high-molecular-weight polyethylene components of 90 retrieved knee prostheses. *J Arthroplasty* 1988;3(suppl):S73-S85.

Ninety prostheses of various designs were retrieved for analysis. Cement-induced abrasion of bone and delamination of the tibial polyethylene was frequently evident. Adverse tissue reaction with inflammation and giant cell formation were noted in membranes formed around the retrieved specimens.

Mintz L, Tsao AK, McCrae CR, et al: The arthroscopic evaluation and characteristics of severe polyethylene wear in total knee arthroplasty. *Clin Orthop* 1991;273:215-222.

Arthroscopic examination was performed in the knees of 33 patients with effusion, pain, or decreased range of motion after porous-coated anatomic knee arthroplasty. Extensive wear on the medial tibial plateau and femoral component abrasion were seen, as well as granulomatous synovial tissue and foreign body giant cell reaction to polyethylene debris in the synovial layers. Arthroscopy enabled the accurate diagnosis of polyethylene wear and facilitated the planning of the revision procedure.

Wright TM, Rimnac CM, Faris PM, et al: Analysis of surface damage in retrieved carbon fiber-reinforced and plain polyethylene tibial components from posterior stabilized total knee replacements. *J Bone Joint Surg* 1988;70A:1312-1319.

Experimental and analytical studies indicate that carbon fiber-reinforced polyethylene has no clear advantage over plain ultra-high-molecular-weight polyethylene for articulations in joint arthroplasty.

Rehabilitation

Johnson DP: The effect of continuous passive motion on wound-healing and joint mobility after knee arthroplasty. *J Bone Joint Surg* 1990;72A:421-426.

Continuous passive motion significantly improved early and late flexion of the knee, reduced duration of the hospital stay, and did not increase the incidence of superficial infection or problems with wound healing. Greater than 40 degrees of knee flexion in the first three postoperative days caused a decrease in the skin oxygen tension. The authors recommended a regimen of continuous passive motion that limits knee flexion to 40 degrees for three days and gradually increases the motion to 90 degrees thereafter.

Maloney WJ, Schurman DJ: The effects of implant design on range of motion after total knee arthroplasty: Total condylar versus posterior stabilized total condylar designs. *Clin Orthop* 1992;278:147-152.

Postoperative range of motion was compared between patients who underwent 51 total condylar arthroplasties and a group who had 53 posterior stabilized total condylar arthroplasties. The postoperative range of motion in both groups was similar, but the total condylar group gained slightly more motion when compared to their preoperative range of motion. Patients in both groups with less preoperative motion gained slightly greater motion postoperatively. The authors could not attribute differences in flexion after total knee arthroplasty to the design of the implant.

Tanzer M, Miller J: The natural history of flexion contracture in total knee arthroplasty: A prospective study. *Clin Orthop* 1989;248:129-134.

Thirty-three patients who underwent 35 total knee arthroplasties were followed for an average of 55 weeks. The mean fixed flexion deformity of the entire group was 12.9 degrees preoperatively, 14.8 degrees immediately postoperatively, and 2.9 degrees at last follow up. In no case did the surgical procedure include excessive bony resection in order to correct a flexion contracture. Treatment emphasized posterior capsular release, posterior femoral osteophyte excision, and postoperative physical therapy. Patients with a preoperative or immediate postoperative flexion contracture greater than 20 degrees corrected to a flexion contracture of 7 to 8 degrees on final follow-up.

Complications

Asp JP, Rand JA: Peroneal nerve palsy after total knee arthroplasty. *Clin Orthop* 1990;261:233-237.

Twenty-five cases of peroneal nerve palsy following 8,998 total knee arthroplasties were identified. Thirteen of the nerve palsies resolved completely and 12, partially. The more severe nerve palsies were associated with a poor knee score postoperatively. Among the patients with an initially partial palsy, 86% eventually recovered fully whereas only 35% of those with initial profound neurologic deficit had complete recovery at one to 11 years.

Beer KJ, Lombardi AV Jr, Mallory TH, et al: The efficacy of suction drains after routine total joint arthroplasty. *J Bone Joint Surg* 1991;73A:584-587.

A prospective study was conducted to assess the effects of postoperative suction drainage on wound healing. Subjects who had closed drainage on one side and not the other included 38 patients who had primary one-stage bilateral total knee replacement and 12 patients who had primary one-stage bilateral hip replacement. There was no difference in wound healing, clinical outcome, rehabilitation, or incidence of deep vein thrombosis between patients who had a postoperative drain and those who did not.

Booth RE Jr, Lotke PA: The results of Spacer Block Technique in revision of infected total knee arthroplasty. *Clin Orthop* 1989;248:57-60.

The results following the revision of 25 severe chronically infected total knee arthroplasty using the spacer block technique are reviewed. The average period of follow up was twenty-five months. The clinical results in 21 patients were excellent, good in two, fair in one, and poor in one. The one failure resulted in a recurrent infection followed by a successful fusion. Modified Hospital for Special Surgery knee score averaged 81.5 postoperatively. An average of 100 degrees of flexion was achieved.

Burger RR, Basch T, Hopson CN: Implant salvage in infected total knee arthroplasty. *Clin Orthop* 1991;273:105-112.

Surgical debridement, antibiotic therapy, and retention of components was attempted in 60 infected total knee arthroplasties. In 18% of the knees, infection was successfully eradicated, after a mean follow-up of 4.1 years. The following factors strongly correlated with successful salvage: (1) short duration of symptoms of infection (less than two weeks); (2) susceptible gram-positive organisms (*Streptococcus* or methicillin-sensitive *Staphylococcus aureus*); (3) absence of prolonged and postoperative drainage or the development of a sinus tract; and (4) no prosthetic loosening or radiographic evidence of infection. The five knees in this series that satisfied these criteria achieved implant salvage with eradication of infection and maintenance of good knee function.

DiGioia AM III, Rubash HE: Periprosthetic fractures of the femur after total knee arthroplasty: A literature review and treatment algorithm. *Clin Orthop* 1991;271:135-142.

The literature of supracondylar femoral fractures after total knee arthroplasty is reviewed. The authors propose a treatment algorithm and a classification system for these fractures based on a modified Neer grading system.

Donley BG, Matthews LS, Kaufer H: Arthrodesis of the knee with an intramedullary nail. *J Bone Joint Surg* 1991;73A:907-913.

Twenty patients underwent an arthrodesis of the knee with an intramedullary nail and were reviewed at an average follow-up of six years. Eight of the 20 patients had infections after total knee arthroplasty. Fusion was achieved in 85% of the patients, and in seven of the eight infected total knee arthroplasties. The operation was lengthy and blood loss was significant. However, the majority of patients were able to bear full weight by the second postoperative week.

Fahmy NR, Chandler IIP, Danylchuk K, et al: Blood-gas and circulatory changes during total knee replacement: Role of the intramedullary alignment rod. *J Bone Joint Surg* 1990;72A:19-26.

Multiple cardiorespiratory variables were measured intraoperatively in patients undergoing total knee arthroplasty. Bone marrow contents and fat were retrieved from samples of blood from the right atrium indicating that embolization of marrow contents had occurred during insertion of the alignment rod. A statistically significant reduction in oxygen saturation occurred after insertion of either a solid or a fluted 8-mm alignment rod through an 8-mm hole in both vented and unvented femoral canals. These changes were eliminated by the use of a 12.7-mm drill hole as the entry site for the 8-mm fluted rod.

Francis CW, Pellegrini VD Jr, Stulberg BN, et al: Prevention of venous thrombosis after total knee arthroplasty: Comparison of antithrombin III and low-dose heparin with dextran. *J Bone Joint Surg* 1990;72A:976-982.

A prospective randomized trial compared the efficacy of a combination of antithrombin III and heparin with that of dextran 40. Venography demonstrated thrombosis in one third of the patients who received a combination of antithrombin III and heparin and in four fifths of those who received dextran. A significantly lower concentration of antithrombin III postoperatively was associated with a higher incidence of venous thrombosis.

Friedman RJ, Friedrich LV, White RL, et al: Antibiotic prophylaxis and tourniquet inflation in total knee arthroplasty. *Clin Orthop* 1990;260:17-23.

One gram of cefazolin administered five minutes before tourniquet inflation resulted in adequate mean soft-tissue and bone concentrations for prophylaxis during total knee arthroplasty with a tourniquet time of less than two hours.

Greene KA, Wilde AH, Stulberg BN: Preoperative nutritional status of total joint patients. *J Arthroplasty* 1991;6:321-325.

Two hundred and seventeen consecutive patients undergoing a primary total hip or total knee arthroplasty were reviewed for preoperative and postoperative nutritional status. A preoperative white blood cell count of less than 1,500 cells per cubic mm was associated with a five times greater frequency of developing a major wound complication, and an albumin level of less than 3.5 g/dl had a seven times greater frequency. Preoperative nutritional assessment is warranted to identify patients at risk for wound healing complications following elective total joint arthroplasty.

Haas SB, Insall JN, Scuderi GR, et al: Pneumatic sequential-compression boots compared with aspirin prophylaxis of deep-vein thrombosis after total knee arthroplasty. *J Bone Joint Surg* 1990;72A:27-31.

A randomized study compared the effectiveness of pneumatic sequential compression boots with that of aspirin in preventing deep vein thrombosis after total knee arthroplasty. Using venography as a diagnostic tool to study 119 patients, the frequency of deep vein thrombosis was 22% for patients who used compression boots compared to 47% for those who received aspirin. Following one-stage bilateral total knee arthroplasty, the frequency of deep vein thrombosis was 48% for the patients who used compression boots, compared to 68% for those who received aspirin.

Hodge WA: Prevention of deep vein thrombosis after total knee arthroplasty: Coumadin versus pneumatic calf compression. *Clin Orthop* 1991;271:101-105.

A nonrandomized prospective study compared the frequency of deep vein thrombosis in patients who received coumadin anticoagulation with those who received pneumatic calf compression. The incidence of deep vein thrombosis ascertained by venography was nearly identical in both groups. Cost analysis showed coumadin to be approximately 50% more expensive than pneumatic boots.

Nichols SJ, Landon GC, Tulos HS: Arthrodesis with dual plates after a failed total knee arthroplasty. *J Bone Joint Surg* 1991;73A:1020-1024.

Eleven patients were treated by arthrodesis with dual compression plates after failed total knee arthroplasty. The reason for failure was infection in seven of the eleven patients. An average of 5.6 months following surgery, all patients had a solid fusion. One patient who had an infected knee arthroplasty had a persistent infection after the initial attempt at fusion, and infection was controlled following removal of both plates with eventual union.

Pedersen JG, Lund B: Effects of gentamicin and monomer on bone. *J Arthroplasty* 1988;3(suppl):S63-S68.

The effect of local gentamicin on bone metabolism was measured in a laboratory model. This test indicated that gentamicin and methylmethacrylate monomer released from antibiotic-impregnated bone cement depressed osteocyte function as measured by the rate of release of calcium-45 and tritiated

proline. This may be significant in the loosening of components fixed with antibiotic-impregnated methylmethacrylate cement.

Pritchett JW, Mallin BA, Matthews AC: Knee arthrodesis with a tension-band plate. *J Bone Joint Surg* 1988;70A:285-288.

A knee arthrodesis was performed in 26 patients using a single anterior, broad, contoured, dynamic compression plate and screws that were applied as a tension band. Arthrodesis was performed as treatment for an infected knee arthroplasty in four of the patients. Bone grafts were not used; no external immobilization was required; and immediate partial weightbearing was encouraged. Clinical union occurred six to 12 weeks postoperatively, and in most patients radiographic union occurred within 16 weeks.

Willemen D, Paul J, White SH, et al: Closed suction drainage following knee arthroplasty: Effectiveness and risks. *Clin Orthop* 1991;264:232-234.

No organisms were isolated from cultures of drain tips when the drains were removed 24 hours after total knee arthroplasty. However, if the drains were removed 48 hours after surgery, cultures of the drain tips were positive in five of 21 drains.

Wilson MG, Kelley K, Thornhill TS: Infection as a complication of total knee replacement arthroplasty: Risk factors and treatment in sixty-seven cases. *J Bone Joint Surg* 1990;72A:878-883.

Sixty-seven infections following 4,171 knee arthroplasties performed during a 15-year period were followed. The risk of infection was significantly increased in patients with rheumatoid arthritis (especially males), patients who had ulcers of the skin, and patients who had a previous operation of the knee. Infection was associated with obesity, recurrent urinary tract infection, and oral use of steroids, although the correlation was not statistically significant.

Windsor RE, Insall JN, Urs WK: Two-stage reimplantation for the salvage of total knee arthroplasty complicated by infection: Further follow-up and refinement of indications. *J Bone Joint Surg* 1990;72A:272-278.

Thirty-eight infected total knee arthroplasties in 35 patients were treated following a two-stage protocol for reimplantation. There was one recurrence of infection, which was due to the original organism. Three patients, all of whom had a compromised immunologic system, developed an infection caused by a new organism. There were 11 excellent, 13 good, six fair, and seven poor clinical results after an average follow-up of four years. Gram-negative infection was successfully treated with this protocol.

Patellofemoral Resurfacing

Bayley JC, Scott RD, Ewald FC, et al: Failure of the metal-backed patellar component after total knee replacement. *J Bone Joint Surg* 1988;70A:668-674.

In a multicenter study, factors contributing to the failure of metal-backed patellar components in 25 knees were obesity and osteoarthritis. Failure occurred from wear, fracture, or dissociation of the polyethylene from the metal backing. Seven different patellar implant designs failed.

Collier JP, McNamara JL, Surprenant VA, et al: All-polyethylene patellar components are not the answer. *Clin Orthop* 1991;273:198-203.

One hundred four retrieved patellar components were analyzed for wear. Significant wear was seen in 65% of the patellas with a metal-backed design and in 78% of the patellas with an all-polyethylene component. Severe wear was seen in 44% of the all-polyethylene components and 39% of the metal-backed components. The incidence of severe wear was significantly less when a congruent design was used than when an incongruent design was used. When testing a dome-shaped incongruent patellofemoral joint, contact stresses measured using pressure-sensitive film exceeded the yield strength of the polyethylene. A congruent geometry was associated with significantly lower stress levels.

Enis JE, Gardner R, Robledo MA, et al: Comparison of patellar resurfacing versus nonresurfacing in bilateral total knee arthroplasty. *Clin Orthop* 1990;260:38-42.

Bilateral knee arthroplasties were performed on 25 patients with advanced patellofemoral degenerative disease. Patellar resurfacing was performed in the right knee, and the left patella was left unresurfaced. The findings suggested that patellar resurfacing provides the patient superior pain relief and strength following knee arthroplasty.

Figgie HE III, Goldberg VM, Figgie MP, et al: The effect of alignment of the implant on fractures of the patella after condylar total knee arthroplasty. *J Bone Joint Surg* 1989;71A:1031-1039.

The results in 36 knees that had a fracture of the patella after total condylar arthroplasty were reviewed. Parameters for neutral radiographic alignment of the knee components were defined. Most patella fractures occurred two years or less after the initial operation. In none of the 36 were the components aligned in the neutral range. The 16 knees that had a minor alignment variation were associated with the least severe fractures and the best overall results. The 20 knees that had major alignment variations were associated with more severe fractures and less satisfactory results. This study indicates that component alignment and sizing during condylar total knee replacement affects the severity of the patella fracture and the result after treatment of the fracture.

Goldberg VM, Figgie HE III, Inglis AE, et al: Patellar fracture type and prognosis in condylar total knee arthroplasty. *Clin Orthop* 1988;236:115-122.

The results of patella fractures following 36 condylar total knee arthroplasties in 35 patients were evaluated with regard to fracture type after an average 4.5-year follow-up period. The overall results indicate that fractures not associated with dislocation of the patella, implant loosening, or complete extensor mechanism disruption usually recover function with nonsurgical management. Knees with implant loosening, patellar dislocation, or complete quadriceps disruption require operative intervention. Outcome following treatment of a patella fracture may be improved by correcting component alignment and position.

Picetti GD III, McGann WA, Welch RB: The patellofemoral joint after total knee arthroplasty without patellar resurfacing. *J Bone Joint Surg* 1990;72A:1379-1382.

One hundred total knee replacements with a total condylar prosthesis and without patellar resurfacing were followed for a minimum of two years. At the most recent follow-up, 29% of knees were still painful in the patellofemoral area. The height and weight of the patient definitely influenced the amount of patellofemoral pain postoperatively. Small patients who had osteoarthrosis were exceptionally free of pain regardless of sex, age, or activity level.

Rhoads DD, Noble PC, Reuben JD, et al: The effect of femoral component position on patellar tracking after total knee arthroplasty. *Clin Orthop* 1990;260:43-51.

A laboratory study evaluated the three-dimensional motions of the patella before and after total knee arthroplasty in fresh cadaveric knees. The patella was displaced medially by an average of 4 mm and tilted medially by an average of 4 degrees after standard total knee arthroplasty. Medial translation or internal rotation of the femoral component further displaced and tilted the patella medially. Lateral translation or external rotation of the femoral component produced patellar tracking patterns closer to those of the intact knee than did any other femoral component positioning.

Shoji H, Yoshino S, Kajino A: Patellar replacement in bilateral total knee arthroplasty: A study of patients who had rheumatoid arthritis and no gross deformity of the patella. *J Bone Joint Surg* 1989;71A:853-856.

Thirty-five patients with rheumatoid arthritis of both knees but no gross deformity of the patella underwent bilateral total knee arthroplasty. In each patient, one knee had a patellar replacement and the other did not. After a minimum follow-up of two years, the results were the same in both knees in terms of relief of pain and improvement of function, arch of motion, and muscle power.

Revision Total Knee Arthroplasty

Elia EA, Lotke PA: Results of revision total knee arthroplasty associated with significant bone loss. *Clin Orthop* 1991;271:114-121.

Forty revision total knee arthroplasties were performed in 38 patients because of aseptic failure associated with significant bone loss. After an average follow-up of 41 months, 75% of the knees were considered excellent or good. There was a 10% failure rate and no infections were reported. The complication rate was 30%; wound complications were most common. Improved results are associated with restoring correct mechanical alignment, filling all bone defects with bone cement or modular spacers, using stems to assist in component support, and achieving soft-tissue balance.

Friedman RJ, Hirst P, Poss R, et al: Results of revision total knee arthroplasty performed for aseptic loosening. *Clin Orthop* 1990;255:235-241.

One hundred thirty-seven revision total knee arthroplasties were performed on 117 patients because of aseptic failure. The mean follow-up was 5.2 years and although function, instability, motion, and pain all improved after revision total knee arthroplasty, these improvements were significantly less than those seen at the primary total knee arthroplasty. The failure rate was 5.8% at 5.2 years, approximately 1% per year. The clinical results of an uncomplicated revision total knee arthroplasty are substantially poorer than those of a primary total knee arthroplasty, but the durability and failure rate are comparable.

Goldberg VM, Figgie MP, Figgie HE III, et al: The results of revision total knee arthroplasty. *Clin Orthop* 1988;226:86-92.

Of 65 total knee arthroplasties revised because of mechanical failure, only 46% had good or excellent results at five years. The most improvement occurred in those knees in which posterior stabilized total condylar replacements were used for the revision. The best results were achieved in those knees in which the component positioning and alignment was restored to normal. The infection rate was 4.5%.

Hanssen AD, Rand JA: A comparison of primary and revision total knee arthroplasty using the kinematic stabilizer prosthesis. *J Bone Joint Surg* 1988;70A:491-498.

Seventy-nine arthroplasties were performed on 66 patients and followed for a mean of 37 months. There were 53 revisions and 26 primary arthroplasties. The Hospital for Special Surgery knee score increased from an average of 56 points preoperatively to 83 points postoperatively in all of the knees. The patients who had had primary arthroplasty had 92% good or excellent results, and the patients who had had revision procedure had 81% good or excellent results.

Hohl WM, Crawfurd E, Zelicof SB, et al: The total condylar III prosthesis in complex knee reconstruction. *Clin Orthop* 1991;273:91-97.

Sixty-one total condylar III prostheses were implanted in 59 patients. The average follow-up was 6.1 years. There were six primary arthroplasties and 29 revisions in this group. The knee scores improved from 22 preoperatively to 74 at last follow-up evaluation. Results were good or excellent in 71% of the patients. The failure rate was 8.6%. Radiolucent lines were present in at least one component in 71% of patients.

Padgett DE, Stern SH, Insall JN: Revision total knee arthroplasty for failed unicompartmental replacement. *J Bone Joint Surg* 1991;73A:186-190.

Twenty-one revision total knee arthroplasties were performed on 19 patients who had a failed unicompartmental knee replacement. The follow-up after the revision ranged from two to ten years. There were 12 excellent, four good, one fair, and two poor results. At the time of revision, a major osseous defect was found in 76%; 62% had a least one radiolucent line. Revision total knee arthroplasty for failed unicondylar arthroplasty is a demanding operation with less predictable results than primary knee arthroplasty.

Bone Defects

Aglietti P, Buzzi R, Scrobe F: Autologous bone grafting for medial tibial defects in total knee arthroplasty. *J Arthroplasty* 1991;6:287-293.

Patients who underwent a total of 17 cemented posterior stabilized knee arthroplasties were followed up for two to eight years. In each case, a large medial tibial bony defect had been filled with autologous bone graft obtained from the same knee and fixed with one or two screws. In 82% of the cases, radiographs demonstrated union between the graft and host bone. Fibrous union occurred in three cases. There was no evidence of graft necrosis or collapse. The importance of meticulous technique and correct component positioning is emphasized.

Laskin RS: Total knee arthroplasty in the presence of large bony defects of the tibia and marked knee instability. *Clin Orthop* 1989;248:66-70.

Twenty-six patients with tibial bone defects were treated by total knee arthroplasty. Bone defects were filled with autogenic bone graft from the local bone resection, which were fixed with either screws or Steinmann pins. The patients did as well clinically as a matched group who underwent total knee arthroplasty without bone grafts. However, four bone grafts demonstrated fragmentation and implant subsidence. Nine grafts that had not fragmented were biopsied one year postoperatively, and in only four of these did microscopy reveal viable osteocytes. The overall success rate at five years was 67%.

Special Cases

England SP, Stern SH, Insall JN, et al: Total knee arthroplasty in diabetes mellitus. *Clin Orthop* 1990;260:130-134.

Fifty-nine total knee arthroplasties in 40 patients diagnosed with diabetes mellitus were studied retrospectively. An overall revision rate of 10%, infection rate of 7%, and wound complication rate of 12% were noted after an average follow-up period of 4.3 years. The authors emphasized caution when performing total knee arthroplasty in diabetic patients.

Figgie MP, Goldberg VM, Figgie HE III, et al: Total knee arthroplasty for the treatment of chronic hemophilic arthropathy. *Clin Orthop* 1989;248:98-107.

The results of 19 knee arthroplasties performed for hemophilic arthropathy were assessed after a minimum of 5.5 years. Four of the seven patients in whom only an 80% level of factor VIII coverage was maintained perioperatively were clinical failures, whereas two of 12 patients in whom a 100% factor VIII level was maintained became clinical failures. Ten of the 19 knees suffered postoperative complications, including one deep infection, six superficial skin necroses, three nerve palsies, seven hemorrhages, and one transfusion reaction. Progressive radiographic lucent lines were evident in 68% of the tibial components.

Gabel GT, Rand JA, Sim FH: Total knee arthroplasty for osteoarthrosis in patients who have Paget disease of bone at the knee. *J Bone Joint Surg* 1991;73A:739-744.

Thirteen patients in whom 16 total knee arthroplasties were performed for pagetic gonarthrosis were followed up for a mean of seven years. Bowing of the tibia or femur related to the disease was associated with multiple intraoperative technical difficulties and in ten limbs with a final position in suboptimum varus or valgus alignment. Paget disease did not affect the amount of blood loss during the operation, the postoperative course, or the loosening of the prosthesis. A preoperative course of calcitonin or diphosphonates was used in four patients to differentiate between pain due to Paget disease or osteoarthritis as the cause of pain. No difference was found between the average amount of intraoperative blood loss in these patients and patients who did not receive preoperative therapy. The mean functional score for all patients improved from 33 points preoperatively to 86 points postoperatively.

Lotke PA, Faralli VJ, Orenstein EM, et al: Blood loss after total knee replacement: Effects of tourniquet release and continuous passive motion. *J Bone Joint Surg* 1991;73A:1037-1040.

The postoperative blood loss in 121 patients who underwent total knee arthroplasty was determined by adding blood in suction drains to the blood loss calculated from the hemoglobin and hematocrit values. These patients lost a mean 1,518 ml of blood. The combination of postoperative continuous passive motion and intraoperative release of the tourniquet to establish hemostasis was associated with a postoperative blood loss of 1,793 ml, significantly more than if either continuous passive motion or tourniquet release was used separately.

Ranawat CS, Padgett DE, Ohashi Y: Total knee arthroplasty for patients younger than 55 years. *Clin Orthop* 1989;248:27-33.

The clinical and radiographic results were reviewed for 93 arthroplasties in 62 patients younger than 55 years of age. After a mean of 6.1 years follow-up, there was a 30% rate of radiolucent lines and an average knee rating score of 87. There was no significant radiographic or clinical difference between the 17 patients with osteoarthritis and the 76 patients with rheumatoid arthritis. The 96% survivorship rate at ten years in these patients is comparable with the long-term results of total knee arthroplasty in older patients.

Smith BE, Askew MJ, Gradisar IA Jr, et al: The effect of patient weight on the functional outcome of total knee arthroplasty. *Clin Orthop* 1992;276:237-244.

Two-year follow-up findings for 109 patients who underwent cemented total knee arthroplasty were analyzed retrospectively. The knee scores for subjects who were less than 10% overweight were significantly higher than scores for subjects 30% or more overweight. However, when the effect of gender was excluded, there was no significant weight-related difference in the postoperative function of patients. The patients without tibial radiolucent lines had a significantly lower mean weight than did those with radiolucent lines.

Stern SH, Insall JN: Total knee arthroplasty in obese patients. *J Bone Joint Surg* 1990;72A:1400-1404.

A total of 182 patients who had undergone total knee arthroplasty were examined retrospectively and grouped into five weight classes according to a percentage of their desired weight. At follow-up, the overall knee scores did not differ substantially between the five weight groups. Symptoms attributable to the patellofemoral joint more common among the heavier patients.

49

Ankle and Foot: Pediatric Aspects

Metatarsus Adductus

Metatarsus adductus is a common foot disorder seen in infancy, probably caused by abnormal intrauterine positioning, although some have speculated it is a result of muscle imbalance. Bilateral deformity occurs about half of the time. The forefoot is medially deviated and slightly supinated. This condition is distinguished from clubfoot by the fact that the heel is never in equinus, although it may occasionally be in a valgus position. Rigid hindfoot valgus, with varying degrees of lateral midfoot shift, combined with forefoot adduction describes a skewfoot, which probably represents an altogether different problem, rather than the most severe form of metatarsus adductus.

The clinical appearance of the foot is that of a C-shaped lateral border with prominence of the base of the fifth metatarsal. A line bisecting the heel pad should pass through the second toe or through the web space between the second and third toes. If this line intersects the third toe or beyond, progressively more severe metatarsus adductus is diagnosed. The forefoot is assessed for flexibility, noting if complete correction is possible by abducting the forefoot against a fulcrum of resistance located at the base of the fifth metatarsal. The presence of a deep medial crease indicates that the foot is likely to need some form of treatment.

Radiographs are not needed for routine metatarsus adductus. However, radiographs are indicated to assess the bony alignment of feet that have resisted correction with casting or, in the older child, that have a rigid deformity. In addition, radiographs of the adducted foot with a short, broad first metatarsal are needed to rule out a congenital malformation such as a bracket epiphysis.

Spontaneous resolution of the deformity occurs in most children (85%). Mild recurrence of the deformity often occurs in children that have had treatment with special shoes, splints, or casts; however, this tends to resolve gradually between the ages of two and four years. Persistent deformity will produce an intoeing gait, and if adduction is pronounced, shoe fitting may be a problem.

The initiation of treatment usually is based on clinical assessment of the degree of flexibility and often is guided by the level of parental anxiety. In general, a passively correctable deformity will not need any formal intervention. The parent can be instructed in stretching exercises and/or straight last shoes may be used. For more rigid feet, or those that have not responded to shoeing, a casting program should be instituted by 3 months of age. Although some feet may respond to one cast, a serial program of two to three casts, changed biweekly, may be necessary. There doesn't appear to be any difference in effectiveness between a short leg and a long leg cast. However, Bleck found the results of cast treatment were significantly better when initiated before 8 months of age. After the casting program, the foot can be controlled with the use of straight last or reverse last shoes. Alternatively, casting can be supplanted with the use of an orthotic splint.

For the child older than 4 years of age who has a fixed deformity, surgical correction of the forefoot may be indicated. Extensive metatarsal-tarsal capsulotomies (Heyman-Herndon release) combined with prolonged casting have been recommended; however, this procedure has many complications and long-lasting results are questionable. The preferred treatment is multiple metatarsal osteotomies, because this treatment provides better correction and produces less postoperative foot rigidity. Care must be taken to avoid damage to the first metatarsal growth plate.

Calcaneovalgus Foot

This frequently seen infant foot disorder (1 per 1,000 live births) is also presumed to be a result of intrauterine positioning. The forefoot is abducted and the ankle severely dorsiflexed. Although the anterior ankle structures may be contracted, the deformity typically is flexible and the foot can passively be placed in the normal position. The fact that the heel can be dorsiflexed helps to distinguish this deformity from congenital vertical talus, in which the foot is stiffer and the heel is in equinus.

Calcaneovalgus deformity also occurs as a result of muscle imbalance, which usually is a result of flaccid paralysis or weakness of the plantarflexors. Myelomeningocele is a typical example, and the problem progresses in severity because of the unopposed action of the anterior tibial and/or extensor tendons.

Most positional deformities resolve spontaneously; however, if there is residual hindfoot valgus the end result is likely to be a flexible flatfoot. Untreated neurologic calcaneovalgus feet generally have forefoot equinus, a large callused heel that is prone to skin breakdown, and cock-up toes.

Occasionally plantarflexion-inversion casting is used in the infant if spontaneous resolution is not seen within the first few months of life. Long-term treatment is not necessary, and orthotics are of no proven benefit. When there is muscle imbalance resulting from paralytic conditions, ankle-foot orthotics can control the foot while the child is small. Once the full extent of muscle function is understood, many children are candidates for tendon transfer (anterior tibialis to the os calcis), and, occasionally, hindfoot stabilization by subtalar fusion is needed. Older children will need a calcaneal elongation osteotomy in addition to tendon transfer and plantar fascia release. Children over 10 years of age may require triple arthrodesis.

Flatfoot

The flexible flatfoot is generally a benign condition that rarely requires treatment. Many infants and toddlers have flattening of the longitudinal arch, forefoot pronation, and heel valgus on weightbearing, the severity of which is quite variable. Ligamentous laxity is apparent, and the degree of abnormality in the bone-ligament complex probably is determined genetically. The flexible flatfoot is rarely symptomatic, and treatment with orthotics or special shoes has not been shown to alter the shape of the foot. Many feet gradually improve as the child ages, at least until 5 to 6 years of age.

The clinical examination is characterized by a hypermobile foot that, when suspended, has a normal appearing arch. In children able to stand on their toes, the arch will reappear and the heel will move out of a valgus position. This is a good indirect test for normal subtalar motion. If the feet are asymptomatic, surgery is not indicated. If the feet are painful and unrelieved by orthotics, medial os calcis sliding osteotomy or opening wedge osteotomy of the lateral calcaneus may realign the hindfoot and relieve symptoms without producing the loss of motion associated with fusions.

If the foot cannot be corrected passively, other conditions should be suspected, such as contracture of the Achilles tendon, peroneal tendon irritability or spasm from a variety of causes (inflammatory subtalar arthritis, os calcis lesions), tarsal coalition, or an occult osteochondral fracture.

Accessory Navicular

The accessory navicular is a frequent finding in the general population (8% to 14% incidence) and often is discovered incidentally on an anteroposterior radiograph of the foot. The bony fragment may be an isolated sesamoid in the posterior tibial tendon, in which case it is rarely symptomatic. More often the fragment is connected closely to the navicular by a fibrocartilaginous union. This lesion can produce pain, either through repeated microtrauma (fracture) and a secondary posterior tibial tendinitis or from direct pressure of the shoe over the prominence. The accessory navicular often is found in combination with a flexible flatfoot.

Conservative treatment consists of three weeks of immobilization in a short leg cast, which may be followed by shoe modification with an orthosis. The most successful surgical treatment is simple excision of the accessory navicular and reduction in the size of the navicular prominence. More extensive operations to treat the flatfoot, such as the Kidner procedure, do not seem to improve the results.

Toe Deformities

Overlapping fifth toe is a familiar condition that is usually bilateral and asymptomatic. The dorsomedial metatarsophalangeal joint capsule and the extensor tendon are contracted. The phalanges are laterally rotated. Occasionally callosities and irritation from shoe wear, as well as cosmetic concerns, prompt treatment of the deformity. Nonsurgical remedies are uniformly ineffective. Surgical correction is maintained best either by partial phalangeal resection combined with syndactylization to the fourth toe or by circumferential incision, allowing for derotation of the toe, and capsulotomy with extensor tendon release.

Congenital curly toe most commonly affects the fourth and fifth toes, is familial, and usually is bilateral. They are rarely symptomatic and 25% improve spontaneously. In children, correction can usually be obtained by long toe flexor release.

Bunions

The bunion, the medial prominence of the first metatarsal head, develops when the intermetatarsal angle exceeds 10 degrees and there is greater than 18 to 20 degrees of hallux valgus. The exact etiology remains obscure but often there is metatarsus primus varus. Ligamentous laxity, forefoot pronation, and shoe wear may be additional predisposing factors. Unlike adults, children rarely have signs of metatarsophalangeal arthritis, and the first metatarsal growth plate is open.

Indications for surgical intervention include pain, deformity, and significant shoewear limitation. Surgical principles entail soft-tissue correction for the hallux valgus (medial capsule plication, lateral capsular release, and recession of the adductor hallucis), removal of the medial prominence, and metatarsal osteotomy if there is an abnormal intermetatarsal angle. The surgical complication rate is high and includes such problems as overcorrection, malunion and nonunion, avascular necrosis, stiffness, and damage to the growth plate. Some reports indicate that the recurrence rate may approach 50%.

Cavus Foot

The cavus foot is characterized by an excessively high arch resulting from a plantarflexed first ray, a pronated forefoot, plantar contracture, and some degree of hindfoot varus. The origin, usually ascribed to muscle imbalance, is not well understood. In over two thirds of cases the cause is neuromuscular, and the initial evaluation should be directed toward elucidating the origin of the problem. This may entail spinal radiographs, magnetic resonance imaging, and nerve conduction studies to rule out spinal cord tumor, tethered cord, diastematomyelia, Charcot-Marie-Tooth, or spinocerebellar disorders. The disorder may also be idiopathic; however, unilateral presentation or a history of late onset and progressive deformity are indicators that there is an underlying abnormality.

Radiographic assessment consists of measuring the angle subtended by a line drawn through the axis of the talus and the first metatarsal (normal = 0 degrees). The foot is evaluated clinically for muscle strength and for flexibility, especially of the hindfoot varus. The deformity is progressive, and rigidity increases over time.

The surgical treatment is based on the rigidity of the foot. Tendon lengthenings and transfers are used for flexible feet, and bony procedures are added for fixed deformities. Most commonly a dorsal closing wedge osteotomy of the first metatarsal base (or the first cuneiform) is combined with a radical plantar release. Rigid heel varus may be corrected by wedge or sliding osteotomy, although triple arthrodesis is the usual method for correction of cavus deformity with rigid heel varus. Claw toe deformity is approached after cavovarus foot correction, if necessary.

Clubfoot

Clubfoot deformity occurs most often in otherwise normal children (1.2 in 1,000 births) but also frequently is associated with such other conditions as myelodysplasia, arthrogryposis, amniotic band syndrome, and diastrophic dwarfism. Idiopathic clubfoot follows a multifactorial system of inheritance, which means that it is influenced by environmental factors (for example, oligohydramnios). When one child has a clubfoot, there is a 2% to 6% chance that the next sibling will be affected similarly; however, if the parent also has a clubfoot, there is a 25% chance that a subsequent offspring will have the same disorder. The condition is bilateral 30% of the time.

The pathoanatomy is remarkable for peroneal muscle atrophy combined with contracture of the Achilles, posterior tibial, and long toe flexor tendons. In addition, there are contractures of the ankle, subtalar, talonavicular, and calcaneocuboid joints, as well as contractures of many of the ligaments in the foot (spring, bifurcate, deltoid, calcaneofibular, talofibular). None of the bones of the midfoot/hindfoot complex have a entirely normal shape, and three-dimensional computer modeling has helped to delineate these positional relationships. The navicular and cuboid are medially subluxated, the calcaneus is in equinus and is rotated internally, the talar neck is plantarflexed and medially deviated, and the forefoot is adducted. Although there is some controversy as to the

position of the body of the talus, recent computer images suggest that it is externally rotated.

The clinical appearance of the foot is a reflection of the pathoanatomy. The calf and foot are smaller than the contralateral extremity, the forefoot is adducted and supinated, the normal space between the navicular and the medial malleolus is not palpable, and there may be a deep medial foot crease that adds to the impression that the longitudinal arch is in cavus. The os calcis is in equinus and varus. However, the intermalleolar axis is generally normal (no internal tibial torsion).

The most reliable roentgenographic view is the lateral projection, usually with the foot in maximum dorsiflexion. In the clubfoot there is no convergence of the talocalcaneal region (parallel alignment), and the tibiocalcaneal relationship reveals equinus.

Treatment of clubfoot usually begins with a program of manipulation and serial casting, which is more effective the earlier it is begun. Most surgeons divide their cast correction into two stages, starting with molding the forefoot out of adduction and the heel out of varus. Later, with the forefoot corrected, the foot is progressively dorsiflexed. Care must be taken not to exert excessive upward force on the metatarsals, because this can result in midfoot break (rocker-bottom deformity). Lateral radiographs are helpful in assessing the quality of cast correction. True, long-lasting success rates with nonsurgical treatment are poorly documented, but are alleged to be between 20% and 40%. Most authorities agree that if satisfactory correction has not occurred by three to six months, and/or progress has plateaued, surgery is indicated.

Surgical release usually is performed somewhere between three and nine months of age, according to the individual surgeon's preference, and a variety of incisions can be used. Many surgeons perform a Cincinnati circumferential incision with the child lying prone, while others use a small medial approach combined with a second posterolateral incision. In any event, the goals are good visualization of the pathoanatomy and protection of the neurovascular structures. The latter is especially important, because in some clubfeet the posterior tibial artery may be the only blood supply to the foot.

As Goldner has suggested, clubfoot release should follow a four-quadrant approach: plantar, medial, posterior, and lateral, modifying the extent of the release according to the severity of the deformity. The plantar quadrant includes the plantar fascia, the short toe flexors, and the long and short plantar ligaments. The medial quadrant involves talonavicular and subtalar release, lengthening of the posterior tibial tendon (often the flexor hallucis longus and flexor digitorum longus are also addressed), and recession of the abductor hallucis origin. It is rarely necessary to cut the interosseous ligament of the subtalar joint. Lengthening of the deltoid ligament may improve ankle range of motion but should be reserved for those familiar with this technique; this surgery is contraindicated when an extensive subtalar release has been performed. The posterior quadrant entails ankle and subtalar capsulotomy, with special attention to the release of the posterior talofibular and calcaneofibular ligaments. The lateral approach involves calcaneocuboid capsulotomy, completion of talonavicular and subtalar release, and, often, sectioning of the peroneal tendon sheath.

The foot is maintained most reliably in a reduced position by pinning the talonavicular joint; many also pin the tibiotalocalcaneal articulation. Postoperative casting is continued for 12 weeks, and pins are removed by six weeks. The use of night splints or special shoes is less common than in the past.

The most common cause of recurrent clubfoot is incomplete initial correction. Occasionally, excessive forefoot adduction persists, and this can be corrected by a combination of lateral column shortening (calcaneocuboid joint resection or fusion) and/or medial column lengthening. Transfer of the anterior tibial tendon to the dorsal aspect of the foot may also help alleviate persistent forefoot varus. Mild to moderate persistent heel varus is corrected by calcaneal closing wedge or lateral displacement sliding osteotomy. Overcorrection of the clubfoot is associated with release of the interosseous ligament, excessive lateral placement of the navicular on the talar head, and overlengthening of the tendon units (especially the Achilles tendon).

Congenital Vertical Talus

Congenital vertical talus is an uncommon rigid flatfoot deformity. The key features are fixed dorsal dislocation of the navicular on the neck of the talus, equinus ankle contracture, and abduction contracture of the foot. The peroneal tendons occasionally are subluxated anteriorly and are shortened as are the anterior tibialis and the toe extensors. Rigid vertical talus infrequently occurs as an isolated problem; rather, it is associated with various chromosomal disorders, neuromuscular defects, arthrogryposis, and myelomeningocele. Diagnosis is confirmed by lateral radiographs in maximum plantarflexion, which demonstrates the irreducible talonavicular joint, and in maximum dorsiflexion, which demonstrates fixed equinus (Fig. 1). A line drawn through the axis of the talus will pass plantar to the metatarsal axis.

Cast correction is not effective except to stretch the lateral and anterior soft tissue in preparation for surgery. The optimal time for surgical intervention is the same as for clubfoot. A single-stage correction is advocated, which consists of Achilles tendon lengthening and posterior ankle/subtalar capsulotomy, peroneal tendon lengthening and calcaneocuboid capsulotomy, anterior tibialis and toe extensor lengthening, and talonavicular capsulotomy with reconstruction of the spring ligament and posterior tibial tendon plication. The talonavicular joint is pinned, and postoperative casting is for 12 weeks.

Children 2 to 6 years of age or those with recurrent deformity should be treated by subtalar fusion at the time of soft-tissue correction. Triple arthrodesis is a salvage procedure reserved for the symptomatic adolescent foot.

Tarsal Coalitions

Tarsal coalition is a congenital failure of segmentation of two or more tarsal bones and may be fibrous, cartilaginous, or bony in nature. Autosomal dominance with variable penetrance is the likely mechanism of inheritance. A synostosis may occur between any of the tarsals; however, the calcaneonavicular bar is the most common, followed by the middle facet of the talocalcaneal joint. Occasionally, more than one coalition pattern can be present in one foot, and the condition is bilateral in 50% of cases.

There is a tendency to progressive ossification of the bar with increasing age, and this often corresponds with the onset of symptoms. Typically, ossification occurs between 8 and 12 years of age for calcaneonavicular bars and between 12 and 15 years for talocalcaneal coalitions. Symptoms usually consist of a vague, aching pain in the region of the subtalar joint, which is aggravated by activity. Other symptoms include frequent ankle sprains and anterolateral calf pain. Subtalar motion is reduced, especially for talocalcaneal bars, and a rigid flatfoot with contracture of the peroneal tendons (peroneal spastic flatfoot) may exist.

The diagnosis is confirmed radiographically: the oblique projection best demonstrates the calcaneonavicular bar (Fig. 2) and the lateral view often has signs suggestive of a coalition. These signs include blunting of the subtalar process, elongation of the anterior calcaneal process, narrowing of the posterior subtalar joint, and talar beaking. Degenerative joint changes rarely are seen in the adolescent; these are not to be confused with ligament traction spurs. The effectiveness of the Harris view for visualizing the subtalar joint is enhanced by measuring the angle of the posterior facet on the lateral radiograph and then adjusting the Harris view to this inclination. Angulation of the middle facet by more than 20 degrees off the horizontal is consistent with a coalition, even if the joint appears open. Computed tomographic scanning provides the clearest imaging of subtalar coalitions and probably should be a routine part of the workup, especially if surgery is anticipated.

The majority of tarsal coalitions are asymptomatic, and evidence indicates that they remain so in adulthood. Symptomatic lesions often are treated initially by immobilization for three to six weeks, followed by an orthosis. Calcaneonavicular bars are very amenable to resection, with a high percentage doing well. Results of talocalcaneal resections are less predictable; more than 50% involvement of the middle facet is a relative contraindication to resection. Persistent hindfoot valgus may also be associated with a poor result, so some recommend me-

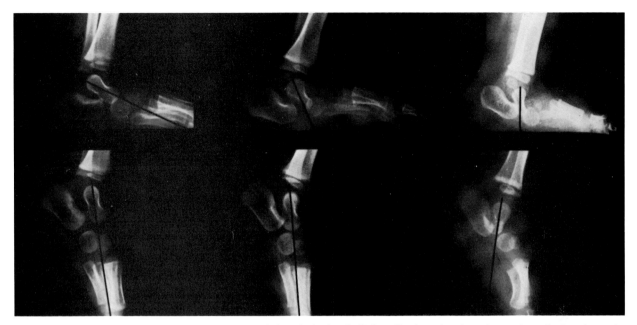

Fig. 1 Roentgenographic differential diagnosis of congenital vertical talus. **Left**, Standing lateral and maximum plantarflexion views of a normal foot. The longitudinal axis of the talus (dark line) remains dorsal to the cuboid and well-aligned with the metatarsal axes in both views. **Center**, Oblique talus. On the standing lateral, the talar axis is not aligned with the metatarsals and falls plantar to the cuboid. A normal configuration is seen with maximum plantarflexion. **Right**, True congenital vertical talus. With maximum plantarflexion, no correction occurs. The axis of the talus falls plantar to the metatarsal axis and the cuboid. (Reproduced with permission from Kumar SJ, Cowell HR, Ramsey PL: Vertical and oblique talus, in Frankel VH (ed): American Academy of Orthopaedic Surgeons *Instructional Course Lectures, XXXI*. St. Louis, CV Mosby, 1982, p 236.)

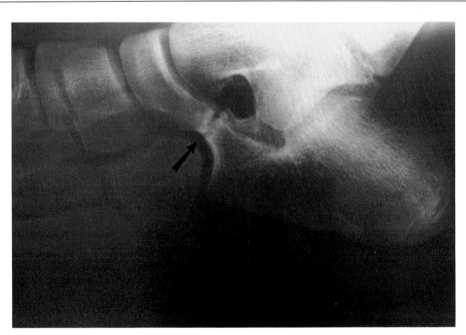

Fig. 2 Calcaneonavicular bar (arrow) in a 9-year-old boy with heel pain, as shown classically on the internal oblique foot film (Slomann view). (Reproduced with permission from Oestreich AE, Mize WA, Crawford AH, et al: The "Anteater nose": A direct sign of calcaneonavicular coalition on the lateral radiograph. *J Pediatr Orthop* 1987;7:709-711.)

dial displacement os calcis osteotomy as an adjunctive procedure. Failed resections are salvaged by subtalar fusion or triple arthrodesis.

Infections

Acute hematogenous osteomyelitis can affect any of the bones in the foot, but it most commonly involves the os calcis. Systemic symptoms often are lacking, and the sedimentation rate may be normal or only slightly elevated. A bone scan may help localize the involved area, which should subsequently be aspirated for culture. A computed tomographic scan may help in the diagnosis of deep infection and will show areas of bony destruction.

Nail puncture wounds occasionally result in the rapid onset of foot infection, despite initial prophylaxis with broad spectrum antibiotics. The swelling is usually dorsal, and there is an advancing cellulitis. If there is pain with motion of the joint or if the puncture wound is in the region of the metatarsal heads, the presence of septic arthritis should be assumed, and prompt surgical drainage should ensue. Pseudomonas, a frequent pathogen (cartilage seeking), responds best to the combination of debridement and appropriate antibiotics. Puncture wounds in the middle of the foot rarely involve the bone or joints, and oral antistaphylococcal antibiotics usually will cure the cellulitis.

Salter-Harris type I and II fractures of the distal phalanx of the great toe are sometimes open injuries, especially if there is evidence of nail bed trauma, and antibiotic prophylaxis should be administered.

Myelomeningocele

Almost every kind of foot condition can occur in this population, and 50% of patients are born with a rigid deformity. Secondary deformities also commonly develop as a result of muscle imbalance and/or spasticity. Because of the invariable lack of sensation in the feet, it is imperative that any treatment should produce and maintain a plantigrade foot. Preferably, this foot is mobile, but arthrodeses are effective if they achieve the goal of a plantigrade surface and a foot that can be braced. In general, complex tendon transfers should be avoided because of the lack of selective muscle control and the tendency to create a new deformity. Of children with this disorder, 85% require lower-extremity bracing on a long-term basis.

Equinovarus deformity requires surgical treatment, and contracted tendons should be resected rather than lengthened. Bracing is needed after correction to prevent a recurrent equinus position. Talectomy rarely is needed initially, but it is effective for revision surgery to return the foot to a neutral position. In younger children, the Verebelyi-Ogston procedure (talar decancellation) may be preferred over talectomy.

Calcaneus position is associated with either a cavus or valgus deformity, and initially is managed with bracing. Progression is usual unless muscle imbalance is corrected early by tenotomy or tendon transfer (for example, anterior tibialis to os calcis). Older children usually require one of a variety of calcaneal osteotomies, depending on the deformity.

Ankle and subtalar valgus deformity is common, especially in ambulatory children, and external tibial torsion often coexists. Fibular shortening contributes to the valgus ankle position. Ankle valgus can be corrected by partial Achilles tenodesis to the fibula if the deformity isn't severe; otherwise, this procedure is combined with medial tibial epiphysiodesis or distal tibial varus osteotomy. If there is associated calcaneus deformity because of unopposed anterior tibialis function, this tendon should be released or transferred to the os calcis. Occasionally subtalar stabilization is needed later to control residual valgus foot, and is accomplished by fusion or by calcaneal osteotomy.

Cerebral Palsy

The pattern of cerebral palsy influences the type of foot and ankle deformity seen in this population, but ankle equinus is the most common problem. In those with diplegia, it is bilateral and almost always flexible (dynamic) in the child under 3 years of age. Ankle position can be controlled with an orthosis until myostatic contracture occurs or when the child is closer to 5 years of age. Overlengthening is to be avoided at all costs, and the condition of the hamstrings should be known. Anterior tibial tendon function determines whether or not the child will be brace-free.

Equinovalgus deformity is more common in children with diplegia and spastic quadriplegia. In ambulatory children, mild deformity can be corrected with peroneal tendon lengthening (transfer of brevis to posterior tibialis is unreliable) combined with Achilles tendon lengthening. If heel valgus is pronounced, a medial displacement os calcis osteotomy can be added. If heel valgus and forefoot pronation are marked, opening wedge osteotomy of the anterior calcaneal process can be performed. If the hindfoot is in rigid valgus, it is best to combine an extra-articular subtalar fusion with the tendon lengthening. The technique of Dennyson and Fulford is very reliable and involves placing a bone screw from the talar neck into the calcaneus. The screw holds the foot in a corrected position while cancellous bone grafting of the sinus tarsi consolidates.

Children with hemiplegia often display an equinovarus foot deformity as a result of posterior tibial tendon dominance, although the anterior tibial tendon is occasionally at fault. Split posterior tibial tendon transfer, combined with heel cord lengthening, works well provided the varus heel is flexible. Split anterior tibialis transfer is used when forefoot supination is predominant, and usually is combined with posterior tibial tendon lengthening. Entire transfer of the posterior tibial tendon to the dorsum of the foot should be avoided unless electromyelograms show that it is active only during the swing phase of gait; tonic activity will produce a calcaneovalgus foot.

For rigid heel varus, a lateral closing wedge osteotomy should be combined with soft-tissue balancing. The triple arthrodesis remains a good alternative procedure for the symptomatic, rigidly deformed foot, especially in the adolescent.

Annotated Bibliography

Bunions

Geissele A, Stanton R: Surgical treatment of adolescent hallux valgus. *J Pediatr Orthop* 1990;10:642-648.

A way to rate the results of bunion surgery is discussed, and some of the potential complications with this surgery are highlighted. The one factor most highly correlated with a decreased recurrence rate of angular deformity and patient satisfaction was reduction of the intermetatarsal angle.

Kalen V, Brecher A: Relationships between adolescent bunions and flatfoot. *Foot Ankle* 1988;8:331-336.

This study evaluates the results of 36 adolescents with 66 hallux valgus deformities for the presence of associated flatfoot. Only 26.6% of these adolescents had an increased intermetatarsal angle and 81% had an abnormal metatarsus varus angle as compared with the published normals. Measurements of pes planus, including talar pitch, calcaneal plantar angle, dorsal plantar talonavicular angle, and lateral talocalcaneal angle, showed the incidence of flatfeet in adolescents with bunions was eight to 24 times greater than expected.

Mann RA: Decision-making in bunion surgery, in Greene WB (ed): American Academy of Orthopaedic Surgeons *Instructional Course Lectures, XXXIX*. Park Ridge, IL, American Academy of Orthopaedic Surgeons, 1990, pp 3-13.

A recognized expert discusses preoperative planning of decision-making in bunion surgery for patients of all ages.

Metatarsus Adductus

Stark JG, Johanson JE, Winter RB: The Heyman-Herndon tarsal-metatarsal capsulotomy for metatarsus adductus: Results in 48 feet. *J Pediatr Orthop* 1987;7:305-310.

A follow-up of 48 procedures revealed a 41% failure rate and 50% incidence of painful dorsal prominence. The authors questioned the benefit of this operation in treating forefoot adduction deformity.

Cavus and Calcaneus Foot

Badelon O, Benasshel H: Subtalar posterior displacement osteotomy of the calcaneus. *J Pediatr Orthop* 1990;10:401-404.

A preliminary report of a new technique for calcaneal osteotomy for calcaneocavus foot deformity is detailed. Geometric analysis of postoperative radiographs showed a 30% to 50% increase in Achilles tendon strength.

Wokuch D, Bowen JR: Long-term study of triple arthrodesis for correction of pes cavovarus in Charcot-Marie-Tooth disease. *J Pediatr Orthop* 1989;9:433-437.

A 12-year follow-up is discussed of triple arthrodesis with an analysis of objective and functional results. The problem of radiographic evidence for degenerative joint disease is noted.

Flatfoot

Staheli LT, Chew DE, Corbet M: The longitudinal arch: A survey of 882 feet in normal children and adults. *J Bone Joint Surg* 1987;69A:426-428.

The authors studied both feet of 441 normal subjects who were asymptomatic. They used a footprint and calculated the arch index, that is, the width of the arch compared to the width of the heel, and plotted this for each age group.

Wenger DR, et al: Corrective shoes and inserts as treatment for a flexible flatfoot in infants and children. *J Bone Joint Surg* 1989;71A:800-810.

A prospective study was performed to determine whether flexible flatfoot in children can be influenced by treatment; 129 children were stratified into four groups. Analysis of radiographs before treatment and at the most recent follow-up demonstrated a significant improvement in all groups (p <0.01), including controls. The authors concluded that wearing corrective shoes or inserts for three years does not influence the course of flexible flatfoot in children.

Accessory Navicular

Bennet G, Weiner D: Surgical treatment of symptomatic accessory tarsal navicular. *J Pediatr Orthop* 1990;10:445-449.

Fifty cases (75 feet) are retrospectively reviewed. Surgery consisted of excision alone with good to excellent results in 90%. A comprehensive review is provided.

Clubfoot

Aronson J, Puskarich CL: Deformity and disability from treated clubfoot. *J Pediatr Orthop* 1990;10:109-119

The authors evaluated 29 patients with unilateral idiopathic clubfoot deformities and 23 controls by comparing morphology, radiography, and performance-testing. The average period following definitive treatment was greater than 10 years. Treatment regimen varied from prolonged casting to early posteromedial release. The most significant average limitations in the treated clubfeet were: (1) a 42% decrease in normal ankle motion, specifically lacking 65% normal dorsiflexion, which was independent of treatment; (2) a 24% decrease in normal plantarflexion muscle strength, which correlated directly to the number of heel cord lengthenings per foot; and (3) a noticeable 10% decrease in calf girth, which was unrelated to total time spent in cast.

Carroll NC: Pathoanatomy and surgical treatment of the resistant clubfoot, in Bassett FH III (ed): American Academy of Orthopaedic Surgeons *Instructional Course Lectures, XXXVII.* Park Ridge, IL, American Academy of Orthopaedic Surgeons, 1988, pp 93-106.

A comprehensive approach to the surgical management of clubfoot (CTEV) deformity is presented.

Cummings RJ, Lovell WW: Operative treatment or congenital idiopathic clubfoot: Current concepts review. *J Bone Joint Surg* 1988;70A:1108-1112.

A well-documented presentation on the management of clubfoot deformity, with input from one of the true giants of pediatric orthopaedics and his colleague, offers a well-thought-out approach to this problem.

Herzenberg JE, et al: Clubfoot analysis with 3-dimensional computer modeling. *J Pediatr Orthop* 1988;8:257-262.

Relative to the bimalleolar axis in the axial plane, the normal talus demonstrated 5 degrees of internal rotation of its body and 25 degrees of internal rotation of its neck. The clubfoot talus showed 14 degrees of external rotation of its body and 45 degrees of internal rotation of its neck. The calcaneus was externally rotated 5 degrees in the normal foot, and internally rotated 22 degrees in the clubfoot. This article is frequently quoted, and until the study is reproduced, will remain the benchmark.

Magone J, et al: Comparative review of surgical treatment of the idiopathic clubfoot by three different procedures at Columbus Children's Hospital. *J Pediatr Orthop* 1989;9:49-58.

Three surgical procedures, the Turco, the Carroll, and the McKay were performed on 76 cases of clubfeet, with subsequent clinical and radiographic analysis. The complications of overcorrection and undercorrection are discussed.

Sodre H, et al: Arterial abnormalities in talipes equinovarus as assessed by angiography and the Doppler technique. *J Pediatr Orthop* 1990;10:101-104.

Preoperative angiography in 30 uncorrected clubfeet demonstrated abnormal vascular patterns in all but two limbs, with hypoplasia or premature termination of the anterior tibial and medial plantar arteries in the remainder. Because the posterior tibial artery usually provides the only arterial supply to the foot, this vessel must be meticulously preserved at surgery and during subsequent ankle dorsiflexion.

Vizkelety T, Szepeis K: Reoperation in treatment of clubfoot. *J Pediatr Orthop* 1989;9:144-147.

One hundred and eighteen operations are evaluated. Relapse was most commonly a result of insufficient primary surgery.

Congenital Vertical Talus

Schrader LF, Gilbert RJ, Skinner SR, et al: Congenital vertical talus surgical correction by a one-stage medial approach. *Orthopedics* 1990;13:1233-1236.

A one-stage procedure for correction of congenital vertical talus using a medial approach is described; the operation was performed on 14 feet with good initial anatomic results in all cases.

Tarsal Coalitions

Gonzalez PK, Kumar SJ: Calcaneonavicular coalition treated by resection and interposition of the extensor digitorum brevis muscle. *J Bone Joint Surg* 1990;72A;71-77.

Seventy-five feet in 48 patients that had calcaneonavicular coalition were evaluated at two to 23 years after resection of the coalition and interposition of the extensor digitorum brevis muscle. The best results were in patients who had a cartilaginous coalition and who were younger than 16 years old at the time of operation.

Olney EW, Asher MA: Excision of symptomatic coalition of the middle facet of the talocalcaneal joint. *J Bone Joint Surg* 1987;69A:539-544.

Excision of a coalition involving the middle facet of the talocalcaneal joint and the interposition of an autogenous fat graft was performed on 10 feet (nine patients). Results were rated as five excellent, three good, one fair, and one poor; incomplete resection was associated with the poor result. The procedure is superior to the triple arthrodesis in adolescents.

Scranton TE Jr: Treatment of symptomatic talocalcaneal coalition. *J Bone Joint Surg* 1987;69A:533-539.

Fourteen feet had a resection of the coalition when symptoms were not relieved by plaster cast immobilization. Indications for resection included failure of conservative treatment, a coalition that is less than one half the surface area of the talocalcaneal joint, and the absence of degenerative changes in that joint. No patient had a poor result. Prerequisites for treatment were absence of degenerative changes and coalition less than one-half the surface area of the talocalcaneal joint. This procedure achieves the best results of 911 tarsal coalition resections.

Myelomeningocele

Georgiadis G, Aronson D: Posterior transfer of the anterior tibial tendon in children who have a myelomeningocele. *J Bone Joint Surg* 1990;72A:392-398.

The technique and indications for this procedure are discussed. Surgical results were best when the child was at least 4 years of age and had a low lumbar or sacral motor level.

Sherk H, et al: Ground reaction forces on the plantar surface of the foot after talectomy in the myelomeningocele. *J Pediatr Orthop* 1989;9:269-275.

Talectomy rarely succeeded in distributing weightbearing forces uniformly over the plantar surface of the foot. This may predispose to neurotrophic ulceration.

Cerebral Palsy

Barnes M, Herring J: Combined split anterior tibial-tendon transfer and intramuscular lengthening of the posterior tibial tendon. *J Bone Joint Surg* 1991;73A:734-738.

A combined procedure is described for the correction of a flexible varus deformity of the foot in patients with cerebral palsy. Other procedures to correct this problem are discussed for comparison.

Crawford AH, Kucharzyk DW, Roy DR, et al: Subtalar stabilization of the planovalgus foot by staple arthroeresis in young children who have neuromuscular problems. *J Bone Joint Surg* 199;72A:840-845.

A new approach was developed for the treatment of planovalgus feet in children who have spastic cerebral palsy and are less than 6 years old. The procedure consists of subtalar stabilization without fusion (arthroeresis) with a vitallium staple. The procedure corrects alignment, restores balance, and allows continued function. Approximately 85% of the results were excellent or good.

Gallien R, Morin F, Marquis F: Subtalar arthrodesis in children. *J Pediatr Orthop* 1989;9:59-63.

A retrospective study of 30 patients (51 feet) with valgus deformity of the feet were treated by three different types of subtalar extra-articular and intra-articular arthrodesis. A combined Grice-Green-Batchelor procedure gave the best results, with 84% excellent and satisfactory results, and bony union in 96% of the feet. The Grice-Green procedure did not yield good results in paralytic flatfeet in children with cerebral palsy. More importantly, one has to rule out ankle valgus versus subtalar valgus. They recommended weightbearing films of the ankles in the anterior-posterior plane as essential to determine the true extent of the deformity in every paralytic child before operation.

Segal L, Mazur J, et al: Calcaneal gait in spastic diplegia after heel cord lengthening: A study with gait analysis. *J Pediatr Orthop* 1989;9:697-701.

The complications of heel cord lengthening are discussed. The authors demonstrate the incidence of overlengthening is higher than expected (30%).

50

Ankle and Foot: Trauma

Soft-Tissue Injuries

Achilles Tendon

The Achilles tendon is susceptible to inflammatory processes, overuse syndromes, and rupture. Inflammatory conditions may precede or accompany complete and incomplete ruptures. Achilles tendinitis generally causes well-localized pain in the heel cord and may be preceded by an alteration in physical activity level. There is some evidence that alterations in footwear during training can cause symptoms in the heel cord. Physical examination may distinguish between inflammation, partial tear, and complete rupture. The inflamed Achilles tendon is treated with rest, anti-inflammatory medications, and the use of a heel lift. After the acute phase, heel cord stretching and a heel lift are helpful. Activity should be restored gradually, beginning below the level at which the symptoms initially occurred and increasing by only about 10% per week. Partial rupture of the Achilles tendon may be difficult to diagnose. The continuity of the tendon, together with inflammation, can obscure smaller defects. Ultrasonography may demonstrate partial rupture. Treatment approaches for partial rupture have not been studied in detail, but may involve immobilization followed by rehabilitation.

Rupture of the Achilles tendon, which is most common in the third to fifth decades of life, often occurs during a forced dorsiflexion against a contracted heel cord. The patient may hear a "pop" followed by difficulty in walking. There may be minimal discomfort. The calf squeeze test is a reliable clinical indicator of rupture. With the patient kneeling on a chair, and the foot hanging free, the calf is squeezed in the middle third just below the region of greatest circumference. Absence of plantarflexion in the foot indicates a ruptured Achilles tendon. Active plantarflexion is a less reliable indicator, as it can be accomplished by intact supplemental foot flexors.

Two other diagnostic methods have been described. A sphygmomanometer may be used as follows: With the patient prone and the knee flexed to 90 degrees and the ankle passively plantarflexed, the cuff is applied to the injured calf and inflated to 100 mm Hg. The ankle is then dorsiflexed. If the heel cord is intact, the pressure will rise approximately 35 to 40 mm Hg. Another clinical text involves the use of a 25-gauge needle. With the patient prone, the needle is passed through the skin into the tendon substance 10 cm above the insertion into the heel cord. The foot is then passively dorsiflexed. If the tendon is intact, the needle will swivel distally, as the intact heel cord moves a greater distance than the skin. If the tendon is ruptured, the needle will move only a small amount as the skin shifts. Ultrasound and magnetic resonance imaging also have been employed and may be helpful in delayed diagnosis or incomplete ruptures when clinical tests are less reliable.

Surgical and nonsurgical treatments are both effective, and long-term comparative studies fail to demonstrate a significant functional difference between them. However, the rerupture rate appears to be higher in patients treated without surgery: rerupture rates of 2% to 7% for surgical treatment and 8% to 35% for nonsurgical treatment have been reported. However, the higher cost and morbidity of surgical treatment must be considered. Nonsurgical treatment involves use of an equinus walking cast for eight weeks, followed by a heel lift for one to two months. Surgery is often recommended for an active person and for one whose lifestyle cannot tolerate the prolonged rehabilitation following rerupture. A postero-medial skin incision is recommended, because it permits access to the plantaris tendon, which may be used to augment the repair. A modified Bunnell-type suture is used, supplemented by a peripheral absorbable suture. The tendon sheath and subcutaneous tissue should be closed separately, if possible, to prevent adhesions of the skin. Careful attention to soft tissues is needed to avoid skin slough and to spare the blood supply that enters the tendon from the ventral paratenon.

Late repair or repair of chronic rupture presents additional problems. It might not be possible to approximate the ends of the tendon, or the ends might be too attenuated to repair. Under these circumstances repair can be supplemented with plantaris tendon, fascia lata, or a strip of fascia turned down from the proximal Achilles tendon. In addition, the repair may be supplemented with the flexor digitorum longus, flexor hallucis longus, or peroneus brevis tendons. The transfers are accomplished by leaving the origin intact and transferring the insertion into the distal heelcord or into the calcaneus itself.

An alternative treatment is percutaneous repair. In theory, this offers the advantages of both methods; low morbidity with good cosmesis together with low rerupture rates and early rehabilitation. Early reports were favorable, but recently injury to the sural nerve and rerupture rates paralleling those occurring after closed treatment have been reported. The use of ultrasound to facilitate tendon healing also has been investigated. Preliminary results suggest that therapeutic ultrasound may provide faster healing and greater tensile strength.

Lateral Ankle Ligaments

Inversion injury to the ankle is the most common injury in sports and one of the most common diagnoses among patients evaluated in the emergency room. The diagnosis of lateral ligament injury is made by history and clinical examination. Inversion of the foot accompanied by pain and a sometimes palpable "pop" suggest a rupture of one or more of the ankle ligaments.

Three ligaments stabilize the lateral ankle: the anterior talofibular, the calcaneofibular, and the posterior talofibular. The anterior talofibular ligament is under increased strain when the ankle is plantarflexed, inverted, and internally rotated. Because injury most often occurs in plantarflexion, it is the ligament most frequently injured. The calcaneofibular ligament is under increased strain when the ankle is dorsiflexed and inverted. It can also be injured during more severe inversion injuries. The posterior talofibular ligament, which is under greatest tension when the ankle is dorsiflexed and externally rotated, is rarely injured.

The injuries are classified as grades I, II, or III. Grade I sprains have minimal tenderness and no measurable instability. Grade II sprains are considered partial tears and may demonstrate some limited instability. Grade III injuries involve a complete tear of the ligament and instability determined by whether one or two ligaments are involved.

Grades I and II injuries can be managed nonsurgically in the acute phase with the rest, ice, compression, and elevation (RICE). This is followed by weightbearing with protective bracing or taping, exercises against resistance, and work on a balance board to reestablish strength and proprioception. Using this functional treatment, a majority of ligaments return to full function. Treatment of grade III injuries is somewhat more controversial, however. There is no prospective randomized study with evidence to suggest that surgical treatment improves outcome, results in earlier return to activity, or prevents recurrence. Surgical treatment of an acute injury may be appropriate when the injury is recurrent, when a large bony avulsion is present, or when ipsilateral limb injury makes traditional methods undesirable or impractical.

When reconstruction is required, a variety of surgical options are available. Primary repair, primary repair reinforced with local tissues, reconstruction with the peroneus brevis tendon, and reconstruction with the plantaris tendon have been advocated. All seem to show equally good results when done for appropriate indications.

Pain at the anterior aspect of the ankle following inversion injuries may be caused by impingement of the talus on the distal fascicle of the anteroinferior tibiofibular ligament. It is not clear whether abnormal anatomy or altered mechanics secondary to instability of the joint is responsible for the clinical syndrome. Also unclear is the long-term consequence of resecting the ligament. The indications for surgical intervention are not clearly defined.

Injuries of the Distal Tibiofibular Syndesmosis

The distal tibiofibular joint is a syndesmosis stabilized by a posterior and an anterior ligament. The posterior ligament is under tension when the ankle is dorsiflexed but relaxes somewhat when external rotation is added. The anterior ligament is under greatest tension with the ankle in dorsiflexion and external rotation. If the anterior ligament is sectioned experimentally, the fibula has greater mobility and allows the talus to rotate laterally in the mortise. Disruption of the entire syndesmosis occurs most often with ankle fractures, but it also can occur with dorsiflexion-external rotation injuries and may present as, or accompany, an "ankle sprain." When the syndesmosis is intact, the distal tibia and fibula bear a consistent relationship to one another that can be expressed in terms of absolute distance between them and in terms of a percentage distance of the distal fibula. This relationship is interrupted when the distal syndesmosis is injured. The "clear space," a cartilage space between the distal tibia and fibula on the mortise view of the ankle, should not exceed 5 mm. The distal tibia and fibula should overlap 6 mm or 42% of the total width of the fibula on the anteroposterior view. A radiograph of the entire tibia and fibula is used to document fractures in the more proximal aspect of the fibula if these criteria are not met on the ankle films. A pure syndesmosis rupture, if complete, requires fixation with a syndesmosis screw. Injuries without diastasis can be treated nonsurgically with a functional rehabilitation program like that used for lateral ligament injuries, but recovery is slower.

Deltoid Ligament

Injuries of the deltoid ligament without fracture are quite uncommon. Cases of avulsed deltoid ligament with attached cartilage or bone trapped in the joint have been reported. A history of severe eversion/plantarflexion coupled with a widened medial ankle joint may reflect this scenario. If tissue is trapped in the joint, arthrotomy is undertaken and the interposed ligament and bone are removed with or without primary repair of the ligament.

Compartmental Syndrome

Compartmental syndromes do occur in the foot and can be isolated to one or more compartments. As in compartmental syndromes elsewhere, a high index of suspicion is the best diagnostic tool. The foot contains between four and nine fascial compartments. The deep posterior compartment of the leg is continuous with the so-called calcaneal compartment in the foot. The geographic and functional separation of the compartments is not as well defined as in the leg, because the compartments are small and muscle mass is meager. Compartments may be released through a combination of dorsal and medial incisions (Fig. 1). Clawing of the toes is a

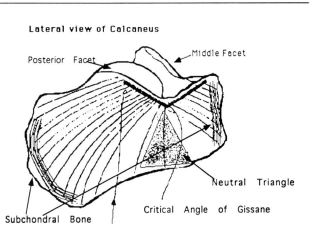

Lateral view of Calcaneus

Posterior Facet
Middle Facet
Neutral Triangle
Critical Angle of Gissane
Subchondral Bone
Thalamic segment

Fig. 1 Thalamic segment and angle of Gissane.

common sequela of compartmental syndrome even with appropriate treatment. Loss of limb has not been reported from missed compartmental syndrome of the foot.

Fractures and Dislocations of the Foot and Ankle

Ankle

Ankle dislocation without fracture is not common. The mechanism of injury appears to be forced inversion and an axial load at the maximally plantarflexed foot. It is most often posteromedial, it occurs in young people, and generalized ligamentous laxity seems to be a predisposing condition. A closed injury is satisfactorily treated with closed reduction and casting for six weeks. An open injury is treated with reduction and primary repair of the lateral ligaments. Syndesmosis rupture is uncommon but should be ruled out.

Ankle fractures involve the medial or lateral malleolus. Treatment of these injuries requires an understanding of the commonly used classification systems. Two classification systems currently in use are based on the concept of an ankle fracture as an indirect injury (Fig. 2). Direct injuries involving the ankle joint (including direct blows and axial loading through the foot, the so-called pilon fracture) defy the classification systems, their impact for treatment, and prognosis for recovery. The Lauge-Hansen classification, described in 1942, was the first widely used system for indirect injuries. It describes the injury using two anatomic words, the first to describe the position of the foot and the second to describe the direction of the applied force. The system was based on studies in cadavers in which injuries were created by forces applied in different directions. The strength of this system is in its usefulness as a guide for the surgeon in the technique of closed reduction. The position and direction of the force are reversed to bring about reduction.

In 1949, Danis described an anatomic classification for surgery. This system was modified by Weber and is now commonly known as the Danis-Weber, or AO, classification. In this system the ankle fracture is divided into three classes—A, B, or C—according to the relationship of the fibular fracture to the syndesmosis and interosseous ligaments. Class A fractures are distal to both the interosseous ligament and syndesmosis. Class B fractures, which occur obliquely through the fibula, involve part or all of the syndesmosis and have an unstable syndesmosis approximately 50% of the time. Class C fractures include fractures of the fibula proximal to the distal tibiofibular ligament and syndesmosis. These fractures are considered to be unstable.

Both systems permit comparisons between different types of injuries. The Lauge-Hansen classification has been criticized for being too comprehensive and difficult to use. The Danis-Weber system, although much easier to use, leaves out important information for treatment evaluation and research. Neither system replaces careful physical examination and an understanding of the anatomy and mechanism of injury.

Comparative studies have assumed a consistent application of these classification systems, but studies have documented the difficulty of staging reproducibility within the four classifications of Lauge-Hansen. However, two studies have demonstrated that participants were able to place the radiographs consistently into the injury types described in the Danis-Weber and Lauge-Hansen classifications.

Treatment of ankle fractures involves reduction and immobilization until healing. Reduction of the fracture appears to be the most important factor that can be controlled by the treating physician. When reduction is obtained by closed means, cast immobilization is an acceptable method of treatment. If closed reduction cannot be obtained, open reduction and internal fixation is required. There seems to be little difference in long-term outcome between methods. Maintaining reduction of unstable ankle fractures is difficult in a cast, however, and the inconvenience and discomfort of a long leg cast, together with the more prolonged rehabilitation involved, commit many patients to surgical treatment. The goals of treatment are to reduce the joint and rigidly fix the fibula to lock the talus in the mortise. The fibula can be fixed rigidly by a lateral plate, lag screws, or an antiglide plate positioned at the apex of the fracture (Fig. 3). Alternative forms of fixation, including intramedullary pins, are not as widely accepted because they afford no rotational control or rigidity.

One drawback to using rigid internal fixation is that a second operation is required in some cases to remove hardware. In theory, an absorbable implant would obviate the need for a second operation. Implants made of polyglycolic and polylactic acid and polydioxanone are used with this in mind. The implants are made in the form of screws and pins, are radiolucent, and are not intended to be removed. They can be cut flush with an

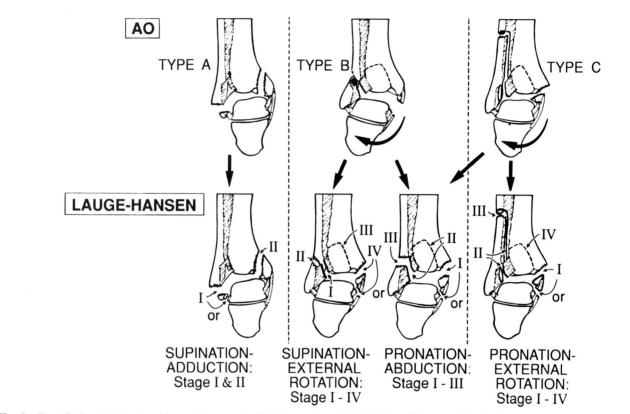

Fig. 2   The AO (Danis-Weber) and Lauge-Hansen classification systems. Note that the AO system includes injuries of different Lauge-Hansen types in one category.

articular surface for small osteochondral fractures. Early reports suggest that the rates of union and complications are similar to those of traditional fixation materials. A small but significant number of sterile abscesses containing breakdown products of the implants and white blood cells have been reported. Removing the remaining implant under these circumstances may be challenging because the implants are radiolucent. These reports, as well as the high cost of the devices, suggest caution in the use of these implants until the clinical performance of the devices is better understood.

When the level of the fibula fracture is above the mortise, the distal tibiofibular syndesmosis may be disrupted. Stabilization of the distal tibiofibular joint with a screw allows the soft tissues to heal in an appropriate position to maintain the integrity of the mortise. The stability of this syndesmotic joint should be visually inspected during surgical stabilization of the fibula. If the medial malleolus is fractured and the deltoid ligament is intact, rigid fixation of fibula and tibia should make syndesmosis fixation unnecessary. When the fracture of the fibula is proximal to the joint and the medial malleolus is intact, syndesmosis fixation often is required. A single 4.5-mm or 3.5-mm screw placed approximately 1 cm proximal to the syndesmosis is the most commonly used technique. Re-

moval of the screw before weightbearing is not mandatory. Breakage of the screw is uncommon, but does occur.

When fixation is performed, cast immobilization may not be necessary. A recent study of three postoperative regimens demonstrated no significant difference in outcome. The patients were treated with a nonweightbearing plaster cast, a plaster walking cast, or no cast or weightbearing. Similarly, Lauge-Hansen SE II injuries were randomized to cast versus removable splint without surgical stabilization. Again, no significant difference in outcome was reported, but patients were happier with brace treatment. Overall, the role of cast treatment of ankle fractures appears to be waning.

Fractures of the Talus

Fractures of the talus may involve the talar dome, the talar body, the neck, the head, or the smaller processes, such as the lateral process or the os trigonum. Lesser fractures are likely to occur with an inversion injury. Osteochondral fractures and lateral process fractures in particular are likely to occur during an inversion injury and are often missed initially. Osteochondral fractures occur at the medial or lateral side of the talar dome. They are

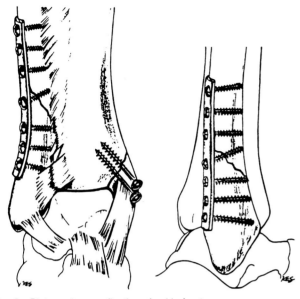

Fig. 3 Plate and screw fixation of ankle fracture.

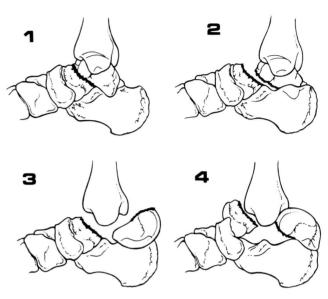

Fig. 4 Talar fracture - Hawkins classification.

classified into four groups: stage 1, a small area of compression; stage 2, a partially detached fragment; stage 3, a completely detached fragment; and stage 4, a displaced osteochondral fracture. Those on the medial dome of the talus are more likely to be on the posterior one third of the dome, those on the lateral side are more likely to be in the middle one third of the dome. Diagnosis of these lesions, particularly those that are stage 1 or 2, requires supplemental cross-sectional imaging. Bone scanning, computed tomography, arthrotomography, and, more recently, magnetic resonance imaging scans have their advocates.

Persistent ankle pain after an inversion injury should suggest to the surgeon that an osteochondral fracture might be present. Medial lesions are less likely to be secondary to trauma and less likely to cause symptoms or require treatment. Lesions that are displaced, whether they are medial or lateral, require surgical excision and early motion without weightbearing.

Lateral process fractures involve the posterior facet of the talocalcaneal joint. These fractures are best visualized using Broden's oblique hindfoot views or cross-sectional imaging techniques, as they may be quite subtle on anteroposterior and lateral radiographs of the foot. Large fractures that are displaced more than 2 mm probably are best treated by open reduction and internal fixation. Treatment of smaller, comminuted fractures must be individualized.

Vertical fractures of the talus can occur through the distal body or through the talar neck. Hawkins classified these talar neck fractures according to the degree of displacement and the prognosis for development of avascular necrosis (Fig. 4). Two issues guide the treatment of the talus fractures. First, because a complex geometric

relationship exists among the articular surfaces of the talus (ankle, subtalar, and transverse tarsal joints), a displaced fracture is disruptive and alters the functions of the various joints. Second, because the talus has no muscular insertions and approximately 60% of its surface is covered by articular cartilage, areas of blood inflow are limited and injuries present a serious threat to the blood supply. The first point dictates that anatomic reduction be restored and maintained until healing. The second mandates that reduction be performed with minimum dissection of the soft tissues that carry the blood supply to the talus. These conflicting requirements of reduction and exposure contribute to the considerable morbidity associated with this injury. A nondisplaced fracture of the talar neck and body may be treated in a nonweight-bearing short leg cast until healing occurs. The surgeon must ensure that the fracture is truly nondisplaced. Even a small amount of displacement may represent an unstable fracture that has returned to a nearly reduced position after the deforming force is removed. Displaced fractures should be treated by open reduction and internal fixation.

The goals of surgery, anatomic reduction and stable fixation, can be achieved by any of a variety of fixation methods: two medial screws, medial and lateral cross screw configuration, posterior to anterior lag screw fixation, and Steinmann pin fixation. Screws provide more rigid fixation than pins and can be left in place for longer periods without concern for pin-tract infection or implant migration.

Osteonecrosis of the talus occurs after a talar neck fracture. There is no convincing evidence that osteonecrosis without collapse requires treatment beyond that to the fracture. If solidly and anatomically healed, a talar neck fracture with osteonecrosis of the body may be entirely asymptomatic. When the body of the talus collapses from osteonecrosis or is severely damaged from the initial impact of the fracture, acceptable results have been achieved using the Blair (modified tibiotalar) arthrodesis.

Fractures of the Calcaneus

The calcaneus is most often fractured by way of an axial load. Methods of classification and treatment are controversial and outcome is variable. The calcaneus is driven upward against the talus. The anterior part of the posterior facet of the talus, which includes the lateral process, acts as a fulcrum across which the calcaneus fractures. A fracture line is created that propagates obliquely across the calcaneus beginning at the lateral wall near the tarsal sinus. It is directed across the posterior facet and out the medial wall posterior to the sustentaculum. This fracture line is quite consistent and has been called the separation fracture or primary fracture line. It divides the tuberosity and lateral wall, along with a variable part of the posterior facet from the sustentacular fragment, along with the middle and anterior facet. The sustentaculum remains relatively nondisplaced; the tuberosity and the lateral wall are shortened and displaced laterally. In addition to this primary fracture line, many secondary fracture lines may occur. The location and number of these lines is determined by the direction and force of impact, as well as by the position of the foot at the time of loading. Several fracture classifications, more recently using computed tomography, have been proposed, but none has been widely accepted and none has demonstrated prognostic capability. The fractures are generally described as nondisplaced or as displaced and extra-articular or intra-articular. In addition to these minor descriptions, Essex Lopresti described two distinct fracture patterns. The first, joint depression type, involves actual depression of the posterior facet. The second, the so-called tongue-type fracture, involves a relative downward rotation of the posterior facet and tuberosity (Fig. 5).

Radiographic evaluation of calcaneus fractures includes the dorsoplantar, lateral, axial, and oblique views of the foot. The lateral view is the most helpful in the assessment of the position of the posterior facet. The dorsoplantar and oblique views demonstrate the calcaneocuboid joint. The axial view provides the direction and displacement of the primary fracture line as well as information about the relationship between the posterior facet and the sustentacular fragment. The axial view also may show fibular abutment and lateral wall displacement. When contemplating surgical treatment, computed tomography is also very helpful. This should be done in two planes—one parallel to the bottom of the foot, known as the transverse plane, and the second perpendicular to the posterior facet, known as the semicoronal plane. The transverse plane shows lateral

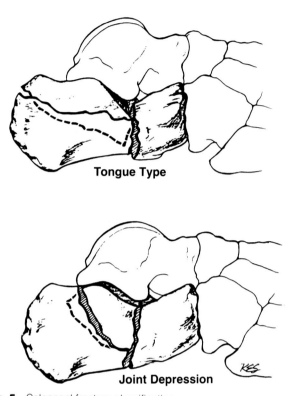

Fig. 5 Calcaneal fracture classification.

and anterior displacement of the tuberosity and displacement of the calcaneocuboid joint. The semicoronal cuts demonstrate injury to the posterior facet, the sinus tarsi and middle facet, and the lateral wall. Sagittal plane reconstruction of computed tomographic cuts may be useful as well.

Fractures of the calcaneus are serious, disabling injuries with prolonged recovery. The goal of treatment is a pain-free functional foot. It has not been established in an objective way that surgical treatment is superior to nonsurgical treatment. Natural history studies demonstrate that almost all patients with displaced calcaneus fractures treated nonsurgically continue to have pain and swelling at long-term follow-up. It is the goal of surgical treatment to improve on this natural history. The options include early motion without reduction, manipulative reduction and casting, or open reduction through the medial, lateral, or the combined medial lateral approaches. The goals of treatment are restoration of the height and of the geometric relationships among the talocalcaneal and calcaneal cuboid joint, and reduction of the joint surface and of the lateral wall to prevent fibular abutment. Significant controversy exists as to the most effective means of achieving these goals. If surgical treatment is elected, the surgeon should be extremely experienced in the technique. The goals of reduction include restoration of the height and length of the os calcis, reduction of the posterior and middle facets, reduction of the calcaneocuboid joint, and restoration of the relationship between the posterior and middle facets. Together, these criteria suggest anatomic reduction of the preinjury shape of the bone. Early results indicate that, in experienced hands, surgical treatment through the lateral or combined medial and lateral approach provides good results in 75% to 80% of patients.

Subtalar Dislocation

Subtalar dislocations can be medial or lateral; lateral dislocations are more likely to be high-energy injuries. Both can be associated with fractures of the posterior talar facet. If no fracture exists, a nonweightbearing short leg cast for three to six weeks following closed reduction is adequate treatment. Lateral subtalar dislocations are frequently open and require surgical reduction and debridement.

Midfoot

The midfoot contains the small tarsal bones—the navicular, cuboid, and three cuneiforms—bound together by a large number of dense ligaments, which permit only limited motion among them. Isolated fractures of the tarsal bones are uncommon. When injuries do occur, they are the result of substantial force. Outcome of treatment from these injuries is rarely excellent but may be functional.

Navicular Fractures

Navicular fractures may involve the tuberosity, the dorsal lip, or the body. Stress fractures also can occur in the navicular. Acute injuries are best evaluated by simulated weightbearing anteroposterior and lateral films, supplemented by an oblique view of the foot. Nondisplaced tuberosity fractures can be treated in a short leg, nonweightbearing cast. When the tuberosity is displaced, the tibialis posterior tendon is nonfunctional. Fixation using a small screw with a soft-tissue washer may bring about a satisfactory result. Avulsion fractures should provoke suspicion that there may be an occult fracture in the lateral side of the foot. Under these circumstances, attention should be paid to the anterior process of the calcaneus and the cuboid. Treatment of undisplaced ligament avulsion is by a short leg cast for six weeks.

Displaced fractures of the navicular body involve the talonavicular and the navicular cuneiform articulation. They are usually the result of high-energy injury and occur in three radiographic patterns. Attempts should be made to reduce the articular surface on both the anteroposterior and lateral views. Failure to restore the relationship of the navicular to the talus alters the relationship of the midfoot and forefoot to the hindfoot and will place additional stress on the already injured joints after

healing. Narrowing of the joint space should be expected. The majority of patients continue to have midfoot stiffness and swelling regardless of treatment. However, those whose talonavicular articulation is restored have an improved prognosis.

Cuboid Fractures

Fractures of the cuboid are most often minimally displaced and they should be evaluated by an oblique view of the foot. Evaluation may be supplemented with cross-sectional imaging of computed tomography, if there is any question about the position of fracture fragments. When compressed, the lateral column of the foot is foreshortened, allowing the forefoot to assume an abducted position. Under these circumstances, treatment requires reduction and bone grafting to maintain length and reduce the intra-articular component. Plantar displacement of the fourth and fifth ray may accompany cuboid fracture. When not reduced, the base of the fifth metatarsal is overloaded during weightbearing.

Lisfranc's Tarsometatarsal Joint

The diagnosis of tarsometatarsal dislocations or fracture dislocations is frequently missed. These injuries may be caused by direct or indirect force. In the latter, radiographs may appear relatively normal, with only a subtle diastasis between the first and second ray. Diagnosis under these circumstances requires an elevated index of suspicion. If plain radiographs are equivocal and the midfoot is swollen and tender, stress radiographs should be performed with the patient under appropriate sedation or anesthesia. If ligament injury is documented in the absence of fracture, reduction and internal fixation should be performed.

Lisfranc level injuries without fracture have a poor prognosis, with late midfoot collapse a common sequela. Fixation should be rigid enough to prevent transverse plane and dorsoplantar motion of the tarsometatarsal joint and maintained for a minimum of 12 weeks (some suggest that four to six months is appropriate). When the diagnosis is delayed for more than six weeks, primary arthrodesis may be required. Similarly, early removal of fixation or early weightbearing can result in collapse that requires salvage by arthrodesis.

The Forefoot

Metatarsal Fractures

Normal functioning of the forefoot requires that weightbearing be distributed evenly beneath the plantar pad. Displacement of tarsal fractures resulting in misalignment can cause uneven weightbearing distribution. If an adequate soft-tissue envelope exists, reduction can be achieved in plaster. Treatment in a well-molded plaster cast is often successful. Metatarsals that cannot be reduced closed, or those associated with severe soft-tissue trauma may require open reduction and internal fixation.

Stress fractures of the fifth metatarsal at the metaphyseal/diaphyseal junction require special treatment. This fracture, the Jones fracture, is associated with significant morbidity: delayed union, nonunion, and refracture. These fractures should be treated in a nonweightbearing cast or with internal fixation and bone grafting. If they are already developed, with widening of the fracture line and sclerosis at the time of initial presentation, cast mobilization is unlikely to be successful.

Overuse Syndromes

Plantar fasciitis, or pain at the plantar surface of the heel, is a common disorder often located at the plantar tuberosity of the calcaneus at the origin of the plantar fascia. Inflammation of the insertion of the plantar fascia and entrapment in the calcaneal branch of the tibial nerve are postulated etiologies. Treatment includes heel cord stretching, elevation of the heel with a special shoe, and nonsteroidal anti-inflammatory medications. University of California/Berkeley-type orthotics may be helpful if lesser means fail. An injection of 0.1 to 0.2 cc of corticosteroid into the tender area may be helpful as a single treatment if physical modalities are unsuccessful after three months. Surgery should be considered in those patients in whom nonsurgical means have been tried for a year without success. The operation includes release of plantar fascia from the medial tuberosity and release of the compressed calcaneal branch of the tibial nerve. Heel pain also may be a presenting symptom for inflammatory arthropathy, such as Reiter's syndrome or psoriatic arthritis.

Calcaneal Stress Fracture

Stress fracture of the calcaneus also may produce plantar heel pain. Under these circumstances, the tuberosity itself is tender, the bone scan is positive, and subsequent radiographs reveal radiodense condensation in the tuberosity. Treatment requires rest, elevation, and range-of-motion exercises.

Navicular Stress Fracture

Stress fracture of the navicular is characterized by insidious onset of midfoot pain. The fracture is usually in the sagittal plane in the middle one third of the bone, where the blood supply is limited. Radiographs are often negative. If the bone scan is positive, computed tomography often will demonstrate this midline fracture. If the fracture margins are not sclerotic, nonweightbearing in a plaster cast for six to eight weeks is usually adequate treatment. When the margins have become sclerotic, open reduction and bone grafting with internal fixation is recommended.

Annotated Bibliography

Anderson EG: Fatigue fractures of the foot. *Injury* 1990;21:275-279.

The author discusses an overview of fatigue fractures in the foot. Such fractures occur more often in the metatarsals and calcaneus than in the tarsal bones, but fatigue fractures can occur in any bone. Specific treatment should be performed for stress fractures that arise from an imbalance in the foot.

Bassett FH III, Gates HS, Billys J, et al: Talar impingement by the anteroinferior tibiofibular ligament. *J Bone Joint Surg* 1990;72A:55-59.

The authors reported on seven patients who had anterolateral ankle pain following an injury and reported that this could be improved by resection of the distal fascicle of the anteroinferior tibiofibular ligament.

Boden SD, Labropoulos PA, McCowin P, et al: Mechanical considerations for the syndesmosis screw: A cadaver study. *J Bone Joint Surg* 1989;71A:1548-1555.

The authors evaluated the results of syndesmosis fixation in 30 cadaver limbs. In one group, the deltoid ligament, syndesmosis, and interosseous membrane were sectioned. In the second group, the same operation was performed except that the deltoid ligament was kept intact, simulating a circumstance in which the medial malleolus is fractured and then rigidly stabilized. In the first group, in which the medial malleolus could not be rigidly stabilized, a force applied through the ankle widened the mortise by 0.5 to 4.5 mm as the fibular level of the simulated fibular fracture rose to 15 cm above the ankle. In the second group, in which the medial malleolus was stabilized and the deltoid ligament remained intact, very little widening occurred when the fibular fracture was proximal to the ankle.

Böstman OM: Osteolytic changes accompanying degradation of absorbable fracture fixation implants. *J Bone Joint Surg* 1991;73B:679-682.

Of 67 patients treated with polyglycolide rods, 17 developed a discharging inflammatory reaction. In more than half the patients, osteolytic foci appeared around the implants; however, in most cases, normal structure of the bone was restored by one year.

Bradley JP, Tibone JE: Percutaneous and open surgical repairs of Achilles tendon ruptures: A comparative study. *Am J Sports Med* 1990;18:188-195.

Of 27 patients wth acute Achilles tendon ruptures, 12 were treated percutaneously and 15 were treated by open reconstruction with a gastrocsoleus fascial graft. There were two reruptures in the first group, but otherwise the differences in results between the two groups were not significant. The authors recommend percutaneous repair for recreational athletes and open repair for high-caliber athletes.

Carr AJ, Norris SH: The blood supply of the calcaneal tendon. *J Bone Joint Surg* 1989;71B:100-101.

The vascular anatomy of the calcaneal tendon was studied in 16 cadaver specimens using an injection technique. The midsection of the tendon had a reduced cross-sectional area of blood vessels compared with the rest of the tendon. Removing the paratenon significantly reduced the number of vessels entering the tendon substance.

Cimino W, Ichtertz D, Slabaugh P: Early mobilization of ankle fractures after open reduction and internal fixation. *Clin Orthop* 1991;267:152-156.

In a prospective study of 51 ankle fractures treated surgically, the effect of a removable ankle-foot orthosis versus casting was studied. At follow-up there was no functional difference in range of motion, nor was there any increased morbidity in terms of loss of fixation with the use of the ankle-foot orthosis.

Colville MR, Marder RA, Boyle JJ, et al: Strain measurement in lateral ankle ligaments. *Am J Sports Med* 1990;18:196-200.

The authors measured strain in intact ankle ligaments as the ankle was taken through range of motion. The anterior talofibular ligament increased its strain when the ankle was moved into plantarflexion, internal rotation, and inversion. The strain in the calcaneofibular ligament increased as the talus was dorsiflexed and inverted. The strain in the posterior talofibular ligament was increased when the ankle was dorsiflexed and externally rotated. The syndesmosis was strained when the ankle joint was dorsiflexed and external rotation increased the strain in the anterior tibiofibular ligament.

Copeland SA: Rupture of the Achilles tendon: A new clinical test. *Ann R Coll Surg Engl* 1990;72:270-271.

Describes use of a sphygmomanometer cuff to detect spontaneous Achilles tendon rupture. This method can also be used to monitor progress following treatment.

Enwemeka CS: The effects of therapeutic ultrasound on tendon healing: A biomechanical study. *Am J Phys Med Rehabil* 1989;68:283-287.

A group of rabbits underwent tenotomy and repair of a right Achilles tendon, and half were treated with daily ultrasound. The tendons in each group were excised and compared with those treated without ultrasound. Those in the treatment group had greater tensile strength and energy absorption capacity than did those treated only by surgical intervention.

Faciszewski T, Burks RT, Manaster BJ: Subtle injuries of the Lisfranc joint. *J Bone Joint Surg* 1990;72A:1519-1522.

The authors retrospectively identified patients whose Lisfranc joint injury had been considered subtle at the time of initial treatment. They found that the true significance of the injury could not be correlated to initial radiographs. Even slight displacement led to significant morbidity 50% of the time.

Finsen V, Saetermo R, Kibsgaard L, et al: Early postoperative weightbearing and muscle activity in patients who have a fracture of the ankle. *J Bone Joint Surg* 1989;71A:23-27.

The authors randomized into three groups their postoperative treatment following fixation of ankle fractures. The first involved no plaster or weightbearing with early range-of-motion exercise of the ankle; the second involved traditional nonweightbearing; and the third involved a weightbearing plaster cast. No adverse effects or advantages could be noted with any of the treatment protocols. These findings suggest that postoperative treatment can be geared to each patient's individual needs.

Fitch KD, Blackwell JB, Gilmour WN: Operation for nonunion of stress fracture of the tarsal navicular. *J Bone Joint Surg* 1989;71B:105-110.

The authors suggest the use of en bloc bone grafting following the resection of the sclerotic margins of tarsal navicular stress fractures. Of these patients, 80% were able to return to satisfactory functional level within 12 months.

Harper MC, Keller TS: A radiographic evaluation of the tibiofibular syndesmosis. *Foot Ankle* 1989;10:156-160.

The width of the tibiofibular "clear space" and the amount of tibiofibular overlap was determined in 12 cadaver specimens. A normal tibiofibular clear space on the anteroposterior and mortise views should be less than 6 mm. Tibiofibular overlap on the anteroposterior view should be 6 mm or more or 42% of the fibular width. Tibiofibular overlap on the mortise view should be greater than 1 mm.

Hirvensalo E: Fracture fixation with biodegradable rods: Forty-one cases of severe ankle fractures. *Acta Orthop Scand* 1989;60:601-606.

Of 41 patients treated by absorbable polyglycolide rods, only three developed foreign body reaction. The results were otherwise comparable to standard methods of internal fixation.

Hopkinson WJ, St. Pierre P, Ryan JB, et al: Syndesmosis sprains of the ankle. *Foot Ankle* 1990;10:325-330.

The authors felt that patients who had syndesmosis injuries at the time of an inversion load took significantly longer to heal than did those patients who were treated for a more traditional ankle sprain. They also suggest that squeezing the calf at midlevel will cause pain in those patients who have an injury to the syndesmosis.

Kaye RA: Stabilization of ankle syndesmosis injuries with a syndesmosis screw. *Foot Ankle* 1989;9:290-293.

When patients are allowed to walk postoperatively after trans-syndesmotic fixation with a screw, radiolucent lines were likely to develop. Screw breakage is uncommon, however, and stability is satisfactory.

Mann RA, Holmes GB Jr, Seale KS, et al: Chronic rupture of the Achilles tendon: A new technique of repair. *J Bone Joint Surg* 1991;73A:214-219.

Seven patients with long-standing rupture of the Achilles tendon were treated by a transfer of the flexor digitorum longus into the os calcis. In an average follow-up of 39 months, the result was excellent or good in six patients and fair in one. Two significant soft-tissue complications were encountered. However, after soft-tissue closure was achieved, both patients had an excellent restoration of function. There were no reruptures.

Myerson M: Diagnosis and treatment of compartment syndrome of the foot. *Orthopedics* 1990;13:711-717.

The author provides a general overview of diagnosis and treatment of compartmental syndromes in the foot.

Sarsam IM, Hughes SP: The role of the anterior tibiofibular ligament in talar rotation: An anatomical study. *Injury* 1988;19:62-64.

The authors evaluated cadaver studies with sectioned ligaments and found that the anterior tibiofibular ligament prevents excessive fibular movement and external rotation of the talus and the ankle joint.

Shereff MJ: Complex fractures of the metatarsals. *Orthopedics* 1990;13:875-882.

The authors provide a general overview of injuries to the metatarsal. This review article suggests that when there is significant displacement of the metatarsal head, reduction and fixation should be performed.

Shereff MJ, DiGiovanni L, Bejjani FJ, et al: A comparison of nonweightbearing and weightbearing radiographs of the foot. *Foot Ankle* 1990;10:306-311.

In comparing weightbearing and nonweightbearing radiographs of human feet, the authors found that forefoot angular measurements change 80% to 90% of the time. Pathologic alterations in the forefoot alter the significance of weightbearing films. More importantly, it was not possible to predict what direction the shift in angular position would take. This suggests that evaluation of abnormalities that occur in weightbearing should be done on weightbearing films.

Stuart PR, Brumby C, Smith SR: Comparative study of functional bracing and plaster cast treatment of stable lateral malleolar fractures. *Injury* 1989;20:323-326.

The authors compare Aircast pneumatic air stirrup with plaster cast fixation. The authors felt that there was an improvement in comfort and swelling and range of motion. Cast was not employed.

Thomsen NO, Overgaard S, Olsen LH, et al: Observer variation in the radiographic classification of ankle fractures. *J Bone Joint Surg* 1991;73B:676-678.

Four people—one orthopaedic consultant, one radiologic consultant, and two orthopaedic trainees—classified 94 radiographs of ankle fractures by the Danis-Weber and Lauge-Hansen classification systems. Overall, there was an acceptable level of agreement for classification into the two types, but poor staging within the Lauge-Hansen classification system. This suggests that studies comparing the outcome within the staging system need to be looked at closely.

Tonnesen H, Pedersen A, Jensen MR,, et al: Ankle fractures and alcoholism: The influence of alcoholism on morbidity after malleolar fractures. *J Bone Joint Surg* 1991;73B:511-513.

The authors used a retrospective case-matched study to evaluate the effect of chronic alcoholism on the outcome of surgical repair of ankle fractures. They found an increased incidence of infection, hematoma, dehiscence, and postoperative medical complications in the alcoholic group.

Weinstabl R, Stiskal M, Neuhold A, et al: Classifying calcaneal tendon injury according to MRI findings. *J Bone Joint Surg* 1991;73B:683-685.

The authors looked at the magnetic resonance image profile of 28 patients with symptomatic calcaneal tendon pathology. They then classified the lesions as inflammatory reaction to generative change, incomplete rupture, or complete rupture. The findings were correlated at surgical intervention.

Winkler B, Weber BG, Simpson LA: The dorsal antiglide plate in the treatment of Danis-Weber Type-B fractures of the distal fibula. *Clin Orthop* 1990;259:204-209.

The authors report the use of the dorsal antiglide plate. The results were similar to those seen with other techniques employed for this injury.

Zeegers AV, vanderWerken C: Rupture of the deltoid ligament in ankle fractures: Should it be repaired? *Injury* 1989;20:39-41.

The authors retrospectively evaluated ankle injuries with the fibula fracture and rupture of the deltoid ligament. In no case was the deltoid ligament repaired. At an average follow-up of 18 months there was no clinical instability or radiographic widening of the ankle joint. The authors concluded that deltoid ligament repair is unnecessary.

51

Ankle and Foot: Reconstruction

Biomechanics of the Foot and Ankle

Clinical biomechanics of the foot and ankle are important in understanding deformity and in planning the surgical correction thereof. Integral to the motion of the foot and ankle is the transverse tarsal joint, which consists of the talonavicular and calcaneocuboid joints. With the hindfoot in varus, the transverse tarsal joint locks and becomes rigid, limiting motion in both itself and the subtalar joint. Hindfoot varus is not a functional position for the forefoot, which now supinates. If hindfoot varus occurs in childhood, the first metatarsal is plantarflexed by the peroneus longus, causing an extremely rigid cavus foot. It is because of this rigidity that the foot is unable to fine tune or compensate for minor stress; therefore, patients with cavus feet are typically more symptomatic than patients with pes planus. In the latter patients, the transverse tarsal joint is "unlocked," and, therefore, the foot can adapt easily to sagittal and horizontal plane stresses.

When considering arthrodesis of the ankle and hindfoot, the position of the midfoot and forefoot is important. Traditionally, arthrodesis is performed with the ankle in neutral dorsiflexion/plantarflexion. However, in the presence of a fixed forefoot equinus, which often occurs following trauma, the ankle may need to be placed in relative dorsiflexion to accommodate for the forefoot position. A fusion in slight plantarflexion is necessary only in the presence of quadriceps weakness; it never should be done to accommodate for heel height in the female patient. Any varus positioning of the foot following a hindfoot arthrodesis is poorly tolerated because the foot is more rigid and less able to compensate. For this reason, 5 degrees of valgus is the optimal position of the hindfoot in any of these fusions. If the subtalar joint is in varus, the weightbearing line of the lower extremity passes lateral to the calcaneus, placing stress on the subtalar joint, and there is pain under the cuboid and the fifth metatarsal. The foot is fused in slight external rotation, in comparison to the opposite extremity. If the foot is placed in too much external rotation, strain is placed not only along the medial border of the foot, but also on the first metatarsophalangeal joint (with valgus stress on the hallux), as well as on the medial aspect of the knee joint.

Hallux Valgus

General Assessment

The hallux valgus deformity consists of lateral deviation of the proximal phalanx on the metatarsal head, resulting in soft-tissue contracture along the lateral aspect of the metatarsophalangeal joint (an adduction contracture), attenuation of the medial capsule, and the formation of a prominent medial eminence. As the first metatarsal deviates medially, the proximal phalanx and hallux deviate further laterally and reciprocally affect one another's position. Because the transverse metatarsal ligament anchors the sesamoids to the neck of the second metatarsal, the sesamoids remain in a constant position, and the first metatarsal head moves off of them. The hallux rotates, and a callous forms at the plantar medial aspect of its interphalangeal joint. Weightbearing under the first metatarsal head is ineffectual because the windlass mechanism is dependent on adequate dorsiflexion of the hallux.

General assessment of the patient involves consideration of that patient's deformity, age and activity level, shoe wear needs, and, particularly, expectations regarding the outcome of any surgery. Adolescents should be counseled, because their expectations are often unrealistic and because conservative care often is the mainstay of treatment in this age group.

During examination the physician should look for the presence of an adduction contracture, mobility and range of motion of the hallux metatarsophalangeal joint, pes planus, hypermobility of the first ray, any circulation problems, and any generalized ligamentous laxity. Weightbearing anteroposterior and lateral radiographs are essential (Fig. 1). On the radiographs, the surgeon should measure: (1) the first-second intermetatarsal angle, (2) the hallux valgus angle, (3) the angulation of the first metatarsocuneiform joint, (4) the generalized metatarsus adductus, (5) the lengths of the first and second metatarsals, and (6) the first talometatarsal angle on the lateral radiograph.

Treatment

Treatment should always begin conservatively. While the cosmesis of the foot is certainly a factor, the shape of the forefoot can always be accommodated by a wider shoe with a broad toe box. The basic premise of all hallux valgus surgery is to realign the hallux, remove the medial eminence, and reduce the intermetatarsal angle. If present, the adduction or lateral soft-tissue contracture must be released. Realignment of the hallux with a closing wedge osteotomy of the proximal phalanx (Akin osteotomy) will fail to correct hallux valgus if it is used instead of an adequate soft-tissue release. Resection of the medial eminence is performed flush with the medial aspect

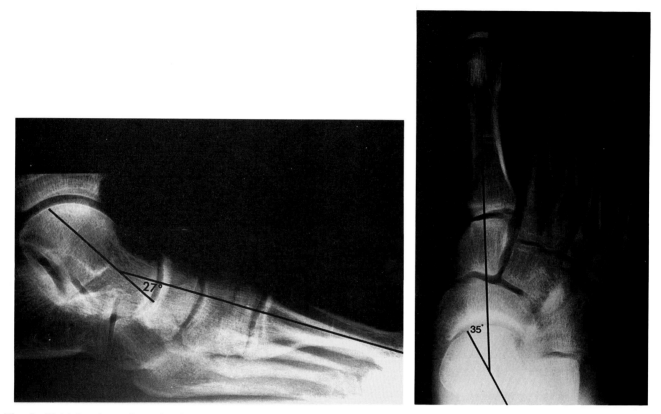

Fig. 1   Weightbearing radiographs of a patient with an acquired flatfoot deformity. Both the lateral (**left**) and anteroposterior radiographs (**right**) demonstrate collapse of the talus, with a change of the talometatarsal angle.

of the metatarsal shaft and not through the sagittal groove, because use of the sagittal groove may result in excessive resection with medial subluxation of the sesamoids. Typically, for distal osteotomies, 1 degree of correction is obtained for each 1 mm of lateral translation of the metatarsal head. The procedure of choice varies for adolescent, middle-aged, and elderly patients. The presence of degenerative changes in the metatarsophalangeal joint necessitates an alternative procedure, preferably arthrodesis; although, in selected elderly patients, resection arthroplasty (the Keller procedure) and Silastic implant arthroplasty are occasionally satisfactory alternatives.

For the mild to moderate deformity (intermetatarsal angle, 9 to 13 degrees), either a soft-tissue procedure (the modified McBride procedure) or a distal osteotomy (chevron or Mitchell type) is satisfactory. The standard Mitchell osteotomy is associated with shortening of the first metatarsal and transfer metatarsalgia to the second metatarsal. Complications such as avascular necrosis following the chevron osteotomy have been reported; however, in a recent study the incidence of avascular necrosis did not increase with the addition of an adductor release through a separate dorsal midline incision.

The blood supply to the first metatarsal head is both extraosseous and intraosseous. The extraosseous supply enters the metatarsal on its dorsolateral aspect approximately 2 cm proximal to the joint. Branches to the lateral capsule are also present and, therefore, significant stripping of both the dorsal and lateral aspects of the distal metatarsal may disrupt the extraosseous blood supply. The intraosseous supply provides additional circulation through both the diaphysis and metaphysis of the metatarsal.

Moderate to severe deformity (13 to 20 degrees) is best treated with a soft-tissue release and a proximal metatarsal osteotomy. This osteotomy may be either closing wedge or dome shaped. The disadvantage of the closing wedge osteotomy is that it is associated with slight shortening of the first metatarsal and potential transfer metatarsalgia. Fixation of the basilar osteotomy is essential, and rigid internal fixation with a compression lag screw is biomechanically more stable and rigid. Inadvertent dorsiflexion of the first metatarsal should be avoided, because this dorsiflexion will cause a dorsal bunion and transfer metatarsalgia to the second metatarsal. A combination of a proximal or distal metatarsal osteotomy with a closing wedge osteotomy of the proximal phalanx of the hallux (Akin procedure) is occasionally required. This procedure may be used in the presence of a congruent deformity of the metatarsophalangeal joint, because straightening the hallux changes this congruity, leading to decreased range of motion. Under these circumstances, the hallux is left in a slight valgus position at the metatarsophalangeal joint after reduction of the intermetatarsal angle with the metatarsal osteotomy, corrected to neutral with the Akin osteotomy.

For severe deformity (intermetatarsal angle greater than 20 degrees), an arthrodesis of the metatarsophalangeal joint may be used. Mann has demonstrated that, during the first year following arthrodesis, reduction of the intermetatarsal angle will occur in proportion to the preoperative intermetatarsal angle. Arthrodesis is indicated in the presence of severe subluxation or degenerative changes in the metatarsophalangeal joint. Moderate or severe deformity associated with hypermobility of the first ray is best treated with arthrodesis of the metatarsocuneiform joint (modified Lapidus procedure). Shortening of the metatarsal will occur if a large biplanar wedge is resected from the joint; therefore, minimal cartilage resection is the optimal technique. The incidence of pseudarthrosis is approximately 15%.

Complications

The most common complication following correction of hallux valgus is recurrence. This is particularly true in adolescents, who have a reported recurrence rate of approximately 30%. Recurrence is usually caused by inadequate soft-tissue release and failure to correct the alignment of the first metatarsal. The optimal correction for this recurrence is an appropriate soft-tissue release combined with a proximal metatarsal osteotomy. Lateral soft-tissue release or excision of the lateral sesamoid may result in hallux varus. It also can recur after overtightening of the medial capsule or after resection of too much of the medial eminence. This hallux varus may be corrected surgically, either by a soft-tissue reconstruction or by arthrodesis. The soft-tissue procedure described by Johnson involves rerouting the extensor hallucis longus underneath the transverse metatarsal ligament and pulling it through a drill hole in the base of the proximal phalanx of the hallux. This procedure is combined with a medial capsulotomy and release of the abductor tendon of the sesamoids.

If a hallux interphalangeal joint deformity is present, then an arthrodesis of this joint is performed along with rerouting of the entire extensor tendon. Alternatively, half of the tendon is rerouted. Salvage following failure of a Silastic implant may be extremely difficult because of fragmentation of the prosthesis, synovitis, and osteolysis of both the proximal phalanx and the metatarsal head. Arthrodesis is the treatment of choice, and the best method is by use of an interposition bone graft that maintains the length of the hallux.

Hallux Rigidus

Degenerative arthritis of the hallux metatarsophalangeal joint associated with decreased range of motion in both dorsiflexion and plantar flexion is termed hallux rigidus. The treatment of choice in the early stage of disease is to avoid high-heeled shoes, and to incorporate a rigid steel shank along the medial border of the shoe with or without a 0.6-cm metatarsal bar or rocker. Cheilectomy is recommended for mild to moderate deformity. The poor results reported with this procedure are caused by insufficient bone resection; at least one third of the dorsal aspect of the metatarsal head should be resected in addition to osteophytes at the base of the proximal phalanx. Range of motion of the hallux should be initiated soon after surgery.

Arthrodesis is the treatment of choice following failed cheilectomy or where advanced degenerative changes are present. The hallux should be fused in 15 degrees of valgus and 25 degrees of dorsiflexion of the hallux with respect to the metatarsal. The optimal position, however, is with the hallux parallel to the plane of support on weight-bearing, because this position takes into account a cavus or planus foot deformity. Excessive dorsiflexion will cause pain over the dorsum of the interphalangeal joint. Fusion in a more neutral position is not tolerated because pain occurs at the tip of the hallux.

Silastic implant arthroplasty is not recommended. Single-stem silicone implants are contraindicated and although double-stem implants may be used, they are neither recommended nor the treatment of choice. These implants are to be used only in elderly patients with low activity levels.

Deformity of the Second Metatarsophalangeal Joint

Although deformities of the second toe and metatarsophalangeal joint are often associated with hallux valgus, they can occur spontaneously. Spontaneous synovitis of the second metatarsophalangeal joint is not uncommon, associated with a long second metatarsal and attritional changes in the volar plate. This problem usually begins with a painful swelling of the second metatarsophalangeal joint. In later cases, medial deviation of the second toe may occur following attritional rupture of the lateral collateral ligament and lateral capsular structures.

Treatment in the initial stages of synovitis and swelling consists of immobilizing or taping the toe into a neutral or slightly plantarflexed position at the metatarsophalangeal joint, giving nonsteroidal anti-inflammatory medication and, occasionally, giving an intra-articular injection of steroids. These modalities invariably help, albeit temporarily. If conservative treatment fails, a synovectomy is indicated.

Subluxation and instability of the metatarsophalangeal joint are often associated with an extension contracture similar to a claw toe deformity. This contracture should be addressed with sequential soft-tissue releases, beginning with an extensor tendon lengthening and dorsal capsulotomy. If the metatarsophalangeal joint is still extended, then a collateral ligament release should be performed on either side of the metatarsophalangeal joint. Following this soft-tissue procedure, the volar plate complex should be inspected. If this complex is ruptured and associated with dorsal instability of the metatarsophalangeal joint, the proximal phalanx should be stabilized with a Girdlestone-Taylor flexor-to-extensor tendon transfer. The flexor digitorum longus tendon is resected off of its insertion on the distal phalanx and then split longitudinally and passed from plantar to dorsal around the base of the proximal phalanx. The tendon is secured to the extensor apparatus over the dorsum of the proximal phalanx with the metatarsophalangeal joint held reduced in the neutral position. The toe should be stabilized with a Kirschner wire introduced across the metatarsophalangeal joint and removed three weeks postoperatively. When instability at the metatarsophalangeal joint is associated with a fixed flexion deformity at the proximal interphalangeal joint, the entire flexor digitorum longus tendon is brought up from plantar to dorsal, without splitting it, as an interposition arthroplasty and is sutured to the extensor apparatus through the proximal interphalangeal resection. When the metatarsophalangeal joint is dislocated, soft-tissue contracture occurs, and when reducing the metatarsophalangeal joint, the neurovascular bundle is stretched, which can cause ischemia of the digit.

The toe cannot be relocated without bone resection. Resection at the base of the proximal phalanx often is associated with dorsal instability of the toe, which is not always addressed satisfactorily with a syndactyly to the third toe. The preferred procedure is arthroplasty at the level of the metatarsophalangeal joint with a shaving or partial resection of the distal portion of the metatarsal head alone. To avoid undue stiffness, the joint should not be immobilized for longer than three to four weeks postoperatively. An alternative procedure for soft-tissue decompression is by shortening of the proximal metatarsal as described for metatarsal osteotomies.

The crossover toe syndrome recently has been brought to focus by Coughlin. This represents a dorsomedial subluxation or dislocation of the second toe. It is caused by attritional rupture of the lateral collateral ligament, lateral capsule, and, occasionally, the lateral dorsal interosseous tendon and a portion of the volar plate complex. The medial aspect of the joint is contracted, including the collateral ligament, capsule, and medial dorsal interosseous and lumbrical tendons. The soft-tissue contracture must be addressed in addition to relocating and stabilizing the toe with a plication laterally. Depending on the severity of the subluxation or dislocation, this procedure should be performed with either a flexor-to-extensor tendon transfer or a metatarsal head arthroplasty as described above.

Claw and Hammer Toes

Although claw and hammer toes differ anatomically, from a functional standpoint, the treatment is similar. A claw toe consists of hyperextension at the metatarsophalangeal joint, and flexion at the proximal and distal interphalangeal joints. A hammer toe is extended at the metatarsophalangeal joint, flexed at the proximal interphalangeal joint, and hyperextended at the distal interphalangeal joint. A mallet toe is in neutral at the metatarsophalangeal and proximal interphalangeal joints but flexed at the distal interphalangeal joint. A curly toe is in neutral at the metatarsophalangeal joint and flexed at both the proximal and distal interphalangeal joints.

Conservative care for claw toe deformity, which includes corn padding, soft metatarsal pads, and a shoe with a high, wide toe box, often succeeds. Surgical correction varies and depends on the magnitude of the deformity, and whether the deformity is fixed or flexible. Soft-tissue releases at the metatarsophalangeal joint should be approached systematically and, at the metatarsophalangeal and proximal interphalangeal joints, sequentially as follows: (1) extensor longus lengthening, (2) extensor brevis lengthening or tenotomy, (3) transverse dorsal capsulotomy, (4) collateral ligament release, and (5) volar plate release.

For mild to moderate deformity, the soft-tissue contracture at the metatarsophalangeal joint is usually corrected through these sequential steps. If the toe still is extended or contracted at the metatarsophalangeal joint, additional contracture is present on both the plantar and the medial lateral joint surfaces. Ideally, the volar plate mechanism needs to be relocated under the metatarsal neck with an arthroplasty. If significant contracture is present, then more extensive soft-tissue release around the metatarsophalangeal joint has to be performed, including lengthening or release of the interossei. These tendons normally pass plantar to the axis of the metatarsal head and insert at the plantar base of the proximal phalanx to act as powerful plantarflexors of the metatarsophalangeal joint.

With severe hyperextension or dislocation, these tendons subluxate dorsal to the axis of the metatarsal head and become extensors of the metatarsophalangeal joint. In these severe deformities, diffuse soft-tissue contracture occurs at both the metatarsophalangeal and proximal interphalangeal joints. In attempting to straighten the toe at other joints, the neurovascular bundle is stretched. The toe can be maximally corrected only with bone shortening at either the proximal interphalangeal or metatarsophalangeal joint. For moderate deformity, bone shortening is easiest to achieve at the proximal interphalangeal joint; for more severe contracture or metatarsophalangeal dislocation, it is best to resect bone from the metatarsophalangeal joint by removing either the base of the proximal phalanx or the distal metatarsal head. Resection of a portion of the base of the proximal phalanx often leads to instability, which is not always corrected by syndactylization to the adjacent third toe, and is not the preferred method of bone resection. The cup and cone shaped articulation at the metatarsophalangeal joint can be preserved by resecting 3 to 4 mm of the metatarsal head, preserving its rounded contour. If the base of the proximal phalanx is still unstable, a flexor-to-extensor tendon transfer is performed using the flexor digitorum longus tendon. In most cases with instability at the metatarsophalangeal joint, temporary fixation with a Kirschner wire is used for three to four weeks postoperatively. Once the metatarsophalangeal joint is dislocated, the result is never entirely satisfactory, and the joint is always slightly stiff.

The deformity at the proximal interphalangeal joint is best treated with a resection arthroplasty, removing the distal one third of the proximal phalanx. Arthrodesis is indicated only in the presence of severe or recurrent deformity, or when associated with neurologic disturbance of the forefoot. When performing arthrodesis of the interphalangeal joint, the toe should be slightly plantarflexed, because this position is better tolerated than a stiff straight toe.

Intractable Plantar Keratosis

Intractable plantar keratosis is the most common cause of metatarsalgia. The differential diagnosis includes interdigital neuroma, a plantar wart, metatarsophalangeal joint synovitis, and, particularly in the elderly, atrophy of subluxation of the metatarsal plantar fat pad. The differential diagnosis of an intractable plantar keratosis and a plantar wart is simple. A wart is painful with side-to-side compression; an intractable plantar keratosis is painful to direct pressure. On paring a callous, the skin markings radiate into and through the callous. These markings stop abruptly at the edge of a wart. Shaving a wart also uncovers small punctate hemorrhage. A plantar callosity is either sharp and focal or diffuse.

The diffuse form of keratosis that extends under more than one metatarsal head should be treated conservatively. The focal intractable plantar keratosis typically results from a prominent metatarsal condyle, while the diffuse variety under one metatarsal head typically is caused by a long or adjacent short metatarsal. Conservative treatment of intractable plantar keratosis is often successful and begins with paring the callous and supporting the metatarsal with a soft pad to spread out the weightbearing surface of the forefoot away from the painful callosity. Surgery is indicated for chronic intractable plantar keratosis.

For the focal keratosis, a Du Vries condylectomy is the treatment of choice. It is important to remove only the prominent condyle, because excessive resection of the base of the metatarsal head can cause a transfer lesion to the adjacent metatarsal.

A chronically painful diffuse callous beneath a single metatarsal head is best treated with a dorsiflexion or shortening osteotomy of the metatarsal. This osteotomy must be done with precision, and internal fixation should be used. A sliding oblique osteotomy of the metatarsal with lag screw fixation achieves this goal. Osteotomies that allow the metatarsal head to float and "seek its own level" are imprecise and are to be avoided. Similarly, excision of portions of the metatarsal are not anatomic or physiologic, and are associated with an unacceptable incidence of transfer metatarsalgia. Diffuse callous below the first metatarsal head is associated with a plantarflexed first metatarsal and, if treated surgically, is best performed with dorsiflexion osteotomy. A diffuse callosity beneath the fifth metatarsal is often associated with a bunionette, and is best treated, in the manner described by Coughlin, with an oblique osteotomy of the metatarsal shaft, to correct both the plantarflexion and lateral deviation of the metatarsal head. Beware of the varus hindfoot causing pain under the fifth metatarsal head. Resection of the fifth metatarsal head is not a satisfactory procedure because it is associated with a floppy short fifth toe and, frequently, a transfer to the fourth metatarsal.

The Acquired Flatfoot in the Adult

The differential diagnosis of the acquired flatfoot deformity in the adult includes: ruptured posterior tibial tendon, old Lisfranc fracture dislocation, inflammatory arthritis of the hindfoot, neuroarthropathic (Charcot) involvement of the midfoot or hindfoot, and idiopathic degenerative osteoarthritis of the tarsometatarsal joint.

Posterior tibial tendon rupture is the most common of these and is a problem because its diagnosis frequently is missed. Early in this condition there is painful swelling along the posteromedial border of the ankle, fatigue, and aching along the medial longitudinal arch of the foot. In later cases, the talonavicular and subtalar joints begin to collapse, the hindfoot drifts into valgus, the midfoot pronates, and the forefoot abducts. In this late stage, pain typically is present laterally, with an abutment between the calcaneus and the fibula. Early treatment should be directed toward the inflammatory tenosynovitis, with nonsteroidal anti-inflammatory medication, a rubber-soled shoe with a quarter-inch medial heel and sole wedge, and, in acutely painful conditions, a period of immobilization in a short leg cast. If symptoms persist or are severe, surgery should be considered.

Early tenosynovitis may be treated by a synovectomy. Although the tendon may appear normal on gross examination, there may be intratendinous tearing, which is not evident grossly. The total excursion of the posterior tibial tendon is approximately 1.5 cm and, therefore, any intratendinous tearing will result in elongation of the tendon with significant mechanical loss. If the tendon is ruptured, the joint is mobile, and no fixed deformity is present, a flexor digitorum longus or flexor hallucis longus tendon transfer to the navicular is performed.

These tendon reconstructive procedures do not correct the flatfoot deformity, and the surgery is performed only for pain relief. In the presence of more severe or long-standing deformity, obesity, or lateral foot pain, an arthrodesis is indicated. If the site of maximal deformity is at the talonavicular joint, an isolated talonavicular or double arthrodesis (talonavicular and calcaneocuboid) may be performed. If more significant hindfoot valgus is present, a subtalar arthrodesis may be indicated. In the presence of fixed valgus deformity of the subtalar joint, a triple arthrodesis would be the treatment of choice.

Posttraumatic Arthritis of the Tarsometatarsal and Subtalar Joints

Arthritis in the tarsometatarsal (Lisfranc joint complex) is not uncommon following injury. The diagnosis frequently is missed in the acute setting, and unfortunately, even adequate initial treatment may not prevent occurrence of arthritis. This pain is poorly tolerated, and the affected joint invariably requires surgical salvage with arthrodesis. Conservative treatment measures should be used initially, including nonsteroidal anti-inflammatory medication and a rigid orthotic support. In planning the arthrodesis, it is useful to evaluate each articulation separately, localizing the source of pain. Invariably, the second metatarsal middle cuneiform joint is involved. Occasionally, the first metatarsal medial cuneiform and the third metatarsal lateral cuneiform segments are involved. The fourth and fifth metatarsocuboid joints are rarely symptomatic, and it generally is not necessary to extend the arthrodesis across these joints. It is important to realign the metatarsals, and fusing the joints in situ should be avoided. Minimal resection of the joint surfaces should be performed with rigid internal fixation. The second metatarsal should be reduced snugly into its mortise, and the fusion may require supplementary autologous bone graft. Complications that occur following arthrodesis include pseudoarthrosis (approximately 15%), injury to the deep peroneal nerve, and metatarsalgia following sagittal plane malunion. Patients are improved following arthrodesis, but rarely are completely asymptomatic.

Subtalar arthritis usually follows injury to the talus or calcaneus, and typically follows calcaneal fractures. Sources of medial pain include tibial nerve entrapment or bony impingement on soft-tissue structures. Lateral pain is caused by subtalar arthritis, peroneal tendinitis, sural neuritis, and calcaneofibular impingement. Diffuse pain may also exist in patients with reflex sympathetic dystrophy, chronic and extensive transtarsal arthritis, or the sequelae of an untreated compartment syndrome of the foot.

All patients should receive an initial course of conservative treatment, including physical therapy, nonsteroidal anti-inflammatory medication, orthotic supports, and possibly the use of a polypropylene ankle-foot orthosis. Selective lidocaine and cortisone injections are also helpful. Electrophysiologic testing of the tibial nerve and its branches should be performed for medial pain. A bone scan and a computed tomographic scan may also help differentiate and localize the source of discomfort. With collapse of the talocalcaneal joint and a decrease in the vertical height of the hindfoot, the talus assumes a more horizontal position. The talar declination angle changes, resulting in an abutment of the tibiotalar joint anteriorly with decreased dorsiflexion of the foot and ankle. The talar declination angle should be restored with a bone block subtalar arthrodesis, which corrects the height and width of the hindfoot as well as the mechanics of the tibiotalar joint. Integral to all surgical procedures for salvage is a lateral calcaneal ostectomy. As the sole procedure, however, this ostectomy fails to substantially improve the patient's symptoms. An in situ arthrodesis is indicated in the presence of subtalar arthritis without decrease in the height of the hindfoot. A triple arthrodesis is indicated rarely, and only when significant and disabling painful arthritis is present in the transtarsal joint.

Posttraumatic Arthritis of the Ankle

Conservative management of degenerative arthritis of the ankle is often successful, with nonsteroidal anti-inflammatory medication, occasional intra-articular steroid injection, and bracing, preferably with a rigid ankle-foot orthosis. The need for surgical treatment is difficult to predict based on the radiographic appearance of the joint, because patients' responses to painful arthritis vary significantly.

Many patients with advanced degenerative changes are relatively asymptomatic, while some with more minor synovitis and arthritis experience debilitating pain. In some patients, the degenerative process is limited to the anterior compartment with anterior tibiotalar osteophytes. If symptomatic, these patients should be treated with an anterior cheilectomy, performed either open or arthroscopically.

For advanced degenerative changes, arthrodesis is the treatment of choice. There is no current role for total ankle replacement. The technique of arthrodesis varies, provided rigid compression is attained. Although internal fixation is the preferred method of treatment, recent studies have demonstrated that triangular external fixation devices have a similar rate of success, albeit with increased morbidity from the transfixation pins. The final position for arthrodesis is ideally 5 degrees of hindfoot valgus, neutral dorsiflexion, external rotation comparable to the opposite extremity, and 0.5 cm of posterior translation of the talus under the tibia. It is essential to position the forefoot perpendicular to the long axis of the tibia. In many patients, repeated immobilization and the trauma from the original injury may be associated with stiffness of the midfoot and forefoot, and positioning the tibiotalar joint in neutral may not bring the forefoot plantigrade. No attempt should be made to accommodate the position of the foot to allow the patient to wear a higher heel, because doing so will cause excessive loading of the transtarsal and midtarsal joints.

Ankle Instability

The treatment of acute and chronic ankle instability is usually conservative. One of the most critical factors in rehabilitation is strengthening the peroneal tendons with the foot in plantarflexion. For evaluation of the lateral collateral ankle ligaments, the ankle should be tested in plantarflexion to assess the talofibular ligament, and in dorsiflexion to assess the calcaneofibular ligament. If both are disrupted, stability is absent in both of these positions. The anterior drawer test for testing stability of the anterior talofibular ligament should be performed with the foot in a neutral position so that the ligament is in a position to maximally resist anterior displacement of the talus.

Following adequate rehabilitation, if the patient has persistent instability, chronic pain, and giving way, surgery may be considered. Options include procedures by Chrisman-Snook, Brostrom, Watson-Jones, and Evans. The latter two do not, however, restore calcaneofibular ligament deficiency and, therefore, do not correct subtalar joint instability. The usefulness of the Brostrom procedure has been demonstrated in athletes and dancers in whom the peroneal tendons should not be sacrificed. Patients who have symptoms of instability with a negative anterior drawer test clinically and radiographically should be evaluated for subtalar joint instability. The most significant stabilizer of the subtalar joint is the talocalcaneal interosseous ligament, with the cervical ligament, the calcaneofibular ligament, and the extension of the extensor retinaculum and capsule providing further stability. Instability is best documented on stress radiographs. Surgical salvage is best achieved with the Chrisman-Snook procedure or a modification thereof.

The Diabetic Foot

It has been demonstrated in numerous studies that patient education alone will reduce the incidence of diabetes-related foot complications. The patient should gain an understanding of neuropathy, circulatory disturbance, shoe wear, and daily routine hygiene and care of the foot. Problems of the diabetic foot include neuropathic plantar ulceration, circulatory disturbance leading to ischemia/infection/gangrene, and neuroarthropathy. The neuropathic ulcer occurs as a result of repetitive minor mechanical stresses on the foot in the setting of neuropathy and deformity and is not the result of ischemia. In the forefoot, this is invariably related to pressure under a metatarsal head, either caused by prior adjacent bone resection or associated with fixed claw toe deformity resulting from motor neuropathy involving the intrinsic muscles. These forefoot ulcers are not usually associated with any acute or active infection and, according to the

Wagner classification, are grades I and II. A grade III ulcer is associated with osteomyelitis, grade IV with gangrene of part of the foot, and grade V with gangrene of the whole foot. Cultures of the wound are not necessary for grades I and II ulcers, because antibiotics are not required. Conservative treatment alternatives, including prolonged bed rest, no weightbearing, and restricted weightbearing with molded shoes, depend on patient compliance and are not as successful as the total contact cast, which is an ambulatory form of treatment. Recent studies suggest a 90% healing rate with minimal morbidity for the total contact cast. Grade III infection requires surgical debridement with metatarsal head or ray resection, and appropriate antibiotic therapy. Grades IV and V ulceration/infection require amputation.

Choice of the appropriate level for amputation is essential. Total lymphocyte count, total protein, and albumin level provide a good indicator of the patient's systemic ability to deal with infection. Local determinants are based on tissue perfusion and include transcutaneous oxygen measurements, Doppler ultrasound flow, temperature, and more sophisticated measurements including xenon washout and laser Doppler flowmetry. The Doppler ultrasound index is obtained by dividing the pressure obtained at either the ankle, metatarsal, or digital level by the brachial systolic pressure. For effective healing in the diabetic patient, the indices should be greater than 0.45 at the level at which the amputation is being planned. Arteriography in the setting of diabetic foot infection is of no use in planning the level of amputation. In the presence of ischemia, vascular consultation should be obtained, because large vessel disease may also be associated with more typical diabetic microangiopathy and small vessel disease.

Revascularization of the extremity will often succeed in salvaging the foot at a more distal amputation level. For gangrene localized to the digits in the presence of healthy digital flow, an isolated amputation of the toe may be performed. A metatarsal ray resection is the treatment of choice for osteomyelitis of the metatarsal with or without ischemia and infection of the toe. When infection is localized to the forefoot, a transmetatarsal amputation is selected and care is taken to reattach the extensor tendons. The Lisfranc and Chopart level amputations are useful and succeed when performed with an Achilles tenotomy and reattachment of the anterior tibial and extensor tendons. The most common complication following midfoot amputation is equinus deformity. Equinovarus deformity may occur following a Lisfranc amputation, because the posterior tibial tendon attachment is intact while the peroneals are disrupted.

A Syme amputation is indicated for infection and ischemia of the midfoot or forefoot when the ischemic index at the ankle is 0.45 or greater. The two-stage Syme amputation is indicated in the presence of active sepsis, and the malleoli are sectioned under local anesthesia six weeks following the first stage. In appropriately selected patients, the success rate of the Syme amputation should approximate 80%.

Diabetic neuroarthropathy occurs in three phases: acute, in which the foot is warm and swollen, and radiographs may show early fragmentation and subluxation of the joint involved; subacute, in which swelling subsides and new bone formation occurs; and chronic, in which no warmth or swelling is present, but the foot is deformed. The primary process in most cases of neuroarthropathy is a ligamentous disruption followed by fragmentation of the joint. Treatment consists of elevation, no weightbearing, and cast immobilization; once the swelling and warmth begin to subside (usually by six to eight weeks), a weightbearing total contact cast is applied. Cast immobilization is continued until the foot is no longer swollen or warm—approximately three to six months. The patient is then placed in the appropriate ankle-foot orthosis for a further six to 12 months. For the hindfoot and ankle, immobilization should be continued until the limb is completely stable. The goal of treatment is to ensure a plantigrade weightbearing surface of the midfoot, and to prevent further structural instability with minimal morbidity from treatment. The indications for surgery in the acute setting are limited. Chronic neuroarthropathy is managed with appropriate shoe wear and bracing. If, however, the deformity is severe, or unbraceable, or if ulceration recurs, surgery is indicated. Limited ostectomy may succeed and is an alternative to arthrodesis or amputation. Arthrodesis is effective for salvage, but is associated with a high complication rate, particularly infection. Pseudarthrosis does not preclude a satisfactory outcome, because most of these are stable. Six to 12 months of immobilization postoperatively is recommended.

Rheumatoid Arthritis

While all joints may be affected, the inflammatory synovitis has a predilection for the talonavicular and metatarsophalangeal joints. The subtalar, ankle, tarsometatarsal, and interphalangeal joints of the lesser toes are less commonly involved. Involvement of the forefoot is common, with painful inflammatory synovitis of the metatarsophalangeal joints in the early stages. A common early symptom is a soft-tissue mass in the second or third web space, which is diagnosed mistakenly as an interdigital neuroma. The radiographic appearance in early stages is typical, with juxta-articular erosions followed by thinning of the cartilage and, finally, dislocation. Early treatment of the synovitis should include appropriate medical therapy and local intra-articular cortisone injections if one or two joints are involved. If diffuse involvement of the forefoot is present, an early synovectomy may halt progression of the disease process.

For the late deformity, the appropriate treatment is resection of the lesser metatarsal heads, performed with an arthrodesis of the hallux metatarsophalangeal joint. Resection of the first metatarsal head or resection arthroplasty of the hallux relieves pain, but is associated with high incidence of recurrent deformity. Additional resection of the bases of the proximal phalanges is rarely necessary. Although implant arthroplasty is recommended by some authors, it is not felt to be as reliable as arthrodesis. Hemiarthroplasty is contraindicated, and, when used, the double-stemmed implant is indicated.

Hindfoot involvement frequently begins at the talonavicular joint; therefore, ankle pain associated with swelling and synovitis should not be confused with talonavicular arthritis. In addition to appropriate medical management, intra-articular joint cortisone injection is useful in alleviating pain and swelling. The hindfoot and ankle joints may need temporary rest and immobilization in a short leg cast if severe synovitis is present. Synovectomy of the ankle, talonavicular, or subtalar joints is indicated in the presence of synovitis refractory to medical management in which advanced joint-erosive changes have not occurred. Arthrodesis is the mainstay of treatment for arthritis and deformity. Total ankle arthroplasty is rarely indicated, and currently available designs are associated with high rates of implant failure. Salvage of failed total ankle replacement with arthrodesis has recently been reported, with satisfactory results but also with a high complication rate.

Annotated Bibliography

Alexander IJ, Johnson KA: Assessment and management of pes cavus in Charcot-Marie-Tooth disease. *Clin Orthop* 1989;246:273-281.

A sequential approach to evaluating the cavus foot is integrated with a description and assessment of various treatment options. The progressive nature of the muscular imbalance causing the deformity is highlighted, emphasizing the need for planned osteotomies and soft-tissue balancing procedures.

Angermann P, Jensen P: Osteochondritis dissecans of the talus: Long-term results of surgical treatment. *Foot Ankle* 1989;10:161-163.

Twenty patients with osteochondritis dissecans of the talus were reviewed nine to 15 years following surgery. Although the short-term results were satisfactory (85% were improved or cured), at follow-up, more than 50% had some pain during activities.

Carr JB, Hansen ST, Benirschke SK: Subtalar distraction bone block fusion for late complications of os calcis fractures. *Foot Ankle* 1988;9:81-86.

These authors present their subtalar fusion techniques for complex hindfoot pathology following os calcis fractures. The pathology is highlighted, including subtalar arthrosis, loss of calcaneal body height, and decreased lateral talocalcaneal angle.

Clohisy DR, Thompson RC Jr: Fractures associated with neuropathic arthropathy in adults who have juvenile onset diabetes. *J Bone Joint Surg* 1988;70A:1192-1200.

Fractures of the ankle and tarsus are described, many of them bilateral. Recommended treatment is nonweightbearing immobilization of the involved extremity with prophylactic immobilization of the contralateral extremity with a cast or orthosis.

Coughlin MJ: Treatment of bunionette deformity with longitudinal diaphyseal osteotomy with distal soft tissue repair. *Foot Ankle* 1991;11:195-203.

A distal longitudinal diaphyseal osteotomy with lateral condylectomy and metatarsophalangeal realignment is described. The advantage of this technique is the potential for biplanar correction of the metatarsal in the presence of plantar keratosis.

Grogan DP, Gasser SI, Ogden JA: The painful accessory navicular: A clinical and histopathological study. *Foot Ankle* 1989;10:164-169.

Simple excision of the accessory bone, the synchondrosis, and the prominent portion of the main navicular is recommended with no attempt to reroute the posterior tibial tendon.

Heilman AE, Braly WG, Bishop JO, et al: An anatomic study of subtalar instability. *Foot Ankle* 1990;10:224-228.

The ligamentous restraints to subtalar instability and radiographic technique to demonstrate it are described.

Johnson JE, Johnson KA, Unni KK: Persistent pain after excision of an interdigital neuroma. *J Bone Joint Surg* 1988;70A:651-657.

Reoperation for pain persisting after excision of a plantar intradigital neuroma (Morton's neuroma) through a longitudinal and plantar incision is described. Sixty-seven percent of patients had complete pain relief, highlighting the difficult nature of recurrent nerve surgery in the forefoot.

Johnson KA, Strom DE: Tibialis posterior tendon dysfunction. *Clin Orthop* 1989;239:196-206.

The clinical findings and staging for posterior tibial tendon dysfunction and the treatment for each stage are described.

Johnson WL, Lester EL: Transposition of the posterior tibial tendon. *Clin Orthop* 1989;245:223-227.

The posterior tibial tendon was rerouted anterior to the medial malleolus in children with dynamic varus deformity resulting from spastic cerebral palsy. This appeared to be a simple and effective procedure for correction in these children.

Leventen EO, Pearson SW: Distal metatarsal osteotomy for intractable plantar keratoses. *Foot Ankle* 1990;10:247-251.

A distal hinged greenstick osteotomy of the metatarsal neck is described for treatment of intractable plantar keratosis.

Mann RA: Hallux rigidus, in Greene WB (ed): American Academy of Orthopaedic Surgeons *Instructional Course Lectures, XXXIX*. Park Ridge, IL, American Academy of Orthopaedic Surgeons, 1990, pp 15-21.

The clinical and radiographic features of hallux rigidus are described, as well as the author's indications for cheilectomy, arthrodesis, resection, and implant arthroplasty.

Mann RA, Katcherian DA: Relationship of metatarsophalangeal joint fusion on the intermetatarsal angle. *Foot Ankle* 1989;10:8-11.

An important study demonstrates a reduction in the first intermetatarsal angle following arthrodesis of the hallux metatarsophalangeal joint, which is directly proportionate to the preoperative intermetatarsal angle. A concomitant proximal first metatarsal osteotomy, therefore, is rarely indicated when a metatarsophalangeal fusion is performed.

Mann RA, Missirian J: Pathophysiology of Charcot-Marie-Tooth disease. *Clin Orthop* 1988;234:221-228.

The components of the cavus deformity including the forefoot equinus associated with contracture of the plantar fascia, varus deformity of the calcaneus, extrinsic and intrinsic muscle weakness are all well described.

Meyer HR, Muller G: Regnauld procedure for hallux valgus. *Foot Ankle* 1990;10:299-302.

Resection arthroplasty for treatment of hallux valgus is described as an alternative to the Keller resection arthroplasty.

Myerson MS, Shereff MJ: The pathological anatomy of claw and hammer toes. *J Bone Joint Surg* 1989;71A:45-49.

The contribution of abnormalities of the skin, tendons, joint capsule, and collateral ligaments to deformity of the metatarsophalangeal and proximal interphalangeal joints are presented. The optimum surgical treatment of claw and hammer toes based on the pathologic anatomy is described.

Roper BA, Tibrewal SB: Soft tissue surgery in Charcot-Marie-Tooth disease. *J Bone Joint Surg* 1989;71B:17-20.

Ten patients with Charcot-Marie-Tooth disease were reviewed 14 years following soft tissue procedures to correct foot deformities. No patient required triple arthrodesis and the overall results were satisfactory. This paper highlights the importance of planned early surgery in these patients avoiding the potential for arthrodesis procedures. Not discussed in this paper is the use of osteotomy of the first metatarsal and calcaneus, which are also successful.

Sammarco GJ, Scioli MW: Metatarsal osteotomy using a double threaded compression screw: An adjunct to revision forefoot surgery. *Foot Ankle* 1989;10:129-139.

The authors describe the use of double threaded (Herbert) screws as internal fixation for metatarsal neck osteotomies with or without bone graft with good results.

Sangeorzan BJ, Veith RG, Hansen ST Jr: Salvage of Lisfranc's tarsometatarsal joint by arthrodesis. *Foot Ankle* 1990;10:193-200.

Posttraumatic arthrosis of the Lisfranc joint with salvage with arthrodesis lag screw fixation is described. Reduction of deformity is recommended combined with arthrodesis. Good results were obtained in 69% of patients.

Wetmore RS, Drennan JC: Long-term results of triple arthrodesis in Charcot-Marie-Tooth disease. *J Bone Joint Surg* 1989;71A:417-422.

Seventy-seven percent of patients experienced a fair or poor result at an average of 21 years following triple arthrodesis for Charcot-Marie-Tooth disease. Failure was attributed to arthrosis of the ankle and progressive muscular imbalance resulting in recurrent cavovarus deformity.

Wredmark T, Carlstedt CA, Bauer H, et al: Os trigonum syndrome: A clinical entity in ballet dancers. *Foot Ankle* 1991;11:404-406.

The posterior impingement syndrome of the hindfoot and ankle is described and treated successfully with excision of the os trigonum or a prominent lateral posterior process at the talus and division of the flexor hallucis tendon sheath if thickened.

Wyss CR, Harrington RM, Burgess EM, et al: Transcutaneous oxygen tension as a predictor of success after an amputation. *J Bone Joint Surg* 1988;70A:203-207.

Preoperative transcutaneous oxygen tension was found to be a more consistent predictor of success or failure of healing of an amputation of the foot than were measurements of systolic blood pressure at the ankle.

Index